Organization of the Text

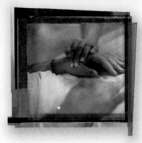

Starting with Unit 2, the chapters of *Nursing Health Assessment* follow a consistent organization to facilitate learning and highlight the key content needed for a full understanding of health assessment in nursing.

Case Study (woven throughout)

Presents a patient with a health concern corresponding to the chapter; ongoing related information, exercises, and details continue throughout the chapter.

Structure and Function Overview

Reviews anatomy and physiology, with additional content on variations according to lifespan and culture.

Acute Assessment

Summarizes emergency signs and symptoms to look for and immediate assessments and interventions.

Subjective Data Collection

Focuses on areas for health promotion and *Healthy People* goals, risk factors, risk assessment and health-related patient teaching, and focused assessments for common symptoms. Questions for risk factors and symptoms are accompanied by rationales. Additional questions associated with lifespan or cultural variations are included, as is sample documentation.

Objective Data Collection

Covers equipment, preparation, techniques, normal findings, abnormal findings, lifespan and cultural adaptations, and sample documentation. Recurring checklists differentiate RN-level from APRN-level practice.

Evidence-based Critical Thinking

Discusses methods for organizing and prioritizing, key laboratory and diagnostic tests, and foundations for diagnostic reasoning.

Tables of Abnormal Findings

Cluster common abnormalities related to the assessment being explored, with compare-and-contrast information on key data points.

Brief Table of Contents

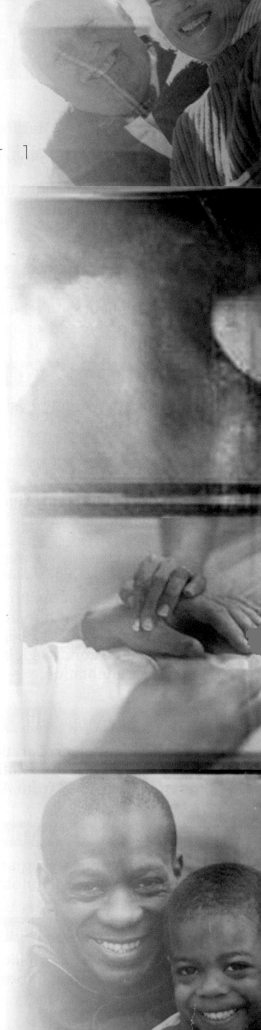

Nursing Health Assessment

A BEST PRACTICE APPROACH

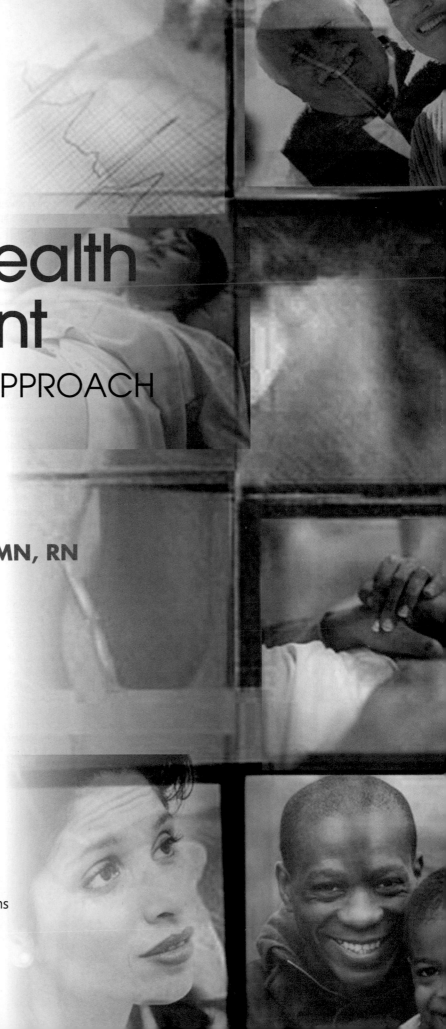

Sharon Jensen, MN, RN

Instructor
School of Nursing
Seattle University
Seattle, Washington

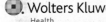 Wolters Kluwer | Lippincott Williams & Wilkins
Health

Philadelphia · Baltimore · New York · London
Buenos Aires · Hong Kong · Sydney · Tokyo

Executive Editor: Elizabeth Nieginski
Product Director: Renee A. Gagliardi
Developmental Editor: Sarah Kyle
Editorial Assistants: Amanda Jordan and Shawn Loht
Design Coordinator: Joan Wendt
Illustration Coordinator: Brett Macnaughton
Manufacturing Coordinator: Karin Duffield
Prepress Vendor: SPi Technologies

Copyright © 2011 Wolters Kluwer Health | Lippincott Williams & Wilkins.

Printed in China

Library of Congress Cataloging-in-Publication Data
Jensen, Sharon, 1955–
   Nursing health assessment : a best practice approach / Sharon Jensen.
      p. ; cm.
   Includes bibliographical references and index.
   Summary: "Nursing Health Assessment: A Best Practice Approach reflects a progressive and modern view of nursing practice. The text combines elements of traditional Health Assessment texts with innovative elements that facilitate understanding of how best to obtain accurate data from patients. It not only includes thorough and comprehensive examinations for each specific topic, but also presents strategies for adapting questions and techniques when communication is challenging, the patient's responses are unexpected, or the patient's condition changes over time. Unique features assist with application and analysis, enhancing critical thinking skills and better preparing all readers for active practice. A real-life approach is introduced at the beginning of each chapter and continued throughout. This includes recurring features that provide related questions, additional data, and variations that challenge one to modify responses. These cases encourage the progressive building and synthesis of knowledge. In addition to the case studies, other distinctive aspects of this text include the following: Emphasis on health promotion, risk-factor reduction, evidence-based critical thinking, and diagnostic reasoning. The end of the chapter demonstrates how to use critical thinking and diagnostic reasoning to cluster data and to analyze findings. End-of-chapter review sections contain questions and critical thinking challenges related to the previously established case study. Additionally, the last section of each chapter focuses on prioritizing and modifying assessment to promote the best care possible, and summarizing multiple findings to create appropriate plans for patient's health"--Provided by publisher.
   ISBN 978-0-7817-8062-9 (hardback : alk. paper)
   1. Nursing assessment. I. Title.
   [DNLM: 1. Nursing Assessment. WY 100.4 J54n 2011]
RT48.J46   2011
616.07′5—dc22
                                                                                                2010023765

LWW.com

9 8 7 6 5 4 3 2 1

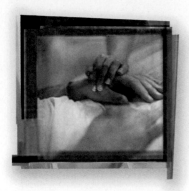

Acknowledgments

The Nursing Education staff at Wolters Kluwer Health is truly invested in nursing and on the frontlines of health care. I would like to thank several specific people:

- **Renee A. Gagliardi** has been a strong supporter and tireless advocate for a book that is based upon current pre-licensure clinical experience, although advanced techniques for fast-track students also are included. She made sure that practice was current and evidence based.
- **Laura Scott** delivered the contracts and kept things organized during busy days.
- **Elizabeth Nieginski, Jane Velker,** and **Margaret Zuccarini** led administrative channels that needed strengthening.
- **Sarah Kyle** helped us finish with consistency with the guidelines and made sure the content was on track.

We truly hope that this text lays out real-life situations so that nurses understand the importance of observation, with subjective and objective assessment as the process on which all nursing is based.

Inspiration

"The most important practical advice that can be given to nurses is to teach them
what to observe."

(Florence Nightingale, *Notes on nursing: What it is and what it is not*, 1860)

Dedication

- To my parents, who instilled in me my strong work ethic and understanding of community.
- To my husband, who has been my most loyal supporter.
- I appreciate the sacrifices of my children, Anna and Eric Jensen.
- To Kathy and Mark and my social network and all of the wonderful faculty and staff at Seattle University, a teaching university forming nursing leaders focused on vulnerable populations in the heart of Seattle.

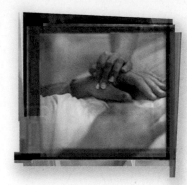

Contributors

Yvonne D'Arcy, MS, CRNP, CNS
Pain Management and Palliative Care Nurse Practitioner
Suburban Hospital
Bethesda, Maryland
Chapter 7: Pain Assessment

Karen S. Feldt, PhD, ARNP, GNP
Associate Professor
College of Nursing, Seattle University
Seattle, Washington
Chapter 30: Older Adults

Cynthia Flynn, MSN, CNM, PhD, ARNP
General Director
Family Health and Birth Center
Washington, DC
Chapter 28: Newborns and Infants

Nan Gaylord, PhD, RN, CPNP
Associate Professor
University of Tennessee, College of Nursing
Knoxville, Tennessee
Chapter 29: Children and Adolescents

Nancy George, PhD, FNP-BC
Assistant Professor (Clinical)
Wayne State University
Detroit, Michigan
Chapter 15: Eyes Assessment

Constance Hirnle, MN, RN, BC
Sr. Lecturer, SON, and Education Specialist
University of Washington Virginia Mason Medical Center
Seattle, Washington
*Chapter 5: Documentation and Interdisciplinary
   Communication*

Kathy Kleefisch, RN
Instructor
Purdue University at Calumet
Calumet, Indiana
Chapter 25: Male Genitalia and Rectal Assessment

N. Jayne Klossner, MSN, RNC
Director, Patient Care Improvement
Baptist Health System
San Antonio, Texas
Chapter 27: Pregnant Women

Margaret Kramper, RN, FNP
Allergy Sinus Nurse Coordinator
Department of Otolaryngology/Head and Neck Surgery
Washington University
St. Louis, Missouri
Chapter 17: Nose, Sinuses, Mouth, and Throat Assessment

Sharon Kumm, RN, MN, MS, CCRN
Clinical Associate Professor
University of Kansas
Kansas City, Kansas
Chapter 23: Musculoskeletal Assessment

Janet Lohan, PhD, RN, CPN
Clinical Associate Professor
Washington State University
Spokane, Washington
Chapter 9: Assessment of Developmental Stages

Amy Metteer-Storer, RN, BSN, MSN
Assistant Professor of Nursing
Cedar Crest College
Bethlehem, Pennsylvania
Chapter 20: Peripheral Vascular and Lymphatic Assessment

Jennifer Mussman, RN, ARNP
Clinical Instructor
Seattle University
Seattle, Washington
Chapter 16: Ears Assessment

Michelle Pardee, MS, FNP-BC
Lecturer
University of Michigan, School of Nursing
Ann Arbor, Michigan
Chapter 15: Eyes Assessment

Debra A. Phillips, PhD, PMHNP
Associate Professor
Seattle University College of Nursing
Seattle, Washington
Chapter 12: Assessment of Human Violence

Margaret S. Pierce, DNP, FNP-BC
Assistant Professor
University of Tennessee College of Nursing
Knoxville, Tennessee
Chapter 14: Head and Neck with Lymphatics Assessment

Barbara Rideout, MSN
Nurse Practitioner
Drexel University College of Medicine
Department of Family, Community, and Preventive
  Medicine
Philadelphia, Pennsylvania
Chapter 22: Abdominal Assessment

Debra Lee Servello RNP, MSN
Assistant Professor of Nursing
Rhode Island College School of Nursing
Providence, Rhode Island
Chapter 6: General Survey and Vital Signs Assessment

Ann St. Germain, MSN, ANP-BC, WHNP-BC
Assistant Clinical Professor
Texas Woman's University, College of Nursing
Houston, Texas
Chapter 26: Female Genitalia and Rectal Assessment

Karen Gahan Tarnow, RN, PhD
Clinical Associate Professor
University of Kansas School of Nursing
Kansas City, Kansas
Chapter 23: Musculoskeletal Assessment

Lisa Trigg, PhD, PMHNP-BC
Instructor
University of Kansas
Kansas City, Kansas
Chapter 23: Musculoskeletal Assessment

Joyce B. Vazzano, MS, APRN, BC, CRNP
Instructor
Johns Hopkins University School of Nursing
Baltimore, Maryland
Chapter 21: Breasts and Axillae Assessment

Deborah Webb, RN (Deceased)
Neurological Clincal Nurse Specialist
Harborview Medical Center
Seattle, Washington
Chapter 24: Neurological Assessment

Mary P. White, MSN, APRN, BC
Clinical Instructor
Director, Campus Health Center
Wayne State University College of Nursing
Detroit, Michigan
Chapter 13: Skin, Hair, and Nails Assessment

Danuta Wojnar, PhD, RN
Assistant Professor
Seattle University, College of Nursing
Seattle, Washington
*Chapter 11: Assessment of Social, Cultural, and Spiritual
  Health*

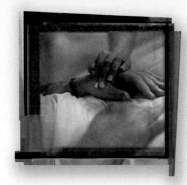

Reviewers

Marianne Adam, MSN, CRNP
Assistant Professor
Moravian College
Bethlehem, Pennsylvania

Colleen Andreoni, MSN, APRN, BC-NP
Instructor, Marcella Niehoff School of Nursing
Loyola University Chicago
Chicago, Illinois

Terri J. Ashcroft, RN, MN
Instructor, Faculty of Nursing
University of Manitoba
Winnipeg, Manitoba

Debra L. Benbow, MSN, APRN, FNP-BC
Assistant Professor of Nursing
Winston Salem State University
Winston Salem, North Carolina

Adrienne Berarducci, PhD, ARNP, CS
Associate Professor
University of South Florida at Tampa
Tampa, Florida

Jayne Bielecki, RN, BSN, MPH&TM
Clinical Instructor
University of Wisconsin at Eau Claire
Eau Claire, Wisconsin

Judy Bornais, RN, BA, BScN, MSc
Experiential Learning Specialist and Lecturer
University of Windsor
Windsor, Ontario

Judith Young Bradford, RN, DNS, FAEN
Associate Professor, School of Nursing
Southeastern Louisiana University
Hammond, Louisiana

Linda M. Caldwell, PhD, APRN
Professor of Nursing
Curry College
Milton, Massachusetts

Celestine Carter, APRN, DNS
Assistant Professor of Clinical Nursing
Louisiana State University Health Sciences Center
New Orleans, Louisiana

Pamella I. Chavis, MSN, RN
Clinical Assistant Professor
North Carolina Agricultural and Technical State University
School of Nursing
Greensboro, North Carolina

Janis Childs, PhD, RN
Professor and Director of Learning Resources and Simulation
Center
University of Southern Maine
Portland, Maine

Michael S. Congemi, ACNP-BC, MSN
Acute Care Nurse Practitioner, Research Scientist and
Clinical Instructor
University of Wisconsin, Milwaukee & Alverno
College
Milwaukee, Wisconsin

Valorie Dearmon, RN, DNP, CNAA-BC
Assistant Clinical Professor
University of South Alabama College of Nursing
Mobile, Alabama

Joseph T. DeRanieri, MSN, RN, CPN, BCECR
Assistant Professor, Faculty of Nursing
Thomas Jefferson University
Philadelphia, Pennsylvania

Holly Diesel, PhD, RN
Assistant Professor
Goldfarb School of Nursing at Barnes Jewish
College
St. Louis, Missouri

Martha A. Donagrandi, BSN, MSN
Faculty of Nursing
Madonna University
Livonia, Michigan

Gloria Ann Jones Taylor, DSN, RNc
Professor of Nursing
Kennesaw State University
Kennesaw, Georgia

Jill Thornton, RN
Suffolk County Community College at Selden
Selden, New York

Nancy Whitman, PhD, RN
Faculty of Nursing
Lynchburg College
Lynchburg, Virginia

Mary Wilby, PhD (c), MSN, RN, CRNP
Assistant Professor, Nursing
LaSalle University
Philadelphia, Pennsylvania

Tamara Wright, RN, MSN
Clinical Instructor
The University of Texas at Arlington
Arlington, Texas

Alice B. Younce, DNP, RN
Associate Professor of Nursing
University of Mobile
Mobile, Alabama

Erica Teng-Yuan Yu, PhD
Assistant Professor, School of Nursing
The University of Texas Health Science Center at Houston
Houston, Texas

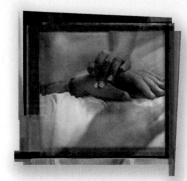

Preface

Nursing Health Assessment: A Best Practice Approach reflects a progressive and modern view of nursing practice. The text combines elements of traditional Health Assessment texts with innovative elements that facilitate understanding of how best to obtain accurate data from patients. It not only includes thorough and comprehensive examinations for each specific topic, but also presents strategies for adapting questions and techniques when communication is challenging, the patient's responses are unexpected, or the patient's condition changes over time. Unique features assist with application and analysis, enhancing critical thinking skills and better preparing all readers for active practice.

A real-life approach is introduced at the beginning of each chapter and continued throughout. This includes recurring features that provide related questions, additional data, and variations that challenge one to modify responses. These cases encourage the progressive building and synthesis of knowledge. They require critical thinking and diagnostic reasoning to analyze data, document, plan for care, and communicate findings. Additionally, other features, ancillary material, and media related to the book build on the in-text cases to reinforce correct elements of subjective data collection, objective data collection, and variations necessary for different problems, age groups, and cultures.

In addition to the case studies, other distinctive aspects of this text include the following:

- **Emphasis on health promotion, risk-factor reduction, evidence-based critical thinking, and diagnostic reasoning.** The book's introductory units provide foundational explanations of these core threads. The emphasis on health promotion, risk factors and related teaching, and prevention reflect the text's forward-thinking attitude and helps underscore the key role of nurses as partners with and advocates for patients. The end of the chapter demonstrates how to use critical thinking and diagnostic reasoning to cluster data and to analyze findings.
- **Distinctions between common techniques and specialty or advanced practice skills.** Recurring features within the Subjective Data and Objective Data sections differentiate focused versus comprehensive techniques, indicating how to modify approaches based on circumstances. The Subjective Data questions include questions about risk factors, health history issues and common symptoms, with follow-up questions for positive responses. A recurring table in the Objective Data section explains which techniques are more commonly performed in routine examinations to distinguish basic from specialty practice. This structure helps users prepare for actual patient interactions, as well as to expect to modify techniques for individual situations.
- **Distinctive two-column format emphasizing not just techniques and findings, but ways to differentiate normal data, normal variations, and abnormalities.** Like many health assessment books, this text uses a two-column presentation to differentiate techniques versus abnormal findings. This text goes another step, however, by differentiating normal responses and variations from abnormalities. Normal findings are italicized in the left column, and abnormal findings are in the right column. Pictures of abnormal findings are generally grouped together in tables at the very end of the chapter. This structure facilitates quick and easy comparison and contrasting of findings and problems.
- **Emphasis on knowledge application and analysis.** End-of-chapter review sections contain questions and critical thinking challenges related to the previously established case

study. Additionally, the last section of each chapter focuses on prioritizing and modifying assessment to promote the best care possible and summarizing multiple findings to create appropriate plans for patient's health.

Organization of the Text

Unit 1, *Foundations of Nursing Health Assessment*, provides in-depth coverage of the basic components of nursing health assessment. The rest of the text builds on and expands the material in this first unit. Chapter 1 explicates the nurse's role in assessment. Chapter 2 reviews the importance of effective communication and interviewing. Chapter 3 explores history taking in subjective data collection, while Chapter 4 outlines the techniques, common equipment, approaches, and process of physical examination for objective data collection. Finally, the unit concludes with information on the important components of documenting findings and sharing them with other health care team members in Chapter 5. Using the correct medical terminology and proper documenting is important, especially avoiding the use of "good" and "normal." This factor is highlighted by italicizing the normal findings in the left column and describing the abnormal findings in the right column.

Unit 2, *General Examinations*, presents those assessments consistently applicable to all patients, regardless of age, medical circumstance, or other specific issue. These topics reflect the holistic nature of nursing health assessment, as opposed to the traditional medical model that generally focuses on the physical domain and "body-systems." Topics in Unit 2 include General Survey and Vital Signs (Chapter 6); Pain (Chapter 7); Nutrition including Medications and Supplements (Chapter 8); Developmental Stages (Chapter 9); Mental Status and Mental Health (Chapter 10); Social, Cultural, and Spiritual Health (Chapter 11); and Safety and Violence (Chapter 12).

Unit 3, *Regional Examinations*, presents individual chapters focusing on assessment of the key areas of the body, beginning with the skin and ending with the genital and rectal examinations. The material focuses primarily on adults; lifespan and cultural variations and considerations are highlighted at crucial points of review.

Unit 4, *Special Populations and Foci*, synthesizes previous discussions for different lifespan groups and presents summational content of assessments for pregnant women, newborns and infants, children and adolescents, and older adults. The content in Units 2 and 3 explicate what is different, unique, or in need of modification for specific age groups when approaching the various assessments discussed. The content in Unit 4 describes how to synthesize and apply these understandings to comprehensive assessments for maternal, pediatric, and geriatric populations.

Unit 5, *Pulling It All Together*, reinforces the book's previous learning by outlining how to complete a full, comprehensive, head-to-toe examination for an adult. This is a summary of the units previously studied in depth.

Chapter Organization and Features

Case Features

Progressive case study material is woven throughout every chapter. From the beginning to the end of the content presentation, readers follow a patient's story and are challenged to apply their reading to the unfolding scenario. A recurring structure serves as a mechanism for supplying more information but also for reinforcing the core assessment foundations of critical thinking, therapeutic communication, documentation, findings analysis, application collaboration, and "pulling it all together."

- **Chapter Opener:** The case begins with a picture, reading, and bulleted list of three to five questions. These elements introduce the patient and generate beginning issues to consider.
- **Therapeutic Dialogue:** These displays provide examples of "less effective" and "more effective" communication with patients. "Critical Thinking Challenges" offer an opportunity to you to consider how the nurse in question might have gathered more information. These dialogues in Units 2 to 5 consistently end the sections on Subjective Data, which are uniquely organized.

- **Analyzing Findings:** The feature focuses on documented summaries of findings related to the case in four areas: Subjective Data (S), Objective Data (O), Analysis, and Plan. The format follows the nursing process, with assessment as the first and most important step.
- **Documenting Abnormal Findings:** This feature summarizes abnormal findings relevant to the case-study patient in the physical examination: Inspection, Palpation, Percussion, and Auscultation. These are the techniques used in objective health assessment. Subjective health assessment techniques are covered previously; some nurses consider subjective to be 80% of the assessment (80% listen, 20% physical).
- **Collaborating With Other Health Care Providers:** This unique feature describes scenarios in which the nurse in the case must coordinate referrals or other advocacy needs for the patient. The feature shows how to organize details using the SBAR framework: **S**ituation, **B**ackground, **A**nalysis (or **A**ssessment), and **R**ecommendations. A Critical Thinking Challenge ends the section, prompting the reader to consider how the nurse might have better communicated findings and recommendations.
- **Pulling It All Together:** A table shows how to bring all the elements of assessment together when arriving at a nursing diagnosis based on previous findings and beginning to develop goals, interventions, rationales, and evaluation criteria.
- **Applying Your Knowledge:** This last case-related feature in the chapter includes summary text and repeats the bulleted questions found at the start of the chapter. This feature shows how assessment generates intervention, evaluation, and collaboration based upon accurate and complete data to generate more effective care.

Other Features
- **Learning Objectives:** These objectives present the most important goals for learning by the time of completing the chapter.
- **Clinical Significance:** This feature highlights content critically related to a point of application. It may appear wherever applicable in the chapter.
- **Safety Alert:** These recurring boxes present important areas of concern or results that require immediate intervention or adjustments. Safety Alert features may be placed wherever applicable in the chapter. Not all acute features are labeled, but the most common ones are highlighted.
- **Equipment Needed:** This box reviews essential equipment that the nurse will want to identify, clean, and gather before entering the patient's room relative to each assessment.
- **Key Points:** Key points are summarized at the end of the chapter to reinforce the most important information.
- **Review Questions:** Each chapter has 10 test questions written as a summary. The case study and related critical thinking questions are a higher level of thinking. They should be discussed with the instructor.
- **Abnormal Findings:** Tables of abnormal findings are summarized at the end of the chapter. Art or tables of normal findings may be integrated into the chapter in the appropriate location, but comparative depictions of abnormal findings generally are found in groups at the end.

Icons
 This designation is used to designate content specifically related to lifespan-oriented issues.

 This icon is found with material specifically related to culturally-oriented issues.

 This icon sets off Abnormality Tables at the end of the chapter.

 This icon clues readers to visit thePoint or their accompanying DVD-ROM to review a corresponding video asset.

 This icon clues readers to visit thePoint or their accompanying DVD-ROM to review a corresponding animation.

 This icon clues readers to visit thePoint or their accompanying DVD-ROM to access an interactive media element.

A Comprehensive Package for Teaching and Learning

To further facilitate teaching and learning, a carefully designed ancillary package is available. In addition to the usual print resources, Wolters Kluwer Health is pleased to present multimedia tools that have been developed in conjunction with the text.

Resources for Students

Interactive DVD-ROM. Packaged with the textbook at no additional charge, this DVD-ROM tests knowledge and enhances understanding of health assessment. It includes:

• More than 500 self-study questions
• Concepts in Action™ Animations
• Watch and Learn™ Videos
• Journal Articles
• Clinical Simulations
• Spanish-English Dictionary with Pronunciation

Laboratory Manual for Nursing Health Assessment. Available at bookstores or at www.LWW.com, this student laboratory manual presents various exercises to reinforce textbook content and enhance learning. It is very helpful for students to complete these exercises before lab.

Pocket Guide for Nursing Health Assessment. Available at bookstores or at www.LWW.com, this clinical reference presents need-to-know information in a concise, easy-to-use, highly visual format. If the course is condensed, this is a good resource.

Resources for Instructors

Instructor's Resource DVD-ROM. The instructor's resource DVD-ROM contains the following items:

• A thoroughly revised and augmented test generator, containing more than 500 NCLEX-style questions
• Sample syllabi
• Strategies for effective teaching
• PowerPoint™ lectures, guided lecture notes, and pre-lecture quizzes
• An image bank
• Discussion topics and assignments
• Case studies

Resources for Students and Instructors

ThePoint* (http://thepoint.lww.com) provides every resource that instructors and students need in one easy-to-use site. Advanced technology and superior content combine at thePoint to allow instructors to design and deliver on-line and off-line courses, maintain grades and class rosters, and communicate with students. Students can visit thePoint to access supplemental multimedia resources to enhance their learning experience, check the course syllabus, download content, upload assignments, and join an on-line study group. ThePoint … where teaching, learning, and technology click!

---

*thePoint is a trademark of Wolters Kluwer Health.

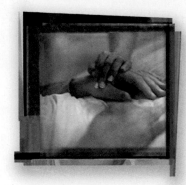

Contents

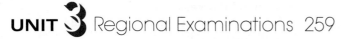

UNIT 3 Regional Examinations 259

UNIT 1

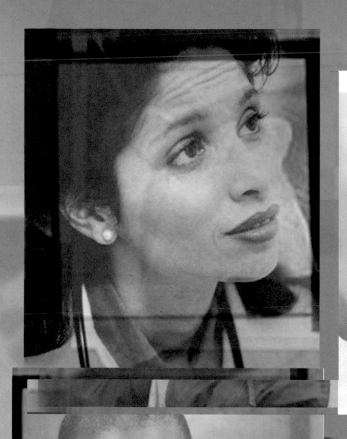

Foundations of Nursing Health Assessment

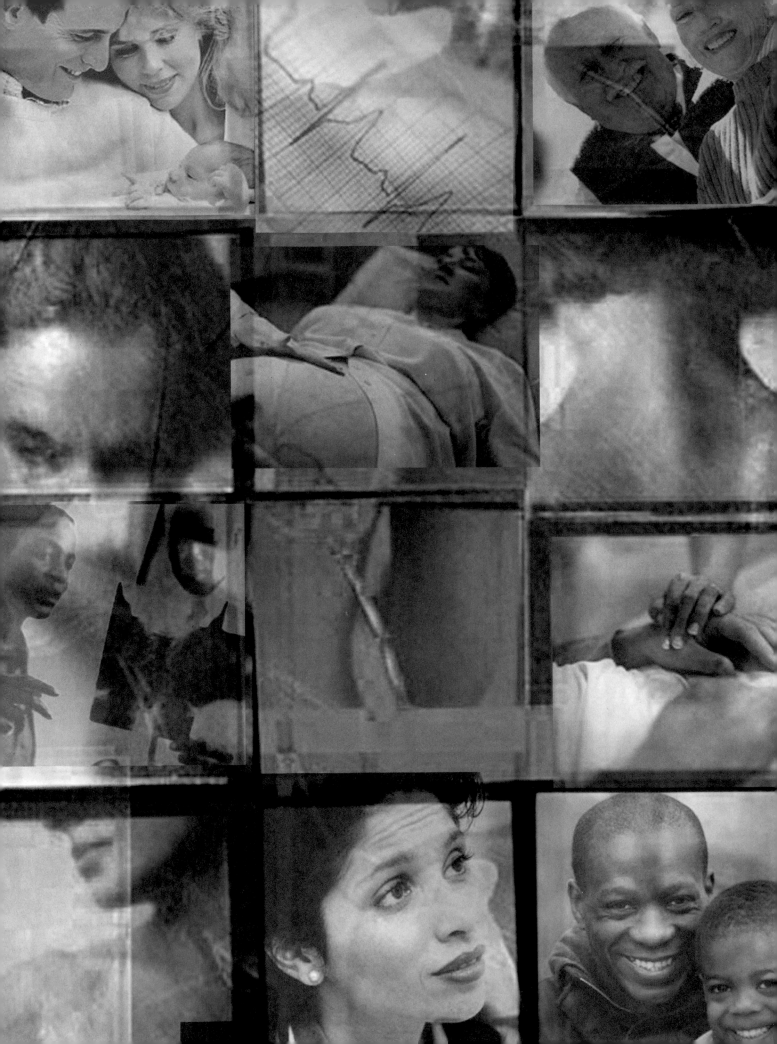

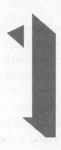

The Nurse's Role in Health Assessment

Learning Objectives

1 Identify the role of the professional nurse in health assessment.

2 State the purpose of health assessment.

3 Describe the relationship of health assessment to health promotion.

4 Identify the roles of the nursing process, critical thinking, and diagnostic reasoning in nursing care.

5 Recognize differences in the types and frequencies of assessments.

6 Identify the components of a comprehensive health assessment.

7 Compare frameworks for collecting health assessment data.

Maria Ortiz, a 52-year-old Mexican American, has a follow-up appointment related to type 2 diabetes mellitus, which was diagnosed 2 weeks ago during an annual physical assessment. Her primary language is Spanish; while her English skills are good, she has difficulty understanding complex medical terminology. Ms. Ortiz has been married for 30 years, and her three grown children live nearby.

Ms. Ortiz is 160 cm tall, weighs 75 kg (body mass index [BMI] 29), and eats a diet high in fats and starches. Her blood glucose levels at home have been elevated. She is otherwise healthy. Current vital signs are temperature 36.5°C tympanic, pulse 82 beats/min, respirations 16 breaths/min, and blood pressure (BP) 138/78 mmHg. Medications include an oral hypoglycemic and a daily vitamin.

You will gain more information about Ms. Ortiz throughout this chapter. As you study the content and features, consider the patient's case and its relationship to what you are learning. Begin thinking about the following points:

- What are potential health-promotion and teaching needs for Ms. Ortiz based on the above information?
- How should the nurse approach a discussion of the patient's diet as related to her diabetes?
- How will the nurse individualize today's health assessment, considering the patient's gender, age, and culture?
- What is the role of the nurse in providing care for Ms. Ortiz during this visit?

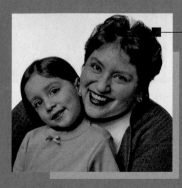

Nursing is a rewarding and challenging profession that requires extensive knowledge and skills. Nurses assess health on many levels, including psychosocial, physical, emotional, spiritual, and cultural. They develop and use skills in communication to provide therapeutic responses to the concerns of patients. Wellness and health are concepts that influence the health beliefs and health behaviors of patients. Nurses explore factors related to such beliefs and behaviors to understand better how to promote health for patients and their families. They use the nursing process to care for patients by assessing completely, making nursing diagnoses, developing outcomes, planning for care, performing interventions, evaluating effectiveness, and revising interventions as needed. The foundation of this collaborative process depends on having accurate and complete assessment data.

Role of the Professional Nurse

According to the American Nurses Association (ANA), "Nursing is the protection, promotion, and optimization of health and abilities, prevention of illness and injury, alleviation of suffering through the diagnosis and treatment of human response, and advocacy in the care of individuals, families, communities, and populations" (2003, p. 6). Four broad goals are within nursing:

1. To promote health (state of optimal functioning or well-being with physical, social, and mental components)
2. To prevent illness
3. To treat human responses to health or illness
4. To advocate for individuals, families, communities, and populations

Nursing: Scope and standards of practice (ANA, 2004) and *Code of ethics for nurses with interpretive statements* (ANA, 2005) further describe nursing and its associated practice standards. Nursing activities to promote health and prevent illness reduce the risk of a disease, reinforce good habits, and maintain optimal functioning (Fig. 1-1). Examples of appropriate nursing interventions include implementation of educational programs, coordination of community resources, and patient and family teaching.

Direct and Indirect Caregiving

Nurses provide direct care to help restore health for ill patients in hospitals, clinics, long-term care facilities, and schools. They work in hospice, rehabilitation centers, and homes to help patients and their families cope with disability and, when unavoidable, to facilitate the most comfortable death for patients. The roles in these areas are primarily as **providers of direct and indirect care** (American Association of Colleges of Nursing [AACN], 2008).

Nurses also have roles as **designers, coordinators, and managers of care**. They gather assessment information that focuses on how a condition influences the patient's functional ability and quality of life. While practitioners of medicine focus on the physical aspects of diseases and prescribe medications or other treatments for them, nurses focus on how diseases are affecting activity levels and abilities to perform tasks as well as how patients are coping with their issues and any related losses of function. While they often work with primary providers on medical diagnoses and collaborative problems, nurses also have an area of independent practice within which they function

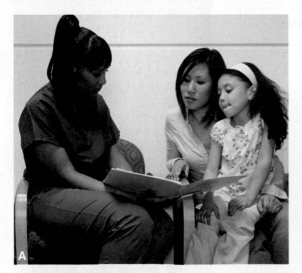
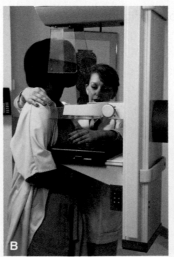
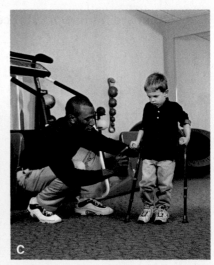

Figure 1.1 Nurses promote health and prevent illness in various ways. **(A)** Family teaching during wellness visits reinforces positive habits and helps parents and children understand behaviors for optimal well-being. **(B)** Conducting regular health screenings with patients, such as scheduled mammograms, is critical to reducing risks for disease. **(C)** Assisting patients with long-term health challenges to restore or maintain optimal functioning is another essential nursing activity.

autonomously. Independent nursing interventions include patient teaching, therapeutic communication, and physical procedures such as turning patients or assisting them with ambulation.

Nurses are constantly making treatment decisions to manage and coordinate care. They are highly respected by patients because often they spend more time with patients and their families and know their issues more completely than do other health care providers (Davis, 2005). Nurses are members of the health care team in this role. They communicate findings to appropriate people and also document data to share information and identify trends. In many chapters, referral of patients to other health care providers (eg, dieticians or speech therapists) is discussed in the SBAR (situation, background, assessment, recommendation) feature. Nurses use interprofessional communication and collaboration to improve patient health outcomes (AACN, 2008).

Advocacy

Nurses are also members of a profession and, in this role, are **advocates for the patient and the profession** (AACN, 2008). Nurses advocate for patients in many ways: keeping them safe, communicating their needs, identifying side effects of treatment and finding better options, and helping patients to understand their diseases and treatments so that they can optimize self-care. Safety is defined as the minimization of "risk of harm to patients and providers through both system effectiveness and individual performance" (Cronenwett, et al., 2007). More than all other health care professionals, nurses can recognize, interrupt, evaluate, and correct health care errors (Rothschild, et al., 2006). Basic organizational and systems leadership for quality care and patient safety is essential (Institute of Medicine, 2004).

As advocates, nurses take responsibility to protect the legal and ethical rights of patients.

Values and ethical principles are beliefs or ideals to which a person is committed. Professional values guide nurses to provide safe, humanistic care (AACN, 2008). Nursing values include altruism, human dignity, autonomy, integrity, and social justice.

- **Altruism** includes a true concern for the welfare of others and is reflected in the desire to understand the patient's perspective and health beliefs.
- **Human dignity** is present when nurses show respect for patients, such as by ensuring privacy and confidentiality.
- Patients have the right to make decisions about their health care; nurses in their role as advocates provide information to patients and their families to promote this **autonomy**.
- Nurses act with **integrity** when providing honest information to patients, documenting care accurately, and reporting errors (Institute for Safe Medication Practices, 2007).
- When nurses work to ensure equal treatment and access to quality health care, they support **social justice**.

The roles as a provider of care, manager, and member of a profession give nursing a unique advantage in understanding and acting on the patient's behalf in the most holistic way.

Scholarship and Research

Nurses also perform **scholarship and research** to provide care based on current evidence. Professional nursing practice is grounded in best practice, critical inquiry, and skilled questioning. Knowledge of patient care technologies and information systems is essential in the management of care. Nurses use systems to influence health care policy, finance, and regulatory agencies. Health promotion and disease prevention are necessary to improve health at both the individual and the population levels (AACN, 2008).

Registered Nurse and Advanced Practice Nurse Roles

Both registered nurses (RNs) and advanced practice nurses fulfill the roles described in the previous section. The RN is licensed nationally and practices independently within the scope of nursing practice and diagnosis. RNs practice wherever people need nursing care, including such common sites as hospitals, homes, schools, workplaces, and community centers. More than half of RNs work in hospitals; other common settings include community or public health, ambulatory care, nursing homes, and nursing education (ANA, 2009a).

Advanced practice registered nurse (APRN) is an umbrella term given to an RN who has met advanced educational and clinical practice requirements, at a minimum of a Master's level, beyond the basic nursing education and licensing required of all RNs and who provides at least some level of direct care to patient populations (ANA, 2009a). APRNs typically also perform more advanced assessments, such as examining the eyes with an ophthalmoscope or performing a gynecologic assessment. The APRN roles include nurse practitioner, midwife, clinical nurse specialist, certified nurse anesthetist, and clinical nurse leader.

There are many opportunities for RNs to advance their education and careers in a way that interests each individual and uses his or her strengths and expertise. The differences between the usual RN and the APRN assessments are included in each chapter of this text.

Purpose of Health Assessment

Health assessment is "gathering information about the health status of the patient, analyzing and synthesizing those data, making judgments about nursing interventions based on the findings and evaluating patient care outcomes" (AACN, 2008). A health assessment includes both a health history and a physical assessment (Fig. 1-2).

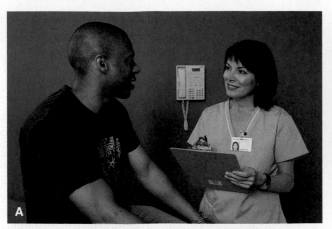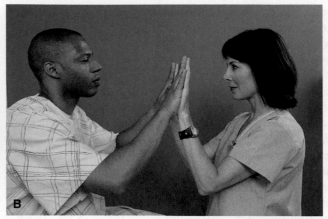

Figure 1.2 Health assessment includes the health history and physical assessment. **(A)** Nurses interview patients during the health history to understand past medical conditions and surgeries; risk factors; current symptoms; perceptions; social, cultural, and spiritual dimensions; growth and development; mental status; nutrition; and environmental and safety issues. **(B)** Specific techniques performed during the physical assessment depend on the patient's acuity, health history, and current symptoms.

The health history includes interviewing to collect the patient's past medical and surgical histories, risk factors, and current symptoms. A comprehensive health history also includes nutrition; development; mental health; social, cultural, and spiritual dimensions; and safety issues. Data that nurses collect during the physical assessment vary depending on a patient's acuity, health history, and current symptoms. In emergencies, nurses collect information that will help pinpoint the source of the issues and treat current conditions. For healthy patients seeking a wellness checkup, the assessment focuses on screening for high-risk conditions (eg, overweight) and teaching and health promotion associated with common issues (eg, nutrition and exercise).

Other purposes of health assessment are to gain further insight into the current condition and to establish a database that subsequent assessments can be measured against. Nurses identify patterns and trends of findings to determine if a patient's condition is improving or worsening. Instead of using one piece of data in isolation, nurses think logically

to analyze how data are related and what interventions may be indicated. They evaluate outcomes, and the assessment becomes a continuous part of the nursing process.

The nursing process begins with a complete and accurate health assessment to promote health at the highest level. Because all future care is based upon the health assessment, it is extremely important that health assessment data are complete and accurate. A health assessment is one of the most important activities of professional nurses.

Wellness and Health Promotion

High-level **wellness** is a process by which people maintain balance and direction in the most favorable environment. The role of nurses is to facilitate this achievement through health promotion and teaching. Most people fall somewhere on a trajectory or continuum of wellness versus **illness** (Travis & Regina, 2004) (Fig. 1-3). The person who moves toward

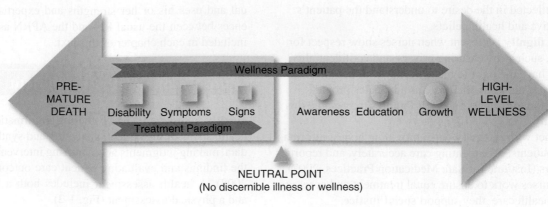

Figure 1.3 The illness–wellness continuum.

high-level wellness focuses on awareness, education, and growth. The person who moves toward illness and premature death develops signs, symptoms, and disability, which, unfortunately, is when most treatment occurs in the current health care system (Satcher, 2006). At the neutral point, there is no discernable illness or wellness; health is more than merely the absence of illness. Nurses collaborate with individuals, families, and communities to promote higher levels of wellness.

The **health belief model** considers the relationship between a person's beliefs and actions (Rosenstock & Kirscht, 1974). The elements of the model include the host (patient), agent (disease), and environment. The three elements interact to explain a person's health beliefs and responses to health care providers. Personal or cultural expectations in relation to health and illness, past experiences with health or illness, age, and developmental state all are patient factors that influence beliefs and actions. For example, a patient who receives the influenza vaccine may subsequently get a cold. This patient may decide not to receive the vaccine again because he or she believes that the injection caused the illness. Pollution, poverty, and external resources are considered environmental factors. Additionally, peer influences, personality characteristics, cultural influences, and age also influence

the individual's perception of and response to illness. For example, an elderly frail client who lives in a nursing home might perceive that he or she is in good health because it is the first time that he or she has ever had someone to nurture and care for her.

The more recent and comprehensive **health promotion model** by Pender, et al. (2005) views individuals as "multidimensional and in interaction with interpersonal and physical environments as they pursue health." Pender's model incorporates many of the elements of previous models, combining individual characteristics and experiences with behavior-specific cognitions and affect as well as with behavioral outcomes (Fig. 1-4). Prior behavioral and personal factors influence the benefits versus barriers to action. Perceived self-efficacy is the judgment of the success of being able to accomplish the action, such as a person believing that he or she will be able to lose weight. Commitment to a plan of action includes not only beginning a single activity but also continuing and reinforcing it. Competing demands can impede completion of the health-promoting behavior, such as stress and financial concerns in a single working mother of four children. Healthy outcomes lead to improvements in functional ability, quality of life, and health. These health beliefs, factors, and experiences

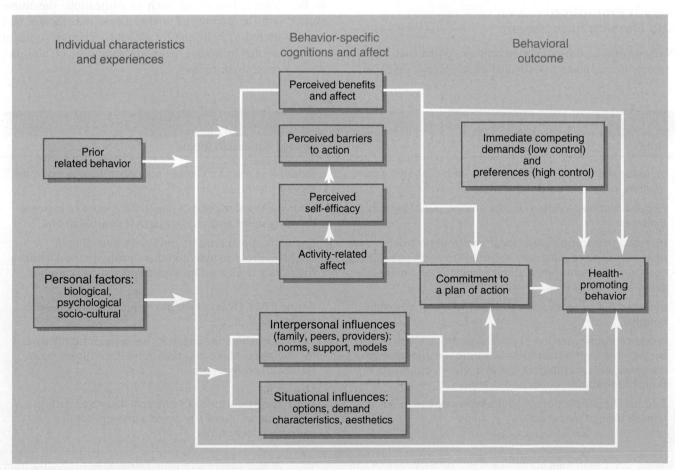

Figure 1.4 Pender's health promotion model.

are ways of explaining who is likely to practice healthy behaviors and why. The model is useful in understanding the perceptions of patients and in developing the most effective nursing interventions.

Healthy People

The U.S. Department of Health and Human Services has developed a national model for health promotion and risk reduction called *Healthy People*. The goals of this project are to increase the length and quality of life for Americans and to eliminate health disparities among different segments of the population. Every 10 years, progress is evaluated and the goals are revised. The 10 leading indicators are physical activity, overweight and obesity, tobacco use, substance abuse, responsible sexual behavior, mental health, injury and violence, environmental quality, immunization, and access to health care. Each of these indicators has specific outcomes, such as "reduce the risk of development of hypertension and colon cancer," "reduce exposure to secondhand smoke," and "reduce health disparities in children who are immunized." Outcomes for each area and associated health teaching are discussed in chapters of this book most directly linked to each indicator. An example related to Ms. Ortiz, the patient presented in this chapter's opening case study, is provided in Table 1-1.

Health Promotion and Nursing Assessment

Nurses assess health-promotion activities of patients, including nutritional intake, activity and fitness levels, psychiatric status, safety and violence activities, and stress and coping measures. They introduce screening questions and ask follow-up questions in the higher risk areas. Rather than addressing all areas associated with healthy behaviors and overwhelming patients, nurses collaborate with them to identify areas in which patients are willing to make changes. Nurses use the principles of health promotion theories (discussed earlier) to identify perceptions, barriers, and positive outcomes.

The National Center for Chronic Disease Prevention and Health Promotion has information about health assessment tools that nurses can use for screening. Organizations such as the American Heart Association (2009) and American Diabetes Association (ADA, 2009) have self-assessment tools and patient education materials. The Centers for Disease Control and Prevention (CDC) also has a Behavioral Risk Factor Surveillance System Survey to assess risk, lifestyle, and stress. Specific tools for various body systems, age groups, and other factors are discussed in chapters throughout this book within the "Risk Assessment" sections.

Sample Health History Taking Related to the Case Study

As part of Ms. Ortiz's assessment, the nurse assesses her risk factors for diabetes to identify factors that contribute to her illness. Following such identification, the nurse works with the patient to modify those risk factors that can be altered to help control diabetes. The questions at the top of the following page are examples of how the nurse assesses risk factors.

Table 1.1	*Healthy People* Goals Related to the Case Study Example	
Goals	**Patient Education Topics**
Increase the proportion of persons with diabetes who receive formal diabetes education.	Refer Ms. Ortiz to diabetes-education courses offered locally.
Reduce diabetes-related deaths among persons with diabetes.	Counsel Ms. Ortiz about health behaviors to prevent microvascular and macrovascular complications.
Increase the proportion of local health departments that have established culturally appropriate and linguistically competent community health-promotion and disease prevention programs.	Ensure that teaching materials are available in Spanish. Provide teaching that considers food choices frequently preferred by Mexican American families.
Increase the proportion of adults who are at a healthy weight.	Counsel Ms. Ortiz on weight-reduction strategies to attain a BMI of <25.
Increase the proportion of physician office visits made by patients with a diagnosis of cardiovascular disease, diabetes, or hyperlipidemia that include counseling or education related to diet and nutrition.	Provide positive feedback for keeping appointments for wellness. Make an appointment for future visits for health counseling.
Reduce the proportion of adults who engage in no leisure-time physical activity.	Teach the importance of physical activity, starting with small and realistic actions and gradually increasing over time.

Source: U.S. Department of Health and Human Services (n.d.). *Healthy People 2010: Diabetes objectives*. Retrieved April 19, 2010, from http://www.healthypeople.gov/hpscripts/KeywordResult.asp?n331=331&Submit=Submit

Questions on History and Risks	Rationales
From the patient's chart, obtain the following data: • Age • Height and weight • Ethnic background • BP • Recent cholesterol level • Any history of the following: gestational diabetes, polycystic ovarian syndrome, impaired glucose tolerance or impaired fasting glucose, cardiovascular disease • Family history	Increased age and being overweight or obese increase the patient's risk of type 2 diabetes. Being Alaska Native, American Indian, African American, Hispanic/Latino, Asian American, or Pacific Islander also increases the risk. Additional risk factors for diabetes include BP above 140/90, high density cholesterol (HDL) (good) cholesterol below 35 mg/dL, triglyceride level above 250 mg/dL, and having a parent or sibling with diabetes (ADA, 2009).
What is your typical daily diet?	A diet low in fat, calories, and sodium is recommended. Fresh fruits and vegetables should replace high-calorie foods (ADA, 2009).
How often do you exercise?	Exercising less than three times a week increases the risk for diabetes. Thirty minutes of exercise five days a week is recommended (ADA, 2009).
Considering your weight, diet, and exercise, which is the most important for you to work on right now?	It is important to identify the issues that the patient is willing to modify and prioritize as most important.

Risk Assessment and Health-Related Patient Teaching

Nurses collaborate with individuals, families, and communities to implement health promotion, risk reduction, and disease prevention strategies. The three levels of interventions to promote healthy change are primary, secondary, and tertiary (Leavell & Clark, 1965).

- **Primary prevention** involves strategies aimed at preventing problems. Immunizations, health teaching, safety precautions, and nutrition counseling are examples.
- **Secondary prevention** includes the early diagnosis of health problems and prompt treatment to prevent complications. Vision screening, Pap smears, BP screening, hearing testing, scoliosis screening, and tuberculin skin testing are examples.
- **Tertiary prevention** focuses on preventing complications of an existing disease and promoting health to the highest level. Diet teaching for patients with diabetes, inhaler teaching for patients with lung disease, and exercise programs for those who have had myocardial infarction are examples.

Assessment in the Nursing Process

The **nursing process** is a systematic problem-solving approach to identifying and treating human responses to actual or potential health problems (ANA, 2009b). It serves as a framework for providing individualized care not only to individuals but also to families and communities. It is patient centered, focusing on solving problems and enhancing strengths. The nursing process is applicable to patients in all stages of the lifespan and in all settings.

Parts of the Nursing Process

The parts of the nursing process include **assessing** the patient, analyzing data and making **diagnoses**, determining patient outcomes or **planning** care, **intervening**, and then **evaluating** the patient's status to determine if interventions were effective (Fig. 1-5). This evaluation is also an assess-

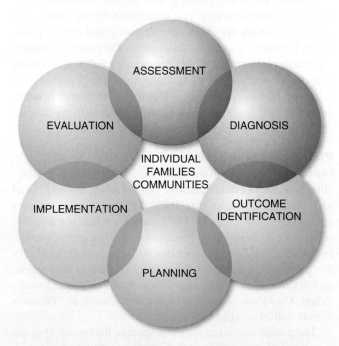

Figure 1.5 The phases of the nursing process are assessment, diagnosis, outcome identification or planning, implementation, and evaluation. Nurses apply these activities to the care of individuals, families, and communities.

ment of how well the patient is meeting the outcomes, as the patient's progress is continually assessed. From this evaluation, interventions may continue or be revised depending on whether the patient is progressing toward the outcomes.

Assess

The nursing process is not linear (progressing step by step). Rather, it is interactive and involves interrelated, sometimes overlapping, steps. As nurses collect assessment data, they provide educational or emergency interventions simultaneously. Nurses also evaluate care during an assessment, such as checking patients for side effects of medications. Nurses set outcomes collaboratively with patients—established priorities guide not only the treatment plan but also the types of future assessments performed. For example, if a hospitalized patient's priority is sleep, the nurse may decide to eliminate taking vital signs every 4 hours during the night if the patient's condition is stable.

Diagnose

Diagnosis is the clustering of data to make a judgment or statement about the patient's problem or condition. The North American Nursing Diagnosis Association (NANDA-I) defines nursing diagnosis as "a clinical judgment about individual, family or community responses to actual or potential health problems/life processes. A nursing diagnosis provides the basis for selection of nursing interventions to achieve outcomes for which the nurse is accountable" (2009, p. 277). NANDA-I has developed some common nursing diagnoses and interventions to provide a specific language and way of thinking. They are helpful for nurses learning about the professional scope of practice. In clinical practice, they are individualized to the patient or family, serving as a foundation for the labeling of problems. Nurses use diagnostic reasoning and critical thinking to formulate diagnostic statements. They use cue clustering, cluster interpretation, and diagnostic validation to ensure accuracy in selecting the correct diagnosis. Diagnoses may be actual problems, risks for developing the problems, possible problems, and wellness oriented. Applicable nursing diagnoses are found throughout the chapters of this text.

Plan Goals and Outcomes

Outcome identification includes the formulation of measurable, realistic, patient-centered goals (ANA, 2009b). Goal identification provides for individualized care as nurses collaborate with patients. For example, when a patient in acute pain is given a pain medication, the nurse assesses the pain level. The nurse collaborates with the patient to identify the pain goal, determines what level of pain is acceptable, and discusses when the patient should take more pain medication. Goals are broader than outcomes, such as "Patient's pain is within acceptable limits."

The patient outcomes are more specific than goals; they are realistic and measurable (Alfaro-LeFevre, 2010). For example, it may not be realistic for a patient to be completely free of pain, but a level of 2 on a 1-to-10 scale (with 10 being the worst) is acceptable to the patient. Because pain is subjective, the nurse gathers this information in addition to measurable

and objective pain indicators such as facial grimace, elevated pulse and BP, or rubbing the affected body part. An example of an outcome is "Pt states pain < 2 on a 1 to 10 scale, without facial grimace, P < 80, BP < 120/80 and appears to be in comfortable position." Outcomes also assist in setting priorities for care, especially with complex issues (Johnson, et al., 2005). The most common nursing outcomes for each system are discussed in each specific chapter.

Plan Care

Care planning activities include determining resources, targeting nursing interventions, and writing the plan of care. In addition to the standard care and physician orders, the nursing care plan requires an analysis about the individual patient and his or her needs. It promotes a higher level of individualized and holistic care in addition to that normally performed. The care plan is communicated verbally and is also documented in the patient's chart so that the next care provider is aware of the plan. Care planning may be documented as a care plan, care map, case note, clinical pathway, teaching plan, or discharge plan. Regardless of format, the care planning document incorporates the parts of the nursing process and critical thinking that nurses are incorporating into the patient care.

Intervene

Nursing interventions are "any treatment, based upon clinical judgment and knowledge that a nurse performs to enhance patient outcomes" (Bulechek, et al., 2007, p. xix). Nursing interventions are used to monitor health status; prevent, resolve, or control a problem; assist with activities of daily living; or promote optimum health and independence (Alfaro-LeFevre, 2010). It is important that nurses are aware of the standards of care within the agency that they work, because these standards define normal activities, such as taking vital signs every 8 hours. Types of nursing interventions include assessment, education, supervision, coordination, referral, support, therapeutic communication, and technical skills. The specific interventions for each system are covered in the appropriate chapters.

Evaluate

The evaluation of care is the judgment of the effectiveness of nursing care in meeting the patient's goals and outcomes based upon the patient's responses to the interventions (Craven & Hirnle, 2009). The purpose of evaluation is to make judgments about the progress of the patient, analyze the effectiveness of nursing care, review potential areas for collaboration and referral to other health care professionals, and monitor the quality of nursing care and its effect on the patient (Alfaro-LeFevre, 2010). Nurses assess both the facilitators of and the barriers to goal attainment. Goals may be completely met, partially met, or completely unmet; additionally, new issues and nursing diagnoses may be developed (Alfaro-LeFevre, 2010).

To effectively evaluate, nurses have knowledge of the standards of care, expected patient responses, and conceptual models and theories. They can monitor the effectiveness of nursing interventions, including interviewing skills for subjective data collection and physical assessment skills for objective data collection. It is also important that nurses are aware of the most current research and use this evidence to direct care. Nurses use critical thinking throughout the nursing process to assess, diagnose, plan, implement, and evaluate care (ADPIE).

Critical Thinking

Critical thinking in nursing (Alfaro-LeFevre, 2010):

- Entails purposeful, outcome-directed (results-oriented) thinking
- Is driven by patient, family, and community needs
- Is based on the nursing process, evidence-based thinking, and the scientific method
- Requires specific knowledge, skills, and experience
- Is guided by professional standards and codes of ethics
- Is constantly reevaluating, self-correcting, and striving to improve

Nurses are frequently involved in complex situations with multiple responsibilities. They are required to think through the analysis, develop alternatives, and implement the best interventions. Critical thinking is the key to resolving problems. Nurses who do not think things through critically deliver incomplete or misdirected care. Additionally, critical thinking is essential to passing the National Council Licensure Examination (NCLEX). Accreditation visitors to colleges of nursing, as well as to health care facilities, look for evidence of critical thinking ability. Critical thinking is a required component of health assessment and nursing care (Alfaro-LeFevre, 2010). Nurses use critical thinking to identify patterns and trends, consider missing or conflicting assessment information, and decide the type and frequency of future assessments.

Diagnostic Reasoning

The process of diagnostic reasoning is based on the nurse's critical thinking. **Diagnostic reasoning** includes gathering and clustering data to draw inferences and propose diagnoses. A seven-step process for diagnostic reasoning can be used in the context of health assessment (Weber & Kelley, 2010). Refer to Figure 1-6.

The first step is to gather assessment data to identify both abnormal findings and patient strengths. During the history and physical examination, nurses collect subjective and objective data. They then cluster data to establish themes, patterns, and common relationships. Additionally, nurses identify data that are inconsistent or missing.

After this clustering, nurses draw inferences or ideas about what the issue is. A wellness diagnosis is appropriate when patients are healthy but would like an improved health state, such as "Readiness for enhanced knowledge" (NANDA-I, 2009). This is considered primary prevention. Patients may also be at risk for a problem, in which an at-risk-for-disease

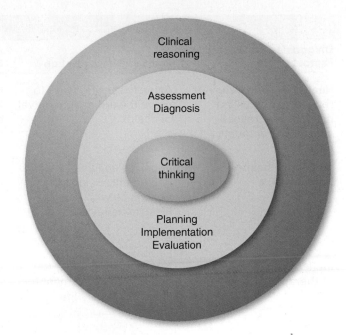

Figure 1.6 The diagnostic reasoning process.

diagnosis is appropriate, such as "At risk for skin breakdown." This can be considered secondary prevention, and interventions are targeted to prevent complications. If patients have a cluster of signs and symptoms that indicate a current problem, nurses identify the diagnoses that fit and compare assessment findings to the defining characteristics (assessments) for the diagnosis. Nurses also review the suggested interventions for each diagnosis (tertiary prevention) to determine which diagnosis is most appropriate. The diagnoses are confirmed or ruled out based on these comparisons. Lastly, nurses document the assessment and diagnoses with the diagnosis, related factors, and assessment in the format of "ineffective airway clearance related to secretions as evidenced by low pitched wheezes, cough, thick yellow sputum and oxygen saturation of 91%" (NANDA-I, 2009). No evidence is documented for the health-promotion or at-risk diagnosis, because patients do not yet have the diagnosis or supporting assessment findings.

Collaborative problems are those that nurses are monitoring but require the expertise of other health care providers for interventions. In the above example, the collaborative problem is written as a "potential complication: pneumonia." The nurse monitors temperature, lung sounds, and sputum carefully for signs and symptoms of pneumonia and notifies the primary provider if present. Although pneumonia itself is not defined as a nursing diagnosis, the collaborative assessments and interventions of the nurse in this situation are equally important. Nurses also perform interventions prescribed by providers, such as medication administration. The nursing role for these prescribed medications includes accurate administration and assessments for both intended effects and side effects. Nurses perform nursing, collaborative, and dependent interventions as part of the diagnostic reasoning process (see Table 1-2).

Table 1.2   Common Nursing Diagnoses Associated with Health

Diagnosis and Related Factors	Point of Differentiation	Assessment Characteristics	Nursing Interventions
Health-seeking behavior related to expressed desire for increased control of personal health	Actively seeking ways to move toward a higher level of health	Expressed desire to seek higher level of wellness, concern about current conditions on health status	Prioritize learner needs based on patient preferences. Emphasize positive health benefits of positive lifestyle behaviors.
Ineffective health maintenance	Impaired abilities to select, implement, or look for assistance with healthy lifestyle behaviors	Lack of health-seeking behavior, lack of resources, lack of adaptive behaviors to changes	Assess feelings, values, and reasons for not following plan of care. Assess family, economic, and cultural patterns that influence plan of care.
Ineffective management of therapeutic regimen	Not regulating and integrating a treatment for illness into daily life	Did not take action to reduce risk factors, difficulty with prescribed regimen for treatment or prevention of complications	Encourage active participation. Review actions that are not therapeutic. Identify the reasons for nontherapeutic actions.
Nonadherence	Behavior that is nonadherent with a health treatment or management plan and may lead to ineffective or undesired outcomes	Failure to adhere to plan or keep appointments, evidence of complications, exacerbation of symptoms	Identify the cause of noncompliance. Monitor the ability to follow directions, solve issues, concentrate, and read. Identify cues that trigger healthy behaviors.

As part of the care planning for Ms. Ortiz, who was recently diagnosed with diabetes, the nurse uses the diagnostic reasoning process to determine which nursing diagnoses best fit with her cluster of symptoms, including her teaching needs. Because she has shown effective management of her treatment thus far, the best diagnosis is health-seeking behavior.

Types of Assessments

Three types of nursing assessments are common: emergency, focused, and comprehensive. Emergency and focused assessments address primarily problem areas. Comprehensive assessments are broad and wide-ranging. The amount and sort of information varies, however, for all types of assessment depending on the patient's needs, purpose of data collection, health care setting, and the nurse's role.

Emergency Assessment

The **emergency assessment** involves a life-threatening or unstable situation, such as a patient in an emergency department (ED) who has experienced a traumatic injury. Staff members at the ED use triage to determine the level of acuity by considering assessments based upon the mnemonic A, B, C, and D:

- A—Airway (with cervical spine protection if an injury is suspected)
- B—Breathing—rate and depth, use of accessory muscles
- C—Circulation—pulse rate and rhythm, skin color
- D—Disability—level of consciousness, pupils, movement

All life-threatening problems identified during the initial assessment require the initiation of critical interventions. The nurse

- Opens the patient's airway
- Assists the patient's breathing
- Provides assistance with circulation (cardiopulmonary resuscitation [CPR] if needed)
- Protects the cervical spine if the patient is injured
- Ensures that the disoriented or suicidal patient is safe
- Provides pain management and sedation

The patient has assessments and critical interventions performed simultaneously as life-threatening problems are treated.

Comprehensive Assessment

The **comprehensive assessment** includes a complete health history and physical assessment. It is done annually on an outpatient basis, following admission to a hospital or long-term care facility, or every 8 hours for patients in intensive care. In primary care, the history may be obtained by having the patient initially complete an in-depth form that includes a family and personal history of illness, medical treatment, and surgeries. Nurses discuss the information with patients and clarify any incomplete or unclear areas. Dates of diagnoses and treatments are important to note along with the rationale for taking medications (eg, if a beta-blocker is taken for high BP or for history of myocardial infarction). A comprehensive history also includes a patient's perception of health, strengths to build upon, risk factors for illness, functional abilities, methods of coping, and support systems.

It is also important to reconcile the medication list with what the patient is actually taking so that patients continue taking their normal medications (Institute for Healthcare Improvement [IHI], 2007a). Because patients may be unable to participate in data collection as a result of the high acuity of the problem, nurses may need to use secondary data sources for information, such as the history in the medical record or the patient's family members.

Nurses assess the patient's health beliefs and discuss health-promotion measures. They conduct health screenings of patients according to national guidelines (eg, bowel cancer screening for a patient who has reached 50 years of age). Nurses answer questions and provide patient teaching in preparation for this diagnostic testing.

A comprehensive physical assessment includes all body systems and areas, usually in a head-to-toe format. This includes an assessment of the skin; head and neck; eyes; ears; nose, mouth, and throat; thorax and lungs; heart and neck vessels; arms and legs; breasts; abdomen; and musculoskeletal and neurological systems. Rectal and genital assessments are completed if necessary. Comprehensive assessment is more in depth when performed by a nurse practitioner. Differences between assessments performed by RNs and APRNs are discussed in each chapter.

Focused Assessment

A **focused assessment** is based upon the patient's issues. This type of assessment can occur in all settings, including the clinic, hospital, and home health. It usually involves one or two body systems and is smaller in scope than the comprehensive assessment but is more in depth on the specific issue(s). An example is a patient who presents to the clinic with a cough. The health history focuses on the duration of the cough, associated symptoms such as wheezing or shortness of breath, and factors that alleviate or worsen the cough. The physical assessment includes an assessment of the nose and throat, auscultation of the lungs, and inspection of sputum. The nurse gathers data to determine the etiology of the cough so that it may be appropriately treated.

Priority Setting

A priority issue assumes the most importance among several issues. **Priority setting** is an important skill in professional nursing practice. Its multidimensional nature and need for solid judgment make it challenging to learn. Priorities depend upon the acuity of the situation. Nurses use clinical experience, knowledge, expertise, and judgment to

determine priorities. Even expert nurses sometimes prioritize in different ways based upon their experiences.

Guidelines to use when prioritizing are to first address life-threatening situations, an issue that needs immediate attention, a concern that is very important to a patient, or something on which the nurse is spending a lot of time. Life-threatening issues always take priority; airway, breathing, and circulation are considered before other things such as elevated temperature. Often, however, priority setting is more subtle, such as deciding what to assess in a patient newly diagnosed with diabetes. In this situation, the things that are more life threatening are assessed first, such as patient knowledge of signs and symptoms of hypoglycemia and what to do when it occurs. This assessment occurs before assessing the knowledge of diet control. An example of a situation that requires immediate attention is a patient at risk for human violence or suicide. Although the patient may not currently have a life-threatening issue, the potential risk requires immediate attention.

An issue of top importance to a patient should also be considered high priority for the nurse. For example, a patient who is seen for an exacerbation of ulcerative colitis might prioritize a painful left knee as highest priority. At times, the patient and nurse may disagree on the priority given to issues. For the postoperative patient, pain or discomfort may be the priority, while the nurse views immobility as the priority because of the potential complications of pneumonia and deep vein thrombosis. In this situation, the nurse works with the patient to control the pain and then implements interventions such as ambulating the patient or coughing and deep breathing exercises. Assessment information is used to direct care in all phases of the nursing process.

Frequency of Assessment

The frequency of assessment varies with the patient's needs, purpose of data collection, and health care setting. A patient in a long-term care setting may need a comprehensive assessment once a month, while a patient in an acute hospital setting may require an assessment once a shift (Fig. 1-7). Patients in intensive care settings have vital signs and a focused assessment hourly. A facility's standards of care often prescribe such time frames, so it is important for the nurse to identify those standards for the unit and facility in which he or she is working. Patients also have focused assessments following treatments to monitor their effectiveness. If a patient who is short of breath is given an inhaler, the nurse listens to lung sounds after the treatment to see if there has been an improvement in wheezing. The nurse also performs assessments to monitor for side effects from interventions, such as assessing for pedal pulses after a cardiac catheterization in which the femoral artery is punctured. Nurses use judgment to collect data at other times based upon a change in the patient's condition.

In the outpatient setting, the frequency of assessment depends upon the course of illness and if the process is

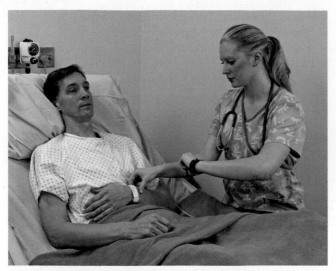

Figure 1.7 The frequency of assessment depends on the acuity of the patient's condition, which is also related to the setting for care. Hospitalized patients may undergo assessments whenever there is a change of shift.

improving or worsening. Patients also are assessed to evaluate the effectiveness of the treatment, such as follow-up for an infection, and for side effects of the treatment, such as immune suppression from chemotherapy.

Well visits are also an important component of health assessment. Periodic health assessment focuses on the most common screening and prevention services for four age groups: (1) birth to 10 years, (2) 11 to 24 years, (3) 25 to 64 years, and (4) 65 years and older. Patients are seen more frequently in the youngest years to monitor growth and development and in later years for treatment of acute and chronic illnesses.

Lifespan Issues

A comprehensive assessment includes cognitive and emotional development in addition to physical growth. Nurses identify expected growth and development patterns, normal variations, and aberrations and deviations. From infancy through adolescence, growth and development are marked by rapid spurts. From adolescence through 25 years, such growth and development proceed more slowly. Motor development occurs rapidly from birth through school age following maturation of the nervous system. Language skills develop rapidly in toddlers and preschool children as vocabulary increases and sentences become more grammatically complex.

Cognitive development follows Piaget's stages from sensorimotor to the age of magical thinking in preschool children to logical reasoning as a school-age child. Although memory may decline in older adults, wisdom remains. Psychosocial development is assessed through Erickson's stages considering trust versus mistrust as an infant and generativity versus self-absorption in the older adult. The actual versus expected stage is compared and differences are identified, such as an

older adult with addictions will have issues remaining from adolescence. Refer to Chapter 9 for more information.

Cultural and Environmental Considerations

Knowledge of cultural diversity is essential for nurses working in all areas and settings of practice. **Cultural competence** refers to the complex combination of knowledge, attitudes, and skills that a health care provider uses to deliver care that considers the total context of the patient's situation across cultural boundaries (Purnell, 2009). Culture is defined as the traits that a group of people shares and passes from one generation to the other, including values, beliefs, attitudes, and customs (Spector, 2009). Subcultures exist within larger cultural groups, so it is important to learn what the patient's specific beliefs or needs are within the larger context. The nurse has to recognize each patient's degree of assimilation into the dominant culture and the extent to which he or she identifies with the culture, considering such variables as dress, food, religion, and customs. An assessment for the effects of spirituality and religion on health is also important. Refer to Chapter 11 for more information.

Components of the Health Assessment

During the interview, the nurse uses communication skills to gather data. Communication includes not only verbal communication but also nonverbal communication observing body position, facial expression, and eye contact. Initially, the nurse introduces himself or herself and explains the purpose of the interview. Confidentiality is important, and the nurse must obtain permission from patients for other people to be present during the assessment or ask those people to step out for a few moments to allow some privacy. More information on the interview is found in Chapter 2.

The purpose of the health history is to collect family and personal histories of risk factors and past issues. The nurse reviews the family history of medical problems or mental health issues with patients. The personal history begins with biographical data on date of birth, primary language spoken, and allergies. A detailed history includes data on all systems, psychosocial and mental health, and functional status. The dates of problems are documented along with treatments and treatment outcomes. More information on the health history is found in Chapter 3.

The primary source in subjective data collection is the patient. **Subjective data** are based on patient experiences and perceptions. The individual describes the feelings, sensations, or expectations to the nurse, who then documents them as subjective data or puts them in quotes. The nurse's role relative to subjective data collection is to gather information to improve the patient's health status and to help determine the cause of the patient's current symptoms.

Remember Maria Ortiz, introduced at the beginning of this chapter. She was seen in the clinic for newly diagnosed diabetes. The following conversations give two examples of communication styles used by different nurses to collect subjective data. One style is more effective than the other. The less effective nurse directs the conversation and misses Ms. Ortiz's concerns about her diet. The more effective nurse asks open-ended questions that provide Ms. Ortiz with an opportunity to express and validate concerns.

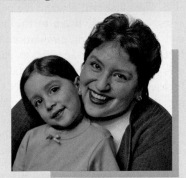

Less Effective

Nurse: It looks like you're coming in today to have your glucose checked and have some diabetic teaching.

Ms. Ortiz: Yes, they told me that I have sugar diabetes 2 weeks ago.

Nurse: It looks like you've already had classes on eating a healthy diet. Did they talk to you about the side effects of your medications and what to do if you have them?

Ms. Ortiz: They told me that I should take a half glass of orange juice if I feel shaky or sweaty because my sugar might be too low. I don't even like orange juice.

Nurse: That's right. And have you had any side effects from the medications?

Ms. Ortiz: No, I just need to learn to eat right.

Nurse: Good. What time of the day are you taking your prescriptions?

Ms. Ortiz: Usually in the morning, just before I eat my breakfast.

Nurse: That's good. When do you check your glucose?

Ms. Ortiz: Right before I take my pill, I check it.

Nurse: That's good. It sounds like you're doing everything right.

Ms. Ortiz: Maybe so.

Nurse: Is there anything else that you need?

More Effective

Nurse: Hello, Ms. Ortiz. How are you doing today?

Ms. Ortiz: Good.

Nurse: Tell me how things have been going for you.

Ms. Ortiz: Well, 2 weeks ago, they told me that I had sugar diabetes. It runs in my family, so I shouldn't be too surprised. I just haven't gotten used to this new diet.

Nurse: Tell me more about your concerns.

Ms Ortiz: Well, my mother was diabetic and she couldn't eat sugar. But they said that I can have a little dessert, just a little though. The dietician seemed to be more concerned about the cheese that I add to my refried beans.

Nurse: All food turns into sugar after you eat it, so having a little bit is OK. The dietician is thinking about the long-term effects of the fat in the cheese, because it contains calories and cholesterol that can damage your blood vessels and lead to a heart attack, stroke, or kidney problems over time. It's a different way of thinking about it than it used to be.

Ms. Ortiz: Yes, it doesn't make sense to me. But things always change. Like this, I didn't think that I would end up with diabetes, too.

Nurse: Yes, it sounds like this is a little overwhelming to you.

Critical Thinking Challenge

- What significance does it have that Ms. Ortiz is saying "sugar diabetes" instead of diabetes mellitus?
- What is the role of the nurse related to health promotion and teaching?
- What would you identify as the priority issue at this time?

The physical assessment follows the history and focused interview and includes **objective data**, which are measurable. The nurse will observe the patient's general appearance; assess vital signs; listen to the heart, lungs, and abdomen; and assess peripheral circulation. Chapters 13 to 26 include focused techniques specific to each body system. Because it is too overwhelming and time consuming to complete all focused techniques at once, only the most important screening assessments are included in the head-to-toe assessment (see Chapter 31). The nurse uses clinical judgment to decide which techniques to perform further based upon the individual patient.

Documentation and Communication

Documentation of both subjective and objective findings is essential for legal purposes and also to communicate findings to others. Accurate documentation provides a baseline so that changes are noted between assessments. Documentation may be in the form of flow sheets, case notes, or care planning. The Health Insurance Portability and Accountability Act (HIPAA, 2003) regulates the security and privacy of information. Confidentiality of documentation is essential, and only information that is pertinent to the care of the patient is shared. More information on documentation is found in Chapter 5. Samples of both normal and abnormal findings are also present in each system chapter.

Communication of assessment data is also shared verbally. Care of the patient is collaborative, and nurses use an organized method when communicating with other health care providers. Commonly, nurses describe the situation, background, and assessment data to make recommendations about the treatment that is indicated—a system known as SBAR (IHI, 2007b). Nurses also use an organized method when giving a report between shifts or transferring (handing off)

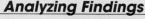

Analyzing Findings

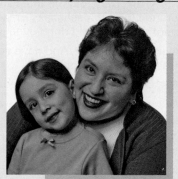

The issues of Maria Ortiz have been outlined throughout this chapter. The initial subjective and objective data collection is complete, and the nurse has spent time reviewing findings and results. This information now needs to be documented. The following nursing note illustrates how subjective and objective data are analyzed and communicated in the form of a SOAPE note (subjective, objective, analysis, plan, evaluation) based on the nursing process.

Subjective: "I just haven't gotten used to this new diet."

Objective: Alert and oriented. Skin pink, warm, and dry. Appears slightly overweight, good personal hygiene, appears stated age. BP 138/78 mmHg, pulse 82 beats/min, and respirations 16 breaths/min. Current medications include an oral hypoglycemic medication and daily vitamin. Expressing concerns about diet and intake of sugar and fat. Typical diet is high in starch and fat and low in fresh fruits and vegetables.

Analysis: Health-seeking behaviors related to new diagnosis and medication.

Plan: Perform teaching on diet and safety related to potential hypoglycemia from oral hypoglycemic medication.

Evaluation: Stated signs and symptoms of hypoglycemia and treatment with 10–15 g of carbohydrate. Given written information on what to do if she becomes hypoglycemic in the future. Stated that she will try using low-fat cheese in her beans and check in at next visit. Will start reading labels for calorie and fat content. Made appointment for clinic visit in 2 weeks. Is enrolled in a diabetes-education class and will bring her questions to the next visit.

P. Miso, RN

Critical Thinking Challenge

- What type of risk assessments will be performed at her next visit?
- What type of physical assessment might be performed at the next visit?
- How might the nurse consider Ms. Ortiz's culture, language, and family in the assessment?

patients to other departments, such as when a patient is sent to the operating room (Joint Commission on Accreditation of Healthcare Organizations, 2007). Examples of SBAR are included in Chapter 5 and also in each individual system chapter.

Frameworks for Health Assessment

There are three major frameworks for organizing assessment data: functional systems, head-to-toe system, and body systems. All these methods provide an organizing framework so that nurses do not inadvertently forget any of the important assessment data. Each type begins with a general survey of the patient, vital signs, and level of distress. Developing a consistent and organized approach is more important than considering which system to use (Table 1-3).

A **functional assessment** focuses on the functional patterns that all humans share: health perception and health management, activity and exercise, nutrition and metabolism, elimination, sleep and rest, cognition and perception, self-perception and self-concept, roles and relationships, coping and stress tolerance, sexuality and reproduction, and values and beliefs (Gordon, 1987). Often, nurses use the functional patterns to collect subjective data following a health history but a head-to-toe system for the physical assessment. Refer to Chapter 3 for more information.

A **head-to-toe assessment** is the most organized system for gathering comprehensive physical data. Because data in one functional area are collected from different parts of the body, it is very inefficient to collect physical data by functional status. For example, peripheral circulation is assessed in both the arms and the legs. Rather than assess the arms and legs and come back to listen to the heart and lungs, it is more organized to proceed from head to toe. When exposing the chest, both the heart and the lungs are auscultated. The chest is covered, then the abdomen is assessed and covered, and the legs and feet are assessed last. This method is more efficient and provides more modesty for patients. See Chapter 31 for more information.

A **body systems** approach is a logical tool for organizing data when documenting and communicating findings. This method promotes critical thinking and allows nurses to analyze findings as they cluster similar data. Data from the functional and head-to-toe assessments are reorganized. When reorganizing data related to the respiratory system, the nurse considers the patient's skin color with lung sounds and any shortness of breath to determine the acuity of the issue and anticipate interventions. The nurse also includes vital signs data including respiratory rate and oxygen saturation. He or she considers data from the general survey, such as posture, shortness of breath, and level of distress. If the patient with shortness of breath is also cyanotic and wheezing, a respiratory issue is suspected. The condition is acute, and the nurse applies supplemental oxygen while contacting a primary care provider. Rather than identifying one piece of data in isolation, a systems approach allows nurses to cluster similar data together to identify issues.

Table 1.3	Comparison of Assessment Frameworks	
Functional Health Pattern	**Head to Toe**	**Body System**
Nutrition and metabolism	Head and neck	Neurological and cardiovascular
Cognitive perceptual		
Cognitive perceptual	Eyes and ears	Neurological
Nutrition and metabolism	Nose, mouth, and throat	Gastrointestinal and respiratory
Activity exercise	Thorax and lungs	Respiratory
Activity exercise	Cardiac	Cardiovascular
Activity exercise	Peripheral vascular	Cardiovascular
Sexuality and reproductive	Breast	Reproductive
Nutrition and metabolism, sexuality and reproductive, elimination	Abdominal	Gastrointestinal, urinary, and reproductive
Activity exercise	Musculoskeletal	Musculoskeletal
Cognitive perceptual	Neurological	Neurological
Sexuality and reproductive	Male or female genitalia	Reproductive
Sexuality and reproductive, elimination	Anus, rectum, and prostate	Gastrointestinal and reproductive
Health perception, sleep, cognition, self-perception, roles, coping, sexuality, values	Functional health status	

Pulling It All Together: Reflection and Critical Thinking

The nurse uses assessment data to formulate a nursing care plan for Maria Ortiz. After these interventions are completed, the nurse will reevaluate the patient and document the findings in the chart to show critical thinking. This is often in the form of a care plan or case note similar to the one below.

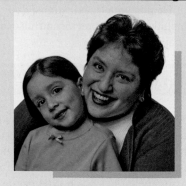

Nursing Diagnosis	Patient Outcomes	Nursing Interventions	Rationales	Evaluation
Knowledge deficit related to new diagnosis and medication	The patient states what to do for symptoms of hypoglycemia.	Discuss signs and symptoms of hypoglycemia. Discuss what to do if hypoglycemic and provide a list of appropriate foods to increase blood glucose level.	Written information reinforces verbal information and can be used as a resource once at home.	Stated signs and symptoms of hypoglycemia. Stated four foods that contain 10–15 g of fast-acting carbohydrate. Will bring questions to next clinic visit.

Evidence-Based Critical Thinking

Evidence-based practice is an approach to patient care that minimizes intuition and personal experience and instead relies upon research findings and high-grade scientific support. **Evidence-based thinking** helps nurses to solve common problems through four steps:

1. Clearly identify the issue or problem based on an accurate analysis of current nursing knowledge and practice.
2. Search the literature for relevant research.
3. Evaluate the research evidence using established criteria regarding scientific merit.
4. Choose interventions and justify the selection with the most valid evidence (Evidence Based Practice, 2007).

Many ways are available for nurses to use research and evidence to provide holistic care to patients. The National Institute for Nursing Research (NINR) (http://www.nih.gov/ninr/), formed in 1986, greatly increased the visibility and funding opportunities for nursing research. The International Honor Society for Nursing, Sigma Theta Tau, has also increased its capacity to support and disseminate nursing scholarships for nursing research (Sigma Theta Tau, 2009). Additionally, McMaster University in Ontario, Canada, has developed extensive resources in teaching and implementing evidence-based practice in nursing and other disciplines (Evidence Based Practice, 2007).

Some evidence is evaluated by performing clinical trials, such as measuring the accuracy of a new oral thermometer against core temperature. If there are several clinical trials, a systematic review of the quality trials becomes the "gold standard." The Cochrane Database is considered the most complete and accurate collection of systematic reviews and is available in most libraries. The National Clearinghouse Guidelines also have recommendations based upon the clinical evidence. PubMed clinical inquiries are another site for obtaining the most current evidence. Many nursing facilities are implementing programs in which nurses develop a clinical question and find the best evidence to plan care. In this way, nurses base individual patient decisions upon the best existing evidence rather than upon their personal experience.

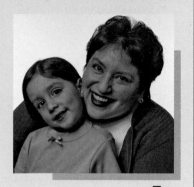

Remember Ms. Ortiz, the 52-year-old patient who is being seen for a follow-up visit for her recently diagnosed diabetes. Consider responses to the questions introduced at the beginning of the chapter. Recognize how the knowledge gained in this chapter can be applied to her case using critical thinking.

• What are potential health-promotion and teaching needs for Ms. Ortiz based on the above information?
• How should the nurse approach a discussion of the patient's diet as related to her diabetes?
• How will the nurse individualize today's health assessment, considering the patient's gender, age, and culture?
• What is the role of the nurse in providing care for Ms. Ortiz during this visit?

Key Points

• The role of the professional nurse is to promote health, prevent illness, treat human responses, and advocate for patients.
• Nurses are providers, designers, managers, and coordinators of care as well as advocates and educators.
• Nursing values include altruism, dignity, autonomy, integrity, and social justice.
• Health can be conceptualized as falling at a point on a trajectory between wellness and illness.
• *Healthy People* is a U.S. initiative to focus on health-promotion and risk-reduction strategies.
• Primary, secondary, and tertiary prevention are used to promote health change.
• Steps of the nursing process include assessment, diagnosis, setting goals and outcomes, planning, intervening, and evaluating.
• Critical thinking is the key to resolving problems.
• Diagnostic reasoning is a process by which nurses use critical thinking to cluster the assessment information and to draw inferences about meaning.
• Types of assessments include emergency, comprehensive, and focused.
• Subjective data are based on the patient's experiences and perceptions.
• Objective data are measurable and usually collected as part of the physical assessment.
• Organizing frameworks for assessment include functional, head-to-toe, and body systems.
• Evidence-based nursing relies upon research findings and high-grade scientific support.

Review Questions

1. A patient is having side effects from a medication. The nurse calls the provider to request a change to the medication order. The nurse is functioning as an/a
A. Educator
B. Advocate
C. Organizer
D. Counselor

2. Nurses advocate for underserved populations to reduce health disparities. This promotes
A. Autonomy
B. Altruism
C. Social justice
D. Human dignity

3. Nurses belong to the ANA as part of their
A. Ongoing professional responsibility
B. Role as manager of care
C. Wellness promotion for patients
D. Cultural education activities

4. The purpose of health assessment is to
A. Obtain subjective and objective data
B. Intervene to correct problems
C. Outline care that is appropriate
D. Determine if interventions are effective

5. The nurse documents the following information in a patient's chart: "cough and deep breathe every hour while awake." This is an example of
A. Evidence-based nursing
B. Priority setting
C. Comprehensive assessment
D. Nursing interventions

6. The nurse provides teaching about smoking cessation to a 20-year-old man. The nurse assesses that the patient is concerned because his father died from lung cancer. Which theory would the nurse most likely use when providing teaching to this patient?
A. Health belief model
B. Diagnostic reasoning model
C. Cultural competence model
D. Body systems model

7. Which of the following processes is the most important when providing nursing care to an ill patient?
A. Writing outcomes
B. Performing a focused assessment
C. Collecting objective data
D. Using critical thinking

8. A patient is admitted to a hospital for surgery for colon cancer. What type of assessment is the nurse most likely to perform upon admission?
A. Emergency
B. Focused
C. Comprehensive
D. Illness

9. Which of the following are components of a comprehensive health assessment?
A. Nursing diagnoses
B. Goals and outcomes
C. Collaborative problems
D. Examination of body systems

10. The nurse conducts the health history based upon the patient's responses to the medical diagnosis. This type of framework is based on the
A. Functional framework
B. Objective framework
C. Coordinator framework
D. Collaborative framework

References

Alfaro-LeFevre, R. (2010). *Applying nursing process: A tool for critical thinking* (7th ed.). Philadelphia: Wolters Kluwer Health/Lippincott Williams & Wilkins.

AACN. (2008). *The essentials of baccalaureate education for professional nursing practice.* Washington, DC: Author.

ADA. (2009). *Nutrition recommendations and interventions for diabetes.* Retrieved April 3, 2009, from http://care.diabetesjournals.org/cgi/content/full/30/suppl_1/S48

American Heart Association. (2009). *Diseases and conditions.* Retrieved April 3, 2009, from http://www.americanheart.org/presenter.jhtml?identifier=1200002

ANA. (2003). *Nursing's social policy statement* (2nd ed.). Washington, DC: Author.

ANA. (2004). *Nursing: Scope and standards of practice.* Washington, DC: Author.

ANA. (2005). *Code of ethics for nurses with interpretive statements.* Washington, DC: Author.

ANA. (2009a). *More about nurses and advanced practice nurses.* Retrieved April 5, 2009, from http://www.nursingworld.org/EspeciallyForYou/StudentNurses/RNsAPNs.aspx

ANA. (2009b). *The nursing process: A common thread amongst all nurses.* Retrieved April 3, 2009, from http://www.nursingworld.org/EspeciallyForYou/StudentNurses/Thenursingprocess.aspx

Bulechek, G. M., Butcher, H. K., & McCloskey Dochterman, J. (2007). *Nursing Interventions Classification* (*NIC*) (5th ed.). St Louis: Mosby.

Craven, R. F., & Hirnle, C. J. (2009). *Fundamentals of nursing: Human health and function* (6th ed.). Philadelphia: Lippincott.

Cronenwett, L., Sherwood, G., Barnsteiner, J., et al. (2007). Quality and safety education for nurses. *Nursing Outlook, 55*(3), 122–131.

Davis, L. A. (2005). A phenomenological study of patient expectations concerning nursing care. *Holistic Nursing Practice, 19*(3), 126–133.

Evidence Based Practice. (2007). Retrieved June 19, 2007, from http://www.fhs.mcmaster.ca/ceb/acts/ebcp.htm

Gordon, M. (1987). *Nursing diagnosis: Process and application* (2nd ed.). New York: McGraw Hill.

HIPAA. (2003). *Standards for privacy of individually identifiable health information.* Retrieved June 15, 2007, from http://www.hhs.gov/ocr/hipaa/privrulepd.pdf

IHI. (2007a). *Medication reconciliation review.* Retrieved June 19, 2007, from http://www.ihi.org/IHI/Topics/PatientSafety/MedicationSystems/Tools/Medication+Reconciliation+Review.htm

IHI. (2007b). *SBAR technique for communication: A situational briefing model.* Retrieved June 19, 2007, from http://www.ihi.org/IHI/Topics/PatientSafety/SafetyGeneral/Tools/SBARTechniqueforCommunicationASituationalBriefingModel.htm

Institute for Safe Medication Practices. (2007). *Medication tools and resources.* Retrieved June 19, 2007, from http://www.ismp.org/Tools/default.asp

Institute of Medicine. (2004). *Keeping patients safe: Transforming the work environment of nurses.* Washington, DC: National Academies Press.

Johnson, M., Bulechek, G. M., & McCloskey Dochterman, J. (2005). *NANDA, NOC, and NIC linkages: Nursing diagnoses, outcomes, and interventions.* St. Louis: Mosby.

Joint Commission on Accreditation of Healthcare Organizations. (2007). *National patient safety goals.* Retrieved June 19, 2007, from http://www.jointcommission.org/PatientSafety/NationalPatientSafetyGoals/ on June 19, 2007.

Leavell, H. R., & Clark, E. G. (1965). *Preventive medicine for the doctor in his community: An epidemiologic approach.* New York: McGraw-Hill.

NANDA-I. (2009). *Nursing diagnoses, 2009–2011 Edition: Definitions and classifications (NANDA NURSING DIAGNOSIS).* West Sussex UK: John Wiley & Sons.

Pender, N. J., Murdaugh, C. L., & Parsons, M. A. (2006). *Health promotion in nursing practice* (5th ed.). Upper Saddle River, NJ: Prentice Hall.

Purnell, L. D. (2009). *Guide to culturally competent health care* (2nd ed.). Philadelphia: F. A. Davis, Co.

Rosenstock, I. M., & Kirscht, J. P. (1974). The health belief model and personal health behavior. *Health Education Monographs, 2,* 470–473.

Rothschild, J. M., Hurley, A. C., Landrigan, C. P., et al. (2006). Recovering from medical errors: The critical care nursing safety net. *Joint Commission Journal on Quality and Patient Safety, 32*(2), 63–72.

Satcher, D. (2006). The prevention challenge and opportunity. *Health Affiliations, 25*(4), 1009–1011.

Sigma Theta Tau. (2009). *Mission and vision.* Retrieved April 3, 2009, from http://www.nursingsociety.org/aboutus/mission/Pages/factsheet.aspx

Spector, R. E. (2009). *Cultural diversity in health and illness* (7th ed.). Upper Saddle River, NJ: Pearson Prentice Hall Health.

Travis, J. W., & Regina, R. S. (2004). *Wellness workbook* (3rd ed.). Berkeley: Celestial Arts.

Weber, J., & Kelley, J. (2010). *Health assessment in nursing* (4th ed.). Philadelphia: Wolters Kluwer Health/Lippincott Williams & Wilkins.

The Jensen suite offers these additional resources to enhance learning and facilitate understanding of this chapter:

• thePoint online resource, http//thepoint.lww.com/Jensen1E
• Student CD-ROM included with the book
• *Laboratory Manual for Nursing Health Assessment: A Best-Practice Approach*
• *Pocket Guide for Nursing Health Assessment: A Best-Practice Approach*

The Interview and Therapeutic Dialogue

Learning Objectives

1 Identify the significance of nonverbal communication.

2 Describe how nurses use active listening, restatement, reflection, elaboration, silence, focusing, clarification, and summarizing in verbal communication.

3 Recognize the less effective results of nontherapeutic responses.

4 Differentiate the preinteraction, beginning, working, and closing phases of the interview process.

5 Describe sensitivity to intercultural communication, including working with patients who have limited English knowledge, working with interpreters, and being sensitive to gender-related issues.

6 Recognize special communication techniques that nurses may use when working with newborns and infants, children, adolescents, and older adults.

7 Identify helpful techniques when working with patients in special situations: hearing impairment, low level of consciousness, cognitive impairment, psychiatric illness, anxiety, crying, anger, drug use, personal questions, and sexual innuendo.

8 Individualize health assessment interview techniques and therapeutic communication considering the condition, age, gender, and culture of the patient.

*M*r. Rowan, a 36-year-old Caucasian man, resides in an assisted-living facility. He was diagnosed with AIDS 2 years ago. He has been nonadherent with his antiretroviral medication regimen, because he dislikes taking "artificial substances" and believes that natural methods (eg, nutrition) are more effective toward controlling his illness. He has been receiving meals and housekeeping as part of his services. The nurse has ongoing contact with him to encourage him to take his medications and to assess his condition and needs.

You will gain more information about Mr. Rowan as you progress through this chapter. As you study the content and features, consider this patient's case and its relationship to what you are learning. Begin thinking about the following points:

- Is it important for the nurse to interview the patient about how he contracted AIDS?
- What is your perceived risk of exposure to HIV/AIDS?
- Which techniques of therapeutic communication might the nurse need to use when talking with the patient?
- How might the nurse's personal beliefs about AIDS and alternative therapies affect communication with Mr. Rowan?
- How can the nurse communicate nonjudgmental care both verbally and nonverbally?
- What cultural, environmental, or developmental issues might you anticipate for Mr. Rowan?

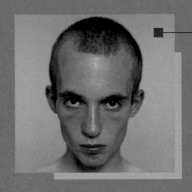

All nursing practice revolves around the **nurse–patient relationship**, which is built upon verbal and nonverbal communication within a specific setting. The nurse–patient relationship differs from personal and social relationships, because its foundation is the therapeutic use of self through verbal and nonverbal communication skills. The nurse has a privileged role as a respected care provider. The relationships with patients are professionally intimate. For example, in some situations, patients disclose information to the nurse that they do not even share with family members. Within the nurse–patient relationship, the nurse learns wide-ranging things about patients—from minute physical details to deep-seated feelings about spirituality, culture, and psychosocial concerns.

Communication Process

Communication is a complex, ongoing, interactive process that forms the basis for building interpersonal relationships (American Association of Colleges of Nursing [AACN], 2008). It is a system of sending and receiving messages, forming a connection between sender and receiver (Fig. 2-1). This continuous and dynamic process is always subject to interpretation. The sender's purpose is translated into a code with verbal language, gestures, facial expressions, and body cues. The receiver decodes the message, making meaning of the verbal and nonverbal messages. Subjective understanding, perceptions, and other variables greatly influence the actual decoding, both correctly and incorrectly. For example, some Native American tribes consider it respectful to shake hands softly; however, Americans of Northern European heritage may incorrectly decode this nonverbal communication as cold or unfriendly.

Once messages are given and decoded, the receiver and sender give feedback and more messages to stimulate further dialogue. Communication ability, culture, and personal experience all influence the interpretation and decoding of messages. Communication ability means having the cognitive and physical faculties to communicate. People who have experienced a cerebrovascular accident (stroke) may have permanent damage to the part of the brain that either elicits

or interprets speech, making it difficult for them to understand (receptive aphasia) or speak (expressive aphasia). For patients with expressive aphasia, the nurse asks questions that facilitate yes or no answers or provides simple choices to ease communication and reduce frustration. For patients with receptive aphasia, the best approach is for the nurse to use short and simple words and sentences.

Additionally, culture can influence a person's understanding of communication. In many Asian cultures, mental health disorders carry great stigma, so patients may describe psychosocial problems instead as a lack of sleep or as feeling tired (Choi & Gi Park, 2006). There are many other situations where culture affects communication.

Both nurses and patients bring perceptions about the relationship with them. A patient who has had positive personal experiences with the health care system may be more open to developing a relationship with a nurse than the one who has had negative experiences. Perceptions of the health care system are important to assess.

Therapeutic communication is a basic tool that the nurse uses in the caring relationship with patients. In therapeutic communication, the interaction focuses on the patient and the patient's concerns. The nurse assists patients to work through feelings and explore options related to the situation, outcomes, and treatments. This skill takes practice but can be learned with attention and awareness. It takes time to learn to listen for messages that might otherwise be unheard, but this careful listening contributes greatly to a therapeutic relationship. Caring and empathy are useful when communicating therapeutically.

Caring encompasses the nurse's empathy for and connection with the patient. It also includes the ability to demonstrate emotional characteristics such as compassion, sensitivity, and patient-centered care (AACN, 2008). The nurse shows warmth, caring, interest, and respect and values patients unconditionally and nonjudgmentally. Patients are more willing to discuss their health issues if they perceive the nurse as caring, understanding, and nonjudgmental.

Empathy means the ability to perceive, reason, and communicate understanding of another person's feelings

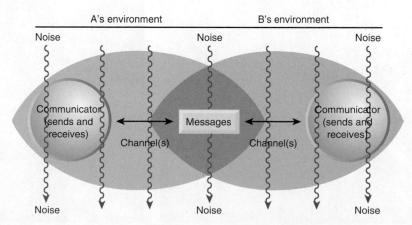

Figure 2.1 Communication is a system of sending and receiving messages, forming a connection between the sender and the receiver. (Source: Adler, R. B., & Proctor, R. F. (2007). *Looking out/looking in* (12th ed.). Belmont, CA: Thomson/Wadsworth.)

without criticism. It is being able to see and feel the situation from the patient's perspective, not the nurse's. When being empathetic, the nurse asks questions that help patients express how they are feeling and what they are thinking so that the nurse understands. The nurse can communicate to patients that he or she accurately appreciates the thoughts, feelings, and experiences. In some situations, such as death of a relative, the nurse may exhibit empathy simply by holding a person's hand or offering a tissue.

The nurse with a comfortable **self-concept** is aware of his or her own biases, values, personalities, cultural backgrounds, and communication styles. He or she builds such awareness through self-reflection and listening to and understanding feedback from others. Self-reflection increases the ability to be genuine, connect with patients, and meet their needs. Having a comfortable sense of self allows the nurse to work with patients of different personalities, cultures, and socioeconomic backgrounds. According to Mezirow (1990), self-reflection includes

> the process of becoming critically aware of how and why our presuppositions have come to constrain the way we perceive, understand, and feel about our world; of reformulating these assumptions to permit a more inclusive, discriminating, permeable and integrative perspective; and of making decisions or otherwise acting on these new understandings. More inclusive, discriminating permeable and integrative perspectives are superior perspectives that adults choose if they can because they are motivated to better understand the meaning of their experience.

Nonverbal Communication Skills

Nonverbal communication is as important as, if not more important than, verbal communication. Physical appearance, facial expression, posture and positioning in relation to the patient, gestures, eye contact, voice, and use of touch are all important components. The nurse should not assume that touch is culturally acceptable. Permission to touch the patient is a courtesy by asking, "Is it OK if I feel your abdomen?"

The physical appearance of the nurse sends a message to patients. Thus, it is important for nurses to ensure that their dress and appearance are professional. Facial expressions should be relaxed, caring, and interested. Facial expressions common in social situations (eg, rolling the eyes, looking bored, or disgusted) reduce trust. The nurse uses gestures intentionally to illustrate points, especially for patients who cannot communicate verbally. The nurse may point with a finger or gesture an action, such as pretending to drink or pointing to the bathroom. Gestures are purposeful rather than distracting from the communication.

To facilitate optimal eye contact, the nurse needs to be at eye level with the patient. Those who stand while patients are in bed will be taller than patients, assuming a position of power. Some patients may interpret the nurse who sits on hospital beds or examining tables as too close or unprofessional, and possibly as infringing on personal space. Also, considering principles of infection control, beds or tables may contain microorganisms or body secretions that the nurse could carry from one room to another (see Chapter 4). For these reasons, the nurse should be seated in chairs at eye level with patients who are in bed during interviews (Fig. 2-2A). For patients seated on examination tables, the nurse will be near eye level when standing (Fig. 2-2B).

Touch is an essential and dominant component of the physical examination. During initial interviews, however, patients may misinterpret touch from the nurse as being too casual. The nurse uses nonverbal skills to communicate messages to patients that facilitate a therapeutic relationship. If a nurse is positioned near the bed, speaks carefully, and maintains good eye contact, the patient feels that he or she is being heard.

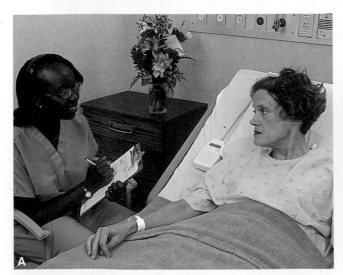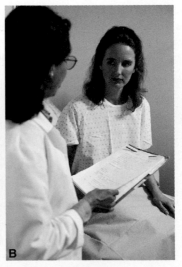

Figure 2.2 **(A)** The nurse working with a patient who is in a hospital bed sits to be at eye level with the patient during the interview. **(B)** The nurse stands to be at eye level with the patient on an examination table.

Verbal Communication Skills

The nurse learns effective interviewing skills through practice and repetition, using these skills to encourage patients to further expand their initial brief answers and also to redirect patients when they wander from the topic.

The nurse's speech is of moderate pace and volume, with clear articulation. A too soft voice might indicate embarrassment or discomfort, while a too loud voice may be powerful and controlling. Speech that is too fast indicates being rushed, while speech that is too slow might send a message that the patient is lacking in cognitive ability. For patients with hearing impairment, the nurse may need to speak loudly and slowly into the better ear or be positioned so that patients can lip read (Fig. 2-3).

For patients with limited English knowledge, the nurse uses simple and clear language but does not need to speak louder. Instead of using complete sentences, the nurse might speak in one or two words, such as "Pain?" The nurse inserts pauses in the conversation to allow patients an opportunity to speak; such pauses facilitate trust, respect, and sharing.

Active Listening

Active listening is the ability to focus on patients and their perspectives. It requires the nurse to constantly decode messages including thoughts, words, opinions, and emotions. For example, if a patient is sad, it is appropriate for a nurse to place a hand over the patient's and to show a facial expression of compassion. If a patient is angry, the nurse listens to the reason for the anger, such as treatment failure. Rather than respond in turn with anger, the nurse attends to the patient's feelings by pulling up a chair and taking the time to listen. He or she tries to uncover the hidden message and reflects appropriate body language.

Talking about difficult feelings helps patients to heal. The nurse is not expected to solve all the problems but instead to therapeutically use the self to assist patients to deal with them.

⚠ *SAFETY ALERT 2-1*

If talking about a situation seems to escalate rather than diffuse a patient's anger, the nurse may redirect the interview. If a patient is abusive or overly aggressive, it may be necessary to take a time-out by saying, "I understand that you're very angry right now. I am feeling a little defensive, so I can either have someone else come in to talk with you or come back in 15 minutes. Which would you prefer?"

Restatement

Restatement relates to the content of the communication. The nurse makes a simple statement, usually using the words of patients. The purpose is to ask patients to elaborate. Restatement provides an opportunity for patients to further understand their communication. For example, the nurse says, "So, you feel like there is a knot in your chest."

Reflection

Reflection is similar to restatement; however, instead of simply restating comments, the nurse summarizes the main themes of communication. The conversation may be longer, in which a patient discusses several elements related to a topic. The nurse listens carefully to the different thoughts expressed and attempts to identify their relationship. With this technique, patients gain a better understanding of the issues that underlie their thoughts, which helps to identify their feelings. The following example illustrates how the nurse can use reflection.

Patient: I really hate getting shots. Do I really need to get the flu shot? My parents never had it and they stayed healthy during the winter.
Nurse: You sound a bit nervous about getting an injection. (Reflection)
Patient: The last shot that I had really hurt.

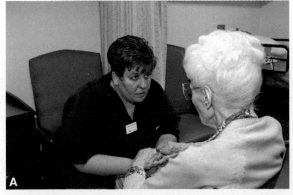
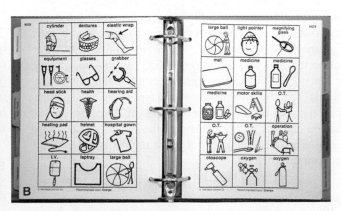

Figure 2.3 The nurse must be creative to communicate with patients who cannot fully interact verbally or who have sensory impairments. **(A)** This nurse is making sure to sit directly in front of the patient and enunciate very clearly for a patient with hearing difficulties. **(B)** Picture boards can be helpful for patients who cannot speak or who cannot communicate in the same language as the nurse.

In the previous situation, the patient was not questioning the need for the injection but was expressing anxiety about it because of previous experience. The nurse now knows to direct the conversation toward dealing with the anxiety rather than teaching about the risk for influenza.

Encouraging Elaboration (Facilitation)

Encouraging elaboration (facilitation) is a technique that assists patients to more completely describe problems. These responses encourage patients to say more and continue the conversation. They show patients that the nurse is interested. The nurse may nod the head or say "Um hum," "Yes," or "Go on" to cue patients to keep talking. Another technique is to let patients know that their thoughts and feelings are common and give them permission to discuss them. The nurse might use a phrase such as, "Sometimes when patients are involved in a car accident, they have flashbacks or bad dreams."

Silence

The nurse uses **silence** purposefully during the interview to allow patients time to gather their thoughts and provide accurate answers. He or she also uses silence therapeutically to communicate nonverbal concern. Silence also gives patients a chance to decide how much information to disclose. For example, patients may be embarrassed to discuss the events that led them to contract sexually transmitted infections. The use of silence by the nurse sends a message that when patients are ready, the nurse will be there to listen. Silence also provides the nurse with an opportunity to decide which direction to take the conversation. He or she can attend to nonverbal language and note whether patients seem like they do not want to continue talking or just need time to gather thoughts and emotions. Be aware, however, that silence may not be appreciated by patients of some cultures and may be perceived negatively.

Focusing

The nurse uses **focusing** when patients are straying from a topic and need redirection. Focusing helps when the nurse needs to address areas of concern related to current problems. An example of focusing is, "We were talking about the reaction that you had to the penicillin. Tell me more about that reaction." This response connects the patient's story to the initial need for information on the type of reaction, which is a safety issue needing further discussion. It keeps the conversation on track without changing the subject and conveys the message that the nurse will assist the patient to provide important information.

Clarification

Clarification is important when the patient's word choice or ideas are unclear. For example, the nurse states, "Tell me what you mean by the evil eye." Another way to clarify is to ask, "What happens when you get low blood?" Such questions prompt patients to identify other symptoms or give more information so that the nurse better understands. The nurse also can use clarification when the patient's history of illness is confusing. Putting data in chronological order or placing events in context can help make the story clearer. For example, a nurse might ask, "When you had chest pain, first you took three nitroglycerin tablets and then you called 911, is that right?"

Summarizing

Summarizing happens at the end of the interview, during the closure phase. The nurse reviews and condenses important information into two or three of the most important findings. Doing so helps ensure that the nurse has identified important information and lets the patient know that he or she has been heard accurately. It gives the nurse and patient future direction as they establish a therapeutic relationship. Summarizing includes the progress made toward problem solving and things to think about later. An example is, "It seems that you are most concerned about your child's appetite and lack of energy. We have talked about adding some low-cost and high-protein foods to her diet. When you come in for your next visit, we can talk about how that worked."

Nontherapeutic Responses

False Reassurance

Often in social situations, people use nontherapeutic casual responses. Probably the most common example is **false reassurance** to minimize uncomfortable feelings. In nurse–patient relationships, giving false reassurance also can minimize the amount of distressing information that the nurse has to handle. Nevertheless, such responses effectively close off communication from the perspective of patients. By providing false reassurance, the nurse unconsciously indicates to patients that their concerns are not worth discussing. This situation enhances anxiety, which can increase a patient's urge to seek further reassurance, and diminishes his or her trust. Examples of false reassurance are, "It won't hurt." or "Don't worry. It will be all right." It would be better to say, "It will hurt a bit when I take off the bandage, but I'll do it quickly." or "It sounds like you're concerned that your cancer might have returned. I want you to know that I will be here when you get your test results tomorrow." This type of reassurance validates the patient's concerns and reassures him or her that the nurse will be there to provide a therapeutic relationship.

Sympathy

Sympathy is feeling what a patient feels from the viewpoint of the nurse. When the nurse is being sympathetic, he or she is not being therapeutic, because the nurse is interpreting the situation as he or she perceives it. By contrast, empathy is feeling what a patient feels from the patient's perspective. The nurse keeps the focus on the patient, allowing his or her complete self-expression.

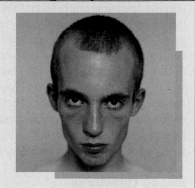

The nurse's role related to interviewing is to gather information to assess the patient's health status and to provide therapeutic communication when indicated. A student nurse is visiting Mr. Rowan, introduced at the beginning of this chapter, to remind him to take his antiretroviral medications and to assess his current needs. The following conversations give two examples of interview styles. One style is more effective than the other.

Less Effective	More Effective
Nurse: Hi, Mr. Rowan. I'm Tom Fritz, a student who is working with your nurse. May I come in?	**Nurse:** Hi, Mr. Rowan. I'm Tom Fritz, a student who is working with your nurse. Betsy said to let you know that she's available if you would rather talk with her.
Mr. Rowan: OK. Do you want a glass of water?	**Mr Rowan:** You're working with Betsy?
Nurse: No, thanks. I just finished my lunch, and I'm full.	**Nurse:** Yes, she's seeing another patient but said that she could come and see you if you would prefer that.
Mr. Rowan: So what do you want?	**Mr Rowan:** No, come on in. Would you like a glass of water?
Nurse: I am here to check your medications by doing a pill count and also to see if you need anything.	**Nurse:** That would be great if it's not too inconvenient.
Mr. Rowan: I already took my pills. You can count them if you want.	**Mr Rowan:** (Gets water) You can sit down.
Nurse: That would be great. Do you have them nearby?	**Nurse:** Thank you so much. Tell me how you're doing today.
Mr. Rowan: They're right here. I don't like taking them, but if I don't, my nurse Betsy tells me that I need to take better care of myself. (Mr. Rowan gets medications.) You can sit down.	**Mr Rowan:** I'm OK—you're here to make sure that I took my medication, aren't you? I already took it—you can count the pills if you want.
Nurse: No thanks. I'm glad that you're taking the medications. The count is right. Do you need anything else?	**Nurse:** We can do that in a minute. I'd just like to talk for a little bit to see how you're feeling and if I can help in any way.
Mr. Rowan: No. I'm just feeling weak and tired. Is there anything else that you want?	**Mr Rowan:** Well, I'd rather be home, but I can't live by myself anymore. Every day I just seem to get weaker.

Critical Thinking Challenge

- Compare and contrast the data collected in the two dialogues. What therapeutic communication techniques were used in each?
- What differences happened at the beginning of each dialogue?
- What interactions occurred in both dialogues that might influence the student nurse's ability to establish trust with Mr. Rowan?
- What were the differences in outcomes at the end of each dialogue?

Unwanted Advice

Giving unwanted advice happens frequently in social situations. It is nontherapeutic in professional relationships, because the advice is usually from the nurse's perspective, not the patient's. It is based upon the experiences and opinions of the nurse, and it may not help patients. Giving advice differs from providing information. For example, if a patient asks, "How do I get rid of the lice in my son's hair?" the nurse answers based on his or her knowledge base and current evidence. A patient who asks, "Do you think that I should have my knee replaced? I don't really know what to do" requires a different type of response. In this situation, when the nurse is using active listening, he or she understands that the patient is asking for an opportunity to discuss options, not what the nurse would want. Instead of responding to the request for an opinion, the nurse might state, "Tell me what you know about the surgery" or "You sound concerned about having knee surgery." Such responses give patients an opportunity to explore choices more fully, clarify any confusing points, and weigh risks versus benefits. They also incorporate the patient's perspective instead of adding potentially confusing or conflicting information or opinions. The nurse takes time to focus on the concerns of patients and help them through decisions by using active listening, reflection, and restatement. In this way, patients reach their own conclusions.

Biased Questions

Using leading or **biased questions** is often an unintentional nontherapeutic response. Biased questions carry judgment and lead patients to respond in the most acceptable way. They also can cause patients to feel guilty or inferior because of unhealthy behaviors. An example of a biased question is, "You don't use drugs, do you?" To obtain a more honest response, the nurse asks objective questions such as, "It is important that we know what recreational drugs you are taking so that we avoid interactions with the medications that we are giving you. Do you use any recreational drugs?" In this way, the nurse places the need for information within the context of health care. Patients understand that the nurse wants to provide the best care, not to judge unhealthy behaviors.

Changes of Subject

Changing the subject may happen when a situation is uncomfortable for a nurse because of personal experiences or coping mechanisms. For example, if the nurse recently experienced the death of a parent, it may be challenging at this time for him or her to talk with a family about a patient who has terminal cancer. Although not therapeutic for the patient, the nurse is using coping mechanisms to protect against emotional distress. The nurse who uses self-reflection is aware when she or he is using less therapeutic communication strategies and seeks to improve them. Options are to control emotions with patients and seek support from others or to be honest with patients and families about the situation. If emotional control is too difficult for the nurse, she or he should refer patients to other health care providers.

The nurse also might change the subject unconsciously when feeling rushed or stressed. In such cases, she or he may not take time to use active listening. As an example, on a busy day, the nurse wants to complete the intake and output record at the end of the shift. When the patient says, "I'm feeling a bit nauseous," the nurse may reply, "What did you have to drink?" instead of "How long have you been nauseous?" Although the nurse constantly strives to use active listening, some situations dictate the type of communication used. The goal is to prioritize and block out times to use active listening when patients need to talk. Part of the plan of care may be, "Allow 15 minutes of uninterrupted time every shift for therapeutic conversation."

Distractions

Distractions in the environment contribute to nontherapeutic communication. Hectic and rushed work environments abound across settings, contributing to patient complaints about depersonalized care (Hurst, 2007). Distractions come from several sources: equipment, other patients, colleagues, pagers, and cell phones. When equipment poses a potential source of distraction, the nurse should silence any alarms and then resolve the problem before initiating a conversation. Equipment alarms indicate an immediate problem that usually takes priority over therapeutic communication. When a patient's roommate is asking for something, the nurse either decides to grant a simple request and then pull curtains and provide for privacy or asks the roommate to wait by saying, "I'm listening to your roommate's lungs right now. I can get you some water in about 5 minutes." The nurse prioritizes the importance of answering pagers or cell phones depending on the intensity of the conversation and point in the interview. Answering a phone during the middle of a conversation is nontherapeutic; some patients may consider it rude. If answering a phone or pager is necessary, the nurse should complete the topic and then ask for permission to answer by saying, "I just received a call about a patient who needs pain medication. Would you mind if I stepped out for a moment to answer?"

Technical or Overwhelming Language

Using too many technical terms or **providing too much information** is another nontherapeutic response. As she or he develops medical vocabulary and knowledge, the beginning nurse must practice translating from medical terminology to lay language. For example, the nurse documents "dysphagia" but asks patients about "trouble swallowing." It also is important to conduct a conversation at the knowledge level of each patient. The nurse may use more technical descriptions with patients who work in health care than with patients who have limited medical knowledge. Complex concepts may best be presented through diagrams and pictures that illustrate points visually (Fig. 2-4). With a new diagnosis, the nurse prioritizes

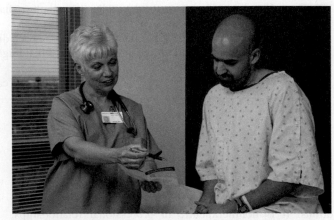

Figure 2.4 Diagrams, pictures, and other instructional materials can greatly assist with the processes of assessment and follow-up teaching related to findings.

information and discusses the most important items first, pacing and spreading out teaching over several sessions. The nurse attends to nonverbal behaviors from patients, such as puzzled facial expressions, that may indicate a lack of understanding.

Interrupting

Talking too much and **interrupting** are two other nontherapeutic ways of communicating. The nurse who exhibits caring behavior is often kinder, gentler, and less vocal than in social situations. Because of the nurse–patient relationship, the nurse in the professional role listens more than talks. Those who might be shy in social situations may exhibit excellent therapeutic communication not by talking but by communicating nonverbally through presence, facial expression, or touch. In health care settings, it is better to listen than to talk and to ask good questions rather than have all the right answers.

Professional Expectations

Learning when to use the various techniques of therapeutic communication is part of both the science and the art of nursing. Because it is easy to overidentify with some patients, especially those who remind the nurse of someone he or she knows, it is important to establish clear professional boundaries. The nurse who becomes too involved with patients experiences burnout and decreased job satisfaction.

Nonprofessional involvement occurs when the nurse crosses the boundaries of professional relationships and establishes social, personal, or economic ties with patients (Holder & Schenthal, 2007). Although social chatting about the weather or current news may put patients at ease, too much personal conversation is unprofessional. Some disclosure may help establish a therapeutic relationship, but the nurse always presents such information with a focus on the patient. For example, the nurse is working with parents of a child who recently was diagnosed with asthma. Coincidentally, the nurse's son also has asthma. The nurse may use that information to say, "I have a child with asthma, too. I noticed that the cough would get worse at night. What was the first thing that you noticed?" The nurse uses personal information to quickly redirect a conversation to focus on patients and their families.

Sexual boundary violation is the clearest example of unprofessional involvement. Sexual contact is never acceptable within the therapeutic nurse–patient relationship. The American Nurses Association (2005) has established professional guidelines about behaviors such as dating or having outside contact with patients: "When acting within one's role as a professional, the nurse recognizes and maintains boundaries that establish appropriate limits to relationships."

Visiting patients beyond the role of the nurse or nursing student also breaks professional boundaries. The nurse recognizes that care continues with other health care professionals and trusts that the health care system exists to meet ongoing needs. Although many times the nurse remembers and becomes more attached to the first patients with whom

she or he works, the nurse must not confuse the privileged intimacy associated with the nursing role with the intimacy involved in a social or personal relationship.

Phases of the Interview Process

The nurse–patient relationship differs from a social relationship because the nurse is in the role of a helper and the focus is on healing patients. In social relationships, the roles and power are closer to equal.

The nurse organizes interviews to use time efficiently and help patients to feel that their needs are met. The nurse is rewarded in the relationship by being able to help others.

Preinteraction Phase

Before meeting with patients, the nurse collects data from the medical record, including the previous history of medical illnesses or surgeries, current medication list, and problem list. She or he uses this information to conduct an interview, already knowing about some of the past problems and responses to treatments (Fig. 2-5). The nurse reviews the record chronologically to detect patterns of illness, such as declining functional status, and to identify how things fit together. For example, a patient who was diagnosed with breast cancer had a mastectomy, developed postoperative infection and lung injury, and now is on home oxygen. The record in this case assists in identifying why this patient with breast cancer has been placed on home oxygen.

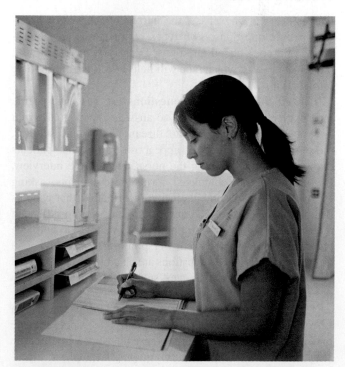

Figure 2.5 The nurse is reviewing data from a patient's medical record before meeting with the patient to conduct the initial interview.

Beginning Phase

The nurse initially introduces herself or himself by name and states the purpose of the interview. An example is, "Hello, my name is Sam, and I am going to be your nurse this evening." At this time, it is appropriate to ask patients by what name they would like to be called. The nurse simply can say, "What name would you prefer me to use?" She or he listens carefully for the correct pronunciation and may ask patients for confirmation that the pronunciation is correct. The nurse shakes hands if that seems comfortable for a patient and is appropriate for the setting.

To relax the patient, the beginning phase may continue with a discussion of some neutral areas, such as the weather, especially if anxiety is noted. The nurse moves through such discussion quickly, however, and introduces the purpose of the interview. For example, "Mrs. Lewis, I will need to ask you some questions about your personal and family history." The nurse also makes some overall remarks based on the observations, such as "You have been in the nurse's office for a cold three times in the last 3 weeks. It doesn't seem like your cold is going away."

Privacy is important, especially considering HIPAA guidelines (U.S. Department of Health and Human Services [USDHHS], 2009) for confidentiality of information (see Chapter 5). The nurse pulls drapes around patients if conducting interviews in hospital rooms or closes doors if working in examination rooms. In community settings where patients are disclosing personal information, the nurse identifies areas where others will not overhear conversations before beginning.

Working Phase

During the working phase, the nurse collects data by asking specific questions. Two types of questions are closed-ended and open-ended questions. Each type has a purpose; the nurse chooses which type will help solicit the appropriate information.

Closed-ended or **direct questions** are best for specific information that yields yes or no answers, such as "Do you have a family history of heart disease?" In clinic settings, these questions commonly appear on forms that patients complete prior to meeting the nurse. During the interview, the nurse reviews completed forms with patients, asking follow-up questions and clarifying information that patients listed as problematic. The nurse also can use closed-ended questions, such as "Is your pain sharp or dull?" to help cue patients who have had difficulty responding to an open-ended question. Closed-ended questions are also helpful for patients with communication challenges, such as those with dementia or limited English knowledge.

Open-ended questions require patients to give more than yes or no answers. They are broad and provide responses in the patient's own words. Sometimes these answers are part of the subjective information and put in quotes. Examples of open-ended questions are, "What does your pain feel like?" and "How are you doing with the low-salt diet?" Patients may find "Why" questions difficult to answer and view such inquiries as

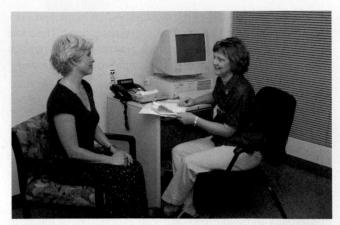

Figure 2.6 This nurse has situated herself so that she can talk and maintain eye contact with the patient while being able to record pertinent findings electronically.

too interrogative or personal. They also may view such questions as accusatory, so the nurse should avoid them. For example, "Why haven't you stopped smoking?" is more threatening than, "Tell me about how difficult it is to stop smoking."

During the working phase, the nurse also charts the patient's history and health problems. The goal is to achieve a balance between listening and documenting. Sometimes documentation is on paper; other times, the nurse records on a computer. When using a computer, ideal positioning is for the nurse to be able to record data while maintaining eye contact with patients and their families (Fig. 2-6). If using paper to document, the nurse may find that a clipboard placed in the lap allows him or her to record information without obstructing eye contact with patients. Usually, the nurse records abnormal findings during the interview and then returns to the form later to note the absence of findings and other descriptions. This method allows the nurse to maintain better eye contact with patients during the interview. It takes practice to achieve a comfortable blend of writing things down and listening.

Closing Phase

The nurse ends interviews by summarizing and stating what the two to three most important patterns or problems might be. She or he might say, "It seems that you are most concerned about control of your pain. Would you agree?" Additionally, the nurse can close by letting patients know the next steps, such as, "I'll make sure to put in your plan of care to ask about your pain level every 4 hours." The nurse also asks if patients would like to mention or need anything else. Doing so gives patients a final opportunity to express their needs and feel that they have been heard. If the nurse is using a checklist, the closing phase is a good time to review it for completeness and to make notes about future interventions.

The nurse thanks patients and family members for taking the time to provide information. She or he acknowledges the commitment of patients to health promotion or disease management appropriately, such as by saying "It was good that you came in to the clinic now, because you caught the infection while it was still early."

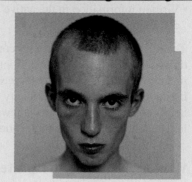

After the initial interview, the student nurse assesses Mr. Rowan, the patient with AIDS from the opening case study. The assessment revealed the following subjective and objective data. Begin to think about how the data cluster together and what additional data the nurse might want to collect. The nurse also uses critical thinking to analyze problems and anticipate nursing interventions. The following nursing note illustrates the use of diagnostic reasoning and nursing process.

Subjective: "I'd rather be home, but I can't live by myself anymore. Every day I just seem to get weaker."

Objective: Appears slightly anxious and weak. Gait slow but steady. Can heat prepared meals in kitchen; housekeeping comes weekly for cleaning. Bathroom with grab bars by shower and toilet. No loose cords or rugs. Environment clean and without clutter. Pill count accurate. Dressing, grooming, and toileting independently.

Analysis: Risk for impaired home maintenance and increasing weakness with disease progression.

Plan: Continue with meal and housekeeping services. Continue to assess for needs related to dressing, grooming, toileting, and meals. Further discuss nutrition and supplements in addition to adherence to the medication regimen.

T. Fritz, SN

Critical Thinking Challenge

- What fears or concerns might the nurse have about visiting this setting or working with this patient?
- What elements should the nurse include when closing the interview process with Mr. Rowan?

Intercultural Communication

During **intercultural communication**, the sender of an intended message belongs to one culture, while the receiver is from another. Cultural differences may exist related to a group or ethnicity, region, age, degree of acculturation into Western society, or a combination of these factors (see Chapter 11). Nonverbal differences in eye contact, facial expression, gestures, posture, timing, touch, and space needs are all culturally influenced. Language differences between patients and the nurse can compound cultural differences and prevent the nurse from understanding the perspectives of patients. Voice volume, vocal tone, inflections, pronunciation, and accents also influence meaning. More than simple language translation, the cultural meanings of health, illness, and treatment are important factors to consider (Murphy, 2007).

Communication etiquette refers to the code of conduct and good manners that show respect for others. Such etiquette varies between and within cultures. The nurse must assess the degree to which each patient identifies with cultural norms. Additionally, many patients identify with multiple cultures. The nurse should avoid assuming that patients follow cultural beliefs and assess the degree to which each individual perceives those beliefs. The nurse can bridge cultural differences by being sensitive to variations and using caring communication techniques. Refer to Chapter 11 for more information.

Limited English

Patients with limited English skills often identify language barriers as frustrating when navigating the health care system (Dysart-Gale, 2007). When possible, an interpreter is used; however, interpreters cannot be involved continuously throughout a patient's care. Thus, the nurse must develop other communication tools. For example, the nurse should cover one concept at a time instead of overwhelming patients with several ideas at once. She or he should use simple words or phrases to facilitate understanding. At times, the nurse can pantomime questions, such as pretending to be in pain or having a questioning look on the face.

When communicating with patients with limited English proficiency, the nurse should remember the following principles:

- Limitations in English are not a reflection of intellectual functioning.
- Patients may be highly literate in another language but functionally illiterate in English.
- Patients tend to think in their native language and translate, delaying their responses.

- Patients interpret the message that reflects their cultural beliefs, often changing the intent.
- Written information in the native language supports verbal communication.

The nurse can use a sheet with common phrases (eg, "I am thirsty," "I need to use the bathroom") if patients are literate in their native languages. Resources with pictures are helpful if patients have good visual acuity but cannot read. It is also helpful for the nurse to know a few key phrases in a patient's language to increase communication and trust.

Working with an Interpreter

The nurse should establish the need for an interpreter during the patient's first contact with the health care agency. Even when a patient's language skills are fluent, a trained medical interpreter may be necessary for discussing sensitive topics, such as end-of-life care or permissions for consent to treatment. In inpatient settings, interpreters may check in with patients daily. In such situations, it is helpful to maintain a list of questions and areas for patient teaching to cluster the most important information during the time that the translator is available (usually for a 30-minute period). Other occasions for using an interpreter are the admission assessment, complex treatments, patient education, informed consent, and discharge planning. Federal law mandates the use of a trained interpreter according to standards established by the Joint Commission (2006). Interpreters are chosen considering language (eg, Mandarin or Cantonese for a Chinese patient), dialect, gender for sensitive subjects, and social status if this is likely to be an issue.

Using children in the family, other relatives, or close friends as interpreters violates privacy laws, because patients may not want to share personal information with others. Additionally, friends and family who are unfamiliar with medical terminology may misinterpret information. When possible, a trained medical interpreter is preferred. Not only are medical interpreters knowledgeable in terminology, but

also they have a health care background. These interpreters also understand cultural health beliefs and practices and can help bridge the gap.

Interpreters are educated to remain neutral. Considering the natural communication process that involves the encoding and decoding of messages, however, interpreters still influence the content and context of communication. Issues can arise when interpreters add their opinion or bias communication. The nurse should pay attention to and look at patients during interviews to keep the focus on them rather than on interpreters. She or he is aware of nonverbal communication that seems inconsistent with the issues being discussed. Tips for communicating through interpreters are in Box 2-1.

Gender and Sexual Orientation Issues

Communication styles vary between and within each gender group. Men commonly prefer more information and facts, whereas women prefer more social and emotional interactions (Seale, 2006). The nurse may need to provide more information and structure for male patients and ask questions that focus more on emotional response, role adjustment, and coping mechanisms for women.

Gender also influences family roles, defined as a "set of beliefs about or expectations of male and female behavior and experiences within the family" (Wright & Leahey, 2009, pp. 71–72). Family roles can become involved in interviewing and history taking when cultural norms influence the nurse–patient relationship. For example, some cultures expect that the eldest male acts as the family leader and communicator. In others, patients may prefer that the husband is spoken with to represent the family. The nurse is aware of these cultural norms and asks patients about their preferences.

The nurse must be aware of societal biases about sexual preference when working with gay, transgender, lesbian, or bisexual patients. She or he takes care to treat all patients with respect and to provide pertinent information, such as safe-sex practices for all patients. Issues related to sexual orientation often become prominent when patients have life-threatening or chronic illnesses. In many cases, their life partners have no legal decision-making capacity. Sometimes, conflicts arise between partners and other family members of patients. Because many companies do not recognize relationships outside of legal marriage, gay and lesbian partners may have limited health care insurance benefits, family leave, or bereavement leave.

Additionally, subtle heterosexual assumptions arise in nursing communication. In many cases, the nurse assumes that patients are heterosexual until the patient does or says something to disprove this mistake. Consider the simple intake question, "Are you single, married, or divorced?" and how patients with unmarried partners would respond. Gays and lesbians may choose to hide their orientations because of the heterosexual assumptions and fear of negative attitudes from health care providers or lack of confidentiality and family conflicts (Hutchinson, et al., 2006). A more inclusive, sensitive, and ultimately better question is, "Do you live alone or

---

BOX 2.1 GUIDELINES FOR INTERPRETER-DEPENDENT COMMUNICATION

- Take time to meet with the interpreter before meeting with the client.
- Allow sufficient time—working with an interpreter may take twice as long as a meeting in which a common language is spoken.
- Speak directly to the client.
- Speak in short sentences and allow the interpreter to interpret.
- Develop alternatives to direct questions.
- Avoid ambiguous language, abstractions, and technical jargon.
- Speak slowly and clearly; use repetition as needed.
- Be aware of nonverbal messages that may require interpretation just as verbal messages.
- Avoid using family members as interpreters.

Adapted from Kennedy, M. G. (1997). Cultural competency. In N. K. Worley (Ed.), *Mental health nursing in the community*. St. Louis: Mosby.

with someone?" because it provides a more direct avenue for finding out about support at home.

Nurses may be afraid of behaving incorrectly when patients have a sexual orientation that differs from their own. This fear can lead to insecurity and cause misunderstandings (Rondahl, et al., 2006). Emotions such as uncertainty may lead to incongruent or "double" messages in communication. As professionals, nurses must become educated about gay patients, same-sex families, and gay culture to learn to communicate naturally and to become aware of the assumptions communicated through language and behavior.

Lifespan Issues

Parents, legal guardians, or other adult representatives serve as primary interview sources of health care information when patients are children. As they age and become more independent, children can participate more fully in interviews.

The nurse should refer to children by their first names and ask parents what name they prefer for address. She or he avoids calling parents "mom" or "dad" to maintain professional communication. The nurse also validates the roles of people bringing children to the attention of the health care facility. For example, a mother may be accompanied by a boyfriend who is not the child's father; a stepparent may bring in a child; or a child of gay parents may have two mothers or fathers.

The nurse should begin by interviewing caregivers and children together. She or he provides toys for children to play with while interviewing parents and observes parent–child interactions. The nurse also observes children in the environment for fine and gross motor skills, attention span, language, and development. If issues that need discussion require separation from parents (especially concerning violence or safety), the nurse asks parents to leave while she or he interviews the child separately (Baren, 2006). Refer to Chapter 12 for more information.

Parents who work outside the home are likely to bring ill children to health care facilities after a call from a day-care provider or babysitter or upon arriving home from work. Such parents may appear distracted or express guilt about not recognizing a symptom earlier. Parents with more than one child may have similar feelings and have difficulty keeping one child's history separate from that of siblings.

Parents of children with developmental delays may be especially sensitive to achievements of developmental milestones. When collecting interview data, it may be helpful to compare a child's progress against past milestones versus against normal findings for the child's age group.

Nonverbal communication is very important with young children, who have limited verbal skills. Toddlers and preschoolers are quick to notice anxiety, pain, distress, or discomfort in either a caregiver or a nurse. Health care settings can be anxiety provoking for children, because many have had immunizations and tests that involved pain or discomfort. It is helpful to have "safe" zones for the interview and physical examination and other areas for drawing blood samples

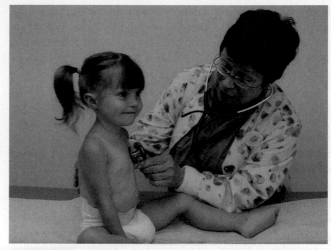

Figure 2.7 Family-practice and pediatric care settings often encourage a relaxed atmosphere and colorful, fun clothing for employees to help create a relaxed and inviting atmosphere for children and their caregivers.

or administering injections. Instead of the formality found in other settings, pediatric and family practice settings usually are colorful, and many care providers there wear playful, bright clothing as well (Fig. 2-7). These environments are child proofed, so parents and providers need to worry less about supervising their child for safety and feel more comfortable and relaxed to provide accurate assessment data.

Newborns and Infants

Families with newborns or infants are undergoing many changes that alter normal patterns and behaviors (see Chapter 28). Parents are often sleep deprived and learning how to feed, dress, and groom their babies while finding time to care for their own needs as well. The excitement of the birth of the infant may make rest difficult. Fatigue is common in the postpartum period from labor, cesarean birth, anemia, breast-feeding, and potentially depression and anxiety. The nurse should acknowledge these issues during the interview and allow time for discussion.

Infants use primarily nonverbal language to communicate. When happy, they appear relaxed, smile, and maintain eye contact. Hungry, tired, or uncomfortable infants become tense, wrinkle the face, and cry. The nurse observes parents as they speak to their infants for encouragement of happy behaviors and comfort for crying. Parental behavior should be appropriate for the situation; a detached or irritable parent is cause for concern. Infants respond to the tone of voice and nonverbal communication, so the nurse speaks softly and with caring. The nurse observes a baby's nonverbal communication, including crooning or smiling.

Children and Adolescents

As children get older, the nurse and other health care providers begin to involve them more directly in aspects of care, including interviewing and history taking (see Chapter 29). They observe whether a child or parent does more of the talking and how the child and parent interact. If both parents are in attendance, one may be more dominant, answering for the child or other partner. Alternatively, a parent may encourage the child to answer questions and become more independent. With development, children can better verbalize symptoms and appreciate information and explanations.

The nurse poses questions to children first and then allows parents to fill in missing information. Verbal and social abilities vary widely in children of all ages, so nurses take cues from each specific child to appropriately direct the conversation. For example, one child may say "Hi" and start talking as soon as the nurse enters the room, while another may hide under the mother's chair. The nurse considers developmental level, personality, social and verbal skills, and parent–child interaction when interviewing the family. Preschoolers and school-age children have varying degrees of modesty and independence. Verbal communication becomes more important, and children can usually make choices.

Adolescents are sometimes capable of mature actions and other times return to a childlike, dependent role. Their developmental task is to achieve independence and separation from family. Increasing value is put on the peer group, which may place strain on family relationships. Adolescent concerns may involve sensitive issues such as sexuality, drugs, and alcohol. Privacy for these patients is especially important; adolescents need an opportunity to discuss health-related issues without parents present. The nurse asks parents for time alone with patients and conveys an attitude of respect toward teens by being honest and treating them maturely. Adolescents may appreciate some brief conversation about hobbies, activities, friends, or school. This establishes more of a relationship in which the nurse is interested in them as a person.

⚠ SAFETY ALERT 2-2

If an interview reveals confidential material, the nurse discloses those things required to be reported by law, such as suicidal thoughts, violence at home, or rape. The nurse informs the patient at the beginning of the interview that he or she must report harm to self or others to get needed assistance. The nurse should notify authorities only after ensuring the victim's safety (Sullivan, 2005).

Older Adults

The nurse begins by introducing himself or herself and addresses the patient according to the patient's preference. She or he also makes sure that the room is free from distractions or interruptions (see Chapter 30). The interview may take longer with older patients who have more complex medical and surgical histories than younger patients. Although it lengthens the process, the nurse allows time for responses and redirects conversation if patients stray too far from a topic.

The nurse avoids rushing the interview, which can frustrate patients and reduce their initiative to provide complete data. It may be necessary to prioritize questions, because older adults become tired more easily than younger people. Thus, the nurse asks the most important questions first. Additionally, the interview might be better accomplished over several

visits rather than all at once. Touch, good eye contact, and clear speech are essential to optimal communication with this population. It is also important to pay particular attention to the temperature of the room, because some older people prefer warm temperatures.

Special Situations

Patients in health care settings may have emotional responses. Fears about illness, results from tests, interactions with health care professionals, and other factors may lead to crying, anxiety, or anger. Sometimes, problems arise related to sexual aggression or the crossing of professional boundaries. Other patients have special situations that require altering the usual approach to interviewing. Examples include hearing impairment, reduced level of consciousness, and the influence of drugs or alcohol. The nurse adapts therapeutic techniques to complete the interview in these special cases.

Hearing Impairment

Approximately 50% of patients with hearing loss are older than 70 years (National Institute on Deafness and other Communication Disorders, 2009). The nurse who suspects that patients have new or previously unsubstantiated hearing loss asks, "Just to be sure that you understand, please repeat what I said." For patients using hearing aids, the nurse makes sure that such devices are turned on and working (Fig. 2-8). She or he should gently touch or use visual signals with patients before speaking to them to verify that patients are paying attention. Closing the door also may help to limit background noise. To ensure understanding from patients, the nurse gives thorough explanations, provides diagrams and pictures, and supplies written information. The nurse asks patients to validate understanding by asking open-ended questions.

Many deaf patients communicate through a combination of methods, such as signing, writing, using speech, and moving the lips. They may sign with larger, quicker, and

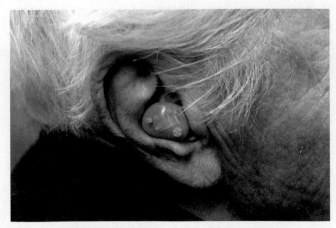

Figure 2.8 Before beginning a conversation with a patient who uses a hearing aid, the nurse should check to make sure the device is working and is turned on.

more forceful motions when expressing urgency, fear, or frustration. They may pantomime or use facial expressions to communicate. The nurse sits closer to patients to facilitate a setting for lip reading. He or she uses regular speech volume and lip movement but may speak slightly more slowly. If a patient does not understand, the nurse uses other wording because the sounds involved may be better decoded.

Low Level of Consciousness

Patients with a low level of consciousness may be unable to communicate to provide answers to interview questions. In this case, the nurse needs to rely on family members and previous documentation. Physical examination and circumstances surrounding the reduced level of consciousness assume more importance until the nurse has obtained a complete history. Refer to Chapter 24 for more information.

Cognitive Impairment

Patients with dementia often have word-finding difficulties. As dementia increases, they may often substitute sound-alike words and sounds, making conversations difficult to track (Acton, et al., 2007). It is important to allow these patients time to process as much as possible to avoid a one-sided conversation. Because it is easy to discount the communication as disordered or unreliable, many patients with dementia have unmet needs. Pain, hunger, thirst, and other basic needs that remain unaddressed may produce behaviors that others interpret as anxious or agitated (see Chapter 7). When these nonverbal behaviors are present, it is essential for the nurse to perform assessments to help identify the source of the problem. Patients with closed-head injuries commonly have difficulties related to attention and social skills (Youse, 2005). They may need redirection and coaching on the organization and appropriateness of their communication.

Mental Health Illness

Patients with mental health illnesses often have difficulty attending to and sequencing communication (Docherty, et al., 2006). The nurse should observe patients for behaviors that indicate distraction, such as looking around the room or appearing to hear noises. Those with mental illness may process communication better if it contains clear, short phrases that require one step in thinking rather than complex directions. It also may be helpful for the nurse to use restatement, reflection, or focusing to redirect conversation to the health topic being assessed (see Chapter 10).

Anxiety

Health care issues can cause great anxiety, which is an expected response to a threat to well-being. Behaviors that indicate anxiety are nail-biting, foot-tapping, sweating, and pacing. A voice may quiver, speech may be rapid, and language or tone may be defensive. These behaviors are an attempt to relieve anxious feelings. A mild level of anxiety heightens awareness of the surroundings and fosters learning and decision making. High levels of anxiety decrease perceptual ability and can progress to panic and immobilizing behavior (Boyd, 2008).

The nurse should use active listening, honesty, and a calm and unhurried manner to reduce anxiety. If anxiety is severe, the nurse teaches patients breathing and relaxation exercises, uses therapeutic touch, and provides structure so that patients know that they will remain safe.

Crying

Health issues are sensitive and sometimes pose sad situations for both patients and the nurse. When sensitive issues arise, the nurse uses therapeutic communication techniques rather than progressing with additional interview questions. If a nurse notices that a patient is sad, he or she may say, "You look sad when talking about your prognosis" to show empathy for the patient. The nurse provides support through silence, acknowledging feelings, or offering a tissue (Fig. 2-9). The nurse avoids giving false reassurance. Crying is therapeutic, and patients usually feel better after having a chance to express the associated emotions. Grief is an expected part of illness; it is therapeutic to express feelings of grief. At times, the nurse may also become emotional; in this case, it is acceptable to tear. However, sobbing or frank expression of emotion is not therapeutic.

Anger

When patients are angry, the nurse listens for the associated themes and avoids becoming defensive or personalizing

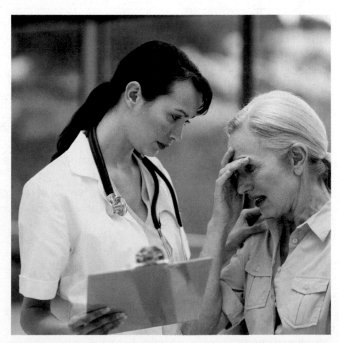

Figure 2.9 The nurse needs to be prepared for emotional reactions to health concerns and challenges from patients and use his or her judgment about the best ways to offer support and caring presence.

the situation. The beginning nurse may think that she or he did something wrong and feel bad, but usually anger from patients does not directly relate to one specific nurse. Such an emotion usually is a response to a situation in which patients have lost control and feel anxious or helpless. The nurse acknowledges the feelings by saying, "I understand that you are upset about being asked this question another time" or "I'm sorry that you're so angry." The nurse validates and encourages patients to express their feelings. The purpose of talking the emotion through is to help patients connect their emotions with related events.

Alcohol or Drug Use

Patients with chemical impairment have difficulty answering complex questions, so the nurse uses direct and simple questions instead. Interview questions include the type of drug, amount ingested, and date and time of the last drink or use. The nurse should explain that this information is important to provide accurate data regarding withdrawal. Patients who have used drugs or alcohol may also provide an unreliable history with a story that changes over time. The nurse is aware that memory may be impaired and drug use and withdrawal can cause confusion. Similar to when working with patients who have reduced consciousness, the nurse will rely more on the circumstances and physical assessment data with patients who have substance use disorders. As patients become sober and family members are available, details about length of use, pattern of use, and related injuries or illnesses can be discussed.

Personal Questions

When interviewing patients, the nurse asks questions within the nursing role. Some patients do not understand the boundaries that define the nurse–patient relationship and instead ask personal questions of the nurse. This situation can be uncomfortable, because the nurse must choose how much (if anything) to disclose. The nurse may briefly provide a response or choose simply to redirect the conversation. The nurse might say, "My husband is a teacher. Tell me more about the occupational hazards that you have" or simply, "I would rather talk about the occupational hazards in your workplace."

Sexual Aggression

Sexual aggression includes inappropriate jokes, flirtatious comments, sexual suggestions, or sexual advances. Patients with low self-esteem may flaunt their sexual prowess as a way to increase feelings of self-worth. The nurse listens for these themes in an attempt to understand why patients are acting this way and, most importantly, set limits on these behaviors. Although the nurse may be shocked, embarrassed, or angry, she or he needs to confront sexual innuendos and be clear that such a behavior is not acceptable. She or he may say, "It makes me very uncomfortable when you tell that type of joke. I would prefer that we talk about other things" or, "Yes, I have a boyfriend. Tell me more about your support systems." If aggression is physical, it may be necessary to set limits, such as, "If you touch me there again, I will need to leave the room."

Applying Your Knowledge

Using the previous steps of diagnostic reasoning, organizing, and prioritizing, consider all the case study findings woven throughout this chapter. When answering the following questions, begin drawing conclusions and see how the pieces of assessment work together to create an environment for personalized, appropriate, and accurate care.

- Is it important for the nurse to interview the patient about how he contracted AIDS?
- What is your perceived risk of exposure to HIV/AIDS?
- Which techniques of therapeutic communication might the nurse need to use when talking with the patient?
- How might the nurse's personal beliefs about AIDS and alternative therapies affect communication with Mr. Rowan?
- How can the nurse communicate nonjudgmental care both verbally and nonverbally?
- What cultural, environmental, or developmental issues might you anticipate for Mr. Rowan?

Key Points

- Nonverbal communication should be congruent with verbal communication.
- Active listening, restatement, reflection, elaboration, silence, focusing, clarification, and summarizing are techniques to facilitate therapeutic communication.
- Nontherapeutic responses include false reassurance, unwanted advice, leading or biased questions, changes of subject, distractions, too many technical terms, and talking too much.
- The phases of the interview process include preinteraction, beginning, working, and closing.
- Intercultural communication requires sensitivity to and knowledge of specific cultures, including language challenges, health beliefs, and gender issues.

- Assessment of newborns, infants, and children includes the care provider and his or her relationship to the patient.
- Privacy and respect are essential when assessing adolescents.
- The nurse may need to collect the health history of older adults over more than one visit because of the length and amount of details involved as well as increased fatigue in these patients.
- Special techniques may be helpful when working with clients in special situations: hearing impairment, low level of consciousness, cognitive impairment, psychiatric issues, anxiety, crying, anger, drug use, personal questions, and sexual innuendo.

Review Questions

1. Nonverbal communication skills include
   A. facial expression and body position
   B. speed of the voice and dress
   C. voice volume and gestures
   D. word choice and questions

2. The nurse talks with the patient and asks, "So tell me more about the chest pain that you had." This is an example of
   A. restatement
   B. reflection
   C. encouraging elaboration
   D. clarifying

3. When the patient says, "I'm so angry that I have to have surgery," the nurse says, "You sound very frustrated." This is an example of
   A. focusing
   B. summarizing
   C. silence
   D. reflection

4. The nurse is gathering the health history data before performing the physical assessment. This phase of the interview process is the
   A. preinteraction phase
   B. beginning phase
   C. working phase
   D. closing phase

5. When working with a medical interpreter, the nurse knows that it is best to
   A. look directly at the patient
   B. speak slightly louder than normal
   C. avoid using medical terms
   D. use close-ended questions

6. When interviewing adolescents, the nurse recognizes that
   A. parents retain strict control
   B. medical authorities have the answers
   C. privacy may be especially important
   D. the peer group has little influence

7. The patient is crying after being given a diagnosis with a poor prognosis. The best response from the nurse is
   A. "Don't cry. It will be OK."
   B. "My mother has the same thing."
   C. "I think that you should have surgery."
   D. "I'll stay with you." (and gets a tissue)

8. An older adult says, "How come you're asking me so many questions?" The best response from the nurse is
   A. "It's all a part of the health history."
   B. "We need a complete understanding of your problems."
   C. "Are you getting tired? I can come back later."
   D. "Why are you asking me that?"

9. When the nurse asks the patient during a health history about mental health problems, the patient responds by saying, "Don't you tell me I'm crazy!" The best response by the nurse is
   A. "I didn't say that you were crazy."
   B. "Having mental health problems is different from being crazy."
   C. "Tell me more about what you mean by that."
   D. "This sounds like a sensitive subject for you."

10. The mother of an infant with severe asthma is extremely anxious. The nurse is treating the patient in the emergency room. When collecting the history, the best response of the nurse is
    A. "You must be extremely worried."
    B. "I'd be in worse shape than you are if it was my baby."
    C. "Is there anyone here that you can talk to?"
    D. "You seem worried, but I need to ask a few questions."

References

Acton, G. J., Yauk, S., Hopkins, B. A., & Mayhew, P. A. (2007). Increasing social communication in persons with dementia. *Research and Theory for Nursing Practice, 21*(1), 32–44.

AACN. (2008). *The essentials of baccalaureate education for professional nursing practice*. Washington, DC: Author.

American Nurses Association. (2005). *Code of ethics for nurses with interpretive statements*. Washington, DC: Author.

Baren, J. M. (2006). Ethical dilemmas in the care of minors in the emergency department. *Emergency Medicine Clinics of North America, 24*(3), 619–631.

Boyd, M. A. (2008). *Psychiatric nursing: Contemporary practice* (4th ed.). Philadelphia: Lippincott Williams & Wilkins.

Choi, H., & Gi Park, C. (2006). Understanding adolescent depression in ethnocultural context: Updated with empirical findings. *Advances in Nursing Science, 29*(4), E1–E12.

Docherty, N. M., Strauss, M. E., Dinzeo, T. J., et al. (2006). The cognitive origins of specific types of schizophrenic speech disturbances. *American Journal of Psychiatry, 163*(12), 2111–2118.

Dysart-Gale, D. (2007). Clinicians and medical interpreters: Negotiating culturally appropriate care for patients with limited English ability. *Family & Community Health, 30*(3), 237–246.

Holder, K. V., & Schenthal, S. J. (2007). Watch your step: Nursing and professional boundaries. *Nursing Management, 38*(2), 24–29.

Hurst, K. (2007). Does workforce size and mix influence patient satisfaction? *Nursing Standard, 21*(46), 15.

Hutchinson, M. K., Thompson, A. C., & Cederbaum, J. A. (2006). Multisystem factors contributing to disparities in preventive health care among lesbian women. *Journal of Obstetric, Gynecologic, and Neonatal Nursing, 35*(3), 393–402.

Joint Commission. (2006). Is your organization linguistically competent? Providing effective interpreter services. *Joint Commission Perspectives on Patient Safety, 6*(4), 1–2, 8.

Mezirow, J. (1990). *Fostering critical reflection in adulthood*. San Francisco: Jossey-Bass.

Murphy, S. T. (2007). Improving cross-cultural communication in health professions education. *Journal of Nursing Education, 46*(8), 367–372.

National Institute on Deafness and other Communication Disorders. (2009). *Statistics about hearing disorders, ear infections, and deafness*. Retrieved April 11, 2009, from http://www.nidcd.nih.gov/health/statistics.hearing.asp

Rondahl, G., Innala, S., & Carlsson, M. (2006). Heterosexual assumptions in verbal and non-verbal communication in nursing. *Journal of Advanced Nursing, 56*(4), 341–344.

Seale, C. (2006). Gender accommodation in online cancer support groups. *Health: An Interdisciplinary Journal for the Social Study of Health, Illness & Medicine, 10*(3), 345–360.

Sullivan, C. M. (2005). Survivors' opinions about mandatory reporting of domestic violence and sexual assault by medical professionals. *Journal of Women & Social Work, 20*(3), 346–361.

USDHHS. (2009). *Medical privacy—National standards to protect the privacy of personal health information*. Retrieved April 11, 2009, from http://www.hhs.gov/ocr/hipaa/ on September 30, 2007.

Wright, L. M., & Leahey, M. (2009). *The nurse and families: A guide to family assessment and intervention* (4th ed.). Philadelphia: F.A. Davis.

Youse, K. M. (2005). Attentional deficits and conversational discourse in closed-head injury. (includes abstract) University of Connecticut, (129 p.) (doctoral dissertation—research).

> **The Jensen suite offers these additional resources to enhance learning and facilitate understanding of this chapter:**
>
> • thePoint online resource, http//thepoint.lww.com/Jensen1E
> • Student CD-ROM included with the book
> • *Laboratory Manual for Nursing Health Assessment: A Best-Practice Approach*
> • *Pocket Guide for Nursing Health Assessment: A Best-Practice Approach*

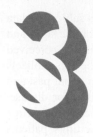

The Health History

Learning Objectives

1 Differentiate primary from secondary data.

2 Compare and contrast emergency, focused, and comprehensive health histories.

3 Identify the components of the comprehensive health history.

4 Gather a complete history of present illness.

5 Complete a family history using a genogram to illustrate family patterns.

6 Perform a functional health assessment using Gordon's nursing framework.

7 Perform a complete review of systems.

8 Identify teaching opportunities for health promotion and risk reduction.

9 Use subjective data to analyze findings and plan interventions.

10 Document and communicate data using appropriate medical terminology.

11 Individualize health assessment considering the condition, age, gender, and culture of the patient.

*E*mma Anderson, a 9-year-old African American girl, was diagnosed with asthma when she was 3 years old. She has carried an inhaler with her for most of her life and uses it when she wheezes during play. She lives in an urban low-income housing area. Her house and school were both built in the 1940s. The house is known to have mold, cockroaches, and dust; her school has old carpets, and rodent droppings have been found there. Emma's mother, a single parent, works two jobs. Three older siblings also are in the household. The family is active in church and has faith that "someday there will be a better life." Today, Emma comes to the school nurse because she thinks that her inhaler might be empty.

You will gain more information about Emma as you progress through this chapter. As you study the content and features, consider this case and its relationship to what you are learning about the health history. Begin thinking about the following points:

- What perceptions do you hold about Emma's situation?
- What personal beliefs could affect communication with Emma?
- What areas of the health history are especially important to focus on with Emma?
- What age-related, cultural, environmental, or developmental issues might you anticipate for Emma?

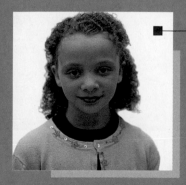

The purpose of the health history is to collect subjective data from patients. **Subjective data** are based on the signs and symptoms that the patient reports; they may not be perceived by observers (Thomas, 2007). Additionally, the nurse collects individual and family histories to obtain data about past and current medical problems, surgeries, and risks for disease. Discussions also include information on health behaviors and activities that promote health. In many settings, patients complete comprehensive forms that the nurse reviews and then asks questions about to add detail during the interview.

Most patients anticipate that the nurse may ask uncomfortable questions, such as those involving bowel habits or sexual practices and activities, because the nursing role focuses on health and screening for potential problems. The health history forms the foundation for care as patterns emerge and problems are identified. It is important because it provides context for the current situation and a more complete picture of how issues are related. The nurse ensures that she or he gathers, records, and analyzes complete data. During history taking and interviewing, the nurse establishes trust with patients.

Through therapeutic communication, the patient and the nurse work together to resolve problems by developing collaborative strategies and solutions (see Chapter 2). As they develop rapport with each other, the patient feels respected and understood. The nurse performs health teaching, based on each patient's needs and priorities, and weaves health promotion and disease prevention into care. For example, a nurse will teach a patient with a history of breast cancer how to perform the breast self-examination (Fig. 3-1).

During health history taking, the nurse uses special techniques and communication skills to gather complete and accurate data about the health state of patients. As the nurse develops and refines his or her interviewing capabilities (see Chapter 2), conversation with patients becomes more comfortable, with smooth transitions from question to question. Each nurse develops a style of communication that suits his or her personality and values, blending together the professional and the personal.

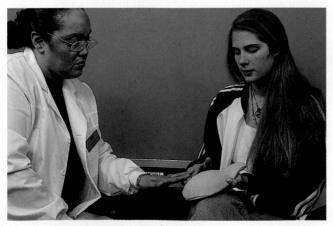

Figure 3.1 During a routine annual physical examination, this nurse uses a prosthetic model of a breast to instruct the patient about self–breast examination.

Primary and Secondary Data Sources

The individual patient is considered the **primary data** source. Charts and family members are considered **secondary data** sources. When possible, patients provide subjective information regarding their health behaviors and problems. Subjective information is from the perspective of the patient. Secondary sources are all other sources of information.

Reliability of the Source

The nurse records the person who provides the information. A **reliable historian** provides information that is consistent with existing records and comprehensive in scope. If information differs from past descriptions, or if details change each time, the patient may be unreliable or considered an **inaccurate historian**. The nurse notes any discrepancies and identifies other sources (such as previous records) to confirm the history.

Components of the Health History

Usually, the nurse collects demographical data first and then elicits from patients a complete description of their reason for seeking care, because that information usually is most important. How much additional data the nurse collects depends on the reason for the visit, pertinence of the data, and time restrictions within the setting. The nurse determines what data to collect beyond the minimum required. Data can be collected in an emergency, during a visit for a specific problem (e.g., shoulder pain), or during a wellness visit. Refer to Table 3-1 to compare and contrast emergency, focused, and comprehensive health histories. The following sections explain the components of the comprehensive health history.

Demographical Data

Depending on the health care setting, personnel at a front desk or admissions department often collect demographical data from patients, including name, address, and billing information (Fig. 3-2). Occupation and insurance may be sensitive issues for some patients. In such cases, the nurse explains the reason for asking about them, such as "Sometimes people are concerned about how they will pay for their care. Do you have any insurance or financial concerns for which you might like help?"

Demographical data include environmental data about exposure to contagious diseases, travel to high-risk areas, and concerns about exposure to pollution, hazards, and allergens. For hospitalized patients, the nurse assesses housing information to identify the level of independence and support needed

Table 3.1	Types of Health Histories		
Type	**Purpose**		**Components**
Emergency	Nurses collect the most important information and defer obtaining details until patients are stable. They elicit the reason for seeking care along with current health problems, medications, and allergies.		Care focuses on gathering information so that interventions can resolve the immediate problem. Assessments and interventions are concurrent.
Focused	The focused health history involves questions that relate to the current situation.		An example is the patient visiting the primary care provider about a cough. In this case, the nurse asks about the length, severity, and timing of the cough and other related factors. During focused health histories, nurses do not perform a complete review of systems (discussed later).
Comprehensive	The comprehensive health history takes place during an annual physical examination, for sports participation screenings, and during a hospital admission.		It includes demographical data, a full description of the reason for seeking care, individual health history, family history, functional status, and a history in all physical and psychosocial areas.

following discharge. Additional considerations for discharge planning and referral to home care services include number of stairs and concerns about structural barriers. The nurse collects occupational information to evaluate the ability of patients to work safely and return to work if an illness is present. She or he assesses any concerns about occupational hazards, personal protective equipment, handicapped access, and adaptive devices.

Reason for Seeking Care

The reason for seeking care is a brief statement, usually in the patient's own words, about why he or she is making the visit. The nurse asks, "Tell me why you came to the clinic today" or "What happened that brought you to the hospital?" He or she records this information in the subjective part of documentation or puts the statement in quotes. If a patient

Demographical Data

Date of Interview: _____

Patient Name: _____

Gender: _____ Date of Birth: _____ Age: _____

Primary Language: _____

Religious Preference: _____

Marital Status: S M W D Other

Address: _____

_____

Type of Dwelling: _____ Transportation:_____

Emergency Contact: _____

_____

Occupation: _____ Insurance: _____

Information obtained from: Patient _____ Other _____

Figure 3.2 A sample of a demographical data form completed during arrival at or admission to a health care facility.

replies by giving a medical diagnosis such as "heart attack," the nurse encourages the patient to describe symptoms such as "shortness of breath and chest pain." When taking the health history, the nurse records the **symptoms**, or subjective sensations or feelings of patients, versus the **signs**, or objective information that the nurse assesses during the physical examination.

History of Present Illness

The nurse collects information about the present illness by beginning with open-ended questions and having patients explain symptoms. A complete description of the present illness is essential to an accurate diagnosis. Additionally, the nurse asks questions about the symptoms in six to eight categories to assist patients to be more specific and complete. For example, if a patient states, "I've been having some abdominal pain," the nurse asks questions to try to find out its source and associated symptoms.

Some providers use a mnemonic to remember the elements that are important to assess for the presenting symptom (Johann, et al., 2007). Some examples of the elements are as follows:

- OLDCARTS (onset, location, duration, character, associated or aggravating factors, relieving factors, timing, severity)
- PQRSTU (provocative or palliative, quality, region, severity, timing, understanding patient perception)
- Location, duration, intensity, description, aggravating factors, alleviating factors, pain goal, and functional impairment (see Chapter 7)

Regardless of the order of the data, the nurse guides the conversation following the cues of patients and uses a mental checklist to ensure that he or she has assessed all categories before the end of history taking. See Chapter 7 on pain for more information.

Location

The nurse asks, "Where does it hurt?" and observes patients' nonverbal cues. If patients have difficulty describing the location, the nurse might ask, "Show me where it hurts" and note not only the location but also nonverbal responses. If a patient points to a location, the area of pain is more specific than if he or she circles with the palm of the hand over a broad area.

Duration

Duration refers to the timing and frequency of the problem. To establish duration, the nurse asks, "When did you first notice the pain?" and records the date and time specifically (month and year) instead of documenting "yesterday." In this way, future health care providers can easily identify the date. Duration also refers to whether the pain is constant or intermittent, how long it lasts, and if it goes completely away or cycles off and on. There are differences in the assessment of acute, chronic, and neuropathic pain (see Chapter 7).

Intensity

The nurse asks, "How bad does it hurt?" Commonly, patients rate intensity on a 0-to-10 scale, with 0 being no pain and 10 being the worst imaginable. Other pain scales use faces and descriptors (see Chapter 7).

Quality/Description

The nurse asks, "What does the pain/discomfort feel like?" If patients cannot describe it, the nurse provides cues by asking, "Is it sharp or dull?" or "Is it stabbing or more achy?" A question for associated symptoms is, "Do you notice anything else when you have the pain?" If patients have difficulty understanding the question, the nurse may ask, "When you have the pain, do you notice any sweating?" which is common with chest pain, or "Do you notice a special feeling before you have a seizure?" to evaluate for an aura (common preceding a seizure).

Aggravating/Alleviating Factors

The nurse asks, "Is there anything that you notice that makes it worse?" regarding aggravating factors. "What were you doing when you noticed the pain?" A possible follow-up question is, "Is there anything that you notice that consistently causes or occurs with the pain?" The nurse assesses for relieving factors when he or she asks, "What things seem to make it better?" or "What have you tried to make it go away?"

Pain Goal

The nurse asks patients, "What is an acceptable level of pain?" or "What do you hope that we can get your pain down to?" This pain goal should be set to allow patients to perform the most important activities easily. Usually, a goal of zero to mild pain (1 to 3 on a 10-point scale) is acceptable.

Functional Goal

Pain can affect the ability to perform common movements and tasks. The nurse assesses the effects of pain on the functional ability by questioning patients about sitting, rising from a chair, standing for periods, climbing stairs, shopping, driving, and participating in sports. Pain is dynamic and increases with activity (Falla, et al., 2007).

Past Health History

The past health history includes an assessment of medical and surgical problems along with the treatment and course. Some problems are acute, others resolve, and others are chronic. Dates of initial diagnosis and surgeries are important to document. For example, the nurse writes, "Appendectomy 2003; testicular cancer 1/2006; orchiectomy 2/2006; chemotherapy with cisplatin, etoposide, and bleomycin 3/2006; currently in remission." He or she also notes any serious accidents and injuries. The nurse charts events chronologically when possible so that future readers can easily identify the sequence. She or he notes current problems on the problem list.

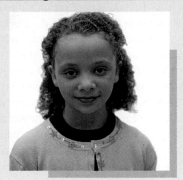

The nurse's role relative to subjective data collection is to gather information to improve the patient's health status and to help determine the cause of current symptoms. Emma, introduced at the beginning of this chapter, has come to the school health clinic to see if her asthma inhaler is working. The following conversations give two examples of different interview styles. One style is more effective than the other.

Less Effective

Nurse: Hi, Emma. It's good to see you. How are you doing?

Emma: I'm good, Nurse Habi. Sara and I were out on the playground and I had to use my inhaler. It doesn't make a sound when I puff it.

Nurse: It's probably empty. How many puffs have you used?

Emma: I don't know. It's new from last year.

Nurse: Let's look at the date on it. Do you still use it with your spacer?

Emma: My spacer takes too much room. I just keep it at home.

Nurse: The date isn't expired. How many times do you use it every day?

Emma: I've been using it a lot when I play.

Nurse: What's a lot?

Emma: Maybe two or three times every day.

Nurse: Can you try to think of when you got it?

Emma: Hmmm.... I think that it was last year in Mr. Tack's class.

Nurse: It's probably old then. I need to let your mom know to get you a new one.

More Effective

Nurse: Hi, Emma. It's good to see you this morning. How are you?

Emma: I'm good, Nurse Habi. Sara and I were out on the playground and I had to use my inhaler. It doesn't make a sound when I puff it.

Nurse: Why did you need to use it, Emma?

Emma: I'm coughing and wheezing. I feel like I'm getting sick.

Nurse: Have you had any trouble breathing or chest tightness?

Emma: Just trouble breathing.

Nurse: How do you know when you need to use your inhaler?

Emma: I can't run and my chest gets tight. I've been using the inhaler a lot, too.

Nurse: How many times a day, Emma?

Emma: About two to three times.

Nurse: Is your chest tightness mild, medium, or really bad now?

Emma: Really bad. I knew that I needed a new inhaler, but my mom said to wait until it didn't puff anymore.

Nurse: We'll see what we can do here at school, and then later we can share the plan with your mom. I know that she's busy taking care of everything.

Emma: Thanks, Nurse Habi.

Critical Thinking Challenge

- What type of assessment does this example represent?
- Compare and contrast the data collected in the two dialogues. What approaches made the second dialogue more effective?
- What components of the history of present illness are important to continue collecting?
- What techniques of therapeutic communication would you use when talking with Emma?

For female patients, the nurse notes the obstetric history, including number of pregnancies (gravida) and number of births (para). If any pregnancies are incomplete, the nurse documents the reason (e.g., spontaneous abortion).

The record should include childhood illnesses with potentially lasting effects (e.g., polio, varicella). Also, the nurse records the date of the most recent immunizations for tetanus; pertussis; polio; measles; rubella; mumps; influenza; hepatitis A, B, and C; and pneumococcus. Refer to Appendix A for a table of recommended immunizations. The nurse also asks about screening tests and the results, such as tuberculin skin test, Pap smear, mammogram, colonoscopy, stool for occult blood, cholesterol, and blood pressure. The nurse documents the date of the last physical assessment.

Current Medications and Indications

The nurse asks patients about current medications including name, dose, and route. He or she identifies the purpose of each medication, because some drugs have more than one use. For example, one patient may take a beta-blocker for blood pressure control, while another may take the same drug to prevent a second myocardial infarction. Additionally, the nurse queries the patient about any over-the-counter medications, supplements, or herbal remedies in use. If confusion

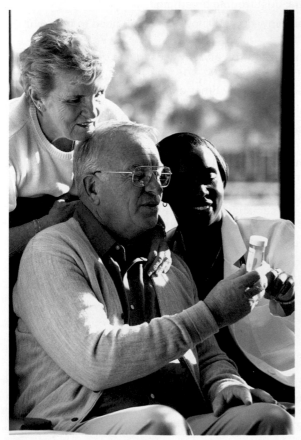

Figure 3.3 It can be helpful for patients who are taking multiple medications, supplements, and over-the-counter drugs to bring these with them to health-assessment appointments.

about any medication exists, the nurse may ask patients or their family members to bring in the pill bottles to be accurate (Fig. 3-3). For hospitalized patients, the nurse must reconcile all medication lists with medications taken regularly at home so that patients continue using the correct drugs (Joint Commission, 2009).

Allergies are verified with patients and compared against their legal records. When asking about allergies, the nurse notes the type of response such as rash, throat swelling, difficulty breathing, or anaphylactic shock. Some patients may confuse a side effect or adverse reaction with an allergy; these should also be noted. For example, a patient may become nauseous when given opiates, but the nurse should note this response as an adverse reaction. He or she would chart a response that includes throat swelling and difficulty breathing as an allergic reaction. It is best to document both the medication and the patient's reaction to it for future reference. Allergies must be appropriately noted in the chart and with a name band in a hospitalized patient.

Family History

The nurse asks the patient about the health of close family members (i.e., parents, grandparents, siblings) to help identify those diseases for which patients may be at risk and to provide counseling and health teaching. The following familial conditions are important to note: high blood pressure, coronary artery disease, high cholesterol, stroke, cancer, diabetes mellitus, obesity, alcohol or drug addiction, and mental illness. Additionally, the nurse obtains the health history of children and identifies patterns of disease that might be genetically transmitted. Ideally, the family history is recorded in a centralized area on a computer and all health care providers can contribute.

A common tool used to understand family patterns is the genogram (Fig. 3-4). This graphic representation allows the nurse to map family structures and compile a large amount of information visually. Genograms make it easier for the nurse to identify the complexity of families and validate patterns pertinent to patients. A complete family history can take as little as 15 minutes or as long as 2 hours. Each family member is represented by a box (male) or circle (female). The patient is noted by using an arrow or doubling the line. Sometimes, the nuclear family is circled. Marriages are identified by lines between people, and divorces are indicated by placing a double slash through the line. Deaths are noted by the use of an X inside the box or circle. Children are linked to parents through a vertical line, beginning with the eldest on the left. The medical history is listed below the symbol. This graphic representation compiles information into a concise pattern of family history.

Functional Health Assessment

Functional health patterns are especially important to nursing because they focus on the effects of health or

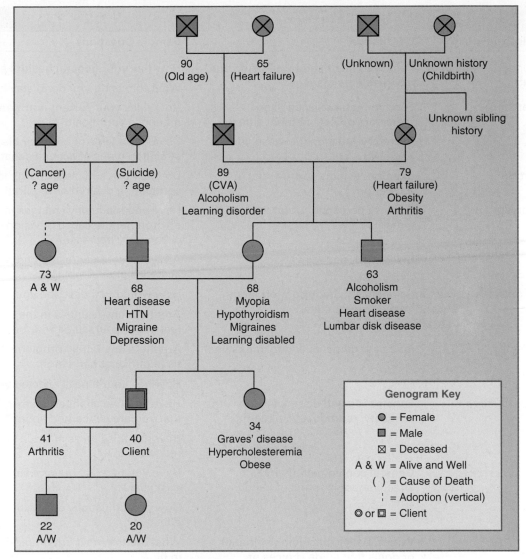

Figure 3.4 An example of a genogram.

illness on a patient's quality of life. By using this approach, the nurse can assess the strengths of patients as well as areas needing improvement (Table 3-2) (Gordon, 1987). Some of the questions are personal and difficult to answer, so it is best to thread the questions throughout the history and address the more personal questions toward the end of the conversation. As the nurse performs care, she or he can integrate these questions into other activities, such as giving the bath or chatting before the next appointment, instead of sitting down and asking the questions in a structured and sequenced order. The nurse identifies issues that may be potential problems for patients and prioritizes to ask those first.

Additionally, the nurse assesses the ability to perform self-care activities, or **activities of daily living (ADLs).** These include behaviors such as eating, dressing, and grooming. The nurse scores these items based on whether patients are totally independent, need assistance from a person or device such as a cane, or are dependent on others. See Box 3-1.

Growth and Development

During the health history with pediatric populations, the nurse observes growth to determine how children compare to peers. He or she assesses physical activities, fine and gross motor skills, and speech. Developmental assessment of infants, children, and adolescents is especially important to determine the achievement of developmental milestones and to gain awareness of deficits to facilitate early intervention and management.

Psychosocial development is part of assessment for all age groups, because even some adults have delays and do not progress as expected. For example, a patient may have problems with drugs and alcohol that interfere with relationships, employment, and housing. This patient may not reach the generativity stage but instead remains self-absorbed. For all patients, the nurse also carefully evaluates the cognitive stage, which becomes especially pertinent for those at each end of the lifespan. The nurse assesses that younger patients are appropriately developing abstract thinking skills, while

Table 3.2 Gordon's Functional Health Patterns

Functional Health Pattern	Description	Sample Questions
Health perception/health management	Perceived health and well-being and how health is managed	How has your general health been? What things do you do to stay healthy?
Nutrition/metabolic	Food to metabolic need and indicators of local nutrient supply	How does your current nutritional status influence your health?
Elimination	Excretory function (bowel, bladder, and skin)	Do your patterns of bowel or bladder habits affect the types of activities that you do?
Activity/exercise	Exercise, activity, leisure, and recreation	Do you have sufficient energy for completing desired or required activities?
Cognition/perception	Sensory perceptions and thought patterns	Have you made any changes in your environment because of vision, hearing, or memory decrease?
Sleep/rest	Sleep, rest, and relaxation	Are you generally rested and ready for activities after sleeping?
Self-perception/self-concept	Self-concept, body comfort, body image, feeling state	How would you describe yourself? Are there any changes in the way that you feel about yourself or your body?
Role/relationship	Role engagements and relationships	Are there any family problems that you have difficulty handling? How has your illness affected your family?
Sexuality/reproductive	Satisfaction and dissatisfaction with sexuality, reproductive patterns	Have you had changes in sexual relations that you are concerned about? How has this illness affected your sexual relationship?
Coping/stress tolerance	General coping pattern and effectiveness in terms of handling stress	Have you had any major changes in the past year? How do you usually deal with stress? Is it effective?
Values/beliefs	Values, beliefs (including spiritual), or goals that guide choices or decisions	What are the most important things to you in life? What gives you hope when times are troubled?

BOX 3.1 ACTIVITIES OF DAILY LIVING

Self-care Activities

Eating
Bathing
Dressing
Grooming
Toileting

Mobility

Walking: miles, blocks, across a room
Climbing stairs, up or down
Balance
Grasping small objects, opening jars
Reaching out, down, or overhead
Use of devices

Home Maintenance

Heavy housekeeping: vacuuming, scrubbing floors, making beds
Light housekeeping: dusting, wiping surfaces, dishes
Washing laundry
Cooking
Shopping
Managing finances
Driving

they evaluate older patients for any signs of memory decline. Refer to Chapter 9 for more complete information on the assessment of growth and development.

Review of Systems

The **review of systems** is a series of questions about all body systems that helps to reveal concerns or problems as part of a comprehensive health assessment. In clinic settings, patients usually fill out forms that give pertinent information, and then the nurse reviews answers with the patient to obtain a more complete and accurate history. The nurse may ask the patient about any symptoms related to each body system, such as a cough in the respiratory system. Other nurses integrate these questions during the physical examination of each region, such as chest pain when listening to the heart. The sequence and format of this review vary with the setting, urgency of the problem, and style of the nurse.

In addition to the problems covered in a review of systems, the nurse also obtains health-promotion practices and provides teaching about areas of interest or concern. Usually, the nurse begins with a general question, such as "How is your appetite?" and progresses more specifically, such as "Have you had any nausea, food intolerances or allergies, or reflux?" For healthy behaviors, the nurse asks, "What types of foods do you eat to stay healthy?" In the review, the nurse documents not only the presence of findings but also the absence of problems or symptoms, such as "No nausea, constipation, or diarrhea."

The nurse logically organizes his or her approach to the review. Most patients are unaware of the order, however, and also might remember other symptoms when talking about another topic. The conversation may be out of order from the usual body systems format. If a patient forgets to mention symptoms associated with the presenting problem, the nurse documents those symptoms with the presenting problem. If the patient forgets to mention major health events, the nurse documents them with the health history. When the nurse arrives at the section of the review that includes the presenting problem, she or he asks only those questions that have not yet been covered. The nurse explains to patients that although the review is lengthy, it is an opportunity to double check for completeness and accuracy of past and current problems. When documenting findings, the nurse reorganizes the information to cluster data regarding a problem together. For example, if a patient is nauseous and vomiting, the nurse may cluster together findings from the nutrition-hydration, skin, and abdominal assessments.

The following information is part of the review of systems; note that the questions are not mutually exclusive. For example, weight gain or loss is part of the general health state, but it also provides information about fluid balance, edema, and appetite. The nurse adapts questions to the patient and directs conversation that is comfortable and logical, rather than asking a set of separate questions. The nurse omits questions that do not apply and adds questions that seem pertinent. Although the form below uses medical terminology, the nurse uses common lay language so that patients better understand the questions; these questions are further explored in each individual chapter.

- **General health state.** Weight gain or loss, fatigue, weakness, malaise, pain, usual activity, fever, chills.
- **Nutrition and hydration.** A history of conditions that increase the risk of malnutrition or obesity. Nausea, vomiting. Normal daily intake, weight and weight change, dehydration, dry skin, fluid excess with shortness of breath, or edema in the feet and legs. Diet practices to promote health.
- **Skin, hair, and nails.** A history of skin, hair, or nail disease. Rash, itching, pigmentation or texture change, lesions, sweating, dry skin, hair loss or change in texture, brittle or thin nails, thick or yellow nails.
- **Head and neck.** A history of high or low thyroid level. Headaches, syncope, dizziness, sinus pain.
- **Eyes.** A history of poor vision or vision problems, glaucoma, cataracts, hearing loss, ear infections. Use of contact lenses or glasses, change in vision, blurring, diplopia, light sensitivity, burning, redness, discharge. Last eye examination.
- **Ears.** A history of ear or hearing problems. Ear pain, change in hearing, tinnitus, vertigo. Last hearing evaluation, ear protection.
- **Nose, mouth, and throat.** A history of mouth or throat cancer. Colds, sore throat, nasal obstruction, nosebleeds, cold sores, bleeding or swollen gums, tooth pain, dental caries, ulcers, enlarged tonsils, dry mouth or lips. Difficulty chewing or swallowing, change in voice. Last dental cleaning.
- **Thorax and lungs.** A history of emphysema, asthma, or lung cancer. Wheezing, cough, sputum, dyspnea, last chest x-ray, last tuberculin skin test.
- **Heart and neck vessels.** A history of congenital heart problems, myocardial infarction, heart surgery, heart failure, arrhythmia, murmur. Chest pain or discomfort, palpitations, exercise tolerance. Results of last screening for cholesterol and triglycerides.
- **Peripheral vascular.** A history of high blood pressure, peripheral vascular disease, thrombophlebitis. Peripheral edema, ulcers, circulation, claudication, redness, pain, tenderness.
- **Breasts.** A history of breast cancer or cystic breast condition. For adolescents, concerns about breast changes. Pain, tenderness, discharge, lumps, last mammogram, frequency and date of last self-examination.
- **Abdominal-gastrointestinal.** A history of colon cancer, gastrointestinal bleeding, cholelithiasis, liver failure, hepatitis, pancreatitis, colitis, ulcer, or gastric reflux. Appetite, nausea, vomiting, diarrhea. Food intolerance or allergy, constipation, diarrhea, change in stool color, blood in stool. Last sigmoidoscopy, colonoscopy, stool for occult blood.
- **Abdominal-urinary.** Renal failure, polycystic kidney disease, urinary tract infection, nephrolithiasis. Pain, change in urine, dysuria, urgency, frequency, nocturia, incontinence. For children, toilet training, bed-wetting.
- **Musculoskeletal.** A history of injury, arthritis. Joint stiffness, pain, swelling, restricted movement, deformity,

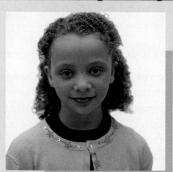

The school nurse completes the health history and physical examination of Emma, reviews findings, and develops a plan of care. She considers age-related, family, developmental, and cultural issues. The following nursing note illustrates how the nurse prioritizes, collects, and analyzes subjective and objective data and develops nursing interventions.

Subjective: "I'm coughing and wheezing. I feel like I'm getting sick. My inhaler doesn't make a sound when I puff it."

Objective: Respiratory rate 40 breaths/min and shallow. Skin color pale. Cheerful and interactive. Lungs with moderate scattered wheezes. Intermittent dry, hacking, nonproductive cough. Peak flow measures 281 mL (70% of personal best). States that she has been using inhaler more frequently, up to two to three times daily with activity.

Analysis: Risk for impaired gas exchange with increased wheezing, most likely because of empty inhaler.

Plan: Provide an inhaler for self-carry as part of her asthma management plan. Obtain spacer for use at school. Contact the patient's mother to talk about how to recognize when the inhaler is empty. Assist Emma with counting doses so that she can recognize when she needs a new inhaler. Ask Emma to come back tomorrow to check in. Talk with the mother to obtain medications for better chronic control if symptoms do not improve. Include a review on proper inhaler use as part of the management plan.

Habi Totsu, RN

Critical Thinking Challenge

- What is the nurse's role in health promotion and asthma control?
- What family history might be important to collect?
- How can the nurse assess how Emma's asthma has affected her functional status?
- Considering the elements of a complete health history, what information will the school nurse collect as a priority?

---

change in gait or coordination, strength. Pain, cramps, weakness.

- **Neurological.** A history of head or brain injury, stroke, seizures. Tremors, memory loss, numbness or tingling, loss of sensation or coordination.
- **Male genitalia.** A history of undescended testicle, hernia, testicular cancer. Pain, burning, lesions, discharge, swelling. Change in penis or scrotum, protection against pregnancy and sexually transmitted infections. Testicular self-examination.
- **Female genitalia.** A history of ovarian or uterine cancer, ovarian cyst, endometriosis, number of pregnancies and children. Pain, burning, lesions, discharge, itching, rash. Menstrual and physical changes, protection against pregnancy and sexually transmitted infections. Last Pap smear.
- **Anus, rectum, and prostate.** A history of hemorrhoids; prostate cancer; benign prostatic hyperplasia; urinary incontinence, pain, burning, itching; for men, hesitancy, dribbling, loss in force of urine stream.
- **Endocrine and hematological system.** A history of diabetes mellitus, high or low thyroid levels, anemia.

Polydipsia, polyuria, unexplained weight gain or loss, changes in body hair and body fat distribution, intolerance to heat or cold, excessive bruising, lymph node swelling. Result of last blood glucose.

Psychosocial and Lifestyle Factors

The nurse may assess psychosocial and lifestyle factors at the end of the interview, because these issues may naturally arise during the review of systems. Because many of these questions are personal, the nurse asks them at the end after the relationship is built and trust is established. Some examples of areas that involve sensitive questions are sexual orientation, risk for domestic violence (see Chapter 12), and drug use (see Chapter 10).

Social, Cultural, and Spiritual Assessment

The nurse assesses overall psychosocial well-being as part of the screening of the functional health patterns, including self-perception/self-concept, role/relationships, and coping/ stress tolerance. The nurse obtains detailed information when patients have a history of psychosocial problems or indicators of current distress (see Chapter 10). The nurse also assesses cultural beliefs and health practices that may influence care. More complete information on cultural assessment is in Chapter 11.

The nurse assesses spirituality and belief systems during the functional health screening questions related to values or beliefs. Additionally, he or she evaluates specific spiritual beliefs, religious preferences, rituals, and practices that improve health status as needed. The nurse uses this information to support the patient during times when hope and guidance are needed. The nurse asks about religious preference so that referrals to pastoral care can be initiated depending upon the patient's preference (see Chapter 11).

Mental Health

If patients are anxious, depressed, or illogical, or if an association exists between current physical status and psychiatric concerns, mental health requires a closer examination. Some potential screening questions that the nurse may ask patients are, "Describe any changes that you have had in your mood or feelings" and "Have you ever been treated for any problems with your mood or behavior?" The nurse notes medications during the initial history and asks follow-up questions regarding the purpose and effectiveness of any psychiatric drugs. Additionally, the nurse may use specific techniques for psychiatric screening, such as a depression screening tool or a full mental status examination. When the primary concern is psychiatric, the nurse performs a complete mental health assessment (see Chapter 10).

The nurse assesses alcohol and drug use by direct questioning and also observation of behaviors that indicate impairment such as slurred speech, nodding off, and unstable gait. Although this may be an uncomfortable area for beginners to ask about, most patients recognize that the nurse needs information to avoid medication interactions, evaluate the effects of use on the current illness or injury, and refer to treatment programs to improve health. The nurse asks, "How many alcoholic drinks are usual for you in 1 week?" or "Do you use any recreational drugs?" To normalize the response, the nurse asks, "A lot of college students like to party. If you party, how much do you usually drink?" The nurse also assesses tobacco use directly by asking, "Have you ever smoked cigarettes, a pipe, or a cigar, or chewed tobacco?" For a complete assessment of drug and alcohol use, see Chapter 10.

Human Violence

Because of the high prevalence of physical abuse in children and women, especially during pregnancy, many nurses routinely question patients about this (Centers for Disease Control and Prevention, 2008). Because of the sensitive nature of the topic, the nurse poses questions so that the patient feels comfortable talking. Examples include, "Some women in your situation have experienced being hurt by someone. Within the past year, have you been hurt either physically or sexually by anyone?" and "Sometimes your mom or dad might get angry with you. What happens when your mom or dad gets mad?"

Abuse is suspected if injuries are inconsistent with explanations, if the story changes over time, if the patient has delayed getting treatment, if there is a past history of injuries or accidents, if there is associated drug or alcohol abuse, or if there is a history of mental illness. Commonly, the patient's abuser is overly protective, may refuse to leave the room, or dominates the interview. Abused children may be overly attentive in an attempt to please the parent. Refer to Chapter 12 for more information.

⚠ SAFETY ALERT 3.1

When abuse is suspected, nurses are obligated to report it to a supervisor and obtain assistance from social work for further assessment. The nurse documents findings objectively in the medical record and avoids judgment (see Chapter 12).

Sexual History and Orientation

The comprehensive history includes sexual history and sexual orientation to establish a baseline for health behaviors and identify the need for education. This may be another uncomfortable area for beginning nurses to ask about, but questions can provide information that allows for health teaching to prevent disease and illness. The nurse considers sexual history and pattern as a topic for health promotion, especially in high-risk patients such as those with multiple partners or having unprotected intercourse. He or she can introduce these questions during discussions of reproductive function or healthy behaviors or during the personal and social histories.

The nurse asks, "As part of your physical examination, we like to provide information on healthy sexual practices. Would you like information about safe sex?" Some other questions are, "Have you had intimate contact, oral sex, or intercourse in the past year?" "How many partners have you had in the past year?" and "What measures do you take to protect yourself from sexually transmitted infections?" The nurse avoids bias about sexual orientation, culture, age, and marital status.

Many nurses provide opportunities for younger children to ask questions about sexuality in an attempt to increase patients' comfort level in discussing sexual topics later in life with health care providers. Refer to Chapters 25 and 26 for more information.

Lifespan Considerations

Pregnant Women

The comprehensive health history is performed at the first prenatal visit. It is important to obtain information about the current pregnancy, previous pregnancies, obstetrical and gynecological history, the family, and psychosocial profile (see Chapter 27). Additionally, the nurse collects information on nutritional history, history of genetically inherited diseases, social and occupational histories, and history of abuse. Patients may be accompanied by family members or their partners. The nurse builds a relationship with support people as part of the process if patients give permission.

Newborns, Children, and Adolescents

The nurse collects the health history for infants and children from parents (Fig. 3-5). As children move into adolescence, the nurse may interview both parents and adolescents. The relationship between the adolescent and the parent determines how the nurse collects data. It may be more comfortable and reliable to ask questions regarding sexual activity and recreational drug use with the parent absent. The nurse may ask parents to step out of the room for a moment.

Health history that is especially important for children includes the pregnancy, birth, and perinatal histories. Immunizations and growth and development are also special areas of attention. Assessment of family structure, function, and home environment is also important. Dietary intake and practices are also important to include because food choices change at each age (see Chapters 28 and 29).

Older Adults

The nurse is aware of the increased risk for sensory deficits that might alter the history taking, such as loss of vision or hearing. Older adults may have more complex histories because of their increased prevalence of disease. It is important to identify the pattern of the illnesses and recognize how they might be related. In addition to the increased risk of illness because of family history, lifestyle choices also begin to influence health later in life (see Chapter 30).

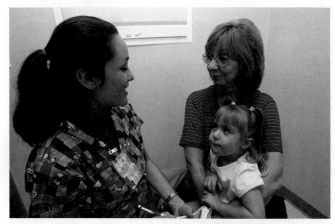

Figure 3.5 The nurse relies on parents and other caregivers to supply health history information for infants and children.

🌐 Cultural and Environmental Considerations

Cultural factors influence the beliefs of patients about their health status. As previously discussed, the nurse considers religious and spiritual, social, political, economic, and educational factors that influence beliefs and care decisions. The nurse is also aware of illnesses that are more common among groups of patients, such as diabetes or genetically inherited diseases. Questions regarding the patient's environment might include safety in the home, transportation issues, or community involvement. The environmental assessment is necessary to evaluate the risk of exposure to hazardous substances. An exposure history includes the agent, length of exposure, and type of exposure. The nurse can use this information to make a referral for further evaluation and follow-up if necessary.

Applying Your Knowledge

Although assessment can be viewed in isolation, it is important to realize that the nurse must be prepared to do something with this information. The reason for completing the assessment is to have data that are accurate and complete so that a plan can be developed with interventions that promote health. All pieces of the nursing process are interdependent and consider patients holistically.

Remember Emma, the 9-year-old girl with asthma. Using the previous steps of diagnostic reasoning, organizing, and prioritizing, consider the case study and its findings, which are woven throughout this chapter. When answering the following questions, begin drawing conclusions and see how the pieces of assessment must work together to create an environment for prioritized, appropriate, and holistic care.

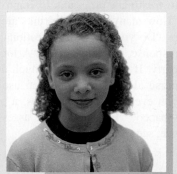

- What perceptions do you hold about Emma's situation?
- What personal beliefs could affect communication with Emma?
- What areas of the health history are especially important to focus on with Emma?
- What age-related, cultural, environmental, or developmental issues might you anticipate for Emma?

Key Points

- Nurses collect primary data from patients. They collect secondary data from other sources such as the chart or family.
- An emergency assessment occurs when the patient's condition is unstable; a focused assessment is more narrow and specific to the presenting problem; a comprehensive assessment covers all body systems for screening and health promotion.
- Components of the comprehensive health history include the reason for seeking care, history of present illness, past health history, family history, functional assessment, growth and development, and review of systems.
- The history of present illness includes assessment of location, intensity, duration, description, aggravating and alleviating factors, functional impairment, and pain goal.
- A complete family history uses a genogram to illustrate family patterns.
- The functional health assessment includes health perception, nutrition, elimination, activity, sleep, cognition, self-perception, roles, sexuality, coping, and values.
- Nurses assess ADLs by asking about feeding, bathing, toileting, dressing, grooming, mobility, home maintenance, shopping, and cooking.
- A complete review of systems assesses the history of all body systems including nutrition/hydration, skin/hair/nails, head/neck, eyes/ears, heart, peripheral vascular, breasts, abdominal, musculoskeletal, neurological, genitalia, rectum, and endocrine/hematological.

Review Questions

1. A patient says that she is having throbbing pain that she rates as 6 on a 10-point scale. This is referred to as
   A. subjective primary data
   B. subjective secondary data
   C. objective primary data
   D. objective secondary data

2. The patient is having crushing chest pain that he rates as 8 on a 10-point scale. His blood pressure is 80/62. The nurse performs which type of assessment?
   A. Emergency
   B. Acute
   C. Focused
   D. Comprehensive

3. As part of the past health history, the nurse collects the following data:
   A. Mother had a history of thyroid disease at 50 years.
   B. Patient uses walker to ambulate at home.
   C. Patient had breast cancer in 2007; treated with chemotherapy.
   D. Child rolls onto stomach; reflexes intact.

4. When gathering the family history, the nurse draws a genogram, using
   A. circles for males and squares for females
   B. the patient on the left to show birth order
   C. lines between parents to show marriage
   D. health problems listed above the symbol

5. The history of present illness includes an assessment of
   A. location, intensity, duration, description, aggravating and alleviating factors, functional impairment, and pain goal
   B. health perception, nutrition, elimination, activity, sleep, cognition, self-perception, roles, sexuality, coping, and values
   C. feeding, bathing, toileting, dressing, grooming, mobility, home maintenance, shopping, and cooking
   D. nutrition/hydration, skin/hair/nails, head/neck, eyes/ears, heart, peripheral vascular, breasts, abdominal, musculoskeletal, neurological, genitalia, rectum, and endocrine/hematological

6. The nurse asks, "What are the most important things to you in life?" to assess the functional pattern related to
   A. role
   B. self-perception
   C. coping
   D. values

7. To assess self-perception, the nurse asks
   A. How would you describe yourself?
   B. Are you having difficulty handling any family problems?
   C. What gives you hope when times are troubled?
   D. How do you usually deal with stress? Is it effective?

8. When the nurse asks about feeding, bathing, toileting, dressing, grooming, mobility, home maintenance, shopping, and cooking, he or she is assessing
   A. whether the patient is a reliable historian
   B. functional health patterns
   C. ADLs
   D. review of systems

9. The nurse assessing the child focuses the health history on
   A. previous pregnancies, obstetrical history, psychosocial factors
   B. birth history, immunizations, growth and development
   C. sensory deficits, illness history, lifestyle factors
   D. religion, spirituality, culture, and values

10. The nurse performs patient teaching after assessing that the nutritional history reveals a patient generally consumes a high-fat, high-calorie diet. This critical thinking

A. uses subjective data to analyze findings and intervene

B. documents and communicates data using appropriate medical terminologies

C. individualizes health assessment considering the age, gender, and culture of the patient

D. uses assessment findings to identify medical and nursing diagnoses

References

Centers for Disease Control and Prevention. (2008). Adverse health conditions and health risk behaviors associated with intimate partner violence–United States, 2005. *Centers for Disease Control and Prevention (CDC) MMWR: Morbidity & Mortality Weekly Report, 57*(5), 113–117.

Falla, D., Farina, D., Dahl, M. K., & Graven-Nielsen, T. (2007). Muscle pain induces task-dependent changes in cervical agonist/antagonist activity. *Journal of Applied Physiology, 102*(2), 601–609.

Gordon, M. (1987). *Nursing diagnosis: Process and application* (2nd ed.). New York: McGraw Hill.

Johann, D., Shapourian, B., & D'Arcy, Y. (2007). Screening for pain. *Nursing Management, 38*(6), 42–44, 46–47.

Joint Commission. (2009). *Discussion brief: Medication reconciliation.* Retrieved October 11, 2007, from http://www.jointcommission.org/NR/rdonlyres/72832B5A-4811-4D63-9FDB-ADBF0043EA6B/0/2_28_Brief.pdf

Thomas, C. L. (2007). *Taber's cyclopedic medical dictionary.* Philadelphia: F.A. Davis.

The Jensen suite offers these additional resources to enhance learning and facilitate understanding of this chapter:

- thePoint online resource, http//thepoint.lww.com/Jensen1E
- Student CD-ROM included with the book
- *Laboratory Manual for Nursing Health Assessment: A Best-Practice Approach*
- *Pocket Guide for Nursing Health Assessment: A Best-Practice Approach*

Techniques of Physical Examination and Equipment

Learning Objectives

1 Identify the four techniques used in physical assessment.

2 Use correct techniques for safety and infection control.

3 Accurately inspect the patient and document findings using medical terminology.

4 Compare light versus deep palpation.

5 Demonstrate the correct technique for percussion.

6 Demonstrate the correct technique for auscultation.

7 Compare the purposes of the four techniques of physical assessment.

*C*hris Chow is a 6-year-old boy visiting the clinic today with a fever and "stuffy nose." He came in with his mother who took the day off from work to stay home with him. His temperature is 38.6°C tympanic, pulse 110 beats/min, respirations 20 breaths/min, and blood pressure 108/66 mmHg. Chris is healthy and meeting developmental milestones, as indicated on the documentation from his well-child visit 2 months ago. He is being seen by an Advanced Practice Registered Nurse Practitioner (ARNP).

You will gain more information about Chris as you progress through this chapter. As you study the content and features, consider Chris's case and its relationship to what you are learning. Begin thinking about the following points:

- How can the nurse facilitate comfort and reduce anxiety when performing the assessment?
- What information does the nurse gain about patients during inspection, palpation, percussion, and auscultation?
- How does the nurse use safety and infection-control principles during an assessment?

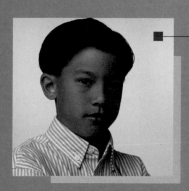

As discussed in Chapters 2 and 3, an accurate and complete health history provides information about which physical assessment data health care providers should collect. Nurses combine objective data from the physical assessment with subjective data from the health history to form a more complete assessment database as well as to develop an impression of the underlying etiology of any health problems.

The four techniques of inspection, palpation, percussion, and auscultation form the basis for physical assessment. *Inspection* means observation of the patient for general appearance and any specific details related to the body system, region, or condition under examination. With *palpation*, the nurse uses the hands to feel the firmness of body parts, such as the abdomen. With *percussion*, the nurse uses tapping motions with the hands to produce sounds that indicate solid or air-filled spaces over the lungs and other areas. He or she uses the stethoscope to perform *auscultation*, in which movements of air or fluid are heard in the body over the lungs and abdomen.

Precautions to Prevent Infection

During assessment, the nurse comes into direct physical contact with patients. Thus, it is essential that nurses follow infection-control principles, including, but not limited to, diligent hand hygiene and standard precautions. Health care environments contain a multitude of organisms that pose threats, especially for those patients with severe diseases, compromised host defenses from underlying medical conditions, a history of recent surgery, or indwelling medical devices (e.g., urinary catheters, endotracheal tubes). Multidrug-resistant organisms including methicillin-resistant *Staphylococcus aureus* (MRSA), vancomycin-resistant enterococci (VRE), and certain Gram-negative bacilli are becoming more prevalent. Treatment of such pathogens is becoming increasingly difficult (Siegel, et al., 2006). Because of these threats, nurses take special measures to prevent the spread of infection before, during, and after conducting assessments.

Hand Hygiene

⚠ SAFETY ALERT 4-1

The single most important action to prevent an infection is hand hygiene. Contact transmission from the hands of all health care providers to patients is the most common mode of transmission, because microorganisms from one patient are then spread to others (Brunetti, et al., 2006).

Patient-to-patient transmission of pathogens requires five sequential steps:

1. Organisms are present on a patient's skin or immediate environment.
2. Organisms are transferred from the patient to the nurse's hands.
3. Organisms survive on the nurse's hands for at least several minutes.

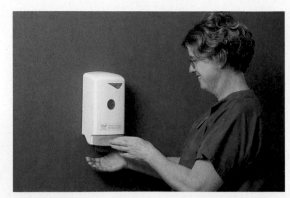

Figure 4.1 The nurse performs hand hygiene in preparation for conducting a physical examination.

4. The nurse omits or performs inadequate or inappropriate hand hygiene.
5. The nurse's contaminated hands come into direct contact with another patient or environment in direct contact with the patient (Pittet, et al., 2006).

Hand hygiene helps prevent the transmission of pathogens and subsequent infections. It includes the use of alcohol-based hand rubs, handwashing, and use of gloves.

Proper technique for using alcohol-based hand rubs is necessary for effectiveness (Fig. 4-1). The nurse applies at least two pumps of the gel to the palm of one hand. He or she then rubs both hands together, making sure to cover all surfaces of the fingers and hands until they are dry (Widmer, et al., 2007).

Soap and water are necessary for visibly soiled hands and when *Clostridium difficile*, a spore-forming bacterium, is in the environment. Patients are cultured for *C. difficile* in cases of suspected infection, such as when a hospitalized patient has diarrhea. The nurse first wets the hands, applies soap, scrubs the hands together vigorously for 15 seconds, rinses the hands, and then turns off the faucet with a paper towel (Centers for Disease Control and Prevention [CDC], 2009). Nails must be trimmed to ¼ in. or shorter; use of artificial nails is not recommended (CDC, 2009).

The CDC (2009) has recommended that the nurse wear gloves to (1) reduce the risk of personnel acquiring infections from patients, (2) prevent the transmission of flora from health care workers to patients, and (3) reduce transient contamination of the hands of personnel by flora that can be transmitted from one patient to another. The nurse wears gloves when touching blood, body fluids, secretions, excretions, and contaminated items. The nurse puts on clean gloves just before touching the mucous membranes and nonintact skin of patients. The nurse should wear gloves when general contact with any "wet" body secretion is anticipated. For example, the nurse does not need to wear gloves when taking an oral temperature, because only the thermometer cover comes in contact with the patient's oral secretions. The nurse would need gloves while assessing the back of a patient with urinary incontinence to avoid contact with any of the patient's urine that might be present. The nurse wears gloves for his or her own protection and also to avoid spreading organisms to other patients or from one body area to another (Fig. 4-2).

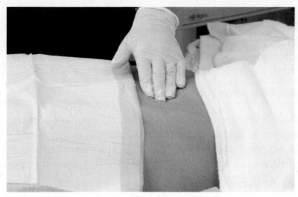

Figure 4.2 Use of gloves is important to protect against the spread of infection in cases in which the nurse could be exposed to a patient's body fluids. This nurse is wearing gloves while examining a patient with problems with urinary and fecal incontinence.

The nurse changes gloves (1) between tasks and procedures on the same patient after contact with a material that contains a high concentration of microorganisms and (2) when going from a contaminated to a cleaner area. Gloves are removed promptly after use, before touching noncontaminated items and environmental surfaces, and before going to another patient. The nurse removes gloves before touching the computer, supply drawers, and some equipment.

BOX 4.1 INDICATIONS FOR HANDWASHING AND HAND HYGIENE

- When hands are visibly dirty or soiled, wash hands with either a nonantimicrobial soap and water or an antimicrobial soap and water.
- If hands are not visibly soiled, use an alcohol-based hand rub for routinely decontaminating hands in all other clinical situations.
- Decontaminate hands before having direct contact with patients and after contact with a patient's intact skin (eg., taking a pulse or blood pressure, lifting a patient).
- Decontaminate hands if moving from a contaminated body site to a clean body site during patient care.
- Decontaminate hands after contact with inanimate objects (including medical equipment) in the immediate vicinity of the patient.
- Decontaminate hands after removing gloves.
- Before eating and after using a restroom, wash hands with a nonantimicrobial soap and water or with an antimicrobial soap and water.
- Wash hands with nonantimicrobial soap and water or with antimicrobial soap and water if an exposure to Bacillus anthracis or Clostridium difficile is suspected or proven. The physical action of washing and rinsing hands under such circumstances is recommended, because alcohols, chlorhexidine, iodophors, and other antiseptic agents have poor activity against spores.

Source: CDC. (2009). *Standard precautions excerpt from the guideline for isolation precautions: Preventing transmission of infectious agents in healthcare settings 2007.* Retrieved July 7, 2010, from http://www.cdc.gov/ncidod/dhqp/gl_isolation_standard.html

Nurses should never wear gloves from the room out into the hallway. Hands are washed immediately after glove removal to avoid transfer of microorganisms to other patients or environments.

Hand hygiene is the single most important element of standard precautions. See Box 4-1 for a summary of the indications for hand hygiene. (See also Table 4-1.)

Standard Precautions

Nurses use **standard precautions** with all patients to reduce the transmission of pathogens in both diagnosed and unknown infections. The intention of standard precautions is to prevent disease transmission during contact with nonintact skin, mucous membranes, body substances, and blood-borne contacts (e.g., needle-stick injury). Because many patients are unaware of being infected, standard precautions serve to help ensure that providers treat all patients equally.

Respiratory hygiene/cough etiquette is another area that the CDC is addressing. Patients and other people with symptoms of a respiratory infection are asked to cover their mouths/noses when coughing or sneezing. Additionally, patients should dispose of tissues directly into receptacles and perform hand hygiene after hands have been in contact with respiratory secretions (CDC, 2009).

The CDC has developed transmission-based precautions for airborne, droplet, and contact routes of transmission. Health care providers combine the use of these specific precautions with standard precautions. The general guideline is for health care providers to wear personal protective equipment whenever they are at risk for coming into contact with body secretions from patients, such as droplet exposure during coughing with tracheal suctioning. Refer to Table 4-2 for a summary of standard precautions.

Latex Allergy

Latex allergy can result from repeated exposures through skin contact or inhalation to proteins in the natural rubber latex. Reactions usually begin within minutes of exposure to latex, but they can occur hours later and produce various symptoms. Nurses are more likely to have latex allergy than the general population (8% to 12% compared to 1%) (Occupational Safety and Health Administration [OSHA], 2009). Nurses exposed to latex show an increased risk of hand dermatitis, asthma, and rhinoconjunctivitis (Bousquet, et al., 2006). Additionally, patients can develop allergies to latex, especially those who are frequently admitted to the hospital.

The best preventive action is to avoid contact with latex when possible. Health care facilities can establish latex-free zones for patients and staff. Nurses should take care to avoid carrying any latex substances into such zones, including stethoscopes, urinary catheters, and vials with rubber stoppers. To avoid increasing exposure to latex and, subsequently, allergy rates, institutions are encouraged to substitute powder-free, low-allergen gloves and latex-free gloves for latex gloves when possible (LaMontagne, et al., 2006).

Table 4.1 Areas for Health Promotion/*Healthy People* (Case Study Example)

As part of routine outpatient visits, the nurse provides information that prevents problems and performs screenings to detect problems early. The following table includes pertinent goals and education topics that the nurse will review with Chris and his mother, who were presented at the beginning of this chapter, based on *Healthy People* goals.

Goals	Patient Education Topics
Reduce the number of courses of antibiotics for ear infections for young children.	Most ear infections resolve spontaneously; antibiotics provide little additional benefit (Glasziou, et al., 2004). Antibiotic use additionally may lead to side effects such as nausea or diarrhea and complicate the issues.
Reduce the number of courses of antibiotics prescribed for the sole diagnosis of the common cold.	Antibiotic overuse had led to the development of antibiotic-resistant strains of organisms. Viruses cause most colds; antibiotics are not effective against viruses (Arroll & Kenealy, 2002). Antibiotics are not recommended unless a specific organism is isolated.
Achieve and maintain effective vaccination coverage levels for universally recommended vaccines among young children.	Vaccinations are important in the prevention of diseases such as measles, mumps, rubella, and hepatitis.
Increase the proportion of persons appropriately counseled about health behaviors.	Lifestyle factors such as healthy eating patterns, exercising, and avoiding smoke are important to achieve high-level wellness.
Increase the proportion of persons who have a specific source of ongoing care.	In addition to seeing a health care provider for illness, it is important to see a provider to promote health and detect problems early, such as with vision and hearing screening.

Source: *Healthy people 2010: What are its goals?* (n.d.). Retrieved May 14, 2010 from http://www.healthypeople.gov/About/goals.htm

Table 4.2 Recommendations for Standard Precautions

Device	Standard Precautions
Mask, eye protection, face shield	Wear a mask and eye protection or a face shield to protect mucous membranes of the eyes, nose, and mouth during procedures and activities that are likely to generate splashes or sprays of blood, body fluids, secretions, and excretions.
Gown	Wear a gown (a clean, nonsterile gown is adequate) to protect skin and to prevent soiling of clothes during procedures and activities that are likely to generate splashes or sprays of blood, body fluids, secretions, or excretions. Remove a soiled gown as promptly as possible and wash hands to avoid transfer of microorganisms to other patients or environments.
Patient care equipment	Ensure that reusable equipment is not used for the care of another patient until it has been cleaned and reprocessed appropriately. Ensure the proper discarding of single-use items.
Environmental control	Ensure that the facility has adequate procedures for the routine care, cleaning, and disinfection of environmental surfaces, beds, bedrails, bedside equipment, and other frequently touched surfaces.
Linen	Handle, transport, and process used linen soiled with blood, body fluids, secretions, and excretions in a manner that prevents skin exposures and contamination of clothing and that avoids transfer of microorganisms to other patients and environments.
Occupational health and blood-borne pathogens	Never recap used needles. Do not remove used needles from disposable syringes by hand; do not bend, break, or otherwise manipulate used needles by hand. Place used disposable syringes and needles, scalpel blades, and other sharp items in appropriate puncture-resistant containers. Use mouthpieces, resuscitation bags, or other ventilation devices as an alternative to mouth-to-mouth resuscitation methods in areas where the need for resuscitation is predictable.
Patient placement	Place a patient who contaminates the environment or who does not (or cannot be expected to) assist in maintaining appropriate hygiene or environmental control in a private room.

Source: CDC. (2009). *Standard precautions excerpt from the guideline for isolation precautions: Preventing transmission of infectious agents in healthcare settings 2007.* Retrieved May 14, 2010, from http://www.cdc.gov/ncidod/dhqp/gl_isolation_standard.html

Skin Reactions

Nurses also have an increased rate of skin reactions because of their increased frequency of hand hygiene. To minimize the adverse effects of hand hygiene, nurses can select less irritating products purchased by institutions and use skin moisturizers after washing hands (Larson, et al.,

2006). Additional measures for reducing exposure to skin irritants include using hand gel instead of soap and water in disinfection procedures when the hands are not visibly dirty and also using gloves for "wet" activities (e.g., bathing patients) to prevent the hands from becoming wet and visibly dirty.

Therapeutic Dialogue: Collecting Subjective Data

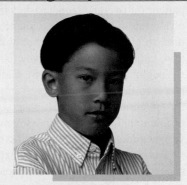

The nurse's role relative to subjective data collection is to gather information to improve the patient's health status and to help determine the cause of the patient's current symptoms. Remember Chris, the 6-year-old boy with a cold who is visiting the clinic with his mother. He is anxious about coming to the clinic, because he received an immunization during his previous appointment. The nurse uses professional communication that is appropriate for the child's developmental level to gather subjective data. The following conversations give two examples of interview styles. One style is more effective than the other.

Less Effective

Nurse: Hi, Mom. How's Chris doing?

Mother: He's had a fever for 2 days along with a sore throat and cold. He just doesn't seem to be getting any better.

Nurse: How high has his fever been?

Mother: It's been up to 102.5°F.

Nurse: What are his other symptoms?

Mother: He's had a runny nose and a little bit of a cough, too.

Nurse: Well, let's take a listen to his lungs.

Chris: What are you going to do to me? I don't want another shot.

Nurse: It won't hurt a bit. I just want to listen to your lungs and look in your mouth and ears.

Chris: Mom, I don't want a shot.

Mother: You've already had your shots. You don't need one today.

Nurse: So if you can pull up your shirt, I'll take a listen to your lungs. When I'm done with that, then I'll look in your mouth and ears. Is that OK?

Chris: (hesitantly) OK.

Nurse: (places the stethoscope on chest) I'm just going to listen to your breathing a minute.

More Effective

Nurse: Hi, Chris. How are you?

Chris: I feel sick. Am I going to have to get a shot today?

Nurse: No, you had your shots last time. Today, I want to listen to your lungs and look in your mouth and ears. Do you want me to listen or look first?

Chris: Mom, I don't want a shot.

Mother: You don't need one today. How about if you come and sit on my lap and Nurse Lesley can listen to your lungs?

Chris: OK. What does that thing do anyway? (points to the stethoscope)

Nurse: I can hear the air moving in your lungs and your heart beating. Would you like to listen first?

Chris: Sure. (The nurse positions the stethoscope for Chris, who smiles as he listens.)

Nurse: So he's had a fever?

Mother: Yes, it's been up to 102.5°F.

Nurse: Are there any other symptoms?

Mother: Yes, a runny nose and a bit of a cough, too.

Nurse: That's the air moving in and out as you breathe (smiles). Can I listen now?

Critical Thinking Challenge

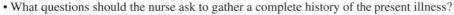

- What questions should the nurse ask to gather a complete history of the present illness?
- Why did the more effective nurse allow Chris to sit in his mother's lap?
- How might the more effective nurse facilitate comfort and reduce anxiety when performing the other techniques and using other equipment such as an otoscope and ophthalmoscope?

Inspection

Perform **inspection** by consciously observing patients for physical characteristics and behaviors and smelling for odors. Inspection is the first technique of the overall general survey and for each body part, because it provides so much information. Inspection is the one technique that is performed for every body part and body system. Initially, observe the patient for overall characteristics including age, gender, level of alertness, body size and shape, skin color, hygiene, posture, and level of discomfort or anxiety. This overall observation, called the general survey, is intentional and conscious for beginners (see Chapter 6). Gather data during this initial phase to determine an overall impression and the acuity of the situation. Additionally, observe cues that might indicate a problem that needs further assessment. Following the general survey, proceed to assess specific body systems and areas.

During inspection, adequate exposure of each body part is necessary. Concurrently, take measures to maintain the privacy of patients through appropriate draping, especially over the breasts in women and genitalia in both men and women (Fig. 4-3). Adequate lighting is essential to observe color, texture, and mobility. Inform patients of the need to look at the body part with the rationale, and ask patients for permission before doing so, especially when assessments involve compromising the patient's modesty. For example, "I need to look at your mastectomy incision to see how it is healing. Is it OK if I lift your gown?"

Sometimes devices limit visibility, such as a splint over a knee. When possible, loosen or remove such devices to adequately observe the skin for any red, inflamed, or infected areas and also for adequate circulation. Examine each body part and use specific descriptions. For example, when inspecting the abdomen, note the shape (whether it is flat or distended), size, skin color and texture, and any bruising, veins, or prominent movements. A common technique is to consider overall shape first and then compare the two sides for symmetry.

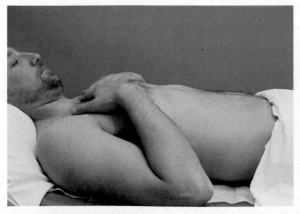

Figure 4.3 Proper draping and gowning are essential to preserving the patient's privacy and building his or her trust. The nurse is careful to expose only those areas pertinent to the immediate examination and to redrape or re-cover the patient upon completion.

In addition to the techniques for each body system, appropriate labeling and documentation of findings are important. One challenge that beginners face is identifying details and subtle differences. Accurate descriptions are essential for legal documentation and communication of findings to others. Each chapter of this book describes associated normal and abnormal findings for various body regions and systems. Associated medical terminology also appears in each chapter.

Paying attention to individual details of inspection, note whether verbal, nonverbal, and inspection data are congruent and identify any preliminary patterns or clusters. If patients appear anxious, note facial expression, nervous gestures, body position or pacing, and voice characteristics. Inspection provides objective data regarding nonverbal communication and also physical data that can lead to an accurate diagnosis and appropriate treatment.

With experience, gathering data from inspection becomes automatic and this information is collected while performing other techniques or interventions. Inspection begins with the initial contact with each patient but continues through each individual body system and with every patient encounter.

Palpation

Palpation is the assessment of the patient through touch to assess texture, temperature, moisture, size, shape, location, position, vibration, crepitus, tenderness, pain, and edema. Before performing this technique, inform the patient of the need to palpate the body part along with the rationale, and ask for permission to use touch. During abdominal assessment, you might say, "I know that you're having some abdominal pain, but I would like to gently feel your abdomen to see if a particular area is firm or tender. Would that be OK with you?" Begin with a gentle and slow technique, while inspecting the patient's face for nonverbal indicators of discomfort such as furrowed brows or grimacing.

Use different parts of the hand depending on the data that you are gathering. The fingers are best for some techniques, while the palms are best for others. Use the finger pads for fine discrimination, because they are the most mobile parts of the hand. Some examples of the need for fine discrimination include locating the pulses, lymph nodes, or small lumps and assessing for skin texture and edema. The palmar surface of the fingers and that of the joints are best for assessing firmness, contour, position, size, pain, and tenderness. The palm of the hand is best during abdominal assessment. The back of the hand (dorsal) is most sensitive to temperature. If a patient complains of being hot, turn the hand over and use this dorsal side to evaluate temperature because the skin there is thinner and more sensitive. Vibratory tremors can sometimes be felt on the chest as the patient speaks; these are best felt with the ulnar, or outside, surface of the hand.

Light Palpation

Begin with light palpation to allow the patient to become accustomed to the touch. If pain is present, you might say,

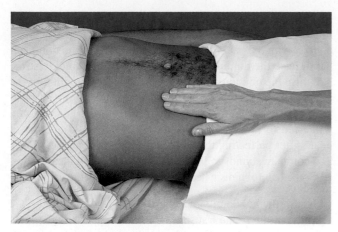

Figure 4.4 Technique for light palpation.

"Let me know if this hurts you" to gain trust and increase comfort. Avoid any tender or painful areas until the end. Ensure correct draping and warm your hands before beginning. It may be necessary to warm the hands under running water or to gently rub them together. Short and smooth nails also are necessary to avoid causing discomfort. Palpation is difficult when patients' muscles are tense, so use a gentle, calm, and easy touch to assist patients to relax.

Light palpation is appropriate for the assessment of surface characteristics, such as texture, surface lesions or lumps, or inflamed areas of skin (e.g., over an intravenous site). Place the finger pads of the dominant hand on the patient's skin and slowly move the fingers in circular areas of approximately 1 cm in depth (Fig. 4-4). Intermittent palpation using this technique is more effective than a single continuous palpation, because your fingers sense the movement of skin and tissue beneath the finger pads. Patients may perceive this gentle light palpation as a light massage in the absence of pain. Communicate concern for patients verbally with conversation during the procedure and nonverbally through this caring touch.

Moderate to Deep Palpation

Use moderate palpation to assess the size, shape, and consistency of abdominal organs. Additionally, note any abnormal findings of pain, tenderness, or pulsations. The same gentle circular motion of light palpation is appropriate, but instead of the finger pads, use the palmar surface of the fingers. Pressure is firm enough to depress approximately 1 to 2 cm. Observe the patient for any guarding, grimacing, or tension during moderate palpation.

During deep palpation, place the extended fingers of the nondominant hand over the dominant hand to use the pressure of both hands. Use the same circular motion to palpate 2 to 4 cm.

⚠ SAFETY ALERT 4-2

Deep palpation should not be used over areas that pose a risk of injuring patients, such as over an enlarged spleen or inflamed appendix.

As with other types of palpation, explain the purpose, touch gently at first, and ask about uncomfortable feelings. With deep palpation, you might say, "I'm going to touch you and push down more deeply than before. It might feel a little uncomfortable. Let me know if you feel pain or want me to stop." As palpation proceeds, continue conversation, asking patients about pain, presenting symptoms, or contributing factors while observing for nonverbal signs of tenderness or discomfort. As a beginner, you may initially be able to concentrate only on the technique. As you gain skill, you will be able to palpate, assess symptoms, and teach all at the same time.

Percussion

The third technique of physical assessment is **percussion** to produce sound or elicit tenderness. You will tap your fingers on the patient, similar to that of a drumstick on a drum. The vibrations that the fingers produce create percussion tones conducted into the patient's body. If the vibrations travel through dense tissue, the percussion tones are quiet; if they travel through air, the tones are loud. The loudest tones are over the lungs and hollow stomach; the quietest are over bones. Two methods of percussion are direct and indirect.

Direct Percussion

With direct percussion, tap with your fingers directly on the patient's skin (Fig. 4-5). An example is percussion of the sinuses in patients with sinus infections or percussion of the thorax in newborns to assess the air-filled lungs. Direct percussion is easier to learn than indirect percussion. For percussion of the sinuses with the hand, the nurse gently taps in the periorbital area for pain that may indicate allergies, congestion, or infection. Percussion that is too weak may not reveal important findings, while percussion that is too strong

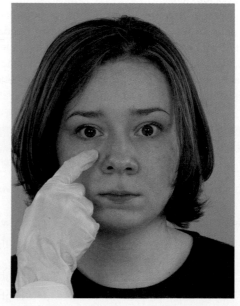

Figure 4.5 Direct percussion of the sinuses.

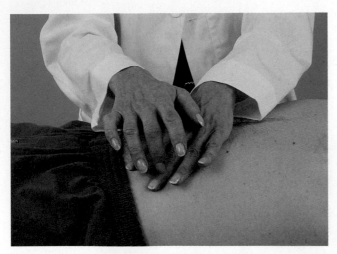

Figure 4.6 Indirect percussion.

may elicit too much pain. Thus, moderate tapping is recommended.

Indirect Percussion

Rather than directly striking a patient, you can use your nondominant hand as a barrier between the dominant hand and the patient. Place your nondominant palm on the patient and initiate a quick moderately strong tap with the dominant hand. Use the ulnar surface of the fist to percuss the kidneys, gallbladder, or liver for tenderness. As with direct percussion, you will practice until you demonstrate a comfortable strength.

The most common and also the most difficult sounds to elicit are the indirect sounds. You can best differentiate among the sounds by moving from area to area and listening to the changes in volume and pitch. It is also easier to hear the difference from resonant to dull. Thus, when you learn indirect percussion, it is easiest to go from the center of the abdomen with tympany and move upward to the liver where dullness is percussed.

This technique requires coordination of both hands. To perform indirect percussion, place your hyperextended middle finger of your nondominant hand firmly over the area to be percussed. Lift the other fingers on that hand from the patient and spread them slightly to avoid contact with the patient and dampening the sound of the striking finger. Then position the

slightly flexed middle finger of your dominant hand approximately 2 to 3 cm above the distal interphalangeal joint in contact with the patient. Using only the wrist of the dominant hand, raise the dominant finger 4 to 5 cm and quickly strike and raise the nondominant joint twice, while listening for the elicited sound (Fig. 4-6). Then move the nondominant hand and strike twice in a new area. As a beginning learner, you will need to practice first to elicit a sound loud enough to hear. After perfecting the technique, you will listen carefully and compare sounds to identify the types of note heard.

Some helpful hints when learning percussion are as follows:

- Most of the nondominant finger should be touching the patient or the sound transmission will be decreased.
- The motion of the striking finger should be quick, forceful, and snappy. The snapping finger must be brisk for a loud sound.
- Because you must use the tip of the finger, nails must be short and smooth to avoid tenderness and to facilitate good contact. Using the pad of the finger dampens the sound.
- The downward motion of the striking hand should be from the wrist, not the finger, elbow, or arm.
- To avoid dampening the sound, immediately withdraw the snapping finger once the nondominant finger is struck.
- The person with small hands and fingers needs to strike more forcefully than the person with large hands.

Percussion Sounds

Four percussion tones in the body have different characteristics. In addition to intensity or loudness, you will listen to the pitch, duration, and quality of sound. Intensity or loudness refers to how soft or loud the sound is. The louder the sound, the louder the intensity and the easier it is to hear. If air fills the structure, there is more ability to vibrate and the sound is louder.

Pitch or *frequency* depends on how quickly the vibration oscillates, similar to music. If the frequency of the sound is fast, the pitch is high; if the frequency of the sound is slow, the pitch is low. Although both the lungs and the hollow stomach are loud, the lungs are low pitched and the stomach is high pitched. See Table 4-3 for a list of percussion tones and their characteristics.

Duration refers to how long the sounds last once elicited. A sound that is freer to vibrate, such as over air-filled spaces,

Table 4.3	Percussion Sounds				
Tone	**Intensity**	**Pitch**	**Duration**	**Quality**	**Location**
Hyperresonant	Very loud	Low	Long	Boomlike	Emphysematous lungs
Resonant	Loud	Low	Long	Hollow	Healthy lungs
Tympanic	Loud	High	Moderate	Drumlike	Gastric bubble (stomach)
Dull	Moderate	High	Moderate	Thud	Liver
Flat	Soft	High	Short	Dull	Bone

has a longer duration. *Quality* means the subjective description of the percussion sound, such as a low-pitched thud of short duration versus a drumlike sound with high pitch and long duration. The process might be compared to the listening skills of a musician: beginners listen to the sound of the overall orchestra, while advanced musicians identify the sounds of the trombone, bassoon, and violin. You will take time to first develop the technique and then develop the listening skills to compare the different types of sounds.

Auscultation

During auscultation, you will listen for sounds produced by the body, usually from movement of organs and tissues. A stethoscope is used to transmit sounds that are normally unheard. Auscultation requires a quiet environment with minimal to no distractions.

Common assessments involving auscultation include blood pressure, lungs, heart, and abdomen. The blood pressure produces sounds that correlate with the bounding of the pulse. Air moving in and out with each breath generates soft and rustling sounds in the lungs. The heart produces the typical lub-dub with the snapping closure of the heart valves. Peristalsis in the abdomen produces typical gurgling or growling sounds. Descriptors vary depending on the body part auscultated; this detail is provided in each individual chapter. Describe sounds in terms of intensity, pitch, duration, and quality (same as percussion). Descriptors for quality are different with auscultation, however, such as knocking, gurgly, or rustling (see Table 4-4).

The stethoscope conducts sound from the patient's body to the listener and also blocks environmental noise to more clearly pinpoint the patient's body movements. It does not amplify sounds—it only conducts them—so listen carefully to the minor differences between sounds that are often very soft.

The stethoscope includes the eartips, earpiece, flexible tubing, and chestpiece. To be effective, the eartips must fit into the ear canal snugly but comfortably. They are tilted slightly forward so that the point on the earpiece is forward in the same direction as the nose (Fig. 4-7). This positioning directs the sound toward the tympanic membrane. Eartips

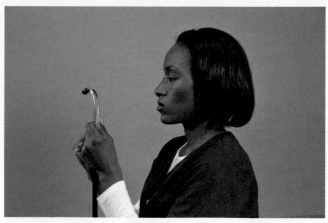

Figure 4.7 Correct positioning of the stethoscope to direct sound toward the tympanic membrane.

come in different sizes and firmnesses, so nurses choose the type that works best depending on personal ear shape and size. Tubing is thick to block environmental noise and short (55 to 69 cm) to increase transmission and reduce distortion of sound. Some pediatric nurses may cover their stethoscopes with colorful fabric or attach a small toy to distract children from touching the tubing during examination.

Most stethoscopes have a diaphragm and bell on the chestpiece (Fig. 4-8). The bell is used with light skin contact to hear low-frequency sounds, while the diaphragm is used with firm skin contact to hear high-frequency sounds. This chestpiece swivels back and forth between diaphragm and bell; when the chestpiece is turned to the bell, the diaphragm does not conduct sound. You may want to place the earpieces in the ears and gently touch the bell or diaphragm before auscultating to ensure that the preferred side of the chestpiece is turned on.

Other stethoscopes have only a diaphragm that changes between bell and diaphragm modes with pressure changes on the chestpiece. Use light contact to hear low-frequency sounds (similar to the bell) and press firmly for high-frequency sounds (similar to the diaphragm). The diaphragm is typically used for most sounds such as lung and heart sounds, although the bell works best for detecting low-pitched heart murmurs. For this reason, heart sounds are usually auscultated with both the diaphragm and the bell.

Table 4.4	Comparison of Auscultation Sounds				
Tone	**Intensity**	**Pitch**	**Quality**	**Duration**	**Location**
Blood pressure	Soft to loud	High	Swooshing or knocking	60–100/min	Arm
Abdominal sounds	Soft to loud	High	Gurgly, intermittent	5–35/min	Abdomen
Heart sounds	Moderate	Low	Lub-dub, rhythmic	60–100/min	Anterior thorax
Lung sounds vesicular	Soft	Low	Rustling, wispy	Inspiration > expiration, 12–20/min	Anterior and posterior thorax

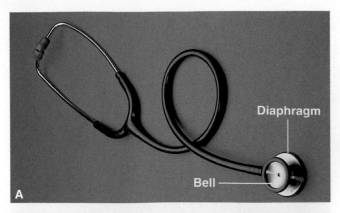

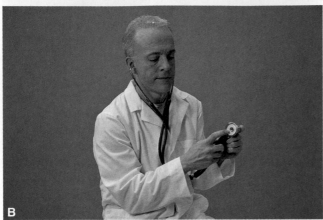

Figure 4.8 (A) The stethoscope. **(B)** Gently tap the bell or diaphragm after placing the stethoscope in the ears to check that the correct piece is on.

Make sure to disinfect the stethoscope between patients to avoid the spread of pathogens. Placement of the stethoscope is directly on the patient's skin so that there is complete contact with the skin surface. If there is a gap, which is common for blood pressures in the antecubital fossa, room noise is conducted and the blood pressure is more difficult to hear. The patient should straighten the arm to optimize contact. The appropriate-sized chestpiece also facilitates good skin contact, so pediatric stethoscopes are best with small children. When holding the chestpiece, place the end piece between the index and the middle fingers, not on top of the stethoscope, which distorts the sound. Position the stethoscope so that tubing is away from objects that might brush against it, which produces extraneous noises that make it difficult for beginners to hear underlying body sounds. If the patient has a large amount of hair on the chest, it may be helpful to moisten the hair to avoid the crackly noises caused when the hair rubs against the stethoscope.

Advanced Techniques

Some physical assessment techniques require special equipment. Examples of such equipment include an ophthalmoscope, visual acuity chart, otoscope, tuning fork, percussion hammer, vaginal speculum, goniometer, and skin-fold calipers. Because many of these tools relate specifically to one body system, they are discussed in the individual appropriate chapters of this book. Equipment discussed in the following paragraphs is included in more than one body system or has complicated instructions.

Ophthalmoscope

The ophthalmoscope is a handheld system of lenses, lights, and mirrors that enables visualization of the interior structures of the eye (Fig. 4-9). The head of the ophthalmoscope attaches to the base, which is both a place to hold on to the ophthalmoscope and a power source with a rechargeable battery. The head contains the system of lights, lenses, and mirrors. When not in use, the base is plugged in for charging, while the head is stored to avoid damage. The head is attached to the base by fitting the adapter of the base into the head and pushing down while turning the head clockwise. Turn on the ophthalmoscope by depressing the on/off switch. For routine use,

---

Documenting Abnormal Findings

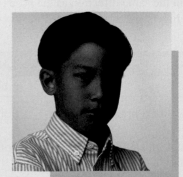

The nurse practitioner has just finished conducting a physical assessment of Chris, the 6-year-old boy with a cold. Review the following important findings that each of the steps of objective data collection for Chris revealed. Begin to think about how the data cluster together and what additional data the nurse might want to collect while thinking critically about the problems and anticipating nursing interventions

Inspection: Somewhat anxious boy, sitting in mother's lap. Face flushed, breathing easily, no shortness of breath. Dry, hacking cough. Oropharynx red without lesions or drainage. Tonsils slightly red and enlarged, graded 3+. Nares red with some clear thin drainage. External canals are clear. Tympanic membranes are pearl gray without perforation. Light reflex and landmarks intact. Hearing intact.

Palpation: No tenderness or swelling over sinuses.

Percussion: Thorax resonant.

Auscultation: Lungs clear, no wheezing or adventitious sounds.

L. Brier, APRN

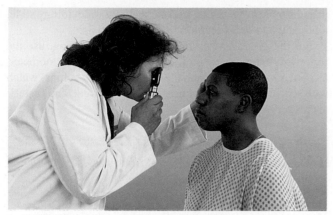

Figure 4.9 Positioning of the ophthalmoscope to visualize the interior structures of the eye.

the aperture commonly selected is the large full spot. Other choices include small light spot for small pupils, a green light to filter out red, a grid used to locate structures and lesions, and a slit used to determine the shape of lesions.

Hold the ophthalmoscope firmly against your face, so that the eye looks directly through the viewing aperture. Both eyes must stay open, but the concentration is on the view through the aperture. The lens selector dial focuses the ophthalmoscope, similar to binoculars. The black numbers (power of + 20 to +140) focus on objects near, while the red numbers (power of −20 to −140) focus on objects far away. In this way, the ophthalmoscope adjusts for nearsightedness (myopia) or farsightedness (hyperopia) in both the nurse and the patient. It does not, however, accommodate for astigmatism.

Darken the room to help dilate the patient's pupils, because the eye is visualized through the pupil. Eyeglasses obstruct visualization, so if you or the patient wears glasses, remove them. Hold the ophthalmoscope in the same hand and use the same eye as the eye being examined to avoid bumping noses with the patient. Starting with zero, adjust the lenses using the index finger to bring the fundus (background) of the eye into focus. Moving the lens selector dial clockwise turns the magnification more positive, or closer, while moving the lens selector dial counterclockwise turns the magnification more negative, or further away. Ask the patient to look at a distant fixation point while you point the light of the ophthalmoscope into the pupil from approximately 25 to 30 cm (10 to 12 in) away, or about an arm's length away, and slightly lateral to the person's line of vision. Visualization of the red reflex is the first step in examination of the eye. The technique, other findings, and more on use of the ophthalmoscope are discussed in Chapter 15.

Otoscope

Similar to the ophthalmoscope, the otoscope directs light into the ear to visualize the ear canal and tympanic membrane. The otoscope head and body connect and are activated in the same way as with the ophthalmoscope. Select the proper-sized speculum, choosing the largest size that fits most comfortably into the patient's ear, and place it on the otoscope. Hold the otoscope base between the thumb and the fingers upside

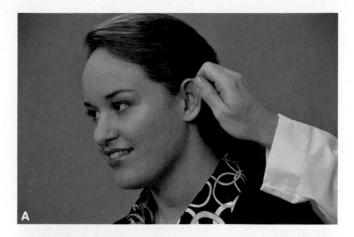

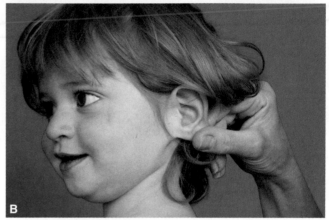

Figure 4.10 Placement of the ear for using the otoscope in **(A)** adults and **(B)** children.

down, and brace the ulnar surface or fingers of the hand against the patient's cheek (Fig. 4-10A). This positioning allows the nurse to move with patients unexpectedly, especially in the case of children with ear tenderness related to an infection. While inserting the speculum, straighten the adult patient's ear canal by gently pulling the auricle up, back, and slightly away from the head. The speculum is inserted gently into the canal, directing it slightly down and forward. You may also ask the patient to tilt the head toward the opposite shoulder to assist with visualization. In the child, pull the pinna down and back to straighten the canal (Fig. 4-10B). The technique and other findings are discussed in Chapter 16.

Tuning Fork

The tuning fork is used with two body systems: to determine vibration sense in the neuromuscular system and to determine conductive versus sensorineural hearing loss in the ears. Depending on their design, tuning forks create vibrations that produce sound waves of low- and high-pitched frequencies. The tuning fork for hearing loss produces a high-pitched tone of 512 to 1,024 Hz, within the range of human hearing (Fig. 4-11). Activate it by briskly squeezing and stroking the outside of the tongs from base to tips, or gently tapping the tongs against the knuckles to produce a soft ringing sound, while holding the fork at the base. Avoid touching the tongs,

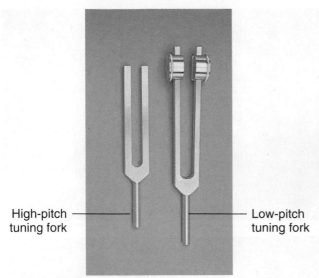

High-pitch tuning fork

Low-pitch tuning fork

Figure 4.11 Tuning forks.

which dampens the sound. If the fork is struck too harshly, the sound is too loud and takes too long to quiet to test the fine threshold of normal hearing. Gentle strokes or taps produce a softer sound for testing (see Chapter 16).

The tuning fork for vibration is at a lower frequency of 128 to 256 Hz. Activate this lower pitched device by tapping it against the heel of the hand. Hold this fork at the base and apply the base to a bony prominence, which the patient feels as a buzzing or tingling sensation (see Chapter 24).

Equipment for a Complete Physical Assessment

Gather all equipment needed for the physical assessment prior to entering the room to avoid interruption and to increase the patient's trust. Appropriate equipment depends on the type of examination. For example, if a patient has an appointment for a full physical assessment and Pap smear, lay out all the materials necessary for a complete physical assessment (Box 4-2),

BOX 4.2	EQUIPMENT FOR COMPLETE PHYSICAL ASSESSMENT
Platform scale with height measure	Tongue depressor
Thermometer	Snellen chart
Blood pressure cuff/machine	Tape measure
Watch with second hand	Reflex hammer
Stethoscope	Cotton swab
Clean gloves	Tuning fork: low pitched
Flashlight or penlight	Coin, paper clip, key, or pen
Ophthalmoscope	Bivalve vaginal speculum
Otoscope	Materials for cytological study
Tuning fork: high pitched	Lubricant
Nasal speculum	Fecal occult blood materials

in addition to a speculum, gloves, material for cytology slide, lubricant, and fecal occult blood test materials.

For the general assessment in a hospital setting, use the following equipment: vital signs equipment (thermometer, alcohol, electronic or manual blood pressure machine, watch with second hand, stethoscope), scale, flashlight, and materials for recording findings.

Lifespan Considerations

Pregnant Women

Most pregnant women provide a urine sample during each visit, so they can empty their bladder before undergoing the abdominal and vaginal examination. Pregnant women may be uncomfortable while lying flat. The nurse can complete most components of the physical examination with the patient sitting. The lithotomy position is necessary for vaginal examination (see Chapter 27).

Newborns and Infants

Positioning of newborns and infants for a physical assessment can be either on an examination table or held against a parent's chest. If the assessment happens on the examination table, you always must be in physical and visual contact with infants to maintain safety. Newborns and infants are comfortable without clothing in a warm environment; however, leaving their diapers on as long as possible is preferable, especially with boys, to avoid contamination of the nurse with urine or feces.

Warm your hands and equipment to avoid startling babies. Once infants can sit, you can perform most of the examination as the infant sits in a caregiver's lap. For sleeping infants, first listen to the heart, lung, and bowel sounds. Perform the most uncomfortable assessments at the end of the examination to prevent an infant's crying from compromising the quality of assessment findings (see Chapter 28).

Children and Adolescents

Active toddlers may be afraid or shy. Ask parents to assist with physical examination by holding or positioning their children as needed. Young children may hesitate to have body parts exposed. An alternative is for a parent to partially undress a child and then cover each body part after it is examined. Many toddlers automatically say "no" to any question asked. To prevent negativism from prolonging the examination, give specific choices, such as "Would you like to sit on the table or on your grandmother's lap while I listen to your heart?" Games also become prominent. Children may better participate if you encourage such activities as "blowing out" the ophthalmoscope light or listening to their own heart and lungs (see Chapter 29).

When working with adolescents, remain aware that their rapidly changing bodies may increase their feelings

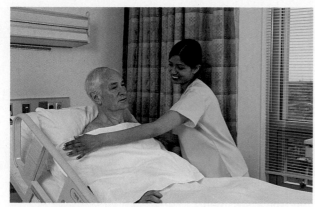

Figure 4.12 Slightly elevating the head of the bed or examination table may help facilitate breathing for older adults. Covering the patient to avoid chilling is another important consideration for patients in this age group.

of modesty or self-consciousness. Draping is especially important for patients of this age group. Additionally, adolescents appreciate explanations of why you are performing assessments, especially any related to or that can affect body image or developmental stage. For example, "I would like to listen to your heart sounds and need to

put the stethoscope on your chest, but I will be careful to keep you covered."

Older Adults

Older adults may chill more easily than younger patients, so you should consider offering them an additional blanket or drape (see Chapter 30). These patients may also fatigue quickly, so it is important to perform the most important assessments in the beginning. When positioning older adults, slight elevation of the head of the bed or examination table may help facilitate breathing (Fig. 4-12).

🌐 Cultural Considerations

Each assessment must be individualized according to the patient's cultural, religious, and social beliefs. Many patients are anxious prior to physical assessment. These feelings may be related to fear of disclosing private or uncomfortable information, embarrassment about being touched or looked at, or worry about abnormal findings. Ask patients about their preferences, such as having a family member in the room or having a same-gender examiner, before starting. Perform less invasive assessments first, such as taking vital signs, and save the most personal assessments for the end (see Chapter 11).

Analyzing Findings

Initial collection of subjective and objective data for Chris Chow is complete. The following nursing note documents the analysis of subjective and objective data and beginning development of nursing interventions.

Subjective: 6-year-old seen for fever, sore throat, and "runny nose." Mother states that patient has had a fever for 2 days; symptoms are not resolving.

Objective: Face flushed, breathing easily, no shortness of breath. Dry, hacking cough. No tenderness or swelling over sinuses. Oropharynx red without lesions or drainage. Tonsils slightly red and enlarged, 1+. Nares red with clear thin drainage. External canals clear. Tympanic membranes pearl gray without perforation. Light reflex, landmarks, and hearing intact. Thorax resonant. Lungs clear, no wheezing or adventitious sounds.

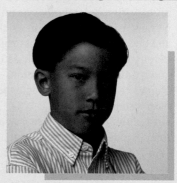

Analysis: Fever, viral rhinitis, and pharyngitis causing impaired comfort.

Plan: Encouraged to drink at least 2 L of fluid a day. Frozen treats and jello may be included in fluid intake. Take acetaminophen as needed for pain relief. Encouraged frequent rest, including naps during the day. Taught measures for infection control including disposal of tissues, covering mouth, and handwashing.

L. Brier, APRN

Critical Thinking Challenge

- What techniques and equipment did the nurse practitioner use during the physical assessment?
- What is the role of a nurse practitioner during this visit? How does this differ from the role of a registered nurse?
- How might the nurse organize the assessment sequentially to include the different body systems in this focused assessment for the child?

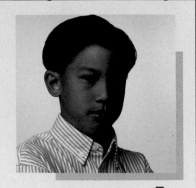

$\bigcup$ sing the previous steps of diagnostic reasoning, organizing, and prioritizing, consider all the case study findings woven throughout this chapter. When answering the following questions, begin drawing conclusions and see how the pieces of assessment must work together to create an environment for personalized, appropriate, and accurate care.

• How can the nurse facilitate comfort and reduce anxiety when performing the assessment?
• What information does the nurse gain about patients during inspection, palpation, percussion, and auscultation?
• How does the nurse use safety and infection-control principles during the assessment?

Key Points

• Hand hygiene is the most important action to prevent nosocomial infections.
• Nurses and other health care providers use standard precautions with every patient because many infections are unknown.
• Latex allergies are more common in nurses and patients frequently hospitalized.
• Nurses wear gloves during anticipated contact with body secretions and remove them when going from contaminated to cleaner areas.
• Inspection, percussion, palpation, and auscultation are the four techniques of physical assessment.
• Inspection relies on vision and smell to assess general status as well as each body system.
• Nurses use light palpation to obtain an overall impression and deep palpation to assess pain, masses, or tumors.
• Percussion sounds vary based on tone, intensity, pitch, quality, duration, and location.
• Nurses commonly auscultate the heart, lungs, and abdomen with a stethoscope.
• An ophthalmoscope, visual acuity chart, otoscope, tuning fork, percussion hammer, vaginal speculum, goniometer, and skin-fold calipers are equipment for advanced techniques used during the complete assessment.

Review Questions

1. Which of the following interventions is most important to prevent nosocomial infections?
A. Proper glove use
B. Hand hygiene
C. Appropriate draping
D. Quiet environment

2. Standard precautions
A. are used on every patient, because many infections are unknown
B. state that hand gel is used for infection with *C. difficile*
C. include the use of gowns, gloves, and masks with all patients
D. recognize that transmission-based precautions are common

3. Latex allergies
A. always result in anaphylactic reactions and shock
B. can be reduced by moisturizing the hands after washing
C. cannot be caused by equipment such as a stethoscope
D. are more common in nurses and frequently hospitalized patients

4. Which of the following is an appropriate use of gloves? Gloves are
A. worn during anticipated contact with intact skin
B. removed when going from clean to contaminated areas
C. worn during anticipated contact with body secretions
D. removed when assessing the back of an incontinent patient

5. Which of the following is an example of inspection?
A. Heart rate and rhythm regular
B. Lungs clear
C. Abdomen tympanic
D. Skin pink

6. The patient is complaining of abdominal pain. What technique is used to form an overall impression?
A. Auscultation
B. Light palpation
C. Direct percussion
D. Deep palpation

7. Tympany is a percussion sound commonly located in the
A. thorax
B. upper arm
C. abdomen
D. lower leg

8. The nurse auscultates which organs as part of the admitting assessment?
A. Heart, lungs, and abdomen
B. Kidneys, bladder, and ureters
C. Abdomen, flank, and groin
D. Neck, jaw, and clavicle

9. What technique facilitates accurate auscultation?
A. Earpieces of the stethoscope are positioned to point toward the back.
B. The tubing of the stethoscope is long and dark in color.
C. The chestpiece of the stethoscope is sealed against the skin.
D. The diaphragm of the stethoscope is used for low-frequency sounds.

10. When assessing the child, the nurse makes the following adaptation to the usual techniques:
A. A pediatric stethoscope provides better contact.
B. The child is seated away from the parent.
C. The room is full of toys for play.
D. The child is undressed, including the diaper.

References

Arroll, B., & Kenealy, T. (2002). Antibiotics for the common cold. *Cochrane Database Systematic Review,* (3):CD000247.

Bousquet, J., Flahault, A., Vandenplas, O., et al. (2006). Natural rubber latex allergy among health care workers: A systematic review of the evidence. *Allergy and Clinical Immunology, 118*(2), 447–454.

Brunetti, L., Santoro, E., De Caro, F., et al. (2006). Surveillance of nosocomial infections: A preliminary study on hand hygiene compliance of healthcare workers. *Journal of Previews in Medical Hygiene, 47*(2), 64–68.

CDC. (2009). *Standard precautions excerpt from the guideline for isolation precautions: Preventing transmission of infectious agents in healthcare settings 2007.* Retrieved April 16, 2009, from http://www.cdc.gov/ncidod/dhqp/gl_isolation_standard.html

Glasziou, P. P., Del Mar, C. B., et al. (2004). Antibiotics for acute otitis media in children. *Cochrane Database Systematic Review* (1):CD000219.

LaMontagne, A. D., Radi, S., Elder, D. S., et al. (2006). Primary prevention of latex related sensitisation and occupational asthma: A systematic review. *Occupational and Environmental Medicine, 63*(5), 359–364.

Larson, E., Girard, R., Pessoa-Silva, C., et al. (2006). Skin reactions related to hand hygiene and selection of hand hygiene products. *American Journal of Infection Control, 34*(10), 627–635.

OSHA. (2009). *Latex allergy.* Retrieved on April 16, 2009, from http://www.osha.gov/SLTC/latexallergy/index.html

Pittet, B., Allegranzi, H., Sax, S., et al. (2006). Evidence-based model for hand transmission during patient care and the role of improved practices. *The Lancet Infectious Diseases, 6*(10), 641–652D.

Siegel, J. D., Rhinehart, E., Jackson, M., et al. (2006). *Management of multidrug-resistant organisms in healthcare settings.* Washington, DC: CDC.

Widmer, A. F., Conzelmann, M., Tomic, M., et al. (2007). Introducing alcohol-based hand rub for hand hygiene: The critical need for training. *Infection and Control in Hospital Epidemiology, 28*(1), 50–54.

The Jensen suite offers these additional resources to enhance learning and facilitate understanding of this chapter:

- thePoint online resource, http//thepoint.lww.com/Jensen1E
- Student CD-ROM included with the book
- *Laboratory Manual for Nursing Health Assessment: A Best-Practice Approach*
- *Pocket Guide for Nursing Health Assessment: A Best-Practice Approach*

Documentation and Interdisciplinary Communication

Learning Objectives

1 Describe multiple purposes of the patient medical record.

2 Discuss the significance of accurate and timely documentation and the relationship between reporting patient assessment data and ensuring patient safety.

3 Compare and contrast various methods of documenting assessment data in the patient's record.

4 Provide a concise, clear handoff report using a template such as SBAR (situation, background, assessment, and recommendation).

5 Discuss ethical and legal considerations when documenting and reporting assessment information into the patient record.

*M*r. Chavez, 29 years old, was admitted to the hospital with a fractured humerus following a motor vehicle collision (MVC) in which he was a passenger wearing his seatbelt. His younger cousin, the driver, suffered a fractured tibia and fibula.

Mr. Chavez was born in Mexico; English is his second language, which he understands and speaks well. His temperature is 37.8°C (100°F) orally, pulse 110 beats/min, respirations 20 breaths/min, and blood pressure (BP) 122/66 mmHg. Current medications include patient-controlled analgesia (PCA) with morphine for pain, an antibiotic, a multivitamin, a stool softener, and medications to be taken as needed for symptoms such as itching and nausea. Initial assessment was in the emergency department (ED); an admitting assessment occurred 4 hours ago upon transfer to acute care. The nurse there is caring for him at the beginning of shift.

As you study the content and features, consider Mr. Chavez's case and its relationship to what you are learning. Begin thinking about the following points:

- What are the differences in the assessment data that nurses collect and document on the admitting assessment, flow sheets, SOAP notes, preoperative checklists, and postoperative assessments?
- How does the collection of data fluctuate between a comprehensive and a focused assessment?
- How do the patient situation and acuity influence the assessment, documentation, and communication of data?

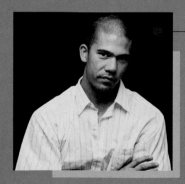

Prompt reporting and recording of patient assessment data are essential to ensuring safe and efficient delivery of care. In 2007, nearly 70% of all serious, often life-threatening, errors in health care (**sentinel events**) reported to the Joint Commission involved failures in communication as the root cause (Joint Commission, 2007). Communication occurs both verbally and in writing. Documentation involves entering patient information into the written or computerized patient record. The patient clinical record contains recorded information from all health care encounters.

All health team members document and retrieve information from the patient record as they plan and provide care. In the last decade, most health care agencies have transitioned the patient medical record from paper to a computerized, electronic form. Whether the patient record is paper or electronic, health care providers are responsible for always maintaining the confidentiality of all patient information.

Nurses use critical thinking and clinical judgment to determine when abnormal assessment data are significant, thus requiring verbal communication to other members of the health care team. Prompt, accurate documentation and reporting help ensure safe delivery and individualization of patient care.

Patient Medical Record

Purposes of the Medical Record

The medical record serves multiple purposes. In addition to being a legal document, the medical record is used for communication among health team members, care planning, quality assurance, financial reimbursement, education, and research.

Legal Document

The patient record serves as a legal document recording the patient's health status and any care he or she receives. The patient record can be used in civil or criminal courts to provide evidence of wrongdoing. Health care agencies have policies and standards that govern documentation that staff members must follow. Documentation helps to ensure that patients pursuing litigation against nurses must demonstrate that nurses did not comply with agency standards and policies or did not act in a manner in which any prudent nurse would have acted under the same circumstances.

⚠ SAFETY ALERT 5.1

The nurse must record normal assessment data, abnormal assessment data, and the time of the assessment. In the legal world, a typical saying is "If it's not documented, it's not done." This reinforces the need to document not only abnormal findings but also normal findings. When listening to the lungs, it is important to note "lungs clear, no shortness of breath" to document that the assessments were performed and that the findings were normal to protect against false litigation. For significant abnormal findings, it is also important to document the name of the primary care provider who was notified, the time of notification, and any interventions. This provides evidence that the nurse communicated and acted on the assessment data to protect against negligence.

BOX 5.1 HIGH-RISK ERRORS IN DOCUMENTATION

- Falsifying patient records
- Failing to record changes in a patient's condition
- Failing to document the notification of the primary provider when the patient's condition changes
- Performing an inadequate admission assessment
- Failing to document completely
- Failing to follow the agency's standards or policies on documentation
- Charting in advance

Source: Adapted from Craven, R. C., & Hirnle, C. J. (2009). *Fundamentals of nursing: Human health and function* (6th ed.). Philadelphia: Wolters Kluwer Health/Lippincott Williams & Wilkins.

Box 5-1 lists high-risk errors in documenting. Notice how many of these potential errors relate to the documentation of assessment data.

Communication and Care Planning

All members of the health care team access the assessment data documented in the patient's record to make care decisions. For example, a primary provider reviews documentation from the patient's pain assessment to determine whether to increase, maintain, or decrease the amount of pain medication prescribed. A social worker reviews the record for evidence of family support or a description of the home environment to plan for discharge. Assessment data provide the basis for the plan of care (POC) that identifies problems, outcomes, and interventions for the patient. The POC helps caregivers coordinate and individualize care until discharge.

Quality Assurance

An **audit** occurs when an agency or outside group reviews the records of a health care facility to determine whether that facility is providing and documenting certain standards of care. During an *internal audit*, the goal is to evaluate the care provided for continual improvement. For example, an agency may audit the record to evaluate whether staff members are charting pain assessments in a timely manner on all patients. The audit might also include if nurses are administering PRN (as needed) pain medication for documented pain levels greater than 4 (on a 0-to-10 scale). Such an audit helps target interventions or education to improve pain management.

Accrediting agencies such as the Joint Commission or state agencies such as Departments of Health can establish standards and audit patient records to evaluate the quality of care provided. Joint Commission accreditation is often required for facilities to obtain Medicare and Medicaid funding, so hospitals are motivated to comply with the standards in documentation and care that the Joint Commission sets. The Joint Commission also requires each hospital to develop an ongoing objective review of patient records for continuous quality improvement and to demonstrate correction of any deficiencies noted during the review. For example, if the standard of care is that postoperative patients have a surgical site check and assessment of vital signs every 15 minutes after surgery, the team conducting the audit will review records to identify if staff members are performing these assessments in a timely manner. Problem solving would occur on a systems level if the standard is not met, such as recommending an increase in unlicensed assistive personnel (UAP) to assist or scheduling surgeries more evenly.

Financial Reimbursement

Medicare, Medicaid, worker's compensation insurance, and third-party insurance companies depend on information in the patient's record to provide reimbursement for care. Documentation can support specific interventions that a care provider ordered (eg, laboratory or diagnostic tests). Diagnostic-related groups (DRGs), a proactive payment system, have become the basis for hospital reimbursement. Detailed information in the patient record helps to support codable diagnoses that insurance companies use to determine the DRG (Fig. 5-1). Detailed charting of assessments

and necessary interventions often can support approval for additional hospital days. Lack of appropriate charting can impact whether financial payment will be authorized. Insurance companies also audit patient records to ensure that billing is accurate and that no fraud has occurred. Accurate assessments are needed to make accurate diagnoses.

Education

Students in various health care disciplines review patient records to enhance clinical learning and to better understand complex clinical situations. They can access and review records during care delivery. At times, students come to the clinical area before their assigned shift to read the patient record and do the necessary research so that they can provide informed and individualized care. Nursing grand rounds or classroom discussions can use specific patient situations to educate nurses and students. For example, an audit of charts from patients who experienced oversedation or respiratory depression from opioid administration may be collected and presented to staff members to help educate nurses about safe pain management. Assessment data are used to identify trends in respiratory rates and to detect early warning signs of clinical deterioration.

Research

Health care practitioners use patient records to obtain data for nursing and medical research. If they obtain such data, they must follow strict policies to protect the privacy and rights of individual patients. They must obtain prior approval by the agency's Institution Review Boards (IRB) before any research study. At times, professionals collect data without IRB approval; however, these studies are limited to internal quality improvement, and data can never be reported to or used by any outside group. The assessments must be performed and documented accurately so that the research outcomes are valid and reliable.

Components of the Medical Record

The patient record is not read like a book, from beginning to end. Instead, each nurse becomes skilled at finding pertinent information quickly. Each agency develops specific forms contained within the medical record and policies governing documentation practice.

Assessment forms include an admitting assessment, flow sheets, and ongoing assessment forms. The patient medical record usually contains the following components:

- Nursing admission assessment
- History and physical examination (H & P) by the primary health care provider
- Primary provider's orders
- POC or clinical pathway
- Flow sheets documenting vital signs, intake and output (I & O), and routine assessments
- Focused assessment sheets (eg, neurological or postoperative reassessment)

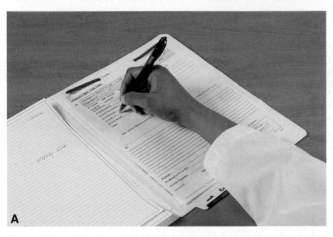

A

DIAGNOSIS				
	722.6	Degenerative Disc Disease	242.90	Hyperthyroidism	V70.3
	276.5	Dehydration	244.9	Hypothyroidism	486
	296.20	Depression	703.0	Ingrown Toenail	V22.2
	250.00	Diabetes	780.52	Insomnia	256.3
	692.9	Eczema/Dermatitis	564.1	Irritable Bowel Syndrome	601.9
	782.3	Edema	785.6	Lymphadenopathy	473.9
	780.79	Fatigue	626.9	Menstrual Disorder	780.2
	780.6	Fever	346.90	Migraine	465.9
se	610.1	Fibrocystic Breast Disease	848.9	Muscle Strain	599.0
	558.9	Gastroenteritis	728.85	Muscle Spasms	616.1
	274.9	Gout	733.00	Osteoporosis	780.4
	784.0	Headache	382.9	Otitis Media	078.1
re	785.3	Heart Murmur	V72.3	Pelvic Exam	
c.	272.0	Hypercholesterolemia	533.90	Peptic Ulcer Disease	
	272.4	Hyperlipidemia	462	Pharyngitis, Acute	
se	401.9	Hypertension	V70.0	Physical Exam, General	
ve)					PREVIOUS

B

Figure 5.1 **(A)** Nurses must take care to document accurately about findings to support specific interventions ordered. **(B)** Such information helps to support codable diagnoses used by insurance companies as well as to get approval for additional hospital days and other treatments required by patients.

- Medication administration record (MAR)
- Laboratory and diagnostic test results
- Progress notes by different members of the health care team
- Consultations
- Discharge or transfer summary

Electronic Medical Record

Most clinical agencies have computerized part or all of the patient's medical record. Software programs allow nurses to enter assessment data quickly, usually by checking boxes and adding free text when appropriate. The electronic medication administration record (eMAR) interfaces medication orders with pharmacy dispensing and allows direct computer charting of medication administration (Fig. 5-2). Computerized provider order entry (**CPOE**) allows providers to enter all orders directly into the computer, electronically communicating orders to the laboratory, pharmacy, and nursing personnel. Appropriate staff members receive a computerized communication (task) when treatments and medications are due during their assigned shift. They also receive a message when the patient requires a reassessment (eg, with assessment of the effectiveness of the pain medication).

Although implementing a computerized system is expensive and requires much planning and education, such systems significantly increase patient safety (Moody, et al., 2004). They allow several health team members to view the patient record simultaneously. For those with special clearance, they enable the off-site viewing of the electronic record to note changes in patient condition or to order necessary laboratory tests, diagnostic studies, or medications. Computerization ensures that all entries are legible and time dated. It enables the graphing of trends in vital signs or assessment data. It minimizes compliance issues, because programs will not let nurses enter data until they have completed all required fields. This ensures a more complete assessment. Some programs create plans of care from entered assessment data.

Computerization of the medical record also permits the use of automated clinical surveillance tools to scan in real time the medical record of all patients to detect assessment data indicating problems. One such tool, the Risk Assessment Report, provides risk scores on sepsis, pressure ulcers, falls, abnormal laboratory reports, and other criteria of interest (Whittington, et al., 2007). This permits early intervention and saves lives. Frequently, patients show clinical signs of deterioration, but health care providers fail to respond for 24 hours before a critical adverse event (O'Neill & Miranda, 2006). A designated

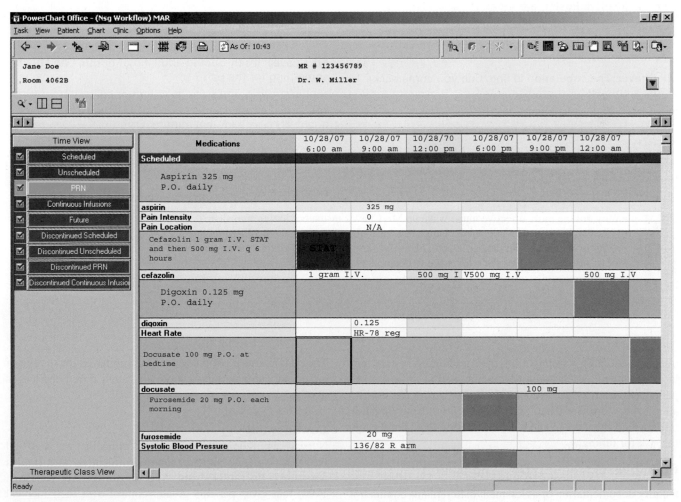

Figure 5.2 An eMAR.

Therapeutic Dialogue: Collecting Subjective Data

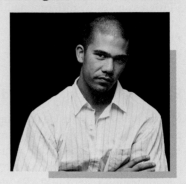

Remember Mr. Chavez, introduced at the beginning of this chapter. The nurse uses professional communication techniques to gather subjective data from Mr. Chavez at the beginning of the shift. The following conversations give two examples of different interview styles. One style is more effective than the other. As you read the conversations, consider the purpose of this data collection.

Less Effective

Nurse: Hi, Mr. Chavez. How are you feeling? (Waits 2 seconds.) (Louder) Mr. Chavez, how are you?

Mr. Chavez: Not too good.

Nurse: Why, what's wrong?

Mr. Chavez: My arm hurts.

Nurse: You fractured it.

Mr. Chavez: It hurts. My arm hurts.

Nurse: You can push the button on your machine to get pain medication. Push the button.

Mr. Chavez: OK. Can you come back later? I hurt now.

Nurse: Well, I need to assess the circulation in your arm.

Mr. Chavez: The circulation is fine. Can you come back in just a little bit?

Nurse: OK. I'll let you sleep.

More Effective

Nurse: Hi, Mr. Chavez. How are you feeling? (Waits 10 seconds.) (Touches patient.) Mr. Chavez, I'm Shannon, your nurse.

Mr. Chavez: Oh, sorry. I was sleepy. Let me sleep.

Nurse: OK, but first I need to look at your arm.

Mr. Chavez: OK (turns over). My arm hurts.

Nurse: Is it OK if I look at it? (Patient nods.) (Nurse notes cool, pale right arm. Pulse is decreased. Capillary refill is slow.)

Nurse: Mr. Chavez, could you please wiggle your fingers? (Patient wiggles fingers.) Tell me what your pain is like.

Mr. Chavez: It's throbbing and kind of numb. Can I have something for the pain?

Nurse: Sure, go ahead and push the button. I'm concerned about your arm and will talk with the doctor about it. I'll be back in a minute. OK?

Critical Thinking Challenge

- Why did the more effective nurse wake up Mr. Chavez instead of letting him sleep?
- How can the less effective nurse change her vocabulary to reduce medical jargon?
- What is the purpose of data collection? How will the nurse organize findings in this case?
- What information does the nurse need to document? Where?

---

nurse can monitor warnings from the surveillance system for large groups of patients and ask the assigned nurse to assess patients to determine if an acute problem exists for those with a high-risk score. See Chapter 13 for a tool for identifying the risk for skin breakdown and Chapter 30 for a tool identifying the risk for falling.

Principles Governing Documentation

Quality documentation of assessment data remains confidential and is accurate, complete, organized, timely, and concise.

The computerized patient record has improved the quality of nursing documentation in some areas and posed challenges in others.

Confidential

Nurses are required legally and ethically to keep all information in the patient record confidential. The **Health Insurance Portability and Accountability Act (HIPAA,** 1996) that gives patients greater control over their medical records became effective in 2003. HIPAA regulates all areas of

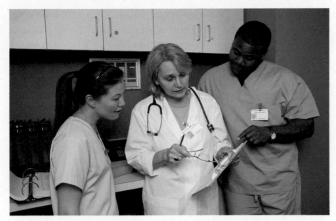
Figure 5.3 Nurses must take all measures to keep information from patients confidential and discuss such information only with other health care professionals directly involved in the patient's care.

Table 5.1	Accurate Documentation Using Medical Terminology
Ambiguous Documentation	**Accurate Documentation**
Vitals normal	T 37°C, P 80, R 12 breaths/min, BP 118/62 mmHg
Neuro status OK	Alert and oriented X Times 3, speech clear
Lung sounds good	Lung sounds clear
Heart sounds good	Heart rate and rhythm regular
Eating well	Ate 60% of regular diet
Voiding well	Voiding 700 mL of clear yellow urine
No problems moving	Moves all extremities with full range of motion and 5/5 strength
Skin color good	Skin color pink
Family was here	Family visiting with appropriate interactions

information management, including reimbursement, coding, and security of records. The HIPAA Privacy Rule requires an agency to make reasonable efforts to limit use of, disclosure of, and requests for protected health information to the minimum necessary to accomplish the intended purpose. Most agencies require students and employees to complete HIPAA training. HIPAA also provides for patient education on privacy protection, patient access to medical records, patient consent prior to disclosing information from the record, and patient recourse if privacy protections are violated.

Confidentiality means keeping information private. This principle applies to computerized and written medical records and any information pertaining to health status or care received (Fig. 5-3). All patient information is confidential and discussed only with other health care professionals directly involved in the patient's care. Nurses should never discuss patients (with or without names) and their situations in public places such as elevators, hallways, or the cafeteria. People who hear conversations can misinterpret information, leading to anxiety or fear. Additional methods of protecting confidentiality include never sharing computer passwords and never leaving a computer with patient information unattended. Forms from the agency should never be taken, even if the patient identification information is removed. Information from the patient's chart should be copied into a notebook without the patient's name.

⚠ SAFETY ALERT 5.2

Health care providers who violate HIPAA may face fines of up to $250,000 or jail time (HIPAA, 1996). Employees have been terminated for breaching HIPAA laws concerning confidentiality.

Accurate and Complete

Assessment information that nurses enter into the patient's record must accurately reflect what they observed, heard, auscultated, palpated, percussed, or smelled. Nurses document subjective data using the patient's exact words whenever possible. Descriptions are as precise as possible. For example, nurses would document the size of a wound as

"6 cm by 9 cm with a 1 cm depth" rather than as "large." Accuracy permits comparison of current findings with future data to detect changes in patient status. Thus, nurses avoid using the words "normal" or "good"; instead, they use correct medical terminologies (eg, "heart rate and rhythm regular," not "normal."). See Table 5-1.

To avoid potential errors, the Joint Commission discourages the use of many abbreviations. It is important to be familiar with abbreviations and to use only those legally accepted. As nurses are learning health assessment techniques, they also should focus on learning the language, labeling the findings, and identifying abbreviations.

Computerization of the patient medical record has greatly increased the legibility of its information. Nevertheless, handwritten entries still occur; when they happen, they must be clear and legible. This is especially true when recording numbers that can easily be confused. Black ink is usually required for written documentation to provide clarity when faxing documentation from the patient record.

Nurses need to correct errors in documentation so that the record is accurate. In the written record, they make corrections by drawing a line through the error and placing initials above the correction (Fig. 5-4). The computerized record

3/1/10	c/o SOB X 15 min. while ambulating.
3:15 pm	error-charted on wrong client S.N. ~~Denies chest pain. BP 126/84, P. 84, R. 16~~
	BP 134/90, P. 86 R. 24. Assisted to bed
	with hob elevated. Notified Dr. Smith.
	———————— Sally North RN

Figure 5.4 A sample of a corrected entry in a written patient record.

permits electronic correction of errors, retaining both the original entry and the correction. Erasing, blacking out information, or using whiteout is not permitted.

Organized

Organized entry of assessment data demonstrates a logical and systematic grouping of information. Flow sheets and documentation systems often cue nurses to a specific organization structure. This encourages nurses to include all areas of assessment and provides an organized report so that other health team members can use the information to make sound clinical decisions. Nurses also should document entries of assessment chronologically so that a picture of the time certain assessments were made is clear. This is especially important if the patient record is used as evidence during litigation.

Timely

Nurses must enter assessment data into the record in a timely manner. Most agencies have policies regarding the frequencies of assessments. For example, on a medical-surgical unit, a complete assessment may occur every 8 hours; in the intensive care unit, it may be every hour; and in the skilled nursing facility (SNF), it might be weekly. Computerized charting automatically reflects the time the entry is made, but nurses can change the documented time to reflect the time of the assessment. Paper charting should also reflect the specific time (eg, 2:04 am) rather than a shift designation (eg, 7-3).

Batch charting (waiting until the end of shift or until all patients have been assessed to document) contributes to many potential errors. Waiting to record may contribute to forgetting important information or charting assessment data on the wrong patient. **Point-of-care** documentation occurs when nurses document assessment information as they gather it, often using a portable computer (Fig. 5-5). This can be done during a home visit, a clinic visit, or in the patient's room during a hospital stay.

Prompt documentation allows health team members to use up-to-date assessment information to make clinical decisions. For example, a change in weight or vital signs might

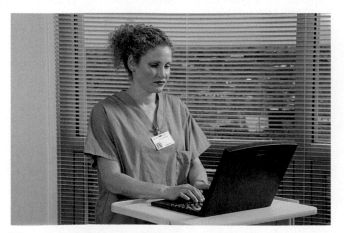

Figure 5.5 The nurse is using a portable computer to carry out point-of-care documentation.

prompt a primary provider to adjust a medication dosage. Computerized documentation systems allow other health team members to review the patient record off-site so that they base decisions on the current record.

> **Clinical Significance 5-1**
>
> Clear documentation that reflects time sequencing is especially important for patients with unstable conditions. If litigation occurs, lawyers use documentation to reconstruct the sequence of events, the time of interventions, and the time that providers were notified. In a code or emergency, the team should designate a single member to document so that entries are accurate and timely.

Concise

Good charting is complete, yet concise. Unnecessary elaboration confuses important issues. Nurses should record the findings, but not how they collected them. For example, the nurse would document "BP (R) 124/78" instead of "BP was auscultated in the right arm at 124/78." Time is a precious health care resource, and long, rambling entries take more time to document and to read. In narrative notes, health care providers use sentence fragments (eg, "alert and oriented") and approved abbreviations instead of complete sentences.

Generally, caregivers chart information in one place and avoid "double charting." An exception is in the care plan or progress note, in which nurses synthesize the most important information to show critical thinking about a problem.

> **Clinical Significance 5-2**
>
> Because assessment requires much critical thinking and clinical judgment and is a professional responsibility, nurses cannot delegate it to UAP.

Critical Thinking and Clinical Judgment

Agency policy governs the precise documentation of assessment data in the patient's record, but nurses continually use critical thinking and clinical judgment to determine the focus, depth, and frequency of assessment documentation. To provide safe individualized care in hospitals, nurses perform a complete nursing assessment for each assigned patient, evaluate the stability of the patient's condition, and determine what monitoring the patient requires during the shift. Nurses obtain assessments as soon as possible after handoff of the patient has occurred, such as after transfer from the ED to the nursing unit, so that a baseline can be determined. Nurses can delegate the monitoring and documenting of specific assessments (eg, vital signs) to UAP; however, nurses always retain the responsibility to interpret delegated assessment data to evaluate the patient's condition.

Based on knowledge and experience, nurses individualize assessments. For example, a middle-aged patient admitted for

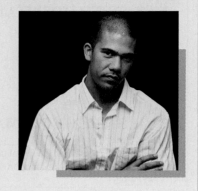

Documenting Abnormal Findings

The nurse has just finished a focused assessment of Mr. Chavez's fractured humerus. Review the following important findings that the relevant steps of objective data collection for Mr. Chavez revealed. Begin to think about how the data cluster together and what additional data the nurse might want to collect as he or she thinks critically and anticipates nursing interventions for the patient.

Inspection: Appears somewhat drowsy with facial grimace from pain. Guarding right humerus. Wiggles fingers, states some numbness and tingling. States 8/10 pain throbbing from above elbow to fingers. Increasing since injury; especially worse in the last 30 minutes. Movement increases pain. Given pain medication 2 hours ago for pain 4/10.

Palpation: Right radial artery 1+; limb pale and cool. Capillary refill 6 seconds. Sensation intact. Left arm pink, warm with 3+ pulse, no pain and intact sensation.

S Cisco, RN

foot surgery may not require a comprehensive neurological assessment if he is alert and can answer questions appropriately. But an intoxicated patient with a head laceration who is admitted following an assault would definitely require a complete neurological assessment, including pupil checks, to promptly detect increased intracranial pressure or alcohol withdrawal (see Chapter 24). Although a primary provider's order determines the minimum frequency of assessments, if a patient's condition appears unstable or deteriorating, nurses independently increase the frequency and documentation of assessments. They also use clinical judgment regarding when to notify the primary provider regarding abnormal findings. They need to document such reporting, including the time of notification and the primary provider's response.

Nursing Admission Assessment

Nurses conduct the *nursing admission assessment*, sometimes referred to as the *nursing history and physical*, to obtain patient history and baseline data so that they can individualize care. In acute care facilities, policy usually requires the completion and documentation of the initial complete nursing assessment within 24 hours of admission. An SNF may require the completion of such an assessment within 3 days of the patient's admission. The agency usually provides separate forms to cue the assessment and standardize the documentation (Fig. 5-6).

The admission assessment provides all future care providers with comprehensive information about the patient's physical, psychological, functional, social, and spiritual abilities and forms the basis for an individualized POC. Care providers can refer to this initial assessment to obtain important baseline information and to detect changes in status.

Flow Sheets

Nurses usually document routine, scheduled assessments on flow sheets. Flow sheets are efficient and standardize the

collected information, permitting easy comparison among assessment data to detect trends or a sudden change in status. Common flow sheets in the patient's record include vital signs, intake and output, routine assessments, and diabetic record. More complex flow sheets are used in critical care, where frequent, extensive physiological assessments are necessary to quickly detect and treat life-threatening problems.

Plan of Care/Clinical Pathway

An assessment of the patient allows for the development of a **POC** that individualizes his or her goals, outcomes, and interventions. The POC is part of the permanent patient record, and nurses update it as the patient's condition changes. A **clinical pathway** is a multidisciplinary tool that identifies a standard plan for a specific patient population (eg, those undergoing total hip replacement). It includes patient problems, expected outcomes, and interventions within an established timeframe. The POC or clinical pathway often provides the structure for shift report handoff.

Progress Note

Multiple health team members (physician, physical therapist, respiratory therapist, social workers, and nurses) document in a **progress note** the patient's progress toward recovery. There has been a movement away from each team member documenting assessments in a discipline-specific section of the patient's record. The current trend is for personnel from different disciplines to consolidate all entries in one place. This permits all team members to quickly locate and read how the patient is progressing and meeting (or not meeting) goals.

Many nurses use progress notes to summarize how the patient is doing, but formats for this type of documentation can vary. Narrative, SOAP, PIE, and Focus notes are common methods of recording assessments, interventions, and patient responses. See Table 5-2 comparing these formats of documentation.

NAZARETH HOSPITAL

NURSING ADMISSION HISTORY

I. GENERAL INFORMATION

ARRIVAL: Date: _9/2/09_   Time: _2:00 PM_

Transportation Method: ☐ Ambulatory ☐ Stretcher ☑ W/C

Admitted Via: ☑ ED ☐ Direct Admission ☐ PACU ☐ SDS**
  ☐ Other:_____

Accompanied By: ☐ Self ☐ Spouse ☑ Daughter ☐ Son
  ☐ Mother ☐ Father ☐ Friend ☐ Other:_____

Correct Name On Identiband? ☑ YES ☐ NO

PATIENT/SIGNIFICANT OTHER ORIENTED TO:
  Call Light at Bedside/in BR : ☑ YES ☐ NO ☐ N/A
  Operation of Bed/Siderails: ☑ YES ☐ NO ☐ N/A
  Phone/TV: ☑ YES ☐ NO ☐ N/A

PATIENT ADVISED HOSPITAL NOT RESPONSIBLE FOR VALUABLES:
  ☑ YES ☐ NO

Does Patient Have Any Valuables? ☑ YES* ☐ NO
  If Yes*, Disposition of Valuables? ☐ Sent Home
  ☐ Security - Envelope #_____
  ☑ Patient Refused Security - Valuables kept with Patient

LIST & DESCRIBE PATIENT'S VALUABLES
  eyeglasses @ bedside
  yellow metal watch on patient
  yellow metal wedding ring on pt.
  sent purse home with daughter

MEDICATION BROUGHT TO HOSPITAL: ☐ YES ☑ NO
  If YES, : ☐ Home ☐ Pharmacy

_____ Date: _____ Time: _____
STAFF SIGNATURE REQUIRED FOR ALL SDS** PATIENTS

INFORMATION GIVEN BY PATIENT: ☑ YES ☐ NO
  IF NO:Name: _____
  Number: _____
  Relationship: _____
  ☐ Unable to obtain history - REASON

_____

REASON FOR ADMISSION ACCORDING TO PATIENT:
  I fell at home this a.m. Couldn't move
  (L) _leg for awhile; headaches_

PATIENT AWARE OF DIAGNOSIS: ☐ YES ☑ NO
FAMILY AWARE OF DIAGNOSIS: ☐ YES ☑ NO
DOES PATIENT HAVE AN ORGAN DONOR CARD? ☐ YES ☑ NO
  If no, & the patient requests further information,   provide
  KIDNEY-1 Number.   1-800-KIDNEY-1
ALLERGIES:
  *****ALLERGY DOCUMENTATION MUST BE COMPLETED AT
  TIME OF ADMISSION ON THE ALLERGY FORM*****
CURRENT MEDICATIONS ☐ NONE
(INCLUDE RX, INHALERS, OVER-THE-COUNTER)

NAME	DOSE	FREQUENCY	LAST DOSE
REASON			
hydralazine	dose ?	OD	yesterday am
for high blood pressure			
aspirin	X 2	prn	noon today- headache
metamucil	1 Tbsp	prn	this am for constipation

HOSPITALIZATIONS/SURGICAL HISTORY ☐ NONE
DIAGNOSIS/REASON

  gallbladder surgery 1985
  hospitalized for ↑BP 2002

FAMILY HISTORY: ☐ NONE
  ☐ Diabetes ☐ Pulmonary ☑ Heart Disease ☑ CA
  ☐ Anesthesia ☐ Other:
  Complication

II.   PAST MEDICAL HISTORY

SKIN: ☑ NEGATIVE HISTORY
  ☐ Scars ☐ Eczema ☐ Psoriasis ☐ Cancer
  ☐ Other: _____
NEUROLOGICAL: ☐ NEGATIVE HISTORY
  ☐ TIA ? ☐ Anxiety ☐ Dementia ☐ Syncope
  (H/A) ☐ Tremors ☐ Parkinson's ☐ Depression

Figure 5.6 A sample admission record.

NAZARETH HOSPITAL

NURSING ADMISSION
HISTORY

Date of LMP: _N/A_

FUNCTIONAL STATUS PRIOR TO ADMISSION

I - Independent   A - Assistance Required   D - Dependent

FEED SELF	☑ I	☐ A*	☐ D*
BATHE SELF	☐ I	☐ A*	☐ D*
DRESS SELF	☐ I	☐ A*	☐ D*
HOUSE CHORES	☐ I	☐ A*	☐ D*
AMBULATE	☐ I	☐ A**	☐ D**
CLIMB STAIRS	☐ I	☐ A**	☐ D**
CHAIR BOUND	☐ I	☐ A**	☐ D**
BED BOUND	☐ I	☐ A**	☐ D**

If * or ** circled, were changes made within past 6 months? ☐ YES* ☐ NO
If YES*, Notify Coordinated Care

III.   PSYCHO-SOCIAL ASSESSMENT

Occupation: _homemaker_   ☑ RETIRED
Marital Status: ☐ Married   ☐ Single   ☐ Separated
☐ Divorced   ☑ Widowed ☐ Common Law *husband died this year
Residential Information: ☐ Home   ☐ ECF   ☑ Other* Just moved
Usual Living Arrangement: ☐ Alone   ☐ Child   ☐ Spouse in with
☑ Other Family   ☐ Parent   ☐ Friend   ☐ S.O.   ☐ ECF   daughter
Contact Person #1: _Barbara Tembra_

Relationship: _daughter_   H#: _215-634-5221_ W#: _____

PRIMARY LANGUAGE:
☑ English   ☐ Polish   ☐ Russian   ☐ German   ☐ Ukrainian
☐ Italian   ☐ Spanish   ☐ Indian   ☐ Korean   ☐ Chinese
☐ Japanese   ☐ Other _____
Does Patient understand English?   ☑ YES   ☐ NO*
   *Contact Person for Translation: _____
   Relationship: _____ H#: _____ W#: _____

ASSISTIVE DEVICES/DURABLE MEDICAL EQUIPMENT: ☑ NONE
☐ Cane ☐ w/pt   ☐ Crutches ☐ w/pt   ☐ Walker ☐ w/pt   ☐ Wheelchair ☐ w/pt
☐ Tub Seat   ☐ Commode   ☐ Grab Bars   ☐ Hospital Bed
☐ Stair Glide   ☐ Other: _____

SPIRITUAL/CULTURAL ASSESSMENT:
Does patient express any spiritual, cultural, or emotional concerns which
may impact on this hospitalization?   ☐ YES*   ☑ NO
   Explain: _____
Does patient express a desire to meet with a Spiritual Care member?
   her own minister   ☑ YES*   ☐ NO
   Priest?   ☐ YES*   ☑ NO   If YES*, notify Spiritual Care.
Coping Mechanisms (How does patient deal with stress?)   ☐ NONE
   Type: _talk with friends, pray * misses husband_
Support Groups   ☑ NONE
   Type: _____
Sleep: _8_ hrs/night   Up at night: _1-2_ times/night
Tobacco: ☐ YES   ☑ NO Amount/day: _____ How Long: _____ ☐
Quit
ETOH: ☐ YES   ☑ NO
Substance Abuse: ☐ YES* ☐ NO   *Type _____
   Has patient been in treatment?   ☐ YES ☐ NO

IV.   EDUCATIONAL ASSESSMENT

Patient Assessed: ☑ YES ☐ NO   Family Assessed: ☐ YES ☐ NO
Patient Responsible for Learning Anticipated Needs: ☑ YES ☐ NO*
   *OTHER: _____ #: _____
Patient's Preferred Method of Learning: ☑ No Preference Stated
   ☐ Hearing   ☐ Seeing   ☐ Reading   ☐ Hands-on

What does patient want to learn about? ☐ Unidentified At This Time
☑ Disease Process   ☐ Diet & Nutrition   ☐ Community Resources
☐ Medication   ☐ Medical Equipment   ☑ Follow-up Care
☐ Pain Management   ☐ Rehab Techniques   ☐ Other: _____

ANTICIPATED EDUCATIONAL NEEDS IDENTIFIED BY STAFF:
☑ Disease Process   ☐ Diet & Nutrition   ☑ Community Resources
☑ Medication   ☐ Medical Equipment   ☑ Follow-up Care
☐ Pain Management   ☐ Rehab Techniques   ☐ Other: _____

ASSESSMENT OF PATIENT'S BARRIERS TO LEARNING:
Motivation: ☑ Good   ☐ Fair   ☐ Poor
Learning Ability: ☑ Good   ☐ Fair   ☐ Poor
Emotional/Mental Factors: ☐ NONE
   ☑ Anxious   ☐ Confused   ☐ Depressed
   ☐ Agitated   ☐ Combative   ☐ Does Not Follow Command
Physical Factors: ☐ NONE
   ☐ Pain   ☑ Age Related   ☐ Language Barrier
   ☐ Fatigue   ☐ Medication Effect   ☐ Limitation of Illness

V.   ADVANCE DIRECTIVE

Patient has an advance directive?   ☐ YES   ☑ NO
Patient would like help to prepare an advance directive? ☑ YES   ☐ NO

VI.   DISCHARGE PLANNING

Return: ☐ Home   ☑ Family   ☐ Rehab   ☐ ECF   ☐ Unknown
Is Patient currently receiving Home Care Services?   ☐ YES* ☑ NO
   *Agency: _____

Were any needs identified requiring notification of Coordinated Care?
                  ☐ YES   ☑ NO

VII. PHYSICIAN NOTIFICATION

ATTENDING: _Dr. Skomar_

9/26/09	2:30 PM	C Tayn RN
DATE	TIME	NOTIFIED BY

HOUSE OFFICER: _____

DATE	TIME	NOTIFIED BY

NURSING ASSESSMENT COMPLETED BY:

9/2/09	2:35 PM	C Tayn
DATE	TIME	RN SIGNATURE

Figure 5.6 (*Continued*)

NAZARETH HOSPITAL

NURSING ADMISSION HISTORY

☑ Falls   ☐ Seizures   ☐ Alzheimer's   ☐ Vertigo
☐ CVA   ☐ Tumor   ☐ Migraines   ☐ Mood
☐ R Hemiplagia   ☐ Benign   ☐ Vertigo   Changes
☐ L Hemiplagia   ☐ Malignant   ☑ Other: _"slightly dizzy"_

Memory Impairment: ☑NONE
☐Acute→ ☐ Short Term ☐ Long Term   ☐Chronic→ ☐ Short Term ☐ Long Term

MUSCULOSKELETAL: ☐ **NEGATIVE HISTORY**
☐ Fractures: _____
☐Arthritis: _____
☐ Amputation: _____
☐ Prosthesis: **TYPE:**_____   ☐R ☐L ☐ WITH PATIENT
☑ Other: ✓ _movement & strength (L) leg_ _____
If **with patient, remind patient hospital not responsible for article.

EENT   _"pins & needles in (L) leg"_
VISION: ☐ **NEGATIVE HISTORY**
   ☑ Glasses ✓ WITH PT   ☐ Contacts ☐ WITH PT   ☐ Prosthesis ☐ WITH PT
   ☐ Nearsighted   ☐R ☐L   ☐R ☐L
   ☐ Farsighted   ☑ Blurred Vision   ☐ Blind
   ☐ Glaucoma   ☐R ☐L   ☐R ☐L
   ☐R ☐L   ☐ Double Vision   ☐ Implants
   ☐ Cataract   ☐R ☐L   ☐R ☐L
   ☐R ☐L

HEARING: ☐ **NEGATIVE**
HISTORY
   ☑ HOH   ☐ Deaf   ☐ Earache
   ☐R ☑L   ☐R ☐L   ☐R ☐L
   ☐ Tinnitus   ☐ Hearing Aid ☐ WITH PT
   ☐R ☐L
   If with Patient, remind patient hospital not responsible for article.

THYROID: ☑ **NEGATIVE HISTORY**
☐ Hypothyroid   ☐ Hyperthyroid   ☐ Surgery
☐ Radiation   → Have large doses of radioactive material been used
       within the last week?   ☐ YES*   ☐ NO
       If YES*, notify Nuclear Medicine Department.

Speech Impairment: ☐NONE   ☐New*   ☐ Old
   If NEW*, notify Coordinated Care.

CARDIOVASCULAR: ☐ **NEGATIVE HISTORY**
☐ MI   ☐ PVD   ☐ Anemia   ☐ Rheumatic H D
☑ HTN   ☐ CHF   ☐ Phlebitis   ☐ Syncope Fainting
☐ CP/Angina   ☐ Palpitations   ☐ Bleeding Problems
☐ Hypotension   ☐ Murmur   ☐ Arrhythmia
☐ Pacemaker   ☐ Internal
Date:_____   Defibrillator   ☐ Other:_____
Plutonium Operated   Date:_____ _____
☐ YES* ☐ NO
If YES*, notify Nuclear Medicine Department.

PULMONARY: ☑ **NEGATIVE HISTORY**
☐ TB   ☐ Hemoptysis   ☐ Cancer
☐ Asthma   ☐ Emphysema   _____
☐ Bronchitis   ☐ Asbestos Exposure   ☐ Other
☐ Pneumonia   _____
☐ Trach   ☐ Exposure to
   ☐ Old ☐ New   Fumes/Smoke
   ☐ Closed

Dyspnea: ☑NONE ☐ Activity ☐ Walking Stairs ☐ #pillows/sleep___
Home O2: ☑NONE ☐ Activity ☐ Night ☐ Day ☐ PRN FlowRate____
GASTROINTESTINAL: ☐ **NEGATIVE HISTORY**
   ☐ Colitis   ☐ Hepatitis   ☐ Diabetes
   ☐ Ulcers   ☐ Heart Burn   ☐ Diet
   ☐ Reflux   ☐ Hiatal Hernia   ☐ Insulin
   ☐ Jaundice   ☑ Hemorrhoids   ☐ PO Meds
   ☐ Nausea   ☐ Hematemesis   ☐ Vomiting within
   ☐ Cirrhosis   ☐ Diverticulosis   last 24 - 48 hrs
   ☐ Cancer _____   ____/day
   ☐ Other: _____
Bowel Pattern:
Last BM: _9/1/09_   ☐ Daily ☐QOD ☐ Q3Day ☑Other: _Q2-3 day_
Bowel Problem: ☐ NONE ☑ Constipation ☐ Incontinence
   ☐ Diarrhea within last 24 - 48 hours _____/day
NUTRITION:
   ☑ Regular Diet   ☐ ↑ Fiber   ☐_____ Calorie ADA
   ☐ ↓ Fat   ☐ Bland   ☐ Fluid Restriction
   ☐ ↓ Chol   ☐ Gluten Free   _____cc
   ☐ ↓ Sodium   ☐ Kosher
   ☐ Other _____
Food Intolerances: ☑NONE ☐ Type: _____
Supplements: ☑NONE ☐ Type: _____
Weight Change: ☑NONE ☐ Gain ☐ Loss
Amount: _____ Time Period: _____ ☐ Intentional ☐ Unintentional*
Intake < 50% in 3 Days: ☐ YES*   ☑NO
Chewing Difficulties: ☐ YES*   ☑NO
If any * above, notify Nutrition Services.

DENTURES: ☑YES* ☐NO   *BROUGHT TO HOSPITAL: ☑ YES ☐ NO
☐ Partial ☐↑ ☐ With Pt   **FIT:** ☐ Loose ☐ Good ☐ Not Worn
         ☐↓ ☐ With Pt   **FIT:** ☐ Loose ☐ Good ☐ Not Worn
☐ Full   ☑↑ ☐ With Pt   **FIT:** ☐ Loose ☑ Good ☐ Not Worn
       ☑↓ ☐ With Pt   **FIT:** ☐ Loose ☑ Good ☐ Not Worn
If with Patient, remind patient hospital not responsible for article

---

Swallowing Difficulties: ☑ NONE ☐ Recent* ☐ Long Term
                          ☐ Solids ☐ Liquids
Coughing During Or After Meals: ☑ YES* ☐ NO
   If any * above, notify Coordinated Care.

GENITOURINARY: ☑ **NEGATIVE HISTORY**
   ☐ Renal Disease   ☐ Kidney Stones   ☐ Prostate Problems
   ☐ Cancer _____   ☐ Other: _____
PROBLEMS URINATING: ☑ NONE
   ☐ Anuria   ☐ Nocturia   ☐ Dialysis
   ☐ Hesitancy   _____/night   ☐ Peritoneal
   ☐ Dysuria   ☐ Self   ☐ Hemo
   ☐ Urgency   Catheterization   Site _____
   ☐ Incontinence   Frequency_____   Schedule_____
   ☐ Frequency   ___   ☐ Other:_____
                ☐ Hematria
   GENITALIA PROBLEMS: ☑ NONE
   ☐ Discharge   ☐ Burning   ☐ Abnormal Bleeding ☐STD
   ☐ **Other:** _____

Figure 5.6 (*Continued*)

NAZARETH HOSPITAL
NURSING ADMISSION
PHYSICAL

V S

BP 184/120 P 88 R I R 18 T 98.2 O R A T
HT 5'2" Actual Estimated WT _____ (Actual) Estimated

P A I N

Current Pain Intensity(0-10): 3
Scale Used: (Numeric Scale) Faces Scale FLACC Scale
Has Patient had pain in the last week? (Yes) No H/A
Unable to obtain information
Complete Initial Pain Assessment Form if Pain Intensity is >5 or if patient has had pain in the last week.

S K I N

Turgor: (Normal) Tenting
Color: Normal (Pale) Flushed Mottled
    Jaundiced Dusky Cyanotic
Temperature: (Cool) Warm Clammy Hot Wet
Integrity: (Normal)

Abrasion _____ Burn _____
Ecchymosis _____ Scar _____
Laceration _____ Wound _____
Rash → _____ Macule _____ Papule _____

Are Multiple Alterations in Skin Integrity or Pressure Ulcers
Present? ☐YES* ☑NO If YES*, Complete Skin Integrity Assessment

Norton Risk Assessment Scale

Circle 1 item for each area, add up total score. Range is 5 - 20. The Lower the total score the greater the risk of developing a pressure ulcer.

Physical		Mental		Activity		Mobility		Incontinent	
Good	4	(Alert)	4	(Ambulant)	4	(Full)	4	(Almost never)	4
(Fair)	3	Apathetic	3	Walk/help	3	Sl. limited	3	Occasionally	3
Poor	2	Confused	2	Chairbound	2	V. limited	2	Usually UA	2
V.Poor	1	Stupor	1	Bed	1	Immobile	1	Both UA/BM	1

Total Score: 19
If <15, implement Potential Risk For Impaired Skin Integrity Care Plan.

N E U R O M U S C U L A R

LOC: (Alert) Lethargic Unresponsive
Mental Status: Pleasant (Cooperative) (Anxious) Agitated
    (Follows Command) Depressed Confused Combative
Oriented: (Person) (Place) (Time)
Pupils: Right (/mm) Left (/mm)
Reaction: (Brisk) (Brisk)
    Sluggish Sluggish
    Non-reactive Non-reactive
Appearance: (Normal) (Normal)
    Dilated Dilated
    Constricted Constricted
    Fixed Fixed
Speech: (Clear) Slurred Garbled Stuttering
    Aphasic → Receptive Expressive
Gait: Steady (Unsteady) Shuffling Limping
    Bedbound
Extremities: (Well Developed) Hypertrophied
    Atrophied Contracted
Tone: (Normal) Rigid Flaccid Spastic
Strength: Strong (Weak) Left leg

E E N T

Eyes: Normal R: (Normal) Red Jaundiced Discharge
    L: (Normal) Red Jaundiced Discharge
Ears: Normal R: (Normal) Discharge Other: _____
    L: (Normal) Discharge Other: _____
Nose: Normal R Nare: (Normal) Discharge/Drainage
    L Nare: (Normal) Discharge/Drainage
Oral Cavity: (Normal) Bleeding Lesions Other: _____
Teeth: Normal (Missing) Dentures

C A R D I A C

Edema: None

Arm:	RU:	+1	+2	+3	+4	LU:	+1	+2	+3	+4
	RL:	+1	+2	+3	+4	LL:	+1	+2	+3	+4
Leg:	RU:	+1	+2	+3	+4	LU:	+1	+2	+3	+4
	RL:	(+1)	+2	+3	+4	LL:	(+1)	+2	+3	+4

Sacral Anasarca Other: _____
Apical Rate: 90 Regular Irregular
Radial Pulse: R: (Strong) Weak Absent Doppler
    L: (Strong) Weak Absent Doppler
Pedal Pulse: R: (Strong) Weak Absent Doppler
    L: (Strong) Weak Absent Doppler
Vascular Dialysis Access: None R L
Type: _____ Bruit: Present Absent N/A

P U L M O N A R Y

Cough: (None) Non-Productive Productive
    Clear White Green Yellow Tan
    Hemoptysis Thick Thin
Breathing Pattern: (Normal) Dyspnea Kussmaul
    Labored Periodic Apnea Cheyne-Stokes Agonal
Breath Sounds: (Clear) **Right Lung** **Left Lung**
    Absent _____ _____
    Diminished _____ _____
    Rhonchi _____ _____
    Rales/Crackles _____ _____
    Insp. Wheeze _____ _____
    Exp. Wheeze _____ _____

G A S T R O

Bowel Sounds:
    RUQ: (Normal) Increased Decreased Absent
    LUQ: (Normal) Increased Decreased Absent
    RLQ: (Normal) Increased Decreased Absent
    LLQ: Normal Increased Decreased Absent
Abdomen: (Soft) Firm Tender Non-tender
Abdominal Tubes/Ostomies: (None) Peg Gastro
    Biliary Jejunostomy Colostomy Illeostomy
    APPLIANCE:

G U

Urinary Device: ☑None ☐Catheter-TYPE _____
    LAST CHANGED _____
Urostomy - APPLIANCE _____
Nephrostomy Tube: ☑None Right Left
Flank Tenderness: ☑None Right Left
Urine Appearance: ☑Not Visualized
    Clear Cloudy Pale Straw Sediment
    Sediment Hematuria Concentrated
Genitalia Appearance: ☑Not Visualized Normal
Other: _____

Does any of the physical assessment findings reflect suspected
elder, domestic or child abuse?
☐YES* ☑NO
If YES, notify Social Worker by consult.*

RN Signature: Carol Tayn, RN
Date: 9/2/09 Time: 2:35 PM

Figure 5.6 (Continued)

	Table 5.2	**Comparing Documentation Formats**		
	Format	**Example**	**Advantages**	**Disadvantages**
Narrative	Information written in phases, usually time sequenced	4/18/08, 15:00: 98.6F, 98 beats/min, 22 breaths/min, 130/82 mmHg. Pt c/o pain 8/10; states he is using his PCA, but it doesn't help. Notified MD of pain level at 14:30. Pain is throbbing from fingers to elbow; has gotten worse over last 30 minutes. Pain increases with movement. Fingers of left hand pink, warm, able to move with strong pulse and no c/o of pain with movement. R hand cool and pale with capillary refill 6 seconds. *S. Roberts, RN*	Easy to learn Easy to adjust length Can explain in detail	Time consuming Difficult to retrieve information May include irrelevant information Possibly unfocused and disorganized
SOAP(IE)	S—subjective data O—objective data A—analysis P—plan I—intervention E—evaluation	4/18/08 15:00 S—States pain 8/10 from elbow to fingertips. Intensity increases with movement, especially over last 30 minutes. PCA does not seem to help. O—98.6F, 98 beats/min, 22 breaths/min, 130/82 mmHg. Rt radial artery 1+, limb pale and cool. Capillary refill 6 seconds. Sensation intact. Left arm pink, warm with 3+ pulse; no pain, intact sensation. A—Reduced tissue perfusion to right hand related to injury and inadequate pain control. P—Contact Dr. Cisco to evaluate patient. Saw patient at 14:30 and indicated no change from baseline; left orders for increased morphine dose. I—PCA morphine increase at 14:35, right hand elevated. E—Evaluate pain effectiveness in 30 minutes and increase CSM checks to hourly. *S. Roberts, RN*	All charting focuses on identified or new problems Interdisciplinary, so all team members chart on same progress note using same format Easy to track progress for identified problems Similar to steps in the nursing process	Specific focus, which makes charting general information difficult without identifying a problem Lengthy and time consuming Repeats assessment data on flow sheets
PIE	P—problem I—intervention E—evaluation	P—Inadequate tissue perfusion and inadequate pain control. I—Dr. Costa contacted at 14:30 to report pain 8/10 and cool, pale right hand with capillary refill of 6 seconds. He saw patient and left orders for increased PCA morphine. Right hand elevated. E—Dr. Costa reports circulation same as admission baseline. Continue hourly CMS checks; evaluate pain effectiveness after 30 minutes. *S. Roberts, RN*	Incorporates POC Includes outcomes, which increases quality assurance Less redundancy Easily adapted to computerized charting	May need to read progress note to determine POC if not on separate document Not multidisciplinary

Table 5.2 Comparing Documentation Formats (*continued*)

	Format	Example	Advantages	Disadvantages
Focus	D—data A—action R—response	D—98.6F, 98 beats/min, 22 breaths/min, 130/82 mmHg. Rt radial artery 1+, limb pale and cool. Capillary refill 6 seconds. Sensation intact. Left arm pink, warm with 3+ pulse, no pain, intact sensation. States pain 8/10 from elbow to fingertips. Intensity increases with movement; has increased especially over last 30 minutes; PCA does not seem to help. A—Dr. Costa contacted at 14:30 to report pain 8/10 and cool, pale right hand with capillary refill of 6 seconds. He saw patient and left orders for increased PCA morphine. Right hand elevated. R—Dr. Costa reports circulation is same as admission baseline. Continue hourly CMS checks and evaluate pain effectiveness after 30 minutes. *S. Roberts, RN*	Broad view, permitting charting on any significant area, not just problems Works well in ambulatory and long-term care	Not multidisciplinary May be difficult to identify chronological order May not relate to POC
Charting by exception	Standards met—sign or check off Standards unmet—write narrative or SOAP note	Abnormal assessments require a note rather than signing off. See above for different note formats.	Efficient No duplicate charting, because most assessments are charted on flow sheets Clearly outlines abnormal assessment	Expensive to develop and educate staff regarding standards Not prevention focused Not useful for ambulatory or long-term care May pose legal problems, because details are often missing

Source: Adapted from Craven, R. C., & Hirnle, C. J. (2009). *Fundamentals of nursing: Human health and function* (6th ed., p. 212). Philadelphia: Wolters Kluwer Health/Lippincott Williams & Wilkins.

Regardless of the format used, the progress note is an evaluative statement summarizing significant problems or improvements. Flow sheets record all collected assessment data, whereas progress notes allow nurses to use critical thinking to document and communicate priority issues to other health team members.

Narrative Notes

Using narrative notes, nurses record, in an unstructured paragraph, relevant assessments and nursing activities during a shift or visit. Usually, the organizing structure is time rather than an identified problem. Historically, narrative notes were very common, but most agencies are moving to more structured documentation formats. The more structured notes assist nurses to use assessment data to analyze findings, critically think about problems, and direct care at a higher level.

SOAP Notes

The SOAP format focuses on a single problem and includes subjective (**S**) assessment findings, objective (**O**) assessment findings, analysis (**A**) of the assessment data to identify a problem or indicate whether the problem is improving or worsening, and plan (**P**) for treating or improving the problem. Some agencies expand SOAP to SOAPIE. In this case, the **I** represents interventions to treat the problem and the **E** represents evaluation of the problem. This text uses examples of the documentation of abnormal findings using the SOAP note format, both in the case below and throughout.

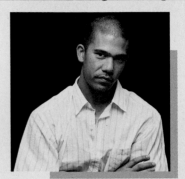

Remember Mr. Chavez, who was admitted to the hospital with a fractured right humerus. The nurse has gathered a more complete assessment, clustered findings, and contacted the physician about concerns over inadequate tissue perfusion to the patient's arm. The following nursing note illustrates how the nurse collects and analyzes subjective and objective data and begins to develop nursing interventions.

Subjective: States pain 8/10 from above elbow to fingertips. Characterized pain as numb and achy. Increased since admission, especially in the past 30 minutes. Morphine less effective now than earlier. Increased by movement.

Objective: Right radial artery 1+, limb pale and cool. Capillary refill 6 seconds. Sensation intact. Left arm pink, warm with 3+ pulse, no pain and intact sensation.

Analysis: Reduced tissue perfusion to right arm related to injury. Increasing pain.

Plan: Contacted Dr. Costa to evaluate limb. Patient seen at 19:30; provider indicated that there was no change from baseline. Patient is on call for surgery for open reduction internal fixation (ORIF) this evening. Orders written to assess circulation, sensation, and movement (CSM) every hour. Morphine PCA orders increased—see orders. Reevaluate the effectiveness of morphine in 30 minutes.

S. Cisco, RN

Critical Thinking Challenge

- How could you evaluate if this assessment is a change from previous findings?
- How should the nurse organize information before contacting the provider?
- What concepts of confidentiality should the nurse use if the patient asks about the status of his cousin or other people with injuries in the collision?
- What further assessments will be important for the nurse to perform and document? Where will the nurse document them?

PIE Notes

The PIE format includes Problem (**P**), Interventions (**I**), and Evaluation (**E**). Its goal is to incorporate the POC into the progress note. Patient assessments are not part of the PIE note but charted on flow sheets. Some agencies adapt the PIE note to an APIE note with (**A**) for Assessment, so documentation reflects pertinent assessment data to support the problem (Craven & Hirnle, 2009).

Focus Note

The focus system of documentation organizes entries by data (**D**), action (**A**), and response (**R**). Documentation can focus on areas of strengths as well as medical problems, family concerns, or nursing diagnoses. Using this chapter's case study as an example, data could include the phone conversation the nurse has with Mr. Chavez's mother who is very worried and trying to get to the hospital to see her son but has younger children who cannot be left alone and no transportation. The data portion contains subjective and objective findings that support the focus of the note. The action section presents interventions and treatments, while the response section reviews how the patient responded or met outcomes (Craven & Hirnle, 2009).

Charting by Exception

Charting by exception (CBE) uses predetermined standards and norms to record only significant assessment data. Clearly identifying the standards and norms and educating all users take time and significant commitment from the agency using CBE. For example, a group may develop the standard of what it considers "normal" in each area of assessment (eg, respiratory, mobility, psychosocial). These norms structure the patient assessment. Norms for respiratory function might include respiratory rate 12 to 18 breaths/min, lungs clear to auscultation with no adventitious breath sounds, oxygen saturation above 93% on room air, and no dyspnea with activity. This cues nurses to assess respiratory rate, auscultate the lungs for adventitious sounds, assess oxygen saturation on room air, and assess whether an activity causes shortness of breath. If the patient's assessment matches the designated norms, the nurse checks a box. Any abnormal assessment findings require additional documentation.

Discharge Note

When a patient is discharged, the nurse enters a discharge note in the chart. The note can be a computer-generated form, paper form, or narrative note in the progress notes. Assessment of the patient should indicate that he or she is stable and has received teaching regarding medications and follow-up care. The discharge note also contains patient discharge teaching, discharge medications, when to contact the provider, condition at discharge, and time of discharge. The nurse gives a copy of the discharge summary with patient teaching and discharge medication to the patient. Assessment information is used to identify necessary resources and strategies for successful home management. This information is useful for social work, physical and occupational therapies, and follow-up care by the nurse and provider when returning to the outpatient setting.

Home Care Documentation

In 2000, the federal government mandated that home care agencies use the **Outcome and Assessment Information Set** (OASIS) in the initial and ongoing assessments of all patients they care for to qualify for Medicare or Medicaid reimbursement. The OASIS tool accurately measures the patient's status at various specified points during an episode of care (Yadgood & Miller, 2005), thus providing the basis for measuring patient outcomes. OASIS data items include sociodemographic data, environmental information, support systems, health status, and functional status of all adult home care patients. Additional education of nurses is necessary because of the complexity of the OASIS system. Assessment is performed initially to reassess the effectiveness of interventions and to measure if the patient is meeting outcomes.

Long-term Care Documentation

The **Resident Assessment Instrument** (RAI) governs documentation in long-term care settings. The RAI tracks goal achievement among long-term care residents and includes (1) minimum data set, (2) triggers, (3) resident assessment protocols, and (4) utilization guidelines. The goal of RAI is to coordinate the efforts of all members of the health care team to optimize the resident's quality of care and quality of life. The care team completes the assessment and planning, with participation from social work, physical therapy, and other disciplines. The RAI is a very comprehensive assessment tool.

Written Handoff Summary

Handoff, or transfer of care for a patient from one health provider to another, significantly increases the risk of errors. Receiving staff must have up-to-date assessment data to safely care for the patient. Traditionally, nurses think of handoff occurring during shift change, but handoff also occurs when a patient is transferred from one area of the hospital to another. For example, handoff occurs when a postoperative patient moves from the postanesthesia recovery unit (PACU) to the surgical floor or back to the medical unit following dialysis or an invasive diagnostic procedure. Transfers also occur when a patient is transferred from one health care facility to another (eg, to a skilled nursing unit or a rehabilitation unit).

To minimize potential errors from lack of information, agencies often provide specific assessments on a written transfer summary in addition to a verbal report. Some agencies have created specific forms for this transfer of information, while others require documentation in the progress notes.

Verbal Communication

Verbal Handoff

A **handoff** occurs anytime one provider transfers the responsibility for the care of a patient to another. Other industries such as aviation, power plants, and the NASA Space Center have studied and standardized handoffs to prevent errors, but only recently has the health care industry started paying attention to handoffs. Effective communication at handoff is critically important to create a shared mental model around the patient's condition, which creates situational awareness (Haig, et al., 2006) and helps to minimize errors. The greater the number of handoffs and the more caregivers involved, the greater the risk for errors (Dracup & Morris, 2008).

In 2006, the Joint Commission developed a National Patient Safety Goal that required agencies to develop a standardized approach to handoff communications, including the opportunity to ask and respond to questions. Box 5-2 lists common handoff situations and strategies for effective handoff communication.

BOX 5.2 HANDOFF REPORTING

Handoff
Occurs anytime the responsibility for care of a patient transfers from one provider to another. Standardized reporting at handoffs promotes continuity of care and prevents errors.

Common Situation Handoffs
- At change of shift, when a new nurse is assigned to care for the patient
- When a nurse leaves for a meal or a break
- When a change in status requires transfer of the patient to another unit such as ICU
- When the surgical patient is transferred from the OR to the PACU or from the PACU to the surgical floor
- When the patient is admitted from the ED to a medical-surgical unit or to the ICU
- When the patient moves to or from a procedural care area for a diagnostic procedure or treatment (eg, cath lab, GI lab, dialysis unit)
- When hospitalists or medical staff members change coverage

Strategies for Effective Handoff Communication
- Use a standardize format such as SBAR for handoffs so that all important information is presented in a predictable, clear manner.
- Communicate with face-to-face verbal update of current status and historical data with interactive questioning.
- Ensure limited interruptions.
- Use "read back" policies to ensure that both parties agree and comprehend.
- Use written documentation to supplement the verbal handoff.
- Cross monitor the handoffs of others with written and verbal communication.

Source: Adapted from Clancy, C. (2006). Care transitions: A threat and opportunity for patient safety. *American Journal of Medical Quality, 21*(6), 414–417.

Reporting

To provide safe patient care, nurses continually communicate with all members of the health care team. Reporting occurs at handoffs, during patient rounds, during patient and family care conferences, and when calling or text paging a provider to report a change in status or provide requested information. Baseline assessment data or significant changes in patient status are crucial elements of most reporting.

In theory, effective communication seems like a simple task. In reality, it is very complex and often suboptimal. The Joint Commission (2007) reported 65% of sentinel events and 90% of root cause analyses conducted at a medical center in the Midwest included problems with communication as a contributing factor. Many barriers potentially contribute to problems in communication:

- Lack of structured format for communication
- Lack of standards and policies for communication
- Uncertainty about who is responsible and should be contacted
- Hierarchy of relationships
- Differences in ethnic background
- Poor clinical decision making regarding what needs to be reported
- Different communication styles of nurses and doctors (Haig, et al., 2006)

Qualities of Effective Reporting

To effectively communicate with members of the health care team, verbal communication needs to be organized, complete, accurate, concise, and respectful. An organizing framework, especially a tool such as SBAR, helps ensure complete and organized reporting. This textbook uses examples of SBAR to illustrate how nurses use and communicate assessment information in clinical settings.

Reporting, because it involves face-to-face communication, is influenced by nonverbal communication as well as the actual spoken words. It is important for nurses to maintain eye contact and to give their undivided attention during

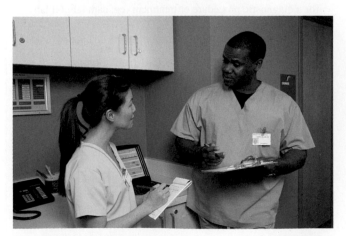

Figure 5.7 During reporting, the nurse should maintain attention, eye contact, and other positive nonverbal indicators.

any reporting situation (Fig. 5-7). Negative nonverbal cues such as lack of respect, inattention, or irritation might negatively affect the quality or completeness of the report. Differences in communication style also influence reporting. Nurses are often instructed to be very descriptive and detailed in their communication, whereas physicians tend to be more concise and to focus on objective facts (Haig, et al., 2006). Providers may become impatient and inattentive with nurses who provide a rambling report. If a nurse, especially a student or a new graduate, experiences a hostile or disrespectful response when giving a report, he or she might hesitate or delay reporting significant information in the future.

SBAR

SBAR, first developed by Kaiser Permanente in Denver and supported by the Institute for Healthcare Improvement (IHI), is a shared mental model for improving communication between and among clinicians. This model organizes communication around Situation, Background, Assessment, and Recommendations. Note that situation, background, and assessment are all based on the collection of complete and accurate assessment data. The last piece, recommendations, encompasses the nurse's suggestions for the next interventions.

- **S**ituation: State concisely why you are communicating.
- **B**ackground: Describe the circumstances leading up to the current situation.
- **A**ssessment: Give objective and subjective data pertinent to the situation.
- **R**ecommendation: Make suggestions for what needs to be done to manage the problem.

Nurses most commonly use this model when contacting a provider regarding a patient issue. SBAR also can serve as a method for structuring communication during handoffs, when delegating care to nursing assistants, or when expressing concern regarding a patient's condition to the charge nurse or manager. Historically, nurses have always attempted to provide concise, organized verbal communication. The SBAR tool, however, gives a standardized format and provides clear articulation of what is desired. Refer to the example in the case study below and in other cases throughout this text.

Reporting to the Primary Health Care Provider

Reporting to the primary care provider can occur face to face, by telephone, by text messaging, or, in some settings (eg, long-term or home care), by fax. First, the nurse needs to identify the appropriate provider to notify by checking the chart to ascertain the primary provider, surgeon, or resident responsible for managing care. This becomes more complex in a teaching center, where multiple providers are involved in care, or during nights or weekends when cross coverage occurs. In these situations, a call schedule helps to determine the appropriate person to contact. Valuable time can be lost if the process and schedule are unclear. Nurses should use an organized

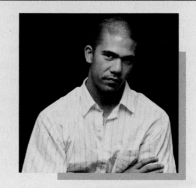

At the change of shift, nurses need to organize information to provide a report on the patient. In this case, Mr. Chavez is still awaiting surgery, so staff members on the evening shift need to report to staff members on the night shift. After a brief introduction, the nurse reviews systems briefly. The nurse should organize pertinent items, including changes, so that the report is efficient and complete. The following report illustrates how the nurse might organize the data and make recommendations about Mr. Chavez.

Situation: I've been taking care of Mr. Chavez for the past 8 hours.

Background: He was admitted with his cousin about 12 hours ago following a MVC. His cousin is in Room 222 with a fractured tibia and fibula. Mr. Chavez fractured his right humerus and is waiting an ORIF tonight.

Assessment: *Neuro:* He is drowsy from the pain medication but oriented. *CV:* His pulse is high at 122, R 20, BP 138/78. I think the BP is elevated because he's in pain. *Pulmonary:* His lungs are clear and oxygen saturation is 96%. *GI/GU:* Abdomen is soft with normal bowel tones. He's voiding in the urinal clear yellow urine, no stool. CSM is normal in both feet and left arm. However, his pulse is 1+ in his right hand, and it's cool and pale. His cap refill is also long at 6 seconds. I contacted the provider, who came and looked at the arm and said that there's no change, just to keep an eye on it. He's on hourly CSM checks now and there hasn't been a change. We also increased his dose of morphine, because he was at an 8/10 but now is down to a 3, which is within his goal. The IV is infusing well with D5NS at 125/hr. It's a new IV from the ER, and I just changed the bag, so you have 1,000 mL hanging. *Psych/soc:* He doesn't have any family in the area and hasn't asked about his cousin yet.

Recommendations: He's been using the PCA more frequently, so encourage him to do that before his pain gets too bad. We're basically just waiting for him to go to the OR to get the repair. He's on call and I think that he's next in line. He's NPO (nothing by mouth) for surgery and his consent has been signed. Everything's in the chart and ready to go. His antibiotic is in the med room. Do you have any questions?

Critical Thinking Challenge

- What is the difference between what the nurse documents in the chart and shares in the report?
- What parts of the nursing process does the report include?
- How does the evening nurse use abbreviations to communicate and document data?
- What is the nurse's role in documenting the patient's immigration and insurance status in preparation for the surgery?

framework such as SBAR to ensure that communications are clear and concise. Beginners learning this skill will be more organized and accurate if they write a draft of what they want to say before contacting the provider.

Telephone Communication

If a significant issue or problem occurs, the nurse may need to phone the primary provider to report this information. The nurse may call the provider's office or page the provider to call back. When talking to a provider over the phone, it is important to have the patient's record and important information available for reference. It is important to document the call, including the time, who was called, what information the nurse gave to the provider, and what information the nurse received. Most agencies now limit the use of telephone orders. For agencies that have CPOE, remote computer access allows providers to enter orders when they are off-site. If a nurse is taking a telephone order, it is important to write the order and then read it back to the provider to make sure it is correct. Students do not take telephone orders—only licensed nurses can do so.

Nurses also communicate via the telephone with other departments to provide or to obtain information. When patients are transferring from one setting to another (eg, from ED or PACU), the nurse may give the handoff report by phone. Nurses often receive laboratory data, especially critical values, by telephone. For any critical values, all health personnel must read back values obtained over the telephone to ensure accuracy and avoid errors.

Patient Rounds and Conferences

Interdisciplinary rounds allow members of different disciplines to share assessment data in an effort to individualize and improve coordination of patient care. When rounds occur at the bedside and include the patient in the dialogue, the nurse facilitates active participation to set goals and plan care. During rounds, nurses present assessment data on nursing issues such as mobility, fluid balance, pain management, and emotional or family issues. Nurses can also help patients articulate questions or concerns. Shift handoffs are increasingly happening in the room with the patient to help communicate and plan the day (Fig. 5-8).

When working with patients with complex problems (eg, end-of-life care), a nurse may request or help facilitate a family care conference. Family members and all members of the health care team meet to discuss how best to provide and coordinate care in challenging situations. Nurses need to plan these conferences in advance to coordinate schedules and to ensure that interpreters are present as needed.

Critical Thinking and Clinical Judgment

Nurses use critical thinking and clinical judgment to determine what assessment data to include in a verbal report, how quickly to report the assessment, the proper team member to receive the information, and what method of reporting (eg, face to face, telephone, text message) is most appropriate. Some reporting is scheduled at specific times, for example, shift change handoff. In other situations, the nurse decides whether an assessment finding or a change in the patient's status requires immediate or routine notification of the provider.

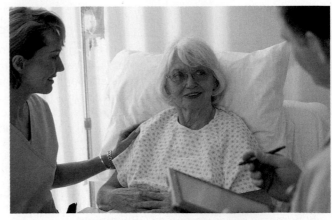

Figure 5.8 During a shift handoff in the patient's room, health care providers can communicate with each other and directly with the patient to plan the day effectively and to ensure that the patient can participate as much as he or she is able.

For example, if a stable patient tells the night nurse that he has not had a bowel movement in 2 days, the nurse waits until the primary provider rounds in the morning to report this and get an order for a laxative. Conversely, if a patient's BP is low and she is NPO for surgery, the nurse contacts the provider for an IV order to prevent severe dehydration. Refer to the Case Challenge toward the end of this chapter for an example of how this is prioritized. If the situation is acute and potentially life threatening, the nurse may activate and report to a Rapid Response Team. In this way, the nurse uses assessment information to take the next steps. Assessment information is never viewed in isolation from other parts of the nursing process.

Applying Your Knowledge

C onsider Mr. Chavez's case and its relationship to what you are learning. Answer the following questions based on his initial injury, impaired tissue perfusion, pain, and the other changes that have occurred during the hours since admission.

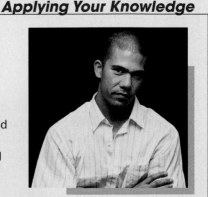

- What are the differences in the assessment data that nurses collect and document on the admitting assessment, flow sheets, SOAP notes, preoperative checklists, and postoperative assessments?
- How does the collection of data fluctuate between a comprehensive and a focused assessment?
- How do the patient situation and acuity influence the assessment, documentation, and communication of data?

Key Points

- In addition to being a legal document, the patient record serves many purposes, namely, communication, care planning, quality assurance, financial reimbursement, education, and research.
- The computerized patient record helps ensure patient safety and enhances communication, because computerized documentation is legible and time dated, increases compliance, permits multiple simultaneous users, and permits surveillance of patient data to identify patients at risk.
- Critical thinking and clinical judgment are important in appropriately communicating and documenting assessment data to keep patients safe.
- Documentation should be accurate, objective, organized, concise, complete, and legible.
- Health care professionals must ensure confidentiality, governed by HIPAA, for all patient information, including what they document in the written or computerized record.
- Nurses can document assessment data in various forms (eg, nursing admission assessment, flow sheets, progress notes, transfer or discharge summaries) in the patient's record. Nurses working in home care and long-term care should follow the specific regulations governing documentation in those settings.
- Formats for nursing progress notes include narrative, SOAP, PIE, DAR, and CBE.
- Handoffs occur when one provider transfers the responsibility for patient care to another provider.
- SBAR (situation, background, assessment, and recommendation) is a mental model for organizing communication.
- Verbal communication of patient status occurs at handoff, over the telephone, via text message, or during rounds.
- Accurate and effective verbal communication and documentation are important to keeping patients safe.

Review Questions

1. Which of the following are advantages of the electronic medical record? Select all that apply.
   A. Nurses can enter data by checking boxes and adding free full text.
   B. It is economical and easy to learn and implement.
   C. It allows primary providers to directly order into the computer.
   D. It cannot be used as a legal document in case of a lawsuit.

2. Which of the following are high-risk assessments for liability? Select all that apply.
   A. Failure to document completely
   B. Inadequate admission assessment
   C. Charting in advance
   D. Bunch charting at the end of shift

3. Which of the following is the purpose of auditing charting?
   A. To enhance nurses' learning and understanding of complex clinical situations
   B. To identify staff members who document completely and counsel those who do not
   C. To determine if staff members are providing and documenting standards of care
   D. To locate data in the chart the evening before a morning clinical

4. Which of the following are acceptable under the HIPAA Privacy Rule? Select all that apply.
   A. Communicate report with the next nurse during change of shift.
   B. Communicate with the primary provider about a patient's change in assessment.
   C. Consult in the hall with the instructor about the patient's abnormal findings.
   D. Describe patient assessment findings to a colleague in the cafeteria.

5. Which of the following is the proper technique for correcting written documentation?
   A. Use whiteout and write over the error.
   B. Completely black out the error with a black marker.
   C. Write over the error in darker ink.
   D. Draw a single line through the error and initial.

6. What do the different formats of progress notes have in common?
   A. All use the nursing process in some form to show nursing thinking.
   B. All identify the patient outcomes or goals to evaluate.
   C. All include head-to-toe assessment data for completeness.
   D. All have a section for evaluation of care so that nurses may revise interventions.

7. What are some strategies for effective handoffs during change-of-shift report?
   A. Tape record the report for efficiency.
   B. Vary the format to individualize to the patient.
   C. Allow an opportunity to ask and answer questions.
   D. Put report in writing so that the next shift provider can get right to work.

8. In the SBAR reporting format, which of the following would be an example of data found in the assessment?
   A. Mrs. Kelly's diagnosis is Stage II breast cancer.
   B. Mr. Imami's lungs sounds are decreased.
   C. Ms. Choi needs to have a social work consult.
   D. Mr. Jones was admitted at 10:30 this morning.

9. Nursing assessment of trends in an unconscious patient's neurological status over time is best recorded on
A. an admission assessment
B. a POC
C. a progress note
D. a focused assessment flow sheet

10. Your patient with a humerus fracture is stating pain of 15 on a 10-point scale. His hand is pale, cool, and swollen. His pain medication is ineffective, and he is at risk for compartment syndrome. What action will the nurse take first?
A. Reassess the pain in 30 minutes and contact the provider if unresolved.
B. Give additional pain medication and reassess the pain in 30 minutes.
C. Document the abnormal findings and give an extra dose of pain medication now.
D. Contact the primary provider and document the findings now.

References

Craven, R. C., & Hirnle, C. J. (2009). *Fundamentals of nursing: Human health and function* (6th ed.). Philadelphia: Lippincott Williams & Wilkins.

Dracup, K., & Morris, P. (2008). Passing the torch: The challenge of handoffs. *American Journal of Critical Care, 17*(2), 95–97.

Haig, K., Sutton, S., & Whittington, J. (2006). SBAR: A shared mental model for improving communication between clinicians. *Joint Commission Journal on Quality and Patient Safety, 32*(3), 167–175.

The Health Insurance Portability and Accountability Act of 1996, Public Law, 104–191. Retrieved October 2, 2009, from http:www.hhs.gov/ocr/hippa

Joint Commission. (2007). *Front line of defense: The role of nurses in preventing sentinel events* (2nd ed.). Oakbrook Terrace IL: Joint Commission Resources.

Moody, L., Slocumb, E., Berg, B., & Jackson, D. (2004). Electronic health records documentation in nursing: Nurses' perceptions, attitudes, and preferences. *Computers Informatic Nursing, 22*(6), 337–344.

O'Neill, A., & Miranda, D. (2006). The right tools can help critical care nurses save more lives. *Critical Care Nursing Quarterly, 29*(4), 275–281.

Whittington, J., White, R., Haig, K., & Slock, M. (2007). Using an automated risk assessment report to identify patients at risk for clinical deterioration. *Joint Commission Journal on Quality and Patient Safety, 33*(9), 569.

Yadgood, M. C., & Miller, P. J. (2005). Solving the mystery: The role of competency assessment in OASIS documentation. *Home Healthcare Nurse, 23*(4), 224–232.

The Jensen suite offers these additional resources to enhance learning and facilitate understanding of this chapter:

- thePoint online resource, http//thepoint.lww.com/Jensen1E
- Student CD-ROM included with the book
- *Laboratory Manual for Nursing Health Assessment: A Best-Practice Approach*
- *Pocket Guide for Nursing Health Assessment: A Best-Practice Approach*

2

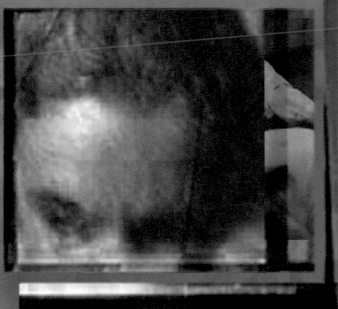

General Examinations

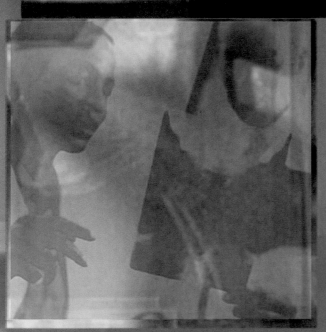

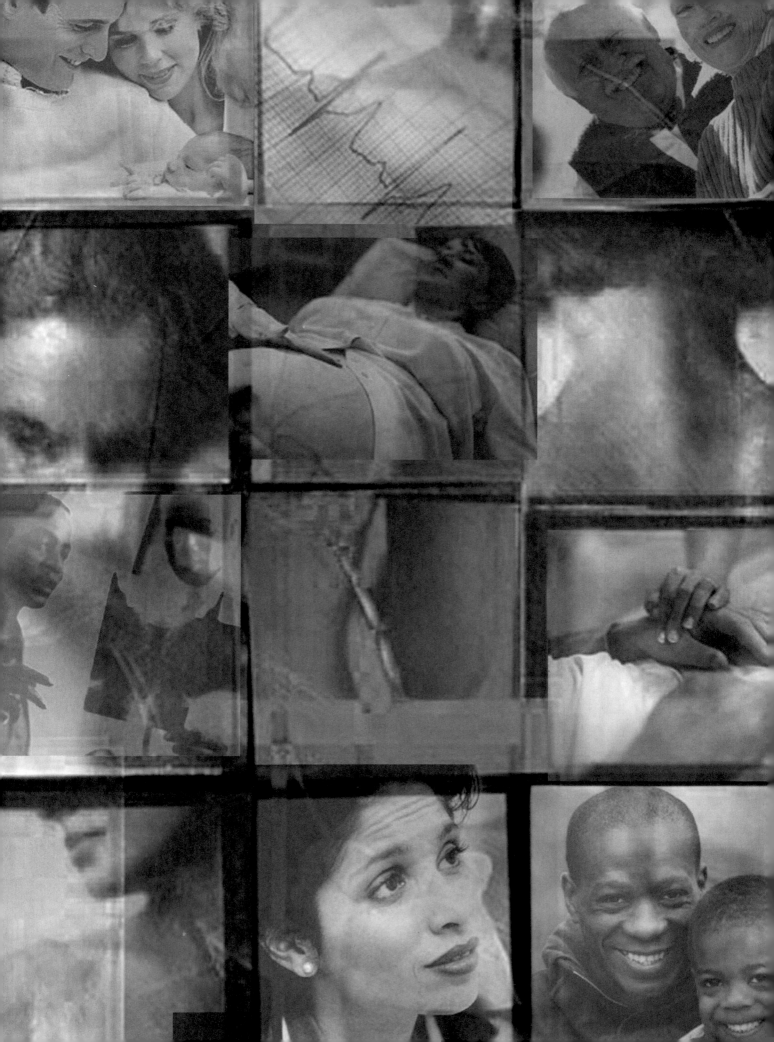

General Survey and Vital Signs Assessment

Learning Objectives

1 Describe the components and importance of the general survey to the comprehensive physical examination.

2 Identify indications for taking vital signs.

3 Use critical thinking to accurately assess vital signs.

4 Describe factors that cause variations in body temperature, heart rate, and respiratory rate.

5 Describe factors that influence blood pressure and its measurement.

6 Identify risk factors for hypertension.

7 Describe nursing responsibilities in assessing vital signs.

8 Incorporate vital signs into the patient's plan of care.

9 Accurately record and report vital sign measurements.

10 Identify age-related variations in vital signs.

11 Identify cultural variations in vital signs.

*M*r. Sanders is a 55-year-old Caucasian man who was admitted to the intensive care unit (ICU) following an episode of rapid heart rate and dizziness. He was monitored in the ICU for 2 days because he had atrial fibrillation (a cardiac dysrhythmia that causes a fast and irregular heartbeat). He was placed on medication to decrease his heart rate; he also is taking an antihypertensive drug for high blood pressure.He was transferred in stable condition yesterday to the acute care medical unit.

You will gain more information about Mr. Sanders as you progress through this chapter. As you study the content and features, consider Mr. Sanders's case and its relationship to what you are learning. Begin thinking about the following points:

- Is Mr. Sanders's condition stable, urgent, or an emergency?
- What immediate health-promotion and teaching needs are evident?
- What are the relationships among the patient's pulse, respirations, and blood pressure?
- How will a comprehensive general survey and vital signs differ from a focused assessment for this patient?

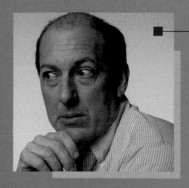

This chapter explores the assessment techniques required to perform the general survey and take vital signs. The general survey begins during the interview phase of health assessment (see Chapter 2). While collecting subjective data, nurses observe patients, develop initial impressions, and formulate plans for collecting objective data from the physical examination. An accurate and thorough physical examination requires keen observational skills. During the physical assessment, nurses use the senses of vision, hearing, touch, and smell.

Vital signs, encompassing temperature, pulse, respirations, and blood pressure (BP) are important indicators of the patient's physiological status and response to the environment. The fifth vital sign, pain, is covered in Chapter 7. Nurses assess vital signs frequently and use findings as guidance for further physical assessment. Thus, being able to differentiate normal from abnormal results is crucial.

Acute Assessment

Indicators of an acute situation include extreme anxiety, acute distress, pallor, cyanosis, and a change in mental status. In cases of such acute or urgent findings, the nurse begins interventions while continuing the assessment. He or she will obtain vital signs including pulse, BP, and oxygen saturation and request help as needed. The nurse may call a rapid response team if he or she has an intuitive sense that something is going wrong with the patient or if the patient displays

- An acute change in mental status
- Stridor
- Respirations less than 10 breaths/min or greater than 32 breaths/min
- Increased effort to breathe
- Oxygen saturation less than 92%
- Pulse less than 55 beats/min (bpm) or greater than 120 bpm
- Systolic BP less than 100 or greater than 170
- Temperature less than 35°C or greater than 39.5°C
- New onset of chest pain
- Agitation or restlessness

Experienced nurses will assist beginners in determining the level of response needed.

Objective Data Collection

Equipment

- Scale
- Height bar
- Stethoscope
- Thermometer
- Watch with second hand
- Sphygmomanometer
- Pulse oximeter
- Tape measure (for infants)

Preparation

Make sure the room is warm, comfortable, and relaxing. Ensure a quiet, well-lit setting that provides privacy. Wash your hands, preferably in the presence of the patient, and cleanse the stethoscope with alcohol to prevent the transmission of bacteria. Have all necessary equipment in reach of the examination area.

Begin the general survey immediately upon meeting the patient and continue it throughout the assessment. Ask the patient to remove shoes and heavy outer garments before taking height and weight. Prior to assessment of vital signs, the patient should rest quietly for 5 minutes. Establish that the patient has not had anything to eat or drink and has not smoked for at least 30 minutes. The patient must remove constricting clothing to above the upper arm to provide access to the brachial artery for measurement of BP. The patient may be sitting or supine for vital signs.

Common and Specialty or Advanced Techniques

The routine screening or registered nurse assessment includes the most important and common techniques. The nurse may add focused or advanced techniques if concerns exist over a specific finding, such as an irregular pulse. Table 6-1 summarizes the differences in techniques used in the screening and focused assessments.

Table 6.1	Common Versus Specialty/Advanced Techniques in General Survey and Vital Signs		
Technique	**Purpose**	**Screening or Registered Nurse Assessment**	**Focused or Advanced Practice Examination**
Assess physical appearance, behavior, and mobility.	Obtain an overall impression.	X	
Obtain height and weight.	Establish baseline.	X	
Obtain temperature, pulse, respirations, and BP.	Screen for abnormal findings.	X	
Evaluate pulse deficit.	Gather information on peripheral perfusion.		X
Obtain oxygen saturation.	Screen for low saturation in hospitalized and respiratory patients.	X	
Assess for orthostatic hypotension.	Identify volume deficit, impaired venous return, and risk for falling.		X

General Survey

The **general survey** begins with the first moment of the encounter with the patient and continues throughout the health history, during the physical examination, and with each subsequent interaction. It is the first component of the assessment, when you make mental notes of overall behavior, physical appearance, and mobility. It helps to form a global impression of the person. Physical appearance and mental status provide valuable clues to overall health. Assessment of these areas requires you to use your senses and observational skills to look, listen, and note any abnormal findings, sounds, or odors.

When you introduce yourself, shake hands with the patient as appropriate to the situation. A handshake not only portrays caring but also allows you to assess the patient. Note if the patient makes eye contact, smiles, and speaks clearly. Some general things to note when first meeting the patient are as follows:

- What is your first impression of the patient? Are there any outstanding features?
- State the patient's name. Does the patient respond immediately?
- Is the patient's hand moist? Did the patient extend the arm completely? Assess the temperature and texture of the skin on the hand. Note muscle strength. Assess for edema, clubbing, malformations, or enlarged joints.
- Observe the patient interacting with others. Can he or she participate in conversation? Does the patient look healthy or ill?

As you proceed through the assessment, note the patient's physical appearance, body structure, mobility, and behavior. Because these characteristics are general overall indicators of health, consider how the data fit together with other systems. Think about what other data you will want to collect to identify patterns. Begin the data collection as soon as you enter the room and continue until you leave.

Technique and Normal Findings	Abnormal Findings
Physical Appearance **Overall Appearance.** Does the patient appear the stated age? Is appearance consistent with chronological age? Are the face and body symmetrical? Are any deformities obvious? Does the patient look well, unhealthy, or in distress? *The patient appears stated age. Facial features, movements, and body are symmetrical.*	Deficiencies in growth hormones may cause patients to appear younger than they are. Severe illness, chronic disease, prolonged sun exposure, and various genetic syndromes may contribute to a premature aging. Facial asymmetry may indicate Bell's palsy or cerebral vascular ischemia. Obvious deformities may indicate fractures or displacements.
Hygiene and Dress. Note hygiene by observing clothing, hair, nails, and skin. What is the patient wearing? Is it appropriate for age, gender, culture, and weather? Is clothing clean and neat or disheveled? Does it fit? Are any breath or body odors noted? Look for the odor of alcohol or urine. Is the patient's skin clean and dry? Are nails and hair well kept, neat, and clean? *Dress is appropriate for age, gender, culture, and weather. The patient is clean and well kempt. No odors are noted.*	Poorly fitting clothes may indicate weight loss or gain. Bad breath can result from poor hygiene, *allergic rhinitis*, or infection (*tonsillitis, sinusitis*). Sweet-smelling breath may indicate *diabetic ketoacidosis*. Body odor may be from poor hygiene or increased sweat-gland activity, which accompanies some hormonal disorders. Previously well-groomed patients who are now disheveled may have *depression*. Eccentric makeup or dress may indicate *mania*. Worn or disheveled clothes may indicate inadequate finances or knowledge.
Skin Color. Observe for even skin tones and symmetry. Note any areas of increased redness, pallor, cyanosis, or jaundice. Observe for any lesions or variations in pigmentation. Note the amount, texture, quality, and distribution of hair. *Skin color is even-toned, with pigmentation appropriate for genetic background and no obvious lesions or variations in color. Hair is smooth, thick, and evenly distributed.*	Pallor, erythema, cyanosis, jaundice, and lesions can indicate disease states (see Chapter 13).
Body Structure and Development. Is the patient's physical and sexual development consistent with expected findings for stated age? Is the patient obese or lean? Is the height appropriate for age and ethnicity? Are body parts symmetrical? Is the patient barrel-chested? Note the fingertips. Are there any joint abnormalities? *Physical and sexual development is appropriate for age, culture, and gender. No joint abnormalities are noted.*	Delayed puberty may indicate a deficiency of growth hormones. Altered growth hormones may lead to markedly short or tall stature. Disproportionate height and weight, obesity, or emaciation can indicate *eating disorders* or hormonal dysfunction.
Behavior Note the patient's behavior. Is he or she cooperative or uncooperative? Is affect animated or flat? Does the patient appear anxious? *The patient is cooperative and interacts pleasantly.*	Uncooperative behavior, flat affect, or unusual elation may indicate a psychiatric disorder (see Chapter 10). Note that mild anxiety is common in people seeking health care.

(text continues on page 94)

Facial Expressions. Assess the face for symmetry. Note expressions while the patient is at rest and during speech and whether they seem appropriate. Are movements symmetrical? Does the patient maintain eye contact appropriate to culture? *Facial expression is relaxed, symmetrical, and appropriate for the setting and circumstances. The patient maintains eye contact appropriate for age and culture.*

Level of Consciousness. Continually assess the patient's mental status throughout all encounters, but pay particular attention to it when gathering the health history. Can the patient state his or her name and location, and the date, month, season, and time of day? Is the patient awake, alert, and oriented to person, place, and time? Note any confusion, agitation, lethargy, or inattentiveness. Is there a change in mental status? If the patient appears confused, ask him or her to respond to the following:

• Tell me your full name.
• Where are you now?
• What is today's date?
• What time of the day is it?

The patient is awake, alert, and oriented to person, place, and time (abbreviated A&O × 3). He or she attends and responds to questions appropriately.

Speech. Listen to the speech pattern. Is the patient speaking very rapidly or very slowly? Is speech clear and articulate? Does the patient use words appropriately? Vocabulary and sentence structure may offer clues to educational level. Also, assess for fluency in language and the need for an interpreter. *The patient responds to questions quickly and easily. Volume, pitch, and rate are appropriate to the situation. Speech is clear and articulate, flowing smoothly. Word choice is appropriate.*

Mobility

Posture. Note how the patient sits and stands. Is the patient sitting upright? When standing, is the body straight and aligned? *Posture is upright while sitting, with the limbs and trunk proportional to the body height. The patient stands erect with no signs of discomfort and the arms relaxed at the sides.*

Range of Motion. Can the patient move all the limbs equally? Are there limitations? *The patient moves freely in the environment.*

Gait. If the patient is ambulatory, observe his or her movement around the room. Note if movements are coordinated. Normally, a person ambulates with arms swinging freely at the sides. Note any tremors or involuntary movements, as well as any body parts that do not move. Does the patient use assistive devices? *Gait is steady and balanced, with even heel-to-toe foot placement and smooth movements. Other movements are also smooth, purposeful, effortless, and symmetrical.*

Inappropriate affect, inattentiveness, impaired memory, and inability to perform activities of daily living (ADLs) may indicate *dementia* (eg, Alzheimer's disease) or another cognitive disorder. A flat or mask-like expression may indicate *Parkinson's disease* or *depression.* Drooping of one side of the face may indicate *transient ischemic attack* or *cerebral vascular accident.* Exophthalmos (protruding eyes) may indicate *hyperthyroidism.*

Confusion, agitation, drowsiness, or lethargy may indicate hypoxia, decreased cerebral perfusion, or a psychiatric disorder. Refer to Chapters 10 and 24.

⚠ *SAFETY ALERT 6-1*
Change in level of consciousness often is the first indication of hypoxia.

Slow, slurred speech can indicate *alcohol intoxication* or *cerebral vascular ischemia.* Rapid speech may indicate *hyperthyroidism, anxiety,* or *mania.* Difficulty finding words or using words inappropriately may indicate *cerebral vascular ischemia* or a psychiatric disorder. Loud speech may indicate hearing difficulties.

Slumped or hunched posture may indicate *depression,* fatigue, pain, or *osteoporosis.* Long limbs may indicate *Marfan's syndrome.* A tripod position when sitting can indicate respiratory disease (see Chapter 18). If the patient is in bed, note the position of the head of the bed or if the patient is lying on the left or right side.

Asymmetrical motion occurs in *stroke;* paralysis may accompany spinal cord injury. Limited range of motion might be present with injuries or degenerative disease.

Tics, paralysis, ataxia, tremors, or uncontrolled movements may indicate neurological disease. Patients with Parkinson's disease may display a shuffling gait. Arthritis may result in a slow, unsteady gait. For patients in bed, note their ability to move and reposition themselves in bed, turn side to side, and sit up. Further evaluate any abnormalities when assessing the neurological and musculoskeletal systems during the comprehensive physical examination (see Chapters 23 and 24).

Anthropometric Measurements

Anthropometric measurements are the various measurements of the human body, including height and weight. Accurate measurements provide critical information about the adult's state of health and the child's growth pattern. They are important parameters for evaluating nutritional status, assessing fluid gain or loss, and calculating medication dosages.

Specific measurements can be compared against standardized charts. The first time a nurse meets a patient, he or she records height and weight as a baseline measurement.

Afterward, the nurse takes measurements at regular intervals, depending on the patient's state of health and agency policy. A series of measurements provide more information than any single measurement. Taking baseline height and weight provides a reference point for weight changes and for assessing body mass index (BMI). The BMI is considered a more reliable indicator of healthy weight than weight measurement alone (see Chapter 8). To obtain accurate height and weight, ask the patient to remove his or her shoes and heavy articles of clothing (eg, winter coat).

Technique and Normal Findings	Abnormal Findings
Height Measure patients older than 2 years, with them standing. Ask the patient to place the heels up against a height bar. Feet should be together, with knees straight and the patient looking forward. Lower the horizontal bar until it touches the top of the patient's head. Read and record the measurement on the height bar (Fig. 6-1). 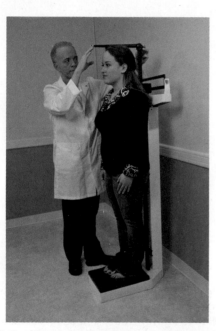 **Figure 6.1** Measuring height in an adult. Sometimes, patients cannot stand up straight for the measurement of height. In such cases, estimate the height by measuring "wingspan." Have the patient hold both arms straight from the sides of the body. Measure from the tip of one middle finger to the tip of the other middle finger. This distance is approximately the same as the patient's height. **Weight** Primary care facilities may use a calibrated balance-beam scale for obtaining weights. Prior to weighing a patient, the nurse must balance the scale by sliding both weight bars to zero. The balancing arm should balance in the center of the gauge. Follow the manufacturer's instructions to balance if needed. Lock the scale if it is	*Chronic malnutrition* may result in decreased height from lack of nutrients for proper growth. Decreased height also may result from *osteoporosis*. Hormonal abnormalities may cause excessive growth, as seen in *gigantism* and *acromegaly*. Deficiency in growth hormone may be seen in *dwarfism*. See Table 6-11 at the end of the chapter. The patient with muscle weakness, *scoliosis*, or neurological disorders may not be able to stand. Excessive unexplained weight loss may result from nutritional deficiencies, decreased intake, decreased absorption, increased metabolic needs, or a combination. Other causes may be endocrine, neoplastic, gastrointestinal, psychiatric, infectious, or neurological. Chronic disease also may contribute to weight loss. Excessive weight

(text continues on page 96)

on wheels. Have the patient stand on the scale. Slide the lower weight bar to the right until the arm drops to the bottom of the gauge (Fig. 6-2).

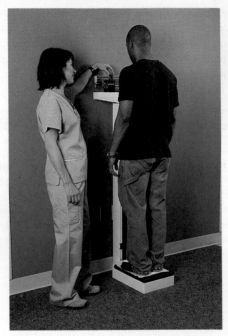

Figure 6.2 Measuring weight in an adult.

Slide the weight bar one notch back. Move the upper weight bar to the right until the arrow is balanced in the center of the gauge. The patient's weight is the total of these two readings. Record the weight. Many facilities use an electronic scale to weigh patients; hospitals may use a scale built into the bed. These scales must be calibrated, or "zeroed," prior to use.

To obtain the most accurate readings when a series of weights are required, weigh the patient at the same time of the day in similar clothing each time.

Calculate BMI by dividing the weight in kilograms by the height in meters squared (or the weight in pounds divided by the height in inches squared and then multiplied by 703). See Table 6.2 for correlations of heights, weights, and BMIs.

gain results when a person consumes more calories than his or her body requires. Overweight may result from endocrine disorders, genetics, or emotional factors such as stress, *anxiety, depression*, or guilt. Drug therapy, especially steroids, may contribute to weight gain. See Table 6-11 at the end of this chapter.

Underweight is BMI < 18.5 kg/m²; overweight is BMI of 25–29.9 kg/m²; obesity is BMI > 30 kg/m²; extreme obesity is BMI > 40 kg/m². *Obesity* poses risks for disease (National Heart Lung and Blood Institute, 2009). See Chapter 8 for more information.

 Vital Signs

Temperature, pulse, respirations, and BP make up the vital signs. Pain, considered the fifth vital sign, is covered in Chapter 7. Oxygen saturation is also collected in hospitalized patients. Nurses must interpret the significance of vital signs within the context of other data from the patient assessment.

Vital signs reflect health status, cardiopulmonary function, and overall body function. They are called vital signs because of their importance as indicators of physiological state and response to physical, environmental, and psychological stressors. Changes in vital signs often indicate changes in health. Assessment of vital signs helps nurses to establish a baseline,

monitor a patient's condition, evaluate responses to treatment, identify problems, and monitor risks for alterations in health.

Assessment of vital signs assists with the process of physical examination. Findings aid in determining specific body systems that need more thorough investigation. For example, if respiratory rate or rhythm is abnormal, the nurse auscultates the patient's lung sounds.

Prior to assessing vital signs, it is important to assess any medications the patient is currently taking. Be aware of the side effects of all medications administered, because many medications alter vital signs. If a medication alters the patient's vital signs, the nurse assesses the effects and provides appropriate teaching to the patient.

Table 6.2   Body Mass Index Table

Height (inches)	Normal						Overweight					Obese										Extreme Obesity										
BMI	19	20	21	22	23	24	25	26	27	28	29	30	31	32	33	34	35	36	37	38	39	40	41	42	43	44	45	46	47	48	49
												Body Weight (pounds)																				
58	91	96	100	105	110	115	119	124	129	134	138	143	148	153	158	162	167	172	177	181	186	191	196	201	205	210	215	220	224	229	234
59	94	99	104	109	114	119	124	128	133	138	143	148	153	158	163	168	173	178	183	188	193	198	203	208	212	217	222	227	232	237	242
60	97	102	107	112	118	123	128	133	138	143	148	153	158	163	168	174	179	184	189	194	199	204	209	215	220	225	230	235	240	245	250
61	100	106	111	116	122	127	132	137	143	148	153	158	164	169	174	180	185	190	195	201	206	211	217	222	227	232	238	243	248	254	259
62	104	109	115	120	126	131	136	142	147	153	158	164	169	175	180	186	191	196	202	207	213	218	224	229	235	240	246	251	256	262	267
63	107	113	118	124	130	135	141	146	152	158	163	169	175	180	186	191	197	203	208	214	220	225	231	237	242	248	254	259	265	270	278
64	110	116	122	128	134	140	145	151	157	163	169	174	180	186	192	197	204	209	215	221	227	232	238	244	250	256	262	267	273	279	285
65	114	120	126	132	138	144	150	156	162	168	174	180	186	192	198	204	210	216	222	228	234	240	246	252	258	264	270	276	282	288	294
66	118	124	130	136	142	148	155	161	167	173	179	186	192	198	204	210	216	223	229	235	241	247	253	260	266	272	278	284	291	297	303
67	121	127	134	140	146	153	159	166	172	178	185	191	198	204	211	217	223	230	236	242	249	255	261	268	274	280	287	293	299	306	312
68	125	131	138	144	151	158	164	171	177	184	190	197	203	210	216	223	230	236	243	249	256	262	269	276	282	289	295	302	308	315	322
69	128	135	142	149	155	162	169	176	182	189	196	203	209	216	223	230	236	243	250	257	263	270	277	284	291	297	304	311	318	324	331
70	132	139	146	153	160	167	174	181	188	195	202	209	216	222	229	236	243	250	257	264	271	278	285	292	299	306	313	320	327	334	341
71	136	143	150	157	165	172	179	186	193	200	208	215	222	229	236	243	250	257	265	272	279	286	293	301	308	315	322	329	338	343	351
72	140	147	154	162	169	177	184	191	199	206	213	221	228	235	242	250	258	265	272	279	287	294	302	309	316	324	331	338	346	353	361
73	144	151	159	166	174	182	189	197	204	212	219	227	235	242	250	257	265	272	280	288	295	302	310	318	325	333	340	348	355	363	371
74	148	155	163	171	179	186	194	202	210	218	225	233	241	249	256	264	272	280	287	295	303	311	319	326	334	342	350	358	365	373	381
75	152	160	168	176	184	192	200	208	216	224	232	240	248	256	264	272	279	287	295	303	311	319	327	335	343	351	359	367	375	383	391
76	156	164	172	180	189	197	205	213	221	230	238	246	254	263	271	279	287	295	304	312	320	328	336	344	353	361	369	377	385	394	402

Source: Adapted from *Clinical Guidelines on the Identification, Evaluation, and Treatment of Overweight and Obesity in Adults: The Evidence Report.*

The patient's physical condition, as well as the situation and agency policies, determine how often to assess vital signs (Box 6-1). Nurses are responsible for determining whether more frequent assessment of vital signs is warranted.

The initial set of vital signs provides a baseline. A series of readings is more informative than a single value, because the series can provide information about trends over time. Additionally, many variables may affect vital signs, including pain, stress, anxiety, and activity. It is imperative that nurses measure vital signs correctly and accurately, understand the data, and communicate appropriately.

Observe the patient for other findings to support or refute your assessment. When encountering an abnormal value, obtain the vital sign(s) again to assess accuracy. Also look at the patient. Does he or she appear to be in distress? Note the color of the skin, respiratory effort, and behavior. Remember that normal readings vary according to age. Furthermore, a normal value for one patient may be abnormal for another. When assessing vital signs, compare the results to normal values for the patient's age and also to the patient's own baseline.

Occasionally, only one vital sign requires assessment. For example, when administering a cardiac medication, the nurse assesses heart rate, BP, or both, but not temperature. If fever is suspected, the nurse may take the temperature only. When administering an antipyretic for fever, the nurse reassesses the effect of the medication by measuring the temperature again.

Temperature

The hypothalamus is the body's thermostat; it functions to maintain a steady temperature throughout the day. This thermostat balances the heat produced from food digestion, exercise, and increased metabolism with the heat lost from evaporation of sweating and environmental exposure. Cellular metabolism requires this steady state of temperature to function properly. Body temperature is most commonly measured either in degrees **Celsius** (*C*) or degrees **Fahrenheit** (*F*) according to the agency's policy. U.S. nurses should be familiar with both scales (Box 6-2).

Normal range of body temperature is 35.9°C to 38°C (96.7°F to 100.5°F), depending on the route used for measurement. Rectal and temporal artery measurements are 0.4°C to 0.5°C (0.7°F to 1°F) higher than oral measurements. Axillary temperatures average 0.5°C (1°F) lower than oral temperatures. No single temperature is normal for all adults. Body temperature varies with diurnal cycle, physical activity, age, gender, and state of health. It also normally fluctuates with activity and time of day. A low temperature usually occurs in the early morning, with temperature peaking in the late afternoon. Temperature may vary as much as 0.5°C (1°F). This variation is called the *diurnal* or *circadian cycle*. Variation according to time of day is somewhat more pronounced in infants and children.

Moderate to hard exercise increases body temperature. In women of childbearing age, increased progesterone secretion that accompanies ovulation causes temperature to rise 0.3°C to 0.5°C (0.5°F to 1°F) and remain elevated until menses. Stress may elevate core (central) temperature as a result of increased production of epinephrine and norepinephrine. These increase both metabolic activity and heat production.

Factors such as age, level of consciousness, and other medical equipment, such as endotracheal tubes, influence the choice of route. Each site has advantages and disadvantages. Nurses determine the safest and most accurate site for assessment. The same site should be used when follow-up measurements are needed for comparisons.

Agency policy and available equipment influence the site to use for temperature assessment; however, nurses are expected to select and use alternative methods when warranted by the patient's condition. Although some routes or devices may be easier than others, they may not be the most accurate.

To ensure accuracy, temperatures must be measured correctly. *Electronic thermometers* are fast, safe, and convenient; they can accurately measure the oral, rectal, and axillary temperatures (Fig. 6-3). Temperature readings can be measured in as quickly as 2 to 60 seconds. Oral (blue-tip) and rectal (red-tip)

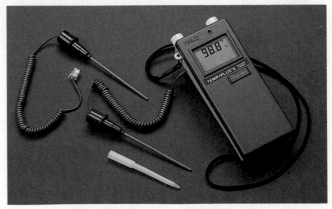

Figure 6.3 Electronic thermometer.

probes are available; they come with disposable, single-use covers. Equipment must be fully charged and correctly calibrated to ensure accuracy. *Disposable, single-use thermometers* can be used for oral and axillary temperature assessment. Readings are available within 1 minute. Disposable thermometers are an effective measure to decrease spread of infection.

Oral. The oral route is common and comfortable for many patients, but it may be contraindicated for others. The sublingual pockets under the tongue are rich in blood supply that responds quickly to changes in the core temperature.

⅃ SAFETY ALERT 6-2

The oral route cannot be used to measure temperature in patients who are unconscious, orally intubated, or confused, or with those who have a history of seizures. Oral temperatures are also contraindicated in cases of postoperative oral surgery or oral trauma. Oral thermometers are not recommended for children younger than 6 years.

Axillary. The axillary route is less common than the oral route. It can be used with infants and young children. It may also be used with patients of other ages who cannot have oral temperature assessed. Electronic or disposable thermometers may be used to access axillary temperatures, which are lower than oral temperatures by 0.3°C to 0.5°C (0.5°F to 1°F). Disadvantages to the axillary route include the need to wait 30 minutes after washing the axilla and that the axillary temperature measures skin surface temperature, which varies and is less reliable than found with other methods (Lawson, et al., 2007).

Tympanic Membrane. The tympanic thermometer uses infrared sensors to detect the heat that the tympanic membrane produces. The tympanic membrane thermometer is noninvasive, safe, efficient, and quick. Because the reading is so quick (2 to 3 seconds), it is commonly used in emergency departments and hospitals. The tympanic temperature should be avoided in patients with ear drainage, ear pain, suspected infection, or scarred tympanic membranes. One disadvantage of tympanic temperature is that reports of accuracy are conflicting. Studies have shown as much as 0.5°C (1°F) variation between tympanic and core pulmonary artery temperatures. The positioning of the probe in the ear canal is inconsistent, which may account for falsely low readings and missed fevers (Mackechnie & Simpson, 2006).

Temporal Artery. Temporal artery thermometers are quick, safe, and convenient, and they do not require contact with mucous membranes. An infrared sensor measures body temperature by capturing the heat emitted from the skin over the temporal artery. This temperature is 0.4°C to 0.5°C (0.7°F to 1°F) higher than an oral temperature. Measurement on either the right or left side of the forehead is equally effective. If a client is in the lateral position, the nondependent side of the forehead should be used. Moving the device too quickly across the forehead or breaking contact with the skin can cause inconsistent results. Another factor to enhance accuracy is to keep the thermometer's infrared lens clean to avoid interference of buildup of skin oil (Lawson, et al., 2007). These thermometers are especially useful in confused or unconscious patients as well as children.

Table 6.3	Advantages and Disadvantages to Various Temperature Routes			
Route	**Normal Temperature Range**	**Appropriate Use**	**Advantages**	**Disadvantages**
Oral	36.5°C–37.5°C (97.7°F–99.5°F)	Older children and adults who are awake, alert, and oriented	Easily accessible and comfortable; provides accurate readings	Do not use with people who have altered mental status. Values may vary because of mouth breathing, oral intake, and smoking. Risk for body fluid exposure is increased.
Axillary	35.9°C–36.9°C (96.7°F–98.5°F)	Infants, young children, and patients with impaired immune systems	Easy to obtain	The nurse must hold the thermometer in place for longer time. Readings reflect temperature of the skin surface, which may be variable. This method may be less accurate than oral or rectal.
Rectal	37.1°C–38.1°C (98.7°F–100.5°F)	Young children and confused or unconscious adults	Very accurate; more reflective of core temperature than other routes	This invasive method should not be used for people with rectal surgery, diarrhea, abscesses, or low white blood cell count. It is contraindicated for newborns and patients with cardiac disease. Risk is increased for exposure to body fluids.
Tympanic	36.8°C–37.8°C (98.2°F–100°F)	All patients except those with ear infection or ear pain	Easily accessible, quick, unaffected by oral intake or smoking	Studies have not proven accuracy. Thermometer is available only in one size. Positioning in children younger than 3 years is difficult.
Temporal	37.1°C–38.1°C (98.7°F–100.5°F)	All patients	Quick and easy to obtain	Diaphoresis or sweat can impair reading.

Rectal. Rectal temperatures, considered one of the most accurate, are taken when other routes are not practical or an accurate core reading is necessary. Adults are usually uncomfortable having a rectal temperature taken.

Adults who cannot close their mouths because of intubation, surgery, change in mental status, or unresponsiveness may require rectal temperatures if tympanic or temporal thermometers are unavailable. Rectal temperatures accurately reflect core temperature changes but are inconvenient, cause discomfort to patients, and are disruptive to normal activity.

Rectal temperatures are 0.4°C to 0.5°C (0.7°F to 1°F) higher than oral temperatures. Electronic and disposable thermometers may be used to measure rectal temperatures. Rectal thermometers are differentiated from oral thermometers by a red color rather than blue. The nurse uses critical thinking to decide on the correct route for temperature. See Table 6-3 for a comparison of routes.

Technique and Normal Findings	Abnormal Findings
Oral Temperature. To ensure accuracy, wait 15–30 minutes after a patient has had anything either hot or cold to eat or drink, smoked, or chewed gum. Turn the thermometer device on. Cover the tip of the probe with a protector. Gloves are unnecessary unless you expect contact with body secretions. Place the thermometer in the sublingual area at the base (back) of the tongue, which has a rich blood supply and corresponds with core temperature. Instruct the patient to keep the lips closed tightly and to breathe through the nose. Hold the probe until it beeps, then remove it. Note the reading and directly dispose of the cover into a wastebasket. Electronic or disposable thermometers have replaced old glass thermometers containing mercury because of toxicity of mercury in the environment. *Oral temperature is 37°C (98.6°F) and ranges from 35.8°C–37.3°C (96.4°F–99.1°F).*	Hypothermia is temperature <35°C (95°F). Prolonged exposure to cold may cause hypothermia. It may be induced purposefully during surgery to reduce the body's oxygen demands. Hyperthermia, also known as *pyrexia* or *fever*, is body temperature exceeding 38.5°C (101.5°F) orally. It occurs during infections caused by toxic bacterial secretions called pyrogens. Another cause is tissue breakdown, as seen in trauma, surgery, *myocardial infarction*, and *malignancy*. Certain neurological disorders, such as *cerebral vascular accident, cerebral edema, tumor,* or cerebral trauma, can affect the thermoregulation of the brain. ⚠ *SAFETY ALERT 6-4* *Fever above 39.5°C (103°F) in adults requires immediate assessment and rapid cooling measures. Monitor rectal temperature constantly during cooling measures to prevent a hypothermic response. Temperature below 35°C (95°F) may require rewarming, according to established protocols.*
Axillary Temperature. Follow the procedure above, except place the electronic thermometer in the axillary fold and have the patient lower the arm. Hold it in place until it reads the temperature. Stay with the patient to ensure correct placement. *Axillary temperature is 36.5°C (97.4°F). It is approximately one degree lower than oral.*	Axillary temperature is the least accurate, so if there are discrepancies, recheck the temperature with another route.
Tympanic Temperature. Turn the unit on and wait for the ready signal. Place a disposable single-use cover on the probe tip. Then, place the tip gently in the patient's ear canal, angling the thermometer toward the patient's jaw. In an adult, pull the pinna up and back to straighten the ear (Fig. 6-4). Take care not to force the probe or to occlude the ear canal. Push the trigger and note the reading. Dispose the cover directly into the wastebasket. Temperature readings are available in 2–3 seconds. *Tympanic temperature is 37.5°C (99°F). It is approximately equal to oral.*	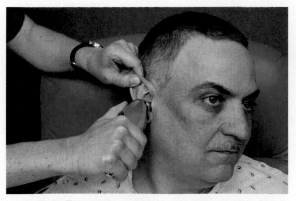 **Figure 6.4** Tympanic temperature assessment. Note placement of the thermometer in the adult's ear.

Temporal Temperature. Position the probe directly on the skin above the eyebrow. Activate the thermometer by depressing and holding the scan bottom. The probe is moved slowly from the forehead, across the temporal artery to level with the top of the ear (Fig. 6-5). Continue to hold the scan button while moving the probe to behind the earlobe. The process requires 5–7 seconds. *Temporal temperature is 37°C (98.6°F). It is approximately equal to oral.*

Studies have shown that the temporal artery measurement using the forehead and behind the ear method is more accurate than temporal artery measurements using just the forehead and is comparable to oral temperature (Lawson, et al., 2007).

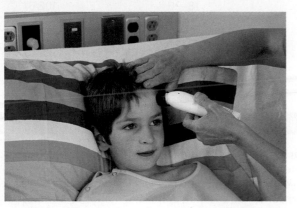

Figure 6.5 Temporal temperature assessment.

Rectal. To assess rectal temperature, ensure that the correct rectal tip is in place. Turn on the unit. Don gloves and cover the probe of the electronic thermometer with a protector. Lubricate the rectal thermometer, and insert the probe 2–3 cm (1 in) into the adult rectum. Hold the thermometer in place and stay with the patient until the temperature is read. Directly dispose the cover into the wastebasket. Using tissue, wipe off any remaining lubricant. Cover the patient and ensure that he or she is comfortable. *Rectal temperature is 37.5°C (99°F). It is approximately 1 degree warmer than oral.*

Avoid placing the probe directly into stool, which may cause an inaccurate reading. The probe should be in contact with the rectal mucosa.

Pulse

Contraction of the heart causes blood to flow forward, which creates a pressure wave known as a **pulse**. The pulse is the throbbing sensation that can be palpated over a peripheral artery or auscultated over the apex of the heart. The pulse reflects the amount of blood ejected with each beat of the heart, which is the stroke volume. The number of pulsing sensations occurring in 1 minute is the heart (pulse) rate.

To assess the pulse, palpate one of the patient's arterial pulse points (usually the radial), noting the rate, rhythm, and strength (amplitude) of the pulse. Also note the elasticity of the vessel.

(text continues on page 102)

Table 6.4   Age-Related Variations in Vital Signs

Age	Heart Rate		Respiration (breaths/min)	Blood Pressure (mm Hg)
	Average (bpm)	Normal Range (bpm)		
Newborn	120	70–190	30–40	73/55
Infant	120	80–160	20–40	85/37
Toddler	110	80–130	25–32	89/46
Child	95	70–115	20–26	95/57
Preteen	90	65–110	18–26	102/61
Teen	80	55–105	12–22	112/64
Adult	70–75	60–100	12–20	120/80
Well-conditioned athlete	May be 50–60	50–100	10–20	120/80

Technique and Normal Findings (continued)

Rate. The normal range of heart rates varies with age. Infants and children have a faster heart rate than adults. Gender, activity, pain, stimulants, emotional state, medications, and disease state also can affect heart rate. *Normal heart rate for an adult is 60–100 bpm. Also see Table 6-4.*

Rhythm. Pulse rhythm refers to the interval between beats. Pulses are described as regular or irregular. A regular pulse occurs at evenly spaced intervals. An irregular pulse has a varied interval between beats. If a pulse is irregular in rhythm, auscultate an apical pulse for one full minute.

A **pulse deficit** provides an indirect evaluation of the ability of each heart contraction to eject enough blood into the peripheral circulation to create a pulse.

Pulse deficits are frequently associated with dysrhythmias. It is essential to recognize a pulse deficit, because it indicates the heart's ability to perfuse the body adequately. When cardiac contractions do not produce enough force or volume to perfuse, a difference exists between apical and peripheral pulses. To assess for a pulse deficit, the beginner nurse and a colleague will at the same time assess the peripheral and the apical pulse rates and compare measurements (see Chapter 19). The more experienced nurse may be able to count the two simultaneously. The pulse deficit is the difference between the apical and radial pulse rates.

Amplitude. The strength of the pulse or *amplitude* indicates the volume of blood flowing through the vessel. It is described on a scale of 0–4 + (Table 6-5).

Normal strength is 2+.

Abnormal Findings (continued)

Tachycardia is a heart rate >100 bpm in an adult. Trauma, *anemia*, blood loss, infection, fear, fever, pain, *hyperthyroidism*, shock, and anxiety can increase pulse rate as a result of increased metabolic demands or low blood volume. In patients with cardiac disease, tachycardia may indicate *congestive heart failure, myocardial ischemia*, or *dysrhythmia*. **Bradycardia** is a heart rate <60 bpm. Medications such as digoxin and beta-blockers decrease heart rate. *Myocardial infarction, hypothyroidism, increased intracranial pressure*, and eye surgery also can decrease heart rate. **Asystole** is the absence of a pulse. *Cardiac arrest, hypovolemia, pneumothorax, cardiac tamponade*, and *acidosis* can cause asystole.

Rhythm may vary with respirations, speeding up during inspiration and slowing with expiration. This is common in children and young adults and is called a **sinus dysrhythmia** or **sinus arrhythmia**.

Table 6.5   Scale for Measuring Pulse

Scale	Description
0	Nonpalpable or absent
1+	Weak, diminished, and barely palpable
2+	Normal, expected
3+	Full, increased
4+	Bounding

Heart failure, hypovolemia, shock, and *dysrhythmias* can cause decreased pulse strength. Bounding pulses are noted with early stages of septic shock, exercise, fever, and anxiety.

Elasticity. The normal artery feels smooth, straight, and resilient. This is known as elasticity of the pulse.

Any artery may be used to assess pulse rate, but the radial and apical are the most common sites because of their accessibility (Fig. 6-6).

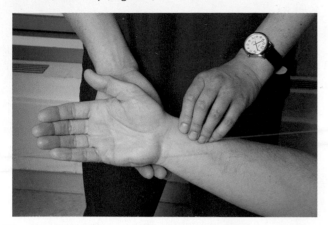

Figure 6.6 Taking a radial pulse.

In cardiac emergencies, the carotid and femoral pulses are assessed. These vessels are larger, closer to the heart, and more accurate in reflecting the heart's activity than are other pulse sites (Table 6-6).

Other sites used to assess circulation include the brachial, ulnar, popliteal, dorsalis pedis, and posterior tibial arteries (see Chapter 20).

The integrity of these peripheral pulses indicates the status of perfusion to the area distal to them.

Vessels become less elastic with increasing age.

⚠ *SAFETY ALERT 6-5*

The carotid pulse should be palpated only in the lower third of the neck to avoid stimulation of the carotid sinus. Never palpate both carotid pulses simultaneously. Palpating both together can significantly decrease cerebral blood flow and cause the patient to lose consciousness.

If a peripheral pulse is diminished or absent, the tissue below may have an inadequate blood supply. This finding indicates the need for further assessment (see Chapter 20).

Table 6.6	Pulse Sites	
Site	**Location**	**Use**
Temporal	Superior and lateral to the eye, anterior to the ear, over the temporal bone	Routinely in infants
Carotid	Medial edge of sternocleidomastoid muscle lateral to trachea	With infants and during shock and cardiac arrest in adults
Apical	Fifth intercostal space, left midclavicular line	To assess pulse deficit and auscultation of heart sounds
Brachial	Proximal to antecubital fossa, in the groove between the biceps and triceps muscles	With cardiac arrest in infants and to auscultate BP
Radial	Thumb side of forearm, at wrist	Routinely to assess heart rate in adults
Ulnar	Ulnar side of forearm, at wrist	To assess ulnar circulation in hand and when performing Allen's test (see Chapter 20)
Femoral	Inferior to the inguinal ligament in the groin	To assess circulation in lower extremities and during cardiac arrest
Popliteal	Behind the knee in popliteal fossa	To assess circulation in the lower extremities and to auscultate leg BP
Dorsalis pedis	Lateral to and parallel with the extensor tendon of the great toe	To assess circulation in the feet
Posterior tibial	Behind the medial malleolus	To assess circulation in the feet

(table continues on page 104)

Assessment. Use the pads of your index and middle fingers. Do not use the thumb, which has pulsations that may interfere with accuracy. Press the patient's artery gently against the underlying bone or muscle until you feel a pulsation. Do not press too hard, because you may obliterate the pulsation. If the pulse is regular in rhythm, count the beats for 30 seconds and then multiply by two to obtain the number of beats per minute. If the rhythm is irregular, auscultate the apical pulse for 1 full minute and assess for a pulse deficit (see Chapter 19). Assess the pulse for one full minute when obtaining a baseline on a patient. When counting, begin with "0" to avoid double counting beats at both beginning and end. *Right radial pulse is 68 beats/min, regular, and 2+/4+.*

To assess apical pulse, place the diaphragm of a stethoscope at the left, fifth intercostal space, midclavicular line and auscultate for one full minute (see Chapter 19). On many patients, it may be easier to auscultate in the second or third intercostal space on the left. This avoids exposing the breast in women, and usually the first and second sounds are heard equally well. *Apical pulse is 60–100 bpm and regular.*

Respirations

Respiration is the act of breathing, which supplies oxygen to the body and vital organs and eliminates carbon dioxide. **Inspiration** occurs when the intercostal muscles and diaphragm contract and expand the pleural cavity, creating a negative pressure for air to flow actively into the lungs. During **expiration** the intercostal muscles and diaphragm relax, decreasing the space in the pleural cavity and passively pushing air out of the lungs.

Rate and depth of respiration change with the demands of the body. Nurses assess for factors that influence respirations. Examples include exercise, anxiety, pain, smoking, positioning, medications, neurological injury, and hemoglobin level.

Observe both inspiration and expiration discretely. Most patients are not aware of their breathing. Do not make the patient aware that you are assessing respirations. Increased awareness may alter normal respiratory pattern. One way to assess respirations is to maintain the position of fingers on the radial artery as if continuing to assess the pulse, while counting respirations. *Normal respirations are relaxed, smooth, effortless, and silent.*

⚠ *SAFETY ALERT 6-6*

Sudden changes in pulse rates or pulse rates >120 bpm or <55 bpm may indicate life-threatening emergencies requiring immediate attention.

⚠ *SAFETY ALERT 6-7*

Absent pulse indicates a need for further assessment. In combination with pain, pallor, or paresthesia, the viability of a limb may be threatened.

Clinical Significance 6-2

Assess patients with dyspnea (difficulty breathing) in the position of greatest comfort to them. Repositioning may increase the work of breathing, which will alter the respiratory rate.

- **Exercise.** Respirations increase in rate and depth to meet additional oxygen demands.
- **Anxiety/pain.** Sympathetic nervous system stimulation increases respiratory rate and depth.
- **Smoking.** Chronic smoking alters pulmonary airways, increasing resting respiratory rate.
- **Positioning.** Slouching impedes the ability of the lungs to fully expand, while standing or sitting erect promotes full expansion.
- **Medications.** Narcotics, anesthesia, and sedatives decrease respiratory rate, while stimulants and bronchodilators increase it.
- **Neurological injury.** Damage to the brainstem inhibits respiratory rate and rhythm.
- **Hemoglobin levels.** Decreased levels of hemoglobin lower the oxygen-carrying capacity of the blood, which in turn increases respiratory rate to increase oxygen delivery.

⚠ *SAFETY ALERT 6-8*

Get help if the respiratory rate is <10 or >32 breaths/min. Such findings may indicate acute distress and prompt the need for a rapid response.

The respiratory rate is a count of each full inspiration and expiration cycle in one minute. Count for 30 seconds and multiply by two to obtain breaths/min. If any abnormalities are noted, assess respiratory rate for one full minute. *Normal respiratory rates for adults are 12–20 breaths/min and regular.*

In addition to rate, observe for the rhythm, depth, and quality of respiration. Is the rhythm regular? As with the pulse, the rhythm refers to the interval between breaths. Regular respiratory rhythm has even intervals. Note the depth of respirations. Is the patient's breath shallow, moderate, or deep? Depth of respirations is a reflection of tidal volume. Also note if the patient uses any accessory muscles while breathing. Normal respiratory effort uses the diaphragm and intercostal muscles. Note the presence of retractions. *Normal respiratory rate, rhythm, and effort are called **eupnea**.*

Oxygen Saturation

Pulse oximetry is a noninvasive technique to measure **oxygen saturation** of arterial blood. Oxygen saturation is the percent to which hemoglobin is filled with oxygen. It does not replace measurement of arterial blood gases for assessment of abnormalities, but it does indicate abnormal gas exchange.

Assess capillary refill and strength of the pulse in the extremity to be used for measuring oxygen saturation. Typically, a finger is used to obtain a reading (Fig. 6-7).

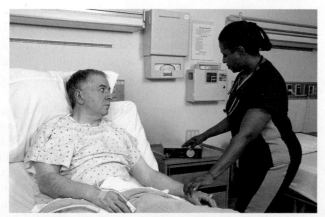

Figure 6.7 Placement of the pulse oximeter in a hospitalized patient.

Tachypnea is a rapid, persistent respiratory rate >20 breaths/min in an adult. It may occur with fever, exercise, **anemia**, or anxiety. Persistent respiratory rate <12 breaths/min is **bradypnea**. It accompanies **increased intracranial pressure**, neurological disease, and sedation. **Dyspnea** is a term used for difficult breathing. Resting respiration that is deeper and more rapid than normal is known as **hyperpnea. Apnea** is the absence of spontaneous respirations for more than 10 seconds.

Hyperventilation is deep, rapid respiration, which may result from hypoxia, **anxiety**, exercise, or **metabolic acidosis. Hypoventilation** is shallow, slow respiration that may be related to sedation or *increased intracranial pressure*. Use of accessory muscles (eg, abdominal or neck muscles) may indicate *respiratory distress*. Also note any cyanosis, retractions, or audible sounds such as wheezing or congestion.

△ SAFETY ALERT 6-9
High-pitched crowing sounds from tracheal or laryngeal spasm, called stridor, may indicate a life-threatening emergency. Any periods of apnea, tachypnea, bradypnea, or irregular respiratory pattern are indications of underlying disease and warrant further assessment.

Accessory muscles include the sternomastoid, rectus abdominis, and internal intercostals. Retractions, or a pulling inward of the soft tissue, are noted in the supraclavicular, intercostal, and costal margin area.

△ SAFETY ALERT 6-10
Get a second opinion if the patient's oxygen saturation is <92%. This finding may require a rapid response.
SpO_2 < 85% indicates inadequate oxygenation to the tissues and may be an emergency.

(text continues on page 106)

Nail polish may also affect the accuracy of pulse-oximetry readings so it should be removed. If circulation is poor, consider using an earlobe or bridge of the nose. A newer oximeter sensor, which attaches to the forehead, has also been useful in patients with poor peripheral perfusion. When compared with arterial blood gases, the forehead sensor is more accurate than the finger probe (Schallom, et al., 2007).

Potential errors in oximetry measurements may result from abnormal hemoglobin value, hypotension, hypothermia, patient movement, or skin breakdown. Falsely low measurements may be associated with cold extremities, hypothermia, and hypovolemia. Falsely high readings may be associated with carbon monoxide poisoning and anemia. *Normal pulse oximetry is SpO$_2$ from 92% to 100%. An SpO$_2$ of 85%–89% may be acceptable for patients with certain chronic conditions such as emphysema.*

Conditions that decrease arterial blood flow may compromise the accuracy of readings, such as *peripheral vascular disease*, edema, and *hypotension*. Patients with *anemia* may have a falsely elevated pulse oximetry reading from circulating hemoglobin containing sufficient oxygen but inadequate hemoglobin to carry adequate oxygen.

Blood Pressure

Blood pressure (BP) is the measurement of the force exerted by the flow of blood against the arterial walls. The pressure in the arteries changes with contraction and relaxation of the heart. Maximum pressure is exerted on the walls of the arteries with contraction of the left ventricle at the beginning of systole. This is known as the **systolic blood pressure** (SBP). The lowest pressure, called the **diastolic blood pressure** (DBP), occurs when the left ventricle relaxes between beats.

Millimeters of mercury (mm Hg) is the standard unit for measuring BP, which is recorded as a fraction with the SBP as the numerator and the DBP as the denominator. Average BP for adults is 120/80 mm Hg, with a range of 100 to 120 mm Hg SBP and 60 to 80 mm Hg DBP. Variations occur normally and are influenced by many factors, including age, gender, ethnicity, weight, circadian cycle, position, exercise, emotions, stress, medications, and smoking.

- **Age.** BP increases gradually throughout childhood into the adult years.
- **Gender.** Prior to puberty, males and females show no discernable difference in BP. After puberty, males show a higher BP measurement than females, but this reverses after menopause, with BP tending to be higher in females than in males.
- **Ethnicity.** Compared with Caucasians, African Americans are 1.5 times more likely to have high BP. American Indians/Alaska Natives are 1.3 times more likely than whites to have high BP (Wallace, et al., 2008).
- **Weight.** SBP elevates 2 to 3 mm Hg and DBP elevates 1 to 3 mm Hg for each 10 kg of extra weight (World Health Organization, 1996).
- **Circadian (diurnal) cycle**. A daily cycle of BP occurs, with it increasing late in the afternoon and decreasing in the early morning.
- **Position.** BP can drop as a patient moves from lying to sitting or standing.

- **Exercise.** Increased activity increases BP, with a return to baseline within 5 minutes of stopping activity.
- **Emotions.** Fear, anger, and pain momentarily increase BP from stimulation of the sympathetic nervous system.
- **Stress.** Patients under continuous tension will experience elevated BP.
- **Medications.** Many medications can lower BP, including antihypertensives, diuretics, narcotics, and general anesthesia.
- **Smoking.** Smoking causes increased vasoconstriction. BP returns to baseline in approximately 15 minutes after cessation of smoking.

A series of BP measurements provides more information than a single measurement. Elevated BP indicates a need for a series of follow-up readings to assess if BP is consistently elevated. Five factors contribute to the BP: (1) cardiac output, (2) peripheral vascular resistance, (3) circulating blood volume, (4) viscosity, and (5) elasticity of the vessel walls. See Table 6-7.

BP is measured using a **sphygmomanometer** and stethoscope. The sphygmomanometer consists of an aneroid or mercury gauge and an inflatable rubber bladder in a cloth covering called the cuff. Many areas have prohibited the use of mercury-containing devices and instead use electronic or automatic BP cuffs.

Cuffs are available in various sizes, ranging from very small for newborns to extra-large arm cuffs for adults and thigh cuffs. It is important to choose the correct cuff size to obtain accurate readings (Table 6-8). The width of the cuff equals 40% of the length of the patient's arm. The length of the bladder equals 80% of the circumference of the limb (Fig. 6-8). If a large cuff is not available in a patient with morbid obesity, blood pressure can be measured on the forearm. The cuff can be placed midway between the elbow and the wrist (Rauen, et al., 2008).

Table 6.7   Factors Contributing to Blood Pressure

1. Cardiac Output. The more blood the heart pumps, the greater the pressure in the blood vessels. For example, BP increases during exercise.

2. Peripheral Vascular Resistance. An increase in resistance in the peripheral vascular system, as happens with people who have circulatory disorders, will increase BP.

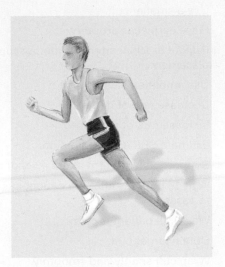

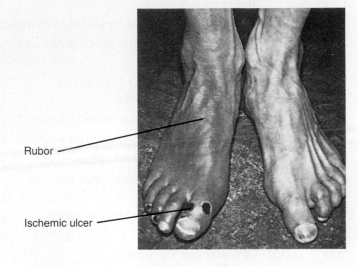

Rubor

Ischemic ulcer

3. Circulating Blood Volume. An increase in volume will increase BP. A sudden drop in BP may indicate a sudden blood loss, as with internal bleeding.

4. Viscosity. When the blood becomes thicker or more viscous (as with polycythemia), the pressure in the blood vessels will increase.

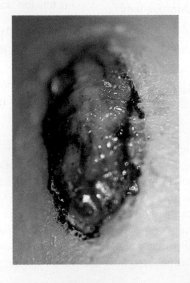

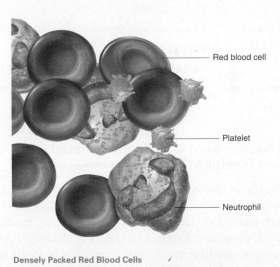

Red blood cell

Platelet

Neutrophil

Densely Packed Red Blood Cells

5. Elasticity of Vessel Walls. An increase in stiffness of the vessel walls (eg, atherosclerotic changes) will increase BP.

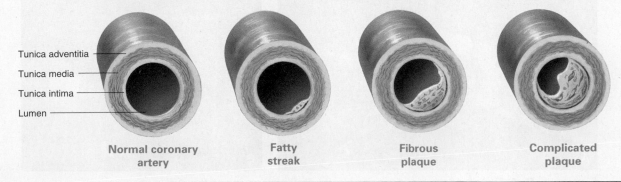

Tunica adventitia
Tunica media
Tunica intima
Lumen

Normal coronary artery   **Fatty streak**   **Fibrous plaque**   **Complicated plaque**

Table 6.8 Common Errors in Blood Pressure Measurement

Error	Contributing Factors	Nursing Action
Falsely low reading	Noisy environment	Maintain a quiet environment during assessment.
	Too large cuff	Use a smaller cuff.
	Improper placement of earpieces of stethoscope	Place earpieces properly.
	Stethoscope not directly over brachial artery	Palpate brachial artery for stethoscope placement.
	Hearing deficit	Use amplified stethoscope.
	Deflating cuff too quickly	Decrease rate of deflation.
	Deflating cuff too slowly (false high diastolic)	Increase rate of deflation.
	Failing to palpate radial artery for estimated SBP	Estimate SBP using palpation.
	Arm position above level of heart	Support patient's arm at the level of the heart.
Falsely high reading	Assessing BP immediately after exercise	Wait 15 minutes after the patient has exercised to assess.
	Assessing anxious or angry patient	Wait until patient is calm.
	Cuff too small	Obtain larger cuff.
	Cuff wrapped too loosely	Wrap cuff snugly and smoothly.
	Reinflation of cuff during auscultation	Deflate cuff, wait 30 seconds, and reassess BP.
	Arm position below level of heart	Support patient's arm at the level of the heart.
	Patient supporting own arm	Support the patient's arm.
	Legs crossed	Uncross legs.
Inaccurate readings	Examiner's eyes not at level of the meniscus	Maintain eye level parallel with meniscus.
	Examiner bias	Do not anticipate or predict what BP should be.
	Defective or inaccurately calibrated equipment	Calibrate equipment regularly.
Other errors	Inflation of cuff too high, causing patient pain	Estimate SBP by palpation.

Risk Assessment and Health-Related Patient Teaching

Teach patients to consistently weigh themselves at the same time of the day, wearing clothing of similar weight. Educate patients about risk factors for hypothermia (ie, frostbite; fatigue; malnutrition; hypoxemia; cold, wet clothing; alcohol intoxication) and hyperthermia (ie, exercising in poorly ventilated areas and hot humid climate, sudden exposures to hot climates, tight-fitting clothing in hot environments, and poor fluid intake before, during, and after exercise).

Patients taking cardiac medications, undergoing cardiac rehabilitation, or starting a new exercise regimen should learn how to take their own pulse rates. Monitoring carotid pulse rate is the most common technique taught to patients. Patients undergoing surgery and those with decreased ventilation should be taught coughing and deep-breathing exercises.

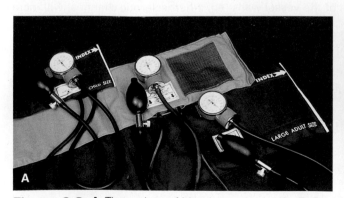 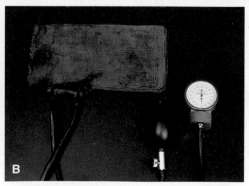

Figure 6.8 A. Three sizes of blood-pressure cuffs. **B.** Bladder is inside the cuff.

Technique and Normal Findings	Abnormal Findings

Arm Blood Pressure. Before assessing BP in the arm, be sure the patient is calm and relaxed and has not eaten, smoked, or exercised for 30 minutes prior to the measurement. It is best to allow the patient to rest for at least 5 minutes prior to assessing BP (Jones, et al., 2003). Measure initial BP in both arms for comparison. A variation of 5–10 mm Hg between arms is normal. If the values are different, use the higher value but record both.

> A difference of 10–15 mm Hg or more between the two arms may indicate arterial obstruction on the side with the lower value.

The patient may be supine or sitting. Support the bare arm at heart level, with palm upward (Adiyaman, et al., 2006). When sitting, the patient's feet are flat on the floor. Crossed legs may falsely elevate BP (Adiyaman, et al., 2007). The back should be supported.

> Do not allow the patient to hold up the arm. Tension from muscle contraction can elevate SBP. Elevating the arm above the heart may result in a false low measurement (Eser, et al., 2006).

Assess the extremity to be used for BP assessment. Do not use an extremity with a shunt, on the same side as a mastectomy, or with an intravenous infusion. Choose the correct size cuff.

> ⚠ SAFETY ALERT 6-11
>
> *Using a cuff that is too narrow causes a falsely high BP reading; using one that is too large causes a falsely low BP reading.*

Palpate the brachial artery above the antecubital fossa and medial to the biceps tendon. Center the deflated cuff approximately 2.5 cm (1 in) above the brachial artery. Line up the arrow on the cuff with the brachial artery. Tuck the Velcro end of the cuff under so that the cuff is snuggly fastened around the arm.

Estimate the SBP by palpating the brachial or radial artery and inflating the cuff until the pulsation disappears. Hold the bulb in your dominant hand. Close the valve on the bulb by turning it away from you but make sure that it will easily release. To control the bulb, it is easiest to brace your fingers against the metal of the valve. Squeeze the bulb to pump air into the bladder. Continue feeling the pulse, and identify when it disappears. Pump the cuff to 20 mm Hg above where the pulse stopped.

> Estimating the SBP will prevent missing an **auscultatory gap**, a period in which there are no Korotkoff's sounds during auscultation. An auscultatory gap occurs in approximately 5% of patients and up to 21% of patients with known vascular disease and hypertension (Cavallini, et al., 1996). Despite this high incidence, only about half of practicing nurses can identify an auscultatory gap (Armstrong, 2002).

Slowly open the valve by turning it toward you to deflate the cuff. Feel for the pulse, noting the number when the pulsation is palpable again and then quickly deflate the cuff completely. This is the estimated SBP. Wait 15–30 seconds before reinflating the cuff to allow trapped blood in the veins to dissipate.

Position the earpieces of the stethoscope in your ears and place the diaphragm or bell of the stethoscope over the brachial artery, using a light touch (Fig. 6-9A). Position yourself so that you can avoid bumping the tubing and can easily see the gauge. Note that you will not hear the tapping of the pulse until the cuff is inflated.

> The bell is designed to pick up low-pitched sounds, such as the turbulent blood flow caused by the BP cuff partially occluding the brachial artery. Some studies have shown that the bell and diaphragm are equally effective (American Heart Association, 2005).

Inflating the BP cuff around the extremity alters the flow of blood through the artery, which generates Korotkoff's sounds (Fig. 6-9B). The sounds are audible with a stethoscope at a pulse site distal to the cuff.

(text continues on page 110)

As pressure against the artery wall decreases from completely occluded blood flow to free flow, nurses can auscultate five distinct sounds (Table 6-9). You will hear sounds only during the period of partial occlusion and not at the top or bottom.

Quickly inflate the cuff to 20–30 mm Hg above the estimated SBP. Then deflate the cuff slowly, approximately 2–3 mm Hg/s, while listening for pulse sounds (Korotkoff's sounds). Note the number when you hear the first Korotkoff's sound, which coincides with the patient's SBP. Be aware of the tendency to round to zero and make sure to read the gauge accurately. Continue deflating the cuff, noting the point of the last pulse sound (Korotkoff IV) and when it disappears (Korotkoff V). Korotkoff V is used to define DPB (see Table 6-9).

Record BP in even numbers as a fraction, with SBP as the numerator and DBP as the denominator. Also record the patient's position, arm used, and cuff size if different from the standard cuff.

Slow or frequent cuff inflations can cause venous congestion. Be sure to deflate the cuff completely after each measurement and wait at least 2 minutes between measurements.

The **pulse pressure** is the difference between the SBP and the DBP and reflects the stroke volume. *Normal pulse pressure is approximately 40 mm Hg.* The **mean arterial pressure** is calculated by adding one third of the SBP and two thirds of the DBP. *A mean pressure of 60 mm Hg is needed to perfuse the vital organs.*

Guidelines from the Joint National Commission on Prevention, Detection, Evaluation, and Treatment of High Blood Pressure (JNC VII) set the standards for diagnosis of high BP (Chobanian, et al., 2003). See Table 6-12 at the end of this chapter. **Hypertension** is not diagnosed on one BP reading alone, but on an average of two or more readings taken on subsequent visits. **Hypotension** is SBP < 90 mm Hg. Some adults have a normal low BP but in most adults, low BP indicates illness.

⚠ *SAFETY ALERT 6-12*

Any sudden change in BP may be an emergency. SBP < 90 or 30 mm Hg below the patient's baseline needs immediate attention. Sudden drop in BP can signify blood loss or a cardiovascular, respiratory, neurological, or metabolic disorder. Sudden, severe rise in BP (above 200/120 mm Hg) is a life-threatening hypertensive crisis.

Decreased elasticity of the arterial blood vessel walls, as well as increased intracranial pressure, can cause the difference between SBP and DBP to increase. This is called a *widened pulse pressure.* Patients with *hypovolemia, shock,* or *heart failure* may exhibit a narrowed pulse pressure. DBP is weighted more heavily because two thirds of the cardiac cycle is spent in diastole.

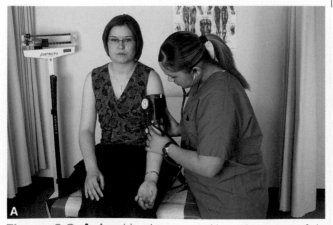
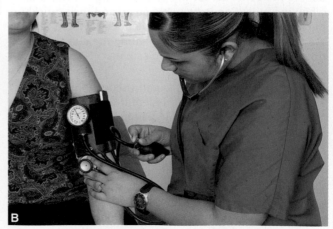

Figure 6.9 A. Arm blood pressure. Note placement of the earpieces of the stethoscope in the nurse's ears as she auscultates over the brachial artery. **B.** Inflating the BP cuff around the arm alters arterial blood flow.

Table 6.9 Korotkoff's Sounds

Phase	Description	Illustration
I	Characterized by the first appearance of faint but clear tapping sounds that gradually increase in intensity; the first tapping sound is the systolic pressure	
II	Characterized by muffled or swishing sounds; these sounds may temporarily disappear, especially in people with hypertension; the disappearance of the sound during the latter part of phase I and during phase II is called the *auscultatory gap* and may cover a range of as much as 40 mm Hg; failing to recognize this gap may cause serious errors of underestimating systolic pressure or overestimating diastolic pressure	
III	Characterized by distinct, loud sounds as the blood flows relatively freely through an increasingly open artery	
IV	Characterized by a distinct, abrupt, muffling sound with a soft, blowing quality; in adults, onset of this phase is considered the first diastolic sound	
V	The last sound heard before a period of continuous silence; the pressure at which the last sound is heard is the second diastolic measurement	

From Taylor, C., Lillis, C., LeMone, P., & Lynn, P. (2011). *Fundamentals of nursing: The art and science of nursing care* (7th ed.). Philadelphia: Wolters Kluwer Health/Lippincott Williams & Wilkins.

Technique and Normal Findings (continued)	Abnormal Findings (continued)
Thigh Blood Pressure. Compare a thigh BP with an arm BP if the arm BP is extremely high, particularly in young adults and adolescents, to assess for coarctation of the aorta. Position the patient prone if possible. Place a large cuff around the lower third of the thigh, centered over the popliteal artery. Proceed as directed for the brachial artery (Fig. 6-10). *The thigh SBP is 10–40 mm Hg higher than the arm SBP, while the DBPs are approximately the same in both sites.*	A thigh or calf may also be used if the patient's arms are unavailable, such as in those with bilateral burns or IVs. *Coarctation of the aorta* (congenital narrowing of the aorta) will produce high arm BP and lower thigh BP as a result of restricted blood supply below the narrowing.

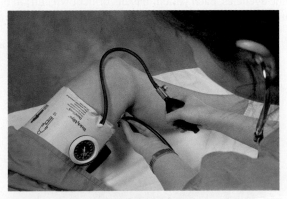

Figure 6.10 Thigh blood pressure.

(text continues on page 112)

Orthostatic (Postural) Vital Signs. These are measured in patients to assess for a drop in BP and change in heart rate with position changes. When a healthy patient changes position, normally the peripheral blood vessels in the extremities constrict and the heart rate increases to maintain adequate BP for perfusion to the heart and brain. Orthostatic changes may indicate blood volume depletion. Some medications can have a side effect of orthostatic hypotension. Additionally, conditions that cause the arterial system to become less responsive, such as immobility or spinal cord injury, can cause orthostatic changes.

Assess BP and heart rate with the patient supine, sitting, and then standing. The patient should rest supine for at least 2 minutes prior to the assessment of the baseline reading. Repeat measurements with the patient sitting and standing, waiting 1–2 minutes after each position change to assess the readings (Lance, et al., 2000). *A drop in SBP of <15 mm Hg may occur and is considered normal.*

Drop in SBP of 15 mm Hg or greater, drop in DBP of 10 mm Hg or greater, or increased heart rate indicates **orthostatic hypotension** and possibly intravascular volume depletion (Calkins & Zipes, 2007). Patients with orthostatic hypotension may exhibit dizziness, lightheadedness, or syncope. *Hypovolemia*, certain medications, and prolonged bed rest may cause orthostatic hypotension. Autonomic dysregulation, as in *Parkinson's disease*, interferes with the normal sympathetic response and may cause orthostasis.

⚠ *SAFETY ALERT 6-13*
Patients with orthostatic hypotension are at risk for falling from dizziness, lightheadedness, and syncope.

Documentation of Normal Findings

Parameters: Temperature and route; pulse rate, rhythm, strength, and site; respiratory rate, rhythm, quality, and depth; pulse oximetry; and BP are recorded on the vital sign flow sheet or other forms per agency policy. Measurements taken after administration of medications or other therapies are documented in the nurse's notes. Strength of peripheral pulses can be documented either as a chart or diagram. When there is a distinct muffling of the Korotkoff's sounds, record both readings (eg, 138/92/72). Abnormal findings are reported to the primary care provider.

Normal Findings: T 37°C orally. R radial P 68 bpm, regular, elastic, 2+/4+. R—14 breaths/min, regular, no use of accessory muscles, no retractions. SpO_2—98%. BP 128/64, right arm, supine. T Roe, RN

Patients should be educated about the risks of hypertension. Risk factors include obesity, cigarette smoking, heavy alcohol consumption, prolonged stress, high cholesterol and triglyceride levels, family history, and renal disease. Primary prevention includes lifestyle modifications such as weight loss, regular exercise, dietary modifications, cessation of smoking, reduction of stress, and reduction of saturated fats and sodium in diet.

Every interaction with a patient is a teaching opportunity. Even patients who are normotensive and have a body weight within normal limits can learn how to maintain a healthy body. The JNC VII published the following recommendations to help maintain controlled BP (Chobanian, et al., 2003):
• If you are more than 10% above ideal body weight, lose weight.
• Limit alcohol to no more than 1 oz of ethanol per day.
• Exercise regularly.
• Limit sodium intake to less than 100 mmol/L/day.
• Quit smoking.
• Reduce dietary saturated fat and cholesterol.

Vital Signs Monitor

Many agencies use a monitor for all vital signs (Fig. 6-11). This portable device usually is on a stand that nurses can wheel from one room to another. It is plugged in when not in use to charge the battery. When taking vital signs with this machine, first unplug it and roll it next to the patient. Attach the cuff. In some agencies, each patient has his or her own cuff; in others, patients share the cuff. Place the cuff on the patient's arm and

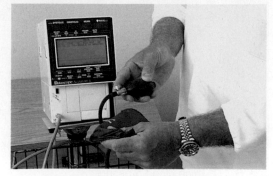

Figure 6.11 Vital signs monitoring device.

press the inflate button. After the display, remove the cuff. The monitor will display the pulse sensed during the BP or SpO_2 reading. Attach the finger clip for the SpO_2. Note the reading that the monitor displays. Load the probe cover on the thermometer. Place the thermometer for the appropriate mode. Note the reading after it is displayed. Eject the probe cover into the wastebasket, using universal precautions. Wash your hands and disinfect the machine according to agency precautions before allowing it to come into contact with the next patient.

⚠ SAFETY ALERT 6-14

When using automatic devices for serial readings, check the patient's cuffed limb frequently to ensure sufficient perfusion to areas distal to the cuff.

Doppler Technique

In some cases, pulse and BP are difficult to auscultate or palpate, such as in patients with shock or poor peripheral circulation. Health care providers use a device called a *Doppler* in this case. This handheld transducer senses and amplifies changes in sound frequency. A whooshing sound similar to the Korotkoff's sounds is audible. The procedure for the assessment of the pulse using Doppler is as follows:

• Apply gel that is specifically for the Doppler to the transducer probe.
• Turn the Doppler on.
• Adjust the volume.
• Touch the probe lightly to the skin at the expected pulse site.
• Hold the probe perpendicular to the skin and move it slowly where you anticipate that the pulse should be until it is located.
• Wipe off the gel and mark the location of the loudest sound with indelible ink.
• Attempt to palpate the pulse in this location.

If you are taking a patient's BP by Doppler, put on the cuff first. Once the pulse is located by Doppler, inflate the cuff until

the sounds go away. Pump up the cuff another 20 to 30 mm Hg. Slowly deflate the cuff and note the reading for the SBP when the whooshing sounds return. Only the systolic pressure is recorded by documenting 88/Doppler.

🔺 Lifespan Variations

Infants, young children, and older adults are more sensitive to environmental temperature than younger adults. Infants and young children have a wider range of normal temperature related to less efficient mechanisms of heat control. Older adults have a lower normal temperature than younger adults, with an average temperature of 36.2°C (97.2°F) (Clark & Baldwin, 2004). They are less likely to mount a fever with the immune response and are more likely to develop hypothermia. Temperature is a less valid indication of infection or inflammation in older adults.

Infants and Children

Although a physical examination consists of painless procedures, it can be scary to children. The use of probes in ears and mouths, a tight BP cuff, and a cold stethoscope can be intimidating. In most cases, allowing the parent of a young child to remain during the assessment is helpful. Young children may feel more secure with their parents present. If appropriate, ask parents to help. Older children and adolescents may prefer not to have parents present. Often it is helpful to allow the child to touch the equipment.

Older Adults

Older adults also have some special considerations relative to the assessment of general survey and vital signs. Remember, do not rush the patient. Allow enough time for him or her to respond to and to ask questions. Do not assume that a patient has a deficit. For example, some but not all elderly patients have a decline in vision or hearing.

Infants and Children

General Survey. As with adults, the general survey begins when the nurse first encounters the child and continues throughout the interaction. What do you see, hear, or smell? Does the child appear well or ill? Never discount your first impression.

Parent–Child Interaction. Observe the interaction between parent and child. Do they mutually respond? Are they warm and affectionate? Remember that children tend to regress developmentally with illness.

Physical Appearance. Observe the same basic components as with an adult, while considering the child's age and developmental stage.

Note hygiene. Are clothes clean? Do they fit appropriately? Are fingernails, hair, and teeth well groomed? Observations provide clues to possible neglect, inadequate finances, or lack of knowledge.

Behavior. Observe the child's response to stimuli and level of alertness. Include personality, level of activity, and interaction with others (especially the primary caregivers) in the assessment.

Mobility. Observe position, posture, and body movement. *A newborn's posture is flexed, with arms and legs tucked in. Toddlers may exhibit slight lordosis (exaggerated curve in the lower back). Preschoolers appear more erect and slender than toddlers. School-age children and adolescents have upright, straight, and well-balanced posture.*

Anthropometric Measurements. Measurements of physical growth in children are essential to assess health status. They include height (length), weight, head circumference, and chest circumference. Values are plotted on growth charts and compared to same-age children.

Length/Height. The term "length" is used when the child is measured in the supine position. Until approximately age 3 years, length should be measured. Because of the infant's normally flexed position, it is important to fully extend the body by holding the head midline, grasping

Note the facial expression and appearance, which may give clues to pain, fear, happiness, or acute illness.

⚠ *SAFETY ALERT 6-15*

Indications of child abuse include the child avoiding eye contact, lack of separation anxiety when appropriate for age, and lack of physical or emotional care. See Chapter 12.

Physical appearance includes an overall impression of the child's state of nutrition, including overweight and wasting.

These observations provide clues of neglect, inadequate finances, unstable housing, or lack of knowledge.

Children with *hearing* or *vision loss* may have a characteristic tilt of the head to see or hear better. Children with low self-esteem may slump.

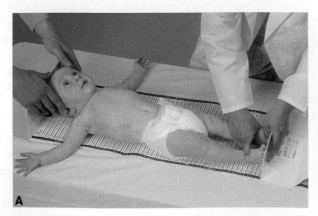 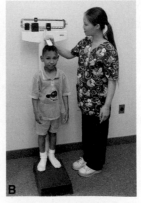

Figure 6.12 **A.** Measuring length of an infant. **B.** Measuring height of a school-age child.

the knees together, and gently pushing down on the knees to extend the legs until they are flat on the table. An assistant or the parent can hold the head while you extend the legs (Fig. 6-12A).

For children older than 3 years, have them stand against the height bar as with adults. Feet are together and heels touch the wall. Encourage the child to stand up straight, looking forward without tilting the head (Fig. 6-12B).

Weight. To weigh an infant, use a platform-style scale. Be careful to watch that the infant does not fall. Nurses may use upright scales starting with children 2–3 years old. Maintain modesty, by older children to continue wearing lightweight clothing. See Fig. 6-13.

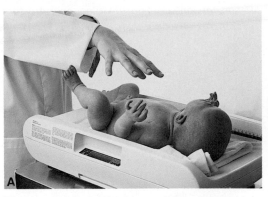
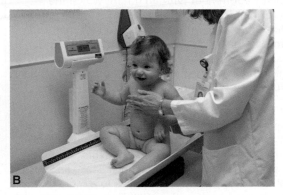

Figure 6.13 **A.** Weighing an infant. **B.** Weighing a toddler sitting up on the scale.

Head Circumference. Head circumference is measured at birth and at each well-child visit up to 2–3 years old. Place a tape measure around the head, encircling the frontal and occipital bones, measuring the largest point across the skull, not including the ears. Plot and compare measurements against expected findings on a standardized growth chart for the age of the infant. A series of measurements is more informative than a single measurement (Fig. 6-14).

Head circumference may be increased with *hydrocephalus*.

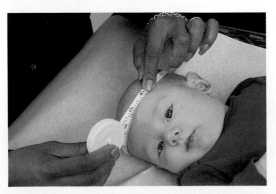

Figure 6.14 Measuring a newborn's head circumference.

Chest Circumference. Measurement of chest circumference is valuable as a comparison to the head circumference, but not by itself. At birth, the newborn's head is approximately 2 cm larger than the chest circumference. The chest grows faster than the cranium,

(text continues on page 116)

and between 6 months and 2 years, the chest and head circumferences are equal. After 2 years, the chest circumference is greater than that of the head.

Vital Signs. When assessing vital signs in infants, obtain respiratory and pulse rates first. Taking a temperature, especially rectal, may cause a child to cry and alter the respiratory and pulse rates. Therefore, assess respiratory rate first, then pulse, and at last, the temperature (Kyle, 2008). Explain the procedure to school-age children and allow them to handle the equipment to promote cooperation. The approach for adolescents is similar to that for adults.

Respirations. Count the respiratory rate in the same manner as for adults, but with an infant, watch the abdomen for respiratory movement. Infant respiration is more diaphragmatic rather than thoracic in nature. Because infants have varying patterns of respirations, assess respiratory rate for one full minute. Infants and young children have a respiratory rate more rapid than that of adults (see Table 6-4).

Pulse. For infants and toddlers younger than 2 years, nurses assess the apical pulse because the radial pulse is difficult to palpate accurately. Assess the apical pulse at the point of maximum intensity (PMI), which for infants is located at the third to fourth intercostal space just above and lateral to the nipple. The PMI moves to a more medial and slightly lower area (fourth or fifth intercostal space, midclavicular line) at approximately 7 years. In children older than 2 years, use a radial pulse for assessment.

Children often have a sinus dysrhythmia, an irregular heartbeat that increases with inspiration and decreases with expiration. Therefore, assess the pulse for one full minute to note any irregularities.

Pulse Oximetry. With infants, the great toe is the recommended site for placement of the pulse-oximetry probe. Cover the patient's foot with a sock to help secure the probe. For an older child, the index finger is the recommended placement.

Tympanic Temperature. The tympanic thermometer is useful with young children who tend to squirm when being restrained for rectal temperature and are not old enough to cooperate with an oral temperature. Measurement with a tympanic thermometer is quick and usually completed before the child is even aware of it. As noted earlier, research studies have not shown conclusively the accuracy of tympanic thermometers (Farnell, et al., 2005).

Inguinal Temperature. The inguinal route is safer than the rectal route. Because of the rich supply of blood vessels in the inguinal area and the ability to form a tight seal around the thermometer, results are closer to the core temperature than the axillary route.

To assess the inguinal temperature, abduct (open) the infant's leg and palpate for the femoral pulse. Place the tip of the thermometer lateral to the pulse site and adduct (close) the leg to create a seal.

Abnormal Findings (continued):

⚠ *SAFETY ALERT 6-16*
Periods of apnea lasting 10–15 seconds are common for infants. Apnea longer than 15 seconds is cause for concern.

Heart rates in infants and children fluctuate more in response to activity, emotions, and illness than do those of adults.

Axillary Temperature. Axillary temperature assessments are safer than those of rectal temperatures, but accuracy in children has been questioned. Axillary temperature is commonly assessed in healthy newborns to avoid the risk of perforating the rectum with the thermometer. When the axillary route is used, place the thermometer well into the axilla and hold the child's arm close to the body.

Oral Temperature. Oral temperatures are contraindicated in children younger than 4 years, sometimes even older. Oral thermometers should be used only when a child can keep the mouth closed around and not bite the thermometer. When possible, use an electronic thermometer because it is less likely to break and yields faster readings.

Rectal Temperature. Rectal temperature is used in infants and other children when other routes are not practical. Position the child supine or sidelying with knees flexed. Insert the lubricated thermo-meter into the rectum no further than 2.5 cm (1 in) and hold the thermometer securely to prevent rectal perforation.

Temporal Temperature. Like the tympanic method, temporal temperature assessment is quick and noninvasive. Allow the child to handle the equipment to decrease fear.

Blood Pressure. BP is assessed annually in healthy children 3 years or older; it is not part of routine assessment for children younger than 3 years. Although BP measurement is generally the same for children as for adults, accurate assessment of BP in children requires some modifications. Because unfamiliar procedures can easily upset children, explain to them what will occur. Tell them what the cuff will feel like. Let them play with the equipment.

Cuff width must cover two thirds of the upper arm, and the bladder must encompass the whole arm. Auscultate using a pediatric end piece on the stethoscope.

Crying may elevate BP; therefore, if possible, allow a crying child to relax for 5–10 minutes prior to assessing BP.

Children younger than 3 years have very small arms, making BP assessment difficult. Electronic BP devices are frequently used in this age group. Refer to Box 6-3 for average SBPs in children.

⚠ *SAFETY ALERT 6-17*
Because of the risk of trauma to the rectal mucosa, rectal thermometers are contraindicated in newborns and infants.

If BP is above the 90th percentile, measurement should be repeated on two other occasions to assess for prehypertension (National Institute of Health, 2007).

BOX 6.3	QUICK FORMULA (USING AUSCULTATION) FOR AVERAGE BLOOD PRESSURE IN CHILDREN

Systolic Blood Pressure	Diastolic Blood Pressure
1–7 years: Age in years +90	1–5 years: 56
8–18 years: (2 × age in years) +83	6–18 years: Age in years +52

(text continues on page 118)

Older Adults

General Survey. By the eighth or ninth decade, physical appearance changes, with sharper body contours and more angular facial features. Posture tends to have a general flexion, and gait tends to have a wider base of support to compensate for diminished balance. Steps tend to be shorter and uneven. Patients may need to use the arms to help aid in balance. Observe normal changes of aging. Assess for any decreasing abilities to function and care for self. Note any changes in mental status.

Height and Weight. People in their 80s and 90s may be shorter than they were in their 70s as a result of thinning of the vertebral discs and postural changes (eg, kyphosis) causing the spinal column to shorten. The proportions of the aging person tend to look different, because the long bones do not shorten but the trunk does. The aging person tends to lose body weight during the eighth and ninth decades from muscle shrinkage and fat distribution changes. Subcutaneous fat is lost from the face and periphery, even with adequate nutrition.

Vital Signs

Temperature. The temperature of older adults is at the lower end of the normal range. Because of changes in the body's temperature regulatory mechanism and decreased subcutaneous fat, aging adults are less likely to develop fevers but more likely to succumb to hypothermia. *Mean body temperature for the older adult is 36°–36.8°C (96.9°F–98.3°F).*

Pulse. Aging adults have a normal range (60–100 bpm). Variation in rhythm may develop. The radial artery may stiffen from peripheral vascular disease. A rigid artery does not indicate vascular disease elsewhere in the body.

The pulse rate of older adults takes longer to rise to meet sudden increases in demand and longer to return to resting state tends to be lower than that of younger adults.

Heart sounds may be more difficult to auscultate and PMI more difficult to palpate.

Respirations. Aging causes rigidity of the costal cartilage, decreasing chest expansion and vital capacity. Decreased vital capacity and inspiratory volume can cause respirations to be shallower and more rapid than that of younger adults, with a normal respiratory rate of 16–25 breaths/min. Decreased efficiency of respiratory muscles results in breathlessness at lower activity levels.

Pulse Oximetry. Placement of the pulse-oximetry probe can present a challenge in older adults. Peripheral vascular disease, decreased carbon dioxide levels, cold-induced vasoconstriction, and anemia may complicate assessment of oxygen saturation on the fingers. Sensors designed for the forehead or bridge of nose may be indicated.

Blood Pressure. Special attention to correct cuff size is necessary when assessing BP in older adults because of loss of upper arm mass, obesity, and decreased arm size. BP tends to increase from atherosclerosis.

Poor hygiene and inappropriate dress may indicate decreased functional ability, medication reactions, infection, dehydration, or malnutrition. Inappropriate affect, inattentiveness, impaired memory, and inability to perform activities of daily living (ADLs) may indicate *dementia* (eg, *Alzheimer's disease*). Changes in mental status may be from poor nutrition, medications, dehydration, underlying infection, or hypoxia.

Kyphosis is an exaggerated posterior curvature of the thoracic spine associated with aging.

Temperatures considered normal for younger adults may constitute fever in older adults.

In older people, both SBP and DBP increase, but SBP more so, leading to a widened pulse pressure (Woodrow, 2004). Elevated BP in older adults is not a normal aspect of aging. Remind older adults to change positions slowly to avoid orthostatic hypotension that increases the risk for falling.

Cultural Variations

During the general survey of every patient, note any cultural influences such as dress, grooming, speech, and nonverbal communication. Some common cultural differences may include the following:

- Mexican American patients expect nurses to show warmth to patients and family members and it should not be strictly business. A nurse should be attentive, take some time, show respect, and, if possible, communicate in Spanish.
- In many Asian cultures, the spoken and written order of the name is last name, then first name with no comma. This often creates confusion in the medical record. Care must be taken to use a consistent format.
- Southeast Asian patients use "krun" to describe a wide range of symptoms including "feeling ill," "feeling hot and cold," or "having a warm body." It may be translated as a fever, although a fever may not be present.
- Patients of Arab cultures may not disclose personal or sexual information.
- Some patients from East African countries apply skin decorations with henna. Black henna causes major errors in oxygen saturation readings, while red henna does not. Use of ear oximetry is recommended if patients have black henna applied to their fingertips (Ethnomed, 2008).

Height varies little among racial groups compared to other anthropometric measures. Height results from genetics, nutrition, and stressors. Mean height varies by gender. In men, Caucasians are tallest, followed by African Americans, and then Mexican Americans (Ogden, et al., 2007). African American women are tallest, followed by Caucasian women, and then Mexican American women. Height is generally not a health concern unless there is more than a 20% variance such as in gigantism or dwarfism (see Table 6-11 at the end of the chapter).

Overall weight of the U.S. population has increased by 24 lbs in the past 40 years, while height has increased by only 1 in; thus, BMI has increased by three units. This same trend is seen in U.S. children and teenagers, whose BMI has increased by 4 units. In women 60 years and older, 61% of non-Hispanic black women are obese compared with 32% of Caucasian women and 37% of Mexican American women. The prevalence of obesity does not differ significantly by race/ethnic group, in men (Ogden, et al., 2007). Reduction of obesity is included in the *Healthy People* goals for the nation (see Chapter 8).

Evidence-Based Critical Thinking

Several nursing diagnoses can be addressed under vital sign assessment. Many are covered in the appropriate body systems chapters of this book, such as respiratory diagnoses in Chapter 18 "Thorax and Lung Assessment." Table 6-10

Table 6.10   Common Nursing Diagnoses Related to Vital Signs

Diagnosis and Related Factors	Point of Differentiation	Assessment Characteristics	Nursing Interventions
Hyperthermia related to prolonged exposure to sun and warm temperature	Temperature > 100°F (37.8°C)	Skin warm to touch, tachycardia, flushed skin, shivering, malaise, fatigue, and loss of appetite	Provide cooling measures, including fans, cooling blankets, fluid replacement, and cool baths (cold baths would cause shivering).
Hypothermia related to prolonged exposure to cold climate	Core temperature < 95°F (35°C)	Tachycardia, peripheral vasoconstriction	Provide warming measures, including warming blankets and warmed IV fluids.*
Imbalanced nutrition, more than body requirements	Body weight > 20% over ideal	Eating response to external cues, sedentary activity level	Determine patient's motivation to loss weight. Observe nutritional intake. Assist with formulation of a food diary and plan for weight loss
Imbalanced nutrition, less than body requirements	Body weight > 20% under ideal	Weakness of muscles, inadequate food intake	Determine healthy body weight for age and height. Assess patient's ability to eat. Consider small frequent meals.
Impaired gas exchange related to immobility	Changes in capillary refill and respiratory rate, rhythm, and effort	Decreased oxygen saturation, fatigue, confusion, tachypnea, tachycardia, and use of accessory muscles for breathing	Administer oxygen.* Teach coughing and deep breathing exercises. Instruct patient in use of incentive spirometer.
Ineffective breathing pattern related to sleep apnea	Changes in respiratory rhythm	Irregular respiratory rate and rhythm, periods of apnea	Encourage weight loss and smoking cessation. Apply continuous positive airway pressure (CPAP).*

*Collaborative intervention.

provides some examples of nursing diagnoses commonly seen in relation to vital signs and general survey. These diagnosis are based on vital sign measurements and supporting data. They are used to label the problem and plan care that is individualized to the patient.

Nurses learn the techniques for assessment of the general survey and vital signs, but use critical thinking to individualize assessments based upon the patient. The nurse collects this data for an initial database, monitors trends in the baseline, and identifies patterns, such as a daily temperature spike in the late afternoon. Additionally, the nurse focuses the assessment based upon the patient situation and current symptoms.

Consider the case of Mr. Sanders, the 55-year-old man admitted to the hospital with a cardiac dysrhythmia. The initial collection of subjective and objective data is complete, and Mr. Sanders is stable. The plan of care includes patient teaching and planning for discharge tomorrow. Unfortunately, Mr. Sanders develops a new onset of symptoms. The following nursing note illustrates how the nurse focuses the assessment, analyzes subjective and objective data, and develops nursing interventions when he is having symptoms.

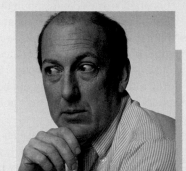

Subjective: "Every once in a while I can feel my heart racing. It doesn't happen very often but it feels like my heart's going to jump out of my chest. It's doing it right now." States no chest pain or pressure.

Objective: Skin color even and pink. Sitting upright, holding chest. Tense facial expression, maintains appropriate eye contact. Talking to his wife in complete sentences. Right radial pulse 122 and irregular, strength 2+/4+, R 22 and regular, BP 136/66 right arm, oxygen saturation 96%. Apical pulse 126 and irregular.

Analysis: Subjective feeling of heart racing may be related to new onset of cardiac dysrhythmia. Pulse deficit of 4 bpm indicates inadequate perfusion of some apical beats. BP lower than normal value may be related to decreased cardiac output with increased heart rate.

Plan: Contact health care provider to inform of new onset of fast and irregular apical pulse. Reassess pulse and BP in 5 minutes. Take apical pulse for one full minute and assess for a pulse deficit. Stay with patient and his wife and assure them that the best care will be provided. Use touch and therapeutic communication to reduce anxiety. Health care provider present and ordered stat 12-lead electrocardiogram that indicated atrial fibrillation with a rate of 126. Consult with provider on collaborative treatment.

T Roe, RN

Critical Thinking Challenge

- How is this focused assessment different from the previous documentation?
- Critique the objective data that the nurse documented. What patterns connect the general survey and vital signs with the focused findings?
- How are the nursing and medical issues similar or different?

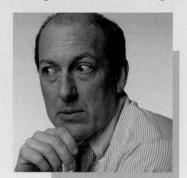

The nurse observes information from the general survey upon each encounter. A complete set of vital signs are taken at the beginning of each shift to establish a baseline. Additionally, the nurse assesses pulse and BP prior to administration of the medications to evaluate effectiveness and side effects, and holds the medications if the pulse or BP is too low. The nurse continually collects assessment data and incorporates it into the care. An accurate and complete general survey and vital signs are the foundation for further assessment and interventions.

You have been studying Mr. Sanders, who was initially admitted to the ICU following an episode of tachycardia and dizziness. He was started on antiarrhythmic medication, stabilized, and transferred to the acute care floor. He developed a new onset of tachycardia and was reassessed by the nurse. The nurse obtained assistance and Mr. Sanders was successfully treated. He will need ongoing assessments related to his problems including hypertension and dysrhythmia.

Using the previous steps of diagnostic reasoning, organizing, and prioritizing, consider all the case study findings woven throughout this chapter. When answering the following questions, begin drawing conclusions and see how the pieces of assessment must work together to create an environment for personalized, appropriate, and accurate care.

- Is Mr. Sanders's condition stable, urgent, or an emergency?
- What immediate health-promotion and teaching needs are evident?
- What are the relationships between his pulse, respirations, and BP?
- How will the general survey and vital signs differ from the focused assessment?

Key Points

- The general survey begins with the first moments of patient encounter, progresses through the history and physical examination, and continues with each subsequent interaction.
- Extreme anxiety, acute distress, pallor, cyanosis, changes in mental status, and changes in vital signs may indicate the need for assistance and a rapid response.
- The general survey includes overall appearance, hygiene and dress, skin color, body structure and development, behavior, facial expression, level of consciousness, speech, mobility, posture, range of motion, and gait.
- Anthropometric measurements include height and weight.
- Vital signs reflect patient health status, cardiopulmonary function, and overall function of the body.
- The nurse assesses the appropriate route of temperature including oral, axillary, tympanic, temporal artery, and rectal.
- The pulse is assessed for rate, rhythm, amplitude, and elasticity.
- Smoking, positioning, medication, neurological injury, and hemoglobin levels affect the respiratory rate.
- An oxygen saturation level less than 92% indicates inadequate oxygenation to the tissues.
- Age, gender, ethnicity, weight, circadian cycle, position, exercise, emotions, stress, medications, and smoking affect the BP.
- The brachial artery is commonly used to measure the BP.
- Width of the cuff size equals 40% of the length, and length of the bladder equals 80% of the circumference of the arm.
- Postural vital signs are taken sitting, lying, and standing; they indicate intravascular volume depletion.
- A vital signs monitor is commonly used in the hospital setting.

- The Doppler is used if the pulse and BP are difficult to auscultate or palpate.
- In children add the length, head circumference, and variations in vital signs to the physical assessment.
- Vital signs change in older adults results from physiological changes in the body.
- Height varies little among racial groups; however, weight in women varies more.

Review Questions

1. Mr. Holmes has come to the clinic for a well-patient visit. When assessing his vital signs, the nurse palpates an irregular heart rate. The nurse must then auscultate for a full minute at the apical pulse site. Locate the apical pulse on the diagram below.

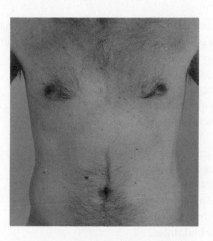

2. What are the four characteristics of a pulse?

3. An unconscious 20-year-old woman arrives at the hospital after drinking large quantities of alcohol. Her vital signs are T 98.2°F, po; P 58; R 9; BP 100/64. What conclusion would the nurse make about this patient's respiratory status?
   A. The patient is experiencing apnea.
   B. The patient is experiencing bradycardia.
   C. The patient is experiencing bradypnea.
   D. The patient's respiratory status is within normal limits.

4. The patient's radial pulse is weak and thready. The nurse would document the finding as
   A. 3+/ 4+
   B. 2+/ 4+
   C. 1+ /4+
   D. Radial pulse absent

5. The nurse is preparing to assess the vital signs of a 62-year-old woman following hip surgery. When the nurse arrives, the patient is sitting in her chair having just finished breakfast. What is the appropriate nursing action?
   A. Take vital signs as planned.
   B. Wait 20 to 30 minutes and then take vital signs.
   C. Ask the patient to lie down in bed to assess vital signs.
   D. Take a rectal temperature.

6. The postoperative vital signs of a 47-year-old man with a ruptured appendix are BP 112/68, pulse 56, R 8, T 37.6°C temporally. The patient is pale and confused, with minimal urine output. The nurse should
   A. recheck the vital signs in 30 minutes
   B. continue with care as planned
   C. administer pain medication
   D. notify the clinician

7. The pulse pressure for a patient with a BP of 144/86 is
   A. 58
   B. 86
   C. 144
   D. 230

8. The nurse is caring for an elderly confused patient. In assessing temperature, the nurse will obtain the reading using
   A. an oral thermometer
   B. a rectal thermometer
   C. a tympanic thermometer
   D. a mercury thermometer

9. The nurse notes an irregular radial pulse in a patient. Further assessment includes assessing the
   A. carotid pulse
   B. apical pulse
   C. femoral pulse
   D. brachial pulse

10. Which actions will result in an accurate BP reading? Select all that apply.
   A. Applying the center of the bladder of the cuff directly over the brachial artery.
   B. Raising the arm to the level of the heart.
   C. Using the bell to assess the BP.
   D. Pumping the cuff 60 mm Hg above the estimated BP.

References

Adiyaman, A., Tosun, N., Elving, L., Deinum, J., & Thien, T. (2007). The effect of crossing legs on blood pressure. *Blood Pressure Monitoring, 12*(3), 189–193.

Adiyaman, A., Verhoeff, R., Lenders, J., Deinum, J., & Thien, T. (2006). The position of the arm during blood pressure measurement in sitting position. *Blood Pressure Monitoring, 11*(6), 309–313.

Armstrong, R. S. (2002). Nurses' knowledge of error in blood pressure measurement technique. *International Journal of Nursing Practice, 8*(3), 118–126.

Calkins, H., & Zipes, D. P. (2007). Hypotension and syncope. In P. Libby, R. O. Bonow, D. L. Mann, et al., *Braunwald's heart disease: A textbook of cardiovascular medicine* (8th ed.). Philadelphia: Elsevier.

Cavallini, M. C., Roman, M. J., Seymour, G., Blank, S. B., et al. (1996). Association of the auscultatory gap with vascular disease in hypertensive patients. *Annals of Internal Medicine, 124*(10), 877–883.

Chobanian, A. V., Bakris, G. L., Black, H. R., et al. (2003). Joint National Committee VII: The seventh report of the Joint National Committee on the Prevention, Detection, Evaluation and Treatment of High Blood Pressure. *Journal of the American Medical Association, 289*, 2560–2572.

Clark, A. P., & Baldwin, K. (2004). Best practices for care of older adults. *Clinical Nurse Specialist, 18*(6), 288–299.

Eser, I., Khorshid, L., Gunes, Y., & Demir, Y. (2006). The effect of different body positions on blood pressure. *Journal of Clinical Nursing, 16*, 137–140.

Ethnomed. (2008). *Clinical topics.* Retrieved April 28, 2008, from http://www.ethnomed.org/

Farnell, S., Maxwell, L., & Tan, S. (2005). Temperature measurement: Comparison of non-invasive methods used in adult critical care. *Journal of Clinical Nursing, 14*(5), 632.

Jones, D. W., Appel, L. J., Sheps, S. G., Roccella, E. J., & Lenfant, C. (2003). Measuring blood pressure accurately. *Journal of the American Medical Assocaition, 289*, 1027–1030.

Kyle, T. (2008). *Essentials of pediatric nursing.* Philadelphia: Wolters Kluwer/Lippincott Williams & Wilkins.

Lance, R., Link, M., Padua, M., Clavell, L., Johnson, G., & Knebel, A. (2000). Comparison of different methods of obtaining orthostatic vital signs. *Clinical Nursing Research, 11*(9), 479.

Lawson, L., Bridges, E., Ballou, I., Eraker, R., Greco, S., Shively, J., et al. (2007). Accuracy and precision of noninvasive temperature measurement in adult intensive care patients. *American Journal of Critical Care, 16*(5), 485–496.

Mackechnie, C., & Simpson, R. (2006). Traceable calibration for blood pressure and temperature monitoring. *Nursing Standard, 2*(11), 42–47.

National Heart Lung and Blood Institute. (2009). *Update: Clinical guidelines on the identification, evaluation, and treatment of* overweight and obesity in adults. Retrieved April 23, 2008, from http://www.nhlbi.nih.gov/guidelines/obesity/obesity2/index.htm.

National Institute of Health. (2007). *Age appropriate vital signs.* Retrieved November 11, 2007, from http://clinicalcenter.nih.gov/ccc/pedweb/pedsstaff/age.html

Ogden, C. L., Carroll, M. D., McDowell, M. D., et al. (2007).t *Obesity among adults in the United States—no statistically significant change since 2003–2004.* Retrieved April 27, 2008, from http://www.cdc.gov/nchs/data/databriefs/db01.pdf

Rauen, C. A., Chulay, M., Bridges, E., et al. (2008). Seven evidence-based practice habits: Putting some sacred cows out to pasture. *Critical Care Nurse, 28*(2), 98–124.

Schallom, L., Sona, C., McSweeney, M., & Mazuski, J. (2007). Comparison of forehead and digit oximetry in surgical/trauma patients at risk for decreased peripheral perfusion. *Heart & Lung, 36*(3), 188–194.

Wallace, M. F., Fulwood, R., & Alvarado, M. (2008). NHLBI step-by-step approach to adapting cardiovascular training and education curricula for diverse audiences. *Previews in Chronic Disease, 5*(2).

Woodrow, P. (2004). Assessing blood pressure in older people. *Nursing Older People, 16*(1), 29–31.

World Health Organization. (1996). *Hypertension control.* Geneva, Switzerland: Author. Tech Rep Ser No 862.

The Jensen suite offers these additional resources to enhance learning and facilitate understanding of this chapter:

- thePoint online resource, http//thepoint.lww.com/Jensen1E
- Student CD-ROM included with the book
- *Laboratory Manual for Nursing Health Assessment: A Best Practice Approach*
- *Pocket Guide for Nursing Health Assessment: A Best Practice Approach*

CHAPTER 6   General Survey and Vital Signs Assessment   123

⚠ **Table 6.11   Abnormal Findings: Anthropometric Measurements**

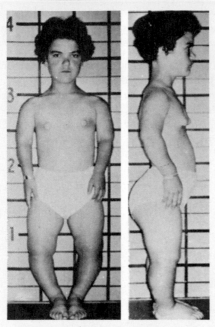

Achondroplastic Dwarfism. Characteristics of this genetic disorder include short stature, short limbs, and a relatively large head. Also note the thoracic kyphosis and lumbar lordosis.

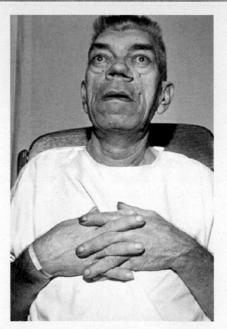

Acromegaly. This condition results from excessive growth hormone secretion during adulthood, after normal body growth has been completed. Overgrowth of bone causes changes in the size of the head, face, hands, feet, and internal organs; height is not affected.

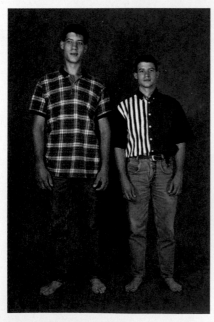

Gigantism. Excessive growth hormone secretion in childhood causes increased height and weight with delayed sexual development. Note the differences in these same-age individuals, one of whom has gigantism and the other whose anthropometric measurements are within expected limits.

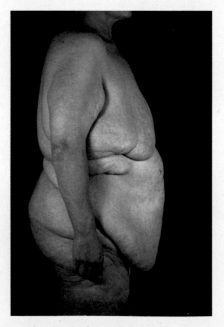

Obesity. Excessive body fat results when calories continually exceed body requirements. It can result from overeating, genetics, endocrine or hormonal disorders, lifestyle issues, or a combination of factors.

Table 6.11   Abnormal Findings: Anthropometric Measurements *(continued)*

Anorexia Nervosa. Severe restriction of caloric intake and disturbance in body image contribute to this psychiatric disorder. Affected patients are clearly emaciated and display other physical findings, such as brittle hair and nails, absent menstruation, delayed puberty, sunken eyes, dry skin, and other manifestations.

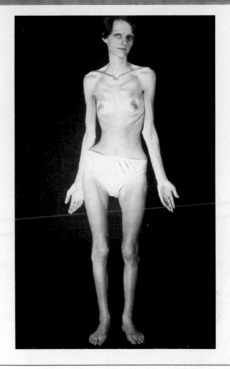

Table 6.12   Abnormal Findings: Blood Pressure in Adults (mm Hg)

Category	Systolic	Diastolic
Hypotension	<90	<60
Normal	<120 and	<80
Prehypertension	120–139 or	80–90
Stage 1 hypertension	140–159 or	90–99
Stage 2 hypertension	>160 or	>100

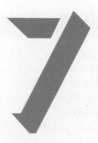

Pain Assessment

Learning Objectives

1 Discuss the basic theories of pain.

2 Identify the elements of pain transmission.

3 Determine the different types of pain.

4 Differentiate musculoskeletal pain from neuropathic pain.

5 Identify the elements of pain assessment.

6 Examine the one-dimensional, multidimensional, and behavioral pain tools for newborns, children, and older adults.

7 Identify issues in assessing pain in special populations such as patients with opioid tolerance or difficulty communicating.

*M*rs. Bond, 42 years old, is visiting the clinic for follow-up care for musculoskeletal pain related to fibromyalgia. She was diagnosed 5 months ago and still has not been able to control her pain to a desirable goal. Her temperature is 37°C orally, pulse 88 beats/min, respirations 16 breaths/min, and blood pressure 112/68 mm Hg. Current medications include a selective serotonin reuptake inhibitor for depression, a benzodiazepine for muscle spasm, and an analgesic for pain. She had a comprehensive assessment documented 5 months ago and has been seen twice since for pain control.

You will gain more information about Mrs. Bond as you progress through this chapter. As you study the content and features, consider Mrs. Bond's case and its relationship to what you are learning. Begin thinking about the following points:

- What is the role of the nurse when assessing Mrs. Bond's pain?
- What subjective information will the nurse gather during today's assessment? What pain tools would be most appropriate?
- What objective data will the nurse assess during the history and interview?
- How will the nurse reassess the effectiveness of interventions?
- What other associated findings would the nurse assess when considering Mrs. Bond's pain?

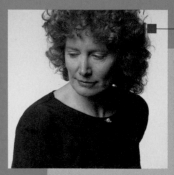

This chapter covers the assessment of pain using reliable and valid pain assessment scales. It presents the basic elements of pain assessment, as well as background information on pain, pain transmission, and assessing pain in difficult-to-assess populations.

Pain is one of the most common reasons patients seek help from health care professionals. Pain does not respect gender, age, or ethnicity. It can occur at any time, to anyone. Pain can profoundly affect quality of life, interactions with family and friends, sense of well-being and self-esteem, and financial resources. For many patients, pain is the result of injury or surgery, but for others, pain has no identifiable cause.

Neuroanatomy of Pain

Peripheral Nervous System

Several different types of nerve fibers that transmit pain are located in the peripheral nervous system. The two main types of nerve fibers are as follows:

1. **A-delta**, large nerve fibers covered with myelin; they conduct pain impulses rapidly. Patients often describe the type of pain impulse that A-delta fibers conduct as sharp or stabbing (Purves, et al., 2004).
2. **C fibers**, smaller unmyelinated nerve fibers; they conduct pain impulses more diffusely and slowly. Patients often describe the pain conducted by C fibers as achy and ongoing, even after the pain stimulus is removed (Purves, et al., 2004).

C fibers release a pain-facilitating substance from nerve endings called substance P. The function of substance P is to quicken the transmission of the pain stimulus up the pain pathway. Bradykinin, another pain-facilitating substance, is released at the site of injury. It is a cellular chemical released from the damaged tissue. The function of bradykinin is to cause continued irritation at the injury site (D'Arcy, 2007a).

These specialized peripheral A and C nerve fibers are referred to as **nociceptors**. They carry the pain signal to the central nervous system.

Central Nervous System

Once the pain stimulus is transferred into the central nervous system via the dorsal root ganglion, it synapses in the substantia gelantinosa in the dorsal horn of the spinal cord and enters the central nervous system. Opening or closing the "gate" to nociception is controlled by the combined effect of both the sum of the pain-facilitating impulse and the facilitating substances and the sum of the pain-blocking impulses and substances as they are received in the substantia gelatinosa. Simplistically, if facilitator impulses predominate, the pain stimulus is passed on; if blocking impulses predominate, the pain stops (Cervero, 2005).

If the pain is allowed to continue, the pain stimulus passes through the spinal cord into the lateral spinothalamic tracts, which lead directly to the thalamus, and then into the limbic system. In the limbic system, the emotions that control pain are produced, and the stimulus is then passed to the cerebral cortex when the sensation is recognized as pain. The whole process takes milliseconds (D'Arcy, 2007a) (see Fig. 7-1).

Two substances are very important to pain transmission at this level. Some nerves use substance P to fire at synaptic junctions. Glutamate is the neurotransmitter responsible for the communication of the peripheral nervous system with the central nervous system (Rowbotham, 2006). An additional function of glutamate is thought to be activation of N-methyl D-aspartate (NMDA) receptors, which can help intensify and prolong persistent pain (Mersky, et al., 2005).

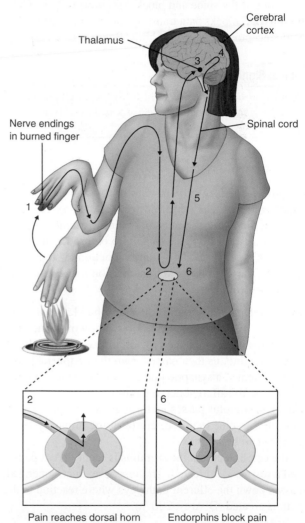

Figure 7.1 (1) Pain begins as a message received by nerve endings, such as in a burned finger. (2) The release of substance P, bradykinin, and prostaglandins sensitize the nerve endings, helping to transmit the pain from the site of injury toward the brain. (3) The pain signal then travels as an electrochemical impulse along the length of the nerve to the dorsal horn on the spinal cord, a region that receives signals from all over the body. (4) The spinal cord then sends the message to the thalamus, and then to the cortex. (5) Pain relief starts with signals from the brain that descend by way of the spinal cord, where (6) chemicals such as endorphin S are released in the dorsal horn to diminish the pain message.

Descending nerve fibers from the locus ceruleus and periaqueductal gray matter transmit the response to the efferent nerve pathways. Substances that can modulate the pain response at this level include opiates, endorphins, and enkephalins. These substances can bind to the opiate receptors in the dorsal horn of the spine and block pain transmission. Gabapentin (GABA) blocks pain transmission by binding to GABA-specific receptors in the dorsal horn (Bennett, et al., 2007).

Gate Control Theory

Currently, the theory of pain with the widest acceptance is the **gate control theory** (Melzack & Wall, 1975). This theory posits that the body responds to a painful stimulus by either opening a neural gate to allow pain to be produced or creating a blocking effect at the synaptic junction to stop the pain (Fig. 7-2). The steps for pain transmission in the gate control theory are as follows:

1. Continued painful stimulus on a peripheral neuron causes the "gate" to open through depolarization of the nerve fiber. This is accomplished by ion influx and outflow.
2. The pain stimulus then passes from the peripheral nervous system at a synaptic junction to the central nervous system up the afferent nerve pathways.
3. The pain stimulus passes up through and across the dorsal horn of the spine to the structures of the limbic system and the cerebral cortex.
4. In the cerebral cortex the stimulus is identified as pain and a response is created. The response, once generated, passes down the efferent pathways where reaction to the pain is created (D'Arcy, 2007a).

Although this theory seems simple, proponents continue to expand and refine it. Recent data suggest that the degree of the stimulus can produce varied responses. Current research focuses on those elements that can affect pain inhibition and stop the pain stimulus. Additionally, pain-facilitating and pain-inhibiting substances that can either help or hinder pain processing have been discovered. Refer to Box 7-1.

Nociception

The most common clinical interpretation of pain transmission is a concept called **nociception**, which means the perception of pain by sensory receptors located throughout the body

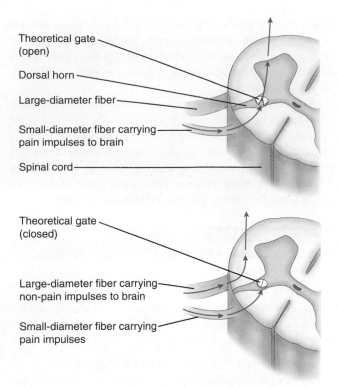

Figure 7.2 The gate control theory.

and called **nociceptors**. These nociceptors can produce pain resulting from heat, pressure, or noxious chemicals, such as those found in the inflammatory process (D'Arcy, 2007a). There are four steps in nociception:

1. **Transduction:** Noxious stimuli create enough of an energy potential to cause a nerve impulse perceived by nociceptors (free nerve endings).
2. **Transmission:** The neuronal signal moves from the periphery to the spinal cord and up to the brain.
3. **Perception:** The impulses being transmitted to the higher areas of the brain are identified as pain.
4. **Modulation:** Inhibitory and facilitating input from the brain modulates or influences the sensory transmission at the level of the spinal cord (Berry, et al., 2006).

Persistent or chronic pain can exist without any identifiable cause and cause the body to adapt or change how it transmits or perceives the pain signal. These changes in transmission (**neuronal plasticity**) can cause the pain to become more severe by activating additional structures for facilitating transmission.

BOX 7.1 SUBSTANCES WITH A ROLE IN PAIN

Pain-facilitating substances
• Substance P
• Bradykinin
• Glutamate
Pain-blocking substances
• Serotonin
• Opioids (both natural and synthetic)
• GABA: gabapentin (neurontin) and pre-gablelin (Lyrica)

Types of Pain

Definitions of pain emphasize that it is an unpleasant experience (Box 7-2). Because pain is so damaging, it is important to understand just how this experience is created. Acute pain is meant to warn the body that some type of insult or injury has occurred. Chronic pain lasts beyond the normal healing period and has no role.

Acute Pain

Acute pain results from tissue damage, whether through injury or surgery. Acute pain is very prevalent in hospital settings and primary care clinics. Following the 73 million surgeries performed each year, 75% of postoperative patients report pain, and 86% of them report pain ranging from extremely severe to moderate (Apfelbaum, et al., 2003).

Pain nociception has various locations. **Visceral pain** originates from abdominal organs, and patients often describe this pain as crampy or gnawing. **Somatic pain** originates from skin, muscles, bones, and joints. Patients usually describe somatic pain as sharp (D'Arcy, 2007a). **Cutaneous pain** derives from the dermis, epidermis, and subcutaneous tissues. It is often burning or sharp, such as with a partial thickness burn. **Referred pain** originates from a specific site, but the person experiencing it feels the pain at another site along the innervating spinal nerve (Fig. 7-3). An example is cardiac pain that a person experiences as indigestion, neck, or arm pain. Phantom

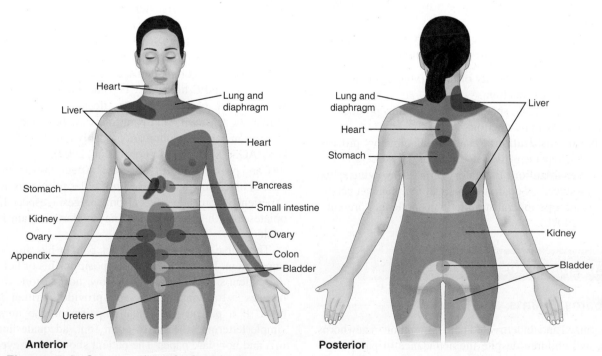

Anterior

Heart — Lung and diaphragm
Liver — Heart
Stomach — Pancreas
Kidney — Small intestine
Ovary — Ovary
Appendix — Colon
— Bladder
Ureters

Posterior

Lung and diaphragm — Liver
Heart —
Stomach —
— Kidney
— Bladder

Figure 7.3 Common sites of referred pain.

pain is pain in an extremity or body that is no longer there (eg, a patient who experiences pain in a leg with an amputation).

Chronic Pain

Chronic pain is also prevalent in U.S. adults, with approximately 40% of them experiencing it daily (Berry, et al., 2006; Cipher, et al., 2006). Estimates of the costs of chronic pain, combining lost income, medical expenses, and worker nonproductivity, are $100 billion/year (Munce, et al., 2007). Because of the stigma associated with chronic pain and its treatment in the health care setting, it is also referred to as persistent pain.

Neuropathic Pain

Once pain becomes a more constant stimulus, the nervous system can modify its function (**neuronal plasticity**) (Rowbotham, 2006). In turn, this can lead to another phenomenon called **peripheral sensitization**, by which peripheral nociceptors are sensitized to pain stimuli. As an example, inflammation can cause peripheral sensitization related to the continued release of inflammatory mediators such as nitric oxide, bradykinin, serotonin (opposite of acute injury), histamine, and adenosine (D'Arcy, 2007a). This irritating process causes cytokines and growth factors to be recruited to the site of injury, prolonging the inflammatory response. Over time, this sensitization produces a condition in which nonpainful touch or pressure becomes painful.

Neuronal windup is produced when repeated assaults on the afferent neurons create enhanced response and increased activity in the central nervous system. Windup can cause tissues in the affected area to become extremely sensitive to pressure in areas not identified usually as painful. Examples of windup include rheumatoid arthritis and osteoarthritis (Rowbotham, 2006).

The following list includes some conditions resulting from physiologic responses to painful stimuli:

- **Neuronal plasticity:** Ability of the nervous system to change or alter its function
- **Windup:** Enhanced response to pain stimulus produced by prolonged pain production
- **Peripheral sensitization:** Result of inflammatory process that creates hypersensitivity to touch or pressure
- **Central sensitization:** Excitatory process involving spinal nerves produced by continued pain stimuli that can persist even after peripheral stimulation is no longer present (D'Arcy, 2007b)

Lifespan Considerations

Newborns, Infants, and Children

Unrecognized and undertreated pain is common in newborns, infants, and children despite the abundance of pain assessment tools. Preverbal newborns and infants are at risk for undertreatment because of myths that they do not experience pain. Additionally, they undergo many painful procedures such as heel sticks, venipuncture, immunizations, vitamin K injection, and circumcision. Many providers have fears about the adverse effects associated with analgesic use.

Much of the research on the physiology of pain has been done in newborns. The number of pain receptors in babies is similar to adults. Connections are present between the peripheral and central nervous systems from 30 weeks' gestation (Anand, 2007). Preterm newborns have an increased sensitivity to pain, compared with older children. This is thought to be because inhibitory neurotransmitters are in insufficient levels until full-term birth. Compared with older children, newborns exhibit more hormonal, metabolic, and cardiovascular responses to pain, and may require higher doses of analgesics for adequate pain control (Anand, 2007). Inadequate pain treatment can lead to a delay in healing and behavioral consequences, such as learning disabilities, psychiatric disorders, and neurodevelopmental problems (Astuto, et al., 2007).

Older Adults

Pain is prevalent in older adults, with 80% of all patients in long-term care facilities and 25% to 50% of community-dwelling elders reporting chronic daily pain (American Geriatric Society [AGS], 2002). Pain is not a normal consequence of aging.

Chronic disease may affect accurate pain assessment, such as with osteoarthritis, peripheral vascular disease, or cancer. Patients who experience surgical or diagnostic procedures may experience acute pain. They may be unable to distinguish if their pain is surgically induced or chronic from preexisting painful conditions. Because the U.S. population is aging proportionately, understanding how to assess pain in older patients is a critical skill for nurses.

Little is known about the effect of increased age on pain perception. No evidence suggests that pain sensation is diminished in older adults, a common misperception. Transmission along the A-delta and C fibers may become altered with aging, but it is not clear how this change affects the pain experience. Studies of sensitivity and pain tolerance have indicated that changes in pain perception are probably not clinically significant (AGS, 2002; Reyes-Gibby, et al., 2007).

Care provider issues also may affect the treatment of pain in older populations. Because older people are likely to experience more side effects from analgesia, especially from opiates, health care providers may undertreat pain in older adults.

The nurse assesses if the older patient has any auditory impairment. If present, the nurse positions his or her face in the patient's view, speaks in a slow, normal tone of voice, reduces extraneous noises, and provides written instructions. If a patient has visual impairment, the nurse uses simple lettering, at least 14-point font, adequate line spacing, and nonglare paper. The patient should wear eyeglasses or a functioning hearing aid if these devices are in normal use, and have adequate time to respond to questions (Herr, et al., 2006a). Because older adults may process information more slowly than younger patients, the nurse allows sufficient time for older adults to respond.

Cognitive impairment, dementia, and delirium are more common in older adults (Linton & Lach, 2007). Accurately assessing pain is more challenging when patients have these conditions. Nevertheless, no evidence shows that patients with cognitive impairment experience less pain. Nurses should not consider pain reports from these patients any less valid than those from other patients. Health care providers may use behavioral observations of pain in patients (eg, restlessness, guarding, pacing) to assess pain, but these observations are not pain specific and may represent responses to other conditions.

Cultural and Environmental Considerations

Health care providers are more likely to rate pain scores lower in patients of racial and ethnic minority groups than in Caucasian patients (Green, et al., 2003). There are also differences in expectations for adequate pain treatment. African Americans, Hispanic Americans, and other patients of racial or ethnic minority heritage receive less pain medication compared to Caucasians across a range of conditions, including cancer pain, acute postoperative pain, chest pain, acute pain presenting in the emergency department, and chronic low back pain (Green, et al., 2003). This disparity may be the result of patient variables such as nociceptive differences, communication processes, or pain behaviors (Green, et al., 2003). In studies of experimentally induced pain, no direct evidence relates biopsychosocial factors to ethnic differences in pain (Reyes-Gibby, et al., 2007). Ethnicity-related differences may exist, however, in willingness to communicate about pain to avoid being stereotyped.

Gender differences in pain exist. Conditions such as fibromyalgia, irritable bowel syndrome, migraines, and temporomandibular joint pain are more prevalent in women than in men (APS, 2007). All patients show an increased physiologic response to pain including heart rate and blood pressure increase. Conditions such as menstrual migraine, a women's pain syndrome, have demonstrated the estrogenic effect of pain (Brandes, 2006). Though considerable attention has been devoted to biological variables such as hormonal influences and genetics, psychological and social factors might also account for gender differences in reporting pain. It is unknown if fundamental, gender-specific differences in basic pain mechanisms exist. A better understanding of the physiological, social, and psychological issues that influence pain is needed.

Nurses need to assess sociocultural variables such as ethnicity, acculturation, and gender that influence pain behavior and expression. They also identify social and contextual variables that may lead to pain disparities among racial and ethnic minorities. For example, the nurse can work closely with the patient and his or her family to identify pain and functional goals that consider the patient's values, resources, and expectations (Green, et al., 2003).

Risk Assessment and Health-Related Patient Teaching

Pain is not a benign experience. It can cause both physical and emotional harm. For nurses caring for patients experiencing pain, adequate treatment is a crucial factor. Acute pain that is not adequately treated can impair pulmonary function, decrease the immune response, and prolong the length of stays in hospitals. For patients with chronic pain, adequate pain management decreases stress and increases the patient's ability to function.

If acute pain is undertreated or untreated, patients are at risk for harder to treat neuropathic pain syndromes, such as CRPS. Continued painful assault on the peripheral nerves results in neuronal plasticity and transfer of the pain stimulus to the central system. These syndromes are very difficult to treat.

Patients who have had surgery or a crush-type of injury are at high risk for developing CRPS. Nurses should be aware that when a patient with such an injury continues to complain of high levels of pain and begins to experience a subsequent loss of function, temperature sensitivity, swelling, or other skin changes (eg, hair loss in the affected area), the patient may be developing CRPS. Nurses should also be alert for the common terms that patients use to report neuropathic pain such as burning, painful tingling, pins and needles, and painful numbness.

Teaching patients about the benefits of controlling pain may help correct misperceptions that some patients have about tolerating pain stoically rather than taking medication to relieve it. Pain has many negative consequences—it is important to help patients understand that reporting pain and treating pain are ways of maintaining a higher level of health and avoiding some chronic pain syndromes. If the patient continues to refuse pain medication, the nurse may consider asking these questions:

• Does the patient have negative biases about taking pain medication?
• Can the patient afford the prescribed medication?
• Are unwanted side effects such as constipation, nausea, or dizzy feelings causing the patient to refuse pain medications?

In some cases, patients can be given antiemetics, laxatives, or dose adjustments that make it easier for them to tolerate pain medications. Above all, if a patient continues to refuse to take pain medication, it is extremely important to understand the root cause of this refusal so that appropriate treatment can take place.

Assessing Pain

Pain is what the patient says it is, and it exists whenever the patient says it does (McAffery & Pasero, 1999). Pain assessment is always subjective. For verbal patients, self-report is the gold standard for assessing pain. Nurses also assess additional pain behaviors, such as grimacing, rocking, or guarding. Increased heart rate and blood pressure are indicators of the physiological response to pain.

Subjective Data Collection

In a basic pain assessment, the nurse asks the patient to rate pain intensity using a simple one-dimensional scale. An example is the numeric pain intensity (NPI) scale with 10 numbers ranked from 0 (no pain) to 10 (worst possible pain). The higher the number, the more severe is the pain.

In addition to pain intensity, other basic elements of a pain assessment are discussed in the following section.

Once you have collected all the data described previously, the most important factor is to accept the patient's rating. It is incumbent on professional nurses to respect the report of pain as patients present them and then act to help relieve the pain. While a nurse may not believe a patient's pain rating, the nurse is obligated to accept the report of pain. The use of in-depth questions to collect all the salient data from the pain assessment will be the biggest help in determining what types of interventions will be most beneficial for providing adequate pain relief to the patient. Using a reliable and valid pain assessment tool can help provide objective criteria for pain assessment.

Questions to Assess Symptoms	Rationales/Abnormal Findings
Location Where is your pain? Ask the patient to point to the painful area. If more than one area is painful, have the patient rate each one separately, and note which area is the most painful.	Note any pain that radiates from the affected area, for example, down the leg with a complaint of low back pain, because such radiation may affect treatment choices.
Duration How long have you had the pain?	This question helps identify onset and duration. Pain for more than 6 months is chronic or persistent.
Intensity How much pain do you have on a 0–10 scale, with 0 being no pain and 10 being the worst possible that you can imagine? • Is the pain worse or better at different times of the day? Does pain medication decrease the intensity?	If the patient cannot use a numeric rating scale, ask the patient if the pain is mild, moderate, or severe. The numbering scale assists in quantifying the pain that the patient is experiencing.
Quality/Description What does your pain feel like? • Describe the quality of the pain. (Allow the patient to describe the pain in his or her own words.) • Is it crampy, gnawing, burning, shooting, sharp, or dull?	Descriptors such as burning, painful numbness, or tingling from patients may alert the nurse to a neuropathic source for the pain.
Alleviating/Aggravating Factors What makes the pain better? What makes it worse? • What methods have you used to manage the pain? Does the application of heat have any effect? • Does a cold pack help relieve any of the pain? • Does activity increase the pain? • Does sitting down make the pain better?	Most patients will try to treat their own pain before they seek health care (DeLuca, 2008).
Pain Management Goal What would be an acceptable level of pain for you? Setting a pain goal is helpful for all patients, but especially for those with chronic pain.	Most patients do not expect to be pain free and are willing to tolerate some discomfort. Ask patients what pain level they think is acceptable, and then tailor interventions to achieve the patient's expectations.
Functional Goal What would you like to be able to do that you can't do because of the pain? (This question is most often used for patients with chronic, persistent pain.) Pain is dynamic and increases with activity (Falla, et al., 2007). • How does the pain interfere with your activities of daily living? • How far can you walk? • Can you care for yourself at home or do you require help? • What does the pain mean to you?	Setting a pain functionality goal with the client allows the nurse to measure the efficacy of pain interventions and adjust the treatment accordingly. Providing maximum pain relief and functionality is the goal of any pain-relief treatment for a patient with chronic pain (Ackley, et al., 2008; ASPMN, 2002; D'Arcy, 2007a; Joint Commission, 2001). Some patients believe that pain is a punishment or worsening of disease.

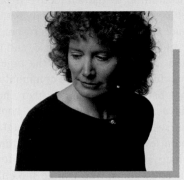

The nurse's role relative to subjective data collection is to gather complete information about the symptoms and to help determine the effectiveness of treatments. Remember Mrs. Bond, who was introduced at the beginning of this chapter. She is 42 years old and was diagnosed with fibromyalgia 5 months ago. Her pain control is less than desired; because this problem is her priority, the nurse will perform a complete assessment. The following conversations give two examples of different questions and different approaches to pain assessment. One style is more effective than the other.

Less Effective

Nurse: Hi, Mrs. Bond. How are you?

Mrs. Bond: Fine, I guess.

Nurse: Good. How's your pain?

Mrs. Bond: My back still hurts.

Nurse: Can you tell me how bad it is?

Mrs. Bond: It seems like it's getting worse instead of better.

Nurse: So if you were to grade it on a 0–10 scale with 10 the worst and 0 at no pain, how would you rate it?

Mrs. Bond: Probably about a 5.

Nurse: What does it feel like—is it sharp or dull?

Mrs. Bond: It's achy.

Nurse: What makes it better or worse?

Mrs. Bond: It's worse when I am tired or stressed out.

Nurse: How does it limit your daily living?

Mrs. Bond: I'm just more tired. I still manage to get things done.

Nurse: So what is your pain goal?

Mrs. Bond: What do you mean?

Nurse: If you used the zero to ten scale again.

Mrs. Bond: Oh, OK. Well I think about a 3.

Nurse: OK, I think that those are all of the questions that I have for you now. Thanks.

More Effective

Nurse: Hi, Mrs. Bond. I see that you were here last month for continued pain. How is that for you today?

Mrs. Bond: It really seems like it's worse instead of better.

Nurse: That must be very frustrating for you. Let's talk a little bit about it. Can you show me where your pain is?

Mrs. Bond: (rubs lower back with her palm) It's here and then it goes down into my bottom and my legs.

Nurse: On a 0–10 scale with 10 being the worst and 0 no pain, how would you rate it?

Mrs. Bond: Probably about a 5.

Nurse: What level of pain would be acceptable to you?

Mrs. Bond: I would be happy with a 3.

Nurse: How would you describe it?

Mrs. Bond: It's an aching pain. In the morning, I'm so stiff that I can hardly get out of bed.

Nurse: Are there other things that you notice with it?

Mrs. Bond: I have trouble sleeping and I just feel tired all of the time.

Nurse: What do you notice makes it worse?

Mrs. Bond: When I'm tired or stressed, it's worse.

Nurse: What makes it better?

Mrs. Bond: If I can get a good night's sleep, it seems better the next day.

Nurse: It seems that being tired is a big part of your pain. How has it influenced your usual activities?

Mrs. Bond: I used to love doing yard work, and I haven't been outside to work for 3 months. I miss that—not the housework, though (laughs)!

Critical Thinking Challenge

- Is there any way to obtain complete information on the pain assessment but shorten the conversation?
- What is the advantage of having Mrs. Bond point to where it hurts first?
- Why is it important to evaluate each item separately rather than combine them, as the less effective nurse did with the alleviating and aggravating factors?
- How does the more effective nurse use listening techniques to help Mrs. Bond to relax?

Objective Data Collection

In addition to the subjective experience of pain, pain has objective effects in other body systems. Acute pain may activate a fight-or-flight stress response in patients. In such an event, blood pressure, pulse, and respirations may increase and the patient will feel the urge to move away from the painful stimulus. These commonly observed responses may not happen with chronic pain, however, because patients have adapted to its ongoing continued stress. Therefore, nurses cannot view a rise in vital signs as an indication of pain level in a patient with chronic pain. They must consider vital signs data in addition to other indicators, because there is no way to isolate the changes with other causes. For example, the patient may be experiencing anxiety for another reason such as fear of needles or a previous bad experience in a health care facility. Assess joints, muscles, the abdomen, and other areas where patients commonly experience pain.

The stress response causes the release of epinephrine, norepinephrine, and cortisol. These hormones have neuroendocrine and metabolic responses. They use stored energy to facilitate the healing of injured tissues. Some effects of these hormones include increases in oxygen consumption, blood glucose and lactate levels, metabolism, and ketones.

Muscle tension may increase; the patient may respond by guarding, or protecting, the affected area. While increased muscle tension helps to protect patients against further pain, chronic tension can contribute to impaired muscle metabolism, muscle atrophy, and delayed return of function.

Inadequately treated pain may contribute to nausea, diaphoresis, and vomiting. Providing pain medication will help alleviate these unwanted effects. Refer to Table 7-1.

In addition to physiological responses, pain manifests with observable behavioral responses. Verbal reports are the most dependable. In patients who cannot verbalize, vocal responses may include moaning or crying. Six pain behaviors indicate pain in patients who cannot verbalize: (1) vocalizations, (2) facial grimacing, (3) bracing, (4) rubbing painful areas, (5) restlessness, and (6) vocal complaints (Feldt, 2000; Feldt, et al., 1998). Many pain assessment tools incorporate the evaluation of these pain behaviors and facilitate accurate detection of pain in various patient populations.

Pain Assessment Tools

Pain tools can be one-dimensional and rate only pain intensity, or multidimensional and include behavioral, affective, and functional domains. Some of the first

Table 7.1	Physiological and Behavioral Pain Indicators
Pain Indicators	**Findings**
Vocalization	Moaning, groaning, grunting, sighing, gasping, crying, screaming
Verbalization	Stated pain, praying, counting, swearing, repeated phrases
Facial expression	Grimacing, clenching teeth, tightly shutting lips, staring, facial mask (flat emotion), wrinkling forehead, tearing
Body actions	Thrashing, pounding, biting, rocking, rubbing, stretching, shrugging, rotating body part, shifting weight
Behaviors	Massaging, immobilizing, guarding, bracing, applying pressure/heat/cold, assuming special position or posture, crossing legs
Neurological	Agitation, restlessness, stillness, irritability, fear, anxiety, fatigue
Cardiac	Tachycardia, increased blood pressure, increased oxygen demand, increased cardiac output
Pulmonary	Hyperventilation with anxiety or hypoventilation with pain, shallow respirations, hypoxia, depressed cough, atelectasis
Gastrointestinal	Nausea, vomiting, decreased bowel tones, stress ulcer
Genitourinary	Reduced urine output, urinary retention
Musculoskeletal	Muscle tension, spasm, joint stiffness, immobility
Skin	Pallor, diaphoresis
Metabolic	Increased catabolism, increased glucose, increased lactate and ketones, impaired immune function, impaired wound healing
Emotional	Depression, excessive sleeping, anxiety, fear, impaired individual or family coping
Social	Isolation, impaired role performance, impaired home maintenance, financial burden if unable to work

multidimensional pain assessment tools were developed for assessing experimentally induced pain, chronic pain, and oncology pain and provide a more comprehensive pain assessment.

One-Dimensional Pain Scales

One-dimensional pain assessment tools measure one element of the pain experience—intensity. Although these tools seem simple and the data they allow examiners to gather are limited, single-item ratings of pain intensity are valid and reliable indicators of pain intensity (Victor, et al., 2008). These scales also help health care providers identify the effects of administered medications on pain intensity. A 2-point or 30% reduction in pain intensity on the NPI scale is a clinically significant improvement in pain level (Farrar, et al., 2001).

Visual Analog Scale (VAS).
The VAS is a 100-mm line with "no pain" at one end and "worst possible pain" at the other end. When using this scale, the nurse asks the patient to mark on the line the intensity of the pain he or she is experiencing. If the patient marks the line at 70 mm, the nurse would note the pain level as 7/10.

This tool is one of the simplest and most basic one-dimensional pain scales. Limitations to the VAS include that some older adults have difficulty marking on the line and place the mark above or below 100 mm (D'Arcy, 2003; Herr & Mobily, 1993).

Verbal Descriptor Scale (VDS).
The VDS uses words such as "mild," "moderate," and "severe" to measure pain intensity. It asks patients to select the word or phrase that best describes their pain. Some patients prefer to use words rather than a number to rate their pain. Limitations to the VDS include that the patient must be able to understand the meaning of the words.

Numeric Pain Intensity Scale (NPI).
The NPI is the most commonly used one-dimensional pain scale (Fig. 7-4). In this 11-point Likert-type scale, 0 means "no pain" and 10 means "worst possible pain." The NPI asks patients to select the number that best fits their pain intensity—the higher the score, the more intense the pain.

In general:

- **Mild pain** is considered in the 1 to 3 range.
- **Moderate pain** is considered in the 4 to 6 range.
- **Severe pain** is considered in the 7 to 10 range.

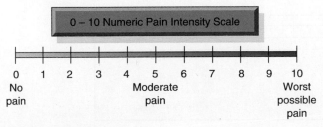

Figure 7.4 NPI scale.

Combined Thermometer Scale.
The combined thermometer scale combines the VDS and the NPI (Fig. 7-5). Some patients respond well to this scale and like its vertical orientation, with numbers that increase from the bottom up.

Multidimensional Pain Scales

Multidimensional scales are also available for the assessment of chronic pain, malignant pain, or complex medical-surgical pain conditions. Figure 7.6 shows an example. Two other commonly used scales are the McGill Pain Questionnaire (MPQ) and the Brief Pain Inventory (BPI). Both have a combination of indices that measure pain intensity, mood, pain location (via body diagram), verbal descriptors, and questions about medication efficacy. They are most often used for research or with patients who are being actively treated for pain over an extended period.

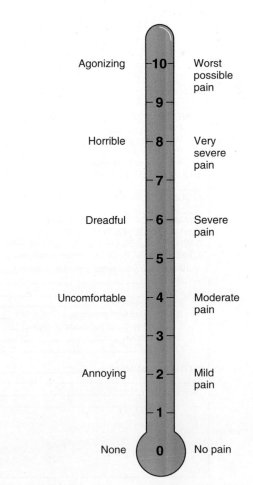

Figure 7.5 Pain distress intensity scale.

McGill Pain Questionnaire (MPQ). The MPQ was developed to measure pain in experimentally induced circumstances, following procedures, and with several medical-surgical conditions. It consists of a set of verbal descriptors used to capture the sensory aspect of pain, a VAS scale, and a present pain intensity rating made up of words and numbers. The tool has been found reliable and valid, and has been translated into several languages (McDonald & Weiskopf, 2001; Melzack, 1975, 1987; Mystakidou, et al., 2004). Limitations include scoring and weighting the verbal descriptor section and difficulty translating the verbal descriptor section into words that indicate syndromes.

Brief Pain Inventory. The BPI was first developed to measure pain in patients with cancer; however, it also has reliability and validity for assessing pain in patients with chronic nonmalignant pain (Daut, et al., 1983; Raichle, et al., 2006; Tan, et al., 2004; Williams, et al., 2006), and has been translated into various languages (Hølen, et al., 2008; Mystakidou et al., 2004). The tool can be administered either through an interview or in a self-report format completed by the patient. The BPI consists of a pain intensity scale, a body diagram to locate the pain, a functional assessment (general activity, mood, walking, employment, housework, relationships, sleep, and enjoyment of life), and questions about the efficacy of pain medications (Fig. 7-7). Limitations

Date ____________

Patient's name ______________________ Age ______ Room ____________

Diagnosis ______________________ Physician ____________

Nurse ____________

1. LOCATION: Patient or nurse marks drawing.

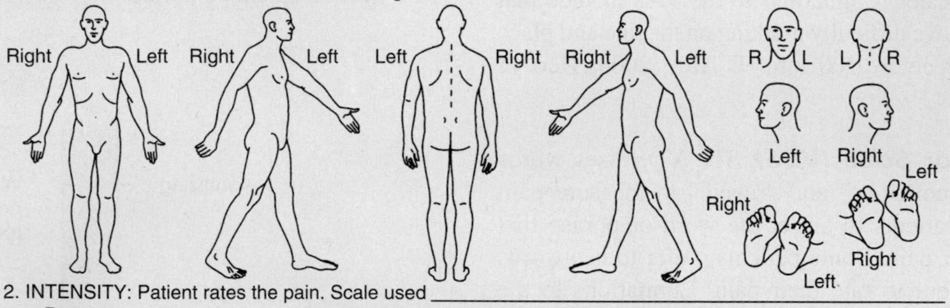

2. INTENSITY: Patient rates the pain. Scale used ____________
   Present: ____________
   Worst pain gets: ____________
   Best pain gets: ____________
   Acceptable level of pain: ____________
3. QUALITY: (Use patient's own words, e.g., prick, ache, burn, throb, pull, sharp) ____________
4. ONSET, DURATION, VARIATION, RHYTHMS: ____________
5. MANNER OF EXPRESSING PAIN: ____________
6. WHAT RELIEVES THE PAIN? ____________
7. WHAT CAUSES OR INCREASES THE PAIN? ____________
8. EFFECTS OF PAIN: (Note decreased function, decreased quality of life.)
   Accompanying symptoms (e.g., nausea) ____________
   Sleep ____________
   Appetite ____________
   Physical activity ____________
   Relationship with others (e.g., irritability) ____________
   Emotions (e.g., anger, suicidal, crying) ____________
   Concentration ____________
   Other ____________
9. OTHER COMMENTS: ____________
10. PLAN: ____________

Figure 7.6 Sample multidimensional pain assessment tool.

_____
DO NOT WRITE ABOVE THIS LINE

Brief Pain Inventory (Short Form)

Date: _____ / _____ / _____   Time: _____

Name: _____ _____ _____
              Last   First   Middle Initial

1. Throughout our lives, most of us have had pain from time to time (such as minor headaches, sprains, and toothaches). Have you had pain other than these everyday kinds of pain today?

1. Yes   2. No

2. On the diagram, shade in the areas where you feel pain. Put an X on the area that hurts the most.

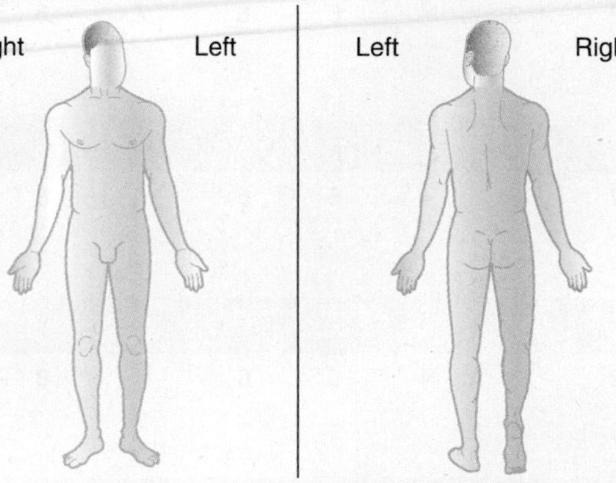

| Right | Left | Left | Right |

3. Please rate your pain by circling the one number that best describes your pain at its **worst** in the last 24 hours.

0   1   2   3   4   5   6   7   8   9   10

No   Pain as bad as
pain   you can imagine

4. Please rate your pain by circling the one number that best describes your pain at its **least** in the last 24 hours.

0   1   2   3   4   5   6   7   8   9   10

No   Pain as bad as
pain   you can imagine

5. Please rate your pain by circling the one number that best describes your pain on the **average.**

0   1   2   3   4   5   6   7   8   9   10

No   Pain as bad as
pain   you can imagine

6. Please rate your pain by circling the one number that tells how much pain you have **right now.**

0   1   2   3   4   5   6   7   8   9   10

No   Pain as bad as
pain   you can imagine

Figure 7.7 Brief Pain Inventory.

7. What treatments or medications are you receiving for your pain?

8. In the last 24 hours, how much relief have pain treatments or medications provided? Please circle the one percentage that most shows how much **relief** you have received.

0%	10%	20%	30%	40%	50%	60%	70%	80%	90%	100%

No relief   Complete relief

9. Circle the one number that describes how, during the past 24 hours, pain has interfered with your:

A. General Activity

0	1	2	3	4	5	6	7	8	9	10

Does not interfere   Completely interferes

B. Mood

0	1	2	3	4	5	6	7	8	9	10

Does not interfere   Completely interferes

C. Walking Ability

0	1	2	3	4	5	6	7	8	9	10

Does not interfere   Completely interferes

D. Normal Work (includes both work outside the home and housework)

0	1	2	3	4	5	6	7	8	9	10

Does not interfere   Completely interferes

E. Relations With Other People

0	1	2	3	4	5	6	7	8	9	10

Does not interfere   Completely interferes

F. Sleep

0	1	2	3	4	5	6	7	8	9	10

Does not interfere   Completely interferes

G. Enjoyment of Life

0	1	2	3	4	5	6	7	8	9	10

Does not interfere   Completely interferes

Figure 7.7 (*Continued*)

of the BPI include that the patient must be able to correlate the questions to their individual pain experience using the various scales.

Brief Pain Impact Questionnaire (BPIQ). Another way to assess pain quickly in patients with chronic pain is to use a set of structured questions, such as those in the BPIQ:

- How strong is your pain, right now, worst/average over the past week?
- How many days over the past week have you been unable to do what you would like to do because of your pain?
- Over the past week, how often has pain interfered with your ability to take care of yourself, for example, with bathing, eating, dressing, and going to the toilet?
- Over the past week, how often has pain interfered with your ability to take care of your home-related chores such as grocery shopping, preparing meals, paying bills, and driving?
- How often do you participate in pleasurable activities such as hobbies, socializing with friends, and travel? Over the past week, how often has pain interfered with these activities?
- How often do you do some type of exercise? Over the past week, how often has pain interfered with your ability to exercise?
- Does pain interfere with your ability to think clearly?
- Does pain interfere with your appetite? Have you lost weight?
- Does pain interfere with your sleep? How often over the last week?
- Has pain interfered with your energy, mood, personality, or relationships with other people?
- Over the past week, have you taken pain medications?
- Has your use of alcohol or other drugs ever caused a problem for you or those close to you?
- How would you rate your health at the present time? (Weiner, et al., 2002).

These questions capture the major elements of pain assessment for patients with chronic pain and are easy to use in the clinical setting. They assist in identifying the effects of pain on the patient's functional abilities and daily life so that the nurse can fully appreciate a holistic perspective on the patient's pain experience.

 Lifespan Considerations

In several patient populations, pain assessment poses significant challenges. Examples include children and older adults. These patients all have a need for adequate pain relief, yet the assessment process can be difficult.

Newborns, Infants, and Children

Assessment of pain in children is complex and challenging. The best practice is to consistently use a scale specific to the patient's age. Pain scales have been developed that are specific to infants and children. Infants in pain may exhibit brow bulge, eye squeeze, nasolabial fold, open lips, stretched mouth, lip purse, taut tongue, chin quiver, and tongue protrusion (Grunau, et al., 1998). The difficulty with these behavioral measures is that they do not discriminate between pain behaviors and reactions from other sources of discomfort, such as hunger. The nurse should assume that if a condition or procedure is painful for an adult, it is also painful for an infant or child.

Infants and children may exhibit physiological responses to pain including increased heart rate, respiratory rate, blood pressure, palmar sweating, cortisone levels, oxygen, vagal tone, and endorphin levels. Because the preverbal infant cannot self-report pain, the nurse relies on these physiological and behavioral indicators.

The two most common tools used to assess pain in children are the Face, Legs, Activity, Cry, Consolability (FLACC) scale and the FACES pain scale. The FLACC scale was originally designed to measure acute postoperative pain in children 2 months to 7 years old. It uses the indicators of facial expression, leg movement, activity, cry, and ability to console the patient. Behaviors include frowning, kicking, arched back, crying, and difficulty consoling. The tool has established reliability and validity.

Children 2 years and older can identify pain and point to its location. Nurses can use a facial expression scale for children starting at approximately 3 years. The FACES scale (Fig. 7-8) uses six faces ranging from happy with a wide smile to sad with tears on the face. The nurse asks

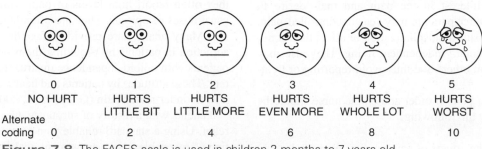

Figure 7.8 The FACES scale is used in children 2 months to 7 years old.

the child to pick the face that best represents the pain he or she is experiencing. FACE zero is very happy because there is "no hurt"; FACE five hurts "as bad as you can imagine." The nurse points to each face, explains the pain intensity, asks the child to choose the FACE that best describes his or her own pain, and records the appropriate number. The young child's thinking is concrete and egocentric, so it is important to use vocabulary such as "no hurt" or "biggest hurt" for the scale. The nurse can also talk with the caregiver to learn vocabulary that the child uses at home to describe pain, such as "owie" or "ouchie." The FACES scale has been tested with concurrent validity established (Wong & DiVito-Thomas, 2006). The scale has also been used to measure pain intensity with children of different ethnicities and with cognitively impaired adults (Wong & DiVito-Thomas, 2006).

Starting between 7 and 10 years, children can use numeric rating scales used with adults. Use of a color-coded scale, such as the combined thermometer, may be helpful (see Fig. 7-5). Additionally, with this scale the child can specify location and quality. He or she might describe the pain experience as horrible, terrible, terrifying, or stabbing.

Pain also affects children in the affective and sensory dimensions. Children may have reduced sleep, appetite, and fitness level, all of which can affect both school and play. Pain can disturb mood, leading to emotional distress, depression, and anxiety. It also can disrupt family functioning and make the child fearful for the future (Eccleston, et al., 2006). An accurate assessment is essential for adequate treatment.

Older Adults

Older patients have some specific circumstances that can lead to problems with pain assessment. Many older patients have chronic illnesses such as osteoarthritis or diabetes that cause pain. Although pain is prevalent in older patients, some of them see pain as just part of natural aging. They may be reluctant to report pain, because they want their providers to consider them "good patients," or they may fear that complaints of pain may lead to costly tests or expensive medications that they cannot afford. The older person may hide expressions of pain and be stoic. Although experiencing pain, their outward reaction to it may hide their discomfort.

When assessing pain in older adults, nurses reassure patients of their interest in the pain and their desire to help manage it. Older patients may fear uncontrolled pain, because it could result in hospitalization or affect their long-term ability to maintain independent living. They also may fear dependency on others and thus avoid reporting or treating pain.

When assessing pain in older adults, the nurse should be sure to also review the following:

• Question about the effects of pain on diet, sleep, and mood. Unrelieved pain may lead to insomnia or depression and seriously affect the patient's quality of life.

• Ask about any comorbidities such as osteoarthritis that may cause pain or have an influence on medication choices.
• Review all medications that the patient is taking, including vitamins and herbal supplements. Older patients may not take medications as ordered or refuse to take drugs that cause side effects such as sedation or constipation.

Assessment of pain leading to effective treatment can improve the quality of life for older adults. Providing adequate pain management for them can occur through care and reassurance and by taking the time to assess pain accurately.

Special Situations

Patients Unable to Report Pain
The Joint Commission instituted pain management guidelines in 2001 that mandated the assessment of pain for all patients. Self-report is the most reliable indicator of pain, but many patients cannot verbally communicate this information. The development of behavioral tools for assessing pain in nonverbal patients is the newest area of pain assessment and a developing science.

When attempting to perform a pain assessment on a patient who cannot self-report pain:

• Attempt a self-report of pain.
• Try to identify any potential causes for pain.
• Observe patient behaviors.
• Ask the family or other caregivers if they have noticed any changes in behavior.
• Attempt an analgesic trial (Herr, et al., 2006b).

Patients With Opioid Tolerance
Patients with a history of opioid tolerance pose difficult challenges to nurses for pain assessment (Jage, 2005). They have an altered physiologic response to the pain stimulus, and the repeated use of opioids causes their bodies to become more sensitive to pain. This sensitivity is called **opioid hyperalgesia** and can occur as soon as 1 month after opioid use begins.

Not only are patients with opioid tolerance more sensitive to pain, they face a high level of bias from health care providers. Because these patients are more sensitive to pain, they often report high levels of pain with little relief from usual doses of opioids. They are often labeled as drug seeking. Many health care providers fear that they will induce addiction in patients by providing them with opioids. Many patients with opioid dependence mistrust the health care system. These attitudes by patients and health care providers can lead to undertreated pain (Grant, et al., 2007).

Patients with a history of substance use are entitled to pain relief. Using a standard reliable pain assessment tool and setting a reasonable pain management goal can help avoid misunderstanding and undertreatment of pain in this group of patients.

Table 7.2   Common Nursing Diagnoses Associated with Pain

Diagnosis and Related Factors	Point of Differentiation	Assessment Characteristics	Nursing Interventions
Acute pain related to actual or potential tissue injury	Sudden and/or severe pain lasting from 1 second to 6 months	Self-report of pain; increased P, BP, R; diaphoresis; guarded position; crying; moaning; nausea; facial grimace	Administer ordered pain medication.* Assess effectiveness of medication. Promote factors that increase pain tolerance (music, distraction). Reduce factors that increase pain, relaxation, breathing, distraction.
Chronic pain	Pain that lasts more than 6 months	Self-report of pain, discomfort, facial mask, weight loss, depression, insomnia, frequent position changes	Assess pain experience and effect on life. Evaluate depression. Collaborate on methods to reduce pain intensity such as relaxation and breathing, pain medication.* Evaluate side effects of medications.

*Collaborative interventions.

Nursing Diagnoses, Outcomes, and Interventions

The nurse assesses the patient's pain level in the initial pain assessment and uses specialized pain tools if indicated. Using the assessment data, the nurse incorporates critical thinking to establish a nursing problem or diagnosis list. Table 7-2 compares two sets of nursing diagnoses, abnormal findings, and interventions commonly related to pain (Johnson, et al., 2005). The assessment data are the basis for the care provided to relieve acute or chronic pain.

Reassessing and Documenting Pain

The Joint Commission has set a standard that states that nurses must assess and reassess pain regularly. Most hospitals set their own standards for assessment such as every shift or every 4 or 6 hours depending on the specific practice area and needs of the patient.

Reassessing pain is similar to reassessing a patient taking blood pressure medication or a patient with diabetes who needs regular blood glucose level testing. For patients taking pain medication, reassessment provides a reliable measure of the drug's efficacy. It allows the nurse to see if pain intensity has decreased since administration—much as blood pressure should be lower once a patient takes blood pressure medication. Most hospitals have a standard time frame for reassessment, such as 1 hour for oral medication and 30 minutes for pain medication given intravenously. They base these time frames on the time it takes a pain medication to provide a noticeable decrease in pain intensity.

Health care facilities are shifting from paper documentation to computerized systems to enter nursing data (see Chapter 5). Figure 7-9 shows examples of documentation of pain intensity for (A) shift assessment and (B) medication administration reassessment. Nurses are legally accountable for the quality of their pain management, including assessment, treatment, and reassessment (Camp & O'Sullivan, 1987).

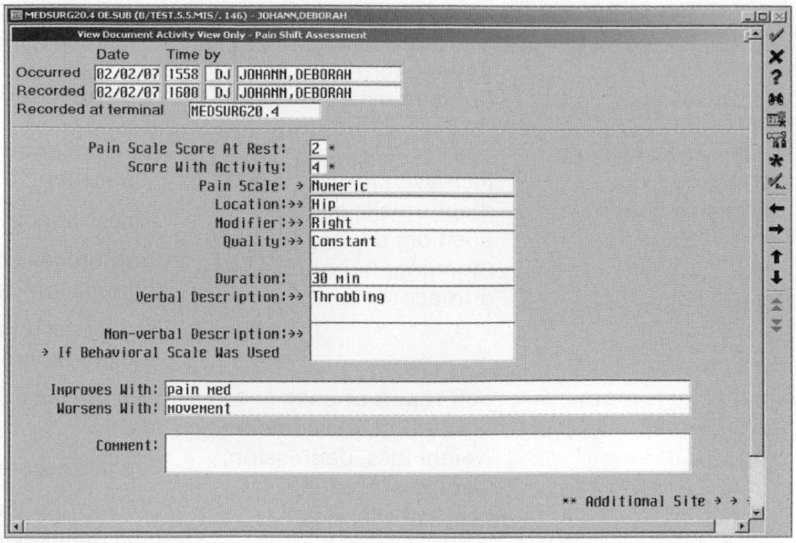

Key:
- Questions with (→) indicate a group reponse is available.
- (→ →) indicates group response with option to write in.
- Questions without an arrow are free text.
- If pain score at rest is elevated, a consult is sent to the Pain Nurse and a care plan is Query linked
- A second page of this intervention is the same as the first, just allowing the RN to document to a site.

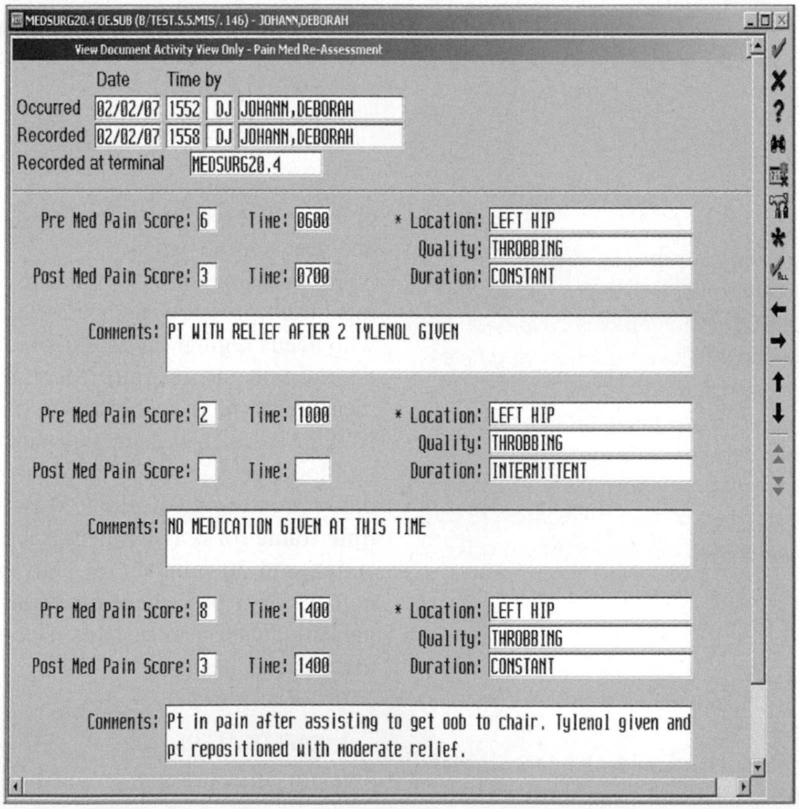

Figure 7.9 A. Example of an electronic pain shift assessment (done every shift). **B.** Example of a post pain medication assessment, completed after medication is given; can have multiple entries.

Barriers to Pain Assessment

Prejudices and bias related to educational, family, or cultural values can affect how nurses perceive the patient's self-report of pain. Studies have shown that nurses have difficulty accepting the patient's report of pain as valid and credible (Berry, et al., 2006; D'Arcy, 2008; Donovan, et al., 1987; Drayer, et al., 1999). It is important to recognize the issues surrounding bias and prejudice and work to minimize their effect on pain management.

When a pain assessment is inaccurate or poor, patients suffer because of incorrect medication and treatment choices. Fear of respiratory depression and addiction affect pain assessment and management (Apfelbaum, et al., 2003; Choiniere, et al., 1990; Donovan, et al., 1987). Focusing on pain relief as the primary end to the assessment process and treatment selection will help control fears and bias that can negatively affect patient care.

⚠ SAFETY ALERT 7.3

Respiratory depression is a side effect of opioid administration. It is essential to observe for side effects and hold the medication if there is evidence of respiratory depression and increasing sedation.

Evidence-Based Critical Thinking

The nurse is responsible for assessing pain and negotiating pain and functional goals with the patient. Based upon those goals, the nurse implements pharmacologic and nonpharmacological interventions. He or she documents the assessment, analysis, interventions, and reassessment in the patient record. Additionally, the nurse may identify pain as a priority problem and consider its broader effects on sleep, activities, and mood. The nurse can analyze and document this information in a SOAP (subjectives, objective, analysis, plan) note that shows this critical thinking.

Analyzing Findings

Remember Mrs. Bond, who was recently diagnosed with fibromyalgia. The nurse has completed the initial data collection, set goals with her, and established a plan of care. The following nursing note illustrates the documentation of subjective and objective data.

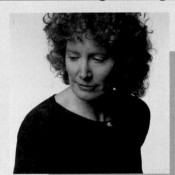

Subjective: States that the pain is getting worse instead of better. Located in lower back and radiates into buttocks and legs. Rates it 5 on a 0–10 scale. Has been present for 5 months since her diagnosis. Described as an achy pain with increased stiffness in the morning. Being tired or stressed out aggravates it. Being well rested alleviates pain. Able to perform functional activities with more effort except that she has not done yard work. Pain goal stated at 3.

Objective: Slightly overweight, appears older than her age. Facial expression fatigued with dark circles under her eyes. Posture slightly slouched in chair, shifting from side to side frequently. Affect flat. Dress appropriate to weather, well groomed. T 37°C, P 112 beats/min, R 20 breaths/min, BP 142/88 mm Hg.

Analysis: Chronic pain related to fibromyalgia.

Plan: Communicate findings to health care provider. Provide patient education on medications and side effects. Discuss ways that patient can get some mild exercise 3–5 times weekly. Evaluate sleep hygiene and recommend routines that promote sleep. Discuss ways that she can make household tasks more efficient to save energy for enjoyable activities, possibly including some light gardening. Provide information about support group for patients with fibromyalgia.

B. Zomas, RN

Critical Thinking Challenge

- Is subjective or objective data collection the higher priority when assessing Mrs. Bond's pain?
- What techniques of physical assessment might the nurse use when assessing Mrs. Bond?
- How do assessments from the general survey cluster with the pain assessment?

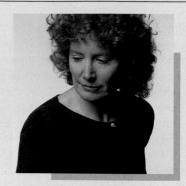

In many facilities, nurses initiate referrals based on assessment findings. In this case, the health care provider ordered a referral to the pain team because Mrs. Bond's pain is not responsive to traditional medical treatment. The nurse communicates the reason for the consult using the following SBAR format. Other results that might trigger a pain consult include history of chronic pain, regular use of opioids for more than 3 months, substance abuse, difficult pain management, patient dissatisfaction with pain relief, high dose requirements, or significant side effects related to pain management.

The following conversation illustrates how the nurse organizes the information to provide necessary details about Mrs. Bond to the pain relief service.

Situation: Hi, this is Belinda and I've been talking with Mrs. Bond about her pain management in the clinic today.

Background: She's 42 years old and was diagnosed with fibromyalgia about 5 months ago. We've been seeing her to help manage her pain. She currently is taking a selective serotonin reuptake inhibitor for depression, benzodiazepine for muscle spasm, and central analgesic for pain.

Assessment: She's reporting a pain level of 5 and really would like to be down to about a 3. Mostly, it's an achy pain that is in her lower back and radiates into her buttocks and legs, the fairly typical type of fibromyalgia pain. She appears to be fatigued and a little depressed and is having difficulty sleeping.

Recommendations: We would like you to see her to see if you have any suggestions about a different medication dose or combination. She's been very patient in working with us on this, and we would like to get something that works for her. She said that she could wait about a half an hour now, or come back to see you for another appointment.

Critical Thinking Challenge

- At what point would you decide to contact other health care providers for more pain medication?
- What is the role of the nurse in working with the pain consult team?
- What parts of the pain treatment are within the nursing domain? Which are within collaborative practice?

Pain is a complex syndrome that involves an accurate and complete assessment. Pain is often a subjective symptom, although there are objective signs of its presence. Many pain tools have been developed for different populations. Pain assessment and its treatment is primarily within the role of nursing practice.

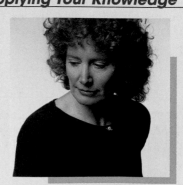

Now that you have completed the reading and case features for this chapter, consider Mrs. Bond's case and its relationship to what you are learning. Answer the following questions.

- What is the role of the nurse when assessing Mrs. Bond's pain?
- What subjective information will the nurse gather during today's assessment? What pain tools would be most appropriate?
- What objective data will the nurse assess during the history and interview?
- How will the nurse reassess the effectiveness of interventions?
- What other associated findings would the nurse assess when considering Mrs. Bond's pain?

Key Points

- Pain can result from various stimuli transmitted via the peripheral nervous system to the central nervous system for processing.
- Pain can be musculoskeletal or neuropathic, depending on the source of the pain stimulus.
- Verbal descriptors that patients use include burning, tingling. Painful numbness or tingling is associated with neuropathic pain.
- A decrease of three points on the NPI scale is considered clinically significant.
- When assessing pain, nurses should use scales designed for the specific population to which the patient belongs (eg, children).
- Patients with chronic pain need more than just a pain intensity rating and require use of a multidimensional scale such as the BPI.
- Nurses must believe the patient's report of pain.
- Avoidance of labeling and stigmatization is important for patients who are dependent on pain medications to control their pain.
- Nurses should always assess a patient's pain. If the patient is nonverbal, the nurse can use a behavioral pain scale designed to identify pain in that particular population.
- Nurses must be aware of the legal implications of pain assessment. Not documenting an assessment means it has not been done.
- Reassessing pain can provide a means of determining the efficacy of an administered pain medication.

Review Questions

1. The patient has pain of a short duration with an identifiable cause. This is referred to as
   A. acute pain
   B. chronic pain
   C. neuropathic pain
   D. complex pain

2. To identify the location of pain, the nurse asks the patient
   A. how long he or she has had the pain
   B. to rate the intensity of the pain on a scale from 0 to 10
   C. to point to the painful area
   D. to describe the quality of pain

3. A patient says that his pain worsens with weight-bearing activity. The nurse would consider this
   A. an alleviating factor
   B. a functional pain goal
   C. quality/description
   D. an aggravating factor

4. Which of the following tools would a nurse use to perform a multidimensional pain assessment?
   A. Visual analog
   B. BPI
   C. NPI
   D. Verbal descriptor

5. For what circumstance would the nurse be most likely to assess pain using the MPQ?
   A. Verbal description
   B. Alleviating factors
   C. Functional status goal
   D. Pain goal

6. Which of the following indicators would be most likely to signify to the nurse that a patient is having pain?
   A. Falling asleep
   B. Rubbing a body part
   C. Relaxed body position
   D. Facial relaxation

7. A patient reports pain, depression, and insomnia. The nurse observes a masklike facial expression and frequent position changes. Which of the following is the nurse most likely to use to describe the patient's findings?
   A. Acute pain
   B. Chronic pain
   C. Neuropathic pain
   D. CRPS

8. With which of the following types of patients is the nurse most likely to use the FACES pain scale?
   A. Children
   B. Patients with dementia
   C. Older adults
   D. Unconscious patients

9. Which of the following is the rationale for the nurse to reassess the patient's pain after treatment?
   A. To pinpoint the pain's location
   B. To measure the pain's duration
   C. To establish the efficacy of medication
   D. To make changes to the patient's pain goal

10. Barriers to pain assessment include that nurses
    A. believe that patients suffer if undermedicated
    B. focus on pain relief as a primary end to the assessment process
    C. choose treatment that will positively affect the patient care
    D. have difficulty accepting the patient's self-report as valid

References

Ackley, B., Ladwig, G., Swan, B. A., & Tucker, S. J. (2008). *Evidence-based nursing care guidelines.* St. Louis: Mosby Elsevier.

AGS. (2002). The management of persistent pain in older persons—The American Geriatric Society Panel on Persistent Pain in Older Persons. *Journal of the American Geriatrics Society, 50*(6), 205–224.

APS. (2003). *Principles of analgesic use in the treatment of acute and cancer pain* (5th ed.). Glenview, IL: Author.

APS. (2007). Are basic pain mechanisms different in women than in men? Retrieved April 20, 2008, from http://www.ampainsoc.org/enews/sept07/.

ASPMN. (2002). *Core curriculum for pain management nursing.* Philadelphia: Saunders.

Anand, K. J. (2007). Pain assessment in preterm neonates. *Pediatrics, 119*(3), 605–607.

Apfelbaum, J., Chen, C., Mehtam, S., & Tong, G. (2003). Postoperative pain experience: Results from a national survey suggest postoperative pain continues to be undermanaged. *Anesthesia and Analgesia, 97*(2), 534–540.

Astuto, M., Rosano, G., Rizzo, G., et al. (2007). Methodologies for the treatment of acute and chronic nononcologic pain in children. *Edizioni Minerva Anestesiologica, 73*(9), 459–465.

Bennett, M., Attal, N., Backonja, M., et al. (2007). Using screening tools to identify neuropathic pain. *Pain, 127*(3), 199–203.

Berry, P. H., Covington, E., Dahl, J., Katz, J., & Miaskowski, C. (2006). *Pain: Current understanding of assessment, management, and treatments.* Reston, VA: National Pharmaceutical Council, Inc and the Joint Commission on Accreditation of Healthcare Organizations.

Brandes, J. L. (2006). The influence of estrogen on migraine. *Journal of the American Medical Society, 295*(15), 1824–1830.

Camp, L. D., & O'Sullivan, P. (1987). Comparison of medical, surgical, and oncology patients' descriptions of pain and nurses' documentation of pain assessments. *Journal of Advanced Nursing, 12*, 593–598.

Cervero, F. (2005). The gate control theory, then and now in the paths of pain. In H. Mersky, J. Loeser, & R. Dubner (Eds.), *The paths of pain.* Seattle, WA: IASP Press.

Choiniere, M., Melzack, R., Girard, N., et al. (1989). Comparisons between patients' and nurses' assessment of pain and medication efficacy in severe burn injuries. *Pain, 40*, 143–152.

Cipher, D. J., Clifford, P. A., & Roper, K. D. (2006). Behavioral manifestations of pain in the demented elderly. *Journal of the American Medical Directors Association, 7*(6), 355–365.

D'Arcy, Y. M. (2003). Pain assessment. In P. Iyer (Ed.), *Medical-legal aspects of pain and suffering.* Tucson, AZ: Lawyers and Judges Publishing Company.

D'Arcy, Y. (2007a). *Pain management: Evidence-based tools and techniques for nursing professionals.* Marblehead, MA: HcPro.

D'Arcy, Y. (2007b). What's the diagnosis? *The American Nurse Today, 1*(4), 29–30.

D'Arcy, Y. (2008). Pain management survey report. *Nursing, 38*(6), 42–49; quiz 49–51.

Daut, R. L., Cleeland, C. S., & Flannery, R. (1983). Development of the Wisconsin Brief Pain Questionnaire to assess pain in cancer or other diseases. *Pain, 17*, 197–210.

DeLuca, (2008). Why chronic pain is a medical emergency. Retrieved May 17, 2010, from http://doctordeluca.com/wordpress/archive/chronic-pain-is-a-medical-emergency/

Donovan, M., Dillon, P., & McGuire, L. (1987). Incidence and characteristics of pain in a sample of medical, surgical inpatients. *Pain, 30*, 69–78.

Drayer, R. A., Henderson, J., & Reidenberg, M. (1999). Barriers to better pain control in hospitalized patients. *Journal of Pain and Symptom Management, 17*(6), 434–440.

Eccleston, C., Bruce, E., & Carter, B. (2006). Chronic pain in children and adolescents. *Paediatric Nursing, 18*(10), 30–33.

Falla, D., Farina, D., Dahl, M. K., & Graven-Nielsen, T. (2007). Muscle pain induces task-dependent changes in cervical agonist/antagonist activity. *Journal of Applied Physiology, 102*(2), 601–609.

Farrar, J. T., Young, J. P., Lamoreaux, L., Werth, J. L., & Poole, R. M. (2001). Clinical importance of changes in chronic pain intensity measured on an 11 point numerical pain rating scale. *Pain, 94*, 149–158.

Feldt, K. S. (2000). The checklist of non-verbal pain indicators (CNPI). *Pain Management Nursing, 1*(1), 13–21.

Feldt, K. S., Ryden, M. B., & Miles, S. (1998). Treatment of pain in cognitively impaired compared with cognitively intact older patients with hip fractures. *Journal of the American Geriatrics Society, 46*, 1079–1085.

Grant, M. S., Cordts, G. A., & Doberman, D. J. (2007). Acute pain management in hospitalized patients with current opioid abuse. *Topics in Advanced Practice Nursing.* Retrieved August 6, 2008, from http://www.medscape.com/viewarticle/557043.

Green, C. R., Anderson, K. O., Baker, T. A., et al. (2003). The unequal burden of pain: Confronting racial and ethnic disparities in pain. *Pain Medicine, 4*(3), 277–294.

Grunau, R. V. E., Oberlander, T. F., Holsti, L., et al. (1998). Bedside application of the Neonatal Facial Coding System in pain assessment of premature neonates. *Pain, 76*, 277–286.

Herr, K., Bjoro, K., & Decker, S. (2006b). Tools for assessment of pain in nonverbal older adults with dementia: A state-of-the-science review. *Journal of Pain and Symptom Management, 31*(2), 170–192.

Herr, K., Coyne, P., Key, T., et al. (2006a). Pain assessment in the nonverbal patient: Position statement with clinical practice recommendations. *Pain Management Nursing, 7*(2), 44–52.

Herr, K. A., & Mobily, P. (1993). Comparison of selected pain assessment tools for use with the elderly. *Applied Nursing Research, 6*(1), 39–46.

Hølen, J. C., Lydersen, S., Klepstad, P., et al. (2008). The Brief Pain Inventory: Pain's interference with functions is different in cancer pain compared with noncancer chronic pain. *Clinical Journal of Pain, 24*(3), 219–225.

Jage, J. (2005). Opioid tolerance and dependence—do they matter? *European Journal of Pain, 9*(2), 157–162.

Johnson, M., Bulechek, G. M., McCloskey Dochterman, J., Maas, M. L. (2005). *NANDA, NOC, and NIC linkages: Nursing diagnoses, outcomes, and interventions.* St. Louis: Mosby.

Joint Commission on Accreditation of Healthcare Organizations. (2001). *Pain assessment and management: An organizational approach.* Oakbrook Terrace, IL: Author.

Linton, A., & Lach, H. (2007). *Matteson & McConnells' gerontological nursing concepts and practice* (3rd ed.). St. Louis, MO: Saunders, Elsevier.

McAffery, M., & Pasero, C. (1999). *Pain: Clinical manual* (2nd ed.). St. Louis: Mosby.

McDonald, D. D., & Weiskopf, C. S. A. (2001). Adult patients' postoperative pain descriptions and responses to the Short Form

McGill Pain Questionnaire. *Clinical Nursing Research, 10*(4), 442–452.

Melzack, R. (1975). The McGill Pain Questionnaire: Major properties and scoring methods. *Pain, 1,* 277–299.

Melzack, R. (1987). The short form McGill Pain Questionnaire. *Pain, 30,* 191–197.

Melzack, R., & Wall, P. (1975). Pain mechanisms: A new theory. *Science, 150*(699), 971–979.

Mersky, H., Loeser, J., & Dubner, R. (Eds.) (2005). *The paths of pain.* Seattle, WA: IASP Press.

Munce, S. E., Stansfeld, S. A., Blackmore, E. R., & Stewart, D. E. (2007). The role of depression and chronic pain conditions in absenteeism: Results from a national epidemiologic survey. *Journal of Occupational and Environmental Medicine, 49*(11), 1206–1211.

Mystakidou, K., Cleeland, C., Tsilika, E., et al. (2004). Greek M.D. Anderson Symptom Inventory: Validation and utility in cancer patients. *Oncology, 67*(3–4), 203–210.

Purves, D., et al. (2004). *Neuroscience.* Massachusetts: Sinauer Associates, Inc.

Raichle, K. A., Osborne, T. L., Jensen, M. P., & Cardenas, D. (2006). The reliability and validity of pain interference measures in persons with spinal cord injury. *Journal of Pain, 7*(3), 179–186.

Reyes-Gibby, C. C., Aday, L. A., Todd, K. H., et al. (2007). Pain in aging community-dwelling adults in the United States: Non-Hispanic Whites, Non-Hispanic Blacks, and Hispanics. *Journal of Pain, 8*(1), 75–84.

Rowbotham, M. (2006). Pharmacologic management of complex regional pain syndrome. *Clinical Journal of Pain, 22*(5), 425–429.

Staats, P. S., Argoff, C., Brewer, R., D'Arcy, Y., Gallagher, R., McCarberg, W., et al. (2004). Neuropathic pain: Incorporating new consensus guidelines into the reality of clinical practice. *Advanced Studies in Medicine, 4*(7B), S542–S582.

Tan, G., Jensen, M. P., Thornby, J. I., & Shanti, B. F. (2004) Validation of the Brief Pain Inventory for chronic nonmalignant pain. *Journal of Pain, 5*(2), 133–137.

Victor, T. W., Jensen, M. P., Gammaitoni, A. R., et al. (2008). The dimensions of pain quality: Factor analysis of the Pain Quality Assessment Scale. *Clinical Journal of Pain, 24*(6), 550–555.

Weiner, D. K., Herr, K., & Rudy, T. (2002). *Persistent pain in older adults: An interdisciplinary guide for treatment.* New York: Springer Publishing Company.

Williams, V. S., Smith, M. Y., & Fehnel, S. E. (2006). The validity and utility of the BPI interference measures for evaluating the impact of osteoarthritic pain. *Journal of Pain Symptom Management, 31*(1), 48–57.

Wong, D., & DiVito-Thomas, P. (2006). *The validity, reliability, and preference of the Wong Baker FACES Pain Rating Scale among Chinese, Japanese, and Thai children.* Retrieved July 18, 2008, from www.mosbysdrugconsult.com/WOW/op080.html

---

The Jensen suite offers these additional resources to enhance learning and facilitate understanding of this chapter:

- thePoint online resource, http//thepoint.lww.com/Jensen1E
- Student CD-ROM included with the book
- *Laboratory Manual for Nursing Health Assessment: A Best Practice Approach*
- *Pocket Guide for Nursing Health Assessment: A Best Practice Approach*

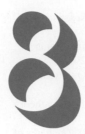

Nutrition Assessment

Karen Pitoci, 15 years old and 88 lb, was recently discharged from the hospital with a diagnosis of anorexia nervosa. This hospital stay was the most recent of three in the past year. Her mother, a full-time homemaker, is very involved in Karen's school and social activities.

The family is being visited today by a home health nurse for a follow-up assessment. The role of the home health nurse is to assess Karen's nutritional status and ability to care for herself at home.

You will gain more information about Karen as you progress through this chapter. As you study the content and features, consider her case and its relationship to what you are learning. Begin thinking about the following points:

- *How might the nurse's previous experiences with patients who have eating disorders influence the assessment of Karen?*
- *What subjective and psychosocial data will the nurse collect?*
- *How will the nurse assess Karen's current nutritional status using objective data?*
- *What adaptations will the nurse make to the assessment based on the patient's condition?*

Learning Objectives

1. Discuss the role of primary nutrients in maintaining health.

2. Outline dietary guidelines based on the Food Guide Pyramid.

3. Discuss developmental, social, cultural, and religious factors affecting the nutritional status of patients.

4. Describe the nurse's role in nutritional assessment.

5. Evaluate the potential effects of medications and nutritional supplements on nutrient intake, absorption, utilization, and excretion.

6. Identify physical signs and symptoms of malnutrition.

7. Differentiate normal from abnormal findings in patients based on the calculation of body mass index (BMI) and ideal body weight, in addition to the consideration of muscle mass and fat distribution.

8. Individualize nutritional assessments for infants, children, adolescents, pregnant and lactating women, and older adults.

9. Document and communicate data from nutritional assessments using appropriate terminology.

10. Use nutritional assessment findings to identify nursing diagnoses and initiate a plan of care.

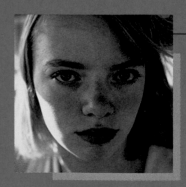

As frontline providers of health care, nurses are involved intimately in all aspects of assessing nutritional status for patients. Determining adequate and appropriate caloric and nutrient intake occurs by analyzing data to identify actual and potential nutritional problems. Because foods rather than nutrients make up the building blocks of a wholesome diet, nurses must be aware of nutrients in whole foods to accurately complete nutritional assessments.

When completing a nutritional assessment, the nurse considers a broad range of influences on the patient's food choices. A complete nutrition assessment includes a history of food intake, weight and height calculations, laboratory data, and the use of specific nutritional tools when indicated.

Nutritional Concepts

Primary Nutrients

Primary nutrients, essential for optimal body function, include carbohydrates, proteins, fats, vitamins, minerals, water, and major electrolytes. Nutrients are the building blocks for tissue maintenance and repair. Furthermore, carbohydrates, proteins, and fats are sources of energy for the body. Fats yield 9 cal/g, while proteins and carbohydrates yield 4 cal/g. Vitamins and minerals also play key roles in cellular function, while water makes up more than half of adult body weight and is essential to supporting life, serving many vital functions within the body.

Carbohydrates

Carbohydrates provide the body's main source of energy. Simple sugars consist of glucose or dextrose, fructose, galactose, sucrose, maltose, or lactose. These simple sugars are absorbed as basic units without undergoing digestion, hence forming a "quick" source of energy. Complex carbohydrates, on the other hand, known as *polysaccharides*, consist of starch, glycogen, and fiber.

Primary sources of carbohydrates are natural and added sugars, starch, fiber, grains, fruits, and vegetables. The recommended daily allowance for carbohydrates varies depending on the activity level; however, the distribution range in a normal healthy diet is 45% to 65% of calories (U.S. Department of Health and Human Services [USDHHS] & U.S. Department of Agriculture [USDA], 2005).

Proteins

Proteins serve important functions in cell structure and tissue maintenance. Amino acids are the building blocks of all proteins. Amino acids and proteins are involved in many essential body functions such as regulating fluid and electrolyte balance and transporting molecules and other substances through the blood. Body tissues such as muscles, bones, teeth, skin, and hair primarily consist of protein. While the body can synthesize most amino acids from nonprotein dietary sources, eight essential amino acids must be obtained through dietary sources.

Lipids

Lipids or **fats** include triglycerides (fats and oils), sterols (eg, cholesterol), and phospholipids (eg, lecithin). Fats help to maintain body functions by providing essential fatty acids (linoleic and linolenic acids) and promoting the absorption of fat-soluble vitamins A, D, E, and K.

Triglycerides. Saturated fats (solid at room temperature) and hydrogenated fats raise levels of low-density lipoprotein (LDL) cholesterol. Saturated fats include those found in animal products such as butter, cheese, and fatty meats. Hydrogenation refers to the chemical processing of animal fats used by food manufacturers to extend the shelf life of products susceptible to rancidity, such as cookies and crackers.

Clinical Significance 8-1

Foods made with hydrogenated fats are particularly harmful to the diet because they are the largest contributors of trans fats. Empirical evidence suggests that trans fats are as damaging to the heart and blood vessels as saturated fats (Mente de Koning, et al., 2009).

Unsaturated fats (liquid at room temperature) are known to reduce LDL levels as well as triglycerides (high levels of which are a major cause of coronary heart disease). Unsaturated fats come in two forms. They are either *omega-3 oils*, found primarily in fish oils and some plant oils such as canola, flaxseed, walnut, and hazelnut, or *omega-6 oils*, found in plant oils such as safflower, sunflower, corn, soybean, and cottonseed (Tangney, et al., 2009). Monounsaturated fats such as canola and olive oils may lower cholesterol if consumed in place of saturated fats.

Cholesterol. Cholesterol is essential to cellular maintenance and repair; however, the body can synthesize sufficient cholesterol to meet its daily requirements. In the typical North American diet, cholesterol primarily comes from meat and egg yolks. Cholesterol ingested in excess of daily requirements contributes to atherosclerosis, stroke, and myocardial infarction (heart attack).

Clinical Significance 8-2

Because of the substantial rise in obesity throughout North America and subsequent increases in incidences of diabetes and heart disease directly attributable to dietary triglycerides and cholesterol, the USDA (2008) and American Heart Association recommend that daily fat intake for adults should not exceed 20% to 35% of total calories (USDHHS & USDA, 2005). In addition, because saturated fats contribute heavily to elevated serum triglyceride and cholesterol levels, they should not exceed 10% of daily calories.

Phospholipids. Phospholipids are emulsifiers that occur naturally in many foods and are used extensively by the food industry. They serve many vital functions such as transporting fat-soluble substances across cell membranes. Lecithin, the best-known phospholipid, is a popular food supplement. Powdered soy lecithin lowers cholesterol absorption and LDL levels when consumed in fat-free foods (Spilburg, et al., 2003).

Vitamins and Minerals

Vitamins play a key role in the metabolism of most nutrients. Light-skinned people obtain vitamin D, also known as the "sunshine vitamin," through exposure to sunlight. People living more than 37 degrees south or north of the equator (roughly above Washington, DC) cannot make adequate vitamin D from sun exposure during winter months, even with sun exposure on the face, hands, and arms (Hemmelgarn, 2009). Additionally, people who use sunscreens in sunny climates and dark-skinned people may require a dietary source to meet daily requirements. Older adults and those who smoke also need added vitamin D, because aging and smoking tend to impair vitamin D synthesis.

⚠ SAFETY ALERT 8.1

Low levels of vitamin D may contribute to falls and fractures; cardiovascular, autoimmune, and infectious diseases; some cancers; type 1 and type 2 diabetes; and reduced muscle strength. Conversely, excessive intake of fat-soluble vitamins may result in toxicity because vitamins A, E, D, and K are stored in adipose tissue (Hemmelgarn, 2009).

Another important vitamin is folate, a B vitamin considered essential to metabolism and cell synthesis. Dietary sources of folate include leafy greens, lentils, seeds, liver, orange juice, grains, cereals, and breads fortified with folic acid. Groups at risk for folate deficiency include patients with alcoholism, older adults, those who follow "fad" diets, and people of low socioeconomic status.

⚠ SAFETY ALERT 8.2

Adequate maternal intake of folate before conception and in the first trimester of pregnancy reduces the incidence of neural tube defects (eg, spina bifida). The U.S. Public Health Service recommends that all women of childbearing age and capable of pregnancy consume 400 mg of synthetic folic acid daily from either foods or supplements (Centers for Disease Control [CDC], 2007).

Vitamin B_{12} and folate need each other to be activated (Dudek, 2010). Vitamin B_{12} is the only water-soluble vitamin not found in plants. In addition to being involved in DNA synthesis and maintaining red blood cells, vitamin B_{12} plays an important role in maintaining the myelin sheath around nerves. Sources of vitamin B_{12} include beef, lamb, organ meats, shellfish, sardines, salmon, canned tuna, catfish, pike and whiting, milk, and dairy products such as yogurt and cheese.

Three **minerals** deserve special consideration in a healthy diet, particularly for vegetarians: iron, zinc (trace element), and calcium (Craig, 2009). Iron and zinc are best absorbed from animal sources; therefore, vegetarians may need to increase their intake of iron and zinc from plant sources, eggs, and dairy products. Vitamin C is required for proper absorption of iron and to meet daily requirements for calcium. The Vegetarian Food Guide recommends eight servings of calcium-rich foods daily such as calcium-fortified orange juice or breakfast cereals and legumes or leafy greens.

Supplements

Patients may not consider food supplements, such as vitamins and herbal remedies, when questioned during a nutritional assessment. Certain drug–herb interactions may be serious and life threatening (Woo, 2008).

Herbs beginning with the letter "g" (eg, garlic, ginger, ginkgo, and grapefruit) are most commonly involved in herb–drug interactions. Drugs prescribed for anticoagulant/antiplatelet activity (eg, warfarin, aspirin) are frequently involved in herb–drug interactions, causing excessive bleeding. Because many herbs adversely affect the liver, there is a potential for interaction with hepatotoxic medications (eg, acetaminophen). St. John's wort reduces the effectiveness of many medications prescribed for heart disease, depression, seizures, some cancers, organ transplant rejection, and oral contraceptives. Fatalities (though rare) have occurred with concurrent ephedra and caffeine use (Woo, 2008).

Fluid and Electrolytes

Water is essential for life. The adult body loses 1,500 to 2,800 mL/day of water through perspiration, exhalation, and excretion of urine and feces. The body requires a minimum fluid intake of 1,500 mL/day to maintain the excretion of metabolic wastes through urine and feces. However, extreme environmental temperatures, high altitude, low humidity, fever, and exercise increase water loss. Therefore, the recommended **adequate intake** (AI) of water varies depending on gender, age, air temperature, activity level, and state of health. Careful consideration of intake and output is warranted in infants and older adults, particularly when vomiting, diarrhea, or fever is present. Other conditions characterized by high water losses include burns, fistulas, hemorrhage, uncontrolled diabetes, and some renal disorders (Dudek, 2010). Nurses caring for anyone requiring fluid and electrolyte adjustments such as those mentioned above are advised to seek additional evidence-based information to guide practice.

Sodium and potassium are major **electrolytes**. Sodium regulates fluid balance and cell permeability, hence the movement of fluid, electrolytes, glucose, insulin, and amino acids across cellular membranes. It serves to regulate acid–base balance, nerve transmission, and muscular irritability (Dudek, 2010). Although there is no recommended daily intake for sodium and wide variation exists between individuals and among cultures, an average North American consumes far more sodium than required for health. As people age, they become more "salt sensitive," and their risk of developing high blood pressure, coronary heart disease, and renal failure increases. This may be problematic to control because approximately 75% of sodium consumed in the average diet comes from salt added by food manufacturers (Dudek, 2010).

Potassium is also implicated in regulating fluid and acid–base balance. In addition, it serves functions in nerve impulse transmission, carbohydrate metabolism, protein synthesis, and skeletal muscle contractility. The AI for potassium is 4.7 g/day; however, on average, North Americans consume only 2.1 to 3.2 g/day (Dudek, 2010). African Americans have a lower than average potassium intake, high salt sensitivity, and increased rate of hypertension. A rule of thumb is that sodium and potassium contents are inversely related: that is, processed foods typically low in potassium tend to be high in sodium, and fresh wholesome foods typically high in potassium are low in sodium.

⚠ SAFETY ALERT 8.3

Potassium levels must be maintained in a very narrow range. A potassium level outside of normal needs immediate correction. Too high or too low potassium level may cause potentially fatal cardiac dysrhythmias.

Many drugs commonly prescribed for people with chronic illnesses such as cardiovascular disease or renal failure interfere with electrolyte balance. In particular, low-sodium or high-potassium foods (or the opposite) may be desirable under such circumstances. Nurses are well advised to consult reliable sources of information on food and drug interactions.

Food Safety and Food Security

Food safety has gained importance in the past decade. Several outbreaks of **food pathogens**, such as salmonella in peanuts and listeriosis in cheeses and processed meats, are contemporary examples of food-borne pathogens affecting the health of large segments of the population. Food pathogens sometimes travel huge distances, making them difficult to trace and thus compromising the health and safety of many people over a matter of days. Despite the best efforts of regulatory bodies and food inspection agencies striving to maintain food safety, food-borne pathogens are becoming increasingly problematic.

Amidst a growing body of evidence showing the link between herbicide and pesticide use in agriculture and certain cancers, many people are seeking organic food sources. Further, the public has also questioned the use of antibiotics and hormones in raising cattle, pork, and poultry. Increased production of genetically modified foods had contributed to a move toward consuming organically grown foods from plant sources (Magana-Gomez & Calderon de la Barca, 2008).

Similarly, public awareness of food security is increasing. Food sources have become highly centralized. Modern urban lifestyles are contrary to people growing and processing their own food. Food sources are sometimes continents away from where foods are consumed, occasionally resulting in sudden, unexpected food shortages. Global climactic and catastrophic events may interfere with water and food production and distribution. Under such circumstances, nurses may be called on to assist in reestablishing food security within communities. They are sometimes also engaged in triage and advocacy to

ensure that the most vulnerable segments of society are not forgotten.

Nutritional Guidelines

The USDHHS and USDA jointly publish guidelines for healthy eating (Fig. 8-1). They revise these guidelines every 5 years to address emerging health issues based on current research pertaining to optimal nutrition. For example, the 2005 guidelines, for the first time, consider gender, age, and activity levels in dietary recommendations. Changes in recommendations also aim at promoting healthy eating habits and reducing obesity, hypertension, heart disease, cancer, and diabetes.

My Pyramid emphasizes the need to select foods from each of the five food groups to meet individual requirements for health while reducing fats, sugars, and sodium. The emphasis is on variety; increased intake of vegetables, fruits, lentils, and grains, particularly from plant sources; and meeting individual nutritional needs while avoiding either deficiencies or excesses in nutrient intake. The overall aim is to gradually promote healthier eating habits among Americans of all ages, lifestyles, classes, and cultures.

🔺 Lifespan Considerations

Pregnant Women

Pregnant and lactating women require special nutritional considerations for healthy outcomes. They need an additional 300 to 500 cal/day, with an emphasis on protein sources, such as milk and meat, to boost tissue building. Whole foods offer the best bioavailable sources of vitamins and minerals and should always be the first choice; however, under certain circumstances, vitamin and mineral supplementation may be required, especially to ensure that daily needs are met for vitamins A and C, folate, iron, calcium, and zinc.

⚠ SAFETY ALERT 8.4

Women who do not meet nutritional requirements of pregnancy are at risk for having premature, low–birth-weight, or small-for-gestational-age infants. Their infants are also at higher risk for disabilities and congenital anomalies including anencephaly, myelomeningocele, meningocele, oral facial cleft, structural heart disease, limb defect, urinary tract anomaly, and hydrocephalus (Wilson, 2007a).

Infants, Children, and Adolescents

More protein is needed for tissue building in periods of rapid growth such as adolescence. Ensuring dietary sources of essential amino acids from protein is critical for children because of their rapid growth (Pencharz, 2010). This is also the case when tissue damage occurs or during prolonged illness.

Infants, children, and adolescents require different nutrients based on developmental and growth factors. For

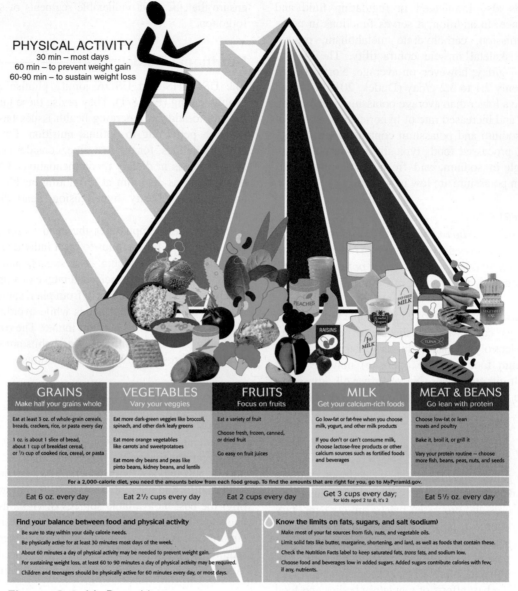

PHYSICAL ACTIVITY
30 min – most days
60 min – to prevent weight gain
60-90 min – to sustain weight loss

GRAINS	VEGETABLES	FRUITS	MILK	MEAT & BEANS
Make half your grains whole	Vary your veggies	Focus on fruits	Get your calcium-rich foods	Go lean with protein
Eat at least 3 oz. of whole-grain cereals, breads, crackers, rice, or pasta every day	Eat more dark-green veggies like broccoli, spinach, and other dark leafy greens	Eat a variety of fruit	Go low-fat or fat-free when you choose milk, yogurt, and other milk products	Choose low-fat or lean meats and poultry
1 oz. is about 1 slice of bread, about 1 cup of breakfast cereal, or ½ cup of cooked rice, cereal, or pasta	Eat more orange vegetables like carrots and sweetpotatoes	Choose fresh, frozen, canned, or dried fruit	If you don't or can't consume milk, choose lactose-free products or other calcium sources such as fortified foods and beverages	Bake it, broil it, or grill it
	Eat more dry beans and peas like pinto beans, kidney beans, and lentils	Go easy on fruit juices		Vary your protein routine — choose more fish, beans, peas, nuts, and seeds

For a 2,000-calorie diet, you need the amounts below from each food group. To find the amounts that are right for you, go to MyPyramid.gov.

| Eat 6 oz. every day | Eat 2½ cups every day | Eat 2 cups every day | Get 3 cups every day; for kids aged 2 to 8, it's 2 | Eat 5½ oz. every day |

Find your balance between food and physical activity
- Be sure to stay within your daily calorie needs.
- Be physically active for at least 30 minutes most days of the week.
- About 60 minutes a day of physical activity may be needed to prevent weight gain.
- For sustaining weight loss, at least 60 to 90 minutes a day of physical activity may be required.
- Children and teenagers should be physically active for 60 minutes every day, or most days.

Know the limits on fats, sugars, and salt (sodium)
- Make most of your fat sources from fish, nuts, and vegetable oils.
- Limit solid fats like butter, margarine, shortening, and lard, as well as foods that contain these.
- Check the Nutrition Facts label to keep saturated fats, *trans* fats, and sodium low.
- Choose food and beverages low in added sugars. Added sugars contribute calories with few, if any, nutrients.

Figure 8.1 My Pyramid.

example, fat intake is crucial to brain development in infants and young toddlers. Therefore, whole milk is recommended for children younger than 2 years. Table 8-1 provides age-related developmental and growth considerations in the diet.

Older Adults

Older adults also require special consideration during assessments of dietary requirements. They may compensate for diminished taste of sweet and salty foods by adding sugar and salt to their diet at a time when they are at increased risk for diabetes, hypertension, and heart disease. Their basal metabolic rate is declining concurrently with reductions in physical activity. When this occurs, caloric needs are significantly reduced. Older adults are also at increased risk for malnutrition as a result of social isolation.

In addition, older adults may need vitamin D supplementation because of changes in nutrient metabolism, particularly when exposure to sunlight is reduced. Older people are advised to ensure AI of vitamin D through dietary sources such as fortified milk and dairy products, fatty fish, and fortified cereals. Other nutrients not likely to be consumed in adequate amounts by older adults include calcium, folate, vitamin B_{12}, and riboflavin (Dudek, 2010).

Older adults may also experience a reduced sense of thirst, thereby increasing their risk for dehydration. They are also at increased risk for osteoarthritis, osteoporosis, dementias, and obesity. This presents unique challenges and increases their susceptibility to dubious claims made by manufacturers of pharmaceutical and nutritional supplements. Social isolation may further compound nutritional problems associated with aging.

Eating alone is particularly problematic for people with reduced mobility, receiving social assistance, or both. They may lack the resources required to maintain a nutritious and appealing diet. Poor dentition may also be an issue. Missing teeth, gum disease, and poor-fitting dentures can all detract

Table 8.1   Recommended Dietary Reference Intakes* for Some Macronutrients

Category	Age or Time Frame (year)	Protein (g/kg)	Energy (kcal/kg)	Calcium (mg/kg)	Phosphorus (mg/kg)	Magnesium (mg/kg)
Infants	0.0–0.5	2.2	108.3	66.7	50.0	6.7
	0.5–1.0	1.6	94.4	66.7	55.6	6.7
Children	1–3	1.2	100.0	61.5	61.5	6.2
	4–6	1.2	90.0	40.0	40.0	6.0
	7–10	1.0	71.4	28.6	28.6	6.1
Males	11–14	1.0	55.6	26.7	26.7	6.0
	15–18	0.9	45.5	18.2	18.2	6.1
	19–24	0.8	40.3	16.7	16.7	4.9
	25–50	0.8	36.7	10.1	10.1	4.4
	51+	0.8	29.9	10.4	10.4	4.5
Females	11–14	1.0	47.8	26.1	26.1	6.1
	15–18	0.8	40.0	21.8	21.8	5.5
	19–24	0.8	37.9	20.7	20.7	4.8
	25–50	0.8	34.9	12.7	12.7	4.4
	51+	0.8	29.2	12.3	12.3	4.3
Pregnant		0.9	4.6	18.5	18.5	4.9
Breastfeeding	First year	1.0	7.9	19.0	19.0	5.4

*These amounts, expressed as average daily intakes over time, are intended to provide for individual variations among most healthy people living in the United States under usual environmental stresses.

Sources: From Food and Nutrition Board, Institute of Medicine of the National Academies. (2005). *Dietary Reference Intakes for energy, carbohydrate, fiber, fat, fatty acids, cholesterol, protein, and amino acids.* Washington, DC: National Academies Press and Food and Nutrition Board, Institute of Medicine of the National Academies. (1997). *DRI Dietary Reference Intakes for calcium, phosphorus, magnesium, vitamin D, and fluoride.* Washington, DC: National Academies Press.

from enjoying meals. Community programs such as Meals on Wheels offer food services to people with disabilities or chronic illnesses who live in social isolation.

Malnutrition and dehydration are also common among residents of long-term care facilities (Simmons, et al., 2007). Commercial supplements aimed at providing added proteins and calories are not advisable over the long term (Dudek, 2010). Rather, nurses should strive to make meal times as enjoyable as possible by encouraging both independent eating and family involvement. It is also advisable to adhere to food preferences as much as possible and to maintain adequate hydration. Other recommendations for maintaining adequate nutrition among long-term care residents include providing clean, comfortable, pleasant surroundings; offering water; providing small, frequent meals; and minimizing distractions during meals. Refer to Box 8-1.

BOX 8.1   FACTORS THAT AFFECT NUTRITION IN THE OLDER ADULT

- Illness or chronic disease, including depression or dementia, which may alter nutrient needs or intake
- Excessive or inadequate intake of a limited variety of
- foods, with missing food groups or compromised by alcohol
- Dental problems (eg, missing or decayed teeth, ill-fitting dentures), which may lead to the avoidance of foods that are difficult to chew (eg, fruits, vegetables, whole grains)
- Low economic status, which can compromise a food budget
- Social isolation—older adults living alone are more likely to experience hunger than households with more than one older adult member
- Use of three or more prescribed or over-the-counter daily medications. Drugs may affect nutritional status by altering appetite; ability to taste and smell; or digestion, absorption, metabolism, and excretion of nutrients. Also, if a large percentage of a fixed income is spent on medications, less money is available for food.
- Significant unintentional weight loss (defined as 5% or more in 30 days, 10% or more in 180 days)
- Self-care deficits that may complicate food purchasing, food preparation, and eating
- Age older than 80 years

Source: Adapted from Dudek, S. G. (2010). *Nutrition essentials for nursing practice* (6th ed.). Philadelphia: Wolters Kluwer Health/Lippincott Williams & Wilkins.

Cultural Considerations

Several factors influence nutritional health including medications, lifestyle choices, socioeconomic status, geographical location, education, and cultural and religious influences. Athletes may require additional protein for muscle building and maintenance. Animal sources of protein include meat, fish, poultry, eggs, milk, and dairy products. Vegetarian diets containing soy protein may also contain essential amino acids if food intake is varied and calories are sufficient, including whole grains, legumes, vegetables, seeds, and nuts.

Some cultural groups believe in the healing properties of foods, while others follow food restrictions during illness. It is important for nurses working with patients from different cultures to assess dietary habits. Box 8-2 outlines items to consider.

The nurse who recognizes that each culture has its own food standards, determining what is edible and what is not, how foods are prepared and when they are eaten, as well as what role foods play in treating illness, is not likely to be ethnocentric when assessing nutritional status. Food preferences are learned, yet they vary depending on tradition, geography, education, income, and employment outside the home. Major US cultural subgroups are Hispanics, Africans, Asians, and Middle Easterners. While each group shares certain eating practices, food choices vary widely within cultural subgroups.

Additionally, food practices may be based on religious beliefs, such as fasting or abstaining from eating certain foods. Some common restrictions include the following (Dudek, 2010):

- Catholicism: Avoid meat on Fridays, mainly during Lent (6 weeks preceding Easter).
- Hinduism: Avoid beef, pork, and alcohol. Many are vegetarians.
- Mormon: Avoid coffee, tea, alcohol, and tobacco.
- Seventh Day Adventist: Many are lacto-ovo-vegetarians.
- Judaism: Eat only Kosher meat and no crustaceans; avoid consuming milk and meat in the same meal.

BOX 8.2 CULTURAL INFLUENCES ON NUTRITION

- What foods are eaten during stress, trauma, or illness? To prevent illness?
- What are the common food preferences? Likes or dislikes?
- In what context is the food purchased, prepared, served, and eaten?
- What are the food nutrients, and what are acceptable versus prohibited foods?
- What are the accepted food combinations (eg, hot and cold or milk and meat together)?
- How do foods facilitate communication and relationships within cultures?
- What geographic or environmental influences exist?

Leininger, M. M., & McFarland, M. R. (2002). *Transcultural nursing: Concepts, theories, research, and practice* (3rd ed.). New York: McGraw-Hill Professional.

- Islam: Avoid pork and birds of prey. Fast during the day during Ramadan.
- Buddhism: Many are lacto-ovo-vegetarians.

Collecting Nutritional Data

Collecting nutritional data is an ongoing process, partly because nutritional intake is an everyday activity. A patient may be seen in the primary care center or may enter hospital care with short- or long-term nutritional deficiencies (eg, a person experiencing complications from liver cirrhosis). At least some malnutrition has been reported in 27% of hospitalized adults (Pirlich, et al., 2006). Additionally, nutritional status does not improve during hospitalization. Malnutrition can be generalized, targeted to specific nutrients, or exist in combination with obesity, cachexia, trauma, or aging.

The responsibility for screening patients to assess their level of nutritional risk and reinforcing dietary counseling is often delegated to the nurse. The nurse's role in the nutritional assessment of patients is complex because of developmental, social, economic, and cultural factors. Nevertheless, nutrition screening is noninvasive, inexpensive, and easy to perform. An example of a simple nutrition screening tool is found in Figure 8-2 on the next page.

Parameters for a complete nutrition screening assessment include a risk assessment, focused history of common symptoms, comprehensive nutritional history, physical examination, calculated measurements, and serial laboratory values (especially during times of high metabolic demand, such as fever, pain, or infection, or during limited nutritional intake).

Acute Assessment

Nutritional deficits are rarely acute—most of them develop over time. During trauma or stress, calorie needs increase. Stress factors that increase the risk for nutritional deficit include surgery, trauma, infection, head injury, and burns. Additionally, the patient may have reduced consciousness or injuries that make it difficult to take in nutrients. In acute illnesses, nutrition assessment and appropriate interventions should be addressed within days of the diagnosis.

Subjective Data Collection

Areas for Health Promotion/*Healthy People*

Table 8-2 includes pertinent goals and education topics based on the *Healthy People* goals related to nutrition. Prevention of obesity and promotion of healthy eating habits are large focal areas for improving the health of the nation. Children are at high risk for obesity, while older adults are at high risk for poor nutrition.

Nutrition History

1. How many meals and snacks do you eat each day?

   Meals _____ Snacks _____

2. How many times a week do you eat the following meals away from home?

   Breakfast _____ Lunch _____ Dinner _____

   What types of eating places do you frequently visit? (Check all that apply)

   Fast-food _____ Restaurant _____ Diner/cafeteria _____

   Other _____

3. On average, how many pieces of fruit or glasses of juice do you eat or drink each day?

   Fresh fruit _____ Juice (8 oz. cup) _____

4. On average, how many servings of vegetables do you eat each day? _____

5. On average, how many times a week do you eat a high-fiber breakfast cereal? _____

6. How many times a week do you eat red meat (beef, lamb, veal) or pork? _____

7. How many times a week do you eat chicken or turkey? _____

8. How many times a week do you eat fish or shellfish? _____

9. How many hours of television do you watch every day? _____

   Do you usually snack while watching television?

   Yes _____ No _____

10. How many times a week do you eat desserts and sweets? _____

11. What types of beverages do you usually drink? How many servings of each do you drink a day?

    Water _____

    Juice _____

    Soda _____

    Diet soda _____

    Sports drinks _____

    Iced tea _____

    Iced tea with sugar _____

    Milk:

        Whole milk _____

        2% milk _____

        1% milk _____

        Skim milk _____

    Alcohol:

        Beer _____

        Wine _____

        Hard liquor _____

Figure 8.2 A nutrition history screening tool.

Assessment of Risk Factors

An assessment of risk factors includes questions about past medical and surgical histories, medication and supplement use, past history, family history, food and fluid intake patterns, and the patient's psychosocial profile (Dudek, 2010). If indicated, the nurse may follow up with a tested and valid tool for screening a specific population for risk factors.

Table 8.2 *Healthy People* Goals Related to Nutrition

Goals	Patient Education Topics
Increase the proportion of treated chronic kidney failure patients who have received counseling on nutrition.	Avoid foods high in potassium; limit fluids if needed.
Increase the proportion of middle, junior high, and senior high schools that provide school health education to prevent unhealthy dietary patterns.	Teach healthy eating patterns in health education courses. Provide age-appropriate materials. The American Dietetic Association has a list of resources.
Increase the proportion of adults with high blood pressure who are reducing sodium intake to help control their blood pressure.	Avoid high-sodium foods, such as canned soups, pickled vegetables, soy sauce, and foods with nitrites.
Increase the proportion of pregnancies begun with an optimum folic acid level.	Schedule prenatal visits that include nutrition counseling. Begin folic acid supplementation before a planned pregnancy.
Increase the proportion of adults who are at a healthy weight.	Provide information on the food pyramid and healthy eating habits.
Reduce the proportion of children and adolescents who are overweight or obese.	Balance high-quality nutrition with exercise and activity.
Increase food security among U.S. households and in so doing reduce hunger.	Provide resources for patients and their families with limited income.

Source: *Healthy people 2010: What are its goals?* (n.d.). Retrieved May 14, 2010 from http://www.healthypeople.gov/About/goals.htm

Questions on History and Risk	Rationales
Medical History	
Do you have a medical condition, such as diabetes or hypertension?	Medical conditions, increased metabolic demand, and malabsorption increase the risk for nutritional deficits. Patients with diabetes or hypertension may benefit from nutrition therapy.
Do you have, or have you recently had, fever, sepsis, thermal injuries, skin breakdown, cancer, AIDS, major surgery, or trauma?	These conditions increase nutritional needs.
Do you have, or have you recently had, malabsorption or certain renal diseases?	These conditions lead to loss of nutrients; special attention to increased nutritional requirements is necessary.
Weight History	
Do you have a history of any problems related to nutrition or weight?	Being underweight, overweight, or obese influences self-perception of health. Such a perception may be distorted or inaccurate, but it is important to know it to address it. Asking how the patient perceives self can be challenging, particularly when the body is visibly outside expected limits (eg, anorexia, obesity).
	Main causes of malnutrition in the United States are poverty, alcoholism, hospitalization, aging, and eating disorders. Other risk factors are poor dentition, chronic illness, multiple medications, social isolation, severe burns, and lack of knowledge.
	Risk factors commonly associated with overweight and obesity include excessive intake of high-calorie foods, typically high in fat and sugar; not enough exercise; alcohol abuse; and lack of knowledge.

Appetite and Taste Changes

- Have you noticed any changes in your ability to smell odors? In the taste of food? If so, what are the changes?
- How would you rate your appetite?
- How does food taste to you?

Senses of taste and smell decrease with aging. Additionally, some medications alter taste and smell. For example, amiodarone, a medication to regulate the heart rhythm, causes food to taste like garlic.

Gastrointestinal Symptoms. Have you ever been diagnosed with a gastrointestinal or other disease that affects nutrition, such as anorexia, heartburn, nausea, diarrhea, vomiting, or pain?

Gastrointestinal diseases may impair appetite and also reduce the absorption of nutrients.

Food Allergy or Intolerance. Have you ever been diagnosed with a food intolerance or allergy?

Note differences between intolerances (nausea, bloating, and flatulence) and allergies (hives, wheezing, and anaphylaxis). Food allergies and intolerances must also be considered when evaluating risk factors for malnutrition because they affect food choices. Patients intolerant to lactose, for example, need sources other than dairy products for calcium. Common food allergens include milk, eggs, soy, peanuts, nuts (eg, cashews, almonds), wheat, fish, and shellfish (Dudek, 2010).

Family History

Do you have a family history of gastrointestinal or other diseases that influence your nutrition?

- Who had the illness?
- What was the illness?
- When did the person have it?
- How was the illness treated?
- What were the outcomes?

A family history of problems such as Crohn's disease, type 2 diabetes, cystic fibrosis, or anemia should be included. Consideration must be given to respecting cultural food patterns and preferences. Gathering information on the patient's family history of obesity, cancer, heart disease, and atherosclerosis may also be useful in developing a nutrition plan.

Food and Fluid Intake Patterns

Eating Patterns. Describe a typical day's eating (include content and amount of meals, meal times, and snacking patterns).

- Are you on a special diet? If so, please describe.
- Are there times of the day when you feel hungry? If so, when? What is satisfying? Are there particular foods that you like? Dislike? If so, please describe.
- Are any foods or food habits important to you? If so, please describe.
- Who shares your mealtimes?

Food habits and intake patterns may vary according to culture, religion, and region. Because variation is wide, it is important to obtain a history for the individual patient.

Fluid Intake Patterns

- How much fluid do you drink each day? (How many glasses and approximate size of glass?)
- Are there particular fluids that you like? Dislike?
- Are there certain times of the day when you drink or refrain from drinking fluids?
- How much coffee, tea, chocolate-, or caffeine-containing beverages do you usually drink in a day? If you do not have any caffeine for a few days, how do you feel (eg, headache, nausea, other sensations)?

Fluid intake may be in excess of needs, causing fluid volume excess. Low fluid intake may cause a fluid volume deficit, or dehydration.

Large consumption of unfiltered coffee such as through a French press may increase LDL levels and the risk for miscarriage (van Dam, 2008).

Psychosocial Profile

Habits

- Does stress affect your eating or drinking habits? If so, please describe.
- Does smoking affect your appetite? If so, describe.

Some patients gain weight with stress, while others lose weight.
Smoking impairs both senses of smell and taste.

(text continues on page 158)

Cooking Ability

- Who does your food shopping?
- Do you have a food budget? If so, could you describe it?
- How often do you eat out? Who prepares your food?
- Does food preparation provide a source of enjoyment for you?
- Could you describe your food preparation facilities?

Functional limitations influence the ability to obtain or prepare food. The nutrition-metabolic pattern does not involve only nutrients ingested each day. It encompasses aspects such as culture, religion, and geography; food and fluid preferences and dislikes; patterns of eating, allergies, digestion, shopping resources, and skills; kitchen facilities; food preparation and eating; meaning of food and feeding; social patterns at meals; and gastrointestinal structures, including dentition. Such information aids in individualizing actions, assisting patients to modify current eating practices, and adopting new eating patterns into everyday life. Knowing what roles a patient plays in groups can aid in prioritizing health problems that relate to the gastrointestinal system. For example, if a patient has primary food preparation responsibilities, he or she may need to relinquish them temporarily or permanently. Should major roles change, the patient will need to be able to assume other roles deemed equally important to maintain a contributing role with the group.

Dietary Lifestyle Changes

- Do environmental or social factors affect your ability to make dietary changes?
- Do you feel that you have sufficient resources to support healthy nutritional intake?

Many social functions revolve around food. If signs, symptoms, or treatments disrupt such functions, social isolation can be a consequence. Asking about such possibilities can be important when assessing a patient's overall health.

Medications and Supplements

Medication Schedule

- What system or systems have you developed to ensure an accurate schedule for your medications?
- Are there particular reminders or methods that are helpful for you? If so, please describe.

A medication history is included because diet and food intake affect medications. For example, dark green leafy foods can decrease the effect of some anticoagulants.

Barriers to Accuracy. Have you experienced any difficulty in getting or taking your medicines as they have been prescribed? If so, please describe.

Remembering to take medications requires intact memory and cognitive skills. If there is any difficulty, the nurse may obtain a medi-set with small compartments for medications for each time of the day.

Adverse Effects. When do you tend to report any adverse effects of your medicines? For example, as soon as you notice; when things get really bad for you; only when they interfere with what you need to do; never.

Patterns of health-seeking behavior vary widely, from patients who visit the provider for health promotion to those patients who defer care until emergently or critically ill.

Resources for Medication-Related Information

- From whom have you received most of your medication information? TV, relatives, neighbors, books, magazines, pharmacist, health store personnel, doctor, nurse, nurse practitioner, others?
- Do you ask questions about your medicines? Do you expect that people helping you with medicines will give you needed information?

Nurses can provide patients with resources for answers. It is important to teach patients to inform providers of side effects, financial concerns, or other health beliefs that affect the ability to take medications as prescribed. An alternative plan can then be developed collaboratively with patients.

Supplements. Do you take any vitamin, mineral, or other nutritional supplements? If so, describe the substance, amount, and frequency.

Approximately one third of patients use some type of supplement, and it is important to monitor for side effects and drug–supplement interactions.

Alcohol and Drug Use

- How much alcohol do you drink?
- Do you feel that you are a "normal" drinker? (By normal, I mean that you drink less than, or as much as, most other people.)

Alcohol can adversely affect the liver and its multiple functions, including protein synthesis. In addition, chronic alcohol exposure can injure the stomach and pancreas. Lack of the digestive enzymes produced by the pancreas can impair the absorption of nutrients including fat.

Questions on History and Risk	Rationales
• [If the person does drink]: How much did you drink yesterday? Is that about usual for you? When did you take your last drink (date and hour)? What is your usual pattern for alcohol intake? If you do not have a drink for a few days, how do you feel? Have you ever gone through alcohol withdrawal? If so, when, and describe the circumstances. Do you go into a DT (delirium tremors) if you do not drink for a few days? See Chapter 10 for the CAGE questionnaire. • Could you tell me about your drug use? (Ask about the substance and quantity after each question.) Do you smoke marijuana? Do you use, or have you used, other's prescription drugs? Sleeping pills? Downers? Uppers? Speed? Ritalin? Cocaine? Meth? Do you use, or have you ever "tripped" or used, hallucinogens?	Alcohol intake can affect the metabolism of nutrients as well as alter the overall nutrient density of the diet. It is common for patients with a high alcohol intake to be deficient in the B vitamins and vitamin K.

Risk Assessment and Health-Related Patient Teaching

Nurses promote healthy nutrition in all settings including health fairs, schools, clinics, and hospitals. Patients often are interested in nutrition as a way to improve their health. Nurses can teach about the Food Pyramid, increasing the intake of fruits and vegetables, and decreasing the intake of foods with low nutrient density. Patients can be taught to read food labels, especially when the intake of a nutrient is limited because of dietary restrictions, such as a low-salt diet. When patients are placed on restricted diets, teaching must be performed. Many organizations, such as the American Diabetes Association, have helpful written materials to reinforce such teaching.

Focused Health History Related to Common Symptoms

Common Symptoms of Altered Nutrition

• Sudden or gradual changes in body weight
• Changes in eating habits
• Changes in skin, hair, or nails
• Decreased energy level

Questions to Assess Symptoms	Rationales/Abnormal Findings
Changes in Body Weight What is your present height and weight? How do these compare with your height and weight 5 years ago? Have there been any changes in your weight over the past year? If so, please describe. How do you feel about your present weight?	Weight can change or remain stable with illness. A patient taking steroids may gain weight, while a patient undergoing cancer treatment may lose weight if nauseous or anorexic. Eating disorders, such as anorexia nervosa and bulimia nervosa, can profoundly affect nutritional health. Typically, patients with anorexia are preoccupied with distorted perceptions of themselves as fat when they are emaciated. They feel "fat" despite being underweight.
Change in Eating Habits Have you experienced a change in a regular diet pattern (number, size, and contents of meals)?	If yes, investigate potential causes (eg, change in appetite, mental status, or mood; ability to prepare meals; ability to chew or swallow; nausea or vomiting). Patients with eating disorders reduce the size and content of meals or may binge and then purge.
Symptoms of Malnutrition • Have you noticed any changes in your hair, nails, and skin? If so, describe. • Would you say that you heal well? Poorly? Other? Do you have any difficulty tolerating hot or cold weather? • How much energy would you say that you have? • Has your energy level changed recently, say during the past year? If so, describe. See Box 8-3 for other symptoms of malnutrition.	Skin, hair, and nails are indicators of nutritional status because those cells turn over rapidly. Thin or brittle hair, thin skin, skin that bruises easily or flakes, and weak or brittle nails are typical symptoms. A malnourished person lacks energy.

Comprehensive Nutritional History

If, after assessing risk factors and common symptoms, data reveal the patient to be at risk for altered nutrition, the nurse takes a comprehensive nutritional history. Commonly used tools include food records, food frequency questionnaires, and direct observations.

Food Records

Food records are integral to nutritional assessment. To ensure accurate and complete data collection, records ought to include all food supplements and drinks consumed over a specified period, including the amount and times they were consumed.

24-Hour Recall. A 24-hour recall consists of asking the patient what he or she had to eat and drink within a 24-hour period. The nurse collects information from patients and their families without appearing judgmental (Fig. 8-3). He or she uses open-ended questions such as "Tell me the first thing that you ate yesterday" or "When was the first time you ate or drank anything yesterday?" The nurse continues by asking, "Did you have anything else to eat or drink at the time?" and then "What was the next thing you had to eat or drink?"

In this method, the patient tends to overestimate low intakes and underestimate high intakes. To control this tendency, it is important for the nurse to use prompts such as "golf-ball size" or "the size of your fist or thumb." Life-size models and digital images of various foods can also be useful in eliciting accurate portion estimates. Also, the nurse cues the patient to include beverages or condiments (eg, "Did you have anything on the toast?"). It is important for the nurse to remember to ask about fortified foods, such as fruit juices and cereals fortified with calcium, other food supplements, and alcohol.

The 24-hour recall is reliable only if the patient or family can recall the type and amount of food eaten. Additionally, the intake over the past 24 hours may not be typical—foods eaten on a weekend may differ from those eaten during the week. Therefore, the 24-hour recall is usually most complete and accurate when the nurse obtains a recall for a weekday and weekend day.

Three-Day Food Diary. To increase accuracy, the nurse may repeat diet recalls, stagger them through several health assessments, or have the patient keep a 3-day food diary. The diary shifts most of the responsibility for data collection from the nurse to the patient. It is best for the patient to write down the intake immediately after eating. This record is not reliant on memory, but the patient may consciously alter the diet during recording. It also is time consuming. For at-risk patients, an analysis of dietary intake is carried out in combination with weight, observation of signs and symptoms of poor nutrition, and consideration of laboratory values that reflect malnutrition.

Food-Frequency Questionnaires. Food-frequency questionnaires help assess the intake of certain required foods for special situations (eg, calcium or folate in pregnancy). Nurses use these questionnaires to track the frequency of intake of a certain food or foods over time, such as each day, week, or month. Food-frequency questionnaires are quick and often combined with the 24-hour recall. They require accurate reporting and intact memory (see Fig. 8-4).

Direct Observation

With hospitalized patients, it is possible to directly observe the amount and types of food they eat. Commonly, nurses describe intake as a percentage of the meal eaten, such as

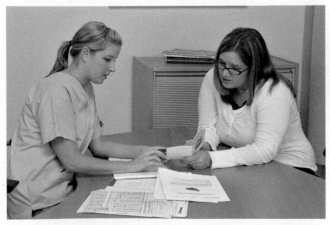

Figure 8.3 The nurse is reviewing a patient's food intake using the 24-hour recall method.

Nutrition Questionnaire

During the past 4 weeks, how often did you
eat a serving of the foods listed here?

Mark only one X for each food

	Last 4 weeks		Each week			Each day			
Number of times	0	1–3	1	2–4	5–6	1	2–3	4–5	6+
Milk						X			
Hot chocolate	X								
Cheese, plain or in sandwiches				X					
Yogurt	X								
Ice cream		X							

0   1   2   3   4   5   6   7   8

Figure 8.4 An example of a food-frequency questionnaire.

50% of breakfast or 75% of dinner. When inadequate intake is suspected, the nurse can count the calories. The nurse records the percentage of each food eaten, and the dietician performs a calorie count based on what is consumed. If intake is inadequate, the patient may need supplements such as high-calorie shakes.

Additionally, the nurse monitors the fluid intake and output for patients receiving intravenous fluids or at risk for fluid volume excess or deficit. The nurse totals the fluids taken in, including orally and intravenously. He or she totals the output by measuring urine output, drainage from tubes or drains, and emesis (vomiting).

Lifespan Considerations

Additional Questions	Rationales/Abnormal Findings
Pregnant Women	
Preconception: How many servings do you eat daily of peas, beans, lentils, asparagus, spinach, papaya, breakfast cereal, or wheat germ? Do you take a supplement with folate?	Neural tube defects are more common in infants of women with low folate intake.
Do you avoid any foods? Are you on a special diet? Do you skip meals?	Any of these practices may lead to nutritional deficiencies.
Do you smoke cigarettes, drink alcohol, or use any recreational drugs?	Stimulants may increase energy requirements and cause inadequate weight gain. The use of alcohol and recreational substances can cause addiction and injury to the fetus.
Do you use any vitamin, mineral, or herbal substances?	Such supplements, including excessive vitamin A, may harm the fetus and should be avoided. Evidence about the safety of herbal remedies is lacking, so a careful history of their use is important when a patient is considering pregnancy, pregnant, or lactating.
How much weight have you gained during the first trimester?	Average total weight gain is only 1–2.5 kg.

(text continues on page 162)

How much weight have you gained during the second and third trimesters?

Nutritional requirements to produce a healthy baby and associated weight gain include increasing intake by about 300 kcal/day in the second and third trimesters, increasing complete protein intake to 60 g/day, increasing elemental iron intake by 27 mg/day, and increasing vitamin intake, especially for women who have multiple fetuses, smoke, or use alcohol or drugs.

⚠ *SAFETY ALERT 8.5*
Women who fail to meet these requirements risk low–birth-weight or intrauterine growth-restricted infants and increased difficulties with breastfeeding.

Do you take an iron supplement?

Beginning with the second trimester, it is recommended that all pregnant women take a supplement of 30 mg of iron (Wilson, et al., 2007).

What is your usual intake of dairy products? Do you take a calcium supplement?

If the diet is low in calcium-rich foods, a supplement with 600 mg of calcium may be needed.

How many servings of fish do you eat weekly?

⚠ *SAFETY ALERT 8.6*
Women who may become or are pregnant or nursing should avoid fish that may be high in mercury, such as shark, tuna, swordfish, mackerel, and tilefish. High mercury levels can harm the fetal or neonatal nervous system.

For the breastfeeding mother: Are you getting adequate calories and fluid to produce milk for your baby?

The recommended intake is an increase of 330 kcal/day for the first 6 months. The mother can use her thirst as a guide for adequate fluids (Lowdermilk & Perry, 2007).

Newborns, Infants, and Children

Are you breast- or bottle-feeding your newborn? How are you and your baby tolerating the feedings?

The healthy term infant who is adequately feeding usually requires no supplements before 6 months of age.

⚠ *SAFETY ALERT 8.7*
Whole cow's milk should not be introduced to infants younger than 1 year of age because of allergies and intolerances.

What solid foods have you added to the infant's diet? Has tooth eruption begun? Can your infant pick up finger foods and feed himself or herself?

⚠ *SAFETY ALERT 8.8*
When solid foods are introduced, beans, grains, and vegetables should be cooked and mashed to avoid choking and aspiration.

How is your preschooler's intake of calcium and fiber?

Milk and dairy products provide major sources of calcium. Preschoolers may change to low- or nonfat milk. For this age group, dietary fiber should include five servings of fruits and vegetables each day.

How many fruit juices does your preschooler drink each day?

An increased intake of fruit juices has been associated with dental caries, gastrointestinal symptoms, and overweight.

Additional Questions	Rationales/Abnormal Findings
Do you eat family meals together?	Maintaining healthy eating for families with busy lifestyles means providing balanced meals at designated times with few distractions such as television. Evidence suggests that people eating from a vehicle or within hearing distance of a television tend to make unhealthier food choices than those who share meals in more traditional family surroundings.

Adolescents

What have you eaten in the past 24 hours? Is this intake typical? What did you drink in the past 24 hours?	Discuss BMI according to the adolescent's gender and age. Intervene with nutritional and activity information early if BMI is ≥85th percentile. Provide nutrition information with the My Pyramid guidelines (USDA, 2005).
What is your typical meal pattern?	Adolescents may have irregular meal patterns or skip meals such as breakfast.
Are you concerned about your weight? Do you think that you are too fat? Too skinny?	Provide information about the nutritional pyramid. Ask and educate about multivitamins with iron for high-risk teens. Ask about food choices at school and assist with wise choices based on the nutritional pyramid.
Do you ever use diet supplements or laxatives or limit calories?	Screen for risk factors for anorexia and bulimia.
Have you ever used any supplements to boost your physical performance?	The use of anabolic steroids or other supplements usually begins in adolescence. Side effects include suppression of testicular function, gynecomastia, hepatotoxicity, mood disorders, elevated blood lipids, and cardiac disease (Snyder, et al., 2009).
What type of physical activity do you get each week?	A healthy diet should be balanced with adequate physical activity.
Do you suspect that you might be pregnant?	A pregnant teen has greater nutritional requirements than adult women, because she is still growing herself. Also, her pelvis may not be fully developed. Teens are at greater risk for pregnancy complications, especially preeclampsia, probably because of inadequate nutrient intake (Lowdermilk & Perry, 2007).

Older Adults

What medications are you taking?	Those taking medications or with diseases that create less saliva or xerostomia are more likely to have problems with taste (Boyce & Shone, 2006).
Use a screening tool to evaluate the risk of malnutrition in the older adult (see Table 8-3).	Financial and transportation issues can limit access to nutritional foods. Functional abilities or sensory losses can affect the ability to physically prepare nutritious foods. Early cognitive losses that impair judgment, planning, foresight, or sequencing of complex tasks may reduce the ability to follow recipes or prepare complete meals. Recent weight loss can cause dentures to fit poorly and interfere with chewing.

Table 8.3 Tools to Evaluate Risk of Malnutrition in the Older Adult

Tool	Description	Validity and Reliability
Mini-nutritional assessment	Perception of health, global assessment, questions about diet, and anthropometric measurements	Widely validated, predictive of poor outcomes
Simplified nutrition assessment questionnaire	Four-item screening tool	Highly sensitive and specific for those at risk for >10% weight loss
Screen II	17-item tool that evaluates food intake, chewing, swallowing, weight change, and social or functional barriers	High sensitivity and specificity, inter-rater reliability, and test-retest reliability
Malnutrition universal screening tool	Includes anorexia, disease, BMI, and percentage of weight loss	Particularly sensitive for undernutrition in hospitalized patients
Determine	Ten-item checklist to increase the awareness of nutritional risk	Commonly used, but criticized for lack of validity; more useful to promote nutrition awareness than to detect malnutrition

Source: Ritchie, C., Schmader, K. E, Lipman, T. O., & Sokol, N. (2009). *Geriatric nutrition: Nutritional issues in older adults*. Retrieved May 4, 2009, from http://www.uptodateonline.com.proxy.seattleu.edu/online/content/topic.do?topicKey=geri_med/8473&selectedTitle=1~150&source=search_result

Therapeutic Dialogue: Collecting Subjective Data

Remember Karen Pitoci, the 15-year-old girl receiving home care following hospitalization for anorexia nervosa. The home health nurse is collecting data to assess the patient's health. The nurse uses professional communication techniques to gather subjective data from Karen. The following conversations give two examples of interview styles used by different nurses. The nurse is interviewing the patient to obtain a 24-hour diet recall.

Less Effective

Nurse: So, Karen, what did you have to eat yesterday?

Karen: I had a sandwich.

Nurse: That's wonderful Karen. A sandwich is very nutritious. What else did you have?

Karen: I had a salad and some soda.

Mrs. Pitoci: It was diet soda.

Nurse: That's OK. The sugar's not good for you anyway. What else did you have?

Karen: Nothing.

Nurse: Well the sandwich is good for you, and you'll get some vitamins from the salad. What else did you have yesterday?

Karen: I had some fruit and yogurt for breakfast.

Nurse: And did you have anything else?

Karen: Some carrots and celery.

More Effective

Nurse: So, Karen, tell me the first thing that you ate yesterday.

Karen: Some fruit.

Nurse: What kind of fruit was it?

Karen: A grapefruit.

Nurse: And did you have anything else with the grapefruit?

Karen: I had a yogurt.

Nurse: And was it the light yogurt or regular?

Karen: Light.

Nurse: How much of the yogurt did you eat?

Karen: (Silent, looks at mother)

Mrs. Pitoci: She only ate half of it.

Nurse: And did you have anything to drink with it?

Karen: Some water.

Critical Thinking Challenge

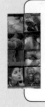

- Who should the nurse be assessing and communicating with—Karen, her mother, or both?
- What made the interview by the second nurse more effective?
- What additional assessment information might the nurse collect in addition to the diet recall?

Technique	Purpose	Screening or Registered Nurse Assessment	Focused or Advanced Practice Examination
Inspect physical status	To take a general survey	X	
Look for signs and symptoms of malnutrition	To assess if the patient appears well or poorly nourished	X	
Review for any weight change	To determine if weight loss is significant	X	
Measure BMI	To compare weight to height to determine underweight or overweight status	X	
Take weight for height calculations	To compare weight against national standards	X	
Measure waist circumference	To determine cardiovascular risk with central obesity		X
Measure triceps skinfold.	To calculate fat stores		X
Measure MAMC	To calculate fat and muscle stores		X

Objective Data Collection

Collecting objective data for a mini-nutritional assessment includes calculating BMI and percentage of weight change. Findings will determine the need for further anthropometric measurements and laboratory tests.

Equipment Needed

- Scale
- Measuring tape
- Growth charts (for children)
- Skin calipers

Preparation

Completing a physical assessment in a hospital, nursing home, or community setting may be embarrassing, especially for overweight or underweight patients. The nurse should reassure the patient of confidentiality and proceed with the examination in a straightforward, nonjudgmental manner while ensuring patient privacy and dignity. Table 8-4 lists common versus specialty techniques for nurses related to nutritional assessment.

Technique and Normal Findings	Abnormal Findings

Physical Assessment

Body Type

Observe body type, which is noted as small build, average build, or large build. *A wide variety of body types fall within the normal range; however, note that muscle tone and mass decrease with age. Aging also causes fat distribution to change. Fat is lost from the face and neck, while it tends to increase in the arms, abdomen, and hips.*

Major causes of morbidity and mortality are linked to poor diet and sedentary lifestyle with associated *obesity*. Obesity is a growing concern. In 2007, 30 states in the United States had adult obesity rates ≥25%; Alabama, Mississippi, and Tennessee had obesity rates ≥30% (CDC, 2009). Lack of subcutaneous fat with prominent bones, abdominal ascites, and pitting edema are other abnormal findings. Amenorrhea is a cardinal symptom of eating disorders; other physical consequences of eating disorders, such as cardiac failure or muscle wasting, can be fatal.

Cachexia means a highly catabolic state with accelerated muscle loss and a chronic inflammatory response. It is a distinct syndrome separate from anorexia with the production of proinflammatory cytokines that contribute to the breakdown of fat and muscle protein, causing loss of both muscle mass and fat stores (Jatoi, et al., 2009). These inflammatory mediators accelerate inflammation, increase the production of C-reactive protein, and reduce albumin levels. Cachexia is common with *cancer, hyperthyroidism,* and *AIDS* and is difficult to treat.

(text continues on page 166)

General Appearance

Observe general appearance. *A healthy adult appears energetic, alert, and erect. Skin, hair, and nails look healthy.*

Clinical findings of malnutrition can occur in many places throughout the body (see Table 8-8 at the end of the chapter). Visible signs include muscle wasting, particularly in the temporal area, and muscle weakness; tongue atrophy; and bleeding or changes in the integrity or hydration status of the skin, hair, teeth, gums, lips, tongue, eyes, and, in men, genitalia (Bellini, et al., 2009). See Box 8-3. *Malnutrition* is less common in developed countries than obesity but can lead to several poor health outcomes including protein-calorie malnutrition, growth retardation, compromised immunity, poor wound healing and muscle loss, and physical and functional decline.

Swallowing

Observe the patient's ability to swallow. *Swallowing is smooth, with no problems with the ingestion of food.*

Difficulty swallowing, known as *dysphagia*, is common in *stroke* and *neuromuscular diseases*.

Elimination

Inspect urine, emesis, and stool. See Chapter 22.

Emesis refers to vomited contents from the gastrointestinal tract. The amount should be described and measured.

Body Mass Index

BMI is a guide for maintaining ideal weight for height. It is also used as a benchmark for obesity or protein-caloric malnutrition. BMI calculation is nonthreatening, noninvasive, and inexpensive. It has one major limitation—BMI can be elevated from large muscles or edema rather than from excess fat.

Calculate BMI as follows: BMI = weight in kg OR weight in lb ÷ height in m² OR height in in² × 703.

BMI of 18.5–24.9 is healthy or normal.

BMI <18.5 or >24.9 is abnormal and a health risk (Table 8-5). Adults with a BMI <17.5 or children and adolescents with a BMI less than the 5th percentile meet the criteria for an eating disorder.

Weight Calculations

Reference standards for height and weight are published, with the most common being the Metropolitan Life Insurance Tables (see Chap. 6). These were made available in 1959 and have not yet been revised. Refer to Table 8-6 for calculations of weight for height based on frame size.

In theory, elbow width or wrist width correlates fairly well with muscle and bone mass. But in practice, frame size is too difficult to use, so instead patients subjectively choose their own categories.

Table 8.5 Classification of Overweight and Obesity by BMI, Waist Circumference, and Associated Disease Risks

	BMI (kg/m²)	Obesity Class	Disease Risk* Relative to Normal Weight and Waist Circumference	
			Men 102 cm (40 in) or Less Women 88 cm (35 in) or Less	Men > 102 cm (40 in) Women > 88 cm (35 in)
Underweight	<18.5		—	—
Normal	18.5–24.9		—	—
Overweight	25.0–29.9		Increased	High
Obesity	30.0–34.9	I	High	Very high
	35.0–39.9	II	Very high	Very high
Extreme obesity	40.0+	III	Extremely high	Extremely high

*Disease risk for type 2 diabetes, hypertension, and cardiovascular disease.
†Increased waist circumference can also be a marker for increased risk even in persons of normal weight.
Source: From NHLBI. (2009). *Classification of overweight and obesity by BMI, waist circumference, and associated disease risks.* Retrieved May 8, 2009, from http://www.nhlbi.nih.gov/health/public/heart/obesity/lose_wt/bmi_dis.htm.

Table 8.6 Calculations and Analysis of Weight for Height

1. "Ideal" weight based on height:

Men: 106 lb for the first 5 ft of height and 6 lb for each additional inch

Women: 100 lb for the first 5 ft of height and 5 lb for each additional inch

Add or subtract 10%, depending on body frame size

2. Use current weight and "ideal" weight to determine the percent ideal body weight:

$$\text{Percentage of ideal body weight} = \frac{\text{Current weight}}{\text{Ideal weight}} \times 100$$

>200%	Morbid obesity
120%–199%	Obese
110%–119%	Overweight
90%–110%	Within normal range
89%–90%	Mild malnutrition
70%–79%	Moderate malnutrition
<69%	Severe malnutrition

Source: From Dudek, S. G. (2010). *Nutrition essentials for nursing practice* (6th ed.). Philadelphia: Wolters Kluwer Health/Lippincott Williams & Wilkins.

Technique and Normal Findings (continued)	Abnormal Findings (continued)
Percentage of Ideal Body Weight The percentage of ideal body weight is based on the ideal and current weight: Percentage of ideal body weight = current weight/ideal weight × 100.	*Mild malnutrition*: 80%–90% of ideal weight *Moderate malnutrition*: 70% to 80% of ideal weight *Severe malnutrition*: <70% of ideal weight
Recent Weight Change Carefully assess the circumstances surrounding any change in weight to determine causes. Cluster weight and weight change with other data to analyze if the change is from fluid, muscle mass, or fat stores. After collecting the usual weight from the history and current weight on a scale (see Chapter 4), calculate the percent weight change (percentage loss of usual weight) as follows: (usual weight − present weight) ÷ usual weight × 100	The following guidelines indicate significant weight loss: • 1%–2% in 1 week • 5% in 1 month • 7.5% in 3 months • 10% in 6 months (Dudek, 2010) Unintentional weight gain or loss is a significant finding. This may occur from a change in fluid volume, such as in *heart* or *kidney failure*, or from a change in nutritional status. Weight gain may result from metabolic issues, such as *hypothyroidism*.
Percent Usual Body Weight Another calculation can be made based upon the current and usual weight. The percentage of usual weight is calculated as follows: Percentage of usual body weight = current weight/usual weight × 100.	*Mild malnutrition*: 85%–95% of usual body weight *Moderate malnutrition*: 75%–84% of usual body weight *Severe malnutrition*: <75% of usual body weight
Waist Circumference —————— Where fat is deposited on the body is a more reliable indicator of disease risk than the amount of fat deposited in the body. Use waist circumference to evaluate the amount of abdominal fat in men and women.	Waist circumference >40 in (102 cm) in men or >35 in (88 cm) in women increases the risk for chronic illness associated with adiposity (National Heart Lungs and Blood Institute [NHLBI], 2009). See Table 8-5.

(text continues on page 168)

The patient should stand straight with the feet together and arms hanging at the sides. Place the tape measure around the waist at the umbilicus. Have the patient take a normal breath and record the measure when the patient breathes out (Fig. 8-5).

The accumulation of abdominal body fat significantly increases the risk for *type 2 diabetes, hypertension,* and cardiovascular disease. Waist measurement provides information about morbidity and relative risk of disease (NHLBI, 2009).

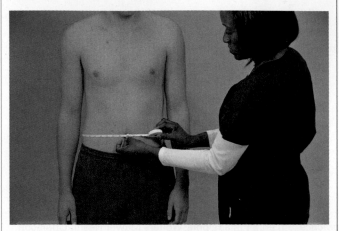

Figure 8.5 Measuring the waist circumference.

Waist-to-Hip Ratio

Assess waist-to-hip ratio to determine body fat distribution as an indicator of risk to health. The waist-to-hip ratio is calculated as follows:

Waist-to-hip ratio = waist circumference ÷ hip circumference (largest point).

Note: *Waist circumference measurement has largely replaced waist-to-hip ratio because it is easier and more accurate to measure* (Bray, et al., 2009).

A waist-to-hip ratio ≥1.0 in men or >0.8 in women indicates upper body (android) obesity, which puts the patient at risk for increased mortality and heart attack (NHLBI, 2009).

Skinfold Thickness

Skinfold thickness is a measure used to indicate subcutaneous fat reserves. It requires an experienced person using a reliable caliper at the correct standardized locations on the body. If this measure is inaccurate, data will be misleading. Measurements of skinfold thickness are much less accurate than measurements of height or

Patients above the 95th or below the 5th percentile are at risk for altered nutritional status.

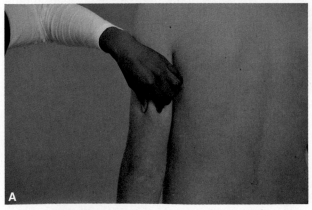
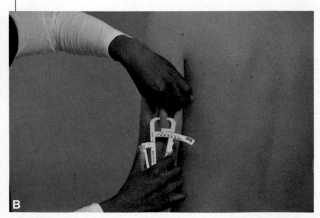

Figure 8.6 Measuring the skinfold thickness. **A.** Gently grasp and pull away a vertical fold of the skin from the muscle. **B.** With the calipers at a right angle to midpoint, apply pressure on the calipers until the spring-loaded level is depressed completely.

weight, especially in obese patients. Thus, it has little practical clinical value unless performed by the same person over a period of time to evaluate trends (Bray, et al., 2009). If performed, a registered dietician (RD) usually takes this measurement.

Measure the skinfold thickness at the triceps, subscapular, biceps, and suprailiac areas. Although the triceps is the most common, it does not accurately represent the adipose tissue of the entire body. For the triceps skinfold (TSF) measurement:

- Locate the mid upper arm point with the arm at 90 degrees.
- Use the fingers to gently grasp and pull away a vertical fold of the skin from the muscle (Fig. 8-6A).
- Apply the calipers at a right angle to the midpoint.
- Apply pressure on the calipers until the spring-loaded level is depressed completely (Fig. 8-6B).
- Take three readings 3 seconds apart and average the values.

Normal findings are according to standardized tables that adjust for age and gender.

Mid Upper Arm Muscle Circumference

The **mid upper arm muscle circumference (MAMC)** is an indirect measure of bone, muscle area, and fat reserves. Measure around the arm, midway between the elbow and the shoulder (Fig. 8-7).

A higher number on the arm circumference indicates both fat and muscle stores. Findings below the 10th percentile are abnormal, indicating loss of muscle. Trends that decrease over time are also significant.

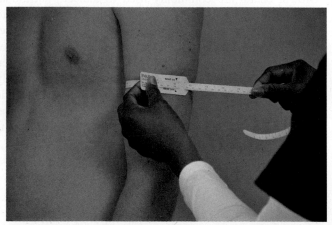

Figure 8.7 Measuring the MAMC around the arm, midway between the elbow and the shoulder.

Derived Measures (Using MAMC and TSF)

The **MAMC and the mid upper arm muscle area (MAMA)** are indicators of muscle and body protein reserves.

MAMC = Mid arm circumference (MAC) − ($\pi \times$ TSF)....

MAMA = (MAC − MAMC)^2 ÷ 4π

A higher number indicates more muscle. These findings are compared to charts with normal values.

Findings below the 10th percentile are abnormal, indicating loss of muscle. Trends that decrease over time are also significant.

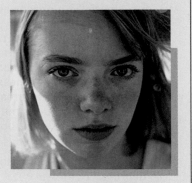

The home health nurse has just completed the physical examination of Karen Pitoci, the 15-year-old girl with anorexia. Review the following important findings revealed in each of the steps of data collection for Karen. Consider the techniques of subjective and objective data collected during the assessment. Notice that the objective data include findings from several body systems.

Subjective: I'm still fat. I don't want to eat because I won't fit into my clothes anymore. 24-hour diet recall: one serving fruit, half yogurt, half sandwich with pickle, celery, carrots, salad, diet soda.

Objective: 15-year-old female is thin and appears older than her age. T 36°C oral, P 88 beats/min, R 20 breaths/min, BP 108/66 mm Hg. Taking fewer than 500 cal/day orally. Weight increased 1.1 lb, BMI 14.8, which is underweight. Ideal weight 125 lb, weighs 71% of ideal weight, moderate malnutrition. Skin pale and dry with some flaking. Appears distressed about eating. No edema, peripheral pulses strong. Nails brittle, skin very thin and dull. Wearing bandana, hair appears dull and thin. Eyes sunken with dark circles. Upper and lower extremities with full range of motion, muscle strength 5/5. Abdomen soft, convex, nondistended, nontender. Heart rate and rhythm regular. Lung sounds clear.

Analysis: Nutrition, less than body requirements related to low calorie intake.

Plan: Continue to encourage nutritious foods with adequate calories and protein. Schedule a visit next week to evaluate weight. Refer to a dietician for further counseling on food choices.

F. Welly, RN

🔺 Lifespan Considerations

Pregnant Women

Vitamin deficiency is rare in developed countries and uncommon among healthy pregnant women (Gillen-Goldstein, et al., 2009). Women who skip several meals each week, have a high intake of soft drinks, snack foods, and fast foods, or both can benefit from nutritional counseling by a RD. Because of financial concerns, some women may require assistance from sources such as the Special Supplemental Food Program for Women, Infants, and Children (WIC) or a social service agency (Gillen-Goldstein, et al., 2009).

The main measure of nutritional health in a pregnant woman is prepregnancy BMI. Prepregnancy body weight and weight gain are associated with both the infant's birth weight and the length of term. Underweight women with low weight gain during pregnancy are at higher risk of having a low–birth-weight infant and preterm birth. Obese women are at increased risk of having a larger than expected infant and late birth.

Recommendations for weight gain during pregnancy are as follows:

- 12.5 to 18 kg for underweight women—BMI < 19.8 kg/m^2
- 11.5 to 16 kg for normal weight women—BMI 19.9 to 26.0 kg/m^2
- 7 to 11.5 kg for overweight women—BMI 26.0 to 29.0 kg/m^2
- At least 6.8 kg for obese women—BMI > 29.0 kg/m^2 (Gillen-Goldstein, et al., 2009).

Infants, Children, and Adolescents

Growth charts are commonly used to indicate nutritional status. One set of charts commonly used from birth to 36 months includes length, weight, and head circumference. See Chapter 6 for measurement techniques. Another set of charts includes height and weight and is used for children 2 to 18 years. Children who should be followed up closely and need a more complete nutritional assessment include those whose height for age is less than the 10th percentile, weight for height is less than the 15th percentile, or BMI is greater than the 85th percentile (Phillips, et al., 2009).

Of particular concern is the prevalence of obesity in children. The percentage of obese children has increased over the past 20 years as follows:

- 2 to 5 years: 5% to 12%
- 6 to 11 years: 7% to 17%
- 12 to 19 years: 5% to 18% (CDC, 2009)

Obese children and adolescents are more likely to have risk factors associated with cardiovascular diseases (ie high blood pressure, high cholesterol, type 2 diabetes) than are other children and adolescents (CDC, 2009). Additionally, poor Hispanic, white, and black children are two to three times more likely to be obese than affluent white children (Singh, et al., 2008). Finally, it is important to remember that obesity and malnutrition are not mutually exclusive. Children with high-fat, high-carbohydrate diets may lack sufficient fruits and vegetables to meet daily requirements for other nutrients such as vitamins.

The physical assessment includes observing for signs of genetic disorders or medical diseases contributing to malnutrition (eg, lack of feeding or vitamin deficiencies) and child abuse or neglect (Kirkland, et al., 2009). The nurse also observes the relationship of the parent to the child and, when able, the parent feeding the child.

Older Adults

In older adults, BMI and weight change are the simplest screening measures. Weight loss in older adults, especially unintentional, is associated with an increased risk of death. It may be difficult to obtain an accurate weight in an older adult. A chair or bed scale that is regularly calibrated may be needed for patients who cannot stand on a scale. Low body weight is defined as <80% of ideal body weight (Ritchie, et al., 2009). Interestingly, loss of as little as 5% of weight over a 3-year period is associated with increased mortality among older adults living in the community. Residents who live in nursing homes have meaningful weight loss if they have lost 5% of usual body weight in 30 days, or 10% in 6 months. Valid and reliable tools have been developed for older adults (see Table 8-4).

Evidence-Based Critical Thinking

Nurses usually complete nutrition assessments in collaboration with dieticians. Often, however, nurses are the first providers to identify patients at nutritional risk. Nutritional issues can affect all body systems, fluid balance, and electrolytes. Undernourished patients may have electrolyte imbalances, delayed healing, and slowed recovery from illness.

Common Laboratory and Diagnostic Testing

No single laboratory test is nutritionally specific. Health-related conditions or treatments can affect each measure. For example, with protracted illness or hospitalization, circulating and nutrient storage pools shift, depending on resources and demands, and body stores of macronutrients and micronutrients may decline to dangerously low levels. Most biochemical measures detect only circulating levels of nutrients; thus, reported values can lead to an incomplete nutritional picture because there is no indication of how much of a measured nutrient is still stored in the body. Therefore, the use of serial tests rather than a single value is suggested to achieve greater accuracy and to discover nutritional trends. Additionally, it is useful to cluster a group of tests and data together to analyze nutritional status.

Serum Proteins

The liver synthesizes several serum proteins. *Albumin* is a prime ingredient of blood oncotic pressure and a carrier protein for many body and pharmacologic substances. The serum protein albumin level is low with liver cell damage, malnutrition, and renal disease. With a low albumin level, interstitial fluid is not drawn back into the vascular system, causing fluid to accumulate in the tissues. Because of the long half-life (18 to 30 days) of albumin, this value is not the best indicator of current nutritional status, although often used. Another circulating protein, *prealbumin*, has a half-life of 2 days. Though less commonly ordered than albumin, prealbumin level is a better indicator of current nutritional status because of its shorter half-life. *Transferrin* has a half-life of 9 days, putting it between prealbumin and albumin. Another serum protein is *creatinine*; however, because the kidneys excrete creatinine, it is more reflective of renal function. Total protein levels measure all circulating body proteins and provide an overview of protein stores.

Hemoglobin and Hematocrit

Low hemoglobin and hematocrit counts may indicate poor iron intake or absorption. Other factors such as bleeding, fluid excess, or low intake of vitamin B_{12} and folate may also decrease these values.

Lymphocyte Count

Severe malnutrition may compromise inflammatory response. An indicator of the ability to mount an immune response is the total lymphocyte (white blood cell) count.

Creatinine Excretion

Creatinine excretion reflects muscle mass, but individual variations are wide. This is a measure of excretion of creatinine in the urine according to the patient's height. A 24-hour urine collection is needed, and there are many sources of error.

Nitrogen Balance

Nitrogen balance reflects total protein mass, but laboratory testing of it is expensive and time consuming. Three consecutive 24-hour measurements of urine are needed because of large variations; there are many potential sources of error.

Skin Testing

Delayed-type hypersensitivity testing is performed by skin testing with common irritants. Theoretically, the immune response will be reduced in the malnourished patient. Skin testing is not commonly performed because it is uncomfortable, and the immune response can be depressed during an acute illness even in the absence of malnutrition (Olendzki, et al., 2009).

Lipid Measurements

Lipid measurements are used to assess the status of cardiovascular health, including total cholesterol, high-density lipoprotein, LDL, and triglyceride levels. Findings are associated with risks for atherosclerosis, heart attack, and stroke.

Other Laboratory Tests

Anemias are associated with iron, vitamin B_{12}, and folate deficiencies. Sodium, potassium, magnesium, calcium, and phosphate are serum electrolytes associated with nutritional status. Because of other factors that can influence these values, they must be considered within a cluster of data rather than independently as a reflection of nutritional status (Olendzki, et al., 2009).

Diagnostic Reasoning

Nursing Diagnosis, Outcomes, and Interventions

Patients may be at risk for fluid volume or nutritional imbalance as listed in the North American Nursing Diagnosis Association (NANDA-I) nursing diagnoses. North Americans are at most risk for imbalanced nutrition: more than body requirements, given that more than two thirds of the population is overweight or obese. The World Health Organization (WHO) states that obesity is a much neglected public health problem and that the world's population is becoming either obese or undernourished (Murray, et al., 2009). North Americans with a lower socioeconomic background, minimal education, or eating disorders are at greatest risk for malnutrition today.

The risk of excess fluid volume is rare. Nevertheless, patients on intravenous therapy may experience fluid overload if fluid replacement is not closely monitored, particularly in cases of cardiac or renal failure. Older adults in care homes run the highest risk of deficient fluid volume. Other possible nursing diagnoses pertaining to nutrition include adult failure to thrive, risk for delayed development, and deficient knowledge. Adult failure to thrive may be linked to an endocrine or metabolic imbalance, whereas delayed development may be related to nutritional deficiencies in pregnancy.

Deficient knowledge is the most pervasive cause of nutritional imbalances. Hence, nurses have a significant role in patient education and follow-up regarding optimal nutrition for people from all sectors and age groups of society. The ongoing proliferation of nutrition information means that nurses must access evidence-based sources of nutrition information regularly to maintain a credible body of knowledge. Table 8-7 compares and contrasts nursing diagnoses, abnormal findings, and interventions related to nutritional care (NANDA-I, 2009).

Nurses use assessment information to identify patient outcomes. Some outcomes related to nutrition include the following:

- Less than body requirements: The patient will show progressive weight gain toward the desired goal.
- More than body requirements: The patient will state pertinent factors contributing to weight gain (Moorhead, et al., 2007).

After outcomes are established, nurses implement care to improve the patient's status. The nurse uses critical thinking and evidence-based practice to develop interventions. He or she evaluates the patient to determine the effectiveness of those interventions and revises the plan as needed.

Table 8.7	Common Nursing Diagnoses Associated with Nutrition		
Diagnosis and Related Factors	**Point of Differentiation**	**Assessment Characteristics**	**Nursing Interventions**
Imbalanced nutrition, less than body requirements	Nutrient intake that fails to meet metabolic needs	Body weight 20% or more below ideal, BMI < 20, lack of interest in food, nausea, vomiting, diarrhea	Weigh the patient daily. Monitor the intake. Provide nutritional supplements. Offer food frequently.
Imbalanced nutrition, more than body requirements	Nutrient intake that exceeds metabolic needs	Body weight more than 20% above ideal, BMI > 30, eating in response to cues other than hunger, triceps skinfold >25 mm in women or >15 mm in men	Keep a food diary and record every food and drink. Teach reading of food labels. Weigh twice a week. Teach an increased intake of vegetables and fruits.
Fluid volume excess	Increased retention of isotonic fluid	Altered electrolytes, elevated creatinine, decreased hematocrit and hemoglobin, weight gain	Monitor the intake and output. Weigh daily at the same time of the day. Evaluate serum sodium, creatinine, and hematocrit.
Deficient fluid volume	Decreased intravascular, interstitial, or intracellular fluid; dehydration	Decreased BP, increased pulse, orthostatic BP changes, thirst, dry skin, sunken eyeballs	Monitor the intake and output. Weigh daily. Provide fluids every 2 hours. Treat causes including nausea, vomiting, or diarrhea.*

*Collaborative interventions.

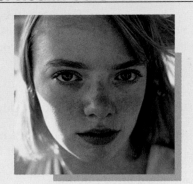

In addition to completing a nutritional assessment, the nurse facilitates the patient's nutritional care by serving as a liaison between the primary provider and the RD. The nurse also confers with colleagues in social work and physical or occupational therapy during discharge planning to ensure that patients benefit from community programs to provide easy-to-prepare food (Box 8-4).

Patients with eating disorders respond best to a highly individualized, multidisciplinary approach to outpatient treatment consisting of nutrition counseling, psychotherapy, and family or group counseling. Treatment plans are designed to foster slow, gradual behavioral changes aimed at maintaining normal eating patterns and promoting long-term maintenance of ideal weight. This can be achieved only by involving the patient in establishing an individualized plan with realistic goals. Patients with eating disorders must be reassessed over time because they often experience chronic problems with eating and exercise as well as weight maintenance.

BOX 8.4   NURSE'S ROLE IN FACILITATING NUTRITIONAL CARE

- Communicate with the RD.
- Serve as a liaison between the physician and the RD.
- Identify patients who may benefit from programs such as Meals on Wheels.
- Request a referral to a speech therapist.
- Confer with the discharge planner, social services worker, and physical or occupational therapist.

From Dudek, S. G. (2010). *Nutrition essentials for nursing practice* (6th ed.). Philadelphia: Wolters Kluwer Health/Lippincott Williams & Wilkins.

In many facilities, nurses initiate referrals for nutrition issues. Assessments that might trigger a nutrition consult include patients who are food or housing insecure, have not eaten in several days, or have wasting syndrome. Additionally, patients with more than three nutrition risk factors or diagnoses that could improve with counseling can be referred to a dietician.

Karen has more than three nutrition risk factors and her health state would improve if she ate more protein and calories. The following conversation illustrates how the nurse might organize data and make recommendations to the RD.

Situation: Hi, I'm Frances Welly, a home health nurse working with Karen Pitoci, a 15-year-old female. She was recently hospitalized for anorexia. I saw her at home today.

Background: She is eating only about 500 cal/day, and I think that she would benefit from a nutrition consult. Although her weight increased 1.1 lb, her BMI is 14.8 and she weighs 71% of ideal weight. She gets distressed about eating and increasing her calorie intake.

Assessment: I am hoping that you might be able to negotiate some food choices that would be good for her.

Recommendations: Would you be able to see her in the next week? Her mother may also want to participate, but I think that you might want to ask Karen for her permission. Thanks so much.

Critical Thinking Challenge

- Why did the nurse leave out most of the physical assessment data?
- How does the nurse use assessment data to make the recommendations?
- How does the assessment performed by the nurse compare to that performed by the dietician?

T he nurse uses assessment data to formulate a nursing care plan for Karen Pitoci. After completing the interventions, the nurse will reevaluate Karen and document the findings in the chart to show critical thinking. This is often in the form of a care plan or case note similar to the one below.

Nursing Diagnosis	Patient Outcomes	Nursing Interventions	Rationales	Evaluation
Imbalanced nutrition, less than body requirements	Gain 10% of body weight, or 9 lb, in next 2 months.	Continue to complete home visits. Assess weight at each weekly visit. Discuss the use of 30 mL of nutritional shake each hour.	Develop a relationship with family. Follow trends of weight over time. Small amounts of intake may be more acceptable.	The patient talks more about anorexia. Weight increased to 9 lb. The patient declined the use of a supplement and will continue to increase the intake.

U sing the previous steps of diagnostic reasoning, organizing, and prioritizing, consider all the case study findings woven throughout this chapter. When answering the following questions, begin drawing conclusions and see how the pieces of assessment must work together to create an environment for personalized, appropriate, and accurate care.

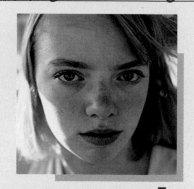

• How might the nurse's previous experiences with patients who have eating disorders influence the assessment of Karen?
• What subjective and psychosocial data will the nurse collect?
• How will the nurse assess Karen's current nutritional status using objective data?
• What adaptations will the nurse make to the assessment based on the patient's condition?

Key Points

• Primary nutrients essential for optimal body function include carbohydrates, proteins, fats, vitamins, minerals, water, and major electrolytes.
• Vitamin D, folate, and B vitamins have important health implications.
• Drug–herb interactions may be serious—even life threatening.
• Three important minerals in a healthy diet are iron, zinc, and calcium.
• Water, sodium, and potassium need to be kept in balance for proper fluid and electrolyte functions.
• Inadequate intake of folic acid during pregnancy is linked to neural tube defects in newborns.
• Newborns and infants have a higher need for proteins and other nutrients than do other age groups.
• My Pyramid emphasizes the need to select foods from each of the five food groups, while reducing fats, sugars, and sodium.

• Risk factors to review in a nutritional assessment include medical history, abnormal weight history, appetite or taste changes, gastrointestinal symptoms, food allergies or intolerances, changes in eating or fluid patterns, poor food habits, inability to cook, poor lifestyle, multiple medications, inappropriate or lack of supplements, and alcohol or drug use.
• Common symptoms that indicate potential nutritional problems include sudden or gradual changes in body weight, eating habits, skin, hair, nails, and energy level.
• Older adults at risk for malnutrition are those who take multiple medications, are socially isolated, or cannot shop, cook, or eat independently.
• The nurse recognizes that each culture has its own food standards, determining what is edible, how foods are prepared, and special foods to eat when ill.
• Comprehensive nutritional screening tools include 24-hour recall, 3-day diet history, and food-frequency questionnaire.

- BMI is calculated as weight in kg divided by height in m^2. BMI of 18.5 to 24.9 is healthy, <18.5 is underweight, 25 to 29.9 is overweight, and ≥30 is obesity.
- Waist circumference is an indicator of accumulated body fat in the abdomen; a high circumference places people at increased risk of obesity-related diseases and early mortality.
- Children who should be followed up closely and need a more complete nutritional assessment include those whose height for age is less than the 10th percentile, weight for height is less than the 15th percentile, or BMI is greater than the 85th percentile (Phillips, et al., 2009).
- Laboratory values related to nutrition include serum albumin, prealbumin, transferrin, total protein, creatinine, sodium, potassium, hemoglobin, hematocrit, total lymphocyte count, and hypersensitivity reaction.
- Nursing diagnoses related to nutrition include imbalanced nutrition, less than body requirements; imbalanced nutrition, more than body requirements; fluid volume excess; and deficient fluid volume.

Review Questions

1. The patient has serum values that are abnormal for sodium and potassium. The nurse recognizes that these values are important to maintain in normal range for proper
   A. tissue oxygenation
   B. tensile strength in the hair
   C. oil production in the skin
   D. fluid and electrolyte function

2. Primary nutrients essential for optimal body function include
   A. carbohydrates, proteins, and fats
   B. folate, vitamin B_{12}, and iron
   C. vitamins A, D, E, and K
   D. iron, zinc, and calcium

3. A patient reports taking St. John's wort along with a medication prescribed for heart disease. Which of the following is the most appropriate response from the nurse?
   A. Never take supplements in addition to prescribed medications.
   B. Supplements act in a very different way from prescribed medications.
   C. Sometimes there might be supplements that interact with your medications.
   D. It is known that St. John's wort interacts with medications for heart disease.

4. A pregnant patient is being screened for AI of calcium and vitamin D. Which of the following tools is most appropriate for the nurse to administer?
   A. 24-hour recall
   B. 3-day diet history
   C. Food-frequency questionnaire
   D. Comprehensive nutrition assessment

5. Which of the following patients has the healthiest eating plans? A plan that
   A. excludes lean meats, poultry, and fish
   B. allows for moderate intake of salt and sugars
   C. emphasizes low-fat milk and dairy products
   D. emphasizes fruits, vegetables, and whole grains

6. A patient has a BMI of 14. Which nursing intervention is indicated?
   A. Provide additional high protein and calorie shakes.
   B. Reduce total fat and calorie intake.
   C. Increase the intake of green leafy vegetables.
   D. Eat complete meals twice a day.

7. The nurse is caring for a child who is at the 95th percentile for weight. Which nursing diagnosis is most appropriate?
   A. Imbalanced nutrition, less than body requirements
   B. Imbalanced nutrition, more than body requirements
   C. Fluid volume excess and deficient fluid volume
   D. Fluid volume deficit and deficient fluid volume

8. From the list below, select the older adult at greatest risk for malnutrition.
   A. A 67-year-old married man with poor dentition
   B. A 73-year-old woman in a nursing home
   C. An 80-year-old widow who lives alone
   D. A 78-year-old widower who receives Meals on Wheels

9. A patient hospitalized 3 days ago has a normal albumin level. The patient is most likely to be
   A. well nourished because albumin is the main protein
   B. moderately nourished because total protein is a better indicator
   C. poorly nourished because hospitalization causes albumin to increase
   D. well nourished 1 month ago but prealbumin is a more current indicator

10. Which of the following patients is at highest risk for complications related to folate deficiency?
    A. A 3-year-old boy who is developmentally delayed
    B. A 15-year-old girl who just started her menses
    C. A 24-year-old woman who is attempting pregnancy
    D. An 82-year-old man living in a nursing home

References

Bellini, L. M., Parsons, P. E., Lipman, T. O., & Wilson, K. C. (2009). Assessment of nutrition in the critically ill. Retrieved May 4, 2009, from http://www.uptodateonline.com.proxy. seattleu.edu/online/content/topic.do?topicKey=cc_medi/17912 &selectedTitle=6~150&source=search_result

Boyce, J. M., & Shone, G. R. (2006). Effects of aging on smell and taste. *Postgraduate Medicine, 82*, 249–251.

Bray, G. A., Xavier Pi-Sunyer, F., & Martin, K. A. (2009). *Determining body composition in adults*. Retrieved April 27,

2009, from http://www.uptodateonline.com.proxy.seattleu.edu/
online/content/topic.do?topicKey=obesity/7584&selectedTitle=
2~150&source=search_result

CDC. (2007). Use of supplements containing folic acid among women of childbearing age – United States, 2007. *MMWR, 57*(01), 5–8.

CDC. (2009). *Overweight and obesity.* Retrieved May 4, 2009, from http://www.cdc.gov/nccdphp/dnpa/obesity/index.htm

Craig, W. J. (2009). Health effects of vegan diets. *American Journal of Clinical Nutrition, 89*(5), 1627S–1633S. Epub 2009 Mar 11.

Dudek, S. G. (2010). *Nutrition essentials for nursing practice* (6th ed.). Philadelphia: Wolters Kluwer Health/Lippincott Williams & Wilkins.

Gillen-Goldstein, et al. (2009). *Prenatal vitamins: Give your baby the best start.* Retrieved May 17, 2010, from http://www.mayoclinic.com/health/prenatal-vitamins/pr00160

Hemmelgarn, M. (2009). Shedding light on vitamin D. *American Journal of Nursing, 109*(4), 19–20.

Jatoi, A., Loprinzi, C. L., Hesketh, P. J., & Savarese, D. M. F. (2009). *Clinical features and pathogenesis of cancer cachexia.* Retrieved May 7, 2009, from http://www.uptodateonline.com.proxy.seattleu.edu/online/content/topic.do?topicKey=genl_onc/4404&selectedTitle=1~77&source=search_result

Kirkland, R. T., Drutz, J. E., Augustyn, M., Motl, K. J., & Torchia, M. M. (2009). Etiology and evaluation of failure to thrive (undernutrition) in children younger than two years. Retrieved May 7, 2009, from http://www.uptodateonline.com.proxy.seattleu.edu/online/content/topic.do?topicKey=gen_pedi/2884&linkTitle=EVALUATION&source=preview&selectedTitle=10~150&anchor=14#14

Lowdermilk, D. L., & Perry, S. E. (2007). *Maternity & women's health care* (9th ed.). St. Louis: Elsevier.

Magana-Gomez, J. A., & Calderon de la Barca, A. M. (2008) Risk assessment of genetically modified crops for nutrition and health. *Nutrition Reviews, 67*(1), 1–16.

Mente, A., de Koning, L., Shannon, H. S., & Anand, S. S. (2009). A systematic review of the evidence supporting a causal link between dietary factors and coronary heart disease. *Archives of Internal Medicine, 169*(7), 659–669.

Moorhead, S., Johnson, M., & Mass, M. (2007). *Nursing Outcomes Classification (NOC)* (4th ed.). Philadelphia: Mosby.

Murray, R. B., Zentner, J. P., Pangman, V., & Pangman, C. (2009). *Health promotion strategies through the lifespan* (2nd Canadian ed.). Toronto: Prentice Hall.

NHLBI. (2009). *Classification of overweight and obesity by BMI, waist circumference, and associated disease risks.* Retrieved May 8, 2009, from http://www.nhlbi.nih.gov/health/public/heart/obesity/lose_wt/bmi_dis.htm

NANDA-I. (2009). *Nursing diagnoses, 2009–2011 Edition: Definitions and classifications.* West Sussex, UK: John Wiley & Sons.

Olendzki, B., Lipman, T. O., & Rind, D. M. (2009). *Dietary and nutritional assessment in adults.* Retrieved May 7, 2009, from http://www.uptodateonline.com.proxy.seattleu.edu/online/content/topic.do?topicKey=nutritio/4489&selectedTitle=8~150&source=search_result

Pencharz, P. B. (2010). Protein and energy requirements for optimal catch-up growth. *European Journal of Clinical Nutrition, 64,* 55–57.

Phillips, S. M., Jensen, C., Motil, K. J., & Hoppin, A. G. (2009). *Indications for nutritional assessment in childhood.* Retrieved May 7, 2009, from http://www.uptodateonline.com.proxy.seattleu.edu/online/content/topic.do?topicKey=nutri_ch/5413&selectedTitle=10~150&source=search_result

Pirlich, M., Schütz, T., Norman, K., Gastell, S., Lübke, H. J., Bischoff, S. C., et al. (2006). The German hospital malnutrition study. *Clinical Nutrition, 25*(4), 563–572.

Ritchie, C., Schmader, K. E, Lipman, T. O., & Sokol, N. (2009). *Geriatric nutrition: Nutritional issues in older adults.* Retrieved May 4, 2009, from http://www.uptodateonline.com.proxy.seattleu.edu/online/content/topic.do?topicKey=geri_med/8473&selectedTitle=1~150&source=search_result

Simmons, S. F., Bertrand, R., Shier, V., Sweeland, R., Moore, T. J., Hurd, D. T., et al. (2007). A preliminary evaluation of the paid feeding assistant regulation. Impact on feeding assistance care process quality in nursing homes. *The Gerontologist, 47*(2), 184–192.

Singh, G. K., Kogan, M. D., Van Dyck, P. C., & Siahpush, M. (2008). Racial/ethnic, socioeconomic, and behavioral determinants of childhood and adolescent obesity in the United States: Analyzing independent and joint associations. *Annals of Epidemiology, 18*(9), 682–695.

Snyder, P. J., Matsumoto, A. M, O'Leary, M. P., & Martin, K. A. (2009). *Use of androgens and other drugs by athletes.* Retrieved May 12, 2009, from http://www.uptodateonline.com.proxy.seattleu.edu/online/content/topic.do?topicKey=r_endo_m/9455&selectedTitle=4~150&source=search_result

Spilburg, C. A., Goldberg, A. C., McGill, J. B., Stenson, W. F., Racette, S. B., Bateman, J., et al. (2003). Fat-free foods supplemented with soy stanol-lecithin powder reduce cholesterol absorption and LDL cholesterol. *Journal of American Dietetic Association, 103*(5), 577–581.

Tangney, C. C., Rosenson, R. S., Freeman, M. W., & Rind, D. M. (2009). Lipid lowering with diet or dietary supplements. Retrieved May 1, 2009, from http://www.uptodateonline.com.proxy.seattleu.edu/online/content/topic.do?topicKey=lipiddis/6831&selectedTitle=17~51&source=search_result.

U.S. Department of Agriculture (USDA). (2008). *Infant Nutrition and Feeding Resource List.*

U.S. Department of Health and Human Services, & U. S. Department of Agriculture. (2005). *Dietary Guidelines for Americans.*

van Dam, R. M. (2008). Coffee consumption and risk of type 2 diabetes, cardiovascular diseases, and cancer. *Applied Physiology of Nutrition and Metabolism, 33*(6), 1269–1283.

Wilson, M. M. G. (2007a). *Nutrition: General considerations.* Retrieved May 5, 2009, from http://www.merck.com/mmpe/sec01/ch001/ch001a.html#BABFCEFH

Wilson, R. D., Johnson, J. A., Wyatt, P., Allen, V., Gagnon, A., Langlois, S., et al. (2007). Pre-conceptional vitamin/folic acid supplementation 2007: The use of folic acid in combination with a multivitamin supplement for the prevention of neural tube defects and other congenital anomalies. *Journal of Obstetrics and Gynaecology Canada, 12,* 1003–1026.

Woo, T. M. (2008).When nature and pharmacy collide: Drug interactions with commonly used herbs. *Advanced Nurse Practitioner, 16*(7), 69–72.

The Jensen suite offers these additional resources to enhance learning and facilitate understanding of this chapter:

- thePoint online resource, http//thepoint.lww.com/Jensen1E
- Student CD-ROM included with the book
- *Laboratory Manual for Nursing Health Assessment: A Best-Practice Approach*
- *Pocket Guide for Nursing Health Assessment: A Best-Practice Approach*

Tables of Abnormal Findings

	Signs	Deficiencies
Hair	Alopecia	Protein-calorie malnutrition
	Brittle	Biotin
	Color change	Zinc
	Dryness	Vitamins E and A
	Easy to pluck	

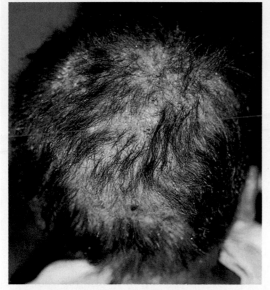

Alopecia (hair loss)

	Signs	Deficiencies
Skin	Acneiform lesions	Vitamin A
	Follicular keratosis	
	Xerosis (dry skin)	
	Ecchymosis	
	Intradermal petechia	
	Erythema	
	Scrotal dermatitis	
	Angular palpebritis	

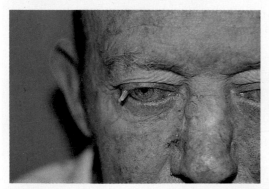

Follicular keratosis

	Signs	Deficiencies
Eyes	Bitot's spots	Vitamin A
	Conjunctival xerosis	Vitamin A

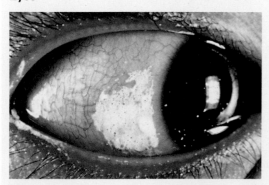

Bitot's spots

(table continues on page 178)

Table 8.8   Physical Signs of Nutritional Deficiency (*continued*)

	Signs	Deficiencies
Mouth	Angular stomatitis	Vitamin B$_{12}$
	Atrophic papillae	Niacin
	Bleeding gums	Vitamin C
	Cheilosis	Vitamin B$_2$
	Glossitis	Niacin, folate, vitamin B$_{12}$
	Magenta tongue	Vitamin B$_2$

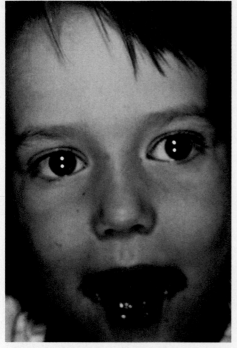

Magenta tongue

Extremities	Genu valgum or varum	Vitamin D
	Loss of deep tendon reflexes of the lower extremities	Vitamins B$_1$ and B$_{12}$

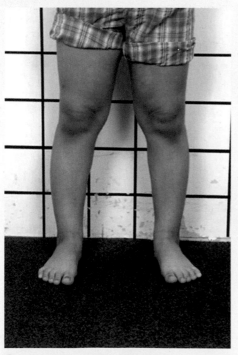

Genu varum

Source: Adapted from Bernard, M. A., Jacobs, D. O., & Rombeau, J. L. (1986). *Nutrition and metabolic support of hospitalized patients*. Philadelphia: W. B. Saunders.

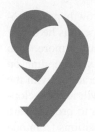

Assessment of Developmental Stages

Learning Objectives

1 Identify physical, psychosocial, and cognitive changes across the life span.

2 Define both individual and family developmental tasks across the life span.

3 Collect subjective and objective data about the patient's adaptation to normal developmental tasks and their relationship to health and wellness.

4 Collect subjective and objective data about alterations in the patient's adaptation to developmental tasks and the wellness risks of those alterations.

5 Use subjective and objective data to analyze findings and plan interventions to promote health and wellness across the life span.

6 Consider the patient's cultural values in planning health-promotion interventions.

*A*mber and Michael Carr have just become first-time adoptive parents to three biological siblings: Emily, 2 months; Jacob, 2 years; and Madeline, 5 years. Amber, a 31-year-old real-estate broker, will be leaving her job to care for the children. Michael, a 35-year-old tax accountant, is enthusiastic about fatherhood but worries about providing for the family's needs with only one income. Both Amber's and Michael's parents, who are in their late 50s and early 60s, are thrilled. They look forward to spending time with their grandchildren and teaching them about outdoor activities, such as camping and hiking.

You will gain more information about the Carrs as you progress through this chapter. As you study the content, consider this family's case and its relationship to what you are learning. Begin thinking about the following points:

- In what stage of psychosocial development are members of the Carr family?
- In what stage of Piaget's cognitive thought are members of the Carr family?
- What nursing diagnoses might be appropriate for members of the Carr family?

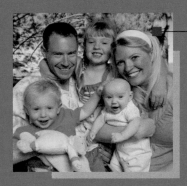

Each unique human experiences physical growth, psychosocial development, and cognitive development as he or she progresses from infancy through old age. Furthermore, each particular life journey varies in unique ways, depending on the person's environmental context and interaction with the world. Understanding the processes of growth and development is essential for nurses. It enables them to provide care and support as patients make inevitable transitions from one life stage to another, become more complex in their thinking and interactivity, and seek to maintain their health.

This chapter summarizes important information about growth and development across the life span. The content serves as a foundational context to support nurses when assessing patients of all age groups and their families. Nurses provide information, anticipatory guidance, role modeling, and protection to individuals, families, and communities to enable optimal, healthy growth and development for children and adults.

Subjective Data Collection

Psychosocial, cognitive, and language **developments** involve qualitative changes in an individual over time. Language acquisition and relationships with others are examples of development (Leifer & Hartston, 2004). Developmental changes are not easily measured with universal tools. Therefore, this chapter covers such material within this section on "Subjective Data Collection."

Areas for Health Promotion/ *Healthy People*

Healthy People contains several goals associated with growth and development. See Table 9-1.

Psychosocial Development

Uri Bronfenbrenner (1979) proposed a frequently cited systems model of development, which describes the individual's development in interaction with the immediate environment (Bronfenbrenner, 1979). In this approach, development is continuous, important at all ages, and an active rather than a passive process.

Erik Erikson (1963) provided another valuable model for viewing individual development over time. His model divides the life span into eight stages, with different psychosocial tasks to complete at each stage (Fig. 9-1). Even if the person does not complete the task, according to Erikson, he or she still must move on to the next stage (which will, in turn, be more difficult because the basis for the new stage has not been established during a previous one).

Infant: Trust Versus Mistrust

The first task for the infant is **trust versus mistrust**. The infant learns that physiologic regulation is linked to a caregiver's provision of comfort. This task depends on consistency, continuity, and sameness of experience; the infant learns that when he or she is uncomfortable, the caregiver comes and provides the appropriate soothing measure. Erikson also says that, by learning to cope with discomfort, the infant learns to trust himself or herself as well.

Toddler: Autonomy Versus Shame and Doubt

The task for the toddler is **autonomy versus shame and doubt**. The toddler learns about "two simultaneous sets of social modalities: holding on and letting go" (p. 251). He or she cannot discriminate between appropriate circumstances that require the choice of retaining or eliminating objects. Caregivers must help toddlers learn how to discriminate and manipulate appropriately. Otherwise, toddlers will overmanipulate themselves and work to repossess the environment in a repetitive fashion.

Preschooler: Initiative Versus Guilt

The preschooler's task is **initiative versus guilt**. According to Erikson, this task has "the quality of undertaking, planning, and 'attacking' a task for the sake of being active

Table 9.1 *Healthy People* Goals Related to Development	
Goals	**Patient Education Topics**
Reduce air toxic emissions to decrease the risk of adverse health effects caused by airborne toxins.	Teach patients to avoid using a cooking stove or heater without ventilation.
Reduce or eliminate indigenous cases of vaccine-preventable diseases.	Encourage timely immunizations.
Reduce the occurrence of developmental disabilities.	Screen for genetically transmitted diseases.
Reduce the occurrence of spina bifida and other neural tube defects.	Provide information on taking folic acid during pregnancy.
Increase abstinence from alcohol, cigarettes, and illicit drugs among pregnant women.	Provide information on the hazards of alcohol, cigarettes, and illicit drugs in pregnancy.
Improve the system for recording and referring infants and children with cleft lips, cleft palates, and other craniofacial anomalies to craniofacial anomaly rehabilitative teams.	Health care providers report and refer infants and children with cleft lips, cleft palates, and other craniofacial anomalies.

Source: *Healthy people 2010: What are its goals?* (n.d.). Retrieved May 15, 2010 from http://www.healthypeople.gov/About/goals.htm

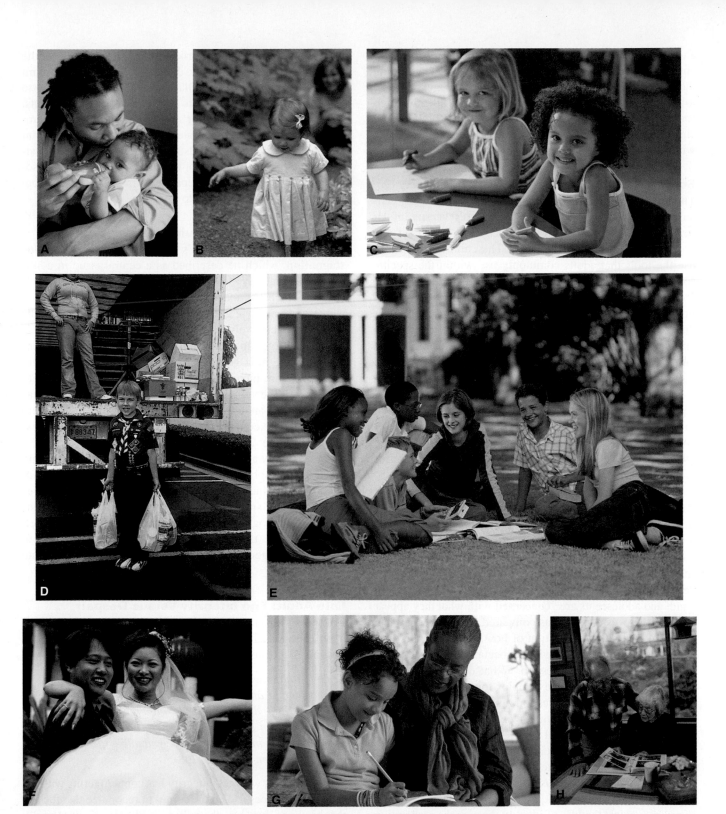

Figure 9.1 Erikson's psychosocial model involves the attainment of different qualities in each of eight life stages. **A.** Infants gain **trust** when caregivers consistently meet their needs. **B.** Toddlers develop **autonomy** as they make simple choices and exert some independent control. **C.** Preschoolers learn **initiative** by engaging in cooperative projects with others. **D.** School-age children develop **industry** by acquiring skills that will assist them in adult roles and responsibilities. **E.** Adolescents achieve **identity** by establishing their own opinions, views, and ideas apart from parents, peers, and other influences. **F.** Young adults achieve **intimacy** by fusing their identity with others. **G.** Middle adults attain **generativity** by sharing their knowledge with younger generations. **H.** Older adults achieve **ego integrity** through acceptance and pride in their life histories.

and on the move" (p. 255). The preschooler is actively engaged in making plans, setting goals, and accomplishing them. Erikson describes the preschooler as "eager and able to make things cooperatively, to combine with other children for the purpose of constructing and planning" (p. 258). The child learns to work with others and can share ideas and plans with peers.

School-age Child: Industry Versus Inferiority

The life of the school age child is, for Erikson, naturally centered on school. His or her task is **industry versus inferiority**. School prepares the child to become "a worker and potential provider" (pp. 258–259). The child must learn to use the tools that adults commonly use within the specific society or environment. At the same time, the school in a literate society has its own culture "with its own goals and limits, its achievements and disappointments" (p. 259). As the child spends more time in the school culture, prepared by teachers for the literate world, the influence of other adults dilutes the role of parents in the child's life. The danger in this stage is that the child will not be able to learn to use the adult tools and will feel a sense of inferiority and inadequacy. It is difficult for the child to be admitted to an adult role in society without the tools to deal with the technology and economy of the culture. If the family has not prepared the child for school, or school does not support the promises of earlier stages of development, the child suffers.

Adolescent: Identity Versus Role Confusion

In Erikson's (1963) model, puberty signals the end of childhood. The task for the adolescent becomes **identity versus role confusion**. With the somatic growth and genital maturity that accompany adolescence, the teen revisits some battles from earlier stages. Adult tasks and roles are now close at hand, and adolescents are "concerned with what they appear to be in the eyes of others as compared with what they feel they are, and with the question of how to connect the roles and skills cultivated earlier with the occupational prototypes" (p. 261) available. The question "What do you want to be when you grow up?" is more complex for the adolescent than for the child. It is now a question not only about a potential career but also about the sort of person the teen wishes to become and his or her social values.

Role confusion in this stage may involve sexual identity but more often involves the teen's struggle to choose an occupational identity. This confusion partially explains why adolescents cling together in cliques and crowds. Doing so helps to protect against the loss of identity through the assumption of a group identity that temporarily defines for the adolescent how to dress, act, and belong. Erikson explained that this behavior will eventually fall away as the individual defines his or her own identity.

Early Adult: Intimacy Versus Isolation

The sixth psychosocial task, occurring in early adulthood, is **intimacy versus isolation**. After the person has navigated the search for personal identity, he or she is willing to fuse with the identity of others. As Erikson (1963) expressed it, the person is "ready for intimacy, that is, the capacity to commit himself [sic] to concrete affiliations and partnerships and to develop the ethical strength to abide by such commitments, even though they may call for significant sacrifices and compromises" (p. 263). By intimate relationships, Erikson meant not only sexual unions but also close friendships and physical expressions. The danger of this developmental task is isolation, in which the person separates himself or herself from others to avoid commitment to intimacy.

Middle Adult: Generativity Versus Stagnation

The seventh stage in Erikson's model is **generativity versus stagnation**, which he described as a central issue in adulthood. Generativity "encompasses the evolutionary development which has made man the teaching, instituting, and learning animal" (p. 266). Erikson argued that when adults focus too exclusively on the dependence of their children, they may forget about the importance of their own dependence on the next generation. The essence of generativity is that "mature man [sic] needs to be needed, and maturity needs guidance as well as encouragement from what has been produced and must be taken care of. Generativity, then, is primarily the concern in establishing and guiding the next generation" (pp. 266–267).

Generativity also involves and includes productivity and creativity. Simply having children does not make an adult generative. In fact, adults who seem to think of themselves as their own "spoiled child" or who demonstrate physical or psychological invalidism have, in Erikson's model, fallen into the trap of stagnation. They have nothing to offer the next generation, even if they wished to contribute something.

Late Adult: Ego Integrity Versus Despair

Erikson's (1963) eighth and last stage applies to late adulthood. The task for the older adult is **ego integrity versus despair**. Ego integrity is difficult to achieve:

Only in him who in some way has taken care of things and people and has adapted himself [sic] to the triumphs and disappointments adherent to being, the originator of others or the generator of products and ideas—only in him [sic] may gradually ripen the fruit of these seven stages (p. 268).

The older adult with ego integrity has come to terms with his or her life choices. He or she comes to recognize that the life that has been lived was the only possible one. If successfully completed, the person is ready to defend against physical or economic threats. If unsuccessful, the person will not come to this understanding of "the one and only life cycle" (p. 269) and will then fear death, which results in despair. "Despair expresses the feeling that the time is now short, too short for the attempt to start another life and to try out alternate roads to integrity" (p. 269). By late adulthood, there is no way to go back and try different paths; choices that were made in life are permanent now.

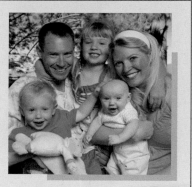

- Emily, 2 months old, is in the trust versus mistrust developmental stage. She must learn to trust that Amber and Michael will care for her.
- Jacob, 2 years old, is in the stage of autonomy versus shame and doubt. His task is to learn to be autonomous.
- Madeline, 5 years old, is in the initiative versus guilt stage; she should be able to plan an activity such as painting a picture and carry out that plan.
- Amber and Michael are in early adulthood. Certainly the addition of three children to their household will call for significant sacrifices and compromises in their marital relationship.
- Amber's and Michael's parents are committing themselves to being grandparents to Madeline, Jacob, and Emily. They want to demonstrate their generativity by teaching the new generation the things they previously taught their children.

Erikson (1963) finished his developmental stage model by relating the circular fashion of the stages. "Trust (the first of our ego values) is here defined as 'the assured reliance on another's integrity,' the last of our values" (p. 269). Erikson further linked the circularity of the relationship between childhood and adulthood in the statement "healthy children will not fear life if their elders have integrity enough not to fear death" (p. 269).

Cognitive Development

Jean Piaget (1952) formulated a theory of cognitive development that begins at birth and continues until adulthood.

Like Erikson's model, Piaget's theory is in stages, and Piaget claimed that the person uses experience to move from stage to stage as thinking becomes more sophisticated and complex in interaction with his or her environment.

Infant: Sensorimotor

The first stage of cognition, the **sensorimotor** stage, is divided into six substages (see Table 9-2).

Toddler and Preschooler: Preoperational

The second stage of Piaget's (1952) cognitive model is **preoperational**, which lasts from approximately ages 2 to 7 years. The preoperational child is forming stable concepts.

Table 9.2	Piaget's Sensorimotor Substages	
Age	**Substage**	**Description and Examples**
Birth to 1 month	Simple reflexes	Behaviors coordinate sensation and action; newborns suck reflexively when a nipple is placed in their mouths; focus is on infant's body
1–4 months	Primary circular reactions	Coordination of sensation and two types of schemes: reflexes and primary circular reactions (reproducing an event that initially happened by chance); main focus is still infant's body; infant sucks on hand differently than on a nipple
4–8 months	Secondary circular reactions	Infant becomes more object oriented, moving beyond being preoccupied with the body; repeats actions that make interesting things happen, such as infant kicks and sees a mobile move and then kicks again to make the mobile move again
8–12 months	Coordination of secondary circular reactions	Infant is beginning to coordinate vision and touch as eye-hand coordination; coordination of schemes and intentionality, such as using one toy to reach another
12–18 months	Tertiary circular reactions	Infant experiments with new behavior; learning about the properties of objects and what they can do; toys can be dropped, pushed, pulled, and used to hit other toys
18–24 months	Internalization of schemes	Infants develop the ability to use simple symbols and form enduring mental representations; the infant sees another child have a tantrum and has one himself or herself the next day

Source: Santrock, J. (2006). *Life-span development* (10th ed.). New York: McGraw-Hill.

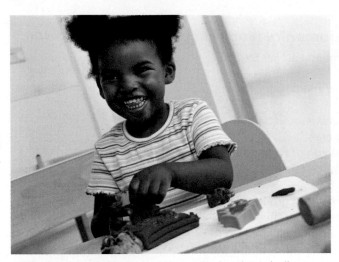

Figure 9.2 Children in the preoperational symbolic function substage rely on pretend play with imagination and creative toys as part of their cognitive development.

Mental reasoning begins, and the child constructs magical beliefs (Santrock, 2006). The child is highly egocentric at the beginning of the preoperational stage but begins, by the end, to be able to consider the perspectives of others. The preoperational child cannot yet think in a well-organized way, but during this period, the child moves from using primitive to more sophisticated symbols (Piaget, 1952).

Piaget divided the preoperational stage into two substages: (1) symbolic function and (2) intuitive thought. The child in the symbolic function substage, which lasts roughly from ages 2 to 4 years of age, can now mentally represent an absent object. For example, he or she can talk about a grandparent's house for many days after a visit. Scribbled designs represent people, houses, cars, clouds, and other objects (Santrock, 2006). Using language and pretend play (Fig. 9-2) are other characteristics of this substage (Santrock, 2006).

While the ability to use symbols greatly increases the child's cognitive abilities, this substage is largely limited because of egocentrism and animism. *Egocentrism* is the inability to distinguish one's own perspective from another person's (Santrock, 2006). The child sees his or her view of the world only. For example, he or she expects that a parent who is away on a business trip still can see what the child sees and know what the child knows, and the child is very confused when the parent does not know what went on at home during the day. *Animism* is the belief that inanimate objects are capable of action and have life-like qualities (Santrock, 2006). Dead leaves blowing down the street are still alive for the child, and objects that cause the child to trip and fall have bad intentions. Imagination and invention are characteristic of children in this substage, and they are as comfortable in the world of make-believe as they are in the world of reality (Santrock, 2006).

The intuitive thought substage occurs from ages 4 to 7 years (Piaget, 1952). These children begin to use reasoning, though it is still very crude. They ask questions constantly and want to know the answers (Santrock, 2006). Piaget (1952) referred to this substage as intuitive because these children seem very sure about *what* they know but cannot tell *how* they know it.

They have not used rational thinking to reach conclusions. An important characteristic of this stage is *centration*, which Piaget defined as the child centering attention on one aspect of a problem and failing to consider other dimensions. It is obvious to an adult that pouring water from a wide and short container to a long and narrow one has no effect on the volume of water. The child in the intuitive substage, however, can see only that the water level is higher in the new container. The child cannot reason that, if the adult poured the water back into the original container, it would be the same volume. This inability to conserve lasts until approximately age 7 or 8 years (Piaget, 1952).

School-age Child: Concrete Operational

Piaget's (1952) next stage of cognitive development is the **concrete operational** stage, which lasts approximately from ages 7 to 11 years of age. Piaget defined *operations* as internalized sets of actions that permit children to do mentally what they once did physically. Concrete operations are reversible mental actions; children now understand conservation and can tell the adult who pours water from one container to another that the volume remains the same and that to prove it, one could just pour the water back into the original container. These children recognize that the original container was short and wide, whereas the new container is tall and thin.

Concrete operational thinkers are also much better able to categorize objects (Fig. 9-3). For example, a school-age child may have a collection of baseball cards carefully organized by team and by each player's position on the team. The child understands that a player can be both a pitcher and a team member at the same time. In addition, children at this stage can reason about relationships between classes, which Piaget called *seriation*. To continue the baseball-card example, the child understands that one team has better players than another team and might organize the cards according to league standings. He or she might then rearrange the cards as

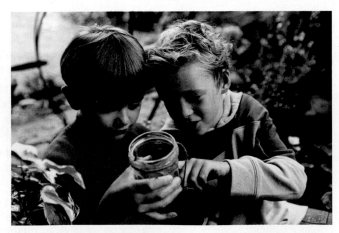

Figure 9.3 A characteristic of concrete operational cognition involves the ability to characterize and sort objects in complex ways. For example, children may have closely catalogued collections of action figures, science specimens, sports materials, or books and spend much time attending to and enhancing such collections.

teams win or lose during a season. Seriation also refers to the ability to arrange objects by quantitative dimensions.

Piaget's concept of *transitivity* refers to the child's ability to consider such problems as if A is greater than B, and B is greater than C, then it must be true that A is greater than C. So the child understands that if John is taller than Jordan, and Jordan is taller than Justin, then John must also be taller than Justin as well.

Adolescent: Formal Operations

The last stage in Piaget's (1952) cognitive theory is **formal operations**. The formal operator uses abstract reasoning far better than the concrete operator and can discuss theoretical concepts that escape younger children. Piaget contended that adolescence is the beginning of formal operations. The adolescent can now talk about "what if…" problems and think logically about abstract solutions. Formal operations also include verbal problem-solving skills. The adolescent who uses formal operations can be presented verbally with "A = B, B = C, A ? C" and substitute the "=" for the question mark without having to see the written problem.

For the first time, those in the formal operations stage can use metacognition (Piaget, 1952), or the ability to "think about thinking." The adolescent also can now think idealistically and consider new possibilities. These abilities lead adolescents to wonder how they could become ideal, and how they compare with role models and heroes. Such insights, however, may have drawbacks. The adolescent who can view world problems in a new light may wonder why those problems have not been solved. Additionally, the teen may find that he or she falls short of the qualities of role models and may then feel inadequate and hopeless about the self.

Formal operations also encompass scientific thinking. The adolescent can now engage in what Piaget referred to as hypothetical-deductive reasoning. He or she can develop hypotheses about problems and deduce the best way to solve them. The concrete operational child uses much less efficient trial-and-error methods of problem solving. Hypothetical-deductive reasoning enables the person to reject some solutions as impractical or inefficient without having to test them and to use logic to arrive at the most likely and feasible solutions (Piaget, 1952).

Adolescent thinking, however, has fundamental shortcomings that result from physiologic changes in the brain. Magnetic resonance imagery studies have shown two main changes before and after puberty. One is the development of myelin in the frontal cortex, and the other is the development of additional synapses (Blakemore & Choudhury, 2006). Because the prefrontal cortex is involved in planning, setting priorities, suppressing impulses, and weighing behavioral consequences (Santrock, 2006), a natural outcome is that adolescents might struggle with these cognitive tasks as the brain undergoes changes in this region. In addition, the amygdala (part of the brain involved in processing emotional information) matures sooner than the prefrontal cortex (Santrock, 2006). This finding may partially explain why teens frequently react emotionally before weighing the consequences of such behavior.

Young Adult: Formal Operations

As the individual moves into young adulthood, Piaget (1952) contended that the person becomes more quantitatively advanced in formal operations. He also believed that the young adult increased knowledge in a specific area (eg, skills regularly used in his or her career). Other developmental theorists have challenged this view.

It may be that the idealism that Piaget considered part of formal operational thinking decreases in early adulthood, because the person moves into the professional world and must face the constraints of reality (Labouvie-Vie, 1986). It is not likely that adults go beyond the scientific thinking methods that accompany formal operational thinking, but that adults surpass adolescents in their *use* of intellect (Schaie & Willis, 2000). While adolescents are more concerned with acquiring knowledge (because they are usually engaged in educational settings or perhaps vocational training), adults move beyond acquisition to application. Pursuing long-term career goals and beginning to achieve professional success (eg, as the person moves from an entry-level to a supervisory position) require much more application than acquisition of knowledge, although certainly the person never stops learning new things.

William Perry (1970, 1999) describes another perspective about changes in adult thinking. His view is that adolescents tend to look at the world in terms of polarities. Things are either right or wrong, people fall into the categories of we and they, and decisions are either bad or good. Such thinking often proves less useful to adults who move into a broader environment and encounter diverse opinions, multiple perspectives, and cultural differences among the people they meet and situations they face. Over time, the reflective, relativistic thinking of adulthood replaces the absolute, dualistic thinking of adolescence. Perry's theory assumes that the individual encounters diverse opinions and values in his or her environment; however, it is possible that a person who isolates himself or herself from new people, situations, and value systems might not move from dualistic to relativistic thinking. Or, the person may simply choose not to accept others' viewpoints, rejecting their belief systems as simply untrue or misguided. The person may even find different ideas threatening instead of evaluating why another person from a certain group or belief system might value the things that are important to that group.

It may be that the changes in thinking that occur as the person moves into young adulthood are qualitatively different than Piaget's (1952) stage of formal operations. Such cognitive development has been termed *postformal thought*. Santrock (2006) explained postformal thought as

> …*understanding that the correct answer to a problem can require reflective thinking, that the correct answer can vary from one situation to another, and that the search for truth is often an ongoing, never-ending process. It also involves the belief that solutions to problems need to be realistic and that emotion and subjective factors can influence thinking* (p. 452).

Middle Adult: Cognitive Expertise

Some people believe that cognitive abilities peak in adolescence or early adulthood and then begin to decline. Research with middle adults, however, shows that this pattern is not at all true. It is important to examine the kinds of intelligence that middle adults use to solve problems at work and in daily living to appreciate what happens with cognition. There are two types of intellectual skills (Craig & Dunn, 2007). The first is *crystallized intelligence*, which is "accumulated knowledge and skills based on education and life experiences" (p. 450) and can

also be referred to as *cognitive pragmatics*; this intelligence is learned and influenced by the individual person's culture. The second type is *fluid intelligence*, which means "abilities involved in acquiring new knowledge and skills" (p. 450) and can also be referred to as *cognitive mechanics*; this intelligence is a reflection of neurological functioning and more likely to be affected negatively by brain damage (Craig & Dunn, 2007). It appears that declines in memory actually do not appear until the last part of middle adulthood or into late adulthood (Santrock, 2006). What may look like memory declines may be attributable to using ineffective memory strategies. When middle adults use organization and imagery to remember things, they can improve their memories.

Another important aspect of intelligence is *expertise*, described by Santrock (2006) as "having an extensive, highly organized knowledge and understanding of a particular domain" (p. 515). Because expertise requires years of experience, learning, and work, middle adults are far more likely to have it compared to young adults. When solving problems, expertise allows the person to rely on past experience, to use automatic processing of information and efficient analysis, to use better strategies and shortcuts, and to be more creative and flexible (Fig. 9-4). The novice must work much harder and less quickly than the expert, because he or she is unfamiliar with the kinds of problems often encountered in a given area.

Older Adult: Wisdom

Cognition is multifaceted, and aging affects some dimensions of intellectual functioning more than others (Craig & Dunn, 2007). Therefore, it is a myth to believe that all older adults are cognitively impaired.

Numerous studies have examined the speed of cognition in older adults, and the results have shown that older adults take about 50% longer than younger adults to do a simple comparison task (Craig & Dunn, 2007). With more complex tasks, older adults take even longer. These differences may partly result from neurological changes that occur with aging, but they may also be linked to the older adult's decreased use of different strategies to perform cognitive tasks (Craig & Dunn, 2007). Older adults may make fewer guesses and try harder to answer items correctly. If older adults are compared with college students, who are more accustomed to doing tests

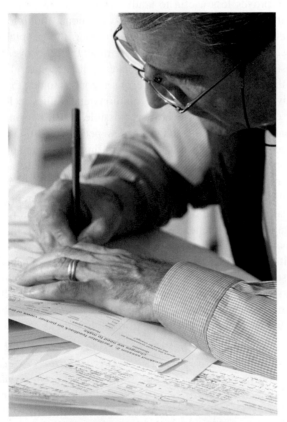

Figure 9.4 Expertise allows middle adults to automatically apply their experience to current situations, which facilitates efficiency and creativity.

Table 9.3	Memory Functions	
Type	**Description**	**Aging Effect**
Sensory memory	Retention of a sensory image for a very brief time	Slight or no decrease
Short-term memory	Memory for things the person is presently and actively thinking about	Slight or no decrease
Working memory	Active processing of information while it is held in short-term memory; active thinking	Decreases, but may use better strategies to limit decrease
Episodic long-term memory	Recollection of past events and personally relevant information	Decreases, but may be from slower processing speed
Semantic long-term memory	Retrieval of facts, vocabulary, and general knowledge	Decreases minimally

Source: Craig, G. J., & Dunn, W. L. (2007). *Understanding human development.* Upper Saddle River, NJ: Pearson Education.

of recall, the older adults will appear less adept at such a test. Older adults may be able to learn new strategies to compensate for their lack of processing speed (Craig & Dunn, 2007).

Memory has been studied by numerous researchers. Table 9-3 shows different memory functions and the effects of aging on those functions.

Despite the small declines in memory in older adults, older adults are wiser comparatively (Craig & Dunn, 2007). *Wisdom* refers to an expert knowledge system comprised of several characteristics:

- Wisdom appears to focus on important and difficult matters often associated with the meaning of life and the human condition.

- The level of knowledge, judgment, and advice reflected in wisdom is superior.
- The knowledge associated with wisdom has extraordinary scope, depth, and balance and is applicable to specific situations.
- Wisdom combines mind and virtue (character) and is employed for personal well-being as well as for the benefit of humankind.
- Although difficult to achieve, wisdom is easily recognized by most people, and it represents the capstone of human intelligence (p. 511).

Although some older adults do not attain wisdom, it is only in older adulthood that the accumulation of life experience results in the acquisition of wisdom.

Cognitive Development for the Carr Family

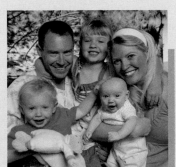

- Emily Carr, 2 months, is in the primary circular reactions stage.
- Jacob Carr is likely to be in the preoperational stage/symbolic function substage. At 2 years, his thinking is still very primitive, and he cannot see the perspectives of his parents or siblings.
- Madeline Carr is in the intuitive thought substage; her thinking is much more sophisticated than is Jacob's. Although she may be very confident about the things she knows, she will not be able to tell her parents how her thought process worked to enable her to know things.
- The stage of postformal thought is still controversial among developmental theorists (Santrock, 2006), but considering some practical problems for the Carr family may demonstrate the challenges a young adult couple faces. Amber and Michael need to learn how to make decisions for their newly adopted children, and they need to consider that they make better decisions when they are not stressed, angry, or upset.
- Amber and Michael's parents, who are in the later years of middle adulthood, will have cognitive expertise. They should be able to expect that their numerical abilities and perceptual speed may have declined somewhat, but their superior abilities to solve practical problems may offset this decline.

Table 9.4	Language Development in Childhood
Age	**Language Skill**
Birth	Crying
1–2 months	Cooing
Middle of first year	Babbling
8–12 months	Gestures such as showing and pointing
10–15 months	Uses first word; has receptive vocabulary of 50 words
18 months	Has expressive vocabulary of 50 words
18–24 months	Uses two-word utterances (telegraphic speech) such as "more milk"
2 years	Expressive vocabulary of 200 words
3–6 years	Learns 5–8 new words a day; works on syntax and meaning
6 years	Expressive vocabulary of 8,000–14,000 words; learns 22 new words per day
7 years	Begins to categorize words by parts of speech; learns comparatives (bigger, longer, etc.) and subjectives ("If you were the school principal....")
6–12 years	Understands and uses more complex grammar; must be able to do this orally in order to read

Source: Santrock, J. (2006). *Life-span development* (10th ed.). New York: McGraw-Hill.

Language Development

All human societies use language as a means to communicate with one another. Language development consists of two parts. *Receptive language* is the understanding of spoken or written words and sentences, and *productive language* is the individual's use of spoken or written words (Craig & Dunn, 2007). Receptive language leads productive language, and throughout the life span, receptive vocabulary tends to be larger than productive vocabulary (Craig & Dunn, 2007). A student who comes across an unfamiliar word while reading a book can relate to this phenomenon. One could stop reading to look up the meaning of the new word, figure out its meaning from the context of the sentence, or simply skip the new word and continue reading. Of course, the choice of options depends on whether the student really wants to understand the meaning of the word,

incorporate the new word into productive vocabulary, or not bother to learn it at all. Using the new word in conversation is risky, however, if the student does not realize its cultural or social connotations before using it in conversation.

Table 9-4 shows the range of ages for the development of language skills in infants and young children.

🌐 Cultural Considerations

Culture profoundly affects individual development. Jean Piaget, Erik Erikson, and Uri Bronfenbrenner all came from Western European backgrounds, and their theoretical frameworks clearly reflect the value their cultures placed on such characteristics as independence, self-motivation, and primacy of the individual. The Western viewpoint, however, is not universally supported. Some cultures value dependence and interdependence over independence.

Language Development for the Carr Family

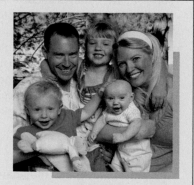

- The Carr family can expect that Emily will make cooing sounds and listen to the language of the people around her.
- Jacob should have a vocabulary of some 50 words, though he may be frustrated when he cannot express all his emotions in words.
- Madeline should be easy for Amber and Michael to understand, and she may be able to translate some of Jacob's words, because she knows Jacob better than his parents do early in the adoption process. Madeline needs to work on her skills with oral language to prepare her for school entry and the development of reading skills.

Through their choices about feeding, carrying, and dressing infants and by sending messages about which temperamental qualities are desirable, parents, families, and communities convey to children which behaviors they consider positive and which they deem as negative or unacceptable (Santrock, 2006). The toddler learns quickly whether independence is more valued than dependence on a caregiver for decision making and exploration. The preschooler may or may not get formal early childhood education, depending on whether his or her parents place value on such preparation for school. Erikson's (1963) emphasis on the school-age child's acquisition of adult tools might mean, for some cultures, learning to read in a classroom, but for others, it might involve following older children to learn livestock herding skills, hunting strategies, or how to care for younger siblings and other domestic skills. Adolescents may be required to stay in school until they are 14 years old, as in Brazil, or until they are 17 years old, as in Russia (Santrock, 2006). What a given culture views as a basic education to acquire the tools needed to enter adulthood clearly varies greatly; the curricula in secondary schools depend on what cultures value as important topics and the time it takes to teach those topics (Santrock, 2006).

In addition, some cultures have rites of passage that mark the transition from childhood to adulthood. Santrock defines a rite of passage as "the avenue through which adolescents gain access to sacred adult practices, to knowledge, and to sexuality" (pp. 415–416). Examples include the Jewish ritual of bar mitzvah for boys and bat mitzvah for girls, Catholic confirmation, and the Hispanic girl's quinceanera (Fig. 9-5). In the United States, these rites do not necessarily give adolescents status as adults in the community outside their faith or ethnic communities. Graduation from high school may or may not lead to adulthood; the graduate may go on to a vocational school, college, or the world of work but may continue to live with or be economically dependent on parents for some years after (Santrock, 2006). The transition to adulthood is a long process for some cultures (particularly those with higher education opportunities) and a very short one in others.

Culture affects intimate relationships in adulthood as well. Desired characteristics in a long-term partner vary across cultures—for example, there are differences in how much people seek out attributes such as chastity, domesticity, spirituality, and age (Santrock, 2006). The ideal age at which to marry is also culturally determined, as is whether it is acceptable to live with a potential spouse before marrying (Santrock, 2006).

By middle adulthood, culture still exerts a large influence on the developing person. Cultures that emphasize parenting as a key role in adulthood may leave the middle adult in an awkward position in a society where the expectation is that children will grow up and leave home; what is the adult's role when parenting is no longer central in his or her life (Santrock, 2006)? Grandparenting may vary greatly depending on cultural expectations for providing childcare, advice, and support to their children and grandchildren (Santrock, 2006).

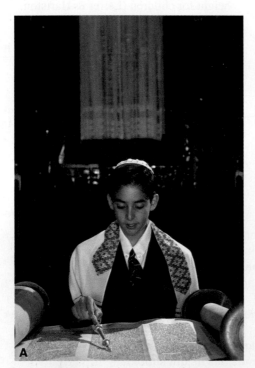 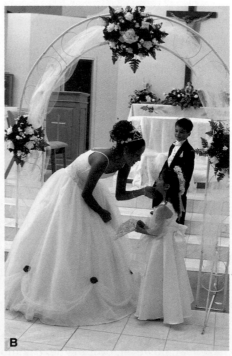

Figure 9.5 Culturally associated rites of passage in Western countries are often symbolic. Often, such occasions are accompanied by large parties with gatherings of family and friends to celebrate. **A.** The bar mitzvah marks that a boy has mastered the fundamental concepts of Judaism and is ready to worship with adults. **B.** The Hispanic quinceanera marks the occasion of a girl's 15th birthday.

Table 9.5	Physical Growth in Childhood and Adolescence
Developmental Stage	**Expected Growth**
Infant	1½ times birth length and triple birth weight by age 1 year
Toddler	½ adult height and quadruple birth weight by age 2 years
Preschooler	2½–3 in and 5–7 lb/year
School-age child	2 in and 5–7 lb/year
Adolescent	Girls: Growth spurt of 2.5–5 in and 8–10 lb Boys: Growth spurt 3–6 in and 12–14 lb

Sources: Leifer, G., & Hartston, H. (2004). *Growth and development across the lifespan: A health promotion focus.* St. Louis, MO: Saunders; Murray, R. B., & Zentner, J. P. (2008). *Health promotion strategies through the life span* (8th ed.). Upper Saddle River, NJ: Prentice Hall.

For the older adult, cultural expectations are important in determining whether or not the individual engages in work and leisure activities. A society's acceptance of older adults may be very limited by ageism and sexism (Santrock, 2006) so that the older adult finds no place in the social order even if he or she had wisdom and experience to share with younger generations. If a woman's role is limited to family maintenance and a man's role to financial productivity, when the older persons are no longer able to fill those roles, they may be defined as no longer useful once their children are grown or they retire from work (Santrock, 2006).

Objective Data Collection

Physical **growth** refers to quantitative changes in a person over time. Increases in height and weight are examples (Leifer & Hartston, 2004). The ways in which nurses measure these changes involve universal tools and metrics (eg, centimeters and kilograms). In addition, nurses can assess motor development more easily through physical examination and use of screening tools. Therefore, this chapter designates physical growth and motor development under the heading "Objective Data Collection."

Physical Growth

Physical growth takes place in an expected pattern, but at a variable pace over time in childhood (Leifer & Hartston, 2004). Table 9-5 shows expected growth patterns in childhood and adolescence. It is important to assess children who are growing more slowly or more rapidly than usual for any potential underlying problems.

There are formulas for estimating potential adult height for children (Leifer & Hartston, 2004). For boys, the formula is

$$\frac{\text{Father's height} + \text{mother's height in inches} + 5 \text{ in}}{2}$$

For girls, the formula is

$$\frac{\text{Father's height} + \text{mother's height in inches} - 5 \text{ in}}{2}$$

Expected Growth for the Carr Family

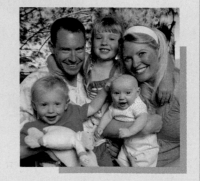

Amber and Michael will need to monitor the growth and nutrition patterns of their three newly adopted children. They need to monitor intake of all the children to ensure that each child consumes high-quality calories and sufficient protein, carbohydrates, and fats to sustain growth (Murray & Zentner, 2008).

- Two-month-old Emily should grow about 1 inch per month and gain two thirds of an ounce per day.
- Jacob, 2 years old, should have quadrupled his birth weight by now. His growth will slow in the next year; however, over the next 12 months, his height should increase by 2.5 to 3.5 in, and he should gain 2 to 4 lb.
- Madeline, 5 years old, should grow 2.5 to 3 in in the next year and gain slightly less than 5 lb.

Table 9.6 Gross and Fine Motor Development: Infancy to Early Childhood

Age	Gross Motor Skills	Fine Motor Skills
0–1 month	Lifts head up off of the bed when prone	Ruled by newborn reflexes
2–4 months	Lifts head and chest up off of the bed when prone, using arms for support	Begins to reach using shoulders and arms
2–4.5 months	Rolls over	Tracks moving objects well
3–6 months	Supports some weight with legs	Begins using hand-eye coordination to reach
5–8 months	Sits without support; some creeping/crawling	Uses visually guided reach; passes object hand to hand
5–10 months	Stands with support	Rolls a ball back and forth to an adult
6–10 months	Pulls self to stand	Looks for a partially hidden object
7–13 months	Walks using furniture for support	Uses pincer grasp to pick up objects
10–14 months	Stands alone easily	Feeds self using spoon and cup, though not neatly
11–14 months	Walks alone easily	
13–18 months	May be able to climb stairs	Stacks 2–4 cubes or blocks, scribbles
19–24 months	Can pedal a tricycle, jumps on both feet, throws a ball	Pours water, molds clay, partially dresses self
2 years	Climbs, pushes, pulls, runs, hangs by both hands	Dresses self; stacks 6–8 cubes or blocks
3 years	Runs and moves smoothly	Builds high block towers, assembles large jigsaw puzzles but often forces pieces into place
4 years	Skips awkwardly, jumps; changes speed while running	Much more precise building and assembling skills
5 years	Skips smoothly, stands on one foot	Draws rectangle, circle, square, and triangle; ties own shoes

Sources: Craig, G. J., & Dunn, W. L. (2007). *Understanding human development.* Upper Saddle River, NJ: Pearson Education; Santrock, J. (2006). *Life-span development* (10th ed.). New York: McGraw-Hill.

Motor Development

Motor development also follows a pattern, but individuals develop at variable rates. Table 9-6 shows gross motor developmental milestones and activities for infants, toddlers, and young children. It is important to recognize that there is a range of ages at which children acquire new skills. Parents concerned about a child's development may need education about the normal range of skill acquisition. Nevertheless, nurses should always take parental concerns about a child seriously so that health care providers can assess delays and intervene quickly, if needed.

Motor Development for the Carr Family

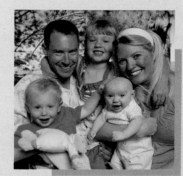

The Carr family should monitor the children's motor development as well as the physical growth.

- Baby Emily will soon be lifting her head off the mattress, although she will not yet be able to reach for objects.
- Toddler Jacob should be very active, learning to pedal a tricycle, jump with both feet, and throw a ball. He may be able to remove clothing and partially dress himself. However, Amber and Michael should not expect Jacob to completely dress himself without help. They will have to closely monitor Jacob, because his ability to climb and run may get him into dangerous situations. Blocks and push or pull toys (eg, wagon, toy lawnmower) are good.
- Five-year-old Madeline should be able to dress herself independently and will run and jump much more easily than Jacob. She should be learning to tie shoes and will be able to draw figures beyond her brother's abilities. Toys could include those that encourage gross and fine motor development (eg, riding toys, toys that she can assemble into shapes).

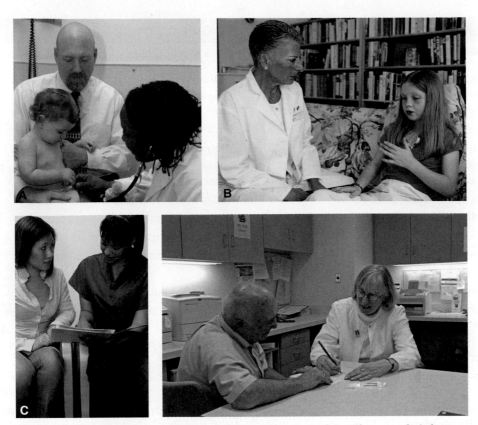

Figure 9.6 Nurses interact with patients at all stages of the life span. **A.** Infants and their caregivers. **B.** Older children. **C.** Young adults. **D.** Older adults.

Evidence-Based Critical Thinking

When making decisions about how a patient is progressing along a developmental trajectory, the nurse needs to use evidence-based knowledge and critical thinking during assessment. Refer to Unit III for more information on pregnant women, infants, children, adolescents, and older adults.

Nurses are concerned with promoting health and wellness in individuals and families across the life span (Fig. 9-6). Healthy children are much more likely to grow into healthy adults, and they need a great deal of support to make healthy and safe choices. Parents also need a great deal of support so that they can choose the healthiest possible lifestyles for themselves and their children. As adults move through the different stages of adulthood,

Evidence-Based Critical Thinking for the Carr Family

Amber and Michael require assistance to help them navigate the major life changes they are facing. They want information that can help them meet the needs of a preschooler, toddler, and infant. Specific concerns include caring for baby Emily, toilet training Jacob and preparing Madeline for school.

In assessing and intervening with the Carr family, the nurse should rely on evidence-based information about childhood growth and development to advise the parents about the best ways to care for their children. It is also important to use accurate information to advise Amber and Michael about how they can make the healthiest choices for themselves. Doing so will help them maintain their relationship and personal wellness so that they are healthy and able to support their children effectively.

Amber and Michael's parents need careful, evidence-based information to guide them as they move through middle adulthood. Health promotion in middle adulthood is important as it sets the stage for health and wellness in older adulthood (Santrock, 2006).

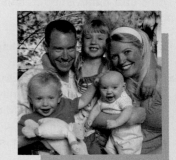

Table 9.7 Common Nursing Diagnoses Associated with Development

Diagnosis and Related Factors	Point of Differentiation	Assessment Characteristics	Nursing Interventions
Risk for delayed child development	At risk for delay in social, cognitive, language, gross motor, or fine motor skills	*Prenatal:* endocrine or genetic disorders, substance abuse *Individual:* adoption, brain damage, chronic illness, congenital disorder, prematurity	*Prenatal:* Avoid exposure to toxins, alcohol, and substances. Teach caregivers appropriate developmental milestone interactions. *Child:* Provide adequate nutrition.
Readiness for enhanced family processes	Family patterns that support overall family unity and the well-being of its members	Activities promote balance between family cohesion and member autonomy. Boundaries are clear and respected. Communication is appropriate. Family adapts to change	Assess the family stress level and coping abilities. Use family-centered care and role modeling. Identify resources. Provide parenting classes. Encourage family meals.
Risk for impaired attachment	Risk for disruption in the normal interactive process that fosters a nurturing relationship	If diagnosed, anxiety, inability to initiate contact or meet personal needs	Encourage mothers to breast-feed. Identify postpartum depression. Offer parents the opportunity to express their childhood experiences.

they also need to make healthy and safe choices for themselves to lead productive, satisfying lives well into old age.

Diagnostic Reasoning

Nurses use the nursing process to assess, diagnose, plan, implement, and evaluate care. Some examples of nursing diagnoses commonly related to growth and development are included in Table 9-7.

Some outcomes that are related to growth and development problems include the following:

• The child will achieve developmental milestones without a delay of 25% or more in one or more areas of social or self-regulatory behavior or cognitive, language, or gross or fine motor skills (Moorhead et al., 2007; Wilkinson & Ahern, 2009).

• The family members will report improvement in their communication, processes, and daily functioning.

Interventions for the Carr Family

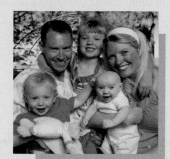

A developmental assessment should be done for each of the Carr children to help identify any developmental delays quickly and begin intervention as early as possible. The nurse can work to decrease the risk for developmental delay in the children by encouraging Amber and Michael to become attached to all of them (especially Emily), by managing the environment to ensure safety (eg, installing gates at stairs in the home, using appropriate car seats for all children, designating safe play areas, supervising children in the bathroom and kitchen, ensuring lead-based paint is not a risk), and by teaching the parents about nutrition and social skills the boy should be acquiring.

The nurse should teach Amber and Michael that Emily needs environmental stimuli (auditory, visual, tactile, vestibular, and gustatory) each day, in short periods when she is awake, and that she must have a parent respond to her vocalizations. Emily needs a comfortable and safe environment to sleep well; Amber and Michael will want to consider factors such as noise, light, temperature, a firm mattress, and appropriate bedding (Wilkinson & Ahern, 2009).

Pulling It All Together: Reflection and Critical Thinking

After completing evidence-based interventions, the nurse reevaluates the Carrs and documents findings in the chart to show progress toward outcomes. The nurse uses critical thinking and judgment to continue or revise the diagnosis, outcomes, or interventions. This is often in the form of a care plan or case note similar to the one below.

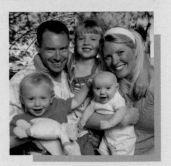

Nursing Diagnosis	Patient Outcomes	Nursing Interventions	Rationale	Evaluation
Risk for delayed child development related to recent adoption	Children will be within 25% of normal limits for growth, motor, and language development.	Teach that Emily needs environmental stimuli each day, in short periods when she is awake. Teach parents to respond to her vocalizations. Consider home health nurse visit to assess the environment for safety and comfort.	Interventions appropriate to developmental stages improve neurodevelopmental outcomes.	Performed screening on all children. Growth, motor, and language development are within normal limits. Continue regular well visits with the family. Allow time for the family members to ask questions as they adjust to the changes.

Applying Your Knowledge

Understanding normal developmental processes is crucial for nurses, so that they can recognize patients who are developing normally and also those who are deviating in some way from a normal developmental trajectory. Using the previous steps of nursing process and diagnostic reasoning, consider all the case study findings about the Carr family woven throughout this chapter. When answering the following questions, begin drawing conclusions and see how the pieces of assessment must work together to create an environment for personalized, appropriate, and accurate care.

- In what stage of psychosocial development are members of the Carr family?
- In what stage of Piaget's cognitive thought are members of the Carr family?
- What nursing diagnoses might be appropriate for members of the Carr family?

Key Points

- Each human experiences physical growth, psychosocial development, and cognitive development.
- Growth refers to changes in height and weight.
- Development refers to changes in motor, language, psychosocial, and cognitive developments.
- Erickson's stages of psychosocial development include (1) trust versus mistrust, (2) autonomy versus shame and doubt, (3) initiative versus guilt, (4) industry versus inferiority, (5) identity versus role confusion, (6) intimacy versus isolation, (7) generativity versus stagnation, and (8) ego integrity versus despair.
- Cognitive development includes sensorimotor, preoperational, concrete operational, and formal operations stages.
- Language development involves receptive and productive language.

- Physical growth takes place in an expected pattern, but at a variable pace.
- Motor development follows a pattern, but individuals develop at variable rates.

Review Questions

1. Caitlyn was 20 in long at birth and weighed 7 lb, 8 oz. At her 1-year well child checkup, the nurse determines that Caitlyn is 26 in and weighs 16 lb. The nurse's reaction to these assessment findings is to be
   A. concerned; Caityln should have quadrupled her birth weight by now.
   B. unconcerned; Caityln is growing in height and weight at a normal pace.
   C. concerned, because Caityln should have tripled her birth weight by now.
   D. unconcerned, because she has slightly more than doubled her birth weight.

2. The nurse's response to Emily's length, which is 26 in now and was 20 in at birth, is to be
   A. concerned, because Emily should have grown 10 to 12 in by now.
   B. unconcerned, because Emily should have grown 6 in by now.
   C. concerned, because Emily should have doubled her birth length by now.
   D. unconcerned, because Emily should have grown 3 to 4 in by now.

3. Jasmyn, who has just had her second birthday, comes to the well-child clinic for an assessment. The nurse reviews her records and discovers that Jasmyn weighed 7 lb at birth. Today the nurse expects that Jasmyn's weight should be
   A. 21 lb
   B. 28 lb
   C. 35 lb
   D. 42 lb

4. Tamika is often in a hurry with her toddler daughter, Samantha, and usually does things for her that Samantha could do herself if given more time. Erikson would say that Tamika's daughter
   A. will develop a healthy sense of autonomy because of her mother's help.
   B. will not develop shame and doubt because of these interactions with her mother.
   C. will develop a sense of autonomy no matter what her mother does.
   D. is at risk of developing a sense of shame and doubt because of her mother's behavior.

5. Oscar, 6 years old, has come to the well-child clinic for a visit. He is 46 in tall today. Assuming that he grows at a normal pace, how tall would the nurse expect Oscar to be at 10 years?
   A. 50 in
   B. 52 in
   C. 54 in
   D. 62 in

6. Mallory, 16 years old, is having difficulty in school and with her friends. She has not decided what she wants to do with the rest of her life after high school. Erik Erikson would say that Mallory is at risk for
   A. industry
   B. inferiority
   C. identity
   D. role confusion

7. At 27 years, Steve is considering purchasing his first house. How might the nurse characterize Steve's cognitive processes now that he has entered into early adulthood?
   A. He will be very optimistic about the purchase regardless of the housing market.
   B. He will use only logical analysis to systematically consider all the pros and cons of the purchase.
   C. He will be less optimistic and more practical, considering the complexities of the situation.
   D. He will be more logical and more optimistic than he would have been a little earlier in development.

8. Nell, 50 years old, is worried about whether her intelligence will change as she continues to advance through middle age. What can the nurse tell Nell about what might happen to her cognitive skills in middle age?
   A. Nell can expect her vocabulary to gradually decrease over time.
   B. Nell can expect to be slightly slower as she does cognitive tasks.
   C. Nell will have great difficulty learning new skills.
   D. Nell will find that her life experience is unhelpful in problem solving.

9. Earl is healthy and vigorous at 68 years. Which of the following will NOT be true of his cognition as he ages?
   A. His long-term memory will definitely be impaired.
   B. His speed of processing information will slow down.
   C. His short-term memory should not be impaired.
   D. His sensory threshold will increase.

10. Amber and Michael Carr need to be taught that 2-month-old Emily
    A. needs stimuli each day, in short periods when she is awake.
    B. will benefit from as much attention as possible.
    C. needs to have stimuli limited to basic needs.
    D. will benefit from long periods of attention with rest.

References

Blakemore, S.-J., & Choudhury, S. (2006). Brain development during puberty: State of the science. *Developmental Science, 9*(1), 11–14.

Bronfenbrenner, U. (1979). *The ecology of human development.* Cambridge, MA: Harvard University Press.

Craig, G. J., & Dunn, W. L. (2007). *Understanding human development.* Upper Saddle River, NJ: Pearson Education.

Erikson, E. H. (1963). *Childhood and society* (2nd ed.). New York: W.W. Norton & Co.

Labouvie-Vief, G. (1986, August). *Modes of knowing and life-span cognition.* Paper presented at the meeting of the American Psychological Association, Washington, DC.

Leifer, G., & Hartston, H. (2004). *Growth and development across the lifespan: A health promotion focus.* St. Louis, MO: Saunders.

Moorhead, S., Johnson, M., & Mass, M. (2007). *Nursing Outcomes Classification (NOC)* (4th ed.). Philadelphia: Mosby.

Murray, R. B., & Zentner, J. P. (2008). *Health promotion strategies through the life span* (8th ed.). Upper Saddle River, NJ: Prentice Hall.

Perry, W. G. (1970). *Forms of intellectual and ethical development in the college years.* New York: Holt, Rinehart & Winston.

Perry, W. G. (1999). *Forms of ethical and intellectual development in the college years: A scheme.* San Francisco: Jossey Bass.

Piaget, J. (1952). *The origins of intelligence in children.* New York: International Universities Press.

Santrock, J. (2006). *Life-span development* (10th ed.). New York: McGraw-Hill.

Schaie, K. W., & Willis, S. (2000). A stage theory model of adult development revisited. In R. Rubinstein, M. Moss, & M. Kleban (Eds.), *The many dimensions of aging: Essays in honor of M. Powell Lawton.* New York: Springer.

Wilkinson, J. M., & Ahern, N. R. (2009). *Nursing diagnosis handbook* (9th ed.). Upper Saddle River, NJ: Pearson Prentice Hall.

The Jensen suite offers these additional resources to enhance learning and facilitate understanding of this chapter:

- thePoint online resource, http//thepoint.lww.com/Jensen1E
- Student CD-ROM included with the book
- *Laboratory Manual for Nursing Health Assessment: A Best-Practice Approach*
- *Pocket Guide for Nursing Health Assessment: A Best-Practice Approach*

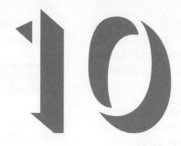

Mental Health Assessment

Learning Objectives

1 Assess for risk factors for mental health conditions and identify appropriate health-promotion measures.

2 Assess for alcohol or substance abuse using the CAGE questions.

3 Assess spirituality and sense of meaning using the HOPE tool.

4 Assess for suicidal ideations.

5 Distinguish normal from pathologic or disease states including auditory and visual hallucinations and delusions.

6 Assess for depression.

7 Assess mental status including appearance, behavior, cognition, and thought processes.

8 Use the Mini-Mental Status Examination (MMSE) to determine mental status.

Mr. Hart, a 75-year-old white man, arrives at the community health care walk-in clinic to have his blood pressure checked. He has been to the clinic several times in the last few weeks for the same purpose. His temperature is 37°C orally, pulse 86 beats/min, respirations 16 breaths/min, and blood pressure 146/82 mm Hg. Current medications include a multivitamin, an antihypertensive, and an antidepressant (citalopram).

You will gain more information about Mr. Hart as you progress through this chapter. As you study the content and features, consider Mr. Hart's case and its relationship to what you are learning. Begin thinking about the following points:

- How are the mental status assessment and mental health history integrated?
- What techniques of mental health assessment will the nurse use to gain the patient's trust and promote respect?
- How will the nurse assess for suicidal ideation, homicidal ideation, and hallucinations?
- What are your experiences with and feelings about patients who have mental health issues or are suicidal?

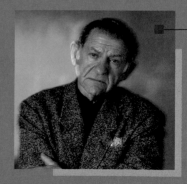

The definition of mental health is important to consider before assessing any patient. In the 1999 report *Mental Health*, the U.S. Surgeon General presented mental health and mental illness as two points on a continuum. In the same report, he defined mental health as

> *a state of successful performance of mental function, resulting in productive activities, fulfilling relationships with other people, and the ability to adapt to change and to cope with adversity (U.S. Department of Health and Human Services [USDHHS], 1999, Chapter 1).*

The World Health Organization (WHO) states

> *There is no health without mental health...it [is a] state of wellbeing in which the individual realizes his or her own abilities, can cope with the normal stresses of life, can work productively and fruitfully, and is able to make a contribution to his or her community...mental health is the foundation for wellbeing and effective functioning for an individual and for a community... (WHO, 2007).*

Based on these definitions, mental health is an integral part of a patient's well-being; thus, the assessment of mental health status is essential. A nurse is often the first health care practitioner whom a patient sees in any health care setting. The patient may be seeking care for a physical problem, and a thorough assessment by the nurse uncovers an underlying mental health problem. It is not uncommon for a patient to have lived with a mental health condition for a long time, even since childhood, and not realize that he or she has a problem. The patient may be self-medicating with alcohol or other substances to feel better.

Common disorders include depression, schizophrenia, and substance abuse. Nursing assessment of mental health consists of screening for preexisting, as well as current, mental health conditions for all age groups. This chapter presents assessment techniques that nurses can use to identify risk factors, assess mental status and mental health, and guide patients in planning care.

Role of the Nurse in Mental Health and Psychiatric Screening

The nurse performs a mental health assessment while considering the patient within the context of his or her own culture. The mental health assessment is based on observation of the patient and his or her responses to the nurse's questions. The nurse determines the extent of the questions based on the clinical setting and ongoing assessment of the patient's needs. Mental health assessment questions are integral to any full medical or nursing examination, even in an examination of a patient without a history of mental illness. Assessment of mental health, unlike assessment of skin or lungs, must be inferred from answers to questions and behaviors because it cannot be observed directly. During the general nursing assessment, the nurse determines whether there is a

need to investigate an area in more depth and may add more assessment questions and observations.

Acute Assessment

An acute mental health assessment includes questions about harm to self or others. Acute situations include a risk for injury with psychotic states, depression, dementia, and delirium. It is important to ask the safety questions first and leave the presenting problem for last. This order prevents the nurse from forgetting to ask about safety. It also allows the nurse to have more time to focus on the presenting problem rather than rushing to ask the safety questions at the end of the interaction when a patient may feel too rushed to speak frankly.

Subjective Data Collection

Subjective data are what the patient says directly to the nurse or is overheard telling someone else or what family and friends have said. The best way to obtain subjective data during an interview is to ask open-ended questions. Doing so encourages the patient to elaborate when answering. It also allows the nurse to assess the patient's cognition processes and understanding of the question. Common practice is to obtain information from family or friends to validate information that the patient provides in the interview. It is best to ask questions that family and friends can validate promptly, especially when assessing for level of memory, accuracy, or perception of the situation.

Assessing mental health is an art as well as a science. The art lies in the nurse's ability to communicate and accurately assess the patient, listening for not only what is said but also what is unsaid. The nurse must be comfortable asking questions about psychosis, suicide, history of abuse, and sexuality. If the nurse is uncomfortable, the patient will sense it and be reluctant to respond. The nurse may even avoid asking relevant questions because of emotions they evoke within himself or herself. It is important to practice asking these types of questions during the laboratory and clinical experiences to increase skill and comfort level. The science lies in the knowledge base that the nurse incorporates in the examination, including the accurate labeling of findings and the precise use of reliable and valid tools that screen for mental health issues.

When assessing a new patient, the nurse establishes rapport first. If there is not much time to establish rapport or the patient is guarded or suspicious, the nurse can say, "The questions I am about to ask you I ask all of my patients" and then proceed. Questions in a mental health assessment are designed to elicit information about various mental health risks and problems.

Patients may use divergent tactics to avoid answering questions. Examples include laughing spontaneously, giving responses that do not follow a logical order, asking the nurse personal questions, or being insulting toward the nurse.

Table 10.1 *Healthy People* Goals Related to Mental Health

Goals	Patient Education Topics
Reduce the suicide rate.	Screen for suicidal ideation.
Reduce the proportion of homeless adults who have serious mental illness (SMI).	Collaborate to find placement for patients with SMI.
Increase the proportion of persons with SMI who are employed.	Collaborate with occupational therapy to find appropriate employment.
Increase the number of persons seen in primary health care who receive mental health screening and assessment.	Screen for depression, anxiety, and illogical thinking.
Increase the proportion of children and adults with mental health problems who receive treatment.	Make referrals and set up appointments for patients with mental health problems.
Increase the proportion of persons with co-occurring substance abuse and mental disorders who receive treatment for both disorders.	Screen for substance use and make appropriate referrals for treatment.

Source: *Healthy people 2010: What are its goals?* (n.d.). Retrieved May 15, 2010, from http://www.healthypeople.gov/About/goals.htm

These tactics will likely disrupt the flow of communication and the nurse's thought processes. Assessing the reasons for such tactics is important. Patients may try to avoid answering questions because they are embarrassed, the topic is too emotionally overwhelming, or they cannot remember and do not want the nurse to realize that. They might also fear being judged or have difficulty concentrating. Being focused on what the patient is saying helps the nurse identify when divergent tactics are being used as well as what is being unsaid.

Areas for Health Promotion/ *Healthy People*

Mental health is one of the 28 focus areas to be addressed in *Healthy People*. Some areas of concern are preventing suicide, especially with the increase in adolescent suicide attempts, addressing serious mental health conditions among homeless adults, employing people with serious mental health conditions, and improving primary care mental health screening and assessment for all age groups. Table 10-1 organizes *Healthy People* foci related to mental health and pertinent patient teaching.

Assessment of Risk Factors

During the MMSE, the nurse is aware that certain situations are considered risk factors for contributing to, or exacerbating, a mental health condition. Factors that cannot be changed include family history, age, and gender. Pregnancy may also exacerbate an existing mental health condition or precipitate postpartum depression.

⚠ SAFETY ALERT 10.1
Women with postpartum depression with psychotic features may harm their infants. The nurse needs to ask specifically if the mother has thoughts of harming her baby.

Environmental factors that may influence mental health include support systems, housing, health care accessibility, and literacy. The nurse also considers metabolic issues and associated physiological processes such as Parkinson's disease, cancer, HIV/AIDS, and other chronic conditions. Identification of the exact risk factors and causes for illness is often complex and interrelated. Nevertheless, identification of these risks helps identify topics for health-promotion teaching.

Questions on History and Risk	Rationales
Biographical Data What is your name? Age? Gender? Race?	Diagnoses early in life may indicate more problems with developmental, cognitive, social, and coping skills. Children are at risk for abuse. Adolescence is a risk because of hormonal changes as well as growth and developmental stage. Older adults are at increased risk for *depression*. Females are more prone to *depression*, and males are more apt to commit *suicide* or *violence*. Suicide rates among U.S. males are highest in American Indians and Alaska Natives. Rates are lowest for African American women (USDHHS, 2009).

(text continues on page 200)

Questions on History and Risk	Rationales

Current Health Status

How are you feeling today?

This generic question opens a conversation about mental health concerns.

Do you have any medical problems?
- Pain
- Thyroid imbalance, diabetes
- Hepatitis, renal disease
- Cerebrovascular accidents, pulmonary diseases, asthma, COPD
- GI distress: irritable bowel syndrome, Crohn's disease
- Potentially terminal illnesses: HIV/AIDS, cancer
- Surgery that has resulted or may result in disfiguring or incapacitating alteration of ability to function

Physiological changes with or emotional responses to illness can affect mental status. Also consider how the medical condition might affect any psychiatric medications, such as causing poor absorption or impaired elimination.

When did you first notice this mental health concern?

Response indicates how long the patient has had a problem. It also can be compared to family perceptions. Identify any possible contributing factors.

- Why do you think it started when it did?
- How often does it occur?
- What changes have you noticed?

Response indicates how it might be affecting functioning. Changes include frequency, intensity, or effects on functioning or well-being.

- Have you ever felt this way before?

This is to assess for any previous episodes, especially if untreated.

- What do you think is causing the problem?

Assess the patient's understanding of the situation and whether it is logical.

- How is this affecting your life now?

Assess implications of how this illness is affecting the patient's life. Assess feelings of self-worth from the patient's responses to the above questions and statements the patient might make about himself or herself or the illness, such as "I don't like feeling this way. I can't be a good mom when I'm feeling depressed."

Describe your typical day.

This helps to identify the ability to perform activities of daily living.

Have you experienced recent weight loss or gain?

Some medications cause weight gain and metabolic issues. Weight changes also may be related to *anxiety*, early *dementia*, *depression*, or *eating disorders*. Physical problems can manifest with mental health issues.

Have you noticed any change in your sleeping habits?

Sleep disorders may be associated with *anxiety, depression, bipolar disorder,* or *substance abuse.*

Medications

What psychiatric medications are you taking? Are you taking them as prescribed?

Do you use, or have you ever used, any alternative treatments, herbs, or other substances? If yes, list the specific treatments or substances.

Consider interactions between medications taken for psychiatric and medical conditions. For example, if the patient has a medical condition such as prolonged QT wave interval (a cardiac problem), the patient should not take or be prescribed some classes of antidepressants. Identify any psychiatric drugs taken, drug interactions, herb–drug interactions, and alternative treatments that might cause psychiatric side effects. Patients may be taking substances to self-medicate. Keep in mind that some patients consider marijuana a natural herb or alternative medical treatment, not a recreational drug.

Past Health History

Have you had any surgeries? If so, please list when and why.

Some patients with mental health conditions present with multiple surgeries and psychosomatic symptoms.

Questions on History and Risk	Rationales

Have you ever been told that you have a mental health problem?
- Have you ever received treatment for a mental health problem before?
- Have you ever been hospitalized for a mental problem before?

Assess for the patient's history of mental health conditions.

Treatment could be outpatient, inpatient, from a general practitioner, or from another health care practitioner. Hospitalization indicates the severity of the condition. It is helpful to get the names of facilities and dates when admitted

Have you ever been physically, sexually, or emotionally abused? If so, did this occur when you were a child?

Assess for situational stressors such as bullying at school, family violence, or war violence (see Chapter 12). People maltreated in childhood are more likely to develop depression or posttraumatic stress disorder and to attempt suicide. Also, abused children develop riskier behaviors (eg, substance use, unprotected sexual activity) as adolescents (Felitti, et al., 1998).

Family History
Has anyone in your family been diagnosed with a mental health condition?

A family history of mental health conditions is a risk factor for the patient.

- If so, which family member(s)?
- What was the diagnosis and treatment plan for each family member diagnosed with a mental health condition?
- Is the treatment plan working well for the particular family member?

Answers may help direct the line of treatment or medication options for the patient.

Psychosocial
Support Network. Do you have a support system?
- Whom do you consider as part of your support system?
- How well does your support system meet your needs?

Assess the patient's coping skills and resources.
Assess members and their effectiveness. Some patients with chronic mental conditions have only their health care providers as a support system.

Do you have a significant other in your life, such as a spouse, partner, or close friend?
- How do you get along?
- How often do you get together with people with whom you do not live?

Assess the stability and effectiveness of the patient's relationships. Patients with high demands often move among relationships as family members, partners, or friends become fatigued.

Stressors. What are some stresses that you have been experiencing?
- Have you experienced a loss recently such as death of a family member or friend or loss of job or income?
- How do you cope with stress?
- How is that working for you now?

Assess for the degree or amount of current stress.

Coping skills are used to deal with stress.
Evaluate their effectiveness.

Are any other factors in your life that may be contributing to your stress level?
- What are your living arrangements?
- How many hours a week do you work?
- Is this affecting your work?
- Is this affecting your level of functioning or thinking?

Factors that contribute to mental health problems include the following:
- Isolation: lives alone or is withdrawn
- Finances: lower socioeconomic status
- Poor or diminished cognitive abilities
- Housing: homeless or unsafe environment
- Health care accessibility: has problems with cost, transportation, or ability to cognitively and safely use public transportation
- Language: cannot speak or understand the predominant language
- Literacy: cannot read or write

Do you have, or have you had, any legal problems? If so, please specify if you were sent to jail or prison for them and when.

Patients with problems of judgment, substance abuse, or anger management may become involved in the legal system.

(text continues on page 202)

Questions on History and Risk	Rationales

Substance Use. Do you drink or use recreational substances? (If you suspect that alcohol use might be a problem, the CAGE is a quick first-step questionnaire to use as an assessment tool. The acronyms are easy for the nurse to remember and use at any time. See Box 10-1.)

- What do you use (ie, beer, wine, hard liquor, and/or recreational substances, such as marijuana, crack, or cocaine)?
- How often do you use each substance?
- How is the use of alcohol or recreational substances affecting your life?

Whenever a patient comes in for treatment of substance use, it is important to be aware of the possibility of an underlying mental health problem. Also, it is very important to know the effects that alcohol and other substances can have on mental health (Table 10-2). When screening for substance abuse, the patient will most likely deny a problem. The CAGE tool is valuable because it addresses this denial.

BOX 10.1   CAGE QUESTIONNAIRE FOR SUBSTANCE USE CAGE

- Have you ever felt the need to **C**ut down on drinking?
- Have you ever felt **A**nnoyed by criticism of drinking?
- Have you ever had **G**uilty feelings about drinking?
- Have you ever taken a drink first thing in the morning (**E**ye-opener) to steady your nerves or get rid of a hangover?

Source: Ewing, J. A. (1984). Detecting alcoholism: The CAGE questionnaire. *Journal of the American Medical Association, 252,* 1905–1907.

Table 10.2 Substances That Can Affect Health	
Substance Used	**Effect on Health**
Injectable drugs	Abscesses, sepsis, endocarditis, pulmonary fibrosis, renal disease
Narcotics	Dependence, addiction, drowsiness, respiratory arrest, overdose
Central nervous system stimulants	Possible dependence, weight loss, tooth decay
Club drugs	Possible loss of memory and subsequent sexual assault
Recreational drugs (specify)	Sherm—formaldehyde-laced marijuana that causes irreversible brain damage
Herbs (specify)	Salvia—a psychedelic that, when misused, can cause errors in judgment, headaches, and vomiting
	Peyote/mescaline hallucinogenic herbs—used in Native American rituals under the guidance of a Shaman; often misused by individuals; visual hallucinations may persist
Misused prescription medicines	
• Taking too much? (sleeping pills, diet pills, painkillers)	Sleeping pills and painkillers to ease emotional distress
• Using prescribed medicine for other purposes?	Patient experiences a "buzz" with no cognitive impairment
• Experimenting with other people's medications (common with teens)?	
• Intentionally taking other people's medications (eg, parent taking a child's Ritalin)?	
• Taking cogentin?	Reported in the news to be common in soldiers serving in Iraq
• Sniffing household chemicals, glue, or car exhaust fumes?	
• Misusing cold medicine or other over-the-counter drugs?	Contain chemical solvents that can cause fatal cardiac arrhythmias, rapid loss of consciousness, and respiratory arrest

BOX 10.2 HOPE ASSESSMENT OF SPIRITUAL BELIEFS

H: Sources of Hope, Meaning, Comfort, Strength, Peace, Love, and Connection

• We have been discussing your support systems. I was wondering, what is there in your life that gives you internal support?
• What are your sources of hope, strength, comfort, and peace?
• What do you hold on to during difficult times?
• What sustains you and keeps you going?
• For some people, religious or spiritual beliefs act as a source of comfort and strength in dealing with life's ups and downs; is this true for you? (*If the answer is "Yes," go on to O and P questions. If the answer is "No," consider asking "Was it ever?" If the answer is "Yes," ask "What changed?"*)

O: Organized Religion

• Do you consider yourself part of an organized religion?
• How important is this to you?
• What aspects of your religion are helpful and not so helpful to you?
• Are you part of a religious or spiritual community? Does it help you? How?

P: Personal Spirituality/Practices

• Do you have personal spiritual beliefs that are independent of organized religion? What are they?
• Do you believe in God? What kind of relationship do you have with God?

• What aspects of your spirituality or spiritual practices do you find most helpful to you personally? (eg, prayer, meditation, reading scripture, attending religious services, listening to music, hiking, communing with nature)

E: Effects on Medical Care and End-of-Life Issues

• Has being sick (or your current situation) affected your ability to do the things that usually help you spiritually? (Or affected your relationship with God?)
• Is there anything that I can do to help you access the resources that usually help you?
• Are you worried about any conflicts between your beliefs and your medical/mental situation/care/decisions?
• Would it be helpful for you to speak to a clinical chaplain/community spiritual leader?
• Are there any specific practices or restrictions I should know about in providing your care? (eg, dietary restrictions, use of blood products)
• If the patient is dying: How do your beliefs affect the kind of medical care you would like me to provide over the next few days/weeks/months?

Source: Anandarajah, G., & Hight, E. (2001). Spirituality and medical practice: Using the HOPE questions as a practical tool for spiritual assessment. *American Family Physician, 63,* 81–89.

Questions on History and Risk	Rationales
Spirituality. Do you have any religious beliefs regarding your illness? Should I be aware of any religious or cultural beliefs while caring for you?	Asking how the patient views the mental health condition in the context of religion and beliefs allows the nurse to provide culturally sensitive nursing care.
Do you have a sense of hope for your future? • What provides you with your emotional support or sense of faith? • What is your religious affiliation? • What are your spiritual beliefs? • What spiritual practices are important to you?	No sense of hope for the future may be an indicator of risk for suicide. The last three questions meet the Joint Commission 2004 standards and recommendations for spiritual assessment. Refer to Box 10-2 for further assessment of spiritual beliefs.

Focused Health History Related to Common Symptoms

Common Symptoms of Altered Mental Health

• Suicidal ideation
• Homicidal ideation and aggressive behavior
• Altered mood and affect

• Auditory hallucinations
• Visual hallucinations

Suicidal Ideation

Do you have any thoughts of wanting to harm or kill yourself? Use the SAD PERSONAS mnemonic to assess for risk of suicide (Box 10-3). This scale facilitates the systematic gathering of patient data and relevant psychosocial history.

Box 10.3 SAD PERSONAS SUICIDE RISK ASSESSMENT

- **S**ex
- **A**ge
- **D**epression
- **P**revious attempt
- **E**thanol abuse
- **R**ational thought loss
- **S**ocial supports lacking
- **O**rganized plan
- **N**o spouse
- **A**ccess to lethal means
- **S**ickness

The presence of each factor is given a point value of one. Total scores range from 0 to 10. Higher scores indicate greater patient suicide risk.

Source: Patterson, W. M., Dohn, H. H., Bird, J., & Patterson, G. A. (1983). Evaluation of suicidal patients: The SAD PERSON Scale. *Psychosomatics*, 24(4), 343–349.

Clinical Significance 10-1

Medical students who received training in SAD PERSONAS showed a greater ability to evaluate suicide risk and make appropriate clinical interventions (Juhnke, 1994). Shea (1999) concludes that the strength of the scale is not as a precise risk predictor but as a way to alert the clinician that the patient may be at higher risk.

Homicidal Ideation and Aggressive Behavior

Do you have any thoughts of wanting to harm or kill anyone?

⚠ SAFETY ALERT 10.3

The nurse assesses for safety of others. If the patient replies "yes," then ask if he or she wants to harm a specific person, and if so, how. Notify the attending primary care provider who will determine if there is a "duty to warn" the other person. The exact nature of the plan for harm and ability to carry it out are an important part of the assessment.

Suicide is the 11th leading cause of death for U.S. citizens of all ages. It may accompany any psychiatric illness or occur without a psychiatric diagnosis. Suicide is one of the five leading causes of death in people 10 to 54 years (Centers for Disease Control and Prevention [CDC] & National Center for Injury Prevention and Control, 2008). U.S. men older than 75 years have the highest suicide rate (38 per 100,000). Men are more than four times more likely to complete suicide than are women (CDC, 2008). In one study, 45% of all suicide victims had contact with a primary care provider within 1 month of killing themselves, while only 20% had contact with a mental health provider in that same period (Luoma, Martin, & Pearson, 2002). Suicidal patients may present in any health care setting with various problems, not necessarily sad mood or suicidal thoughts. They may hint or joke about suicide or wanting to die to test the nurse's comfort with discussing the subject. In many cases, patients do not want to talk, but despondent behaviors indicate that they are suicidal. Failure to ask if these patients have had suicidal thoughts would be a lost opportunity to assist them.

A patient is considered to have very "lethal" suicidal ideation if he or she has a history of suicide attempts, a specific plan, and access to the means (eg, owns a gun, has medications).

⚠ SAFETY ALERT 10.2

The nurse assesses for safety. Some patients are not suicidal but perform self-mutilation, often to release pain. The above question covers both suicidal and parasuicidal gestures. Identifying parasuicidal thoughts is important because patients can accidentally kill themselves while releasing pain.

Risk factors for aggressive behavior include male gender, history of violence, and substance abuse. Ethnicity, diagnosis, age, marital status, and education do not reliably identify this behavior (Moore & Pfaff, 2008). Patients with a history of violence are more likely to inflict serious injuries. Typically, the patient becomes angry, resists authority, and finally becomes confrontational. A violent behavior may occur without warning, however, especially when caused by medical problems or dementia. The nurse should always trust his or her "gut feeling" about the potential for violence. The nurse considers an obviously angry patient potentially violent. It is important to take actions to avoid injury.

Signs of violence include the following:
- Provocative behavior
- Angry demeanor
- Loud, aggressive speech
- Tense posturing (eg, gripping side rails tightly, clenching fists)
- Frequently changing body position, pacing
- Aggressive acts (eg, pounding walls, throwing objects, hitting oneself) (Moore & Pfaff, 2008)

Questions to Assess Symptoms	Rationales

Altered Mood and Affect

What has your mood been like?
Normal mood is pleasant.

Mood is a sustained emotion. Assess the intensity, depth, and duration of altered mood.

On a scale of 0 to 10, with 10 being most intense, how depressed do you feel now?

Patients may use descriptors to describe mood, such as sad, tearful, depressed, angry, anxious, grandiose, or fearful. Mood inappropriate to the situation is abnormal.

Assess the patient's affect. Affect is an objective observation of how the patient expresses his or her feelings and mood. Assess whether affect matches what the patient says. *Normal affect is congruent with the situation.*

Affect may be temporary and changing compared with mood. Bland, apathetic, dramatic, bizarre, constricted, blunted, flat, labile, and euphoric are descriptors of altered affect. See Table 10-5 at the end of the chapter.

Auditory Hallucinations

Do you hear voices that others do not hear? (Ask this question while closely observing the patient.)

A patient may answer "no" even though he or she is actually experiencing auditory hallucinations. The patient may not realize that others do not hear voices or not want to tell the nurse for fear of ramifications, such as continued hospitalization or starting medications. If the answer is "yes," alert the primary provider; the patient may need more supervision if it seems that he or she cannot resist "command" hallucinations.

Assess the nature of auditory hallucinations.
• Does the voice tell you what to do?
• Must you listen or do what the voice says or does?

⚠ *SAFETY ALERT 10.4*

If the patient confirms auditory hallucinations, it is important to ask about their nature. Are they hostile or critical? Do they "command" or tell the patient to do things such as harm self or others?

Visual Hallucinations

Do you see things that other people do not see?

Common causes of visual hallucinations include side effects from medications, alcohol withdrawal, and *Parkinson's disease.*

Other Hallucinations

If there is a history of hallucinations or assessment indicates otherwise, continue to ask questions about other types of hallucinations such as olfactory and tactile.

Some patients with *psychotic disorders* smell smoke or feel someone touching them.

Do you smell things that other people do not smell?

Brain tumors, toxins, and hallucinogens are common causes of olfactory hallucinations.

Do you have any unusual sensations on your skin such as bugs crawling?

Hallucinogen and methamphetamine use is associated with tactile hallucinations.

Documentation of Normal Findings

> Denies suicidal or homicidal thoughts. Mood pleasant, affect appropriate to situation. Denies visual, auditory, olfactory, or tactile hallucinations. *J. O'Placey, RN*

Compare these normal findings with the assessment of Mr. Hart, the 75-year-old man at the clinic who has come to have his blood pressure checked.

> *Documentation:* Making some inappropriate comments, such as asking personal information. Denies thoughts of harming self or others. Mood is anxious, affect is labile. Hearing mumbling conversations with several people talking. The voices are telling him to run away and they frighten him. He states that he can tell the difference between what the voices are saying and what is real. He knows that running away would not be good and that he needs to be here to get better. Talking to others usually makes the voices go away. Denies visual hallucinations. *P. Terris, RN.*

Lifespan Considerations

Additional Questions	Rationales/Abnormal Findings

Pregnant Women

Are you feeling blue? Risk factors include prior psychopathology, poor marital relationship, lack of social support, and stressful life events in the past 12 months (O'Hara & Swain, 1996).

Pregnancy is associated with relapse in psychotic disorders, and women with a history of depression are at highest risk for an episode during pregnancy or postpartum (Cohen, et al., 2006). Pregnant women experience hormonal changes and also may need to stop psychiatric medications because of side effects in the fetus.

Have you used alcohol or other drugs during this pregnancy?

Substance abuse during pregnancy is a concern for the mother and the fetus.

Children and Adolescents

How are you adjusting to the changes in your body?

Adolescence may be difficult because of hormonal changes as well as growth and developmental stage. The onset of menarche and puberty can contribute to *depression*.

Have you ever thought of harming yourself?

Suicide is the fourth leading cause of death in all U.S. children and the third leading cause in U.S. children 10 to 19 years. Rates of suicide consideration are greater in adolescent girls than boys (21%–31%, versus 13%–20%). However, the rate of suicide is greatest among white adolescent males (Kennebeck & Bonin, 2009).

⚠ *SAFETY ALERT 10.5*

Previous history of suicide attempt is an indicator for future possible suicide completion.

Do you feel like you "belong" or are part of your school? How are you getting along with your friends?

Social stress and isolation can contribute to *depression* leading to suicide.

Are firearms in your home? Other weapons? Prescription drugs?

The risk of risky behavior leading to accidental death is increased in adolescents.

⚠ *SAFETY ALERT 10.6*

Be aware of firearms in the home.

Have you or any of your friends used alcohol or other drugs?

Adolescents may experiment with substance use, causing impaired judgment.

Older Adults

Have you felt sad lately? Risk factors to assess include the following:
- Female gender
- African American or Hispanic background
- Social isolation
- Widowed, divorced, or separated marital status
- Lower socioeconomic status
- Comorbid medical conditions
- Uncontrolled pain
- Insomnia
- Functional impairment
- Cognitive impairment (Hirsch, et al., 2009)

Females are at higher overall risk for *depression*. Older men and older African American and Hispanic adults are at higher risk for unrecognized *depression*. Assess for poor cognitive performance, sleep problems, and lack of initiative (Craven & Hirnle, 2009).
Older adults may also have physical health changes or end-of-life issues (Randall, et al., 2008). People who lose interest in work or hobbies, sleep too much, or live alone may be at risk for social isolation. Those experiencing financial pressure may have increased stress and potential depression.

Use the Geriatric Depression Scale to assess for the risk of depression in older adults (Box 10-4).

The more "yes" answers the patient gives, the more depression is likely.

To family: have you noticed any memory lapses or confusion?

Delirium, dementia, and depression are more common in older adults (Wasynski, 2007).

Box 10.4 GERIATRIC DEPRESSION SCALE: SHORT FORM

Choose the best answer for how you have felt over the past week:

1. Are you basically satisfied with your life? YES/**NO**
2. Have you dropped many of your activities and interests? **YES**/NO
3. Do you feel that your life is empty? **YES**/NO
4. Do you often get bored? **YES**/NO
5. Are you in good spirits most of the time? YES/**NO**
6. Are you afraid that something bad is going to happen to you? **YES**/NO
7. Do you feel happy most of the time? YES/**NO**
8. Do you often feel helpless? **YES**/NO
9. Do you prefer to stay at home, rather than going out and doing new things? **YES**/NO
10. Do you feel you have more problems with memory than most? **YES**/NO
11. Do you think it is wonderful to be alive now? YES/**NO**
12. Do you feel pretty worthless the way you are now? **YES**/NO
13. Do you feel full of energy? YES/**NO**
14. Do you feel that your situation is hopeless? **YES**/NO
15. Do you think that most people are better off than you are? **YES**/NO

Answers in **bold** indicate depression. Score 1 point for each bold-faced answer.

A score >5 points is suggestive of depression. A score >10 points is almost always indicative of depression. A score >5 points should warrant a follow-up comprehensive assessment.

Source: Yesavage, J. A., Brink, T. L., Rose, T. L., Lum, O., Huang, V., Adey, M., et al. (1982). Development and validation of a geriatric depression screening scale: A preliminary report. *Journal of Psychiatric Research, 17,* 37–49.

Cultural Considerations

Using an Interpreter for a Patient with a Mental Health Condition

When using an interpreter, the nurse greets him or her first without the patient being present. If an interpreter has not been trained to work with psychiatric patients, the nurse will need to address a few preliminary points. First is confidentiality. The interpreter cannot discuss any part of the communication with anyone other than the health care providers working with the patient. Even if the interpreter translated for that patient at another time, the interpreter cannot share information about how the patient is currently doing with primary providers or nursing staff members who previously cared for the patient.

Also, the interpreter can tell no one that the patient has some mental health issues. This can be a very difficult concept for patients from very community-oriented cultures in which people band together to assist one another in times of need. If the interpreter has interpreted for other family members or friends in the community, he or she should not divulge that information to the patient. The interpreter may think such disclosure is a way of connecting and establishing rapport, when in reality it could cause the patient to feel uncomfortable or worry that the interpreter will share information with others. Be aware if the interpreter seems to not be providing all the information the patient is stating. If the interpreter has little experience dealing with patients with mental illness, he or she may feel embarrassed that someone of his or her culture is acting this way and would want to provide a better picture than what is really being presented.

After the interview, walk out of sight of the patient and, in a private area, ask the interpreter about the communication style and context. Did the patient make sense? Were sentences structured properly and completely? Did the patient have difficulty expressing himself or herself? Was the patient oriented to reality? Are there any cultural practices or beliefs to be aware of? Be sure to include the interpreter's name in the nursing documentation of the interview.

Additional Questions	Rationales/Abnormal Findings
In what racial, cultural, or ethnic group do you identify?	Patients from different groups tend to selectively express or present symptoms in culturally acceptable ways. For example, Asian patients may be more likely to report physical (eg, dizziness) but not emotional symptoms (USDHHS, 2009). Attitudes and beliefs that a culzture holds influence whether a patient considers an illness "real" or "imagined" and if it is of the body or mind (or both). Cultural meanings of illness have real implications for whether people are motivated to seek treatment, how they cope with symptoms, how supportive families and communities are, and where they seek help (mental health specialist, primary care provider, clergy, and/or traditional healer).
Do you have an inherited family pattern of mental concerns?	The prevalence of *bipolar disorder* and *panic disorder* is higher in parts of Asia, Europe, and North America (USDHHS, 2009). Poverty, violence, and other stressful social environments increase risks for *depression.*
Are you concerned about seeking health care because of issues related to your living situation? Have you experienced traumatic situations in your life?	Traumatic experiences are common for combat veterans, inner-city residents, and immigrants from countries at war, placing them at risk for posttraumatic stress disorder.

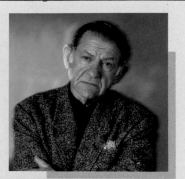

The nurse's role relative to subjective data collection is to gather information to improve the patient's health status and to help determine the cause of the patient's current symptoms. Remember Mr. Hart, introduced at the beginning of this chapter. This 75-year-old man has come to the health care walk-in clinic to have his blood pressure checked on several occasions. He is currently taking a prescription antidepressant.

The nurse uses professional communication techniques to gather subjective data from Mr. Hart. It is important to assess for suicidal ideations. The following conversations give two examples of different interview styles. One style is more effective than the other.

Less Effective	More Effective
Nurse: Hi, Mr. Hart. How are you feeling?	**Nurse:** Hi, Mr. Hart (pauses and smiles).
Mr. Hart: Fine. Are you married?	**Mr. Hart:** You're cute. Are you married?
Nurse: No, why do you ask?	**Nurse:** I'm sorry but the hospital policy is not to disclose personal information. I would like to talk to you today.
Mr. Hart: You're cute. Do you want to go out?	
Nurse: No, I'm your nurse. That would be outside of my professional boundaries.	**Mr. Hart:** Where do you live?
	Nurse: I'm sorry but I can't tell you that. How is that book that you're reading?
Mr. Hart: Where do you live?	
Nurse: I live in Chase. Where do you live?	**Mr. Hart:** It's good. I like to read novels that have some mystery in them.
Mr. Hart: I live in Chase, too. Where do you live in Chase?	**Nurse:** (nods head and smiles) Reading is a good way to relax.
Nurse: Mr. Hart, I can't talk about that. I need to ask you a question.	**Mr. Hart:** I don't have much time for relaxing. They keep us all busy with therapy and groups. I wish that I could rest more.
Mr. Hart: Yeah, you want to know where I live, right?	
Nurse: No, I was wondering if you have any thoughts about suicide.	**Nurse:** You're here so that you can be safe. Do you have any thoughts of wanting to harm or kill yourself?
Mr. Hart: No. Do you?	**Mr. Hart:** No. I did when I came here but not now.

Critical Thinking Challenge

- Did any elements in the conversations make you feel uncomfortable?
- How can the nurse provide an environment so that Mr. Hart will feel comfortable and safe talking about feelings?
- What are some other ways that the nurse can ask either directly or indirectly about suicidal ideation?

Objective Data Collection

The nurse obtains objective data by observing the patient and the patient's behavior, which includes not only how the patient communicates and responds to questions but also physical presentation. A patient's physical presentation may be the first indication of toxicity, underlying medical problem, or psychosis. Collecting objective data is an ongoing process throughout the time the nurse spends with the patient. Data for the objective assessment are usually organized by **A** (appearance), **B** (behavior), **C** (cognitive function), and **T** (thought process), plus the MMSE.

A: Appearance

Overall Appearance

Observe the overall physical appearance including noticeable physical deformities, weight, and asymmetrical movements. *The patient appears stated age, is normal weight, and shows symmetrical movements without obvious deformity.*

There may be evidence of cutting or self-harm. Physical problems such as stroke or dementia may exacerbate some mental health conditions. Cradle cap around the face of adults indicates long-term lack of care and is often seen in patients with schizophrenia.

Posture

Assess the posture. *Posture is erect but relaxed.*

Abnormal postures are rigid (indicates *anxiety*) or slouching (indicates *withdrawal*). A rigid posture might indicate that the patient is trying to hide, either from a real person or from his or her thoughts.

Movement

Assess baseline and additional movements. Observe their pace, range, and character. *Movements are voluntary, deliberate, coordinated, smooth, and even.*

Immobility (or tremor) might indicate *Parkinson's disease* or *schizophrenia.* The patient may walk a lot to distract from "voices." He or she may feel the need to keep physically occupied to avoid having to deal with emotional thoughts. The patient might have a tic or tardive dyskinesia.

Assess the gait for steadiness and rhythm. *Gait is steady and even.*

Abnormal gaits include limping, fast or slow speed, pacing, shuffling, and stiff. The gait is altered in some patients who take antipsychotic medications. Arm movements are lost with some gait abnormalities and in patients who have taken antipsychotic medications.

Observe the activity level. Is it under voluntary control? Do posture and motor activity change with topics under discussion or with activities or people around the patient? *Activity is moderately paced and relaxed.*

The activity level may be altered from *hypomania* or *ADHD*, side effects of medications, or internal *anxiety*. Activity may be hypoactive, hyperactive, rigid, restless, agitated, gesturing, posturing, with inappropriate mannerisms, hostile or combative, or unusual. See Table 10-6 at the end of the chapter.

Hygiene and Grooming

Note hair, nails, teeth, skin, and, if present, beard. Observe hygiene and grooming, including body odor and hair. If the patient is unwashed or unkempt, estimate for how long. Note a change in appearance in a previously well-groomed patient. Compare one side of the body with the other. *Patient is well groomed and has no unusual body odors.*

Poor hygiene may be from *paranoia* of water, homelessness, severe *depression*, or incapacitation as a result of mental illness. Risk of lice increases with poor grooming. Excessive fastidiousness may accompany *obsessive-compulsive disorder* (OCD). One-sided neglect may result from *stroke*, brain trauma, or physical injury. An unkempt state might indicate *depression* or *psychosis*.

Observe for makeup and how it is worn. *Makeup is appropriate to weather, age, gender, culture, and social situation.*

Garish makeup with bold colors and outside the lines may indicate *mania*. Inappropriate makeup may also indicate a decline in mental status.

Observe the hands for coloration, cleanliness, tremors, pill rolling, or clubbing of the nail bed. Look for any signs of itching or scratching.

Hands may provide indicators of health problems, smoking status, drug withdrawal, low blood glucose level, or side effects of medications. Clubbing is seen in patients with emphysema or who use recreational drugs with talc in them; poor oxygenation affects cognition. Itching or scratching may be related to hallucinations, crystal methamphetamine use, or self-harm.

Dress

Observe how the patient is dressed. Is clothing clean, pressed, and fastened properly? How does it compare with clothing worn by people of comparable age and social group?

Clothing style and color may indicate an identified social group (eg, gangs, Goth).

(text continues on page 210)

Is clothing worn correctly such as right side out, not backward, shirt buttoned in alignment? How many layers is the patient wearing? *Clothing is clean and appropriate for culture and weather.*

Unfastened or incorrectly worn clothes might indicate physical difficulty, cognitive deficits, or altered mental status. Clothing may be slovenly, unkempt, overly meticulous, disheveled, inappropriate, provocative, unusual, inappropriate for weather, or with multiple layers. A patient wearing five shirts and three pairs of pants at once may be cold, homeless (and wearing so many clothes because there is nowhere to store them), or irrational.

B: Behavior

Level of Consciousness
Is the patient awake and alert? To assess if the patient is arousable, gently shake the bed or chair that the patient is in; do not directly shake the patient.

Abnormal findings include drowsy, hyperalert, somnolent, intermittent alertness, or stupor. If the patient is not arousable, assess for breathing, stupor, or psychosis. This addresses the patient's ability to remain safe.

• Note if the patient is aware of surroundings and environmental situations.
• Is the patient aware of self?
• Does the patient respond appropriately to stimuli?

The patient is awake and alert, responding appropriately to voice cues.

Abnormal findings are a lack of awareness of own physical needs and emotional responses. Refer to Chapter 24 for more information on neurological assessment and the Glasgow coma scale.

⚠ *SAFETY ALERT 10.7*
The patient's ability to correctly interpret the environmental cues and respond accordingly addresses safety.

Eye Contact and Facial Expressions
Assess eye contact. *The patient converses with eyes open and maintains eye contact.*

Abnormal findings are eyes closed, avoiding eye contact, staring, looking vacantly ahead, or twitching to side when discussing a traumatic event. A patient who looks away may be responding to voices or easily distracted by the environment. Poor eye contact may indicate low self-esteem, shame, embarrassment, *depression*, or a cultural trait.

Observe facial expressions at rest and when the patient is interacting with others. Watch for variations in facial expression with topics under discussion. Are they congruent? Is the face relatively immobile throughout? *The patient is calm, alert, and expressive. Facial expressions are congruent with subjects.*

Facial expressions indicate the emotional state. Abnormal expressions are perplexed, stressed, tense, dazed, grimacing, and lacking in expression. Facial expressions may give clues to *depression, anxiety*, hallucinations, physical injury, *mania*, side effects of medications, or possible extrapyramidal symptoms.

Speech
Assess speech for

• Rate. *The rate is moderately paced.*

Slow, fast, latent, pressured, monotone, or disturbed rates are abnormal. Determine if causes are anxiety, depression, or auditory hallucinations.

• Rhythm. *The rhythm has normal fluctuations.*

Rhyming, slurring, mumbling, or unusual rhythm is abnormal. Determine if the cause is a hearing problem, anger or agitation, or *mania*.

• Loudness. *Speech is audible with moderate loudness.*

Note if barely audible or too loud. Determine if the cause is a hearing problem, auditory hallucination, or speech problem.

• Fluency. *Speech is fluent.*

Note any lengthy pauses, hesitancy, or stuttering (specify the frequency). Determine if these are from difficulty speaking (aphasia) or hallucinations.

• Quantity. Does the patient respond only to direct questions? Assess for voluminous speech, poverty of speech, talkativeness, silence, or spontaneity. *There is usually a flow of conversation with pauses.*

Too much speech may be covering feelings of discomfort, embarrassment, not knowing answers, or avoiding questions. Too much or too little speech may indicate auditory hallucinations. Too little speech may indicate poverty of thought or developmental delay.

• Articulation. *Speech is articulate with words clear and distinct.*

Note difficulty expressing self or finding words. See also Chapter 24.

- Content. *Content is organized and congruent with behavior or nonverbal communication.*

- Pattern. *There is a pattern of exchange in conversation*

Disorganized, nonsensical, judgmental, religiously preoccupied, or sexually preoccupied speech may indicate impaired judgment and illogical thinking. Note if the patient uses fragmented sentences, circuitous speech (talks in circles and cannot answer questions), confabulation (makes up answers to cover for loss of memory), or intellectualization (uses intellectual analysis to avoid dealing with emotions). Frequent or inappropriate laughter may indicate hallucinations or disordered perception. See also Table 10-7.

C: Cognitive Function
Orientation
Assess orientation through the following questions.

- Tell me what day of the week, month, and year it is now.
- Where are you right now?
- What is your name (first and surname)?
- Why are you here right now?

The patient is alert and oriented, which is commonly written as A&O × 3—alert and oriented times 3. It is also written as A&O × 4 indicating the additional information that the patient is aware of current situation (eg, why hospitalized).

Note any inconsistencies regarding orientation. Determine if the patient is new to the area and might not know the place. If a woman provides her maiden versus her married surname when questioned, determine if she retained her maiden surname or is confused. A confused patient will lose time first, then place, and lastly name. As confusion clears, the patient will regain knowledge in the reverse order (name, place, and time). If the patient is aware of person and time but not place (out of normal sequencing order), it is indicative of an organic process for the confusion. Refer to Chapter 24 for more information.

Attention Span
Can the patient follow the conversation? Is the patient easily distractible? *The patient can follow conversation and events.*

Attention span indicates the current level of cognitive functioning. Note if altered attention span is from restlessness, poor focus, ADHD, or hallucinations.

Memory
Assess memory using the MMSE or Mini-Cog (Box 10-5).
- Does the patient have short-term memory?
- Does the patient have long-term memory?

Short- and long-term memories are intact.

Short- and long-term memories indicate the current level of cognitive functioning. Altered memory may be from *dementia, Alzheimer's disease,* or other processes. Refer to Chapter 24 for more information on the assessment of memory.

Judgment
Assess judgment by noting the patient's responses to family situations, employment, interpersonal conflict, and use of money. Ask direct questions such as

- How will you get home if you have no money?
- What will you do if you feel the urge to use alcohol again (in patients with alcoholism)? (They might respond with answers such as seek help, call my AA sponsor, or talk myself out of it.)
- What will happen if you hit someone you love, a neighbor, or someone else?
- What is your part in this conflict? Or how might you have contributed to this situation?

The patient makes good judgments and takes responsibility for own actions.

Assess the patient's ability to solve problems.
Assess the patient's ability to choose among alternatives based on reality.

Assess the patient's ability to understand the consequences of behavior and take responsibility for actions.
Note if the patient has poor insight, poor judgment, or poor impulse control and what these findings might indicate.

T: Thought Processes and Perceptions
Assess thought processes. *They are easy to follow, logical, coherent, relevant, goal directed, consistent, and abstract.*

Illogical, incoherent, irrelevant, wandering, inconsistent, or concrete thought processes are abnormal indications that the patient is thinking less efficiently. Refer to Table 10-8 at the end of the chapter.

(text continues on page 212)

Box 10.5 THE MINI-COG

Administration

The test is administered as follows:

1. Instruct the patient to listen carefully to and remember three unrelated words and then to repeat the words.

2. Instruct the patient to draw the face of a clock, either on a blank sheet of paper or on a sheet with the clock circle already drawn on the page. After the patient puts the numbers on the clock face, ask him or her to draw the hands of the clock to read a specific time.

3. Ask the patient to repeat the three previously stated words.

Scoring

Give 1 point for each recalled word after the clock-drawing test (CDT) distractor.

Patients recalling none of the three words are classified as demented (Score = 0).

Patients recalling all three words are classified as non-demented (Score = 3).

Patients with intermediate word recall of 1-2 words are classified based on the CDT (Abnormal = demented; Normal = non-demented)

Note: The CDT is considered normal if all numbers are present in the correct sequence and position, and the hands readably display the requested time.

Source: Borson, S., Scanlan, J., Brush, M., Vitallano, P., & Dokmak, A. (2000). The Mini-Cog: A cognitive 'vital signs' measure for dementia screening in multi-lingual elderly. *International Journal of Geriatric Psychiatry, 15*(11), 1021–1027. Copyright John Wiley & Sons Limited. Reproduced with permission.

Technique and Normal Findings (continued)	Abnormal Findings (continued)
Mini-Mental Status/Mini-Cog Assess cognitive function by using the MMSE or Mini-Cog (Box 10-5). The self-explanatory MMSE has 11 questions about time and place orientation, serial 7s (subtract 7 from 100 and continue to subtract 7 from each subsequent remainder), naming objects (eg, pencil), repeating phrases (eg, "No ifs, ands, or butts"), following a 3-step direction, reading and responding, writing a sentence, and drawing intersecting pentagons (Folstein, et al, 1975). It takes 10 to 15 minutes to administer. The Mini-Cog takes about 3 minutes to administer and is perceived as less stressful. It includes recall and the clock drawing test. Registration is the ability to immediately state three words; recall is the ability to state them 3 minutes later. Recall is tested in both.	The MMSE and Mini-Cog are both scored tests. A score of 23 or lower on the MMSE indicates cognitive impairment (Folstein, et al., 1975). For more information on this copyrighted tool, contact Psychological Assessment Resources, Inc., 16204 North Florida Avenue, Lutz, Florida 33549. Unsuccessful recall of three items or an abnormal clock drawing test indicates dementia on the Mini-Cog.

Documentation of Normal Findings

Appears stated age and normal weight, no obvious deformity. Posture is erect and relaxed. Movements are symmetrical, voluntary, deliberate, coordinated, smooth, and even. Gait is steady and even. Activity is moderate and relaxed. Patient is well groomed with no unusual body odors. Makeup is appropriate to culture and social situation. Clothing is clean and appropriate for gender, age, culture, and weather. Patient is awake, alert, calm, and expressive, responding appropriately to voice cues. Patient converses with eyes open and good eye contact. Facial expressions are congruent with subjects. Speech is of moderate pace and volume, fluent with normal fluctuations, and articulate with clear and distinct words. Speech is organized and congruent with behavior and nonverbal communication. A&OX 3. Patient follows conversation and events; attention span is normal. Short- and long-term memory intact. MMSE completed with no deficits. Patient makes good judgments and takes responsibility for actions. Thought processes are easy to follow, logical, coherent, relevant, goal directed, consistent, and abstract. *J. O'Placey, RN*

Assessment of Dementia, Confusion, Delirium, and Depression

Dementia is more common in older adults. It is usually a gradual process over months to years. Delirium generally has an underlying medical cause that, once treated, results in the delirium resolving.

Some cues that the patient may have dementia include the following:

- Seems disoriented
- Is a "poor historian"
- Defers to a family member to answer questions directed to the patient
- Repeatedly and apparently unintentionally fails to follow instructions
- Has difficulty finding the right words or uses inappropriate or incomprehensible words
- Has difficulty following conversations (Waszynski, 2007)

Delirium, dementia, and depression can also be acute situations. Delirium usually has an acute onset, and the disorganized thoughts can place the patient at risk for injury. The risk of suicide increases with depression. Refer to Table 10-3 for a comparison of findings.

Evidence-Based Critical Thinking

Nursing Diagnoses

When formulating nursing diagnoses, it is important to use critical thinking to cluster data and identify patterns that fit together. Table 10-4 compares and contrasts nursing diagnoses, abnormal findings, and interventions commonly related to mental health assessment (Johnson, et al., 2005). Note that altered thought processes and sensory perceptions are also related to the neurological system (see Chapter 24). Some coping behaviors are also relevant to other body systems and how patients cope with the effects of physical problems.

Patient Outcomes

Nurses use assessment information to identify patient outcomes. Some outcomes related to mental health problems include the following:

- The patient does not harm self.
- The patient demonstrates appropriate social interactions.
- The patient identifies personal strengths (Bulechek, et al., 2008).

Nursing Interventions

Once outcomes are established, the nurse implements care to improve the patient's status. The nurse uses critical thinking and evidence-based practice to develop interventions. Some examples of nursing interventions for mental health challenges are as follows:

- Assess for risk of harm to self or others.
- Provide a safe environment by removing items that might cause harm.
- Identify support systems and involve them in care (Bulechek, et al., 2008).

Table 10.3 Comparison of Delirium, Dementia, and Depression

	Delirium	Dementia	Depression
Onset	Acute over a few hours, lasting hours to weeks. Occurs in the context of medical illness, substance abuse or withdrawal	Slow, lasting months to years	Slow
Description	Impaired recent and remote memory	Impaired remote memory	Impaired memory
	Fluctuating attention	Attention preserved	Attention intact
	Thoughts disorganized	Thoughts impoverished	Impaired concentration
	Change in cognition	Global impairment of intellect	If psychosis is present, it is usually systematized and with normal emotional response
	Clouding of consciousness	Alert	
	Perceptual disturbances—usually disorganized	Aware	Perceptual disturbances
	Does not usually present with mood components		Sad affect or mood

Sources: Adapted from Sadock, B. J., Sadock, V. A., & Kaplan, H. I. (2004). *Kaplan & Sadock's comprehensive textbook of psychiatry* (8th ed.). Philadelphia: Lippincott Williams & Wilkins and Edwards, N. (2003). Differentiating the three D's: Delirium, Dementia, and Depression. *MEDSURG Nursing, 12,* 347–358.

Table 10.4   Common Nursing Diagnoses Associated with Mental Health

Diagnosis and Related Factors	Point of Differentiation	Assessment Characteristics	Nursing Interventions
Risk for suicide	At risk for potentially fatal, purposefully self-inflicted injury	States desire to die, hopelessness, impulsiveness, loneliness	Establish a relationship. Assess for suicide risk. Refer for counseling. Remove lethal medications and weapons from the environment.
Risk for self-mutilation	At risk for deliberately injuring oneself to relieve stress and tension, but not to end one's life	Cuts or scratches on body, picking at wounds, self-inflicted burns, insertion of objects into body orifices	Establish trust. Provide medical treatment for injuries.* Assess for depression, anxiety, impulsivity, and suicide. Secure a contract to notify staff when experiencing a desire to mutilate.
Altered thought processes	Alterations or disruption in cognition, thinking, and associated activities	Perceiving or interpreting one's surroundings incorrectly, nonreality-based thinking	Reorient as needed. Use concrete, nontechnical words and short phrases. Assess for hallucinations. Convey that you would like to understand what the patient is trying to say, but make sure that the patient does not follow through on harmful processes.
Sensory-perceptual alterations	Disturbances in and inappropriate responses to incoming stimuli	Poor concentration, auditory or visual hallucinations, irritability, agitation, change in behavior	Validate that the patient is the only person hearing or seeing the hallucination. Provide a safe environment. Encourage expression of responses to hallucinations. Encourage the use of alternate coping strategies, such as singing or wearing headphones.
Ineffective individual coping	Impairments in the way one appraises, responds to, or uses resources to deal with stressors	Substance abuse, ignoring problems, lack of concentration, sleep disturbances	Assess for causes. Build on the patient's strengths. Set realistic goals. Listen and avoid false reassurance.
Self-esteem disturbance	Negative self-evaluation; long-term view of self or self-capabilities that is focused on negative aspects	Does not believe or trust positive feedback from other people, exaggerates or fixates on negative feedback, displays shame or guilt	Listen to and respect the patient. Assess strengths and coping abilities. Reframe difficulties as learning opportunities.
Impaired social interaction	Engagement with others that is insufficient in frequency, lacking in quality, or both	Feeling ill-at-ease during social situations; interactions with peers, family, or others that are limited or result in negative consequences (eg, arguments, poor communication)	Assess the social support system. List behaviors associated with being disconnected and alternative responses. Role play social interactions and appropriate responses.

*Collaborative interventions.

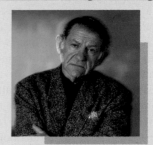

Remember Mr. Hart, whose problems have been outlined throughout this chapter. Initial subjective and objective data collection is complete, and the nurse has spent time reviewing findings and other results. The following nursing note illustrates how subjective and objective data are collected and analyzed and nursing interventions are developed.

Subjective: "I'm scared when the voices tell me to run away. I know that I should stay here to stay safe."

Objective: A&O × 3. Some inappropriate comments, such as asking personal information. Denies thoughts of harming self or others. Hearing mumbling conversations with several people talking. He states that he can tell the difference between what the voices are saying and what is real. Talking to others usually makes the voices go away. Denies visual hallucinations. Somewhat distracted during initial conversation but attends more as conversation progresses.

Analysis: Altered auditory sensory perception. Risk for suicide.

Plan: Continue involuntary treatment hold. Monitor for effectiveness and side effects of medications. Encourage participation in both individual and group therapies. Assess for suicide and hallucinations every shift and as needed. Avoid asking questions about the past and focus on teaching skills to remain safe. Allow time to build a trusting relationship. Assist with problem solving. Avoid disclosing personal information.

P. Terris, RN

Critical Thinking Challenge

- What things will the nurse observe during the assessment of Mr. Hart?
- What other assessments might be indicated?
- What other nursing diagnoses might be considered?

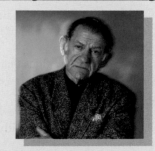

Using the previous steps of nursing process, consider all of the case study findings woven throughout this chapter. When answering the following questions, begin drawing conclusions and see how the pieces of assessment must work together to create an environment for personalized, appropriate, and accurate care.

- How are the mental status assessment and mental health history integrated?
- What techniques of mental health assessment will the nurse use to gain the patient's trust and promote respect?
- How will the nurse assess for suicidal ideation, homicidal ideation, and hallucinations?
- What are your experiences with and feelings about patients who have mental health issues or are suicidal?

Key Points

- During a mental health assessment, the nurse assesses the patient and family history, including gender, age, race, current health status, history of mental health concerns, functional status, weight gain or loss, sleeping difficulties, and medications.
- Risk factors for mental health conditions include abuse, family history, poor support network, stressors, substance abuse, and loss of hope.
- The nurse assesses for alcohol or substance abuse using the CAGE tool.
- The nurse assesses spirituality and sense of meaning using the HOPE tool.
- Suicidal ideation is assessed by asking, "Do you have any thoughts of wanting to harm or kill yourself?"
- Homicidal ideation is assessed by asking, "Do you have any thoughts of wanting to harm or kill anyone?"
- Altered moods include sad, tearful, depressed, angry, anxious, grandiose, and fearful.
- Altered sensory perceptions include auditory, visual, tactile, and olfactory hallucinations.
- Depression may be assessed using the SAD PERSONAS.
- Assessment of mental status includes **A**ppearance (posture, movement, hygiene, and dress), **B**ehavior (level of consciousness, eye contact, facial expressions, speech), **C**ognitive function (orientation, attention span, memory, judgment), and **T**hought processes.
- The MMSE tool measures cognitive function and includes orientation, registration, attention and calculation, recall, and language to determine mental status.
- Common nursing diagnoses include risk for suicide, risk for self-mutilation, altered thought processes, sensory-perceptual alterations, ineffective individual coping, self-esteem disturbance, and impaired social interaction.

Review Questions

1. A nurse is working with a new patient. To establish rapport, the nurse would use which of the following statements?
   A. "These are questions that I ask all my patients."
   B. "Don't worry because we are working with crazy patients."
   C. "We're here because we want to help psych people."
   D. "These questions are silly, but I have to ask them."

2. The patient's family should not be present during the interview with the patient requiring a translator because
   A. the patient may feel uncomfortable speaking openly with a relative present, especially if that person is contributing to the patient's stress
   B. the translator may not ask questions related to the family member and could be perceived as insensitive or inappropriate

C. the family member may be ashamed or embarrassed by the patient's actions or statements and try to withhold or change the facts
   D. all of the above

3. "Do you have any thoughts of wanting to kill or harm yourself?" is a common question to assess for suicidal ideation because it
   A. is blunt and patients cannot refuse to answer
   B. will cover both suicidal and parasuicidal thoughts
   C. is subtle and patients will not know how to answer
   D. will encourage patients who perform self-harm to stop cutting

4. When charting general appearance and behavior, documentation may include
   A. alert and oriented × 3
   B. thought logical
   C. judgment intact
   D. clothes disheveled

5. Abnormal movements from medications might be described as
   A. voluntary
   B. deliberate
   C. uncoordinated
   D. smooth and even

6. Normal speech is audible is a normal finding describing which quality of speech?
   A. Fluency
   B. Quality
   C. Loudness
   D. Articulation

7. A 90-year-old patient has a drooped body position, appears sad, and says that she has seasonal affective disorder. What tool would the nurse use to assess her?
   A. MMSE
   B. CAGE
   C. HOPE
   D. Geriatric Depression Scale

8. Which of the following represents the nurse's documentation of a patient with normal mood?
   A. Pleasant or appropriate to situation
   B. Grandiose or strongly confident
   C. Fearful but mildly humble and meek
   D. Sad and tearful during conversation

9. Patients may laugh spontaneously, provide inappropriate responses, ask the nurse personal questions, or insult the nurse. These are examples of
   A. perseveration
   B. auditory hallucinations
   C. divergent tactics
   D. altered mood

10. The MMSE is used to assess for severity in orientation, registration, attention and calculation, recall, and language. For which of the following patients would the MMSE be most appropriate?

A. Women during the postpartum period

B. Adolescents struggling with sexual orientation

C. Various cultural groups not tested by other tools

D. Adults to assess for cognitive impairment and the severity

References

Borson, S., Scanlan, J., Brush, M., Vitallano, P., & Dokmak, A. (2000). The Mini-Cog: A cognitive "vital signs" measure for dementia screening in multi-lingual elderly. *International Journal of Geriatric Psychiatry, 15*(11), 1021–1027.

Bulechek, G. B., Butcher, H. K., & McCloskey Dochterman, J. (2008). *Nursing Interventions Classification (NIC)* (4th ed.). St. Louis: Mosby.

CDC. (2008). *Suicide facts at a glance.* Retrieved October 16, 2009, from http://www.cdc.gov/ncipc/dvp/suicide/suicide_data_sheet.pdf

CDC & National Center for Injury Prevention and Control. (2008). *WISQARS leading causes of death reports, 1999–2005.* Retrieved October 16, 2009, from http://webappa.cdc.gov/sasweb/ncipc/leadcaus10.html

Cohen, L. S., Altshuler, L. L., Harlow, B. L., et al. (2006). Relapse of major depression during pregnancy in women who maintain or discontinue antidepressant treatment. *JAMA, 295,* 499.

Craven, R. C., & Hirnle, C. J. (2009). *Fundamentals of nursing: Human health and function* (6th ed.). Philadelphia: Wolters Kluwer Health/Lippincott Williams & Wilkins.

Felitti, V. J., Anda, R. F., Nordenberg, D., et al. (1998). Relationship of childhood abuse and household dysfunction to many of the leading causes of death in adults: The adverse childhood experiences (ACE) study. *American Journal of Preventive Medicine, 14*(4), 245–258.

Folstein, M. F., Folstein, S. E., & McHugh, P. R (1975). "Mini-mental state." A practical method for grading the cognitive state of patients for the clinician. *Journal of Psychiatric Research, 12*(3), 189–198.

Hirsch, J. K., Duberstein, P. R., & Unützer, J. (2009). Chronic medical problems and distressful thoughts of suicide in primary care patients: Mitigating role of happiness. *International Journal of Geriatric Psychiatry.* 2009 Jan 14. [Epub ahead of print] PMID: 19145577 [PubMed—as supplied by publisher].

Johnson, M., Bulechek, G. M., McCloskey Dochterman, J., & Maas, M. L. (2005). *NANDA, NOC, and NIC linkages: Nursing diagnoses, outcomes, and interventions.* St. Louis: Mosby.

Juhnke, G. (1994). SAD PERSONS Scale review. Measurement and evaluation in counseling and development. *27*(1), 325–327.

Kennebeck, S., & Bonin, I. (2009). *Epidemiology and risk factors for suicidal behavior in children and adolescents.* Retrieved October 17, 2009, from http://www.uptodateonline.com.proxy.seattleu.edu/online/content/topic.do?topicKey=adol_med/7847&linkTitle=EPIDEMIOLOGY&source=preview&selectedTitle=3~6&anchor=2#2

Luoma, J. B., Martin, C. E., & Pearson, J. L. (2002). Contact with mental health and primary care providers before suicide: A review of the evidence. *American Journal of Psychiatry, 159,* 909–916.

Moore, G., & Pfaff, J. A. (2008). Assessment and management of the acutely agitated or violent patient. Retrieved February 1, 2009, from http://www.uptodateonline.com.proxy.seattleu.edu/online/content/topic.do?topicKey=ad_symp/6273&selectedTitle=2~6&source=search_result

O'Hara, M. W., & Swain, M. (1996). Rates and risk of postpartum depression: A meta-analysis. *International Review Psychiatry, 8*(1), 37.

Randall, T., Espinoza, R. T., & Unützer, J. (2008). Diagnosis and management of late-life depression. Retrieved February 1, 2009, from http://www.uptodateonline.com.proxy.seattleu.edu/online/content/topic.do?topicKey=psychiat/12560&selectedTitle=1~150&source=search_result

Shea, S. C. (1999). *The practical art of suicide assessment. A guide for mental health professionals and substance abuse counselors.* Hoboken, NJ: John Wiley and Sons, Inc.

USDHHS. (1999). *Mental health: A report of the surgeon general.* Rockville, MD: U.S. Department of Health and Human Services, Substance Abuse and Mental Health Services Administration, Center for Mental Health Services, National Institutes of Health, National Institute of Mental Health.

USDHHS. (2009). *Culture counts: The influence of culture and society on mental health, mental illness.* Retrieved May 25, 2009, from http://mentalhealth.samhsa.gov/cre/ch2_culture_of_the_patient.asp

Waszynski, C. M. (2007). How to try this: Detecting delirium. *American Journal of Nursing, 107*(12), 50–59.

WHO. (2007). *Fact Sheet # 220 mental health: Strengthening mental health promotion.* Retrieved October 16, 2009 from *http://www.who.int/mediacentre/factsheets/fs220/en/*

The Jensen suite offers these additional resources to enhance learning and facilitate understanding of this chapter:

- thePoint online resource, http//thepoint.lww.com/Jensen1E
- Student CD-ROM included with the book
- *Laboratory Manual for Nursing Health Assessment: A Best-Practice Approach*
- *Pocket Guide for Nursing Health Assessment: A Best-Practice Approach*

Table 10.5 Abnormal Findings: Mood Disorders

Euphoria	Excessive sense of emotional and physical well-being inappropriate to the actual situation or environmental stimuli
Flat affect	No emotional tone or reaction
Blunted affect	Severe reduction in emotional expressiveness (often confused with flat affect)
Elation	High degree of confidence, boastfulness, uncritical optimism, and joy accompanied by increased motor activity
Exultation	Reaction extending beyond elation and accompanied by feelings of grandeur
Ecstasy	Overpowering feeling of joy and rapture
Anxiety	A feeling of apprehension or worry, especially about the future
Fear	An emotional reaction to an environmental threat
Ambivalence	Having two opposing feelings or emotions at the same time
Depersonalization	Feeling that oneself or one's environment is unreal
Irritability	Feeling of impatience, annoyance, and easy provocation to anger
Rage	Furious, uncontrolled anger
Lability	Quick change of expression of mood or feelings
Depression	Feeling characterized by sadness, dejection, helplessness, hopelessness, worthlessness, and gloom

Source: Adapted from Department of Health. (2008). *Psychiatry*. Retrieved November 1, 2008, from http://www.doh.gov.ph/zcmc/index.php?option=com_content&task=view&id=101&Itemid=26

Table 10.6 Abnormal Findings: Motor Movements

Akathisia	Motor restlessness, inability to remain still; can also be a subjective feeling
Akinesia	No movement or difficulty with movement
Dystonia	Muscle spasms, spastic movements of the neck and back, can be painful or frightening
Parkinsonism	Slow, shuffling gait; masklike facial expression; tremors; pill-rolling movements of the hands; stooping posture; rigidity
Tardive dyskinesia	Involuntary and abnormal movements of the mouth, tongue, face, and jaw, may progress to the limbs; irreversible condition; may occur in months after antipsychotic medication use
Neuroleptic malignant syndrome	Develops as a potentially lethal side effect of antipsychotic medications, with muscle rigidity, tremors, altered consciousness, and incontinence; first warning signs are usually hyperthermia and hypertension, tachycardia. May be referred to as "lead-pipe" rigidity
Choreiform movements	Irregular, involuntary actions of muscles of face and extremities
Waxy flexibility	Holding body posture that is imposed by another person for a long time
Hyperkinesias	Excessive movement; destructive or aggressive activity
Compulsive	Unwanted repetitive actions
Automatism	Not consciously controlled, automatic, undirected motor activity
Cataplexy	Temporary loss of muscle tone precipitated by strong emotions
Catalepsy	Trancelike state with loss of voluntary motion
Stereotypy	Repetitive imitation of another person's movements
Psychomotor retardation	Decreased, slowed activity
Catatonic stupor	Extreme underactivity
Catatonic excitement	Extreme overactivity
Impulsiveness	Outbursts of unpredictable and sudden activity
Tics and spasms	Involuntary twitching and jerking of muscles, usually above the shoulders

Source: Adapted from Department of Health. (2008). *Psychiatry*. Retrieved November 1, 2008, from http://www.doh.gov.ph/zcmc/index.php?option=com_content&task=view&id=101&Itemid=26

Table 10.7 Abnormal Findings: Speech Patterns

Verbigeration	Repetitive, meaningless expression of sentences, phrases, or words
Rhyming	Interjecting into conversation regular, recurring, corresponding sounds at the ends of phrases or sentences, as in poetry
Punning	Interjecting clever and humorous uses of a word or words
Mutism	No expression of words or lack of communication over a period of time
Selectively mute	Mostly mute with intermittent periods of verbal expression
Aphasia	Partial or total loss of the ability to express self through language or to understand the verbal communication of another person
Neologisms	Words created by the patient that are either not easily understood by others or unintelligible
Spontaneous	Communication initiated by a patient with others
Circumlocutions	Phrases or sentences substituted for a word that the person cannot think of (eg, "what you write with" for a pen)
Paraphasias	Malformed, wrong, or invented words

Source: Adapted from Department of Health. (2008). *Psychiatry*. Retrieved November 1, 2008, from http://www.doh.gov.ph/zcmc/index.php?option=com_content&task=view&id=101&Itemid=26

Table 10.8 Abnormal Findings: Thought Processes

Thought blocking	Sudden cessation of flow of thought and speech related to strong emotions
Flight of ideas	Rapid conversation with logically unconnected shifting of topics
Word salad	Disconnected and incoherent combination of phrases, words, and sentences
Perseveration phenomena	Repetitive behaviors such as lip licking, finger tapping, pacing, or echolalia
Circumstantiality	Interjection of great detail and incidental material with no primary significance to the central idea of the conversation
Tangential	Deviation from the central theme of conversation
Echolalia	Repetitive imitation of another person's speech
Delusion	False belief kept despite nonsupportive evidence
Phobia	Strong, persistent, abnormal fear of an object or situation
Obsession	Persistent, unwanted, recurring thoughts
Compulsions	Repetitive mental act or physical behavior that a patient feels driven to perform to reduce distress, prevent a dreaded event or situation, or respond to an obsession
Hypochondriasis	Morbid concern for one's health and feeling ill without any actual medical basis
Psychosis	Disorderly mental state in which the patient has difficulty distinguishing reality from internal perceptions
Thought broadcasting	Delusion that others can hear one's thoughts
Thought control	Delusion that others can control a person's thoughts against one's will
Thought insertion	Delusion that others have the ability to put thoughts in a person's mind against one's will
Neologisms	Creating and using new words
Loose associations	Changes of conversation in an unrelated, fragmented manner
Incoherent	Not making any sense
Confabulation	Making up answers to cover for not knowing. Demonstrates the ability to think and reason with only short-term memory present. Symptom of Korsakoff's syndrome
Ideas of reference	Perception that others or the media are talking to or about the patient
Ruminating	Getting "stuck" on, worrying, or thinking about an idea repetitively

Source: Adapted from Department of Health. (2008). *Psychiatry*. Retrieved November 1, 2008, from http://www.doh.gov.ph/zcmc/index.php?option=com_content&task=view&id=101&Itemid=26

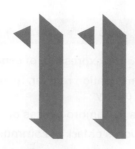

Assessment of Social, Cultural, and Spiritual Health

Learning Objectives

1 Identify the purpose of the *National Standards for Culturally and Linguistically Appropriate Services in Health Care*.

2 Identify "models of health" and how they relate to social, cultural, and spiritual assessment.

3 Identify the components of social assessment for individuals, communities, and societies.

4 Review questions considered in the transcultural assessment and how to individualize it.

5 Identify the components of the core community assessment.

6 Identify the components of the Community as Partner Assessment Model.

7 Define *culture* and its attributes.

8 State the four goals of a cultural assessment.

9 Identify the attributes and behaviors of a nurse practicing effective care within the patient's cultural context.

10 Seek understanding of one's culturally based health care practices, because each culture has its own traditional values and beliefs about health and illness that may affect individuals' adherence to treatments.

11 Define *spirituality* and how it influences patient care in health care settings.

12 Discuss why it is important to be aware of the roles of religions and places of worship in sustaining patient development, national identity, and survival.

13 Discuss how spirituality often takes central position during life transitions, such as loss of loved ones, accidents, or serious illnesses.

14 Identify nursing diagnoses related to social, cultural, and spiritual nursing assessments.

Mr. El-Kebbi, a 54-year-old Somalian Muslim immigrant, is being seen in an outpatient clinic for follow-up care related to his type 2 diabetes. He works in maintenance at a local hospital during the day and also has a part-time job selling used goods at auction in the evening. He takes an oral hypoglycemic, Metformin, for diabetes, and is otherwise healthy. A focused assessment was documented during his last clinic visit 6 months ago.

You will gain more information about Mr. El-Kebbi as you progress through this chapter. As you study the content and features, consider Mr. El-Kebbi's case and its relationship to what you are learning. Begin thinking about the following issues:

- How might Mr. El-Kebbi's social network influence his healthy lifestyle?
- How will the nurse assess this patient's cultural needs?
- What effect might religion have on Mr. El-Kebbi's diabetes management?

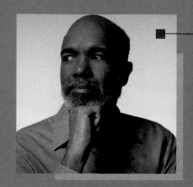

Given the multicultural composition of the United States and the steady influx of new and diverse immigrants, assessing patients' social and cultural backgrounds and spiritual beliefs becomes imperative, as does incorporating findings into plans of care. The American Nurses Association, Joint Commission, American Psychological Association, and other accrediting agencies direct nurses to acknowledge and address the biopsychosocial and spiritual needs of patients. This is because the composition of the United States is multicultural. To facilitate this process,

the Office of Minority Health of the Federal Cabinet of Health and Human Services published the *National Standards for Culturally and Linguistically Appropriate Services in Health Care* (Box 11-1). The agencies mandated that the standards must be upheld in every health care setting.

Many health care professionals already understand the importance of social, cultural, and spiritual assessments or are actively pursuing educational opportunities to enhance their knowledge. This chapter presents basic principles

---

BOX 11.1 NATIONAL STANDARDS FOR CULTURALLY AND LINGUISTICALLY APPROPRIATE SERVICES IN HEALTH CARE (CLAS)

The CLAS standards are primarily directed at health care organizations; however, individual providers are also encouraged to use the standards to make their practices more culturally and linguistically accessible. The principles and activities of culturally and linguistically appropriate services should be integrated throughout an organization and undertaken in partnership with the communities being served.

The 14 standards are organized by themes: Culturally Competent Care (Standards 1–3), Language Access Services (Standards 4–7), and Organizational Supports for Cultural Competence (Standards 8–14). Within this framework, there are three types of standards of varying stringency: mandates, guidelines, and recommendations as follows:

CLAS **mandates** are current Federal requirements for all recipients of Federal funds (Standards 4–7).

CLAS guidelines are activities recommended by OMH for adoption as mandates by Federal, State, and national accrediting agencies (Standards 1–3, 8–13).

CLAS recommendations are suggested by OMH for voluntary adoption by health care organizations (Standard 14).

Standard 1: Health care organizations should ensure that patients/consumers receive from all staff member's effective, understandable, and respectful care that is provided in a manner compatible with their cultural health beliefs and practices and preferred language.

Standard 2: Health care organizations should implement strategies to recruit, retain, and promote at all levels of the organization a diverse staff and leadership that are representative of the demographic characteristics of the service area.

Standard 3: Health care organizations should ensure that staff at all levels and across all disciplines receive ongoing education and training in culturally and linguistically appropriate service delivery.

Standard 4: Health care organizations must offer and provide language assistance services, including bilingual staff and interpreter services, at no cost to each patient/consumer with limited English proficiency at all points of contact, in a timely manner during all hours of operation.

Standard 5: Health care organizations must provide to patients/consumers in their preferred language both verbal offers and written notices informing them of their right to receive language assistance services.

Standard 6: Health care organizations must assure the competence of language assistance provided to limited English.

proficient patients/consumers by interpreters and bilingual staff. Family and friends should not be used to provide interpretation services (except on request by the patient/consumer).

Standard 7: Health care organizations must make available easily understood patient-related materials and post signage in the languages of the commonly encountered groups and/or groups represented in the service area.

Standard 8: Health care organizations should develop, implement, and promote a written strategic plan that outlines clear goals, policies, operational plans, and management accountability/oversight mechanisms to provide culturally and linguistically appropriate services.

Standard 9: Health care organizations should conduct initial and ongoing organizational self-assessments of CLAS-related activities and are encouraged to integrate cultural and linguistic competence-related measures into their internal audits, performance improvement programs, patient satisfaction assessments, and outcomes-based evaluations.

Standard 10: Health care organizations should ensure that data on the individual patient's/consumer's race, ethnicity, and spoken and written language are collected in health records, integrated into the organization's management information systems, and periodically updated.

Standard 11: Health care organizations should maintain a current demographic, cultural, and epidemiological profile of the community as well as needs assessment to accurately plan for and implement services that respond to the cultural and linguistic characteristics of the service area.

Standard 12: Health care organizations should develop participatory, collaborative partnerships with communities and utilize a variety of formal and informal mechanisms to facilitate community and patient/consumer involvement in designing and implementing CLAS-related activities.

Standard 13: Health care organizations should ensure that conflict and grievance resolution processes are culturally and linguistically sensitive and capable of identifying, preventing, and resolving cross-cultural conflicts or complaints by patients/consumers.

Standard 14: Health care organizations are encouraged to regularly make available to the public information about their progress and successful innovations in implementing the CLAS standards and to provide public notice in their communities about the availability of this information.

Source: Office of Minority Health. (2001). *National standards for culturally and linguistically appropriate services in health care.* Retrieved June 4, 2009, from http://www.omhrc.gov/templates/browse.aspx?lvl=2&lvlID=15

of conducting social, cultural, and spiritual assessments and ways to incorporate findings into plans of care for patients.

Models of Health

Across times and cultures, the concept of *health* has been defined from various perspectives (see Chapter 1). In the Western world, several models of health emerged in the 20th century. The most prominent, the **biomedical model**, views health as the absence of disease (Boyd, 2000; Wade, 2004). From the biomedical standpoint, health is restored by prompt diagnosis of illness, prevention of complications, and elimination of pathology. Social, cultural, and spiritual dimensions of health are not central to the biomedical perspective, being generally considered private matters (Wade, 2004).

The traditional biomedical model continues to serve as the philosophical basis for Western medical care. In recent years, however, a trend in the biomedical community has emerged to consider the social, cultural, and spiritual aspects of health during decision making about treatment regimens (Davies, 2005; Wade, 2009; Wilkinson, 2005).

The **complementary and alternative medicine (CAM) model** of health, which emerged in the later 20th century, has been defined largely in relation to the biomedical perspective. The CAM therapies used instead of conventional treatments to restore health are often termed *alternative*, while CAM therapies used with conventional medicine are often labeled *complementary* (Barrett, et al., 2003). The evolving process of integration between the two perspectives evokes a new conceptual framework, which considers the complex interplay of mind, body, and spirit and offers opportunities to explore ways to facilitate healing (Berman, 2006; Caspi, et al., 2003). Although the CAM model is said to view health in a considerably more holistic way than the biomedical model, research is needed to evaluate the effectiveness of numerous CAM therapies before skeptics will become open to incorporating CAM treatments into plans of care (Eisenberg, et al., 1998).

This notion of wholeness is not a new concept to nursing. Florence Nightingale, the matriarch of modern nursing, described the nurse's duty as putting the patient in the best condition for nature (God) to act upon him or her (Nightingale, 1860/1992). She maintained that healing can occur only in an environment equipped with proper ventilation, adequate temperature, pure air and water, efficient drainage, cleanliness, light, and diminished noise. These environmental features are as important to health and healing today as they were to Nightingale in the 19th century. Evidence that care that embraces the patient's biopsychosocial and spiritual dimensions is important to health is also growing, because it puts the patient's life context and perceived needs first and offers healing for both body and spirit (Burkhardt, 2009; Romeo, 2000). This holistic approach to care results in more favorable outcomes than conventional treatments alone (Bradwell, 2009; Burkhardt, 2009; Kerwin, 2009; Liu, et al., 2008;

McCaffrey, 2008; Morad, 2008; Palmer & Ward, 2007; Vance, et al., 2008). Nursing must embrace the wholeness of individuals to properly manage the resources and constraints in their internal (biological, mental, and spiritual) and external (social and cultural) environments (Barker, 2002; Leininger & McFarland, 2005; Swanson 1993; Swanson & Wojnar, 2004; Watson, 1999).

In addition to the biomedical and CAM models, several models of health emerged in nursing. **Roy's adaptation model** was one of the earliest conceptualizations (Roy & Andrews, 1999). Roy refers to health as the patient's ability to adapt, compensate, manage, and adjust to physiologic–physical health-related setbacks (Hobfoll, 2001). The adaptation model holds that a person is a set of parts connected to function as a whole. The goal of nursing care is to assist the patient to attain an optimal level of

- *Physical health*: also described as physiological processes involved in the proper functioning of a living organism
- *Self-concept*: mental health
- *Role function*: ability to adequately perform in roles occupied in society
- *Interdependence*: satisfying interpersonal relationships (Roy & Andrews, 1999)

The healing environment is one that addresses symptoms of disease, supports bodily functioning, and sustains life by infection control, good oxygenation and nutrition, proper balance between activity and rest, and protection of the individual from harm (Roy & Andrews, 1999). The optimal level of adaptation is accomplished by educating the patient about the management of illness and health-promotion activities (Swanson & Wojnar, 2004).

Another broadly used nursing model is **Gordon's functional health model** (Gordon, 2006). Gordon posits that people are considered healthy if they can fulfill their social roles by contributing to family and society in meaningful ways. She emphasizes the importance of personal role fulfillment. The primary focus of the functional health model is the use of the person's skills and talents to their full potential and avoidance of the risks associated with losing independence.

Gordon identified 11 categories of **functional health patterns**, which she refers to as behaviors that occur sequentially across time: (1) health perception–health management; (2) nutrition-metabolic; (3) elimination; (4) activity-exercise; (5) sleep-rest; (6) cognitive-perceptual; (7) self-perception–self-concept; (8) role-relationship; (9) sexuality-reproductive; (10) coping-stress tolerance; and (11) value-belief. Chapter 3 discusses these patterns within the context of the patient's health history in detail. From the functional health perspective, an optimal healing environment would sustain life to a level expected for and desired by the patient, using various treatment modalities (Swanson & Wojnar, 2004).

The **eudaimonistic model of health** (Smith, 1981) emphasizes that wholeness of the individual is essential to maintaining good health. Basic dimensions of wholeness include biopsychosocial and spiritual well-being. In this model, biopsychosocial and spiritual health enables the person to achieve happiness and joy, in which he or she uses aspirations as a measure of the value of each human act. This model opens the possibility for ongoing growth, learning, maturity, and positive transformation. The optimal healing environment is one in which providers of care respond to the patient's unique physical, psychosocial, and spiritual needs to promote the unity of mind, body, and spirit, which leads to restoration, maintenance, or promotion of good health (Swanson & Wojnar, 2004, p. 46).

Social Assessment

Social assessment refers to identifying the social context influencing the patterns of health and illness for individuals, communities, and societies. Basic variables of social assessment include gender, age, ethnicity, race, marital status, occupational class, shelter, employment status, and education level. It is important to understand how these variables interact with the broader sociocultural environment. Knowledge obtained from social assessment helps nurses understand and address issues of equity and social justice related to health. It also helps providers to create new ways to improve patients' access to resources (Anderson & McFarlane, 2011; Anderson, et al., 1999; Kaplan, 2006; Marmot & Wilkinson, 2006).

Social assessment is integral to quality nursing care at every level. It emphasizes the interconnectedness of physical, psychosocial, and spiritual dimensions of health for individuals, communities, and populations studied. It helps health care providers and health-policy makers to refrain from compartmentalizing or making sweeping generalizations not grounded in data about individuals and communities. Though on the surface social assessment might appear simple, it is a daunting task that requires knowledge, creativity, and skill to make the connections among the assessment variables and to interpret data accurately before incorporating them into plans of care.

There are three levels of social assessment: individual, community, and societal.

Social Assessment of the Individual

Social assessment of the individual is intended primarily to inform nurses about the patient's physical and mental health as related to the patient's existing resources, constraints, and demands. Resources might include education, income, housing, and support systems; constraints might be unemployment, single-parent family, minority status, unsafe neighborhood, and lack of social support; demands might involve struggling to live on a fixed income or caring for aging parents (Leape, et al., 2002; Seid, 2008). Although information obtained from an individual's social assessment may not be necessary to diagnose illness or initiate treatment, it is essential for planning long-term management of illness as well as evidence-based

health-promotion activities for that patient (Melnyk & Fineout-Overholt, 2004).

Methods for individual social assessment predominantly entail personal interviews. Depending on assessment goals, interview questions vary from open-ended to specific, often guided by agency-designed assessment forms. A specific example of a comprehensive nursing assessment that attends to both social and cultural dimensions is the transcultural assessment shown in Figure 11-1. Because the list of suggested questions is extensive, it is recognized that nurses cannot conduct a complete assessment on admission to inpatient or outpatient care for every patient. Instead, the nurse must determine which questions are most relevant based on the patient's symptoms and learning needs. He or she also must consider any potential effects of culturally based practices on health.

Social Assessment of the Community

At the community level, the scope of social assessment is broader and more complex than at the individual level. Community social assessment involves gathering data to identify community resources, constraints, and high-priority health concerns (Anderson & McFarlane, 2011; Green & Kreuter, 1999).

Ideally, the process begins with the assessment of various social, economic, environmental, and quality-of-life health indicators and their relationship with the community's health concerns. Examples of findings from a community social assessment include the relationship between social determinants of health (family income, level of education, social support, and living conditions) with family violence (Bonomi, et al., 2009; Romito, et al., 2009), chronic illness (Lipstein, et al., 2009; Seid, 2008), and teen pregnancy (Crittenden, et al., 2009). This knowledge is invaluable for planning community-based health-promotion campaigns; yet, one must keep in mind that every community is unique with different strengths, weaknesses, and concerns. Hence, ongoing community assessments are essential to tailor interventions to each community's unique needs (Basara & Yuan, 2008).

Community-level social assessment techniques range from interviewing key informants through focus groups and mailed surveys to analyzing global housing situations, environmental concerns, and general access to health services. An example of a systematic community assessment framework is Kretzmann and McKnight's (1993) "asset mapping." Core community assessment variables include the gender, age, ethnicity, race, marital status, housing, employment status, and education of members. Data generated from the assessment are grouped into three categories: **primary, secondary**, and **potential building blocks**. Formal institutions in the area, such as local businesses, schools, libraries, parks, police, and fire stations, constitute the primary building blocks (Kretzmann & McKnight, 1993). Secondary building blocks include agencies designed to serve the community that have outside overarching corporations that manage and

Affiliations

- With what culture does the patient self-identify?
- To what degree does the patient identify with the cited cultural group?
- What is the patient's place of birth?
- Where has the patient lived? When? (If the patient is a recent U.S. immigrant, ask about or research prevalent diseases in the country of origin.)
- What is the patient's current residence?
- What is the patient's occupation?

Values

- How does the patient view birth and death?
- What is the patient's view of health versus illness?
- How does the patient regard health care providers?
- How does culture affect the patient's body image and any changes resulting from illness or treatment? For example, what emphasis does the patient's culture place on appearance, beauty, and strength?
- Is cultural stigma associated with any of the patient's illnesses or conditions?
- How does the patient view work?
- What is the patient's perspective on leisure?
- What are the patient's views on education?
- How does the patient feel about/perceive change?
- What effects on lifestyle do health, illness, treatments, and surgery pose for the patient?
- What is the patient's perspective on privacy? Courtesy? Touch? Age? Class? Gender?
- What perspective does the patient have regarding biomedical/scientific health care?
- How does the patient relate to those not from his or her culture?

Cultural Sanctions/Restrictions

- How do members of the patient's culture typically express emotion and feelings?
- How do they view dying, death, and grieving?
- How do men and women show modesty? Does the culture place expectations on male-female relationships? The nurse-patient relationship?
- Does the patient have restrictions related to sexuality, body exposure, or type of surgery?
- Are there restrictions about discussing the dead or fears related to the unknown?

Communication

- What is the patient's primary language? What other languages does the patient speak or read? In what language would the patient prefer to communicate with the nurse?
- What is the patient's level of fluency in English (written and spoken)?
- Does the patient need an interpreter?
- How does the patient prefer to be addressed?
- How does the patient's culture influence expectations about tempo of conversation, eye contact, topical taboos, confidentiality, and explanations?
- How does the patient's nonverbal communication compare with those from other cultural backgrounds? How does it affect the health care relationship?
- How does the patient view health care providers from different cultural backgrounds?
- Does the patient prefer to receive care from a nurse of the same cultural background, gender, or age group?
- What are overall cultural characteristics of the patient's language and communication?

Health-Related Beliefs/Practices

- To what cause(s) does the patient attribute illness and disease (eg, punishment from God, imbalance in hot/cold or yin/yang)?
- What are the patient's beliefs about ideal body size and shape?
- What name does the patient give to his or her health-related conditions?
- What does the patient believe promotes health (eg, certain foods, amulets)?
- What is patient's religious background (if any)?
- Does the patient rely on cultural healers (eg, curandero, shaman, spiritualist, priest)?
- Who influences the patient's choice/type of healer and treatment?
- In what types of cultural healing practices does the patient engage (eg, herbal remedies, potions, massage, talismans, healing rituals, incantations, prayers)?
- How does the patient perceive biomedical/scientific health care providers? Nurses? Nursing care?
- What comprises appropriate "sick" behavior? Who determines what constitutes symptoms? Who decides when the patient is no longer sick? Who cares for the patient?
- How does the patient's culture view mental disorders? Are there differences in acceptable behaviors for physical versus psychological illnesses?

Nutrition

- How does the culture influence the patient's nutritional factors?
- What is the meaning of food and eating for the patient?
- With whom does the patient usually eat? What is the timing and sequencing of meals?

Figure 11.1 Sample of a comprehensive cultural nursing assessment inventory.

- What does the patient define as food? What is "healthy" versus "unhealthy" eating?
- Who shops for food? Where are groceries purchased? Who prepares the meals? How are foods prepared at home?
- Has the patient chosen a specific practice (eg, vegetarianism, abstinence from alcohol)?
- Do religious beliefs/practices influence the patient's diet? Does the patient abstain from certain foods regularly, on specific dates determined by the religion, or at other times?
- If the patient's religion mandates or encourages fasting, what does "fast" mean (eg, refraining from certain types or quantities of foods, eating only during certain times)? For how long does the patient fast?
- While fasting, does the patient refrain from liquid? Does the religion allow exemption from fasting during illness? Does the patient believe the exemption applies to him or her?

Socioeconomic Considerations

- Who comprises the patient's social network (family, friends, peers, and cultural healers)? How do they influence health or illness status?
- How do members of the patient's social support network define caring (eg, being continuously present, doing things for the patient, providing material support, looking after family)?
- What is the role of various family members during health and illness?
- How does the patient's family participate in health promotion (eg, dietary modifications, exercise) and nursing care (eg, bathing, feeding, touching) of the patient?
- Does the cultural family structure influence the patient's response to health or illness? Does one key family member especially influence health-related decisions?
- Who is the principal wage earner in the family? What is the total annual income? (Note: This is a potentially sensitive question.) Is there more than one wage earner? Are there other sources of financial support?
- What insurance coverage does the patient have?
- What effects does economic status have on lifestyle, residence, living conditions, and ability to obtain health care? How does the home environment influence nursing care?

Organizations Providing Cultural Support

- What influences do ethnic/cultural organizations have on the patient?

Educational Background

- What is the patient's highest educational level obtained?
- Does the patient's educational background affect his or her knowledge of the health care delivery system, how to obtain needed care, teaching-learning, and any written material that he or she receives from health care providers?
- Can the patient read and write English, or is another language preferred? Are materials available in the other language?
- What learning style is most comfortable/familiar? Does the patient prefer to learn through written materials, oral explanation, or demonstration?

Religious Affiliation

- How does the patient's religious affiliation affect health and illness?
- What is the role of religious beliefs and practices during health and illness? Are there special rites or blessings for those with serious or terminal illnesses?
- Does the patient believe that any healing rituals or practices can promote well-being or hasten recovery from illness? If so, who performs these?
- What is the role of significant religious representatives during health and illness? Are there recognized religious healers?

Cultural Aspects of Disease

- Are there any specific genetic or acquired conditions more prevalent for the patient's cultural group (eg, hypertension, sickle-cell anemia, Tay Sachs)?
- Are socioenvironmental diseases more prevalent among a specific cultural group (eg, lead poisoning, alcoholism, HIV/AIDS, ear infections)?

Biocultural Variations

- Does the patient have distinctive physical features characteristic of a particular ethnic or cultural group?
- Does the patient have any anatomical variations of a particular ethnic or cultural group (eg, body structure, height, weight, facial shape and structure)?
- How do anatomic, racial, and ethnic variations affect the physical examination?

Developmental Considerations

- Do any developmental characteristics vary based on the patient's culture(s) (eg, bone density)?
- What developmental factors are culturally influenced (eg, expected growth, age for toilet training, feeding practices, gender expectations, methods of discipline)?
- What is the cultural perception of youthfulness?
- How does the culture view older adults?
- What are culturally acceptable roles for older adults?
- Are older adults isolated from culturally relevant supportive people?

Figure 11.1 (Continued)

operate these agencies. An example is a community's small primary care clinic that belongs to, and shares the values and mission of, a national corporate health care system. Potential building blocks are programs and services designed by an individual or agency outside the community to improve some aspect of community well-being. An example is a federally funded participatory action research study aimed at improving the cardiovascular health of a given community with an increased incidence of heart disease. Using the participatory action research approach, an investigator who is an "outsider" to the community strives to address and evaluate intervention outcomes by actively engaging with community members and facilitating change in a culturally sensitive way (McKnight & Kretzmann, 1977; Merzel & D'Afflitti, 2003).

Another example of a community assessment framework is Anderson and McFarlane's (2011) **Community as Partner Assessment Model** (Fig. 11-2). It has been

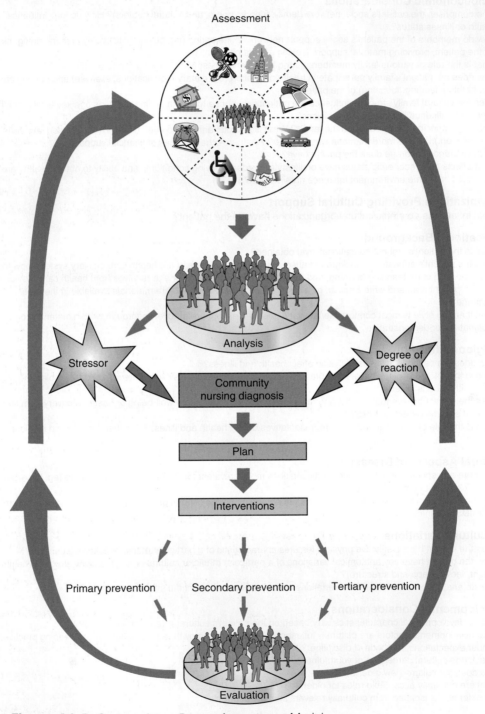

Figure 11.2 Community as Partner Assessment Model.

designed to help nurses thoroughly assess the demographics of a given community, including its values, beliefs, and history. It also assesses how resources (ie, recreation, physical environment, education, safety and transportation, politics and government, health and social services, communications, and economics) affect and influence the community. This information is used to define community nursing diagnoses and to plan and implement interventions in collaboration with community members. Anderson and McFarlane's model mandates that every community assessment and intervention include systematic evaluation to identify the effects of interventions.

Social Assessment at the Societal Level

At the societal level, social assessment is intended to generate information about societal trends and relationships among the social variables and prevalent health concerns. Data collected through society-wide assessments are used to inform healthy public policy and broad health-promotion initiatives. One specific example of societal-level social assessment is the recently conducted population vulnerability analyses to identify areas of highest concern (Capistrano, et al., 2005; Cernea & McDowell, 2000). Not surprisingly, regions with high concentrations of low-income households, non-English speaking immigrant families, and indigenous settlements emerged as areas of highest public health concern with respect to health vulnerabilities.

Collecting data and analyzing findings at the societal level are very complex. Social assessments are conducted to identify human and material assets, social networks, and the norms and sanctions that govern character, which, in turn, influences health behavior and values. Societal-level social assessment can also be used to identify, for example, ecological risks, disaster preparedness, or posttraumatic stress. Social assessment at the society level can be conducted using diverse research methods ranging in complexity from mailed surveys, telephone assessments, Internet-based questionnaires, opinion polls, to focus groups in multiple locations. Data analyses include summary statistics from complex samples, population stratification, associations between variables, and predictions.

Cultural Assessment

Cultural health assessments and related care are known to promote health and healing. Hence, nurses have an ethical, moral, and professional responsibility to conduct cultural assessments and create safe, culturally congruent physical and emotional environments in which patients and their families feel cared for and well supported.

Characteristics of Culture

At the most basic level, **culture** can be defined as a shared, learned, and symbolic system of values, beliefs,

and attitudes that shape and influence how people see and behave in the world (Hofstede, 1997). Major influences that shape worldview, and the extent to which people identify with their culture of origin, are called *primary and secondary characteristics* of culture (Purnell & Paulanka, 2005). Primary characteristics include age, gender, nationality, and ethnicity. Secondary characteristics include cultural values, religious beliefs, morals, occupation, socioeconomic status, immigration status, reasons for migration, and beliefs about health held as important to life and healthy living. All people's cultural beliefs about health are important and often powerfully influence health practices. Health professionals, like their patients, add a unique dimension to the complexity of culturally based care (Purnell & Paulanka, 2005).

Aims of Cultural Assessment

From a holistic perspective, people of different cultures have the right to receive **cultural assessment** and have their health beliefs, values, and practices acknowledged and incorporated into plans of care, provided there are no safety concerns. Cultural assessment refers to systematic assessment of individuals, families, and communities regarding their health beliefs and values (Leininger & McFarland, 2005). The specific aim of cultural assessment is to provide an all-inclusive picture of the patient's culture-based health care needs by

1. Gaining knowledge about the patient's cultural beliefs and practices, including food and eating rituals, daily and nightly personal hygiene rituals, and sleeping habits
2. Comparing culture care needs of the specific person with the general themes of those of similar cultural background
3. Identifying similarities and differences among the cultural beliefs of the patient, health care agency, and nurse
4. Generating a holistic picture of the patient's care needs, upon which a culturally congruent nursing care plan is developed and implemented (Leininger & McFarland, 2005)

Based on the comprehensive body of knowledge drawn from anthropology and nursing, Madeline Leininger developed the Theory of Culture Care Diversity and Universality (Leininger & McFarland, 2005). She proposed essential areas of assessment to better understand the relationship between one's culture and health. Leininger's theory identifies the relationships between cultural variables (ie, cultural values and beliefs, religion and personal philosophy of life and spiritual beliefs, educational and economic background, relationship with family and friends, views on and use of technology, politics, and the patient's legal status) and health, and highlights the nursing behaviors and skills necessary to carry out effective cultural assessment.

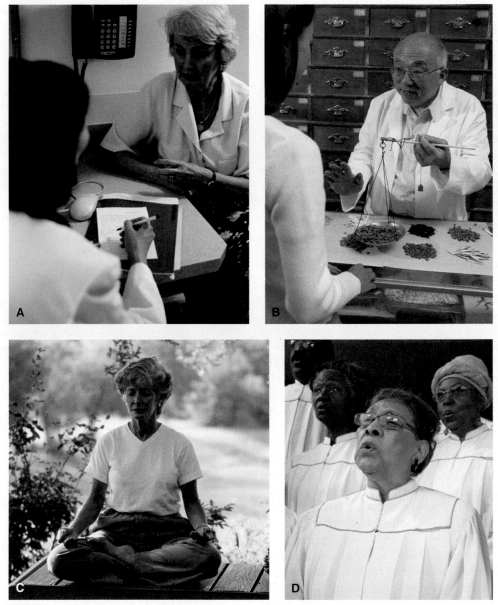

Figure 11.3 **(A)** Patients benefit when nurses discuss with them cultural or spiritual practices they follow that may influence their health. Examples include **(B)** Chinese medicine, **(C)** meditation/relaxation, and **(D)** participation in religious services.

Leininger suggests that the attributes and behaviors of a nurse practicing effective care within the patient's cultural context include the following:

- Genuine interest in a patient's culture and personal life experiences
- Active listening, and awareness of meanings behind the patient's verbal communication (story telling)
- Nonverbal communication (body language, eye contact, facial expressions, interpersonal space, and preferences regarding touch)
- Acknowledgement that the nurse's own beliefs and prejudices might create barriers to providing culturally sensitive care.

Consideration of patients' cultural background and incorporating their health beliefs and practices in care plans

contribute to enhanced patient experiences with health care and improve health outcomes (Berry, 1999; Higgins, 2000; Lumberg, 2000; Sellers, et al., 1999). Because of the comprehensive body of research showing the benefits of culturally based care, the mandate from accrediting professional organization, and the core values of nursing profession, nurses have an obligation to skillfully conduct cultural assessments and to incorporate findings into plans of care without bias, prejudice, or discrimination. See Figure 11-3.

Cultural Health Beliefs and Practices

At the core of culturally based care is the assessment of the patient's health beliefs and practices (Box 11-2) and, when no safety concerns arise, incorporation of the patient's beliefs and practices into the plan of care. Seeking

1. In what prevention activities do you engage to maintain your health?
2. Who in your family takes responsibility for your health?
3. What over-the-counter medicines do you use?
4. What herbal teas and folk medicines do you use?
5. For what conditions do you use herbal medicines?
6. What do you usually do when you are in pain?
7. How do you express your pain?
8. How are people in your culture viewed or treated when they have mental illness?
9. How are people with physical disabilities treated in your culture?
10. What do you do when you are sick? Stay in bed, continue your normal activities, etc.?
11. What are your beliefs about rehabilitation?
12. How are people with chronic illnesses viewed or treated in your culture?
13. Are you adverse to blood transfusions?
14. Is organ donation acceptable to you?
15. Are you an organ donor?
16. Would you consider having an organ transplant if needed?

Source: Adapted from Purnell, L. D., & Paulanka, B. J. (2005). *Guide to culturally competent health* care (p. 18). Philadelphia: F. A. Davis.

an understanding of patients' culturally based health care practices is essential to nursing because each culture has its own traditional values and beliefs about health and illness that may affect individuals' adherence to treatments. For example, for some individuals health care services may not be affordable or culturally relevant, especially when dietary habits and preferences are not taken into consideration when treatments are ordered. Others, because of the unequal distribution and underrepresentation of ethnic minorities in health care, may reluctantly decide to seek conventional care from a provider that does not represent their own culture after traditional healing remedies prove unsuccessful. Some examples of traditional health and illness beliefs and practices of people from various minority groups are reviewed in Table 11-1.

Cultural Food and Nutrition Practices

Food and nutrition are an important part of cultural nursing assessment because they represent an expression of peoples' culture and, as such, their consumption may affect individuals' physical health. People all over the world use food to celebrate special events or religious holidays. In some cultures, food represents wealth and health; others use food as an offering to gods or a special gift to guests. All cultures relish ethnic dishes as symbols of identity or cultural expression that they often pass from generation to generation. Nurses must be sensitive about the meaning of food to people. They must be careful about not refusing food that accompanies special events such as childbirth or infant circumcision performed in hospitals for religious reasons, because patients

might perceive such refusal as personal rejection (Purnell & Paulanka, 2005).

In many cultures, ideal body weight is higher than medical experts recommend. Such cultures may not consider "dieting" healthy. People may prefer to consume foods high in fat, salt, and cholesterol, and low in fruit and vegetables because they believe it is best for their health (Purnell & Paulanka, 2005). Others may have awareness that the ideal diet should be well balanced and rich in different nutrients, but they cannot afford this. Likewise, new immigrants may have difficulty finding ethnic food stores that carry healthy foods with which they are familiar and unknowingly select unhealthy foods in nearby supermarkets based on affordability. It is therefore very important that nurses provide facts about the nutritional value of various foods and help patients make choices that promote health and are congruent with their cultural background and personal preferences.

Cultural Beliefs and Practices of Pregnancy and Childbirth

Cultural beliefs and practices surrounding pregnancy care and childbirth are powerful and cannot be ignored. Many culture-specific taboos are believed to promote well-being and prevent bad outcomes for mother and child (Enang, et al., 2002). For example, some women claim that the fetus signals what he or she wants them to consume via cravings and that if they do not eat the foods they are craving, their children will be birth-marked for that particular food.

SAFETY ALERT 11.1

Certain cravings in pregnant women may be unhealthy. Nurses need to provide evidence-based information about the benefits of a well-balanced diet and avoiding substances that might harm mother and fetus.

Women in many cultures believe that buying infant clothing before birth is bad luck and may contribute to a stillbirth. Hence, they might arrive at the hospital for childbirth without infant clothing. In these situations, nurses must seek information about beliefs regarding pregnancy and childbirth rather than making assumptions that the baby is unwanted or the mother "doesn't care" (Purnell & Paulanka, 2005).

Across cultures, childbirth is a time of celebration. Relatives and friends might congregate in a hospital or house where childbirth is occurring. While some cultures permit their presence in birthing rooms, others might forbid even the father to visit the mother until after the baby is born. Understanding and accepting cultural differences and preferences surrounding childbirth help to alleviate interpersonal barriers between nurses and clients, make families feel more at ease to discuss their beliefs and needs, and help to enhance the experience (Enang, et al., 2002).

Culturally based postpartum practices are also diverse. Generally, most cultures recognize that, after childbirth, women must rest, take care of the baby, and "eat for two" when breastfeeding. In some cultures, people may believe

Table 11.1	Health Characteristics of Minority Populations			
Characteristic	African Americans	American Indians/ Alaska Natives	Asian Americans/ Pacific Islanders	Hispanics/Latinos
Demographics	14% of U.S. population (second largest minority). Many live in the South	1.6% of U.S. population. 60% live in metropolitan areas	Consists of people of Far Eastern, Southeast Asian, or Indian subcontinent descent. 5% of U.S. population	Largest U.S. minority group. Consists of people of Cuban, Mexican, Puerto Rican, South or Central American, or other Spanish culture or origin
Educational Attainment	Fewer blacks earn a high school diploma than whites. More black women than black men earn a bachelor's degree.	76% have a high school diploma. 14% have a bachelor's degree	62% of Vietnamese, 50% of Chinese, 24% of Filipinos, and 23% of Asian Indians are not fluent in English. 86% have a high school diploma. 50% of Asian Americans compared to 28% of total U.S. population have a bachelor's degree. 45% are professional compared to 34% of total.	Language fluency varies among subgroups; nationally, 12% of Mexicans speak Spanish at home. 81% have a high school diploma. 13% have a bachelor's degree.
Economics	Average family income is $34,000 compared to $55,000 for white families. 25% of families live at poverty level. Rate of unemployment is twice that of whites.	Median family income is about $34,000. 26% work in professional occupations. 25% live at poverty level.	Median family income is $55,600, higher than the national income.	25% work in service occupations, compared to 14% of whites. 17% work in professional occupations, compared to 40% of whites.
Insurance Coverage	About 50% of African Americans have health insurance, compared to 66% of whites. Twice as many African Americans are uninsured, compared to whites.	36% have insurance; 33% have no health insurance	Public insurance rates vary according to subgroup, from 76% to 84%. Overall insurance coverage is 84% compared to 90% of whites.	Hispanics have the highest uninsured rates of any U.S. racial or ethnic group. Uninsured rate ranges from 23% to 38%.
Cancer	African American men are more likely to have new lung, prostate, and stomach cancer. African American women are less likely to be diagnosed with stomach and breast cancer, but 34% more likely to die from breast cancer and 2.4 times more likely to die from stomach cancer.	Men are twice as likely to have liver and bowel cancer. Native Americans have higher rates of stomach, liver, kidney, and pelvic cancers.	Asian men are 40% less likely to have prostate cancer. Women are 30% less likely to have breast cancer. Asian Americans have three times the incidence of liver, bowel, and stomach cancers as whites.	Hispanic men are 16% less likely to have prostate cancer. Women are 33% less likely to have breast cancer. They have higher rates of stomach, liver, and cervical cancer than whites.

		American Indians/	**Asian Americans/**	
Table 11.1	**Health Characteristics of Minority Populations** (*continued*)			
Characteristic	**African Americans**	**American Indians/ Alaska Natives**	**Asian Americans/ Pacific Islanders**	**Hispanics/Latinos**
Diabetes	African Americans are twice as likely to be diagnosed with diabetes. They are about twice as likely to die from complications of diabetes.	American Indians are 2.3 times more likely to be diagnosed with diabetes and twice as likely to die from it. They are more likely to be obese and have hypertension.	Native Hawaiians have twice the rate of diabetes and are six times more likely to die from it.	They are twice as likely to have diabetes. Hispanics are more likely to have treatment for end-stage renal disease and die from diabetes.
Heart Disease	African American men are 30% more likely to die from heart disease. African Americans are 1.5 times as likely to have high blood pressure. Women are 1.7 times more likely to be obese.	They are more likely to have heart disease, smoke cigarettes, be obese, and have high blood pressure.	Asian adults are less likely to have heart disease and die from it than whites.	Hispanics are 10% less likely to have heart disease and 30% less likely to die from it.
HIV/AIDS	Although African Americans make up only 14% of the population, they have almost 50% of cases of HIV/AIDS.	American Indians are more likely to have AIDS. Women have twice the AIDS rate of white women.	They have lower AIDS rates than whites and are less likely to die from it.	Hispanic men have almost three times the AIDS rate as whites. Women have almost five times the rate as whites. Hispanics are 2.5–3 times more likely than whites to die from AIDS.
Immunization	Older adults are 30% less likely to receive the flu shot and 40% less likely to receive the pneumonia shot.	Children were immunized at the same rate as white children They are more likely to die from sudden infant death syndrome (SIDS), low birth weight, and congenital malformations.	Older adults are 40% less likely to receive the pneumonia shot. Children reached the Healthy People goal for immunizations.	Older adults are 10% less likely to receive the flu shot and 50% less likely to receive the pneumonia shot. Children have comparable rates of immunization.
Infant Mortality	African Americans have 2.3 times the infant mortality rate of whites. They have higher rates of SIDS, low birth weight babies, and failure to receive prenatal care.	American Indians have 1.4 times the mortality as whites. They are 3.7 times as likely to begin prenatal care in the third trimester.	SIDS is the fourth leading cause of mortality. It is higher for babies born to mothers younger than 20 years.	Infant mortality varies among subgroups from 4.4–8.3 compared to 5.8 for whites. Puerto Ricans have 1.4 times the infant mortality rate of whites.
Stroke	African Americans are 1.7 times more likely to have a stroke and 60% more likely to die from it.	American Indian adults are 60% more likely to have a stroke. Women have twice the rate of stroke.	Adults are less likely to die from stroke, be overweight or obese, have hypertension, or smoke.	Hispanic men and women are 15%–25% less likely to die from stroke than whites.

Source: http://minorityhealth.hhs.gov/templates/browse.aspx?lvl=2&lvlID=9

that a fat baby is a healthy baby and new parents might be advised to offer their baby a bottle after breastfeeding to ensure that the infant is "not starving" and "puts some meat on the bones fast." In these situations nurses must provide facts about infants' nutritional needs and weight-gain patterns, as well as health risks associated with infant formula consumption and overfeeding (Riordan & Auerbach, 2005).

In some situations, adhering to culture-based postpartum practices is difficult. For example, women who are practicing Muslims are expected to rest, eat well, take care of the baby, and stay at home for 40 days. Traditionally, they are cared for by other women in the community and not expected to have demands put on them during this time. This may be difficult, if not impossible, when they arrive in the United States as new immigrants and give birth before they make new friends or have a community network. In such cases, nurses might help by making arrangements for visitations of volunteer women in the community (Purnell & Paulanka, 2005).

Cultural Beliefs and Expressions of Illness and Pain

In some cultures, the roles of men and women, young and old, can vary greatly. Also, it is important to consider differences in culture and religion—for example, a U.S.-born Muslim may have a different kind of cultural orientation than a Muslim who has immigrated to the U.S. While many U.S. immigrants transition to Western medicine, some maintain their roots in traditional healing practices, and others mix traditional and Western therapies to restore health. When a nurse conducts cultural health assessment, he or she might find that an African American patient mentions already consulting the *Farmers' Almanac* with limited success. Patients of Hispanic background may mention that they have already turned for help to a "*curandero(a)*" spiritualist, herbalist, or traditional healer. Asian patients may report that they received care from a herbalist, acupuncturist, or bone setter (Andrews & Boyle, 2003; Purnell & Paulanka, 2005).

⚠ SAFETY ALERT 11.2

It is imperative that the nurse asks patients whether they are currently using any traditional remedies to better understand their perspectives on health and illness and to impress upon them the potential for antagonistic reactions when some traditional and conventional therapies are used at the same time.

Pain assessment is an integral feature of culturally based health assessment. For example, many people perceive pain as a sign of disease. In the absence of pain, they may decide to not take prescribed medications or take them only when they feel discomfort, which could have grave consequences. Others believe that pain is an inevitable part of being human and endure pain in silence. This belief might contribute to a high pain tolerance or complete refusal of pain medication.

Therefore, nurses must rely both on patients' verbal and nonverbal manifestations when assessing and treating pain (Purnell & Paulanka, 2005).

Some cultures believe that praying and laying on of hands or using holy water and religious symbols will free the person of all pain and suffering. Hence, in some circumstances, sick patients who still report pain may be considered to have little faith. In contrast, other cultures encourage sick patients to be pampered and to express pain freely. Whatever the situation, nurses must display a nonjudgmental attitude, provide facts, and use a culturally specific approach when administering prescribed treatments. They must never interpret patients' inactivity and dependence as apathy, depression, or "being difficult" without first conducting a cultural assessment and gaining insight into the patient's medical diagnosis and behavior.

Spiritual Assessment

Spirituality, in the most fundamental sense, pertains to matters of the human soul, be it a state of mind, a state of being in the world, a journey of self-discovery, or a place outside the five senses (Holt, et al., 2005). In general, spirituality emphasizes a notion of a path to achieve better understanding and connectedness with nature, inner harmony, other people, or an improved relationship with the divine (Fig. 11-4). Spirituality is also considered an integral part of one's religion or self-directed path modeled after several different religions. In all cases, spirituality is concerned with matters of the soul rather than the world of senses and material things (Borysenko, 2005). Similar to social and cultural assessments, spiritual assessment involves understanding the relationship between spirituality and health (Borg, et al., 2003).

To be meaningful, spiritual care within the health care context must be congruent with the patient's spiritual beliefs (Thomas-McLean, 2004). Just as with social and cultural assessment, making assumptions or generalizations about a patient's spiritual needs based on ethnic or religious affiliation is almost certain to be an oversimplification. Nevertheless, it is important to be aware that for people of many cultures, church and religion play important roles in sustaining their development, national identity, and survival and must be treated as such. For example, patients of Polish descent may identify the Catholic Church as a symbol of their national identity and sustainability, because it helped the nation to survive and maintain native language and culture for more than 150 years of foreign occupation (Pease, 1991). Similarly, Black Churches played a major role in the development and survival of African American culture. Hence, many African Americans make no distinction between the Black Church and the black community (Pinn, 2002). These specific examples are not isolated. Having faith in God and participating in organized religious life are important to

An example would be to assess the cultural background of Mr. El-Kebbi, whom is mentioned at the beginning of this chapter, to address his concerns related to diabetes care during the Muslim religious holiday of Ramadan. Through therapeutic dialog, nursing assessment seeks to incorporate the patient's social, cultural, and spiritual dimensions of health. One method is more effective than the other.

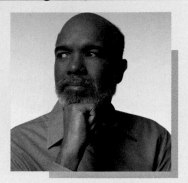

Less Effective

Nurse: Hello, Mr. El-Kebbi. How are you doing today? (extends right hand and shakes)

Mr. El-Kebbi: Very well, thank you.

Nurse: How are you doing with managing your diabetes?

Mr. El-Kebbi: I think, well. I am going to fast during Ramadan and want to know if I should do anything special with my diabetes management.

Nurse: You don't need to fast during Ramadan; you can get an exception because you have diabetes.

Mr. El-Kebbi: I would like to fast with my family.

Nurse: But you shouldn't if it creates hardship because of your diabetes.

Mr. El-Kebbi: Allah will take care of me.

Nurse: But fasting when you are a diabetic can cause your blood sugar to fluctuate and you can get hypoglycemia, hyperglycemia, or become dehydrated.

Mr. El-Kebbi: I want to fast in order to be closer to Allah.

Nurse: Do you exercise? If you exercise, you should do it after you eat.

Mr. El- Kebbi: Yes, I can do that. I want to keep my body healthy.

Nurse: The best way to keep your body healthy is by not fasting during Ramadan. Your spiritual leader will give you an exception.

Mr. El-Kebbi: It is important for me to experience this fasting to feel closer to Allah.

Nurse: Well, then, you do what you need to do.

Mr. El-Kebbi: Thank you.

More Effective

Nurse: Hello, Mr. El-Kebbi. How are you doing today? (smiles)

Mr. El-Kebbi: Very well, thank you.

Nurse: How are you doing with managing your diabetes?

Mr. El-Kebbi: I think, well. I am going to fast during Ramadan and want to know if I should do anything special with my diabetes management.

Nurse: I am glad that you came in to talk to us about it. We may need to make some changes in your medication and diet regimen. (smiles)

Mr. El-Kebbi: Allah will take care of me.

Nurse: When do you usually take your metformin? We may need to adjust the timing.

Mr. El-Kebbi: In the morning.

Nurse: How do you usually break your daily fast?

Mr. El-Kebbi: We have a big meal together after sunset.

Nurse: You might want to have a few small meals after sunset instead. And what is your typical daily exercise?

Mr. El-Kebbi: I go for a 30-minute brisk walk after work on most days.

Nurse: During Ramadan, you may want to exercise a few hours after eating so that you don't get hypoglycemia. We can talk with your doctor about making adjustments so that your diet, exercise, and medication management all fit together during Ramadan.

Mr. El-Kebbi: Thank you so much.

Critical Thinking Challenge

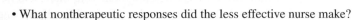

- What nontherapeutic responses did the less effective nurse make?
- What might be the social, cultural, or spiritual influences on Mr. El-Kebbi's decision to fast?
- What is the role of a nurse when counseling a patient making this decision?

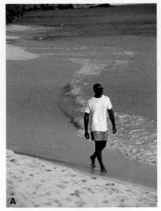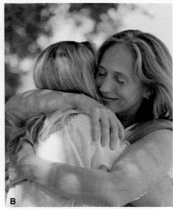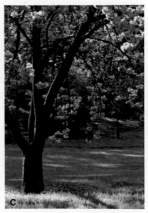

Figure 11.4 A sense of spirituality can be manifested through a relationship with **(A)** oneself, **(B)** other people, or **(C)** transcendent forces, such as God or nature.

people of diverse cultures and ethnicities and are often seen as a source of inner strength and spirituality. It is therefore important to assess the meaning of the church and organized religion in the patient's life and how it might best be incorporated in the plan of care to promote health and healing. An example of spiritual assessment is presented in Box 11-3.

During spiritual assessment, a nurse might learn that a practicing Muslim wishes to combine conventional bio-medical treatments with spiritual nourishment consisting of daily prayers and reading or listening to the Qur'an. He or she may request to have a hospital bed turned to face Mecca and have a hospital gown changed and a basin of water placed near the bed for ritualistic washing of hands before praying. By making simple accommodations, nurses can create environments in which Muslim patients may not only have their spiritual needs met but also experience a general sense of respect and understanding (Purnell & Paulanka, 2005).

For practicing Jews, observance of Jewish Holidays and participating in religious rituals are also important to health and healing. Some Jews may want to pray three times a day and bring their prayer items such as Yarmulke or kippah, tallit, tzitzit, and tefillin to the hospital. They may refuse medical or surgical procedures on the Sabbath or other holidays unless the situation is life threatening. A nurse may also find many visitors in the patient's room because, among other reasons, visiting the sick is a social obligation for Jews. It is important that nurses and others are accommodating and respectful of the patient's wishes and create an environment in which the physical and spiritual healing of the client occurs concurrently (Robinson, 2000).

For many practicing Hindus, spirituality and religion are also closely related. Those who live far away from temples often pray, sing, recite scriptures, and repeat the names of deities at home or other places. Shrines that represent symbols of one or more deities may therefore be set up in the back of the house or even by the sick person's bedside in the hospital. It is important that nurses assess the extent to which the patient who discloses Hinduism as his or her religion practices it and how beliefs relate to health and illness and to daily religious prayer. Assessing the spiritual needs of these patients may assist nurses in accommodating their need for prayer in privacy (Jambunathan, 2003).

Even when daily prayers or other religious practices are not a routine part of a patient's life, they often take central position during life transitions, such as loss of a loved one, accident, or serious illness (Hudson & Rumbold, 2003; Rumbold, 2003). Assessment of spiritual needs might reveal that the use of blood products or modern technologies to sustain life may not be congruent with their beliefs. On the other hand, another patient's spirituality allows aggressive medical treatments until the end of life. In each instance, imposing the values of the health care provider may be stress provoking and counterproductive (Holt, et al., 2005). Thus, individual patient assessment and incorporation of spiritual assessment findings into plans of care are essential to promote acceptance and spiritual well-being of individuals across the lifespan.

BOX 11.3 SPIRITUAL ASSESSMENT

1. What is your religion?
2. Do you consider yourself deeply religious?
3. How many times a day do you pray?
4. What do you need in order to say your prayers?
5. Do you meditate?
6. What gives strength and meaning to your life?
7. In what spiritual practices do you engage for your physical and emotional pain?

Source: Adapted from Clancy, C. (2006). Care transitions: A threat and opportunity for patient safety. *American Journal of Medical Quality, 21*(6), 414–417.

Diagnosis and Related Factors	Point of Differentiation	Assessment Characteristics	Nursing Interventions
Social interaction impaired related to knowledge/skill deficit, isolation, sociocultural misfit, physical or communication barriers, altered thought processes	Engagement with others that is insufficient in frequency, lacking in quality, or both	Failure to maintain eye contact (as culturally appropriate); minimal verbal communication; decreased interaction with friends, neighbors, family, work, and groups	Assess cause of discomfort. Use listening skills. Encourage feelings. Role play situations. Use humor as appropriate.
Social isolation related to problems with cognition or mental status, decreased relationships, unacceptable social behaviors	Loneliness experienced as a negative condition	Hostility, withdrawal, lack of communication, inappropriate activities for age, rejection of others, expressions of loneliness	Discuss causes of isolation. Recommend support groups. Identify support system. Offer choices of activities. Provide physical activities.
Spiritual distress related to challenged belief and value system or separation from religious or cultural ties	Disruption in big life concepts that integrate the meaning of life	Expresses concern with meaning of life or death, questions the meaning of suffering, questions the meaning of own existence, and expresses anger toward higher power	Assess sources of support and make appropriate referrals. Ask how to be most helpful. Listen to feelings. Assist with providing appropriate religious materials. Provide privacy for praying.
Readiness for enhanced spiritual well-being	Developing of inner strengths to understand life's purpose and harmony with all	Expresses feelings of hope; recognizes inner strength; states purpose of life; feels at peace with self, others, and higher power	Assess spiritual or religious preferences. Make referrals when indicated. Promote support from friends and family. Allow time for praying, talking, or journaling. Provide music.

Evidence-Based Critical Thinking

Nursing Diagnoses, Outcomes, and Interventions

Table 11-2 compares and contrasts nursing diagnoses, abnormal findings, and interventions commonly related to social, cultural, or spiritual assessment (NANDA-I, 2009). Note the differences between the two diagnoses for social interaction and spirituality.

Nurses use assessment information to identify patient outcomes. Some outcomes related to social, cultural, and spiritual issues include the following:

- The patient will express a sense of connectedness with self, others, arts, music, or power greater than oneself.
- The patient will express meaning and purpose in life.
- The patient will initiate interactions with others (Moorhead, et al., 2008).

Once the outcomes are established, nursing care is implemented to improve the patient's status. The nurse uses critical thinking and evidence-based practice to develop the interventions. Some examples of nursing interventions for the social, cultural, and spiritual domains are as follows:

- Monitor and promote supportive social contact.
- Integrate family into spiritual practices as appropriate.
- Offer visits with spiritual or religious advisors (Bulecheck, et al., 2008).

The nurse then evaluates care according to the patient outcomes that were developed, therefore reassessing the patient and continuing or modifying the interventions as appropriate. An accurate and complete nursing assessment is an essential foundation for holistic nursing care. Even as a beginner, the nursing student can use the patient assessment to implement new interventions, evaluate their effectiveness, and make a difference in the quality of patient care.

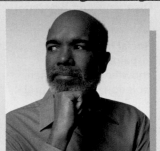

Remember Mr. El-Kebbi, the patient with diabetes who was planning on fasting for Ramadan. Initial subjective and objective data collection is complete, and the nurse has spent time reviewing findings with the primary provider. The following nursing note illustrates how subjective and objective data are collected and analyzed and nursing interventions are developed.

Subjective: Mr. El-Kebbi, a 54-year-old Somali immigrant man seen in clinic for 6-month follow-up appointment related to type 2 diabetes. Plans on fasting for Ramadan next month. Asks for advice on how to best manage diabetes during this time. Usually, takes metformin in the morning and exercises on a treadmill after work in the evening. States that he has a large family with seven children and that some of his children live away from home. During Ramadan, his entire family gathers together at his home to break the fast each night. Prays to Allah five times daily and attends mosque weekly and on holidays. Allah is a source of strength for him and he reads the Qur'an daily. He is involved in a community of Somali immigrants in the Somali Community Services agency. He is also very much involved in a Sunni mosque in the central district of town. He feels well supported and connected to others.

Objective: Wearing Western clothing, well groomed with good personal hygiene. Conversing appropriately, maintaining distance because of gender roles. Affect appropriate, interested, and animated. T 36.8°C tympanic, P 78 beats/min, R 16 breaths/min, BP 112/68 mm Hg. Height 157 cm, weight 66 kg, BMI 26.8. Skin with pink undertones, erect posture, and breathing easily.

Analysis: Health-seeking behaviors related to anticipated fast for Ramadan.

Plan: Consult with physician to establish risk for fasting and modifications to usual routine. May need adjustments in medication, diet, and activity, to prevent glycemic complications and dehydration. Further assess types of food eaten and nutritional content to promote a healthy diabetic diet. Assess knowledge of symptoms of hypoglycemia and hyperglycemia and the actions that should be taken.

P. Fritz, RN

Critical Thinking Challenge

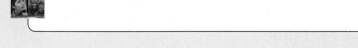

- What are your beliefs about a diabetic fasting? How might such beliefs influence care provided?
- What information on the social, cultural, and spiritual practices of Mr. El-Kebbi is needed to provide culturally competent care?
- How will Mr. El-Kebbi recognize if his fasting has been successful?

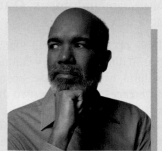

In many facilities, nurses initiate referrals to social or spiritual care based on assessment findings. Results that might trigger a consult include patients and families expressing social concerns, cultural concerns, or spiritual concerns; death; receiving a terminal diagnosis; comfort care; family conferences; and families in crisis (Interdisciplinary Plan, 2007). It is important to assess if the patient or family is interested in receiving social or spiritual care. Because of the personal nature of religion and the meaning of spirituality, an open-ended question such as, "How would you feel about talking to someone about your spiritual needs?" or "Tell me about whether you want someone to talk or pray with you?" can offer support. Follow-up questions, such as "Do you have a religious preference?" or "Would you like to have someone important from your church to visit with you?" can help identify the most appropriate person to contact. Many patients appreciate spiritual guidance, especially during challenging times. Social issues may be referred to social workers who have knowledge of resources that can be gathered during times of need. Cultural understandings can be learned through Web sites such as Ethnomed or through the Office of Minority Health. It is especially important to interpret these issues within the context of the individual patient, family, and community.

Using the previous steps of diagnostic reasoning, organizing, and prioritizing, consider all the case study findings woven throughout this chapter. When answering the following questions, begin drawing conclusions and see how the pieces of assessment must work together to create an environment for personalized, appropriate, and accurate care.

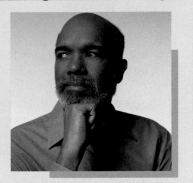

• How might Mr. El-Kebbi's social network influence his healthy lifestyle?
• How will the nurse assess this patient's cultural needs?
• What effect might religion have on Mr. El-Kebbi's diabetes management?

Key Points

• *National Standards for Culturally and Linguistically Appropriate Services in Health Care* mandate the standards to be upheld in every health care setting.
• CAM therapies used instead of conventional treatments to restore health are often termed alternative, while CAM therapies used with conventional medicine are often labeled complementary.
• Social assessment refers to identifying the social context influencing the patterns of health and illness for individuals, communities, and societies.
• With the transcultural assessment, the nurse must determine which questions to ask based on the patient's symptoms, learning needs, and potential effects of the patient's culturally based practices on health.
• Core community assessment variables include gender, age, ethnicity, race, marital status, housing, employment status, and education of community members.
• The Community as Partner Assessment Model has been designed to help nurses thoroughly assess the demographics of a given community and its values, beliefs, and history, and to determine how the community is affected and influences resources (recreation, physical environment, education, safety and transportation, politics and government, health and social services, communications, and economics).
• Culture can be defined as a shared, learned, and symbolic system of values, beliefs, and attitudes that shapes and influences the way people see and behave in the world.
• The goal of cultural assessment is to provide a picture of the patient's culture-based health care needs by (1) gaining knowledge about the patient's cultural beliefs and practices including food and eating rituals, daily and nightly personal hygiene rituals and sleeping habits; (2) comparing culture care needs of the specific individual with the general themes of persons from similar cultural background; (3) identifying similarities and differences between the cultural beliefs of the patient, health care agency, and the nurse; and (4) generating a holistic picture of the patient's care needs, upon which culture congruent nursing care plan is developed and implemented.

• The attributes and behaviors of a nurse practicing effective care within the patient's cultural context include genuine interest in culture and personal life experiences, active listening, and effective nonverbal communication.
• Seeking understanding of one's culturally based health care practices is essential to nursing because each culture has its own traditional values and beliefs about health and illness that may affect patients' adherence to treatments.
• Spirituality pertains to the matters of human soul—be it a state of mind, state of being in the world, journey of self-discovery, or place outside of our five senses.
• For people of many cultures, church and religion play important roles in sustaining their development, national identity, and survival.
• Even when daily prayer or other religious practices are not part of a patient's life routine, they often take central position during life transitions, such as loss of a loved one, accident, or serious illness.
• Common nursing diagnoses related to social, cultural, and spiritual assessments include impaired social interaction, social isolation, spiritual distress, and readiness for enhanced spiritual well-being.

Review Questions

1. *National Standards for Culturally and Linguistically Appropriate Services in Health Care* mandate that the standards
   A. should be applied in private offices
   B. may be used in public settings
   C. should be used in hospitals
   D. be upheld in every health care setting

2. CAM therapies used instead of conventional treatments to restore health are often termed
   A. alternative
   B. advantaged
   C. complementary
   D. conventional

3. The social context influences the patterns of health and illness for individuals, communities, and societies. An example is
   A. assessment of the patient's health beliefs and practices
   B. assessment of focus groups in multiple locations
   C. assessment of culturally based postpartum practices
   D. assessment of the religious practices of the patient

4. The purpose of comparing culture care needs of the specific individual to the general themes of people from similar cultural background is to
   A. identify the dietary needs of a specific religious preference
   B. determine if the patient needs a spiritual consultation
   C. provide a picture of the individual's culture-based health care needs
   D. consider how closely the patient follows his or her religion

5. With transcultural assessment, the nurse must
   A. ask all the questions for completeness
   B. determine which questions to ask
   C. include all the questions as part of an admitting assessment
   D. wait until the relationship is established to ask questions

6. A shared, learned, and symbolic system of values, beliefs, and attitudes that shapes and influences the way people see and behave in the world is defined as
   A. society
   B. community
   C. culture
   D. spirituality

7. Even when daily prayers or other religious practices are not a part of a patient's life routine, they often take central position during life transitions, such as loss of a loved one, accident, or serious illness. A related nursing diagnosis might be
   A. spiritual distress
   B. impaired social interaction
   C. readiness for enhanced spiritual well-being
   D. social isolation

8. It is important to identify similarities and differences among the cultural beliefs of the patient, health care agency, and the nurse to
   A. get the proper diet
   B. perform a spiritual consult
   C. communicate with family
   D. avoid making assumptions

9. Seeking understanding of one's culturally based health care practices is essential to nursing because each culture has its own traditional values and beliefs about health and illness that
   A. has things that need to be avoided
   B. affect the body image and overweight habits
   C. may affect patients' adherence to treatments
   D. use various health methods that might be harmful

10. What is the nurse's best response when a Muslim patient has a basin of water on his bedside stand that he does not want emptied?
    A. Tell him that the water is a health hazard.
    B. Empty it because it could spill and get the bed wet.
    C. Talk with him about why he should not have it there.
    D. Support and accommodate his preference.

References

Anderson, L. M., Fullilove, M., Scrimshaw, S., Fielding, J., Normand, J., Zaza, S., et al. (1999). A framework for evidence-based reviews of interventions for supportive social environments. In N. E. Adler, M. Marmot, B. S. McEwen, & J. Steward (Eds.), *Socioeconomic status and health in industrial nations: Social, psychological and biological pathways.* New York: New York Academy of Sciences.

Anderson, E. T., & McFarlane, J. (2011). *Community as partner. Theory and practice in Nursing* (6th ed.). Philadelphia: Lippincott Williams & Wilkins.

Andrews, M. M., & Boyle, J. S. (2003). *Transcultural concepts in nursing care* (4th ed.). Philadelphia: Lippincott Williams & Wilkins.

Barker, P. (2002). The Tidal Model: The healing potential of metaphor within the patient's narrative. *Journal of Psychosocial Nursing, 40*(7), 42–50.

Barrett, B., Marchand, L., Scheder J., Plane, M. B., et al. (2003). Themes of holism, empowerment, access and legitimacy define complementary, alternative and integrative medicine in relation to conventional biomedicine. *Journal of Alternative and Complementary Medicine, 9*(6), 937–948.

Basara, H. G., & Yuan, M. (2008). Community self assessment using self organizing maps and geographic information systems. *International Journal of Health Geography, 7*(1), 67.

Berman, B. M. (2006) Cochrane Complementary Medicine Field. About The Cochrane Collaboration (Fields), Issue 1. Art. No.: CE000052.

Berry, A. (1999). Mexican American women's expressions of the meaning of culturally congruent prenatal care. *Journal of Transcultural Nursing, 10*(3), 229–236.

Bonomi, A. E., Anderson, M. L. Cannon, E. A., Slesnick, N., & Rodriguez, M. A. (2009). Intimate partner violence in Latina and non-Latina women. *American Journal of Preventive Medicine, 36*(1), 43–48.

Borg, J., Andree, B., Soderstrom, B., & Farde, L. (2003). The serotonin system and spiritual experience. *American Journal of Psychiatry, 11*, 965–969.

Borysenko, J. (2005). *Healing and spirituality: The sacred quest for transformation of body and soul.* Carlsbad, CA: Hay House Audio.

Boyd, K. (2000). Disease, illness, sickness, health, healing and wholeness: Exploring some elusive concepts. *Med Humanit, 26,* 9–17.

Bradwell, M. (2009). Survivors of childhood cancer. *Pediatric Nursing, 21*(4), 21–24.

Bulecheck, G. B., Butcher, H. K., & McCloskey Dochterman, J. (2008). *Nursing interventions classification (NIC)* (5th ed.) St Louis: Mosby.

Burkhardt, M. A. (2009). Commentary on "Existential and spiritual needs in mental health care: An ethical issue. *Journal of Holistic Nursing, 27,* 43–44.

Capistrano, D., Samper, C., Lee, M., & Raudsepp-Hearne, C. (2005). *Ecosystems and human well being: Multi-scale assessments.* Maryland, MD: Island Press.

Caspi, O., Sechrest, L., Pitluk, H. C., Marshall, C. L., Bell, I. R., & Nichter, M. (2003). On the definition of complementary, alternative, and integrative medicine: Societal mega-stereotypes vs. the patients' perspectives. *Alternative Therapies in Health and Medicine, 9*(6), 58–62.

Cernea, M. M., & McDowell, C. (2000). *Risks and reconstruction: Experiences of resettles and refugees.* Washington, DC: The World Bank.

Crittenden, C. P., Boris, N. W., Rice, J. C., Taylor, C. A., & Olds, D. L. (2009). The role of mental health factors, behavioral factors, and past experiences in the prediction of rapid repeat pregnancy in adolescence. *Journal of Adolescent Health, 44*(1), 25–32.

Davies, P. (2005). Biomedical models and healthcare systems: Tangible pathology has great validity. *British Medical Journal, 330,* 419–420.

Eisenberg, D. M., Davis, R. B., Ettner, S. L., Appel, S., Wilkey, S., Van Rompay, M., et al. (1998). Trends in alternative medicine use in the United States, 1990–1997: Results of a follow-up national survey. *Journal of American Medical Association, 280,* 1569–1575.

Enang, J., Wojnar, D.., & Harper, F. (2002). Childbearing among diverse populations. How one hospital is providing multicultural care. *Lifelines, 6*(2), 153–158.

Gordon, M. (2006). *Manual of nursing diagnosis* (11th ed.). Boston, MA: Barnes & Noble.

Green, L. W., & Kreuter, M. W. (1999). *Health promotion planning: An educational and ecological approach* (3rd ed.). Mountain View: Mayfield Publishing.

Higgins, B. (2000). Puerto Rican cultural beliefs: Influence on infant feeding practices in western New York. *Journal of Transcultural Nursing, 11*(1), 19–30.

Hobfoll, S. E. (2001). Social and psychological resources and adaptation. *Review of General Psychology, 6,* 307–324.

Hofstede, G. (1997). *Cultures and organizations: Software of the mind.* New York: McGraw Hill.

Holt, C. L., Lewellyn, L. A., & Rathweg, M. J. (2005). Exploring religion-health mediators among African American parishioners. *Journal of Health Psychology, 10*(4), 511–527.

Hudson, R., & Rumbold, B. (2003). Spiritual care. In M. O'Connor & S. Aranda (Eds.), *Palliative care nursing* (2nd ed.). Melbourne: Ausmed Publications.

Interdisciplinary Plan. (2007). *Interdisciplinary plan for assessment/reassessment and care planning.* Retrieved August 26, 2007, from https://hmcweb.washington.edu/ADMIN/APOP/Administration/5.20.htm

Jambunathan, J. (2003). People of Hindu heritage. In L. Purnell & B. Paulanka (Eds.), *Transcultural care: A culturally competent approach* (2nd ed., chapter on CD). Philadelphia: F. A. Davis.

Kaplan, G. (2006). Book review: *Social determinants of health* (2nd ed.). In M. Marmot & R. Wilkinson (Eds.). Oxford. *International Journal of Epidemiology, 35*(4), 1111–1112.

Kerwin, R. (2009). Connecting patient needs with treatment management. *Acta Psychiatrica Scandinavica, 438,* 33–39.

Kretzmann, J. P., & McKnight, J. L. (1993). *Building communities from the inside out: A path toward finding and mobilizing a community's assets.* Evanston, IL: Institute for Policy Research.

Leape, L. L., Berwick, D. M., & Bates, D. W. (2002). What practices will most improve safety? Evidence-based medicine meets patient safety. *Journal of American Medical Association, 288,* 501–507.

Leininger, M. M., & McFarland, M. (2005). *Culture care diversity and universality: A worldwide nursing theory* (2nd ed.). Boston: Jones & Bartlett.

Lipstein, E. A., Perrin, J. M., & Kuhlthau, K. A. (2009). School absenteeism, health status, and health care utilization among children with asthma: Associations with parental chronic disease. *Pediatrics, 123*(1), e60–e66.

Liu, C. J., Hsiung, P. C., Chang, K. J., Liu, Y. F., Wang, K. C., Hsiao, F. H., et al. (2008). A study on the efficacy of body-mind-spirit group therapy for patients with breast cancer. *Journal of Clinical Nursing, 17*(19), 2539–2549.

Lumberg, P. (2000). Culture care of Thai immigrants in Uppsala: A study of the effects of transcultural nursing in Sweden. *Journal of Transcultural Nursing, 11*(4), 274–280.

Marmot, M. G., & Wilkinson R. G. (2006). *Social determinants of health* (2nd ed.). Oxford: Oxford University Press.

McCaffrey, R. (2008). Music listening: Its effects in creating a healing environment. *Journal of Psychosocial Nursing and Mental Health Services, 46*(10), 39–44.

McKnight, J. L., & Kretzmann, J. P. (1977). Mapping community capacity. In M. Minkler (Ed.), *Community organizing and community building for health.* New Brunswick, NJ: Rutgers University Press.

Melnyk, B., & Fineout-Overholt, E. (2004). *Evidence-based practice in nursing and healthcare. A guide to best practice.* New York: Lippincott Williams & Wilkins.

Merzel, C., & D'Afflitti, J. (2003). Reconsidering community-based health promotion: Promise, performance, and potential. *American Journal of Public Health, 93*(4), 557–574.

Moorhead, S., Johnson, M., Mass, M. L., & Swanson, E. (2008). *Nursing outcomes classification (NOC)* (4th ed.). Philadelphia: Mosby.

Morad, M. (2008). Focus on holistic care for children and adolescents with diabetes. *International Journal of Adolescent Med Health, 20*(4), 387–388.

North American Nursing Diagnosis Association. (2009). *Nursing diagnoses, 2009–2011 Edition: Definitions and classifications (NANDA NURSING DIAGNOSIS).* West Sussex, UK: John Wiley & Sons.

Nightingale, F. (1860/1992). *Notes on nursing: What nursing is, what nursing is not.* New York: Lippincott Williams & Wilkins.

Palmer, D., & Ward, K. (2007). 'Lost': Listening to the voices and mental health needs of forced migrants in London. *Medicine, Conflict, and Survival, 23*(3), 198–212.

Pease, N. (1991). Poland and the Holy Sea, 1918–1939. *Slavic Review, 50*(3), 521–530.

Pinn, A. H. (2002). *Fortress introduction to Black Church history.* Minneapolis: Augsburg Fortress.

Purnell, L. D., & Paulanka, B. J. (2005). *Guide to culturally competent health care.* Philadelphia: F. A. Davis.

Riordan, J., & Auerbach, K. (2005). *Breastfeeding and human lactation.* Boston: Jones & Bartlett.

Robinson, G. (2000). *Essential Judaism: A complete guide to beliefs, customs, and rituals.* New York: Pocket Books.

Romeo, J. H. (2000). Comprehensive versus holistic care. *Journal of Holistic Nursing, 18*(4), 352–361.

Romito, P., Turan, J. M., Neilands, T., Lucchetta, C., Pomicino, L., & Scrimin, F. (2009). Violence and women's psychological distress after birth: An exploratory study in Italy. *Health Care for Women International, 30*(1–2), 160–180.

Roy, C., & Andrews, H. (1999). *The Roy Adaptation Model* (2nd ed.). Stamford, CT: Appleton & Lange.

Rumbold, B. (2003). Caring for the spirit: Lessons from working with the dying. *Australian Medical Journal, 179*(6 Suppl), S11–S13.

Seid, M. (2008). Barriers to care and primary care for vulnerable children with asthma. *Pediatrics, 122*(5), 994–1002.

Sellers, S. C., Poduska, M. D., Propp, L. H., & White, S. I. (1999). The health care meanings, values and practices of Anglo American males in the rural Midwest. *Journal of Transcultural Nursing, 10*(4), 320–330.

Smith, J. A. (1981). The idea of health. A philosophic inquiry. *Advances in Nursing Science, 3*, 43–50.

Swanson, K. M. (1993). Nursing as informed caring for the well-being of others. *Image, 25*(4), 352–357.

Swanson, K. M., & Wojnar, D. M. (2004). Optimal healing environments in nursing. *Journal of Alternative and Complementary Medicine, 10*(1), 43–48.

Thomas-MacLean, R. (2004). Understanding breast cancer stories via Frank's narrative types. *Social Science and Medicine, 58*(9), 1647–1657.

Vance, D. E., Struzick, T. C., & Raper, J. (2008). Biopsychosocial benefits of spirituality in adults aging with HIV: Implications for nursing practice and research. *Journal of Holistic Nursing, 26*(2), 119–125.

Wade, D. T. (2004). Education and debate: Do biomedical models of illness make for good healthcare systems? *British Medical Journal, 329*, 1398–1401.

Wade, D. T. (2009). Goal setting in rehabilitation: An overview of what, why and how. *Clinical Rehabilitation, 23*, 291–295.

Watson, J. (1999). *Postmodern nursing and beyond.* New York: Churchill Livingstone.

Wilkinson, S. R. (2005). Biomedical models and healthcare systems: Developmental perspective may elucidate argument. *British Medical Journal, 330*, 419–419.

The Jensen suite offers these additional resources to enhance learning and facilitate understanding of this chapter:

- thePoint online resource, http//thepoint.lww.com/Jensen1E
- Student CD-ROM included with the book
- *Laboratory Manual for Nursing Health Assessment: A Best Practice Approach*
- *Pocket Guide for Nursing Health Assessment: A Best Practice Approach*

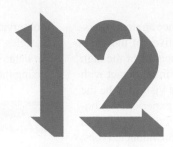

12

Assessment of Human Violence

Learning Objectives

1 Identify types of human violence.

2 Recognize the scope of the human violence problem.

3 Identify physical, mental, psychosocial, and environmental health effects of human violence.

4 Collect subjective and objective data on violence.

5 Analyze subjective and objective findings from assessment of patients victimized by human violence to plan effective interventions.

6 Document assessment findings related to human violence and safety concerns.

7 Identify the basics of a safety plan.

8 Identify key differences among various forms of human violence and how these differences affect assessment and intervention.

*S*ue Brown is a 24-year-old, middle-class Caucasian woman being interviewed by a psychiatric nurse practitioner at a day-treatment substance-abuse program. Sue, who tells the nurse that she prefers to be called by her first name, is dependent on opiates to treat chronic back pain from a car accident. When Sue was a child, her father traveled for work frequently; her mother stayed at home. Sue was an athlete in high school and attended 1 year of college before dropping out. She has seen health care professionals throughout her life for routine examinations, injuries, sexually transmitted infections (STIs), and dental care. Sue lives with her parents and brother and works part time as a grocery checker.

Across the various forms of human violence are commonalities in signs and symptoms (red flags), effects, appropriate assessment techniques, interview strategies, documentation, and resources for nurses and patients. As you study the content and features of this chapter, consider Sue's case and its relationship to what you are learning. Begin thinking about the following points:

- Based on Sue's history, what red flags might prompt health care providers to perform a complete safety assessment?
- How do Sue's symptoms and behaviors cluster together?
- What is the role of the nurse in assessing safety?

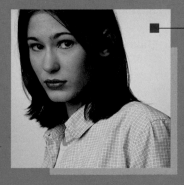

Men, women, and children perpetrate violence against others, the effects of which ripple through the lives of individuals, families, communities, and societies. Because of the high prevalence of human violence, nurses come into contact with victims and perpetrators daily. A health care visit may be the first time that a patient discusses a violent experience. Conversely, many people, including nurses, are unaware of or in conscious or unconscious denial about the prevalence, types, and effects of human violence. Appropriate, compassionate, and sincere awareness and assessment are crucial to stopping violence and to assisting those victimized by it toward safety and recovery, thereby preventing ongoing consequences.

This chapter provides basic information on human violence related to assessment, safety, prevention, and recovery. It describes many different types of violence, their prevalence rates, and physical and psychological effects. The chapter explores important screening and assessment techniques, such as observation for signs and symptoms of violence and interview strategies, both of which are used to collect subjective and objective data. The last part of the chapter provides information on nursing interventions related to safety, recovery, and healing.

Types of Human Violence

Almost half of all people (44%) report experiencing human violence (Plichta & Falik, 2001). The following paragraphs discuss various forms of violence in detail; Table 12-1 summarizes and defines them.

Family Violence

A crime is considered **family violence** if the victim is biologically related to the offender or is or was related to him or her

Table 12.1	Types of Human Violence
Type	**Definition**
Family violence	All types of violent crime committed by an offender who is related to the victim either biologically or legally through marriage or adoption
Child maltreatment	Covers a wide range of abusive and neglectful behaviors toward children; figures are based primarily on reported cases of child abuse and neglect investigated by CPS
Polyvictimization	Experiences of more than one type of violence
Sibling violence	Not frequently taken seriously in the United States; it often comes under the rubric of sibling rivalry or roughhousing
Intimate partner violence (IPV)	Between spouses or nonmarital partners, threatened or actual physical or sexual violence or psychological/emotional abuse, coercive tactics, or both when there has been prior physical and/or sexual violence
IPV in pregnancy	Violence between spouses or nonmarital partners during the prenatal, intrapartum, or postpartum period
Punking and bullying	Aggression in which (1) the behavior is intended to harm, (2) the behavior occurs repeatedly over time, and (3) there is an imbalance of power, with a more powerful person or group attacking a less powerful one
School violence	Crimes at school including theft, simple assault, and serious violent crime
Sexual violence	Forced sex in dating and marital relationships, gang rape, sexual harassment, inappropriate touching or molestation, sex with a patient, and forced prostitution and/or exposure to sexually explicit behavior
Violence against older adults	Intentional or unintentional acts such as physical, sexual, psychological, and financial abuse and neglect against older adults
Violence against adults with developmental disabilities	Intentional or unintentional acts such as physical, sexual, psychological, and financial abuse and neglect against adults with developmental disabilities
Hate crimes	Crime in which a victim is selected based on a characteristic such as race, ethnicity, sexual orientation, age, and the like and for which the perpetrator provides evidence that hate prompted him or her to commit the crime
Human trafficking	The recruitment, transportation, transfer, harboring, or receipt of people by threats, force, coercion, or deception
War and violence victimization	Witnessing the killing of human beings including friends and fellow service people, intentionally killing and injuring other humans, and being intentionally injured or potentially killed by another human

through marriage, adoption, or legal guardianship. The term family violence often is used interchangeably with *domestic violence, intimate partner violence (IPV)*, and *male violence against women*. It is best to ask the patient for clarification and specifics if he or she uses any of these terms.

Types of family violence include child maltreatment, sibling violence, IPV, and elder abuse. The nurse may encounter all these types during patient assessments. From 1998 to 2002, approximately 9.2 million people sustained injuries from family violence (U.S. Department of Justice, Bureau of Justice Statistics, 2005a,b,c). Only 41% of victims received medical attention for their injuries. Some patients never disclose that they have been hurt or seek assistance from police, health care professionals, counselors, or lawyers.

Child Maltreatment

Child maltreatment covers a wide range of violent behaviors against children. Prevalence rates, however, have focused primarily on abuse of children by parents and are based mainly on reported cases of abuse investigated by Child Protective Services (CPS). Violent practices rarely occur as isolated incidents; often, children have more than one victimization experience (Finkelhor, et al., 2005, 2006). Polyvictimization is highest in children who report rape and dating violence (Finkelhor, et al., 2007). About 25% of children experience four or more different kinds of victimization (Finkelhor, et al., 2007). Trauma symptoms such as anxiety, depression, anger, and aggression are "red flags" of polyvictimization.

Sibling Violence

Historically, violence between and among siblings has not been taken seriously. It often has been considered within the realm of normal sibling relationships and represented by such terms as *sibling rivalry, roughhousing*, and *sibling competition* (Phillips, et al., 2009). Nevertheless, sibling violence is among the most common type that children experience (Finkelhor, et al., 2006).

Intimate Partner Violence

IPV has been defined as behaviors between spouses or nonmarital partners involving threatened or actual physical or sexual violence, psychological/emotional abuse, and/or coercive tactics when there has been prior physical or sexual violence (Saltzman, et al., 1999). Nonmarital partners include those in adolescent and adult dating relationships and in long-term, committed, intimate, heterosexual or homosexual relationships.

No group is immune to IPV—it occurs in all cultures and populations and across all ages, ethnicities/races, education levels, and socioeconomic statuses (Moracco, et al., 2007). Perpetrators of IPV are most often male. Of women who report being raped, physically assaulted, or stalked since age 18 years, approximately two thirds are victimized by a current or former husband, cohabiting male partner, boyfriend, or date (RAINN, 2008). Abusive and controlling behaviors and practices by perpetrators of IPV are described in Table 12-2.

Table 12.2 Methods of Power and Control in IPV	
IPV Behaviors and Practices by Perpetrators	**Descriptions**
Intimidation	Making victims afraid by using looks, actions, gestures; smashing things; destroying property; abusing pets; displaying weapons
Coercion and threats	Making and/or carrying out threats to do something to hurt victims; threatening to leave, commit suicide, report victims to welfare; making victims drop charges or do illegal things (ie, take drugs)
Emotional abuse	Putting down victims or making them feel bad about themselves; calling victims names; making victims think they are crazy; playing mind games; humiliating or making victims feel guilty
Isolation	Controlling what victims do or read, whom they see or talk to, or where they go; limiting their involvement outside the home; using jealousy to justify actions
Minimizing, denying, and blaming	Making light of abuse and not taking concerns of victims seriously; saying abuse did not happen; shifting responsibility for abusive behavior; saying victims caused it
Using children	Making victims feel guilty about children; having children relay messages; using visitation to harass victims; threatening to take children away; using children as spies
Privilege	Treating victims like servants; making all big decisions; acting like the "master of the castle"; being the one who defines men's and women's roles
Economic abuse	Preventing victims from getting or keeping a job; making victims ask for money or giving them an allowance; taking money; not letting victims know about or have access to family income

Source: Adapted from the Domestic Abuse Intervention Project, Duluth MN 55306 (DAIP, 2008).

IPV Among Immigrants and Refugees. Female U.S. immigrants and refugees, particularly those who do not speak English or have U.S. legal documents, are especially vulnerable to IPV (Family Violence Prevention Fund, n.d.). Rates of IPV may be higher in female immigrants than in female U.S. citizens for several reasons. Some cultures more visibly accept violence against women than does the U.S. culture. In addition, U.S. immigrants who attempt to escape IPV face significant barriers. For example, they may not have access to bilingual safety shelters, financial assistance, food, or other support services. It is also unlikely that they have assistance from certified interpreters during court proceedings, when reporting complaints to police, or even when acquiring information about their rights and the legal system. Lastly, perpetrators of IPV may use their partners' immigration status as a tool of control and force women to remain in the relationship, making it difficult for victims to escape the violence.

⚠ SAFETY ALERT 12.1

Murder, homicide, or femicide (murder of a female) is IPV when perpetrated by a current or ex-intimate partner. Most femicides are preceded by a history of IPV before the woman's death (Campbell, 1992; Campbell, et al., 2000). Similar to statistics that show males as perpetrators of most IPV, males also commit 91% of femicides (U.S. Department of Justice, Bureau of Justice Statistics, 2000).

IPV in Pregnancy. IPV in pregnancy is a serious and widespread problem. Of women abused during pregnancy, more than half also experienced IPV before pregnancy. Between 4% and 32% of women from nonindustrialized countries are abused during pregnancy, a much greater percentage than in the United States and industrialized countries (Campbell, et al., 2004). For nurses working with U.S. citizens, immigrants, and refugees, the high rates of abuse demonstrate that an assessment for violence in the prenatal, intrapartum, and postpartum periods is essential. See also Chapter 27.

Elder Abuse

Maltreatment of older adults can be in the form of abuse, neglect, financial exploitation, or abandonment. Abuse includes intentional actions by a caregiver or other person who stands in a trust relationship to a vulnerable elder that cause harm or create a serious risk to him or her (Fulmer, 2008). Examples include kicking, punching, slapping, or burning. Factors that put older adults at risk include dependency, cognitive decline, strained mental or physical health of caregivers, and financial issues. A commonly used tool to screen for maltreatment in older adults is the Elder Assessment Inventory (Fulmer, 2008).

Violence Against Adults with Disabilities

Violence against vulnerable adults, such as those with physical and mental disabilities, includes harmful acts of commission (abuse) or omission (neglect). Physical, sexual, psychological, and financial abuse and neglect may be intentional or unintentional (NCEA, 1998; Sengstock, et al., 2004). Adults with disabilities are more likely to experience severe and long-term abuse, be victims of multiple violent episodes, and be abused by many perpetrators. In addition, sexual assault is exceptionally high in women with developmental disabilities—they are four to eleven times more likely to be sexually assaulted than women without disabilities (Schaller & Lagergren Fieberg, 1998; Stromsness, 1993).

⚠ SAFETY ALERT 12.2

In 2003, 565,747 reports of elder and vulnerable adult abuse were filed with Adult Protective Services, a 20% increase from the previous 2000 survey (NCEA, 2004). Findings showed that older women are far more likely than older men to suffer from abuse or neglect. Two of every three victims of elder abuse were women; more than two in five victims were 80 years or older.

"Youth" and School Violence

Many young people witness, perpetrate, and are victimized by violence in and around their schools and neighborhoods. This includes daily nonfatal crimes, such as theft and simple assault, as well as serious violent crime (National Center for Education Statistics, 2007). Violent practices include being slapped, hit, or punched at school; beaten or mugged in neighborhoods; and being shot, shot at, or stabbed. Rates of recent witnessing of violence range widely from 5% to 72% (Singer, et al., 1995).

Punking and Bullying

Punking and bullying are common among middle- and high-school males, usually resulting in shame, humiliation, and anger. Similar to bullying and sometimes used interchangeably, *punking* is a practice of verbal and physical violence, humiliation, and shaming, usually done in public or with an audience (Phillips, 2007). Bullying in the form of verbal violence is common among middle- and high-school girls (Beaty & Alexeyev, 2008; O'Moore & Hillery, 1989).

Sexual Violence

Sexual violence includes forced sex in dating and marital relationships, gang rape, sexual harassment, inappropriate touching, molestation, sex with a patient, forced prostitution, and forced exposure to sexually explicit behavior. Child sexual abuse and adult rape are two relatively common types. Marital rape is not a crime in all countries; in fact, it has been illegal in the United States only for 20 years. Strongly patriarchal societies, cultures, and religions are strictly organized around the supremacy of the father as head of the family or clan, with wives and children dependent (legally and otherwise) on him. Many women in some countries do not have the right or a voice to say "no" to sex in such patriarchal relationships.

Hate Crimes

The U.S. Department of Justice, Bureau of Justice Statistics (2005a,b,c), defines a **hate crime** as one in which a perpetrator chooses a victim because of a characteristic such as race, ethnicity, gender, sexuality, or religion and provides evidence that hate motivated the crime. Psychological and emotional violence are the most common forms of hate crimes, which include practices such as racism, homophobia, and discrimination. Nurses and other health professionals often meet people who have experienced hate crimes; however, such violence may never be disclosed by patients or asked about by professionals.

⚠ SAFETY ALERT 12.3

Race "motivates" approximately 50% of all hate crimes, while ethnicity is the reason in 25% of cases.

Human Trafficking

The United Nations (2008) defines **human trafficking** as the recruitment, transportation, transfer, harboring, or receipt of people through threats, force, coercion, or deception. Misleading or false advertising (eg, offers of good wages and "legitimate" work abroad) may entice women attempting to escape unemployment in their home countries. After responding to such advertising, these women may be abducted, bonded, or sold into indentured servitude. Reasons people are trafficked include sexual exploitation, forced marriage, and cheap labor for domestic or commercial purposes. Those who own and manage commercial "sex trade" businesses (ie, forced prostitution, stripping, pornography, live-sex shows) are the major perpetrators of human trafficking (U.S. DHHS, 2006). *Labor exploitation* includes domestic servitude, sweatshop factories, and migrant agricultural work.

War-Related and Military Violence

A relatively common form of violence is related to military combat. War-related fighting can involve witnessing killing, including of friends and fellow service people; intentionally killing and injuring other humans; and being intentionally injured or potentially killed. People who have experienced war violence include veterans of all ages, families of veterans who are traumatized vicariously by living with them, and people of all ages who witness war and its violence. This group also includes those who escaped war, spent time in a "camp" before coming to the United States, or both.

The escape or camp experience may have been traumatic and included actual or witnessed violence. Rates of IPV perpetration are increased in veterans with posttraumatic stress disorder (PTSD) related to combat exposure (Gerlock, 2004; Prigerson, et al., 2002).

Importance of Violence/Safety Assessment

Many of those who receive care for violence-related trauma do not disclose the cause of their injuries. When a patient presents with any injury, screening and assessing for violence as the cause are parts of a complete nursing assessment.

Clinical Significance 12-2

Like Sue, nearly all child and adult victims of violence have contact with health care professionals throughout their lives. Although violence frequently is undetected, patients often seek care for many different related reasons. Victims of violence often have increased health problems, health care visits, and financial burdens (Dube, et al., 2005; Felitti, 2002; Felitti, et al., 1998).

Routine assessment for violence and safety is important during every encounter with patients because of the high prevalence of human violence and its short- and long-term effects on health, relationships, and well-being. Community-based entry points for such screening and assessment include home visits and immunization, school, and Woman/Infant/Children (WIC) clinics. Other entry points are nursing homes, primary care offices and clinics, mental health services, substance-abuse services, and medical emergency services. Any health care or community setting with a nursing presence is an appropriate point for such assessment, however.

Violence assessment can range from brief screening questions for all patients to a thorough history and head-to-toe physical examination for those who disclose violence or present with violent injuries. See Box 12-1.

Subjective Data Collection

The pace and extent of safety assessment should be geared to the patient's needs. The nurse provides the safe opportunity and environment for disclosure as well as the skills and attitude needed to support the patient through what can be a difficult process. Sometimes a nurse is the first person to "bear witness" to the truth of the patient's story of violence victimization. Validating the importance and difficulty of disclosure is essential. Conversely, some patients deny the seriousness of violence or consider it "normal." They may feel this way because many people in their family have also experienced violence or because most women or men or a specific group in their culture commonly experience it.

BOX 12.1 ABUSE ASSESSMENT SCREEN

1. **Within the last year**, have you been hit, slapped, kicked, or otherwise physically hurt by someone? YES NO
   If YES, by whom? _____
   Total number of times ____

2. **Since you've been pregnant**, have you been hit, slapped, kicked, or otherwise physically hurt by someone? YES NO
   If YES, by whom? _____
   Total number of times ____

3. **Within the last year**, has anyone forced you to have sexual activities? YES NO
   If YES, by whom? _____
   Total number of times ____

Score each of the following incidents according to the following scale. If any of the descriptions for the higher number apply, use the higher number.

1 = Threats of abuse including use of a weapon
2 = Slapping, pushing; no injuries and/or lasting pain
3 = Punching, kicking, bruises, cuts, and/or continuing pain
4 = Beating up, severe contusions, burns, broken bones
5 = Head injury, internal injury, permanent injury
6 = Use of weapon; wound from weapon

Developed by the Nursing Research Consortium on Violence and Abuse. Readers are encouraged to reproduce and use this assessment tool.

When a nurse asks about violence, some patients decide that the time, setting, or health care professional is not a comfortable fit for them to disclose their story. In such cases, violence-screening questions provide an opportunity for the nurse to let patients know about the high prevalence of human violence so that they do not feel singled out or alone. During these encounters, the nurse also can teach about the health effects of violence, review safety and resources, and connect and establish rapport.

Most women, regardless of victimization status, are comfortable being screened for IPV; in fact, approximately 80% of female victims disclose IPV when asked (Plichta, 2007). They are unlikely to disclose abuse, however, without being asked (Plichta, 2007).

Some health professionals are inhibited from asking about, screening for, or assessing for violence (Fahey, 2007; Plichta, 2007). There are many reasons why health professionals, including nurses, do not ask about violent experiences. Examples include a lack of education about such assessment, deficient knowledge about resources to provide to patients who disclose violence, and discomfort with this discussion. Health professionals need to ask questions and be prepared for patients who disclose childhood or adult experiences of violence. This statement has several implications. Being prepared to hear that "Yes, my partner raped me" or "My father molested me" requires that nurses hear what patients are saying and not deny, discount, ignore, disconnect, judge, or be overly solicitous.

Largely as a result of work of the Nursing Network on Violence Against Women International and the Nursing Research Consortium, screening and assessment of violence against women have become more common practices (Harley, 2006; Hindin, 2006; Plichta, 2007). Nevertheless, bearing witness to disclosures of violence can be particularly difficult for nurses and other health care professionals who have experienced and/or witnessed human violence themselves. In such cases, nurses need to recognize unresolved aspects of their lives and move forward on recognition, healing, and resolution so that they can do their professional work and uphold standards of care.

Similar to other sensitive or difficult topics (eg, constipation, flatulence, disfigurement), asking about violence breeches social taboos and may seem to some nurses as "too personal" or "none of my business." While this may be true in nonprofessional relationships, nurses must remember that they are in professional, therapeutic relationships with patients. Their assessments need to include questions about intimate body functions, intimate relationships, and negative life experiences—including human violence—that cause physical and mental health consequences.

Areas for Health Promotion/ *Healthy People*

In 1995, U.S. costs related to injury and violence were estimated at more than $224 billion/year. These costs include direct medical care and rehabilitation as well as productivity losses to the nation's workforce. A focus area for *Healthy People* is injury and violence prevention, which greatly affects the health of individuals and communities (USDHHS, 2000). *Healthy People* identifies risk factors for violence as poverty, discrimination, lack of education, and lack of employment opportunities. See Table 12-3 for specific goals and patient education topics related to human violence.

Interviewing Patients About Human Violence

Asking patients about personal experiences of violence is a key aspect of assessment. Of utmost importance is how such assessment is conducted. First and foremost in every nurse's mind should be the patient's physical and emotional safety. A universal rule is that patient interviews are done in private—including without significant others or anyone who may be or could represent the perpetrator (eg, friend, mother-in-law). Nurses should not assume who may or may not be a perpetrator or have power over the patient and prevent her or him from talking freely and safely.

Asking about violent experiences works best when it is a normal and natural part of nursing assessment, similar to asking about sleep or activity problems or dietary or sexual concerns. It is important to try to establish a connection with the patient first. In general, nurses should listen to patients more than they talk, using an 80% to 20% guideline (80% patient, 20% nurse). The possible exception is during patient education.

Table 12.3 *Healthy People* Goals Related to Human Violence	
Goals	**Patient Education Topics**
Reduce firearm-related deaths.	Assess for depression, suicide, domestic violence, and community violence.
Reduce the proportion of persons living in homes with loaded and unlocked firearms.	Teach firearm safety.
Reduce nonfatal firearm-related injuries.	Assess individual and family firearm use. Teach firearm safety.
Reduce maltreatment and maltreatment fatalities of children.	Assess for human violence and neglect. Assess individual and family weapons use.
Reduce the rate of physical assault by current or former intimate partners.	Assess for physical assault, controlling behaviors, and isolation. Teach about safety and healthy relationships.
Reduce the annual rate of rape or attempted rape.	Assess for sexual assault or rape. Teach about healthy boundaries, relationships, communication skills, and safety planning.
Reduce sexual assault other than rape.	Assess for red flags that may indicate child sexual abuse. Teach children about safe touch, healthy relationships, and safety.
Reduce physical assaults.	Assess for safety and red flags of physical abuse. Teach about healthy communication and safety plans.
Reduce physical fighting among adolescents.	Assess for signs of bullying and punking. Teach about healthy communication skills, bullying, and safety.
Reduce weapon carrying by adolescents on school property.	Assess safety. Teach about gun violence and safety. Report cases of weapons in schools.

Source: U.S. Department of Health & Human Services (DHHS). (2000). *Healthy People 2010: 15 Injury and violence prevention.* Retrieved May 17, 2010, from http://www.healthypeople.gov/Document/HTML/Volume2/15Injury.htm

Nurses can also encourage rapport, connection, and patient participation by using a narrative approach in their interactions. In the narrative approach, a patient of any age tells her or his story, whether it involves abdominal pain, sore throat, headache, or experiences of bullying or other violence. As the patient provides the account, the nurse collects data and listens for aspects of the story that need clarification, elaboration, or both. Taking time to listen in a nonjudgmental, nondirective way and to ensure confidentiality helps create a safe, supportive atmosphere (Plichta, 2007).

Basics for nurses to review when assessing for violence include the following:

• Perform assessment and screening only when the patient is alone in a safe, private environment.
• Establish rapport and connection by showing interest in the patient and by listening.
• Be very patient as the patient talks.
• Move from general, open-ended questions to specific questions.
• Demonstrate compassion, not judgment.
• Use interpreters if there is any question about understanding on the patient's or nurse's part. Clarify and reflect back to the patient what he or she says and what you understand.
• Maintain comfortable and neutral body language.
• Remain close to and at eye level with the patient, but not in her or his "personal" space.

• Use a relaxed and calm tone of voice at medium volume, with pacing appropriate to the patient's developmental level and level needed for clear understanding.
• Do not ask a patient if he or she wants to press charges against the perpetrator. This decision is up to a prosecutor and is not part of a violence assessment.
• Often, the best way to ask a patient about violence is simple and direct.

These above points are generalizations. Nurses should always ask a patient if she or he is comfortable with the approach taken and the physicality of the interview space. Open-ended questions, such as "What would you like to know?" "How can I help you understand?" or "What would you like me to know?" are especially helpful if a patient appears uncomfortable.

Nurses can prepare patients for sensitive or difficult questions about violence by prefacing comments with statements such as, "Now is the point in the interview where I ask patients about relationships in their family. Who lives in your home with you? How do you feel in that relationship?" It is also common to ask, "Because violence is so common for so many people, I routinely ask all patients about violent experiences—in the past and currently? I wonder if you have experienced or are experiencing violence?" See Box 12-2 for other ways to phrase questions about violence.

Another way to begin assessment about controlling behaviors or emotional and psychological abuse is to assess daily routines. Examples of questions include, "Tell me what you

Assessing Violence Victimization Sample Questions (See Also Box 12-1)

• "Because violence is so common in many people's lives, I ask all patients about it routinely."
• "Are you in a relationship with a person who physically or sexually hurts or threatens you?"
• "Did someone cause those injuries? Who?"
• "Injuries like yours could have been caused by someone hurting you. Did someone hurt you?"
• "Sometimes when people feel the way you do, it's because they have been hurt or abused at home. Is that happening to you?"

• "Many of the adults (children, teens) I work with have experienced violence in their past, and some are experiencing it in their current lives. I wonder if you have any experiences of violence."

Assessing Violence Perpetration

• "Some people think that under certain circumstances it's OK to hit a person you love. What are your thoughts about that?"
• "If you were faced with overwhelming stress (eg, losing your job, spouse/partner leaving you), what behaviors might you display?"
• "Have you ever physically hurt someone in your family?" (Ask for specifics and think safety first.)
• "Have you ever physically hurt someone?"

Therapeutic Dialogue: Collecting Subjective Data

Until her current interview sessions, Sue never told anyone about her experiences of sibling violence or IPV by former boyfriends. Growing up, she assumed that violence was normal, despite being asked about it in other health care encounters. The following conversation occurs near the end of the fifth session.

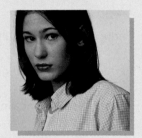

Less Effective

Nurse: So I was just looking at your history. You've had a lot of injuries.

Sue: Yeah, I'm accident prone.

Nurse: It really looks like you have ruptured eardrum, broken arm, bruises, and black eyes. How did all of those happen?

Sue: Well, I'm just clumsy I guess.

Nurse: Do you think it's because of your opiate use? Does that make you dizzy?

Sue: Yeah, my head is a little foggy, and sometimes I just bang into things.

Nurse: That's no good.

Sue: I'm tough, though. It takes a lot to get me down. I'm pretty independent and can get through almost everything.

Nurse: You're lucky that way then.

Sue: Yeah, I don't really need a lot of people around me. My brother and I are close, and I've had a lot of boyfriends.

Nurse: That's good in some ways, but it looks like you have had frequent STIs. That's not so good.

Sue: At least I'm getting them treated.

More Effective

Nurse: You've had other injuries—ruptured eardrum, broken arm, bruises, and black eyes.

Sue: Yeah, I'm accident prone.

Nurse: I know that I asked you before, but I routinely ask all patients about past and current violent experiences. I wonder if you have experienced or are experiencing violence?

Sue: (hesitates) Well, my brother and I are close, but sometimes we get a little rough.

Nurse: What would you like me to know?

Sue: I'm beginning to think that my relationships aren't healthy. My brother and I are very physical, and he has thrown me against walls and punched me.

Nurse: (Silent, nonverbal active listening)

Sue: It's hard to talk about (pause). I just assumed that getting hit was normal. My brother has ADHD. He's been kicked out of school for being so aggressive.

Nurse: (Silent, nonverbal active listening)

Sue: I just got used to being hit and learned to fight back. Maybe that's why I get involved in relationships where I get hurt.

Critical Thinking Challenge

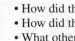

• How did the more effective nurse build a relationship so that Sue felt comfortable disclosing?
• How did the more effective nurse weave the violence assessment into the conversation?
• What other questions should the nurse ask before ending the interview?

did today from the time you got up until the time you got here" or "Describe your last 3 days." Sometimes asking patients about their daily lives and routines reveals detailed information about victimizing behaviors and isolation, even when abuse is by a sibling, peer, or parent. In addition, this approach gives the patient a chance to share her or his story, connect with the nurse, and display strengths. It also provides the nurse opportunities for teaching, providing resources, affirming strengths, and giving support.

Include questions about adverse childhood and family events and about current living context; these questions may elicit information about adverse experiences. Psychosocial histories often include violence assessment, but they can be very sensitive areas for patients to discuss (see Chapter 10). Moving into this area of assessment toward the end of the patient history allows time to build rapport and to ask less sensitive questions first.

Nurses should be patient and not pressure patients to disclose, leave their partners, or otherwise make decisions that patients are not ready for, all of which can cause disconnection in the nurse–patient relationship. This outcome may lead a patient not to return for follow-up care and, thereby, possibly be less safe and with fewer resources. The nurse's responsibility is to screen for and identify controlling and abusive behaviors, provide information about safety and resources, and report when mandatory reporting is required (see later discussion). Normally, patient information is confidential, which remains true when patients report violence, but with some exceptions.

Objective Data Collection

While performing physical assessments, a nurse may find signs of violence in patients. The nurse assesses nonverbal behaviors, such as the patient's eyes scanning the environment or the patient jumping or startling when a door slams. A nurse may notice that a child is very clingy to the person accompanying him or her, has a flat affect, or does not establish eye contact.

The following signs are indicators of possible abuse or neglect:

• Injuries not consistent with the story of their cause
• Sexual activity in a child younger than 14 years
• Inadequate supervision
• Serious injury
• Failure to seek timely medical care
• Multiple hospital or clinic visits for injuries
• Multiple previous fractures
• Bruises in multiple stages of healing

If any of the above occurs, the nurse should perform a complete physical assessment to evaluate for other manifestations of violence.

Many additional indications, or "red flags," alert nurses to the possibility of past or current human violence (Edwards, et al., 2007; Felitti, 2002) (Fig. 12-1). Common psychological red flags are mood and behavior changes from normal for

---

Child Abuse Assessment Red Flags

✓ Mood changes, anger, isolating, sullenness
✓ Critical of self and/or others
✓ Risky behaviors
✓ Behavior changes
✓ Friend changes
✓ School troubles
✓ Short temper, difficulty getting along with others
✓ Verbal and physical violence with siblings, parents, peers
✓ Weight gain or loss
✓ Quiting teams and activities

IPV Assessment Red Flags

✓ Physical injury (facial fractures, dental, neurological, soft tissue, internal, "falls")
✓ Chronic pain (back, abdomen, chest, head)
✓ Fibromyalgia, chronic irritable bowel
✓ Hypertension, smoking
✓ Unintended pregnancy, adolescent pregnancy
✓ Abortion
✓ Anal and vaginal tearing, painful intercourse
✓ Depression

Sexual Abuse Assessment Red Flags

✓ Bruising or scratching around breasts, genitals
✓ Unexplained venereal or genital infections (children should not have STDs)
✓ Unexplained vaginal or anal bleeding
✓ Torn, stained, bloody underclothes
✓ Victim reports being sexually assaulted
✓ Victim withdrawn, personality changes, behavior changes

General Assessment Red Flags

✓ New-onset behaviors or change in behavior
✓ Withdrawal, depression
✓ Agitation, hyperarousal
✓ New displays of anger, noncompliance
✓ Sexualized behavior
✓ Bowel or bladder problems
✓ Sleep problems
✓ Unexplained and/or "curious" injuries

Elder/Vulnerable Adult Violence Assessment Red Flags

✓ Frailty, cognitive impairment
✓ Psychiatric disorder, depression, anxiety
✓ Alcohol abuse
✓ Decreased social network
✓ Shared living arrangements
✓ External stressors on family
✓ Vague excuses for missing activities, therapy
✓ Untrimmed, dirty nails
✓ Inadequate or absent assistive devices
✓ History of family violence
✓ Unexplained injuries
✓ Explanation not consistent with findings
✓ Recurrent UTIs or other infections
✓ Poor hygiene, poor oral hygiene, dirty clothes
✓ Weight loss/lack of interest in meals
✓ Recurrent or worsening pressure ulcers, dehydration

Abuse/Neglect Assessment Red Flags

✓ Bruises, welts, cuts, scratches, restraint-marks
✓ Open wounds, punctures, untreated sores, maggots
✓ Sprains, dislocations, internal injuries
✓ Victim changes in behavior
✓ Caregiver refuses to allow visitors to see the victim
✓ Victim reports being hit and/or maltreated
✓ Soiled clothing or linens
✓ Overall bad hygiene, poor oral hygiene
✓ Dehydration, malnutrition, extreme weight loss

Violence in Pregnancy Assessment Red Flags

✓ Late or inconsistent prenatal care
✓ Preterm bleeding and/or labor
✓ Abruption placentae–especially more than one time/with more than one pregnancy
✓ Low birth weight
✓ Unexplained fetal death
✓ Suicide attempts during pregnancy
✓ Postpartum depression
✓ Injuries during pregnancy
✓ Poor weight gain during pregnancy
✓ Partner unwilling to leave woman's side during prenatal visits, labor and delivery, and/or postpartum
✓ Partner speaks for woman and/or condescending to woman
✓ Partner makes negative comments about woman's appearance
✓ Woman speaks less or is very quiet especially when partner around, poor eye contact
✓ Partner oversolicitous with care providers

Figure 12.1 General assessment of violence.

the specific patient. Depression and anxiety can manifest as a flat, quiet, and sullen affect (emotional dullness), withdrawal, or irritability and impulsive anger (see Chapter 10), which can further manifest as acting-out behaviors (eg, impulsive aggression toward others, risky and dangerous behaviors). Some violence victims use substances such as alcohol, marijuana, methamphetamines, cocaine, and narcotics to feel better while simultaneously numbing feelings of anxiety, low self-worth, sadness, and fear. Nevertheless, a link between human violence and mental health problems is usually hidden, and health care providers may overlook opportunities for healing interventions frequently.

Mental health effects associated with human violence that can be assessed during patient visits include depression, PTSD, panic disorders, dissociative symptoms, relationship and marital problems, acting out violently, and sexual and substance abuse (Basile, et al., 2004; Chu & Dill, 1990; Dube et al., 2005; Steel, et al., 2004; Stein et al., 2004; Winfield, et al., 1990). Symptoms common during assessment are easily triggered anxiety and panic episodes, isolation and social withdrawal, numbing or shutting down feelings, spacing out and forgetfulness, and difficulty focusing.

Assessment findings are similar and different among violence survivors. Differences in how each person experiences and is affected by violence depend on the type and severity and the lived experiences of a person in her or his family, community, and society. Age, ethnicity, socioeconomic status, education, sexual orientation, religion, urban or rural living, culture, and relationships can be highly influential on outcomes. Thus, it is very important not to make assumptions but to use open-ended questions such as, "How are you coping?" and "What has your experience been?"

Documentation

Documentation is an important aspect of violence assessment. Close listening and keen observation skills are necessary to capture key details. It is important to reassure adults that their patient records are available only with their consent and may be useful someday if needed for legal action. Nurses should document subjective data in quotes as much as possible (eg, "pt states…").

When documenting objective data, it is important to be detailed, be descriptive, and note findings without bias. Box 12-3 outlines basic information about forensic evidence and documentation.

Mandated Reporting

Nurses and other health care professionals are "mandated reporters" when child, elder, or vulnerable-adult abuse or neglect is disclosed, assessed, or suspected (Sheridan, 2004). Mandated reporters must call the protective services hotline when they suspect abuse or neglect. Provided the report is done in good faith and without malice, the nurse and other professionals mandated by the state to report are protected by the state.

Clinical Significance 12-3
Nurses need to be aware of the mandatory reporting laws in the state where they practice. They also need to be aware of their institution or agency's policies and procedures regarding disclosure of violence perpetration and/or victimization and its appropriate documentation.

In addition to documenting findings from the patient assessment on forms approved by the health professional's institution, the nurse should document the call to the protective services hotline in the patient's file, including the reason for the call, time of the call, full name of the person who took the call, and response of the worker. State laws on reporting domestic violence in adults or IPV vary from no mandatory reporting to requiring providers to report to a state agency (eg, state health department, police).

Lifespan Considerations

Pregnant Women
Pregnant women constitute a population group at particularly high risk for IPV. Some of these patients also may have experienced adverse childhood experiences (Felitti, 2002;

BOX 12.3 FORENSIC EVIDENCE AND DOCUMENTATION

Written Documentation: Use Verbatim Subjective Data (ie, "pt states…")

Photographs: "Rule of Thirds" for each injury

- Take photos before the patient is cleaned or clothes are changed.
- Take an overall image of the patient plus three photographs of each injury.
  - First: Several feet away, injury clear, in context of patient
  - Second: Distance cut by 1/3, photo more focused on injury
  - Third: Distance cut by another 1/3, 2 ft from actual injury

Injury Maps: Locations, Measurements of Bruises, Incisions, Lacerations, Punctures, Hematomas

- Assess mouth and teeth.
- Do not throw away evidence even if badly soiled or ruined.
- Do not cut through clothing, undergarments, or bedding where evidence is visible.
- Store items, such as clothes, in paper bag (not plastic).
- Label evidence: patient's name, ID number, date of birth, date and time of documentation/photo.

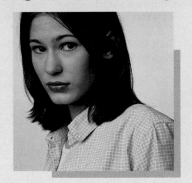

The nurse has finished a physical assessment of Sue Brown. Note the following unexpected findings.

Inspection: Appears anxious, scanning environment visually. Fearful when touched. Multiple bruises in various stages of healing, including two 5 × 7.5 purple ecchymoses on buttocks, one yellow 2.5-cm ecchymosis on forearm, and three 3 × 3 blue and yellow ecchymoses on legs. See attached photographic documentation. 2 × 3 scar present on left forearm from previous repair of fracture.

Palpation: Area over buttocks is tender, painful. Lesions on legs and arms are nontender, nonraised. Full range of motion and strength on left arm.

Parker, et al., 1994). In addition to assessing for human violence, nurses need to assess for physical and mental health effects and specific effects related to pregnancy. Potential effects against pregnant women include increased chance of low–birth-weight infants, decreased maternal weight gain, and late prenatal care. Pregnant women who have or are experiencing IPV are also at increased risk for alcohol, tobacco, and street drug use throughout pregnancy when compared to women who have not experienced IPV in pregnancy (Hindin, 2006).

Infants, Children, and Adolescents

Of all age groups, infants are the most likely to be abused. Too often, health care providers do not suspect or report suspected abuse. Long-term psychological and emotional sequelae from abuse are cumulative. When a nurse reports suspected abuse and, thereby, prevents future violent episodes, he or she has made a significant difference in the health of a child for the rest of his or her life.

In addition to the common red flags (see Fig. 12-1), red flags for infants, children, and adolescents include the following:

- The story keeps changing or is inconsistent between partners or over time.
- No history of trauma is given, but signs of trauma are present.
- Parent changes physicians, health care facilities, or both frequently.
- Infants have bruises before they are walking.
- Injuries resemble objects, such as cigarette burns, burns in the shape of an iron, loop marks, etc.
- Grab, slap, or human-bite marks are evident.
- There is evidence of immersion burns, which are usually well demarcated and bilateral (eg, both hands or feet) or occur on the buttocks and feet.

Any fracture in an infant who is not walking should raise the index of suspicion for abuse, unless there is a verifiable cause (eg, motor vehicle collision, documented bone disorder predisposing to bone fragility) (Kemp, et al., 2009). Bleeding, bruising, or redness in the genital area, anus, or both is cause to suspect sexual abuse. In the general survey and vital measures, symptoms and signs include poor hygiene, infant dressed in clothing inappropriate for the weather, evidence of tissue wasting, signs of poor nutrition, failure to gain weight, or an untreated illness (see Chapter 6). Symptoms of shaken baby syndrome include subdural hematoma, retinal hemorrhages, rib fractures, and bilateral bruising in the rib cage area. See also Chapter 28.

Older Adults

Many older adults are vulnerable to abuse by family members. Continued abuse may be compounded because of nondetection by professionals, in part because elderly patients often do not report violence. Many victims are isolated; some have shame, guilt, embarrassment, and self-blame. In addition, some elders experience fear of reprisal, retribution from caregivers, or losing their home or independence. Others are pressured by relatives not to report.

🌐 Cultural Considerations

Cultural differences between patients and caregivers may lead to an erroneous suspicion of abuse. For example, a nurse might observe a patient and caregiver having an aggressive conversation that includes shouting. Some cultures consider such behavior acceptable, whereas others consider it verbal abuse. Views on financial or personal autonomy of patients, their right to make decisions independently, or the amount of respect they deserve may also differ among cultural or socioeconomic groups (Fulmer, 2008). More information is needed about the influence of culture on disclosure of abuse and fear of retribution (Montalvo-Liendo, 2009). The social stigma attached to human violence may vary among cultures. For example, a patient from a neighborhood with a high rate of violent crime may feel less stigmatized because it is a common occurrence.

Table 12.4 Common Nursing Diagnoses Associated with Human Violence

Diagnosis and Related Factors	Point of Differentiation	Assessment Characteristics	Nursing Interventions
Risk for violence directed at others	Potential to act in ways that can harm others physically, emotionally, sexually, or in all these ways	Risk behaviors	Monitor environment and situations that could become violent, and intervene early to de-escalate the situation. Know and follow policies and procedures concerning violence.
Impaired parenting related to abuse	Failure of a parent or guardian to establish, enforce, or sustain an environment that nurtures and protects children	Abandonment, abuse, neglect of attachment or health care, harsh punishments, hostility between spouses or other relatives	Examine the characteristics of parenting style and behaviors. Institute abuse/neglect projection measures.* Assess maternal depression. Appraise the parent's resources and support systems.
Dysfunctional family processes related to child neglect	Change in family relationships, functioning, or both	Changes in assigned tasks, availability for emotional support, communication patterns, or all of these	Establish rapport with families. Acknowledge the emotions experienced during stressful times. Encourage members to list their strengths.
Rape-trauma syndrome	Long-term psychological, emotional, and physical consequences following one or more episodes of sexual abuse, sexual assault, or both	Use of drugs or alcohol, anger, aggression, anxiety, problems in relationships, confusion, embarrassment, fear, guilt, humiliation, loss of self-esteem	Stay with the patient. Explain the rationale for interventions. Warn before touching the patient in advance. Observe for signs of physical injury. Document according to forensic standards.
Risk for posttrauma syndrome	Potential to experience long-term maladaptive consequences following one or more traumatic, overwhelming events	Risk factors include poor self-esteem, chronic duration, minimal or ineffective social support	Assess history; question about sleep, bad dreams, and reexperiencing the event.

Evidence-Based Critical Thinking

Nursing Diagnoses, Outcomes, and Interventions

After the nurse assesses for violence, he or she can establish one or more nursing diagnoses. A nursing diagnosis labels the findings and suggests potential interventions. Table 12-4 compares nursing diagnoses, abnormal findings, and interventions commonly related to human violence (NANDA-I, 2009).

The nurse establishes and develops realistic and measurable outcomes with the patient. These outcomes must be based on respect for autonomy and recognition of patient safety. Some outcomes related to human violence include the following:

- The patient maintains social safety.
- The patient demonstrates personal safety behaviors.
- The patient avoids injury.
- Abuse ceases.

- The patient exerts abusive-behavior self-control (Moorhead, et al., 2007).

Nurses need to ask about adverse childhood experiences, especially violence (Felitti, 2002). This type of assessment and subsequent interventions can assist the patient to find treatment for "root" causes of physical and mental health problems and prevent years of treating symptoms while underlying causes go undetected. RNs and APRNs are on the frontlines to assess for adverse health consequences and to intervene in ways that decrease suffering and promote healing. Figure 12-1 shows many specific physical and mental health red flags for which nurses can intervene. Table 12-5 describes even more basic ways to begin providing support and advocacy for all victims.

Patient needs following violent experiences can be categorized as immediate, transitional, and long term (Box 12-4). Safety planning is key to intervention. If a patient is in an unsafe or potentially unsafe situation, nurses must suggest and encourage a safety plan. The first step is to ask the patient what he or she has done in the past to be safe and then build on this.

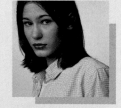

Nursing assessment at each point includes assessing verbal and nonverbal behaviors. These include what the patient says (responses to questions and spontaneous comments or silence), how he or she appears (physical signs and symptoms), and his or her behaviors. The following note describes important information from Sue Brown's interview and physical assessment.

Subjective: "I'm beginning to think that the relationships that I have aren't very healthy. My brother and I are very physical, and he has thrown me against walls and punched me. It's hard to talk about. (pause) I just assumed that getting hit was normal. My brother has ADHD. He's been kicked out of school for being so aggressive and impulsive. I just got used to being hit and learned to fight back. I think that might be part of why I'm getting involved in relationships where I get hurt."

Objective: Appears anxious, scanning environment visually. Withdraws when touched. Multiple bruises in various stages of healing, including two 5 × 7.5 purple ecchymoses on buttocks, one yellow 2.5-cm ecchymosis on forearm, and three 3 × 3 blue and yellow ecchymoses on legs. See attached photographic documentation. Area over buttocks is tender, painful. Lesions on legs and arms are nontender.

Analysis: Risk for posttrauma syndrome related to sibling abuse

Plan: Needs abuse protection support to prevent infliction of physical and emotional harm. Call in report to get assistance in analyzing how to proceed with this difficult case.

L. Linn, RN

Critical Thinking Challenge

- What challenges are involved with this case?
- What strengths does Sue bring? How will the nurse assess for them?
- What dilemmas does the nurse face when working with Sue?

Sue has been seeing the APRN for five sessions. She has disclosed some reportable information. The following conversation illustrates how the nurse might organize data and make recommendations about Sue's situation.

Situation: "I've been seeing Sue Brown for five sessions now. Over the course of several interviews, she has disclosed abuse by her older brother throughout her childhood and adolescence, and it is continuing at this time."

Background: "He repeatedly has beaten her, kicked her, thrown her down and against walls, punched her, broke her arm, and made verbally humiliating and derogatory comments to her."

Assessment: "Sue's brother was diagnosed with ADHD and conduct disorder. She reports that her brother's signs and symptoms include acting out aggressively; severe physical, verbal, and psychological violence against her; and repeated expulsions from schools because of violence toward peers, teachers, and property. He has also been treated for self-injury (Phillips, unpublished data, 2009). Sue reports that her parents, neighbors, and friends witnessed her brother's violence, and the police did not assess for this violence when contacted (Phillips, et al., 2009). In addition to disclosing this information to me, Sue has physical signs of injury including bruising in multiple stages of healing."

Recommendations: "I am calling to report this situation to you. I want to get help with protecting Sue."

Critical Thinking Challenge

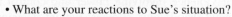

- What are your reactions to Sue's situation?
- How might your reactions influence your assessment of her situation?
- Describe the issues related to the victimization. What type of violence is described?

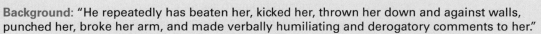

Table 12.5 Part of the Solution

Advocacy Practices	Descriptions
Respect confidentiality.	Discussions must be private with no other family members present; this is essential to building trust and ensuring the patient's safety.
Believe and validate his or her experiences.	Listen to the patient and believe; acknowledge her or his feelings and let the patient know that she or he is not alone; many other people have similar experiences.
Acknowledge the injustice.	Violence perpetrated against the patient is not her or his fault; no one deserves to be abused.
Respect her or his autonomy.	Respect the patient's right to make decisions when ready; she or he is the expert at her or his life.
Help the patient plan for future safety.	What has the patient tried in the past to stay safe? Is it working? Does she or he have a place to go if escape is necessary?
Promote access to community services.	Know resources in your community; is there a hotline and shelter for victims of violence?

Source: Adapted from "The Medical Power & Control Wheel," developed by the Domestic Violence Project in Kenosha, WI 53143. Based on the "Power & Control and Equality Wheel" developed by the Domestic Abuse Intervention Project, Duluth, MN 55306.

Basic components of safety plans usually include the following:

- Charged cell phone with preprogrammed emergency phone numbers (or these numbers readily available but not necessarily identifiable to the perpetrator) for police, support people, and safe housing
- Copies of important or difficult-to-replace documents such as birth certificate or insurance papers stored in a safe place (possibly with support person)

- Change of clothes for self (and children) packed and hidden
- Extra set of house and car keys
- Transportation plan
- Extra money hidden in a safe location
- Escape plan from potential house or apartment exits
- Escape locations/safe places

Each patient will have individualized safety needs. It is very important for the nurse to explain to the patient that research shows that danger of violence is particularly high when victims leave or have left a relationship with a perpetrator (Campbell, et al., 2006). This fact makes patient teaching and safety planning even more essential aspects of nursing interventions.

Sometimes nurses and other health professionals contribute to victims failing to ask for and receive assistance or perpetuate attitudes that reinforce violent practices. Six methods of "medical power and control" should be avoided: (1) violating confidentiality, (2) trivializing and minimizing violence and abuse, (3) blaming the victim, (4) not respecting autonomy, (5) ignoring the victim's safety, and (6) normalizing victimization. Each of these can cause victims to feel an increased sense of entrapment and could potentially escalate the danger of a current violent situation.

Nurses should be especially careful not to pressure patients to make decisions about the violence, perpetrator, relationship, or particular interventions. Contrary to experiences of violence involving power and control in which victims have few, if any, choices, patient decisions about their care, interventions, and future are just that: patient decisions. Nurses should be explicit and patient about this—because making decisions and having choices may be new experiences for those who experienced violence in the past or present.

BOX 12.4 PATIENT SAFETY NEEDS

Immediate

- Safety and support
- Medical stabilization
- Psychological and emotional stabilization
- Collect forensic evidence

Transitional

- Safety and support
- Connect to resources: financial, parenting, health, housing, immigration, legal
- Teaching: safe and healthy coping skills, social skills, positive relationships
- Promote sense of mastery

Long Term

- Safety and support
- Healing: trauma psychotherapy
- Support systems/resource building
- Physical rehabilitation/physical therapy
- Long-term health needs

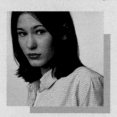

Assessment data help nurses to formulate nursing care plans. Outcomes are specific to the patient, are realistic, are measurable, and have a time frame for completion. The nurse performs interventions based on evidence and practice guidelines. He or she also charts progress toward patient outcomes. See a sample care plan related to Sue Brown below.

Nursing Diagnosis	Patient Outcomes	Nursing Interventions	Rationale	Evaluation
Risk for posttrauma syndrome related to sibling abuse	The patient discloses abuse. The patient states that she is not to blame for the events.	Provide support person to stay with the patient; explain protocols; determine any cuts, bruises, bleeding, lacerations, or other signs of injury. Assess for past experiences and symptoms.	Evidence must be collected as soon as possible, although it may be difficult for the patient. Dissociation, avoidant behavior, hypervigilance, and reexperiencing are ongoing symptoms.	Photos are taken of bruises in multiple stages of injury. No bleeding, lacerations, or other signs of acute injury are evident. Will interview about mood and behavior changes. ∎

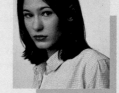

Using the previous steps of diagnostic reasoning, organizing, and prioritizing, consider all case study findings throughout this chapter. When answering the questions, begin drawing conclusions and see how the pieces of assessment must work together to create an environment for personalized, appropriate, and accurate care.

• Based on Sue's history, what red flags should prompt health care providers to conduct a complete safety assessment?
• How do Sue's symptoms and behaviors cluster together?
• What is the role of the nurse in assessing safety?

Key Points

• Types of human violence include family violence (which encompasses child maltreatment, sibling violence, IPV, and elder abuse), violence against vulnerable populations, youth and school violence, sexual violence, hate crimes, human trafficking, and war/combat violence.
• IPV in pregnancy is a serious and widespread problem.
• Elders are vulnerable to continued abuse, partly as a result of nondetection by professionals.
• The patient's physical and emotional safety is a key aspect of assessment.
• The nurse moves from general to specific questions about violence.
• Open-ended versus closed questions about violence are best.
• Phrasing to normalize questions about the experience of violence is "Because violence is common in so many people's lives, I ask all patients about it routinely."

• One safety assessment question is "Tell me what you did today from the time you got up until the time you got here."
• Red flags of violence victimization include mood and behavior changes.
• Nurses are mandated reporters when child, elder, or vulnerable adult abuse or neglect is disclosed, assessed, or suspected.
• Documentation is an important aspect of nursing assessment and intervention.
• Human violence has psychological, mental, physical, emotional, and social consequences.
• Nursing diagnoses associated with violence experiences include risk for other-directed violence, impaired parenting, dysfunctional family processes, and rape-trauma syndrome.

Review Questions

1. Child maltreatment, sibling violence, bullying, elder abuse, hate crimes, and war/combat violence are types of
   A. punking
   B. sexual violence
   C. intimate partner violence
   D. human violence

2. Intimate partner violence in pregnancy is
   A. a serious and widespread problem
   B. associated with unwanted pregnancy
   C. a serious but uncommon situation
   D. usually the fault of the mother

3. Older adult abuse
   A. usually occurs when the caregiver is tired
   B. is usually not detected by health care providers
   C. usually occurs once and then stops
   D. is usually detected by social work or legal services

4. When questioning a patient about violence, it is best to
   A. ask to get the police involved to collect evidence
   B. have the perpetrator present to assess behaviors
   C. move from general to specific questions
   D. ask the patient what he or she did to provoke the violence

5. When child, elder, or vulnerable adult abuse or neglect is disclosed, nurses
   A. must contact a physician
   B. may get family involved
   C. might consider referral
   D. are mandated reporters

6. Red flags of signs and symptoms of violence include which of the following?
   A. Stating that everything is just fine
   B. Displaying mood and behavior changes
   C. Expressing sadness over loss
   D. Wanting to have family involved

7. A patient is seen in the emergency department for a fracture that is inconsistent with the description of the cause of it. Which question would be best in this situation?
   A. "Because violence is so common for so many people, I routinely ask all patients about experiences of violence—in the past or currently. I wonder if you have experienced or are experiencing violence?"
   B. "Sometimes people fall because someone hurt them. Your injury looks like someone might have done this to you on purpose. Do you have a violent boyfriend?"
   C. "Your injury doesn't look like what you described. It looks to me like someone might have intentionally done this to you. With whom do you live?"
   D. "It's common for women to get shoved, kicked, or beaten. You seem like you might be in this situation. Who would you do this to?"

8. The patient's physical and emotional safety is
   A. a key aspect of assessment
   B. discussed in the interventions section
   C. considered during outcomes
   D. written up in interventions

9. It is best to ask questions about violence that are
   A. reflective
   B. focused
   C. closed ended
   D. open ended

10. Interventions that might be appropriate for victims of violence include which of the following?
    A. Maximizing protective influences
    B. Involving police and pressing charges
    C. Getting placement in a shelter and telling them to leave home
    D. Calling parents of victims to provide support

References

Basile, K. C., Arias, I., Desai, S., & Thompson, M. P. (2004). The differential association of intimate partner physical, sexual, psychological, and stalking violence and posttraumatic stress symptoms in a national representative sample of women. *Journal of Trauma and Stress, 17*(5), 413–421.

Beaty, L. A., & Alexeyev, E. B. (2008). The problem of school bullies: What the research tells us. *Adolescence, 48*(169), 1–11.

Campbell, J. C. (1992). "If I can't have you, no one can": Power and control in homicide of female partners. In J. Radford & D. E. H. Russell (Eds.), *Femicide: The politics of woman killing* (pp. 99–113). New York: Twayne.

Campbell, J. C., Garcia-Moreno, C., & Sharps, P. (2004). Abuse during pregnancy in industrialized and developing countries. *Violence Against Women, 10*(7), 770–789.

Campbell, J. C., Koziol-McLain, J., Glass, N. E., et al., (2006). *Validation of the danger assessment: Results from the 12 city femicide study.* National Institute of Justice Briefs.

Campbell, J. C., Sharps, P. W., & Glass, N. E. (2000). Risk assessment for intimate partner homicide. In G. F. Pinard & L. Pigani (Eds.), *Clinical assessments of dangerousness: Empirical contributions* (pp. 136–157). New York: Cambridge University Press.

Chu, J. A., & Dill, D. L. (1990). Dissociative symptoms in relation to childhood physical and sexual abuse. *American Journal of Psychiatry, 147*(7), 887–892.

Domestic Abuse Intervention Project (DAIP). (2008). *The power and control wheel.* Retrieved July 20, 2008, from http://www.theduluthmodel.org/pdf/PhyVio.pdf

Dube, S. R., Anda, R. F., Whitfield, C. L., et al. (2005). Long-term consequences of childhood sexual abuse by gender of victim. *American Journal of Preventitive Medicine, 28*(5), 430–438.

Edwards, V. J., Anda, R. F., Gu, D., Dube, S. R., & Felitti, V. J. (2007). Adverse childhood experiences and smoking persistence in adults with smoking-related symptoms and illness. *Permanente Journal, 11*, 5–7.

Fahey, J. (2007). Unpublished research. Seattle University College of Nursing: Seattle, WA.

Family Violence Prevention Fund (endabuse.org). (n.d.). *The facts on immigrant women and domestic violence.* Retrieved July 20, 2008, from http://www.endabuse.org/userfiles/file/Children_and_Families/Immigrant.pdf

Felitti, V. J. (2002). The relation between adverse childhood experiences and adult health: Turning gold into lead. *Permanente Journal, 6*(1), 44–51.

Felitti, V. J., Anda, R. F., Nordenberg, D., et al. (1998). Relationship of childhood abuse and household dysfunction to many of the leading causes of death in adults: The Adverse Childhood Experiences (ACE) Study. *American Journal of Preventive Medicine, 14*(4), 245–258,

Finkelhor, D., Ormrod, R. K., & Turner, H. A. (2005). The victimization of children and youth: A comprehensive, national survey. *Child Maltreatment, 10*(1), 5–25.

Finkelhor, D., Ormrod, R. K., & Turner, H. A. (2007). Poly-victimization: A neglected component in child victimization. *Child Abuse & Neglect, 31*, 7–26.

Finkelhor, D., Turner, H., & Ormrod, R. (2006). Kid's stuff: The nature and impact of peer and sibling violence on younger and older children. *Child Abuse & Neglect, 30*, 1401–1421.

Fulmer, T. (2008) Screening for mistreatment of older adults. *American Journal of Nursing*, 108 (12), 52–60 ISSN: 0002-936X PMID: 19033914.

Gerlock, A. A. (2004). Domestic violence and post-traumatic stress disorder severity for participants of a domestic violence rehabilitation program. *Military Medicine, 169*(6), 470–474.

Harley, A. M. (2006). Domestic violence screening: Implications for surgical nurses. *Plastic Surgery Nursing, 26*(1), 24–28.

Hindin, P. K. (2006). Intimate partner violence screening practices of certified nurse-midwives. *Journal of Midwifery and Women's Health, 51*(3), 216–221.

Kemp, A. M., Dunstan, F., Harrison, S., Morris, S., Mann, M., Rolfe, K. I., et al. (2009). Patterns of skeletal fractures in child abuse: systematic review. *Child: Care, Health & Development, 35*(1), 141–142 & 1365–2214.

Montalvo-Liendo, N. (2009). Cross-cultural factors in disclosure of intimate partner violence: an integrated review. *Journal of Advanced Nursing, 65*(1), 20–34.

Moorhead, S., Johnson, M., & Mass, M. (2007). *Nursing Outcomes Classification (NOC)* (4th ed.). Philadelphia: Mosby.

Moracco, K. E., Runyan, C. W., Bowling, J. M., & Earp, J. L. (2007). Women's experiences with violence: A national study. *Women's Health Issues, 17*(1), 3–12.

National Center for Education Statistics. (2007). *Indicators of school crime & safety: 2007.* Retrieved May 12, 2008, from http://www.ojp.usdoj.gov/bjs/pub/pdf/iscs07.pdf

National Center on Elder Abuse (NCEA). (1998). *The national elder abuse incidence study: Final report.* Madison, WI: Publisher.

National Center on Elder Abuse (NCEA). (2004). Abuse of adults aged 60+: 2004 Survey of adult protective services. Retrieved May 12, 2008, from http://www.ncea.aoa.gov/NCEAroot/Main_Site/pdf/2-14-06%2060FACT%20SHEET.pdf

North American Nursing Diagnosis Association. (2009). *Nursing diagnoses, 2009–2011 Edition: Definitions and classifications (NANDA NURSING DIAGNOSIS).* West Sussex UK: John Wiley & Sons.

O'Moore, A.M. & Hillery, B. (1989). Bullying in Dublin schools. *Irish Journal of Psychology, 10*, 426–441.

Parker, B., McFarlane, J., & Soeken, K. (1994). Abuse during pregnancy: Effects on maternal complications and birthweight in adult and teenage women. *Obstetrics and Gynecology, 84*(3), 323–328.

Phillips, D. A. (2007). Punking and bullying: Strategies in middle school, high school, and beyond. *Journal of Interpersonal Violence, 22*(2), 158–178.

Phillips, D. A., Phillips, K. H., Grupp, K., & Trigg, L.J. (2009). Sibling violence silenced: Rivalry, competition, wrestling, playin', roughhousing, benign. *Advances in Nursing Science, 32*(2), E1–E16.

Plichta, S. B. (2007). Interactions between victims of intimate partner violence against women and the health care system: Policy and practice implications. *Trauma Violence Abuse, 8*(2), 226–239.

Plichta, S. B., & Falik, M. F. (2001). Prevalence of violence and its implications for women's health. *Women's Health Issues, 11*(3), 244–258.

Prigerson, H. G., Maciejewski, P. K., & Rosenheck, R. A. (2002). Population attributable fractions of psychiatric disorders and behavioral outcomes associated with combat exposure among US men. *American Journal of Public Health, 92*(1), 59–63.

Rape, Abuse & Incest National Network (RAINN). (2008). Who are the victims? Retrieved July 20, 2008, from http://www.rainn.com/get-information/statistics/sexual-assault-victims

Saltzman, L. E., Fanslow, J. L., McMahon, P. M., & Shelby, G. A. (1999). Intimate partner violence surveillance: Uniform definitions and recommended data elements, version 1.0. Atlanta, GA: National Center for Injury Prevention and Control, Centers for Disease Prevention.

Schaller, J., & Lagergren Frieberg, J. (1998). Issues of abuse for women with disabilities and implications for rehabilitation counseling. *Journal of Applied Rehabilitation Counseling, 29*(2), 9–17.

Sengstock, M.C., Ulrick, Y. C., & Barrett, S. A. (2004). Abuse and neglect of elderly in family settings. In J. Humphreys & J. C. Campbell (Eds.), *Family violence and nursing practice* (pp. 97–149). Philadelphia: Lippincott Williams & Wilkins.

Sheridan, D. J. (2004). Legal and forensic nursing responses to family violence. In J. Humphreys & J. C. Campbell (Eds.), *Family violence and nursing practice* (pp. 385–406). Philadelphia: Lippincott Williams & Wilkins.

Singer, M. I., Anglin, T. M., Song, L. Y., & Lunghofer, L. (1995). Adolescents' exposure to violence and associated symptoms of psychological trauma. *JAMA, 273*(6), 477–482.

Steel, J., Sanna, L., Hammond, B., Whipple, J., & Cross, H. (2004). Psychological sequelae of childhood sexual abuse: abuse-related characteristics, coping strategies, and attributional style. *Child Abuse Neglect, 28*(7), 785–801.

Stein, M. B., Lang, A. J., Laffaye, C., Satz, L. E., Lenox, R. J., & Dresselhaus, T. R. (2004). Relationship of sexual assault history to somatic symptoms and health anxiety in women. *General Hospital Psychiatry, 26*(3), 178–183.

Stromsness, M. M. (1993). Sexually abused women with mental retardation: Hidden victims, absent resources. *Women & Therapy, 14*(3–4), 139–152.

United Nations. (2008). *What is human trafficking?* Retrieved May 12, 2008, from http://www.ungift.org/ungift/en/humantrafficking/index.html

U.S. Department of Health & Human Services (DHHS). (2000). *Healthy People 2010: 15 Injury and violence prevention.* Retrieved July 20, 2008 from http://www.healthypeople.gov/Document/HTML/Volume2/15Injury.htm

U.S. Department of Health & Human Services (DHHS). (2006). *HHS fights to stem human trafficking.* Retrieved May 12, 2008, from http://www.hhs.gov/news/factsheet/humantrafficking.html

U.S. Department of Justice, Bureau Justice of Statistics. (2000). *Intimate partner violence.* Retrieved May 20, 2008, from http://www.ojp.usdoj.gov/bjs/pub/pdf/ipv.pdf

U.S. Department of Justice, Bureau Justice of Statistics. (2005a). *Human trafficking.* Retrieved May 12, 2008, from http://www.ojp.usdoj.gov/ovc/ncvrw/2005/pg5l.html

U.S. Department of Justice, Bureau Justice of Statistics. (2005b). *Family violence statistics: Including statistics on strangers & acquaintances.* Retrieved May 5, 2008, from http://www.ojp.usdoj.gov/bjs/pub/pdf/fvs.pdf

U.S. Department of Justice, Bureau Justice of Statistics. (2005c). *Hate crime reported by victims and police.* Retrieved May 12, 2008, from http://www.ojp.usdoj.gov/bjs/pub/pdf/hcrvp.pdf

U.S. Department of Justice, Bureau Justice of Statistics. (2006). *Criminal victimization, 2006.* Retrieved July 20, 2008, from http://www.ojp.usdoj.gov/bjs/pub/pdf/cv06.pdf

Winfield, I., George, L. K., Swartz, M., & Blazer, D. G. (1990). Sexual assault and psychiatric disorders among a community sample of women. *American Journal of Psychiatry, 147*(3), 335–341.

The Jensen suite offers these additional resources to enhance learning and facilitate understanding of this chapter:

- thePoint online resource, http//thepoint.lww.com/Jensen1E
- Student CD-ROM included with the book
- *Laboratory Manual for Nursing Health Assessment: A Best-Practice Approach*
- *Pocket Guide for Nursing Health Assessment: A Best-Practice Approach*

Regional Examinations

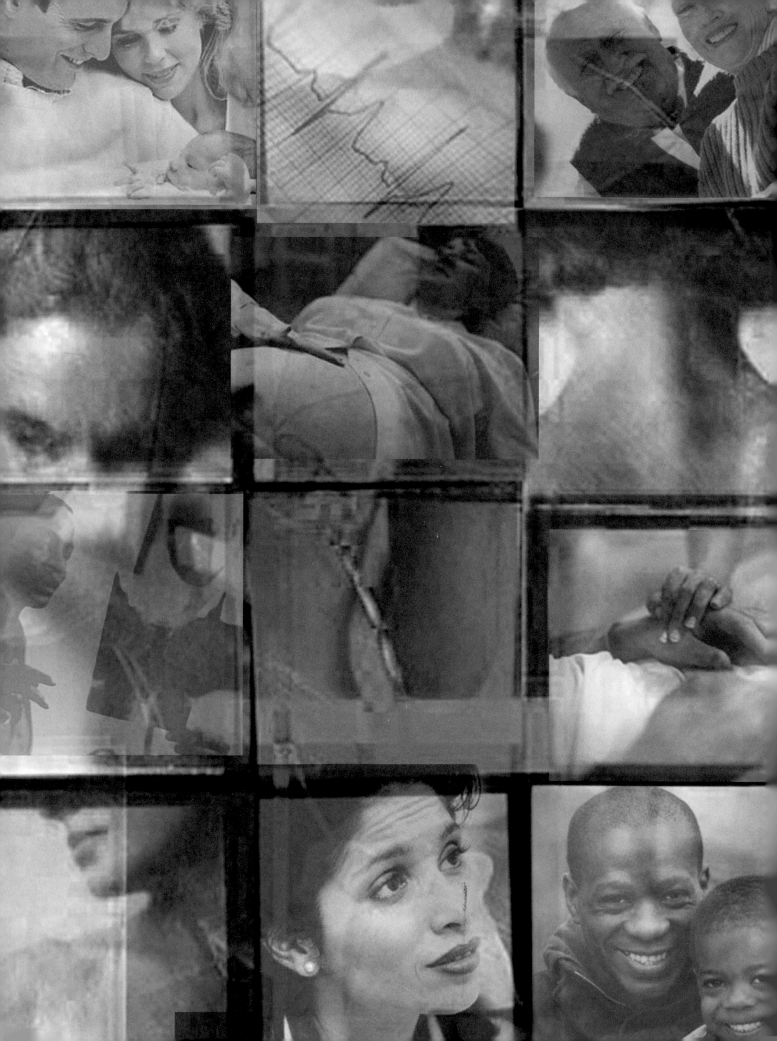

Skin, Hair, and Nails Assessment

Learning Objectives

1 Identify the structures and functions of the integumentary system.

2 Identify teaching opportunities for integumentary health promotion and risk reduction.

3 Collect subjective data relating to various skin lesions and risk factors for altered skin integrity (eg, cancer, pressure ulcer).

4 Collect objective data on the skin, including turgor, temperature, color, and moisture.

5 Differentiate normal from abnormal skin conditions, including the location, size, distribution, and configuration of any lesions.

6 Differentiate normal from abnormal findings of the nails and hair.

7 Identify variations of normal from abnormal skin lesions.

8 Use subjective and objective data from integumentary assessment to analyze findings and plan interventions.

9 Document and communicate integumentary data using appropriate medical terminology.

10 Individualize assessment of the integumentary system, considering the patient's condition, age, gender, and culture.

11 Use integumentary assessment data to identify diagnoses and initiate a plan of care.

*M*r. Stoli, a 65-year-old Russian immigrant, has been on an acute care unit since yesterday for a venous ulcer. He is scheduled to have a wound vacuum applied later today. Current medications include a thiazide diuretic for high blood pressure, platelet inhibitor for peripheral vascular disease (PVD), and insulin for type 2 diabetes mellitus. The nurse documented assessment findings last shift. Mr. Stoli's temperature was 37.4°C orally, pulse 92 beats/min, respirations 16 breaths/min, and blood pressure 142/78 mm Hg.

You will gain more information about Mr. Stoli as you progress through this chapter. As you study the content and features, consider the patient's case and its relationship to what you are learning. Begin thinking about the following points:

- How will the nurse assess and document Mr. Stoli's wound and peripheral circulation?
- What information will the nurse collect to assess risk for skin breakdown related to hospitalization?
- In what circumstances would the nurse refer Mr. Stoli to a wound care nurse? How would the nurse communicate information to the wound care nurse?
- Once the patient is discharged, what data would a nurse performing follow-up home care need to collect? How would that nurse assess if the wound was healing?

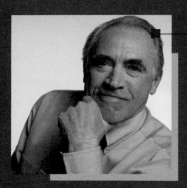

The integumentary system—skin, hair, nails, and sweat glands—provides vital information about a patient's health status and whether functioning of the thermoregulatory, endocrine, respiratory, cardiovascular, gastrointestinal, neurological, urinary, and immune systems is adequate. Integumentary findings also reflect the patient's hydration, nutrition, and emotional status and help direct the nurse about other systems or organs that may be compromised. For example, cyanosis in a patient's lips may prompt the nurse to further evaluate the respiratory and circulatory systems. Skin assessment is ongoing, and nurses integrate such assessment into the examination of other body areas.

This chapter reviews normal anatomy and physiology of the skin, hair, and nails. It presents common variations of normal integumentary findings, as well as findings that relate to systemic disorders. It outlines data collection strategies related to common skin lesions, alterations in skin integrity, risk factors for skin cancer (eg, excessive sun exposure, inadequate skin protection), current health-promotion practices, and wound assessment. It presents a systematic method for skin assessment and strategies for interweaving such assessment with examination of other systems. This chapter discusses approaches for accurately documenting integumentary subjective and objective findings and presents information relating to health promotion and disease prevention, such as skin self-assessment, dry skin care, pressure-ulcer prevention, and skin protection.

Structure and Function Overview

Skin

The skin is comprised of three layers with distinct and separate functions: the epidermis, dermis, and subcutaneous layer (Fig. 13.1).

Epidermis

As the outermost skin layer, the **epidermis** serves as the body's first line of defense against pathogens, chemical irritants, and moisture loss (Revis & Seagle, 2006). The five layers of the epidermis are (1) *stratum corneum*, (2) *stratum lucidum*, (3) *stratum granulosum*, (4) *stratum spinosum*, and (5) *stratum germinativum*. The stratum germinativum contains keratinocytes and melanocytes. *Keratinocytes* are composed chiefly of keratin, a tough protein providing resistance against friction and trauma. Keratinocytes differentiate over time and move through the more superficial strata, become anuclear, and eventually are shed from the stratum corneum. *Melanocytes* produce two types of melanin, *eumelanin* and *pheomelanin*, which contribute to integumentary variations based on their amounts and proportions in each person. Larger amounts of eumelanin produce darker skin and hair, whereas larger amounts of pheomelanin are responsible for lighter skin and hair (Ortonne, 2002). The absolute number of melanocytes, however, is consistent in all people (Barsh, 2003).

The epidermis contains specialized cells responsible for perception of pain, light touch, vibration, and temperature, as well as detection of foreign antigens (Kamel, 1998). In other words, the epidermis is the first part of the body to initiate the immune response. Thickness of the epidermis remains constant throughout the lifespan and across genders.

Dermis

The second layer, the **dermis**, supports the epidermis. The dermis contains blood vessels, nerves, sebaceous glands, lymphatic vessels, hair follicles, and sweat glands, which support the nutritional needs and protective function of the epidermis (Revis & Seagle, 2006). The two layers of the dermis are papillary and reticular. The *papillary dermis*, composed primarily of loose connective tissue and elastin, contains capillaries, smaller blood vessels, and nerve endings. It connects

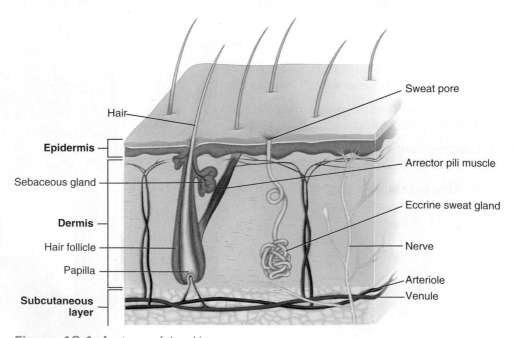

Figure 13.1 Anatomy of the skin.

directly to the epidermis, facilitating exchange of oxygen, nutrients, and waste products with it. The deeper *reticular dermis*, composed of collagen and elastin, provides the resilience, distensibility, elasticity, and turgor of the skin.

Variations in skin thickness result from changes in dermal thickness, with the thinnest example being the eyelids and the thickest being the palms and soles. Dermal thickness varies across the lifespan and with gender. Skin is thinnest at birth but gradually increases until the fourth or fifth decade of life, when thickness begins to decline. Men have consistently thicker skin than women as a result of their greater number of androgens (Zouboulis, et al., 2007).

Subcutaneous Layer

The **subcutaneous layer** provides insulation, storage of caloric reserves, and cushioning against external forces. Composed mainly of fat and loose connective tissue, it also contributes to the skin's mobility.

Clinical Significance 13-1

The integumentary system is a window to other body systems. Changes in skin, hair, or nails may be the first clue to other health problems. See Table 13-9 at the end of this chapter.

Hair

Hair is an appendage of skin. It protects various body areas from debris and invasion, provides insulation, enables the conduit of sensory stimulation to the nervous system, and contributes to gender identification.

Vellus hair is fine, short, hypopigmented, and located all over the body (Alaiti, 2007). **Terminal hair** is darker and coarser than vellus hair. It varies in length and is generally found on the scalp, brows, and eyelids. In postpubertal people, terminal hair also is found on the axillae, perineum, and legs; on postpubertal males, it appears on the chest and abdomen.

Hair, composed of keratin, is produced by hair follicles located deep in the dermis. Hair follicles are present in all body areas except the palms and soles. Follicular activity is cyclical, with approximately 30% of follicles in a resting state at any given time (Brannon, 2006).

Shape of the hair shaft determines the curliness of hair, with oval shape producing curlier hair than rounded shape. The amount and proportion of eumelanin and pheomelanin produced by melanocytes in the hair bulb influence hair color. Arrector pili muscles attached to each hair follicle contract in response to environmental and nervous stimuli, causing erection of the hair and follicle. Sebaceous glands supporting each follicle secrete sebum, maintaining hair moisture and condition. Sebum production declines with increasing age (Fig. 13.2).

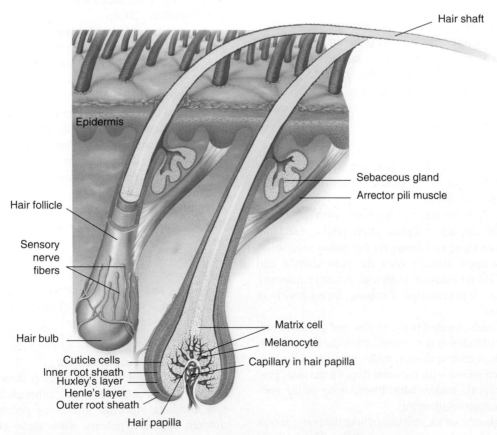

Figure 13.2 Anatomy of hair.

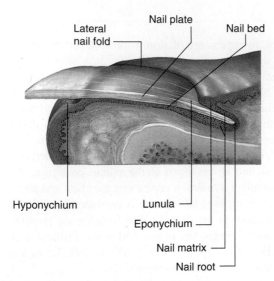

Lateral nail fold
Nail plate
Nail bed
Hyponychium
Lunula
Eponychium
Nail matrix
Nail root

Figure 13.3 Anatomy of nails.

Nails

Another epidermal appendage, the *nails* arise from a nail matrix in the epidermal layer, near the distal portions of each finger and toe. The nail plate, comprised of hardened keratin, grows at varying rates, with fingernails growing faster than toenails. The highly vascular nail bed is visible as a pink color through the transparent nail plate. Lateral folds of skin on each side and a proximal fold of skin at the base border each nail plate (Fig. 13.3).

Some systemic diseases and infectious processes affect the growth rate and thickness of nails (Fawcett, et al., 2005). Changes caused by disease or infection generally are not visible for some time after the incident. See Table 13-24 at the end of this chapter for more information.

Sweat Glands

Sweat (cutaneous) glands function to maintain normal body temperature by controlling the evaporation and resorption of water. The two types of sweat glands are eccrine and apocrine (Revis & Seagle, 2006).

Eccrine glands cover most of the body, with the exception of the nailbeds, lip margins, glans penis, and labia minora. They are most numerous on the palms and soles. Eccrine glands open directly onto the skin surface and secrete a weak saline solution known as *sweat* in response to environmental or psychological stimuli. Sweat assists in thermoregulation.

Apocrine glands, located in the axillae and genital areas, open into hair follicles and become active during puberty. Apocrine glands secrete a thicker, milky sweat into the hair follicle that, once mixed with bacterial flora on the skin, produces a characteristic musky odor. Functioning of the apocrine glands decreases with aging.

Sebaceous glands are located throughout the body, except the palms and soles, and open into hair follicles. These glands secrete sebum, an oil-like substance that assists the skin with moisture retention and friction protection (Fig. 13.4).

⚠ Lifespan Considerations

Pregnant Women

During pregnancy, increased levels of progesterone, estrogen, and melanocyte-stimulating hormone cause increased pigmentation in body areas that normally have higher pigmentation (ie, areolae, nipples, axillae, vulva, inner thighs; American Pregnancy Association, 2008). *Melasma*, increased pigmentation of the face in response to the hormonal changes of pregnancy, occurs mainly on the chin, cheeks, and upper lip. It generally resolves postpartum but can be permanent. *Linea nigra* is a darkened line extending from the umbilicus to the pubic area. See also Chapter 27.

Both sweat and sebaceous glands may become hyperactive during pregnancy, causing worsened acne and increased sweating. Hair loss usually decreases, because increased hormonal levels influence the retention of hair entering the resting phase of growth. After childbirth, retained hairs as well as those just entering the resting phase fall out quickly, giving the appearance of accelerated hair loss.

Newborns and Infants

Skin structures begin to develop at 4 weeks' gestation. The fetus attains adult epidermal thickness at 32 weeks' gestation and develops most subcutaneous fat during the third trimester (AWHONN, 2006).

At birth, an infant's skin can be red or ruddy. It is usually smooth and may be covered with *vernix*, which is a cheese-like substance comprised of shed epithelial cells and sebum. Vernix protects the infant's skin from the effects of prolonged exposure to amniotic fluid. Postterm infants have little if any vernix. Fine hair called *lanugo* may cover the newborn. Vellus hair replaces lanugo over the first few months after birth, and terminal hair begins to grow on the scalp and eyebrows. Physiologic jaundice can occur within the first 48 hours postnatally, giving the skin, mucous membranes, and conjunctiva a yellowish hue.

The skin of a preterm infant may be translucent or gelatinous. In contrast to a full-term newborn, the preterm baby has less dermal collagen and elastin, increased visibility of vascular structures (contributing to a ruddy appearance), thinner subcutaneous fat, more lanugo (dependent on gestational age), and increased risk for inadequate thermoregulation, skin injury, and edema (Lowdermilk & Perry, 2007). See also Chapter 28.

Children and Adolescents

Skin thickness continues to develop throughout childhood. Eccrine glands produce sweat, although in lower amounts than in adults. Apocrine glands are generally inactive until children approach puberty when these glands enlarge. At puberty, increased sebaceous activity results in the secretion

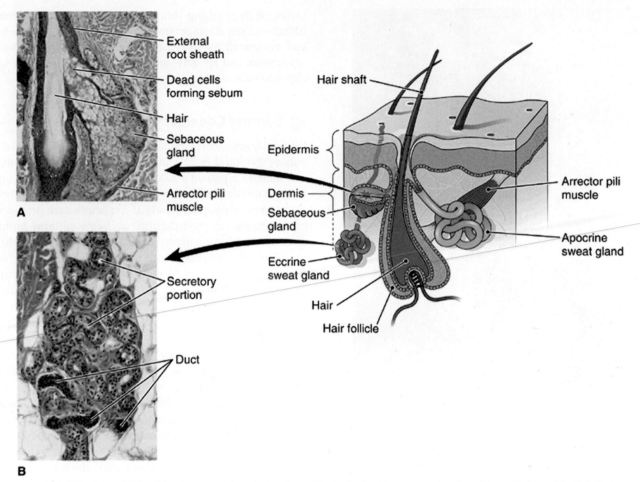

External root sheath

Dead cells forming sebum

Hair

Sebaceous gland

Arrector pili muscle

A

Secretory portion

Duct

B

Hair shaft

Epidermis

Dermis

Sebaceous gland

Eccrine sweat gland

Hair

Hair follicle

Arrector pili muscle

Apocrine sweat gland

Figure 13.4 Portion of skin showing associated glands and hair. **A.** A sebaceous gland and its associated hair follicle. **B.** An eccrine (temperature-regulating) sweat gland.

of large amounts of sebum into the hair follicles of the face, neck, chest, and back. Anything impeding sebum secretion onto the skin surface may result in the formation of closed comedones and ultimately acne (Fig. 13.5). Adolescents continue to develop additional terminal hair in the axillae and perineal areas; male teens develop such hair on the face, chest, and abdomen.

Older Adults

As skin ages, it gradually loses elastin, collagen, and subcutaneous fat, resulting in overall thinner skin (Merck Manual of Geriatrics, 2006). Effects of these changes include decreased resilience, sagging and wrinkling of skin structures, and increased visibility and fragility of superficial vascular structures. Elders are prone to increased bruising and shearing injury.

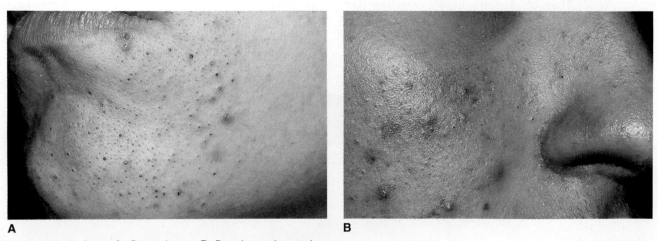

A

B

Figure 13.5 Acne. **A.** Comedones. **B.** Papular and pustular acne.

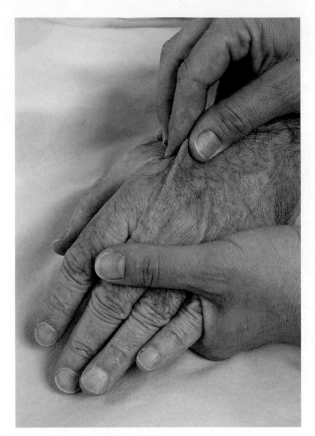

Figure 13.6 Assessing skin turgor.

Turgor, a measure of skin elasticity, decreases as a result of thinning of the dermis and reduced elastin production. The patient's hydration status also can affect skin turgor (Fig. 13.6). Replacement of the epidermal layer decreases with aging, resulting in rougher skin texture and prolonged time for wound healing. These changes affect thermoregulation, resulting in increased hypothermia and increased risk for heat stroke. Function of the eccrine and apocrine glands is reduced, causing increased skin dryness. Decreased melanin production in the hair matrix and epidermis results in gray or white hair and increased risk for the damaging effects of ultraviolet (UV) radiation (Ortonne, 2002). Hair follicles atrophy, with resultant hair loss. Influences from both genetics and hormones may result in androgenic hair loss (Fig. 13.7). Nail growth

slows, with resulting thinning and increased brittleness. Effects of sun damage are more apparent in older adults and evidenced by increased wrinkling, yellowing, leathery texture and atrophy, and uneven pigmentation of sun-exposed skin.

Cultural Considerations

Culturally sensitive assessment includes consideration of the patient's cultural beliefs and practices. Cultural variations can include a patient's refusal to remove a head covering and a requirement for the presence of a chaperone during skin examination, particularly if the health care provider is of a different sex than the patient. Some cultures prohibit directly touching a patient, requiring a nurse to wear gloves to avoid skin-to-skin contact. Becoming familiar with such cultural practices facilitates communication, accurate assessment, and necessary patient education. When a nurse is working with a patient from an unfamiliar culture, inquiring about cultural practices and norms is appropriate prior to beginning.

Common integumentary findings in African Americans include keloid formation, traction alopecia, pseudofolliculitis, folliculitis barbarae, and perineal follicularis (Juckett, 2005). African American women have increased incidence of melasma in pregnancy; Mongolian spots are fairly common in African American newborns. Curly hair in these patients tends to be coarser than in Caucasians because of a decreased ability of secreted sebum to travel along the hair shaft to the skin. Skin is commonly dry, resulting in ashy dermatitis. Pityriasis rosea, which presents as a macular hyperpigmented viral dermatitis in Caucasians, commonly presents with papular, maroon or purple lesions in African Americans. Skin cancers are more common on the palms, soles, and nailbeds in African Americans than in other groups (Hemenway, 2006).

Southeast Asian men have less body and facial hair than patients of other genetic heritages. Tattoos, body piercings, and other skin adornments are common in various Asian cultures (Ethnomed, 2008). Skin discolorations from cupping or coining may be found. Pigmentary disorders such as vitiligo or melasma in darker-skinned Asian populations carry a higher degree of psychosocial and emotional distress than in Caucasian patients (Parsad & Kumarasinge, 2006).

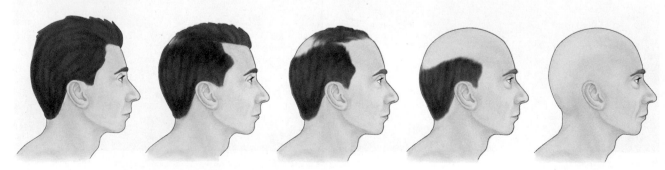

Figure 13.7 Common hair loss patterns in men.

Other lesions rarely found outside Asian populations include Hori's nevus and nevus of Ota. Other common lesions include solar lentigo, dark eye circles, postinflammatory hyper/hypopigmentation, ashy dermatoses, and melanocytic nevi. Many Asian men request removal of nevi from body parts for cultural rather than cosmetic reasons (Ethnomed, 2008).

Henna tattoos are common in Arabic and Indian females. Newborns of Arabic descent commonly have Mongolian spots, café au lait spots, and congenital nevi (Kahana, et al., 1995).

Acute Assessment

Skin findings indicating dehydration, cyanosis, or impaired skin integrity (acute lacerations) require prompt evaluation and intervention with fluids, oxygen administration, skin repair, or a combination. Most skin findings are nonemergent but require nurses to report them to other health care providers for further evaluation and management.

Concern about cancer can be anxiety-provoking. If a patient has a suspicious lesion, the primary care provider needs to assess and biopsy the site. To minimize stress for the patient, the nurse facilitates these actions in a timely manner.

A patient may present with infections or infestations that necessitate use of gloves or, in the case of measles, isolation. Rash and fever in a patient should raise suspicion of an infectious process (McKinnon & Howard, 2000). The patient should avoid contact with others to avoid infecting them.

Acute trauma and burns may require immediate attention, depending on severity (Hettiarachi & Papini, 2004). With large lacerations, the nurse must control bleeding and then work with colleagues to manage the wound. Patients with burns can lose large amounts of fluid through their wounds, so rapid fluid replacement is a necessity. Both large wounds and burns are acute and potentially life-threatening situations that require advanced interventions.

Subjective Data Collection

During subjective data collection, nurses have the opportunity to integrate health teaching with history taking. For the integumentary system, a major focus of such teaching relates to prevention of skin cancers, including melanoma. Table 13-1 reviews pertinent integumentary goals and education topics based on *Healthy People*.

Assessment of Risk Factors

Risk factors increase the probability that a patient will experience health concerns. Exposure of patients to knowledge of such risk factors can help the nurse identify areas of potential understanding and self-care deficits. Identifying concerns directs the implementation of therapeutic interventions, education for prevention, management of related issues, and documentation of status in the patient record.

When assessing general skin condition in patients without an identified concern, the nurse gathers information about general health, including nutritional status, which may identify any potential causes for skin disorders. In patients at high risk for skin alterations, such as immobile or bed-bound patients, additional information related to potential alterations in skin integrity is necessary.

Clinical Significance 13-2

If a patient has a specific concern about his or her skin, inspect the area/lesion first and ask other questions second. Often, once the nurse has identified the type of lesion (inflammatory, infectious, tumor, or altered integrity), he or she can focus questions to address the specific type of lesion. For instance, if a patient is scratching a deep pink scaly lesion on his elbow, the nurse may want to inquire about atopic illness or contact irritants instead of about melanoma.

Table 13.1 *Healthy People* Goals Related to Integumentary Health	
Goals	**Patient Education Topics**
Reduce the rate of melanoma cancer deaths.	Teach the patient early signs of melanoma.
Increase the proportion of persons who use at least one of the following protective measures that may reduce the risk of skin cancer: avoid the sun between 10 AM and 4 PM, wear sun-protective clothing when exposed to sunlight, use sunscreen with a SPF of 15 or higher, and avoid artificial sources of UV light.	Teach the patient to use sunscreen with an SPF of 15 or higher, avoid peak exposure, wear sun-protective clothing, and avoid UV light.

Source: *Healthy People 2010: What are its goals?* (n.d.). Retrieved May 20, 2010, from http://www.healthypeople.gov/About/goals.htm

Family History

Do you have any first-degree family members (parent, sibling, child) with a history of melanoma?
• Who had the problem?
• Do any first-degree relatives have multiple dark, irregular moles?

Having one or more first-degree relatives with a history of **melanoma** increases the patient's risk (American Cancer Society [ACS], 2008). Two or more first-degree relatives with a history of melanoma and a personal history of one or more dysplastic nevi increase risk for melanoma by 50% (ACS, 2008). Approximately 10% of all patients with melanoma have a family member with melanoma.

Past History

Do you examine your skin for new lesions or changes in current lesions monthly? When was your last clinical skin examination?

Determining if the patient performs regular skin screenings or seeks at least annual professional examinations assists in providing appropriate education and reinforcement. Give the patient information related to identifying potentially serious skin lesions by teaching what changes warrant further evaluation. A simple method is to use the *ABCDE*s of melanoma detection:
• Asymmetry
• Border irregularity
• Color
• Diameter of more than 6 mm
• Evolution of lesion over time
See Table 13-2 for more information.

Do you have any pigmented skin lesions?
• How many lesions?
• Where are they located?
• Are any larger than a pencil eraser?
• Have any lesions changed (itching, bleeding, nonhealing, color change, size change, change in borders)?

Any **dysplastic nevi** (Fig. 13.8) or more than 50 normal moles increases risk for melanoma. These moles can be in sun-exposed or sun-protected skin areas. Melanomas are most common on the face, shoulder, and upper arms for both genders, back for men, and legs for women, most likely related to sun exposure (Bulliard, et al., 2007). Evolving changes in moles that warrant further evaluation are changes in size, color, texture, or shape, onset of itching or bleeding, and nonhealing wounds.

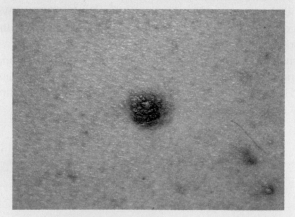

Figure 13.8 Dysplastic nevus.

Did you ever have severe sunburn, particularly during childhood or adolescence? How long can you be in the sun before your skin begins to turn red?

Melanoma on the trunk, arms, or legs is associated with severe (blistering) sunburn during childhood or adolescence. Fair-skinned people who turn red after minimal exposure to sunlight have less melanin, with less protection from the sun's harmful UV rays, and are at increased risk for melanoma (American Academy of Dermatology, 2008).

(text continues on page 270)

Table 13.2　ABCDEs for Assessment for Melanoma

A: Asymmetry

Does one half look like the other half?

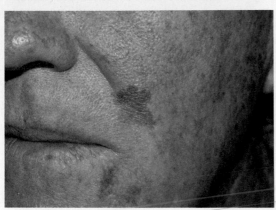

B: Border irregularity

Is the border ragged or notched?

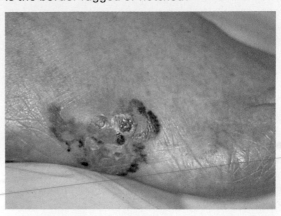

C: Color

Does the mole have a variety of shades or different colors?

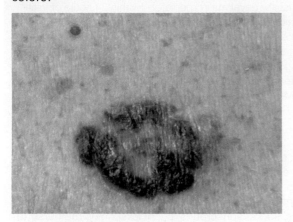

D: Diameter

Is the diameter >6 mm (pencil eraser)?

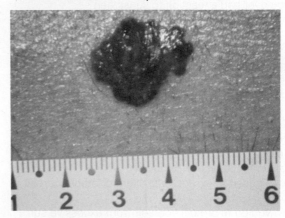

E: Evolution
Has the lesion evolved or changed over time?

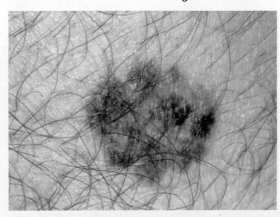

Questions to Assess History and Risks	Rationales

Have you ever had skin cancer?
- When did you have skin cancer?
- Where was it located?
- How deep was it?
- How was it treated?

Prior history of any skin cancer (squamous cell, basal cell, or melanoma) significantly increases the risk of developing additional cancerous skin lesions (NCI, 2003). Deeper melanoma lesions indicate advanced staging and increased risk for metastases. Prior treatment may have caused additional skin problems, such as burns from radiation or extensive scarring or disfigurement from surgical excision.

Do you have a history of organ transplant, HIV/AIDS, chemotherapy, or radiation therapy?

A weakened immune system increases the risk for developing melanoma (ACS, 2008).

Medications

Are you taking any medications, including herbal or nutritional supplements, vitamins, or over-the-counter medications?
- Have you recently begun a new prescription or nonprescription medication/supplement? Which one(s)?
- Do you use topical medicated creams?
- Do you have allergies to medications, latex, nuts, bees, or other items?
- What was your reaction to the allergy?
- Have you ever had a reaction to sunscreen?

Certain medications (Table 13-3), sunscreens, perfumes, cosmetics, and topical skin creams can cause **photosensitivity** reactions (Barrett, 2008; Guthrie Ambulatory Health Care Clinic Pharmacy, 2008), which usually present with rash following sun exposure. Other medications stimulate **phototoxicity**, a reaction caused by a drug's molecules absorbing energy from a particular UV wavelength and then damaging surrounding tissues. The result is marked and severely tender sunburn (Eustice & Eustice, 2007). Phototoxicity usually develops immediately (within 24 hours of initial ingestion of the photoreactive medication) and resolves readily upon removal of the offending substance, UV exposure, or both. **Photoallergy** manifests with blisters and redness on exposed skin, occurs only after repeated exposure to an offending substance, and persists for some time after removal of the offending substance, UV exposure, or both.

Lifestyle, Occupational History, and Personal Behaviors

- What is your occupation? Hobbies?
- Are you exposed to excessive sunlight or other sources of radiation?
- What do you do to protect yourself from excessive sun exposure?

Work or hobbies involving excessive exposure to sunlight, especially during intensive midday hours, increase risk for melanoma. Determining what protection the patient uses (eg, gloves, hats, long-sleeved shirts, pants, shoes, socks, sunscreens, sunblocks) helps the nurse to ascertain the patient's risk level for melanoma.

- How often do you shower or bathe?
- What is the water temperature?
- Do you apply moisturizer after you bathe?

Excessive dry skin may result from frequent bathing and inadequate moisturizing. Showering or bathing more than once daily in the normal adult causes excessive loss of skin oils. Elderly patients need to bathe less often, usually every 2–3 days. Using hot water to bathe increases loss of skin oils. Bathing should be with warm water only and for the shortest time necessary to cleanse all body areas. Use of moisturizing creams (not lotions) immediately after toweling dry decreases the effect of loss of skin oils from bathing.

Determine risk for skin breakdown.
- Are you confined to bed?
- Do you have a cast, brace, or other immobilizing device on any body part?
- Can you change your body position or position of the immobilized body part?
- How often are you changing position or shifting weight from one part of your body to another?

Immobility of the body or a body part increases risk for pressure ulcers. The National Pressure Ulcer Advisory Panel (2007) defines a **pressure ulcer** as a "localized injury to the skin and/or underlying tissue usually over a bony prominence, as a result of pressure or pressure in combination with shear and/or friction." Casts, splints, or other immobilizing devices may exert pressure on bony prominences of an immobilized extremity or part and increase risk for pressure ulcer. This risk is amplified in patients with decreased sensory perception of the immobilized

Questions to Assess History and Risks	Rationales
• Do you have any problem with loss of sensation or position sense of any part of your body? • Do you have diabetes mellitus, PVD, or any known sensory loss? • How is your nutritional intake? • What is your age? • What is your weight?	extremity or body part (eg, in diabetic neuropathy, venous insufficiency, other sensory deficits), because they cannot sense discomfort associated with decreased circulation to an area caused by prolonged pressure. Elderly patients are at increased risk for pressure ulcers from age-related loss of subcutaneous fat and decreased cushioning. Thin patients have less subcutaneous fat to cushion the skin against pressures exerted on it (see Table 13-20 at the end of the chapter).

Table 13.3 Medications That Cause Photoreactions

Antimicrobials	Psychotropics and Other Psychiatric Agents	Cardiovascular Agents	Herbals and Topicals
Azithromycin	Alprazolam	Amiloride	Bergamot
Chloroquine	Amitriptyline	Amiodarone	Bitter orange peel
Ciprofloxacin	Clomipramine	Captopril	Cedar
Doxycycline	Chlordiazepoxide	Chlorothiazide	Celery
Griseofulvin	Desipramine	Digitoxin	Citron
Mefloquine	Doxepin	Dilitazem	Dong quai
Minocycline	Haloperidol	Enlapril	Lavender
Naldixic acid	Imipramine	Fosinopril	Motherwort
Ofloxacin	Isocarboxazid	Furosemide	Musk
Oxytetracycline	Maprotiline	Hydrochlorothiazide	PABA esters
Pyrvinium pamoate	Nortriptyline	Methyldopa	Parsley
Quinine	Prochlorperazine	Metolazone	Peppermint oil
Sulfonamides	Resperidone	Nifedipine	St. John's wort
Sulfasalazine	Sertraline	Quinapril	Sandalwood
Tetracyclines	Thiothixine		Wormwood
Trimethoprim	Thioridazine		
	Trazodone		
	Venlafaxine		

Antihistamines	Disease-Modifying Agents	Chemotherapeutic Agents	Hypoglycemics
Cetirizine	Dapson	Dacarbazine	Chlorpropamide
Cyproheptadine	Gold	Fluorouracil	Glimepiride
Dimenhydrinate	Hydroxychlorquine	Methotrexate	Glipizide
Diphenhydramine	Methotrexate	Procarbazine	Glyburide
Hydroxyzine	Sulfasalazine	Vinblastine	Tolbutamide
Loratadine			Tolazamide
Promethiazine			

Other Agents	Topical Agents	NSAIDs	
Carbamazepine	Benzocaine	Diclofenac	
Gabapenitin	Benzoyl Peroxide	Etodolac	
Interferon beta	Bithionol	Ibuprofen	
Oral contraceptives	Coal tar	Ketoprofen	
Zolpidem	Hexachlorophene	Nabumetone	
	Isotretinoin	Naproxen	
	Psoralens	Oxaprozin	
	Tretinoin	Piroxicam	

Risk Assessment and Health-Related Patient Teaching

As mentioned previously, risk assessment identifies areas of concern and provides direction for patient education. Excessive UV radiation is the most important focus area for the integumentary system, because exposure to it has been shown to cause skin cancers, particularly melanoma.

Self-Skin Examination (SSE) assists patients with identifying potentially problematic lesions through the detection of moles (Fig. 13.9). The nurse educates the patient that a normal mole has the following features (American Academy of Dermatology, 2008):

- A solid tan, brown, black, or skin-toned color
- Size smaller than 6 mm in diameter (approximately the size of a pencil eraser)
- Well-defined edges
- Usually round or oval shape with a flat or dome-like surface
- Emergence before 30 years of age.

The nurse emphasizes to the patient the following steps of the SSE:

1. Get fully undressed and stand in front of a full-length mirror.
2. Carefully scan the entire body, using a hand-held mirror to look at areas difficult to see (eg, soles of feet).
3. When examining the scalp, use a comb or blowdryer to part the hair and examine the scalp section by section.
4. Report any suspicious lesion to the health care provider.

Both natural and artificial forms of UV light are carcinogenic, and exposure to UV light directly increases risk for skin cancer (American Academy of Dermatology, 2007a). Short ultraviolet B (UVB) waves are more likely than ultraviolet A (UVA) waves to cause sunburn. UVB waves are directly linked with skin cancers, especially basal cell and squamous cell cancers. Longer UVA waves have deeper skin penetration than UVB (EPA, 2008). UVA waves are responsible for some melanomas, but are chiefly responsible for the effects of photo-aging, specifically wrinkling and leathering

of the skin. Intensity of UV waves is greatest during midday, and exposure between 10 AM and 4 PM increases potential damaging effects. Reflection of UV waves off of sand, concrete, snow, and water doubles UV exposure and its damaging effects.

Nurses can simplify the education of patients about decreasing UV light exposure by teaching the phrase "Slip! Slop! Slap!…and Wrap!" Coined by the ACS (2008), it reminds people to slip on a shirt, slop on sunscreen, slap on a hat, and wrap on sunglasses to increase protection against UV exposure. Sunburn protection from clothing depends on how much skin is covered, fabric color, and fabric weave. Dark colors reflect UV rays better than light colors, and tightly woven fabrics afford less penetration by harmful UV rays. Some fabrics provide less protection than sunscreen with sun-protective factor (SPF) of 15 or higher. Wearing a hat with a wide all-around brim protects the face, neck, and ears; common sites for skin cancer (American Academy of Dermatology, 2007b).

The SPF is defined as the amount of time a product protects the skin from reddening, as compared to the amount of time for unprotected skin to redden (US FDA, 2006). If it normally takes 10 minutes for unprotected skin to redden, use of a product with SPF 15 would protect the skin from reddening for 150 minutes. Applying sunscreen 15 to 30 minutes prior to exposure enhances absorption of the sunscreen into the skin and increases protection. Sunscreen application needs to happen every 2 hours for maximum benefit. **Sunscreens** absorb harmful UV rays; **sunblocks** deflect rays from absorption. People also should apply lip balm with SPF repeatedly during sun exposure to protect the lips. To be effective when extended sun exposure is anticipated, sunglasses should have at least 99% UVA and UVB protection.

Another helpful reminder to limit excessive UV exposure is "short shadow seek shade" (US EPA, 2009). Sun that is overhead casts a shadow shorter than the actual person and should serve as an alert to seek more shade for protection. As a shadow lengthens, it signifies decreased UV intensity and thus a need for less protection. Changes

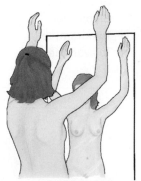 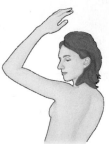 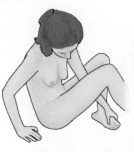 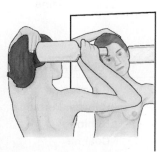 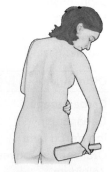

1. Examine the body front and back in the mirror, then the right and left sides, with the arms raised.

2. Bend the elbows, looking carefully at the forearms, back of the upper arms, and palms

3. Next, look at the back of the legs and feet, the spaces between the toes, and the soles of the feet.

4. Examine the back of the neck and the scalp with a hand-held mirror. Part the hair to lift.

5. Finally, check the back and buttocks with a hand mirror.

Figure 13.9 Self-skin examination.

Table 13.4 Ultraviolet Light Index and Skin Protection Recommendations

UV Index	Level	Minutes to Reddened Skin			Recommended Skin Protection
		Fair Skin	*Medium Skin*	*Dark Skin*	
0–2	Low	44–120+	74–120+	120+	Wear sunglasses when it is bright outside.
					Wear sunscreen, especially fair-skinned patients and those who burn easily.
3–5	Moderate	26–43	44–71	77–120	Wear sun-protective clothing.
					Follow "Short Shadow Seek Shade."
6–7	High	18–26	31–43	55–76	Unprotected skin can burn quickly.
					Wear SPF ≥ 15 sunscreen or sunblock, protective clothing, sunglasses, shade, hat.
					Reduce exposure between 10 AM and 4 PM.
8–10	Very high	13–18	22–31	38–54	Risk of harm from unprotected sun exposure is high.
					Wear SPF ≥ 15 sunscreen or sunblock, protective clothing, sunglasses, shade, and hat.
					Reduce exposure between 10 AM and 4 PM.
11+	Extreme	9–13	14–21	25–38	Avoid UV exposure if possible.
					Use liberal application of SPF ≥ 15 sunscreen or sunblock.
					Wear protective clothing, sunglasses, shade, and hat.
					Reduce exposure between 10 AM and 4 PM.

Source: Environmental Protection Agency. (2008). *UV index.* Retrieved May 20, 2010, from http://epa.gov/sunwise/uvindex.html

in the weather, seasons, and ozone layer affect the intensity of UV rays (WHO, n.d.). The *UV Index* (Table 13-4), published daily, uses a scale from 0 to 11 or higher to indicate the degree of predicted UV radiation based on weather, season, and ozone layer changes. The higher the number, the greater the risk, and the greater degree of protection required.

Focused Health History Related to Common Symptoms

Common Integumentary Symptoms

- Pruritis
- Rash (multiple lesions)
- Single lesion or wound

Questions to Assess Symptoms	Rationale/Abnormal Findings
Tell me about your skin problem.	This question encourages the patient to present his or her view and perceptions of the problem.
Pruiritis (Itching) Do you have a problem with itching? • How long have you had the problem? • Where do you itch? • (If there are signs of a rash) Did you first have itching followed by rash, or did the rash come first? • What makes the itching worse? What makes it better? • Does itching disrupt rest and sleep? • Have you tried any remedies for the itching? What was the result? • What do you think the problem is?	Skin lesions or conditions are pruritic, occasionally pruritic, or never pruritic. Pruritus frequently precedes atopic lesions but follows inflammatory lesions. Recent pruritis may indicate toxic exposure, insect bites, parasite infestations, or viral xanthems such as *varicella*. Localized pruritis may indicate infestation, insect bite, allergic reaction, or toxic exposure. Generalized pruritis is common in medication or food allergies. Severe pruritis interfering with sleep is frequently from *scabies. Psoriasis* is occasionally pruritic. Moles usually do not itch. Noting what, if any, remedies the patient tried and their effectiveness may help identify cause.

(text continues on page 274)

Rash

Where is/are the lesion(s) located?
- Do you have a single lesion or are there several lesions?
- Is the rash all over or just in one area?
- Does the rash appear to have a pattern?

Lesions from *contact or allergic dermatitis* are usually on the body part exposed to an irritant or allergen (Hogan, 2007). Lesions over the entire body, including palms and soles, may be linked to *syphilis. Seborrheic dermatitis* is often found on the face, head, and hair-covered body areas. *Herpes zoster* follows a dermatome and is often found on the chest, back, abdomen, and face and rarely on the extremities. Genital lesions are commonly from sexually transmitted infections. Single lesions could be *cancer;* multiple lesions could indicate an infection.

Has the rash changed since you first noticed it?

Varicella begins with macular lesions, progresses to papular, then vesicular, and ultimately superficial ulcers. Lesions changing in size, color, or other characteristics may indicate *cancer. Pityriasis rosea* begins as a single large macular lesion on the trunk and progresses to multiple macular lesions of similar shape but smaller size distributed predominately over the chest and back. *Contact dermatitis* spreads from initial point of contact; in severe cases, lesions appear in unexposed areas.

Have you been exposed to anything that would cause itching or the rash?
- Have you been exposed to any chemicals, either at work or play?
- Do you have pets or frequent contact with animals?
- Have you worked in the yard recently?
- Have you had any close contacts with people with a similar skin problem?
- Have you started any new medications, vitamins, or herbal/nutritional supplements recently?
- Have you eaten unusual foods recently?
- Have you recently traveled, especially foreign travel?
- Have you shared clothing, hats, bed linens, or sleeping bags, or slept in someone's house on sofa/upholstered furniture recently?
- Do you live in a community dwelling?

Skin exposure to an allergen releases histamine from mast cells, resulting in pruritis. Scratching causes additional histamine release, stimulating further pruritis. This prompts further scratching, and develops into a persistent cycle of itching and scratching. Determining recent occupational and leisure activities, animal or plant contacts, and outdoor activities may identify exposures to poison ivy, insects, microbials such as dermatophytes or bacteria, chemicals, and pesticides. Medications, vitamin or herbal supplements, and foods new to the patient may be causes for *allergic dermatitis.* Insect bites or contact with foods or other products not found in the patient's home country may cause lesions that present during or shortly after travel. Wearing another person's clothes, sleeping in someone else's bed, or living in communal dwellings may expose the patient to *scabies* or *lice.*

How would you describe your rash?
- Flat?
- Raised?
- Blister like?
- Pus-filled?
- Looks like thickened skin?

Macular lesions could be ecchymosis, pressure point, or *tinea versicolor.* **Papular** lesions may indicate *acne, warts,* nevi, insect bites, or early *varicella.* **Pustular** lesions include *acne,* furuncles, and carbuncles. **Vesicular** lesions may be *herpes simplex, varicella,* or *impetigo.* **Plaque** lesions are commonly *psoriasis* or *lichen simplex.* (See Table 13-10 at the end of the chapter.)

Do you have any other symptoms related to this rash or skin lesion?
- Have you had a recent illness?
- Any fever, chills, or headache?

Fevers and chills often accompany infectious skin disorders such as *measles, rubella,* and *varicella* (McKinnon & Howard, 2000). Headache often accompanies *mumps* and *meningitis.*

Single Lesion or Wound
- Is this wound acute or chronic?
- Is it related to medical, surgical, or traumatic causes?
- Would any factors delay healing, such as malnutrition, impaired circulation, immune suppression, obesity, smoking, diabetes mellitus, or infection?

Obtain additional information about the wound, when it first appeared, if it has increased or decreased, and associated symptoms. If the wound is related to an injury, evaluate the nature of the events leading to the trauma. If the patient provides vague or suspicious explanations, be alert to the possibility of abuse and make appropriate referrals (Craven & Hinrle, 2008). Also ask about any treatments including natural and over-the-counter remedies.

Documentation of Normal Findings

Patient denies pruritis, skin lesions, excessive dryness of skin. Denies changes to existing moles. *M. Olson, RN*

Additional Questions	Rationales/Abnormal Findings
Pregnant Women What skin changes have you noticed since becoming pregnant?	Hormonal changes in pregnancy produce multiple effects on the skin. Striae appear as the skin stretches to accommodate the growing fetus. They do not completely disappear after pregnancy but may fade to a light silvery color. Fingernails may grow at an accelerated rate.
Do you have a problem with acne?	Women with a history of acne before pregnancy may experience a resurgence of acne lesions during pregnancy (American Pregnancy Association, 2010).
Do you have a problem with itchy skin?	Itchiness is common in the second and third trimesters and results from stretching of the skin, particularly on the abdomen and breasts, to accommodate the growing fetus and milk production. Severe itchiness may indicate *intrahepatic cholestasis of pregnancy*; it may be associated with nausea, vomiting, fatigue, jaundice, and decreased appetite and warrants further evaluation.
Do you have a problem with excessive skin oiliness?	Hormonal changes increase the oil secretion of sebaceous glands, contributing to the "glow of pregnancy." Another contributor is increased circulation and the development of superficial capillaries that brighten the skin.
Have you noticed color changes on your face or body?	Pigmentary changes of pregnancy include **linea nigra** (darkened line from umbilicus to pubis) and **melasma** (blotchy facial discoloration known as the "mask of pregnancy").
Have you had problems with skin tags?	Hormonal changes also may cause these small growths of skin that extend from the epidermis anywhere on the body. Skin tags do not resolve spontaneously after pregnancy, but require removal.
Newborns, Infants, and Children Does your child have any problems with frequent or persistent bruising? • What safety measures do you have at home to prevent accidental injuries? • Has you child been ill recently?	Certain infections, hematologic problems, or coagulopathies present with **ecchymoses**. Accidental trauma resulting in bruising warrants evaluation of the child's coordination or the absence of safety precautions. Bruises in various stages of healing require careful questioning to determine if nonaccidental trauma has caused them.
Does your child have a rash? • Is the rash associated with fever, nausea, or vomiting? • Has your child been treated with antibiotics or other medications lately? Which one(s)? • Do you have any pets in your home? • Has your child recently visited an outdoors area that he or she rarely or has never visited?	Many bacterial, fungal, and viral infections cause *dermatoses*. The papulovesicular lesions and honey-colored crusting of *impetigo* results from staphylococcal or streptococcal infection. *Tinea cruris, capitis*, or *corporis* is fungal. Exposure to tinea is frequently from animals. *Roseola, varicella*, and *herpes* are viral causes of dermatitis. Rash that follows recent antibiotic use may be a drug reaction or *Stevens-Johnson syndrome* (penicillins, sulfa, ciprofloxacin, some seizure medications; Parrillo, 2008). This serious and even lethal syndrome causes the skin to slough off, similar to a burn.
Adolescents Do you have a problem with acne? • Do certain foods worsen your acne? • What have you tried to clear your acne? • (In females) Do you tend to break out more before or during your monthly period?	Diet generally does not influence acne, but in some people certain foods or a high glycemic load tend to be associated with an increased number or severity of acne lesions (Smith, et al., 2007). Hormonal influences can affect or increase acne lesions. Identifying what remedies the patient has tried will help determine what other therapeutic regimens may help resolve the acne.

(text continues on page 276)

Additional Questions	Rationales/Abnormal Findings
Do you have cuts or sores on your skin?	"Cutting" is the self-inflicted act of using a razor, knife, or other sharp instrument to make "cut marks" on the extremities. This manifestation of mental illness often begins in late childhood or adolescence, and is frequently associated with depression.
Do you have any piercings or tattoos? • How long have you had it? • Have you had any problems with swelling, redness, or tenderness at the piercing site? • How are you keeping the pierced area clean? • Did you have any reaction to the tattoo such as redness, swelling, tenderness, or itching? • Did your tattoo practitioner use sterile, single-use needles and dyes?	Tattooings and piercings of various body parts frequently begin in adolescence. Improper postpiercing care can lead to infection, scarring, and possibly **keloid** (Mayo Staff, 2008). Swelling, redness, or tenderness at a piercing site may indicate infection or allergic reaction to the inserted metal stud, ring, or rod. Dyes used in tattooing may cause an allergic reaction and result in swelling, redness, and tenderness at the tattoo site (American Academy of Dermatology, 2004). Tattoo dyes are not FDA approved for injection into the skin and may contain pigments suitable for automobile paints and other chemicals (Cronin, 2003). Tattoos applied without known sterile equipment or single-use dyes increase risk for bloodborne diseases (eg, *hepatitis B, HIV*).
Older Adults Do you have problems with easy or excessive bruising? Does your skin tear or split easily?	Multiple ecchymoses may be from repeated trauma (falls), clotting disorder, or physical abuse. Aging causes the junction between the dermis and epidermis to flatten, increasing the tendency of the skin to tear. Decreased eccrine gland function results in a decreased sweat response. Nerve endings in skin decrease with age, causing decreased sensation to 2-point discrimination, touch, and vibration.
Are your nails brittle or splitting?	Nail growth decreases with aging, leading to the formation of concave, flat, or dry and brittle nails. Pigmented nail bands present earlier in life are more pronounced in aging patients.

🌐 Cultural Considerations

• What are some treatments you use at home for this skin problem?
• What would your parents do for you if you had this skin problem?
• Do practitioners in your culture apply any health or beauty aids directly to the skin?
• Why do you think this skin problem began when it did?
• What do you think caused this problem?
• What kind of treatment do you think you need to correct the skin problem?
• What do you fear the most about this skin problem?

More than half of all patients are likely to self-treat a skin lesion or dermatitis with what is culturally familiar to them before seeking assistance from a health care professional. Inquiring about cultural practices and home remedies provides insight into the patient's specific culture and assists in designing appropriately sensitive therapeutic interventions. A common practice among Southeast Asians is *coining*, in which they rub a coin or other object across the skin in a specific manner to treat various health concerns (Fig. 13.10). Coining frequently results in bruising and abrasions and is often mistaken as a sign of physical abuse. Cupping involves placement of a cup on the skin surface, applying heat to form a vacuum. This practice often leaves circular bruises on the skin. The patient's perception of the cause, reason for onset, type of treatment needed, and fears related to any illness will affect the approach and effectiveness in treating the patient's skin condition. Another common cultural practice is the application of henna tattoos in an array of patterns and at specific locations to represent a particular occasion in the patient's life and culture (Ethnomed, 2008).

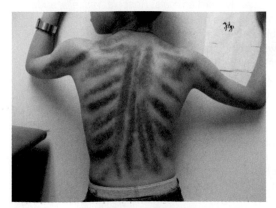

Figure 13.10 Effects of coining.

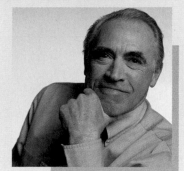

Therapeutic Dialogue: Collecting Subjective Data

Remember Mr. Stoli, the patient described at the beginning of this chapter, who was admitted to the hospital with a venous ulcer. The nurse uses professional communication techniques to gather subjective data from Mr. Stoli. The following conversations give two examples of interview styles. One style is more effective than the other.

Less Effective

Nurse: Hi, Mr. Stoli. I'm Lilin, and I'm going to be your nurse today. How are you feeling?

Mr. Stoli: Fine.

Nurse: I need to check your foot, OK?

Mr. Stoli: It's fine.

Nurse: Your chart says that you have an ulcer on your right foot, so I need to check your foot, OK?

Mr. Stoli: I guess so.

Nurse: It's a good thing you came to the hospital to get this wound treated, isn't it?

Mr. Stoli: I was doing fine at home. I don't know why my doctor—he tells me to come to the hospital. My wife was taking care of me just fine.

Nurse: Well, your doctor must have thought that things were getting worse and that you needed to come here to take a little better care of your foot. I don't think that he would tell you to come here if you didn't need to.

Mr. Stoli: I would be better if I could get up and move around. Sitting is bad for you.

Nurse: Right now getting up and moving around is the worst thing for you. If you get up all the time, the wound will never heal. You need to keep your foot up and not walk on it for it to get better. Let's have a look at the foot and see what's happening.

More Effective

Nurse: Hello, Mr. Stoli. I'm going to be your nurse today. My name is Lilin. (smiles, pauses) How are you feeling?

Mr. Stoli: Fine.

Nurse: Your chart says that you came to the hospital because of your foot. Is that right?

Mr. Stoli: Yeah, I have kept it up at home, you know, but the doctor wanted me to come here.

Nurse: What other things did you do to get it better?

Mr. Stoli: My wife, she told me to stay home. I didn't do that.

Nurse: It sounds like you really like to be active.

Mr. Stoli: I don't like being here. I can take care of my foot myself, you know.

Nurse: You sound like you like being independent. It must be hard for you to be in the hospital.

Mr. Stoli: (silent)

Nurse: Can I look at your foot? Maybe we can talk about how it has changed. I know that it's difficult to have us help you, but we really want to help you to get better (smiles). Perhaps we can talk about other things you can do at home to help your foot improve and prevent further problems requiring hospitalization.

Critical Thinking Challenge

- How might the more effective nurse's nonverbal communication promote a therapeutic relationship?
- How might the patient's Russian heritage influence his perceptions, values, and beliefs about his diagnosis and healing?
- What is the role of the nurse in giving advice versus listening to the patient's perspective?

Objective Data Collection

Equipment Needed

- Examination gown
- Tape measure
- Adequate light source
- Magnifying glass

Preparation

Ensure a comfortable room temperature. Wash your hands thoroughly. Apply clean gloves if you anticipate contact with a skin lesion and during inspection of the scalp. Examination of the skin involves inspection and palpation. Expose only areas being directly examined to facilitate privacy, decrease the patient's anxiety, and show consideration for possible cultural concerns.

Common and Specialty or Advanced Techniques

Objective assessment of the skin is performed in a head-to-toe format if the patient is seeking a complete skin assessment, usually in a dermatology clinic for cancer screening. More commonly, the nurse assesses skin with inspection of each body area, such as abdominal skin when inspecting the abdomen. General skin assessment includes color, texture, moisture, turgor, and temperature. Additionally, the nurse might assess a specific problem, such as rash on the thorax. The nurse assesses and describes wounds, lesions, rashes, and hematomas separately during the focused assessment. Table 13-5 summarizes comprehensive assessment techniques, and additional examinations may be added if indicated by the clinical situation.

Comprehensive Skin Assessment

First, the nurse assesses the overall skin appearance and inspects the face and exposed skin surfaces for color and pigmentation. The nurse needs to move bedbound patients to visualize all body surfaces. If a patient cannot help with the movement, additional help may be necessary to position the patient safely.

Bedridden patients require frequent detailed inspection of dependent areas, especially bony prominences, to detect early evidence of skin breakdown. Additionally, it is important to evaluate skin folds for infection or irritation, especially under the breasts, in the groin, and in the abdominal pannus.

Individual lesions may be generally categorized as primary or secondary. *Primary lesions* arise from previously normal skin and include maculae, papules, nodules, tumors, polyps, wheals, blisters, cysts, pustules, and abscesses. Primary lesions may be further described as nonelevated, elevated-solid, or fluid-filled. *Secondary lesions* follow primary lesions (eg, scar tissue, crusts from dried burns). Review the tables at the end of this chapter for more details.

The language of the integumentary system can be very complex and intimidating. Remember it is best to describe lesions if you are unsure about how to label them. A complete and accurate description can be used to identify if the patient is healing.

Table 13.5	Comprehensive Versus Focused/Advanced Techniques in Integumentary Assessment		
Comprehensive Assessment Technique	**Purpose**	**Screening or Registered Nurse Assessment**	**Focused or Advanced Practice Examination**
Inspect skin with each body area	To collect data on rashes, lesions, wounds	X	
Inspect entire body thoroughly	To screen for cancer or other conditions		X
Inspect fingernails and toenails	To assess hygiene, circulation	X	
Inspect hair	To look for lesions, nits		X
Inspect wounds	To evaluate wound and wound healing	X	
Palpate skin	To assess temperature, turgor, vascularity	X	

Technique and Normal Findings	Abnormal Findings
Inspection If performing a complete skin assessment, inspect all body areas, beginning at the crown of the head, parting the hair to visualize the scalp, and progressing caudally to the feet. Make sure to assess the undersides of the feet and to separate the toes. Note general skin color. *Pigmentation is consistent throughout the body. Patients with dark skin may have hypopigmented skin on the palms and soles.*	Note changes in pigmentation in any areas. ***Vitiligo*** is characterized by areas of no pigmentation. Other abnormal color changes include ***flushing, erythema*** (redness), ***cyanosis*** (bluish discoloration), ***pallor*** (paleness), ***rubor*** (dependent redness), ***brawny*** (dark leathery appearance), and ***jaundice*** (yellow discoloration of skin and sclerae). The tongue, lips, nail beds, and buccal mucosa are less pigmented areas and may be the best indicators of pallor or cyanosis ***Uremic frost*** is a whitish coating noted with severe kidney failure. See Table 13-9 at the end of this chapter.
Inspect for any lesions. If observed, identify the configuration, pattern, morphology, size, distribution, and exact body location. *Common benign lesions include freckles, birth marks, skin tags, moles, and cherry angiomas.*	Configurations may be annular, arciform, iris, linear, polymorphous, punctuate, serpiginous, nummular/discoid, umbilicated, filiform, or verrucaform. Patterns include asymmetric, confluent, diffuse, discrete, generalized, grouped, localized, satellite, symmetric, or zosteriform. Lesion morphology is a key determinant in identifying a skin disorder. Primary morphology is the type. Secondary morphology includes shape, size, arrangement, and distribution, which further defines the underlying problem (or normal variant). *Vitiligo*, a miscellaneous lesion, causes skin depigmentation. See Tables 13-10–13-13 at the end of this chapter.
Identify any infections. Be sure to use infection-control principles if infection is suspected.	Infections include *acne, cellulitis, impetigo, German measles* (rubella), *herpes simplex* (cold sores), *measles* (rubeola), *pityriasis rosea, roseola, warts, candida, tinea corporis,* and *tinea versicolor*. See also Table 13-14.
Note any inflammatory lesions.	These include *psoriasis, eczema, urticaria, contact dermatitis*, allergic drug reaction, insect bites, or seborrhea (Merck Manual of Diagnosis and Therapy, 2005). See Table 13-15.
Assess for any infestations.	Lice (*pediculosis*), scabies, or ticks may infest the skin and produce lesions. See Table 13-16.
Observe for growths, tumors, or vascular or other miscellaneous lesions.	Growths and tumors include moles or nevi, skin tags, *lipoma, lentigo, actinic keratosis, basal or squamous cell carcinoma, malignant melanoma,* and *Kaposi's sarcoma*. Vascular lesions include *hemangiomas, nevus flammeus* (port-wine stain), *spider or star angiomas,* and *venous lake*s. See also Table 13-17.
Inspect any wounds or incisions. If observed, note the shape and measure the length, width, and depth with a ruler. If a wound is deep or tunneled, insert a cotton applicator to measure depth. Wounds can be intentional (surgical) or unintentional (trauma); open or closed; acute or chronic; superficial or deep; and clean, contaminated, or infected (Table 13-6). Wound assessment involves some knowledge of the healing process, which is divided into inflammatory, proliferative, and remodeling phases (Mercandetti & Cohen, 2008).	*Partial-thickness wounds* involve the epidermis; *full-thickness wounds* involve the dermis and subcutaneous tissue. Healthy-healing tissue appears pink to red; necrotic tissue may be yellow, white, brown, or black (eschar; Wound Care Information Network, 2008). Pale tissue may indicate poor circulation and may be slow to heal. The surrounding area may be inflamed and red or pale with poor circulation. See Table 13-18 at the end of this chapter.
Describe any wounds related to trauma. Assess status of the blood supply to the skin, making note of any bleeding or ecchymosis (bruising).	Lesions from trauma may be *petechiae, purpurae, ecchymoses, hematomas, lacerations, abrasions, puncture wounds,* or *avulsions*. See also Table 13-19.

(text continues on page 280)

Table 13.6 Wound Classification

Wound Healing Phase	Description
Inflammatory Phase: Begins within 30 minutes of injury; lasts 2–3 days	Upon injury, vasoconstriction, platelet aggregation, and release of thromboplastin promotes *hemostasis*. An *inflammatory* reaction follows, initially through polymorphonuclear cells to cleanse the wound of debris and kill bacteria. Mononuclear cells follow and become macrophages to further cleanse the wound of debris, dead bacteria, and spent neutrophils.
Proliferative Phase: Begins at end of inflammatory phase; may last up to 4 weeks	Fibroblasts migrate into the wound bed to deposit collagen and secrete growth factors. Macrophages now produce enzymes to stimulate tissue growth and generate blood vessels. The wound bed has the appearance of *granulation*. As the wound bed continues to regenerate, the wound edges begin to *contract* and move centrally to close the defect. Finally *epithelial regrowth* closes the defect.
Remodeling Phase: Begins at end of proliferative phase; may last as long as 2 years	Once deposition of new collagen is maximized (at approximately 3 weeks), macrophages stimulate a gradual replacement of the new, rapidly replaced collagen with mature collagen, which greatly increases the tensile strength of the wound.

Wound Classification	Description
Clean	Made under sterile conditions and not at risk for infection. Usually skin or vascular incisions
Clean-contaminated	Made under sterile conditions but involving the respiratory, gastrointestinal, genital, or urinary tracts without unusual contamination. Includes appendectomies, hysterectomies, cholecystectomies, and oropharyngeal surgeries
Contaminated	Exposed to contents of the gastrointestinal tract or infected fluids from the genitourinary systems. Also includes open, traumatic wounds such as lacerations, puncture wounds, and open fractures
Infected	Exposed to contaminants or exhibiting evidence of infection prior to surgery. Includes any traumatic wound because of the high risk for foreign body, bacteria, and chemical or other organic contaminant

Technique and Normal Findings (continued)	Abnormal Findings (continued)
Identify risk for skin breakdown, which is especially important in hospitalized or inactive patients. Many health care facilities use the Braden scale (Table 13-7) to assess risk in patients, with interventions based on the total score (Bergstrom, et al., 1987). Alternatively, the similar Norton scale includes incontinence and other variables (Norton, 1989).	The Braden scale scores patients from 1 to 4 in each of six subscales: sensory perception, moisture, activity, mobility, nutrition, and friction (Braden & Bergstrom, 1989). The Norton scale rates patients from 1 to 4 in each of five subscales: physical conditi on, mental condition, activity, mobility, and incontinence. A score <14 on the Norton scale or from 14 to 18 on the Braden scale indicates a high-risk of pressure ulcer development.
Classify the wound as partial or full thickness; if a pressure ulcer is present identify the stage. When assessing any ulcer, it is important to observe and document the size in depth and diameter, margins, condition of surrounding tissues, any varicosities or telengectasias, status of granulation tissue and epithelial growth, and any drainage, odor, or necrotic tissue. Describe the color and texture of the tissue. Identify the amount, color, consistency, and odor of exudate (drainage). Describe the location using appropriate landmarks. Use an objective tool to measure associated pain (see Chapter 7).	Pressure ulcers may be deep tissue, Stage I, Stage II, Stage III, Stage IV, or unstagable (Black, 2007). Stages I and II are partial thickness into the dermis. Stages III and IV are full thickness. Wound drainage is classified as serous (clear), sanguineous (bloody), serosanguineous (mixed), fibrinous (sticky yellow), or purulent (pus). Note any signs or symptoms of infection. See also Table 13-20 at the end of the chapter.

(text continues on page 282)

Table 13.7 The Braden Scale for Predicting Pressure Sore Risk

Patient Name: _____ Room Number: _____ Date: _____

Sensory Perception	1. Completely Limited	2. Very Limited	3. Slightly Limited	4. No Impairment	Indicate Appropriate Numbers Below
Ability to respond meaningfully to pressure-related discomfort	Unresponsive (does not moan, flinch or grasp) to painful stimuli, due to diminished level of consciousness or sedation. OR limited ability to feel pain over most of body surface.	Responds only to painful stimuli. Cannot communicate discomfort except by moaning or restlessness. OR has a sensory impairment which limits the ability to feel pain or discomfort over 1/2 of body.	Responds to verbal commands, but cannot always communicate discomfort or need to be turned. OR has some sensory impairment which limits ability to feel pain or discomfort in one or two extremities.	Responds to verbal commands. Has no sensory deficit which would limit ability to feel or voice pain or discomfort.	
Moisture	**1. Constantly Moist**	**2. Very Moist**	**3. Occasionally Moist**	**4. Rarely Moist**	
Degree to which skin is exposed to moisture	Skin is kept moist almost constantly by perspiration, urine, etc. Dampness is detected every time patient is moved or turned.	Skin is often, but not always, moist. Linen must be changed at least once a shift.	Skin is occasionally moist, requiring an extra linen change approximately once a day.	Skin is usually dry. Linen only requires changing at routine intervals.	
Activity	**1. Bedfast**	**2. Chairfast**	**3. Walks Occasionally**	**4. Walks Frequently**	
Degree of physical activity	Confined to bed.	Ability to walk severely limited or non-existent. Cannot bear own weight and/or must be assisted into chair or wheelchair	Walks occasionally during day, but for very short distances, with or without assistance. Spends majority of each shift in bed or chair	Walks outside the room at least twice a day and inside room at least once every 2 hours during waking hours.	
Mobility	**1. Completely Immobile**	**2. Very Limited**	**3. Slightly Limited**	**4. No Limitations**	
Ability to change and control body position	Does not make even slight changes in body or extremity position without assistance.	Makes occasional slight changes in body or extremity position but unable to make frequent or significant changes independently	Makes frequent though slight changes in body or extremity position independently	Makes major and frequent changes in position without assistance	
Nutrition	**1. Very Poor**	**2. Probably Inadequate**	**3. Adequate**	**4. Excellent**	
Usual food intake pattern	Never eats a complete meal. Rarely eats more than 1/3 of any food offered. Eats two servings or less of protein (meat or dairy products) per day. Takes fluids poorly. Does not take a liquid dietary supplement. OR is NPO and/or maintained on clear liquids or IVs for more than 5 days.	Rarely eats a complete meal and generally eats only about 1/2 of any food offered. Protein intake includes only three servings of meat or dairy products per day. Occasionally will take a dietary supplement. OR receives less than optimum amount of liquid diet or tube feeding.	Eats over half of most meals. Eats a total of four servings of protein (meat, dairy products) each day. Occasionally will refuse a meal, but will usually take a supplement if offered. OR is on a tube feeding or TPN regimen which probably meets most of nutritional needs.	Eats most of every meal. Never refuses a meal. Usually eats a total of four or more servings of meat and dairy products. Occasionally eats between meals. Does not require supplementation.	
Friction and Shear	**1. Problem**	**2. Potential Problem**	**3. No Apparent Problem**		
	Requires moderate to maximum assistance in moving. Complete lifting without sliding against sheets is impossible Frequently slides down in bed or chair, requiring frequent repositioning with maximum assistance. Spasticity, contractures or agitation lead to almost constant friction.	Moves feebly or requires minimum assistance. During a move, skin probably slides to some extent against sheets, chair restraints, or other devices. Maintains relatively good position in chair or bed most of the time, but occasionally slides down.	Moves in bed and in chair independently and has sufficient muscle strength to lift up completely during move. Maintains good position in bed or chair at all times.		

NOTE: 1. Bed and chairbound individuals or those with impaired ability to reposition should be assessed upon admission for their risk of developing pressure uclers. Patients with established pressure ulcers should be reassessed periodically. 2. Patients with a total score of 16 or less are considered to be at risk of developing pressure ulcers (15 or 16 = low risk; 13 or 14 = moderate risk; 12 or less = high risk). TPN, total parenteral nutrition; NPO, nothing by mouth.

Total Score: _____

Assess for nonpressure ulcers; note the characteristics of the wound.

Burns are classified based on depth of tissue destruction and percentage of total body surface area (TBSA) affected. Depth involves assessing vascular and sensory status and appearance and blanching of the burn. Assess blanching by applying pressure with a sterile cotton-tipped applicator and observing capillary refill time. Calculate the percentage of TBSA affected using the Wallace Rule of Nines (Fig. 13.11) or the Lund and Browder chart (Fig. 13.12).

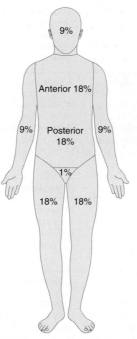

Figure 13.11 Wallace Rule of Nines to estimate percentage of TBSA burned in adults. Different areas are sectioned into numerical values related to nine (9). Note that the anterior and posterior head equate to 9% each.

Inspect each fingernail and toenail. Assess for color, thickness, and consistency. *Nails are smooth, translucent, and consistent in color and thickness. Longitudinal ridging is common in aging patients. Longitudinal pigmentation in dark-skinned patients is a normal variant.*

Have the patient place the fingernails of both index fingers together to assess the nail angle. *A diamond-shaped opening is visible between the two fingernails, indicating a nail angle of at least 160 degrees.*

Inspect the hair, noting color, consistency, distribution, areas of hair loss, and condition of the hair shaft. *Hair is equally and symmetrically distributed across the scalp. Hair shafts are smooth, shiny, of even consistency, and without evidence of breakage.*

Examples include neuropathic, venous (vascular), and arterial (vascular) ulcers. See Tables 13-21 and 13-22 at the end of this chapter.

Superficial burns involve the epidermal layers, superficial dermal burns involve the epidermis and part of the dermis, deep dermal burns involve the epidermis and all of the dermis, and total thickness burns involve all layers of the skin and may extend into the supportive fascia below (Hettiarachi & Papini, 2004). See also Table 13-23.

Relative percentage of body surface areas (% BSA) affected by growth

	0 yr	1 yr	5 yr	10 yr	15 yr
a—½ of head	9½	8½	6½	5½	4½
b—½ of 1 high	2¾	3¼	4	4¼	4½
c—½ of 1 lower leg	2½	2½	2¾	3	3¼

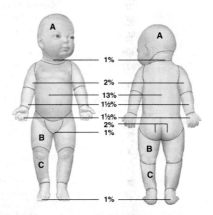

Figure 13.12 The Lund & Browder burn estimation chart. This chart and method for assigning percentage of burns are commonly used in pediatric populations.

Dietary deficiencies lead to splitting of nail tips (Fawcett, et al., 2005). Thickened nails may be from fungal infection. Discoloration of the nailbed may indicate trauma, fungal infection, or melanoma.

Clubbing of the nails indicates chronic hypoxia. Clubbing is identified when the angle of the nail to the finger is more than 160 degrees (see Table 13-9). Also see Table 13-24 at the end of the chapter for common nail abnormalities.

In female patients, ovarian dysfunction may be characterized by hair on the beard area, abdomen, upper back, shoulders, sternum, and inner upper thighs.

Note areas of decreased or absent hair. Parting the hair enables visualization of the scalp skin. Note any lesions or color changes there. *Scalp skin is of consistent color with the rest of the body.* Observe hair shafts near the root for lice or nits.

Brittle or broken hair shafts may indicate endocrine or metabolic dysfunction. Lice or their nits (eggs) may be on the hair shaft. The closer to the scalp the nit is located, the more recent the infestation. Excessive dryness and scaling of the scalp is often present in *seborrheic dermatitis*. See Table 13-25 at the end of this chapter.

Palpation

Using the dorsal surface of the hands, assess skin temperature. *Skin temperature is consistently warm or cool and appropriate, considering the environmental temperature.*

Further assess any areas of increased temperature for lesions, swelling, and color changes.

Using the palmar surface of the fingers and hands, assess for skin moisture and texture. *Moisture is consistent throughout, with evenly smooth skin texture.*

Excessive dryness may be from frequent bathing or *hyperthyroidism*. Excessive moisture may signify a problem with temperature regulation. Cracked or fissured skin may indicate hydration disorders, infections, or chemical injuries.

Assess skin turgor. Gently grasp a fold of the patient's skin between your fingers and pull up. Then, release. This is easiest performed on the dorsal surface of the patient's hand or lower arm, but the most accurate reflection of turgor in the adult is on the anterior chest, just below the midclavicular area (Dains, et al., 2007). *The skin promptly recoils to its normal position.*

A persistent pinch, or **tenting**, indicates dehydration.

Assess for vascularity by applying direct pressure to the skin surface with the pads of your fingers. This will cause the skin to blanche, or pale, in comparison with surrounding skin. *On releasing your finger, color promptly returns to normal.*

Decreased vascular supply is often initially found in the extremities, particularly the hands and feet. Delayed return of skin color to normal after direct pressure indicates decreased circulation. Altered circulation can result in pallor or rubor of an extremity.

Palpate lesions for tenderness, mobility, and consistency. Apply gentle pressure and attempt to move the skin under your finger. *Skin shifts slightly without adherence.*

Tenderness of a lesion or dermatitis may indicate infection. Lesions seemingly fixed in place may be cancerous. Consistency of skin lesions will assist in diagnosis of the problem.

Palpate each fingernail and toenail. *Nails are smooth, nontender, and firmly adherent to the nail bed. Lateral and proximal folds are nontender and nonswollen.*

Swelling, redness, or tenderness in the lateral or proximal folds may indicate *paronychia*. Sponginess of the nail bed may indicate clubbing.

Palpate the hair. *Hair is smooth.* Grasp 10–12 hairs and gently pull. *Just a few hairs are in your hand.*

Note excessive hair loss (more than six hairs) and then assess for presence or absence of the hair bulb. Absent hair bulb may indicate chemical damage to the hair shaft (excessive coloration). Presence of the hair bulb may indicate endocrine dysfunction.

Documentation of Normal Findings

Skin evenly colored, smooth, soft, consistently warm, with intact turgor. No suspicious lesions. Nails smooth and translucent, lateral and proximal folds without swelling or erythema. Hair smooth texture, symmetrically distributed on the scalp, consistent coloration and hydration, without evidence of excessive breakage or loss. Scalp with consistent pigmentation, no lesions noted. *M. Olson, RN*

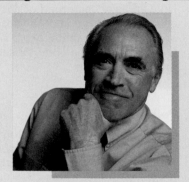

The nurse has just finished a physical examination of Mr. Stoli, the 65-year-old patient with a venous ulcer secondary to PVD. Unlike the samples of normal documentation previously charted, Mr. Stoli has abnormal findings. Review the following important findings revealed in each step of objective data collection for Mr. Stoli. Consider how these results compare with normal findings. Note that inspection is the major technique used in wound assessment.

Inspection: A 6 × 8 cm wound on left lateral ankle above the medial maleolus. Irregular wound margins with some pallor at the edges. Wound is partial thickness with 80% beefy red and 20% yellow. Large fibrinous exudate on dressing. Left leg skin hyperpigmented and ruddy. Some flaking is present, no hair on leg. 3+ edema, capillary refill 4 seconds. Full range of motion present, strength 2+ and slightly decreased.

Palpation: Leg is cool, sensation decreased.

L. Lee, RN

 Lifespan Considerations

Pregnant Women

Common skin findings in pregnant women include *melasma, striae gravidarum* (stretch marks), *spider telangiectasias, and hyperpigmentation* (American Pregnancy Association, 2008). Others include enlargement of preexisting keloids; edema of the face, legs, and hands; rapid nail growth; and increased nail brittleness (March of Dimes, 2008). During pregnancy, women may report rapid hair growth; during the postpartum period, they may experience excessive hair loss (March of Dimes, 2008).

Abnormal skin findings in pregnancy include *pyogenic granuloma, erythema nodosum,* and *pruritic urticarial papules and plaques of pregnancy* (PUPPP) (Hebel, 2006) (Fig. 13.13). Pyogenic granuloma commonly arises during the late second or third trimester and develops rapidly over a few weeks (Pierson & Pierson, 2006). In pregnancy, it usually appears on the oral mucosa or lips as a glistening red papule or nodule that bleeds easily if traumatized. *Erythema nodosum* presents as 2- to 6-cm tender, red, painful nodules usually on the extensor surfaces of the lower extremities. The lesions usually resolve postpartum. *PUPPP* is a benign disorder of the third trimester, usually in first or multiple-gestation pregnancies, and is characterized by intensely pruritic reddish papules and plaques within striae gravidarum.

Newborns, Infants, Children, and Adolescents

Evaluation for cyanosis is part of the Apgar scoring done at 1 and 5 minutes after birth (see Chapter 6). The more cyanotic the appearance, the lower is the score and thus the greater indication of compromised circulation. Cyanosis on the hands and feet that persists for several days after birth can be a normal response to cool environmental temperatures. Bluish mottling of the skin, known as *cutis marmorata,* is from chilling or stress. Some newborns exhibit a harlequin color change, usually seen when lying on the side, with the dependent half

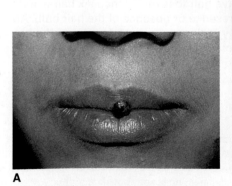
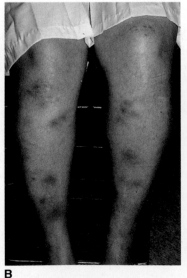
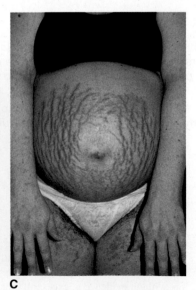

A   **B**   **C**

Figure 13.13 **A.** Pyogenic granuloma. **B.** Erythema nodosum. **C.** PUPPP.

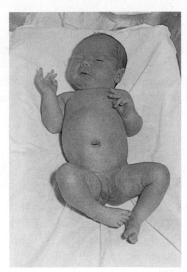

Figure 13.14 Jaundice.

of the body a darker pink color while the upper half is paler (AWHONN, 2006). Jaundice may be evident within 24 hours of birth from the immature liver's inability to breakdown bilirubin for excretion. Jaundice disappears once the liver can process bilirubin effectively (usually 5 to 10 days after birth) (Lowdermilk & Perry, 2007). To verify jaundice, apply light pressure to the skin to cause blanching. Jaundice does not blanche, while yellowish skin tones from other causes turns white. *Physiologic jaundice* occurs after 24 hours and persists approximately 72 hours. Jaundice is always considered pathologic if it appears in the first 24 hours of birth (Fig. 13.14).

Pigmented lesions (eg, *nevus flammeus, cavernous hemangioma, strawberry hemangioma, capillary hemangioma*) are common in newborns. Café au lait spots larger than 3 cm or more than six café au lait lesions are associated with severe illness. See also Chapter 28.

At birth, a newborn's skin is flushed and appears a deep red. By the second day of life, the skin becomes pink, flaky, and dry. Skin is usually thin and almost transparent, especially in premature newborns. Vernix or lanugo may appear, depending on gestational age. *Milia* are tiny white papules on the cheeks, chin, and nose of newborns. They result from distended sebaceous glands, and generally resolve spontaneously in a few weeks or months. *Erythema toxicum* is a pink papular, vesicular, and occasionally pustular rash on the trunk and extending outward. Lesions of erythema toxicum are surrounded by an erythematous, blotchy halo and usually resolve spontaneously. Ecchymoses may be from birth trauma. It is common to observe edema of the eyes, scrotum, and labia in neonates. See also Chapter 28.

△ SAFETY ALERT 13.1

Cyanosis in a newborn lasting longer than 20 minutes after birth is a critical indicator of increased risk for morbidity and mortality. Progressive jaundice, pallor, cracked or peeling skin, café au lait spots larger than 3 cm or more than 6 in number, or stiff, immobile skin (sclerema) are indications of greater risk for morbidity and mortality.

Assessing hydration status in infants and children should not rely on turgor evaluation alone. It is best to assess capillary refill, turgor, and respiratory pattern. Turgor in newborns, infants, and young children is best evaluated by gently pinching a fold of abdominal skin and watching the skin recoil to its normal state (Steiner, et al., 2004). Turgor in the older child or adolescent can be assessed on the medial aspect of the lower forearm or on the infraclavicular area as in an adult. Capillary refill is assessed by applying just enough pressure to the nail bed to cause blanching. Normal capillary refill occurs in less than 2 seconds.

△ SAFETY ALERT 13.2

Capillary refill requiring more than 4 seconds indicates severe dehydration.

Infants and young children with yellowish palms, soles, and face, but not sclerae, may have carotenemia from excessive ingestion of yellow or orange vegetables or chronic renal disease. Skin findings in children are commonly the result of an infectious process, such as varicella, roseola, rubella, measles, or erythema infectiosum. All these conditions present with systemic symptoms and skin lesions (O'Connor, et al., 2008). See Table 13-9 for commonly observed lesions related to viral, bacterial, or fungal infections.

Pubertal adolescents will have maturation of the apocrine glands in the axillae and genitalia areas with production of malodorous sweat. Sebaceous gland secretion increases, as does the predisposition to acne lesions.

Older Adults

As discussed earlier, common skin assessment findings for older adults include decreased elasticity, thinness, excessive dryness, and lesions associated with aging such as seborrheic *keratosis, actinic keratosis,* and *lentigines* (Merck Manual of Geriatrics, 2006). In addition, they are at increased risk for skin cancer, abnormal ecchymoses or purpuric lesions, and trauma.

Evidence-based Critical Thinking

Integumentary findings often reflect the status of other systems (see Table 13-9). Nurses must constantly observe the skin while assessing other systems and interpret skin findings in conjunction with other systemic findings to determine underlying function. Interpreting these findings assists in planning appropriate interventions and making necessary referrals.

Common Laboratory and Diagnostic Testing

Once a dermatologic problem has been identified, inspected, and palpated, one of several laboratory tests may be indicated to determine the most effective treatment. A superficial scraping of disordered skin for microscopic examination may help to identify type of lesion. If exudate or signs of infection are present, a culture and sensitivity test may reveal specific organisms. For suspected fungal infections, a culture using a preparation of potassium hydroxide (KOH) may confirm diagnosis. The Wood's light test may diagnose scalp infections caused by a particular group of spore-producing microorganisms. The spores, located on hair strands, fluoresce apple green under the Wood's light. Special skin tests (eg, patch tests) may detect sensitivity to allergens.

Biopsy of skin tissue is indicated for those disorders that manifest changes in color, size, or shape. Nonhealing lesions, abnormal growths, or tumors are also biopsied. Nursing responsibilities include preprocedure discussion with the patient regarding the reason for the biopsy, procedure involved, and time required for results. The nurse also ensures that the patient signs consent forms. He or she assists with procedures, ensures samples are appropriately labeled, applies necessary dressings, and gives postoperative instructions to the patient.

Diagnostic Reasoning

Nursing Diagnosis, Outcomes, and Interventions

When formulating a nursing diagnosis, it is important to use critical thinking to cluster data and identify patterns that fit together. The nurse compares these data clusters with defining characteristics (abnormal findings) for the diagnosis to ensure the most accurate labeling and appropriate interventions. See Table 13-8 (NANDA, 2009).

Nurses use assessment information to identify patient outcomes. Some outcomes related to integumentary problems include the following:

• Skin and mucous membranes are intact.
• Patient reports no altered sensation or pain at site.
• Patient demonstrates measures to protect and heal the skin (Moorhead, et al., 2007).

Once outcomes are established, interventions are enacted to improve the patient's status. The nurse uses critical thinking and evidence-based practice to develop them. Some examples for integumentary care are as follows:

• Assess skin and risk for skin breakdown.
• Change dressing as ordered with topical agent that promotes a moist healing environment.
• Evaluate for specialty mattress (Bulechek, et al., 2007).

Table 13.8	Common Nursing Diagnoses Associated with the Integumentary System		
Diagnosis and Related Factors	**Point of Differentiation**	**Assessment Characteristics**	**Nursing Interventions**
Impaired skin integrity	Alterations in or damage to one or more layers of the skin	Wound, surgical incision, break in skin integrity	Classify wound as partial or full thickness (stage I or II). Document wound assessment. Assess for risk of skin breakdown. Apply appropriate dressing. Evaluate for use of specialty mattress. Avoid positioning over bony prominences.
Impaired tissue integrity	Damage to tissues of the subcutaneous layer of the skin, mucous membrane, cornea, or all of these	Damaged or destroyed subcutaneous, muscle, bone, mucous membrane, or corneal tissues	Determine size and depth of wound (stage III or IV), skin around wound, continence status, tube/incision placement. Apply appropriate dressing. Collaborate with physician on necessary débridement and surgical intervention.*
Pain related to tissue injury and treatments	An unpleasant sensory and emotional experience directly related to skin or tissue damage	Self report of pain is subjective. Expressions are variable and include facial grimace, guarding, muscle tension, tachycardia, tachypnea, and nausea (see Chapter 7).	Use pain scale to identify current pain intensity and effectiveness of medication. Develop pain goal with patient. Provide pain medications as ordered.* Provide alternatives such as distraction, breathing, and relaxation.
Risk for infection	At risk for pathogenic organisms from break in the skin or tissue, the body's primary defense	Break in skin integrity, tubes and procedures, exposure to pathogens, malnutrition, inadequate immunity, chronic disease	Practice frequent handwashing and universal precautions. Protect wound with dressing. Monitor for fever, elevated WBCs, wound drainage, or erythema. Discontinue tubes as soon as possible. Encourage adequate nutrition.

*Collaborative interventions.

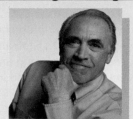

Analyzing Findings

Mr. Stoli's problems have been outlined throughout this chapter. Initial subjective and objective data collection is complete, and the nurse has spent time reviewing findings and results. The following note illustrates how the nurse collects and analyzes subjective and objective data and develops interventions.

Subjective: States throbbing 4/10 pain that increases when legs are dependent and with ambulation, decreases when lying in bed. Refuses medication for pain. States "Those pills make me sleepy, and I don't like that."

Objective: Grimacing with movement. Ambulates in room to bathroom, sits in chair for meals with legs elevated. A 6 × 8 cm wound on left lateral ankle above the medial maleolus. Irregular wound margins with some pallor at the edges. Tissue 80% beefy red and 20% yellow. Large fibrinous exudate on dressing. Left leg skin hyperpigmented and ruddy. Some flaking is present, no hair growth. 3+ edema, capillary refill 4 seconds. Leg is cool, sensation decreased. Full range of motion, strength 2+ and slightly decreased.

Analysis: Impaired skin integrity related to venous impairment as evidenced by ulcer on left lateral ankle. Pain related to ulcer.

Plan: Hydrocolloid dressing changed. Consult with wound care nurse about placement of wound vacuum. Elevate legs when awake. Monitor temperature every 4 hours. Monitor wound for signs of infection, drainage, increased pain, and erythema. Encourage 1 L of fluid a day and 50% of meals.

Critical Thinking Challenge

- What type of ongoing assessment would you predict?
- How should the nurse address the issue of pain assessment and management?
- What teaching should the nurse provide related to venous stasis, ulcer, and treatment?

Collaboration with Other Health Care Providers

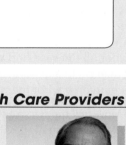

In many facilities, nurses initiate referrals based on assessment data. Findings that might increase urgency of a referral include decreased vascularity, new infection, and increased pressure/shearing forces (Gorst, et al., 2008). Wound and ostomy nurses are available for consultation on complex wounds, ostomy management, and monitoring for pressure ulcers.

A wound care consult is indicated for placement of the wound vacuum. The following conversation illustrates how the nurse might organize data and make recommendations about Mr. Stoli when the wound care nurse arrives.

Situation: Hello. I'm taking care of Mr. Stoli. He's 65 years old and was admitted yesterday for placement of a wound vacuum because his left ulcer isn't healing.

Background: He has a history of PVD, high blood pressure, and diabetes. Blood pressure and diabetes have been under fairly good control. He's had the ulcer for about 3 months, and the physician would like a wound vac applied. Mr. Stoli can potentially go home with it tomorrow.

Assessment: The wound doesn't look infected. It's fairly clean and about 6 × 8 cm just above his left medial maleolus. He's fairly independent and eager to get home. He also doesn't like taking pain medications because they make him drowsy.

Recommendations: When you place his wound vac, I think that you might discuss how he can manage with it at home. His wife should be there, so that will be a good teaching opportunity. He's really anxious to get back home, so if you can work with him to get prepared, he'll appreciate it. He prefers to be as independent as possible.

Critical Thinking Challenge

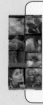

- Why is the information on the wound assessment summarized in this verbal communication versus the level of detail in the documentation?
- What other assessments might be performed related to the patient's history?
- What further assessment information might need collection before discharge?

Pulling It All Together: Reflection and Critical Thinking

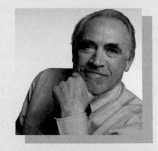

The nurse uses assessment data to formulate a nursing care plan with patient outcomes and interventions for Mr. Stoli. After interventions are completed, the nurse reevaluates Mr. Stoli and documents findings in the chart to show progress. The nurse uses critical thinking and judgment to continue or revise diagnoses, outcomes, or interventions. This is often in a form similar to the one below.

Nursing Diagnosis	Patient Outcomes	Nursing Interventions	Rationales	Evaluation
Impaired skin integrity related to venous stasis as evidenced by ulcer on left lateral malleolus	Patient demonstrates understanding of the plan to heal skin and prevent reinjury.	Teach care for wound vacuum. Initiate home care consultation. Teach patient signs of healing, infection, and complications. Involve wife in care.	Knowledge of the function and purpose of the wound vacuum promotes patient autonomy. He should know when to call the physician if the wound is worsening.	Patient and wife asked multiple questions about wound vacuum at home; especially related to mobility. Wife appreciates home health visit and looks forward to patient returning home.

Applying Your Knowledge

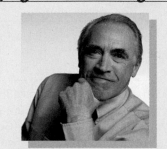

Using the previous steps of diagnostic reasoning, organizing, and prioritizing, consider all the case findings woven through this chapter. When answering the following questions, begin drawing conclusions and see how pieces of assessment work together to create an environment for personalized, appropriate, and accurate care.

- How will the nurse assess and document Mr. Stoli's wound and peripheral circulation?
- What information will the nurse collect to assess risk for skin breakdown related to hospitalization?
- In what circumstances would the nurse refer Mr. Stoli to a wound care nurse? How would the nurse communicate information to the wound care nurse?
- Once the patient is discharged, what data would a nurse performing follow-up home care need to collect? How would that nurse assess if the wound was healing?

Key Points

- Skin assessment findings reflect overall health, hydration, and nutritional status.
- Skin color variations largely result from the amounts and proportions of eumalanin and phemoalin produced by the melanocytes.
- Skin changes during pregnancy include melasma, linea nigra, increased sebaceous and cutaneous gland function, and hair loss following pregnancy.
- Loss of elastin, collagen, and subcutaneous fat result in decreased resilience, sagging, wrinkling, and increased fragility of the skin in the older adult.
- The ABCDEs of melanoma detection include Asymmetry, irregular Border, Color, Diameter of more than 6 mm, and Evolution of the lesion over time.

- Skin self-examination assists patients to identify problematic lesions.
- Common integumentary symptoms include pruritis, rash, and lesions or wounds.
- Coining and cupping are self treatments performed as cultural home remedies.
- Skin assessment involves inspection of general color, texture, moisture, turgor, and temperature and focused inspection and palpation of rashes, lesions, or wounds.
- When assessing a lesion, identify configuration, pattern, morphology, size, distribution, and exact body location.
- Assess a wound for location, size, color, texture, drainage, margins, surrounding skin, and healing status.
- Depth of a burn can be superficial, superficial-dermal, dermal, or full thickness.

- Assessment of the nails and hair is performed as a part of the skin assessment.
- Abnormal skin findings include infection, inflammation, infestation, growths and tumors, trauma, and ulcers.
- Common nursing diagnoses related to the integumentary system include impaired skin integrity, impaired tissue integrity, pain, and risk for infection.

Review Questions

1. The nurse is admitting a 75-year-old man with a 50-year history of smoking one pack of cigarettes per day. Among the patient's concerns is his chronic shortness of breath. One nail finding that demonstrates chronic hypoxia is
   A. pitting
   B. thickening and discoloration of the nailbed
   C. clubbing
   D. brittleness and cracking of the nails

2. All of the following skin lesions are papular except
   A. warts
   B. acne
   C. moles
   D. herpes zoster

3. The ABCDs of melanoma identification include all of the following except
   A. A (asymmetry): one half does not match the other half
   B. B (birthmark): recently changed in appearance
   C. C (color): pigmentation is not uniform; there may be shades of tan, brown, and black as well as red, white, and blue
   D. D (diameter): greater than 6 mm

4. A nurse observes a skin lesion with well-defined borders on the upper left thigh. It is 1.5 cm in diameter, flat, hypopigmented, and nonpalpable. What is the correct terminology for this lesion?
   A. Patch
   B. Plaque
   C. Papule
   D. Macule

5. When assessing hydration in an infant, the nurse would
   A. pinch a fold of skin on the medial aspect of the forearm and observe for recoil to normal.
   B. pinch a fold of skin on the abdomen and observe for recoil to normal.
   C. pinch a fold of skin just below the midpoint of one of the clavicles and allow the skin to recoil to normal
   D. pinch a fold of skin on the head and allow for skin to recoil in children.

6. A fair-skinned, blonde, 18-year-old woman is at the clinic for a skin examination. She reports that she always turns red within 10 minutes of going outside. She is planning a trip to Mexico and wants to avoid getting sunburned. What would the nurse teach the patient?
   A. Excessive exposure to UVA and UVB rays increases risk of sunburn and skin cancer.
   B. Apply a sunscreen or sunblock at least 15 to 30 minutes prior to sun exposure.
   C. Avoid sun exposure between 10 AM and 4 PM to reduce UVA and UVB exposure.
   D. All of the above.

7. An 8-year-old patient presents to the clinic with erythematous vesicles on the face and chest. Some vesicles have broken open, revealing a moist, shallow ulcerated surface; some have scabbed over. The nurse suspects which of the following infectious illnesses?
   A. Varicella
   B. Measles
   C. Roseola
   D. Herpes simplex

8. A 24-year-old patient reports an itchy red rash under her breasts. Examination reveals large, reddened, moist patches under both breasts in the skin folds. Several smaller, raised, red lesions surround the edges of the larger patch. What is the correct terminology for the distribution pattern of these smaller lesions?
   A. Satellite
   B. Discrete
   C. Confluent
   D. Zosteriform

9. A 22-year-old patient presents to the clinic with a large firm mass on her left earlobe. She had her ears pierced approximately 3 weeks ago. The mass began as a small bump and progressively enlarged to its current size of approximately 1 inch in diameter. It is not tender, reddened, or seeping any drainage. What is the term used to describe this secondary skin lesion?
   A. Crust
   B. Lichenification
   C. Keloid
   D. Scale

10. An 83-year-old woman is undergoing a routine physical examination. Which of the following assessment findings would the nurse consider an expected age-related variation?
    A. Thinning of the skin
    B. Increased skin turgor
    C. Hypopigmented, flat macules and patches over sun-exposed areas
    D. Multiple purplish bruises on the arms and legs

11. A patient has several red, inflamed, superficial, palpable lesions containing a thickened yellowish substance. How would the nurse document this lesion?

A. Papule
B. Pustule
C. Cyst
D. Vesicle

References

AWHONN. (2006). *Module 5: The newborn skin and skin care.* Retrieved March 27, 2008, from www.awhonn.org/awhonn/binary.content.do?name=Resources/Documents/pdf/NOEP/NOEP_Mod5_Preview.pdf

Alaiti, S. (2007). *Hair anatomy.* Retrieved January 20, 2008, from http://www.emedicine.com/ent/TOPIC10.HTM

American Academy of Dermatology. (2004). *Tattoos, body piercings, and other skin adornments.* Retrieved May 31, 2008, from http://www.aad.org/public/publications/pamphlets/cosmetic_tattoos.html

American Academy of Dermatology. (2007a). *Skin cancer: A fact of life in skin of color.* Retrieved March 20, 2008, from http://www.skincarephysicians.com/SkinCancerNet/skin_of_color.html

American Academy of Dermatology. (2007b). *Be sun smart.* Retrieved March 20, 2008, from http://www.aad.org/public

American Academy of Dermatology. (2008). *Skin self examination.* Retrieved March 20, 2008, from http://www.skincarephysicians.com/skincancernet/skin_examinations

American Cancer Society. (2008). *Detailed guide: Skin cancer—melanoma.* Retrieved March 30, 2008, from http://www.cancer.org

American Pregnancy Association. (2010). *Skin changes during pregnancy.* Retrieved May 23, 2010, from http://www.americanpregnancy.org/pregnancyhealth/skinchanges.html

Barrett, S. (2008). *A sensitive subject: Defining photosensitivity.* Retrieved March 20, 2008, from http://www.sun-wellness.com/articles/251column1.html

Barsh, G. (2003). What controls variation in human skin color? *PLoS Biology, 1*(1). Retrieved March 30, 2008, from http://biology.plosjournals.org/perlserv/?request=get-document&doi=10.1371/journal.pbio.0000027

Bergstrom, N., Braden, B. J., Laguzza, A., & Holman, V. (1987). The Braden Scale for predicting pressure sore risk. *Nursing Research, 36,* 205.

Black, J., Baharestani, M., Cuddigan, J., et al. (2007). National Pressure Ulcer Advisory Panel's updated pressure ulcer staging system. *Dermatological Nursing, 19*(4), 343–349.

Braden, B., & Bergstrom, N. (1989). Clinical utility of the Braden scale for predicting pressure sore risk. *Decubitus, 2*(3), 44–51.

Brannon, H. (2006). *The biology of hair. Your guide to skin & beauty.* Retrieved January 21, 2008, from http://dermatology.about.com/cs/hairanatomy/a/hairbiology.htm

Bulechek, G. B., Butcher, H. K., & McCloskey Dochterman, J. (2007). *Nursing interventions classification (NIC)* (4th ed.). St. Louis, MO: Mosby.

Bulliard, J.-L., De Weck, D., Fisch, T., Bordoni, A., & Levi, F. (2007). Detailed site distribution of melanoma and sunlight exposure: Aetiological patterns from a Swiss series. *Annals of Oncology.* Advance Access accessed on September 17, 1008.

Craven, R., & Hirnle, C. (2008). *Fundamentals of nursing: Health and human function* (6th ed.). Philadelphia: Lippincott Williams & Wilkins.

Cronin, T. (2003). Tattoos, body piercings and other skin adornments. *Skin & Aging, 11*(4), 48–52.

Dains, J., Baumann, L., & Scheibel, P. (2007). *Advanced health assessment and clinical diagnosis in primary care* (3rd ed.). St. Louis, MO: Mosby.

Environmental Protection Agency. (2008). *UV index.* Retrieved March 20, 2008, from http://epa.gov/sunwise/uvindex.html

Ethnomed. (2008). *Self teaching module for the influence of culture on skin conditions in children.* Retrieved September 17, 2008, from http://ethnomed.org/ethnomed/clin_topics/dermatology/pigmented_main.html

Eustice, C., & Eustice, R. (2007). *Sun sensitivity can be side effect of some medications.* Retrieved March 20, 2008, from http://arthritis.about.com

Fawcett, R., Linford, S., & Stulberg, D. (2005). Nail abnormalities: Clues to systemic Disease. *American Family Physician, 69*(6), 1417–1424.

Gorst, R., Bagg, G., Albert, M., & Couture, N. (2008). *The interdisciplinary urgency tool – A comprehensive wound-care referral form.* Retrieved July 15, 2008, from http://www.cawc.net/open/wcc/1-1/gorst.html

Guthrie Ambulatory Health Care Clinic Pharmacy. (2008). *Sunless sunburn.* Retrieved March 20, 2008, from http://www.drum.amedd.army.mil/CLINIC/Pharmacy/sunless_sunburn.htm

Healthy People 2010: What are its goals? (n.d.). Retrieved January 7, 2007, from http://www.healthypeople.gov/About/goals.htm

Hebel, J. (2006). Erythema nodosum. *eMedicine.* Retrieved July 4, 2008, from http://www.emedicine.com/derm/topic138.htm

Hemenway, M. (2006). Skin cancer: Skin color doesn't matter. *EastWest Magazine.* Retrieved June 8, 2008, from http://www.eastwestmagazine.com/content/view/39/40

Hettiarachi, S., & Papini, R. (2004). Initial management of a major burn: II-assessment and resuscitation. *British Medical Journal, 329,* 101–103.

Hogan, D. J. (2007). Contact dermatitis, irritant. Retrieved September 17, 2008, from http://www.emedicine.com/DERM/topic85.htm

Juckett, G. (2005). Cross-cultural medicine. *American Family Physician, 72*(11), 2267–2274.

Kahana, M., Feldman, M., Abudi, Z., & Yurman, S. (1995). The incidence of birthmarks in Israeli neonates. *International Journal of Dermatology, 34*(10), 704–706.

Kamel, M. (1998). Anatomy of the skin. In *The electronic textbook of dermatology.* Retrieved January 20, 2008, from http://www.telemedicine.org/anatomy/anatomy.htm

Lowdermilk, D. L., & Perry, S. E. (2007). Maternity & women's health care (9th ed.). St. Louis, MO: Elsevier.

March of Dimes. (2008). *Pregnancy & newborn health education center: Skin changes.* Retrieved May 10, 2008, from http://www.marchofdimes.com/pnhec/159_15294.asp

Mayo Staff. (2008). Tattoos: Risks and precautions to know first. Retrieved May 10, 2008, from http://www.mayoclinic.com/health/tattoos-and-piercings/MC00020

McKinnon, H., & Howard, T. (2000). Evaluating the febrile patient with a rash. *American Family Physician, 62*(4), 804–816.

Merck Manual of Diagnosis and Therapy. (2005). *Contact dermatitis.* Retrieved March 31, 2008, from http://www.merck.com/mmpe/sec10/ch114/ch114c.html

Merck Manual of Geriatrics (2006). *Age-related changes in skin structure and function.* Retrieved May 10, 2008, from http://www.merck.com/mkgr/mmg/sec15/ch122/ch122b.jsp

Mercandetti, M., & Cohen, A. (2008). Wound healing, healing and repair. *eMedicine*. Retrieved July 6, 2008, from http://www.emedicine.com/plastic/TOPIC411.HTM

Moorhead, S., Johnson, M., & Maas, M. (2007). *Nursing outcomes classification (NOC)* (4th ed.). St. Louis, MO: Mosby.

National Cancer Institute. (2003). *What you need to know about melanoma*. Retrieved June 8, 2008, from http://www.cancer.gov/cancertopics/wyntk/melanoma/page7

National Pressure Ulcer Advisory Panel. (2007). *Updated staging system*. Retrieved July 4, 2008, from http://www.npuap.org/pr2.htm

North American Nursing Diagnosis Association. (2009). *Nursing diagnoses, 2009–2011 Edition: Definitions and classifications (NANDA NURSING DIAGNOSIS)*. West Sussex, UK: John Wiley & Sons.

Norton, D. (1989). Calculating the risk: Reflections on the Norton scale. *Decubitus, 2*, 24.

O'Connor, N., McLaughlin, M., & Ham, P. (2008). Newborn skin: Part 1. Common rashes. Retrieved March 27, 2008, from http://www.aafp.org/afp/20080101/47.html

Ortonne, J. (2002). Photoprotective properties of skin melanin. *British Journal of Dermatology, 146*(Suppl. 61), 7–10.

Parrillo, S. (2008). *Steven-Johnson syndrome*. Retrieved May 10, 2008, from www.emedicine.com/emerg/topic555.htm.

Parsad, D., & Kumarasinge, S. (2006). *Psycho-social implications of pigmentary disorders in Asia*. Retrieved June 8, 2008, from http://paspcr.med.umn.edu/Commentary/Parsad_Kumarasingecommentary.pdf

Pierson, J., & Pierson, D. (2006). *Pyogenic granuloma (lobar capillary hemangioma)*. Retrieved July 4, 2008, at www.emedicine.com/derm/topic368.htm.

Revis, D., & Seagle, M. (2006). *Skin, anatomy*. Retrieved January 16, 2008, from http://www.emedicine.com/plastic/TOPIC389.HTM

Smith, R. N., Mann, N. J., Braue, A, et al. (2007). A low-glycemic-load diet improves symptoms in acne vulgaris patients: A randomized controlled trial. *American Journal of Clinical Nutrition, 86*(1), 107–115.

Steiner, M., DeWalt, D., & Byerley, J. (2004). Is this child dehydrated? *Journal of the American Medical Association, 291*(22), 2746–2754.

U.S. Environmental Protection Agency. (2009). *Sunwise program*. Retrieved March 30, 2008, from http://www.epa.gov/sunwise

U.S. Food and Drug Administration. (2009). Retrieved May 23, 2010, from, http://www.fda.gov/RadiationEmittingProducts/RadiationEmittingProductsandProcedures/Tanning/ucm116445.htm

World Health Organization. (n.d.). *Ultraviolet radiation and the INTERSUN Programme*. Retrieved March 30, 2008, from http://www.who.int/uv/intersunprogramme

Wound Care Information Network. (2008). *Phases of wound healing*. Retrieved July 6, 2008, from http://medicaledu.com/phases.htm

Zouboulis, C. C., Chen, W. C., Thornton, M. J., Qin, K., & Rosenfield, R. (2007). Sexual hormones in human skin. *Hormone and Metabolic Research, 39*(2), 85–95.

The Jensen suite offers these additional resources to enhance learning and facilitate understanding of this chapter:

- thePoint on line resource, http//thepoint.lww.com/Jensen1E
- Student CD-ROM included with the book
- *Laboratory Manual for Nursing Health Assessment: A Best Practice Approach*
- *Pocket Guide for Nursing Health Assessment: A Best Practice Approach*

Tables of Abnormal Findings

Integument Finding	Associated Disorder	Other Considerations/Depictions
Cardiovascular		
Flushing	Increased permeability of the peripheral capillaries, as with *fever*	May be normal with exercise
Pallor (shown)	Decreased arterial blood flow of *arterial insufficiency*	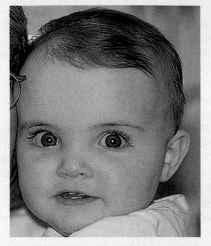
Rubor and brawny skin	Decreased venous return in *venous insufficiency*	Skin is cool or cold over areas of decreased circulation.
Cyanosis (shown)	*Circumoral cyanosis* in *congestive heart failure* or *chronic obstructive pulmonary disease* *Peripheral cyanosis* in areas of impaired circulation with oxygenated blood	Bluish skin discoloration occurs in areas of decreased blood flow or poor blood oxygenation. Cyanosis in dark-skinned patients is not readily observed on the skin, but can be assessed in buccal mucosa or conjunctivae. 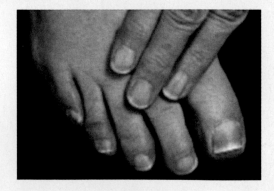
Fingernail clubbing	Disease states with prolonged hypoxia (eg, *emphysema*)	
Gastrointestinal		
Thinning of the skin, hair, and nails and hair loss	Nutritional deficiencies, inadequate absorption of vitamins A, B$_6$ (riboflavin), and C	

Table 13.9 **Manifestations in Integument of Systemic Disorders** (*continued*)

Integument Finding	Associated Disorder	Other Considerations/Depictions
Jaundice (yellow discoloration of the skin, sclera, or buccal mucosa; shown)	Liver disease	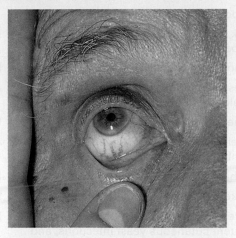
Pigmented macules (shown)	Peutz-Jeghers' disease	Pigmented areas may be on hands, lips, or buccal mucosa. 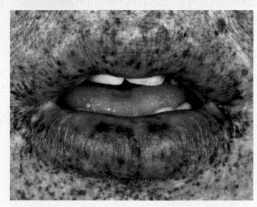
Facial flushing	Gastrointestinal cancers	
Genitourinary		
Uremic frost	Marked renal failure	Results from precipitation of renal urea and nitrogen waste products through sweat onto skin
Hirsutism (shown)	Polycystic ovarian syndrome	Affected women show male-pattern hair distribution, usually on face, chest, abdomen, or genital area. 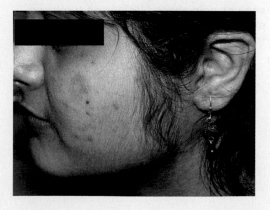

(table continues on page 294)

Table 13.9 Manifestations in Integument of Systemic Disorders *(continued)*

Integument Finding	Associated Disorder	Other Considerations/Depictions
Endocrine		
Thick, coarse hair, dry skin, and cool skin temperature	Hypothyroidism	See Chapter 6.
Smooth skin, thin, silky hair, and brittle nails	Hyperthyroidism	See Chapter 6.
Excessive hair growth or thinning; development of or worsening of acne	Androgen disorders	
Striae	Cushing's syndrome	
Hyperpigmentation of skin and mucous membranes; nevi	Addison's disease	
Flushing	Pheochromocytoma	
Thickened skin	Pituitary tumor	
Decreased sweating (hypohidrosis), frequent cutaneous yeast infections, and hair loss on distal extremities	Diabetes mellitus	
Acanthosis nigricans (hyperpigmentation)	Diabetes mellitus and many other endocrine disorders	
Neurological		
Neuropathic ulcers on distal extremities	Peripheral neuropathy in diabetes	Decreased sensation of any body area increases risk for injury, including burns and pressure ulcers.
Café au lait macules (shown)	Neurofibromatosis	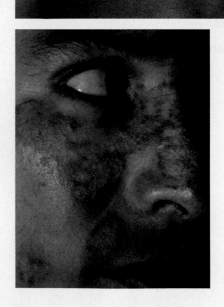
Musculoskeletal		
Photosensitivity, ***malar rash*** (red macular lesions distributed over forehead, cheeks, and chin, resembling a butterfly, as shown), coin-shaped lesions on trunk and extremities, and apthous ulcers on buccal mucosa	Systemic lupus erythematosus	

Table 13.9   **Manifestations in Integument of Systemic Disorders** (*continued*)

Integument Finding	Associated Disorder	Other Considerations/Depictions
Annular erythema (shown)	Sjörgen's syndrome	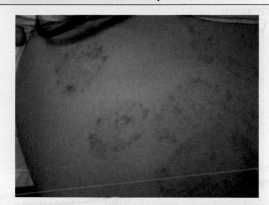
Pallor of fingers and toes in response to cold (shown)	Raynaud's phenomenon	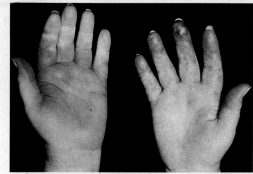
Erythema and increased temperature over a joint	Sepsis or acute inflammation of the joint	
Heme/Lymph		
Generalized pallor	Anemia	
Pruritis	Polycythemia, mastocytosis, lymphoma, or leukemia	
Spooning of nails	Iron deficiency states	
Psychiatric		
Patchy alopecia on the scalp or body, as well as missing or sparse eyelashes and eyebrows	Trichotillomania (compulsive hair pulling)	
Small linear cuts on patient's arms, legs, or anterior torso	"Cutting"	This self-injury coping method occurs in patients with borderline personality disorder, depression, and other psychiatric states.

Table 13.10 Primary Skin Lesions

Macule

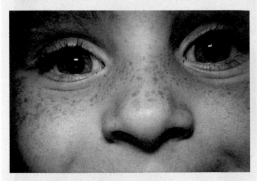

Flat, circumscribed, discolored, <1 cm diameter

Examples: Freckles (shown), tattoo, stork bite

Patch

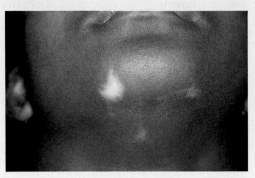

Flat, circumscribed, discolored, >1 cm diameter

Examples: Vitiligo (shown), melasma, tinea versicolor

Papule

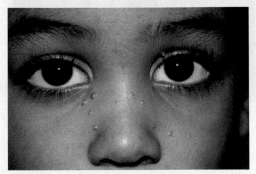

Raised, defined, any color, <1 cm diameter

Examples: Wart, insect bite, molluscum contagiosum (shown)

Plaque

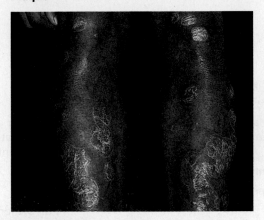

Raised, defined, any color, >1 cm diameter

Examples: Psoriasis (shown), lichen sclerosus

Wheal

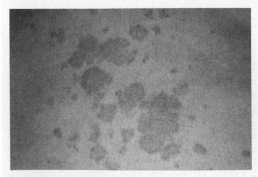

Raised, flesh-colored or red edematous papules or plaques, vary in size and shape

Example: Urticaria (shown)

Nodule

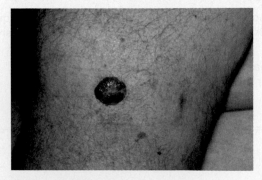

Solid, palpable >1 cm diameter, often with some depth

Example: Basal cell carcinoma (shown)

Table 13.10 **Primary Skin Lesions** *(continued)*

Tumor

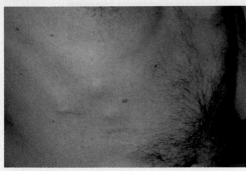

Large nodule

Examples: Large nevus, basal cell carcinoma, lipoma (shown)

Vesicle

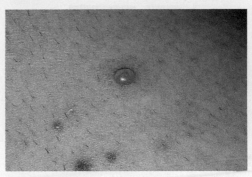

Fluid-filled, <1 cm diameter

Examples: Herpes simplex, chicken pox (shown)

Bulla

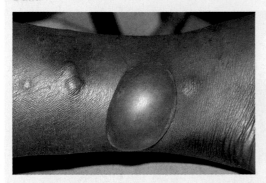

Fluid-filled, >1 cm diameter

Examples: Second-degree burns, bullous impetigo (shown)

Pustule

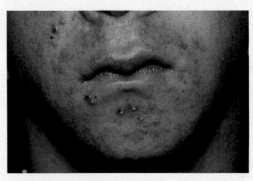

Purulent, fluid-filled, raised of any size

Examples: Pustular acne (shown), folliculitis

Cyst

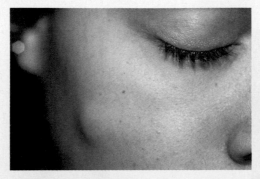

Distinct and walled-off, containing fluid or semi-solid material, varied in size

Examples: Epidermal cysts (shown), cystic acne

Table 13.11   Secondary Skin Lesions

Atrophy

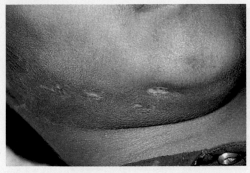

Thinning of skin from loss of skin structures

Examples: Steroid-induced atrophy, scleroderma (shown)

Keloid

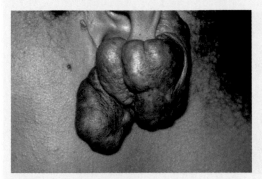

Excessive fibrous tissue replacement resulting in enlarged scar and deformity

Scale

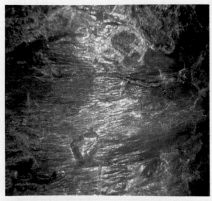

Rapid turnover of epidermal layer resulting in accumulation of and delayed shedding of outermost epidermis

Examples: Psoriasis (shown), tinea corporis

Scar

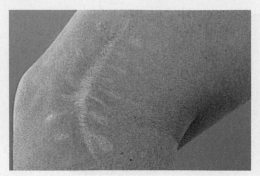

Fibrous replacement of lost skin structure

Example: Surgical scar (shown)

Crust

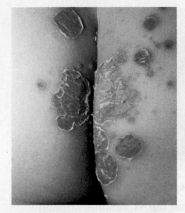

Dried secretions from primary lesion

Example: Impetigo (shown)

Lichenification

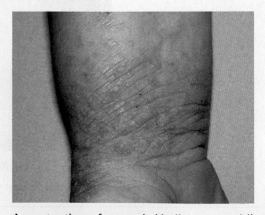

Accentuation of normal skin lines resembling tree bark, commonly caused by excessive scratching

Examples: Lichen simplex chronicus (shown), psoriasis, chronic contact dermatitis

Table 13.11 Secondary Skin Lesions *(continued)*

Excoriation

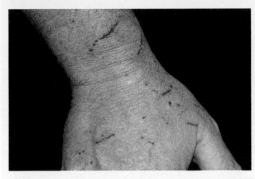

Lesion resulting from scratching or excessive rubbing of skin

Example: Cat scratches (shown)

Fissure

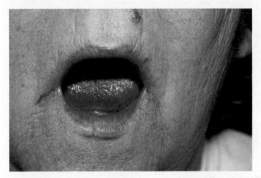

Linear break in skin surface, not related to trauma

Examples: Cheilitis, angular stomatitis (shown)

Erosion

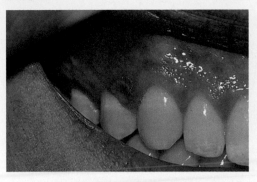

Loss of epidermal layer, usually not extending into dermis or subcutaneous layer

Examples: Apthous stomatitis (shown), varicella

Ulcer

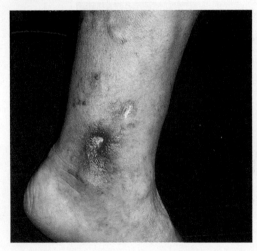

Loss of skin surface, extending into dermis, subcutaneous, fascia, muscle, bone, or all

Examples: Pressure ulcers, vascular ulcers, neuropathic ulcers (shown)

Table 13.12   Configurations of Lesions

Annular

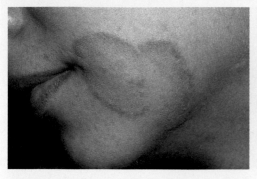

Ring-like, circular

Example: Tinea corporis (shown)

Iris

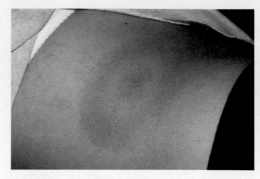

Bull's eye

Examples: Lyme disease (shown), erythema nodosum

Linear

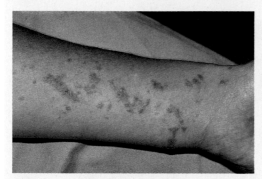

Line shape

Example: Contact dermatitis (shown)

Polymorphous

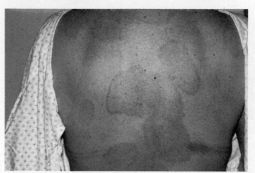

Several different shapes

Examples: Urticaria, tinea corporis (shown)

Punctuate

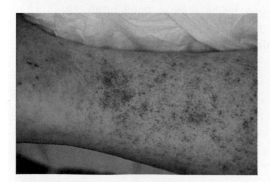

Small, marked with points or dots

Examples: Petechiae, Rocky Mountain spotted fever (shown), meningococcemia, vasculitis

Serpiginous

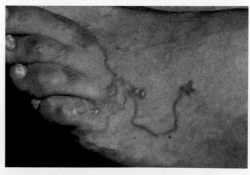

Curving, snake-like

Examples: Cutaneous larva migrans (shown), scabies

Table 13.12 Configurations of Lesions *(continued)*

Nummular/Discoid

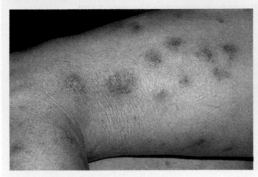

Coin-shaped

Examples: Nummular psoriasis, nummular eczema (shown)

Umbilicated

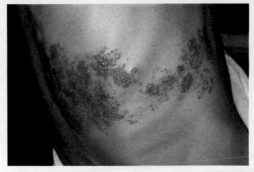

Central depression

Examples: Herpes zoster (shown), basal cell carcinoma

Filiform

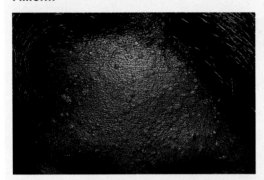

Papilla-like or finger-like projections (similar to tongue papillae)

Example: Warts (shown)

Verrucaform

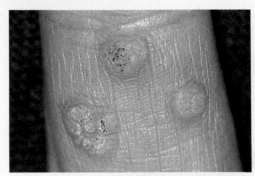

Circumscribed, papular with rough surface

Example: Warts (shown)

Table 13.13   Distribution Patterns of Lesions

Asymmetric

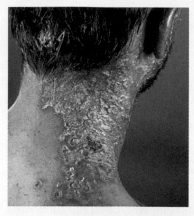

Distributed solely on one side of body

Examples: Contact dermatitis (shown), herpes zoster

Confluent

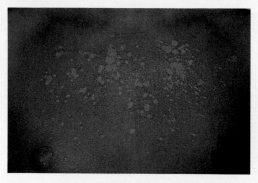

With enlargement or multiplication, begin to coalesce to form larger lesion

Examples: Urticaria, tinea versicolor (shown)

Diffuse

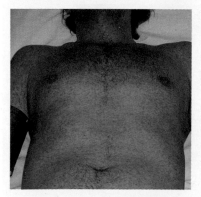

Distributed widely across affected area without any pattern

Examples: Drug reaction (shown), rubella, rubeola

Discrete

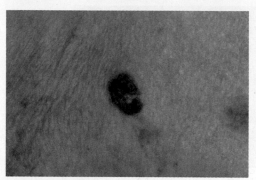

Single, separated, well-defined borders

Examples: Malignant melanoma (shown), wart

Generalized

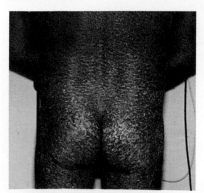

Distributed over large body area

Examples: Psoriasis (shown), acne vulgaris, exfoliative dermatitis

Grouped

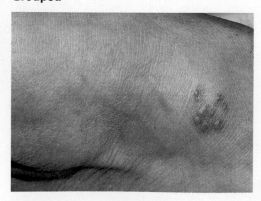

Clustered

Examples: Herpes simplex (shown)

Table 13.13 Distribution Patterns of Lesions (*continued*)

Localized

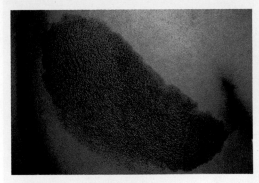

Located at distinct area

Examples: Giant nevus (shown), contact dermatitis, vitiligo

Satellite

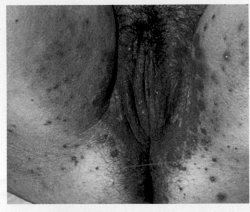

Single lesion(s) in close proximity to larger lesion, as if "orbiting"

Example: Cutaneous candidiasis (shown)

Symmetric

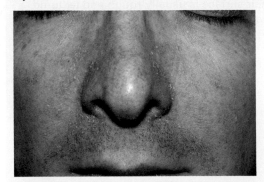

Distributed equally on both sides of body

Examples: Pityriasis rosea, freckles, seborrheic dermatitis (shown)

Zosteriform

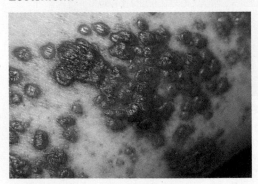

Distributed along dermatome

Example: Herpes zoster (shown)

Table 13.14 Common Skin Infections

Acne

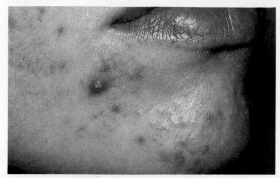

Pustular acne

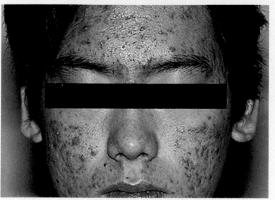

Cystic acne

Acne presents as an inflammatory and noninflammatory skin disorder characterized by one or a combination of the following lesions: comedone, papule, pustule, or cyst. Distribution of acne is frequently on the face, neck, torso, upper arms, and legs, although lesions may occur in other areas.

Warts

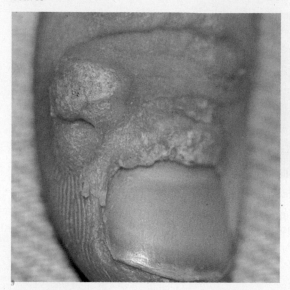

Warts are flesh-colored papules commonly caused by viruses. Their surface is usually rough and textured without scale.

Cellulitis

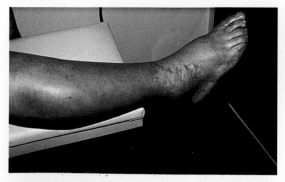

Cellulitis is a bacterial infection of deep skin tissues, often preceded by a minor wound to the area allowing bacteria to invade the tissue. Cellulitis can occur anywhere and is characterized by swelling, redness, warmth, and tenderness or pain.

Impetigo

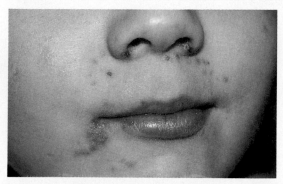

This highly contagious superficial skin infection commonly results from *Staphylococcus aureus* or group A beta-hemolytic streptococci. It is characterized by vesicles or bullae that eventually rupture and ooze serous fluid that forms the classic honey-colored crust.

Table 13.14   Common Skin Infections (*continued*)

Herpes Simplex (Cold Sores)

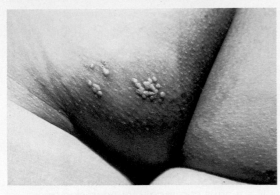

The herpes simplex virus is characterized by grouped vesicles on an erythematous base. These lesions can appear anywhere. Generally lesions on or around the mouth are *herpes labialis*, lesions in the genital regions are *herpes genitalis*, and lesions elsewhere are *cutaneous herpes*.

Measles (Rubeola)

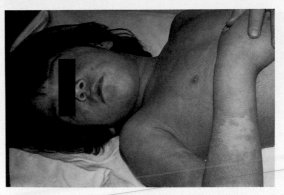

Commonly called the hard measles, rubeola is a virus characterized by pinkish, erythematous macules and papules initially on the face, with progressive caudal spread. In 3–4 days, the rash becomes brownish with a fine desquamation.

Pityriasis Rosea

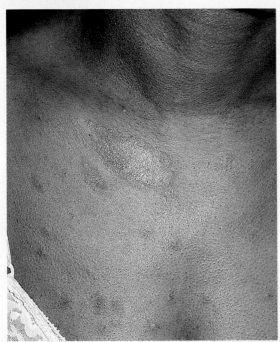

This viral infection is initially characterized by a "herald patch"—a large oval hyperpigmented lesion with a fine scale, usually on the chest or back. Over subsequent days, additional similar but smaller lesions develop and are distributed generally over the torso and extremities, with the face usually spared.

German Measles (Rubella)

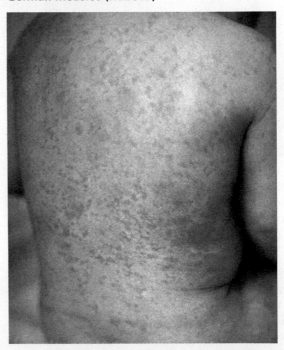

Commonly called the 3-day measles and largely vaccine-preventable, this viral illness presents as a pinkish discrete macular and papular rash covering the entire body. It usually resolves in 3 days.

(table continues on page 306)

Table 13.14 **Common Skin Infections** (*continued*)

Roseola

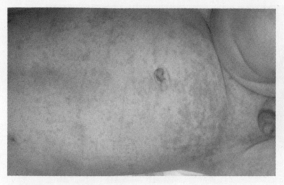

Roseola is a viral illness whose rash appears as the fever resolves. The rash of roseola is described as discrete macules and papules, usually no more than 1–5 mm diameter, with an area of pallor surrounding each lesion.

Candida

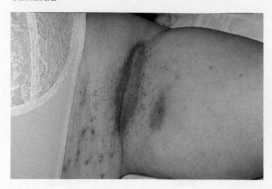

Candida is a fungus commonly found in skin folds or generally warm and moist areas. Commonly affected sites are the axillae, inframammary areas, and groin. Satellite pustules commonly surround the erythematous macules.

Tinea Corporis

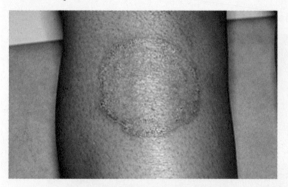

Commonly called *ringworm*, this dermatophyte skin infection results in an erythematous, commonly pruritic, annular lesion with a raised border and central clearing.

Tinea Versicolor

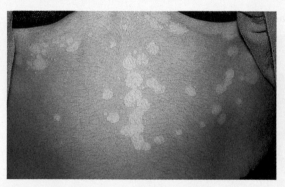

This dermatophyte infection caused by normal skin flora results in hypopigmented patchy lesions generally distributed on the upper chest, upper back, and proximal extremities. It rarely occurs on the face and legs.

 Table 13.15 **Inflammatory Skin Lesions**

Psoriasis

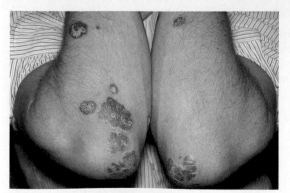

This chronic skin disorder is commonly characterized by reddish-pink lesions covered with silvery scales. It occurs on extensor surfaces (eg, elbows and knees), but can appear anywhere on the body.

Eczema

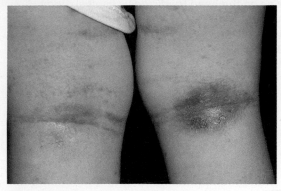

Also known as *atopic dermatitis*, eczema is characterized by itchy, pink macules or papules, commonly on flexural areas (eg, inner elbows and posterior knees). Eczema can occur anywhere on the body.

Urticaria

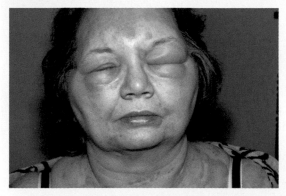

Commonly called *hives*, urticaria is the accumulation of fluid in the dermal layer of the skin as a direct result of histamine release.

Insect Bites

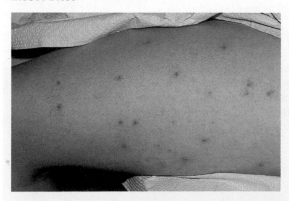

Insect bites usually cause an inflammatory and pruritic response at the site. Lesions are usually erythematous and papular with a visible puncta at the central part.

Contact Dermatitis

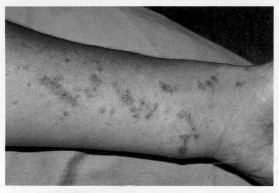

This inflammatory response to an antigen that has contact with exposed skin initially causes stimulation of the histamine receptors, which results in the classic erythematous and pruritic lesions.

Allergic Drug Reaction

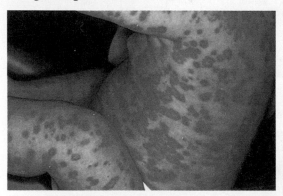

Drug allergies can occur immediately or have a delayed response after exposure to the offending agent.

Seborrhea

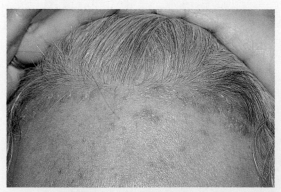

Seborrhea (seborrheic dermatitis) is an inflammatory skin disorder characterized by macular pink, red, or orange-yellow lesions that may or may not have a fine scale. Distribution is usually on the face, scalp, and ears.

Table 13.16   Skin Lesions From Infestations

Lesion	Description
Lice (Pediculosis) 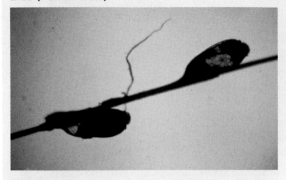 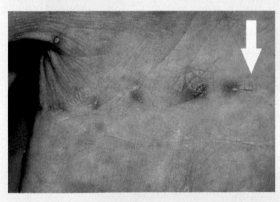	Infestations on the head (*pediculosis capitis*), body (*pediculosis corporis*), or genitals (*phthirus pubis*) are frequently characterized by the secondary lesions resulting from scratching. Visualization of the louse is common, and eggs on the hair shaft also indicate infestation in the absence of visualization.
Scabies 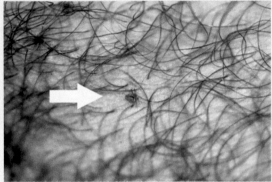	Scabies is caused by a mite that burrows into the epidermis and deposits eggs and waste materials as it progresses, resulting in a hypersensitivity reaction of erythema and pruritis.
Ticks 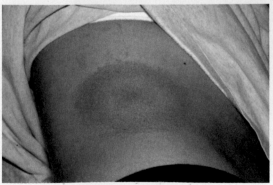	Tick bites frequently resemble simple insect bites. Nevertheless, certain ticks cause systemic illness, with a characteristic erythematous target lesion that appears at the site of the bite, and require prompt medical evaluation.

Table 13-17 Skin Tumors and Growths

Moles or Nevi

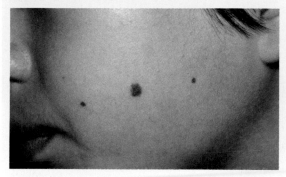

Nevi (moles) are normal variants. They can be macular or papular and distributed anywhere. They are congenital or acquired. *Congenital nevi* exist from birth and are commonly referred to as "birth marks." *Acquired nevi* occur most commonly in childhood and adolescence.

Skin Tags

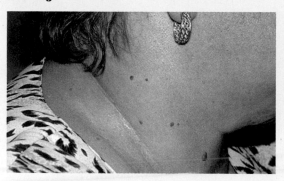

These normal papules are generally <1 cm and commonly distributed on the neck, axillae, inframammary area, and groin. Skin tags are common in pregnancy and in aging skin.

Lipoma

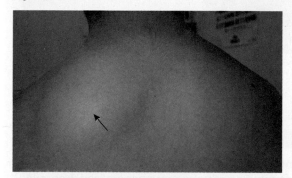

Lipomas are tumors comprised of fat cells and commonly located on the back of the neck, torso, arms, and legs. Though benign, some varieties are painful. Lipomas occur singly and multiply, ranging in size.

Lentigo

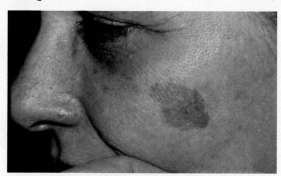

Lentigines are benign, acquired, circumscribed, pigmented macules found generally on sun-exposed skin.

Actinic Keratosis

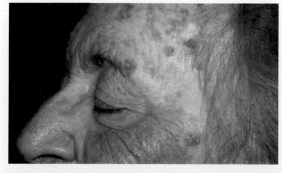

Also commonly called solar keratosis, they usually are found on sun-exposed skin, and are thought to result from UV damage. These macular or papular lesions are discrete, with a rough or scaly surface.

Basal Cell Carcinoma

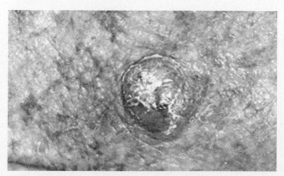

This nodular or popular lesion appears shiny with a rolled pearly border, and typically has telangiectases (small spider veins) on its surface. This skin cancer grows slowly and rarely metastasizes.

(table continues on page 310)

Table 13-17 Skin Tumors and Growths (continued)

Squamous Cell Carcinoma

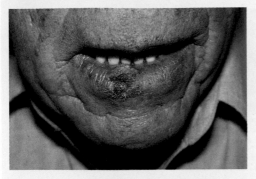

The second most frequently found skin cancer is related to actinic keratosis and sun exposure. Lesions are typically papular, nodular, or plaques located on sun-exposed skin surfaces.

Malignant Melanoma

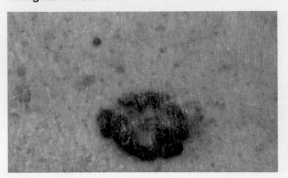

Malignant melanoma is identified by the ABCDEs of skin cancer detection (see Table 13-2).

Kaposi's Sarcoma

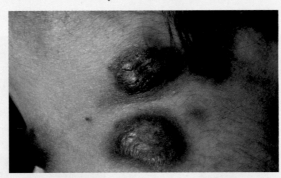

This opportunistic skin infection is a consequence of impaired immune status, as with AIDS. Lesions generally occur on the nose, penis, and extremities, though with advanced HIV, distribution may be more generalized. Improved immune status may cause resolution.

Table 13-18   Common Vascular Lesions

Hemangioma

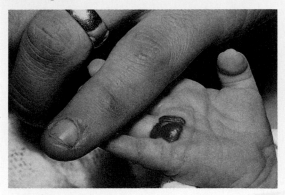

These vascular lesions, present at birth, rapidly develop and grow, but spontaneously resolve by age 9 years. Comprised of endothelial cells that form caverns and fill with blood, they blanch with applied pressure.

Nevus Flammeus (Port Wine Stain)

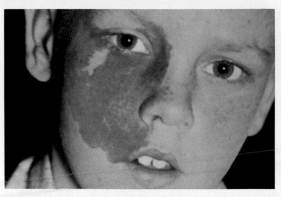

Malformation of superficial dermal blood vessels is present at birth. The lesion grows with the child and never resolves on its own.

Spider or Star Angioma

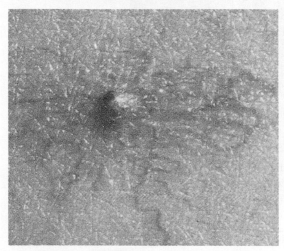

This vascular lesion arises from a central dermal arteriole with multiple extensions forming the appearance of spider legs. Distribution can be anywhere, but is commonly found on the face, arms, and torso.

Venous Lake

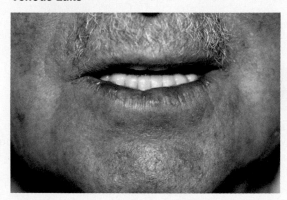

This papular bluish to purple lesion blanches on pressure, and is generally found on the face, especially on the lips or ears. It is benign, and often associated with sun exposure.

Table 13.19 Acute Wounds and Lesions From Trauma

Petechiae

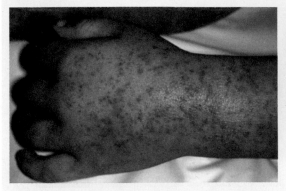

These small reddish to purple macules or papules can develop anywhere on the body in response to physical trauma.

Ecchymosis

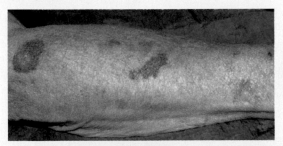

Physical trauma to the skin damages capillaries and allows blood to seep into surrounding tissues. As blood is gradually resorbed, color of ecchymoses changes and can be purple, blue, green, yellow, or brown.

Laceration

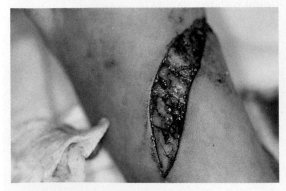

Tears in the skin can be superficial or deep, short or long, and frequently require suturing to heal correctly.

Purpura

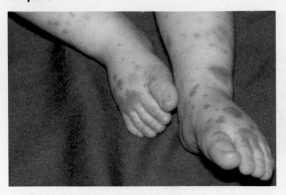

Purplish macules or papules result from bleeding under the skin secondary to inadequate clotting mechanisms.

Hematoma

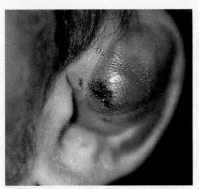

Collection of blood under the skin usually results from blunt-force trauma. Hematomas are palpable lesions, and coloration mimics that of ecchymoses.

Abrasions

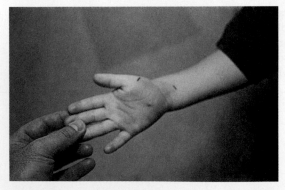

Abrasions are caused by shear force or friction against the skin, removing several layers and exposing the dermis.

Table 13.19   Acute Wounds and Lesions From Trauma (continued)

Puncture Wound

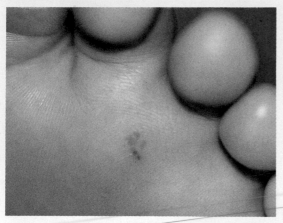

A sharp object pierces the skin, causing a wound with greater depth than width.

Avulsion

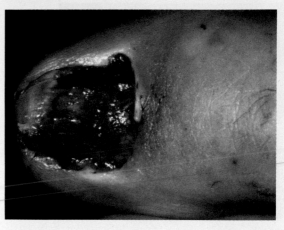

Trauma forces the skin to separate from underlying structures, leaving an open ragged wound.

Table 13.20   Pressure Ulcers

Suspected Deep Tissue Injury (not shown)

Purple or maroon localized area of discolored intact skin or blood-filled blister from damage to underlying soft tissue as a result of pressure, shearing, or both. The area may be preceded by tissue that is painful, firm, mushy, boggy, warmer, or cooler as compared to adjacent tissue. Deep tissue injury may be difficult to detect in people with dark skin. Evolution may include a thin blister over a dark wound bed. The wound may further evolve and become covered by thin eschar. Evolution may be rapid, exposing additional layers even with optimal treatment.

Stage I

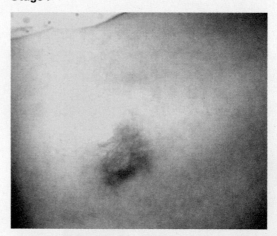

Intact skin with nonblanchable redness of a localized area, usually over a bony prominence. Darkly pigmented skin may not have visible blanching; its color may differ from the surrounding area. The area may be painful, firm, soft, warmer, or cooler as compared to adjacent tissue. Stage I may be difficult to detect in people with dark skin. May indicate "at risk" people (a heralding sign of risk).

(table continues on page 314)

Table 13.20   Pressure Ulcers (continued)

Stage II

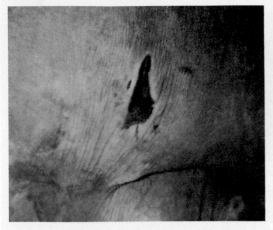

Partial thickness loss of dermis presenting as a shallow open ulcer with a red pink wound bed, without slough. May also present as an intact or open/ruptured serum-filled blister. Presents as a shiny or dry shallow ulcer without slough or bruising (indicates suspected deep tissue injury). This stage should not be used to describe skin tears, tape burns, perineal dermatitis, maceration, or excoriation.

Stage III

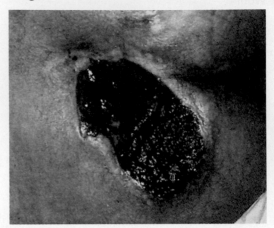

Full thickness tissue loss. Subcutaneous fat may be visible, but bone, tendon, or muscle is not exposed. Slough may be present but does not obscure the depth of tissue loss. May include undermining and tunneling. The depth of a stage III pressure ulcer varies by anatomical location. The bridge of the nose, ear, occiput, and malleolus do not have subcutaneous tissue, and stage III ulcers can be shallow. In contrast, areas of significant adiposity can develop extremely deep stage III pressure ulcers. Bone/tendon is not visible or directly palpable.

Stage IV

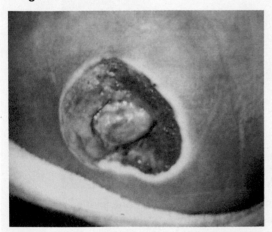

Full thickness tissue loss with exposed bone, tendon, or muscle. Slough or eschar may be present on some parts of the wound bed. Often include undermining and tunneling. Depth of a stage IV pressure ulcer varies by anatomical location. The bridge of the nose, ear, occiput, and malleolus do not have subcutaneous tissue and these ulcers can be shallow. Stage IV ulcers can extend into muscle, supporting structures (eg, fascia, tendon, joint capsule), or both, making osteomyelitis possible. Exposed bone/tendon is visible or directly palpable.

Unstageable (not shown)

Full thickness tissue loss in which the base of the ulcer is covered by slough (yellow, tan, gray, green, or brown), eschar (tan, brown, or black), or both. Until enough slough or eschar is removed to expose the base of the wound, true depth, and therefore stage, cannot be determined. Stable (dry, adherent, intact without erythema or fluctuance) eschar on the heels serves as "the body's natural (biological) cover" and should not be removed.

Source: National Pressure Ulcer Advisory Panel. (2007). *Updated staging system*. Retrieved May 20, 2010, from http://www.npuap.org/pr2.htm

Table 13.21   Nonpressure Ulcers

Neuropathic Ulcer

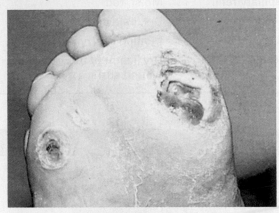

Loss of sensation in an extremity impairs the patient's ability to detect pressure on the feet. Sustained pressure or friction results in lost skin surface, which often remains unnoticed because the patient is not detecting pain. Diabetes is a common cause of this type of ulcer. Use the Wagner's classification to determine grade (severity) (see Table 13-22).

Venous Ulcers (Vascular)

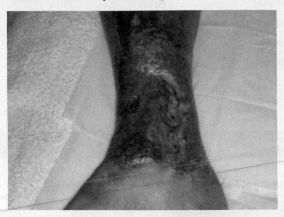

Venous ulcers develop from chronic pooling of blood in the extremity. See Chapter 20. Venous ulcers usually occur between ankle and knee in a "gaiter" distribution. Wound edges are ragged and irregular; the base is beefy red with evident granulation tissue. There is large exudate. Some ulcers can be deep. These ulcers are generally painless. The surrounding tissue commonly is hyperpigmented.

Arterial Ulcer (Vascular)

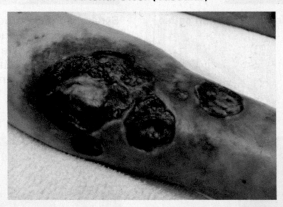

Arterial ulcers result from chronic ischemia as a consequence of impaired arterial circulation to an extremity. See Chapter 20. Arterial ulcers are usually located distally, such as at the ends of the toes or fingers. Wound edges are sharply defined; the base is pale when elevated and appears ruddy when dependent. These ulcers may be deep, frequently infected, and painful; they exhibit minimal granulation tissue.

 Table 13.22   Wagner's Classification of Ulcers

Grade	Classification
0	Preulcerative lesion, healed ulcers, presence of bony deformity
1	Superficial ulcer without subcutaneous tissue involvement
2	Penetration through the subcutaneous tissue (may expose bone, tendon, ligament, or joint capsule)
3	Osteitis, abscess, or osteomyelitis
4	Gangrene of the forefoot
5	Gangrene of the entire foot

Depth of Burn	Bleeding	Sensation	Appearance	Blanching
Superficial	Brisk	Pain	Rapid capillary refill	Moist, red
Superficial-dermal	Brisk	Pain	Slowed capillary refill	Dry, pale pink
Dermal	Delayed	No pain	No capillary refill	Mottled cherry red color
Full thickness	None	No pain	No blanching	Dry, leathery or waxy hard wound surface

⚠ Table 13.24   Nail Findings

Longitudinal Ridging

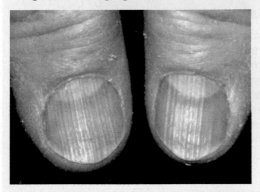

Normal variation, especially in elderly. Common cause is normal aging.

Onycholysis

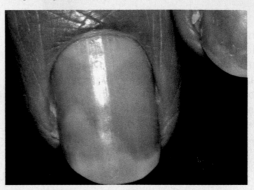

Separation of a portion of the nail plate from the nail bed; results in opaqueness to the affected part of the nail, appearing white to yellow to green. Common causes include trauma, fungal infections, topical irritants, psoriasis, and subungual neoplasms or warts

Koilonychia (Spoon Nails)

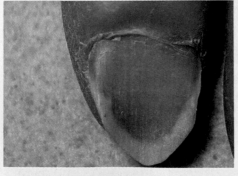

Transverse and longitudinal concavity of the nail, giving the appearance of a spoon. May be normal in infants (usually resolves in few months). Other causes include trauma, iron-deficiency anemia, and hemochromatosis

Pitted Nails

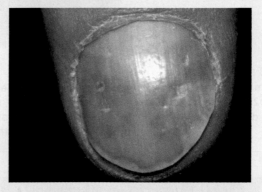

Lesions from psoriasis; arise from nail matrix that cause pitting on the nail plate as it grows

Table 13.24 Nail Findings (continued)

Beau's Lines

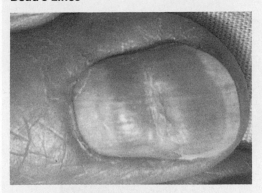

Results from slowed or halted nail growth in response to illness, physical trauma, or poisoning

Clubbing

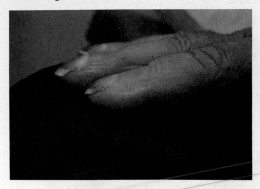

Results from chronic hypoxia to distal fingers, such as with emphysema or congestive heart failure

Yellow Nails

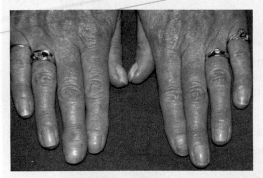

Slowly growing nail, without cuticle, and onycholysis resulting in thickening of nail and yellowish appearance. Causes include lung disorders and lymphedema.

Half-and-half Nails

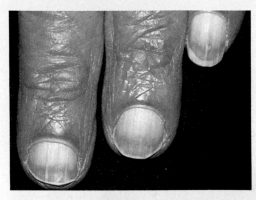

Color changes associated with chronic renal failure; proximal portion of nail is white, distal portion is pink or brown

Dark Longitudinal Streaks

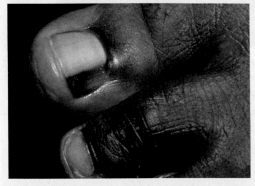

Often a normal variant in dark-skinned patients from junctional nevus of nail matrix. Suspicious for malignancy if the streaks blur, spread, or are not solid the full length of the nail.

Splinter Hemorrhages

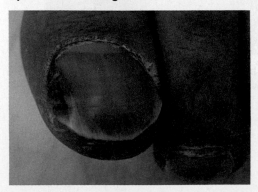

Brownish red longitudinal lines in the direction of nail growth that result from damage to capillaries (eg, endocarditis, vasculitis, antiphospholipid syndrome) supplying the nail matrix caused by microemboli

Alopecia Areata

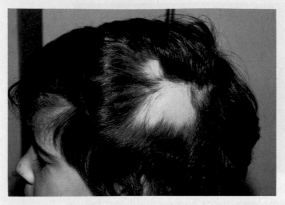

This autoimmune disorder results in noninflammatory loss of hair in a circumscribed distribution.

Hirsutism

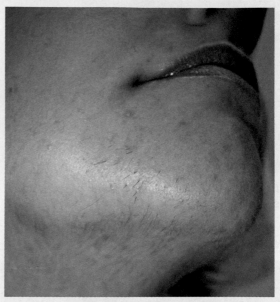

Excessive androgenic hormones in a female patient can cause masculine changes including hair in male distribution patterns (beard, chest, back, upper thighs).

Traction Alopecia

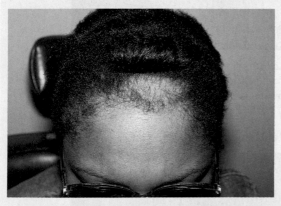

Tight hair braiding practices exert traction force on the hair bulb with subsequent hair loss.

Trichotillomania

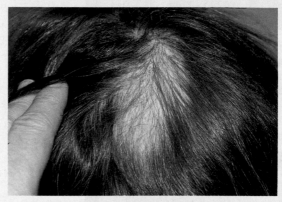

Compulsive hair pulling causes breakage of hair and thinned or balding areas on scalp, although some hair remains present and visible in the affected area.

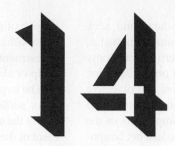

Head and Neck with Lymphatics Assessment

Learning Objectives

1 Identify the structures and functions of the head, neck, and associated lymphatics.

2 Identify teaching opportunities for health promotion and risk reduction related to the skull, thyroid, and lymphatics of the head and neck.

3 Differentiate subjective data collected for headache, head trauma, neck pain, neck masses, and thyroid dysfunction.

4 Collect objective data about the scalp, cranium, facial structures, and neck, including lymphatics and thyroid.

5 Identify normal and abnormal findings from inspection and palpation of the head and neck.

6 Use subjective and objective data of the head and neck to analyze findings and plan interventions.

7 Document findings from head and neck examinations using appropriate terminology.

8 Individualize health assessment of the head and neck considering the age, gender, race, and culture of the patient.

9 Use findings from assessment of the head and neck to identify nursing diagnoses and to initiate a plan of care.

_F_aye Davis-Pierce, 21 years old, is visiting her college clinic for the first time with reports of fatigue and weight gain of 20 lb over the past 3 months. She is also concerned because her hair has been falling out. Her temperature is 36.8°C orally, pulse 64 beats/min, respirations 12 breaths/min, and blood pressure 98/66 mm Hg. Her height is 5 ft 8 in, weight is 208 lb, and BMI is 31.6 (obese). Current medications include an oral contraceptive and a multivitamin.

You will gain more information about Faye as you progress through this chapter. As you study the content and features, consider Faye's case and its relationship to what you are learning. Begin thinking about the following points:

- How might Faye's physical issues relate to her psychosocial health, including potential issues related to her age and status as a college student?
- What other physical findings might be present, and what other body systems might be involved?
- What type of follow-up care and reassessment might the patient need at subsequent visits?

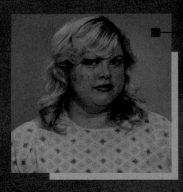

This chapter describes assessment of the head and neck regions, which include the scalp, cranium, lymphatics, parathyroid, and thyroid gland. It explores pertinent anatomy and physiology, as well as variations based on age, gender, and culture. Methods for collecting subjective and objective data related to skull or scalp injury, lymphatic function, and thyroid function are included. Other key components of the chapter include the signs and symptoms of headache, lymphadenopathy, and parathyroid and thyroid imbalances; correct techniques for inspection and palpation of the structures of the head and neck; and descriptions of common normal and abnormal findings.

Structure and Function Overview

Structures of the head and neck interact with multiple body systems—integumentary, neurologic, musculoskeletal, respiratory, vascular, gastrointestinal, lymphatic, and endocrine. Knowledge of important information for accurate determination of normal and abnormal function is included.

The Head

The head includes the cranium and facial skeleton, which together encompass 22 bones that support and contain soft-tissue organs, including the eyes (see Chapter 15), ears (see Chapter 16), and brain (see Chapter 24; Ellis, 2002). The bones of the cranium are the *frontal, parietal, occipital*, and *temporal* (Fig. 14-1). **Sutures** join these bones together. The major sutures are the *coronal*, which crosses the top of the scalp from ear to ear, *sagittal*, which crosses the skull from anterior to posterior, and *lambdoidal*, which separates the parietal and occipital bones (see Fig. 14-1). Fetal sutures are not tightly joined, which allows the skull to mold and pass through the maternal birth canal more easily. The sutures remain somewhat loose during childhood to facilitate

growth of the head and brain, but eventually knit together by approximately 12 to 18 months. When documenting physical assessments, nurses must take care to describe the location of scalp or skull findings according to the bones and sutures.

The largest facial bones are the *maxilla, mandible, nasal, lacrimal palliative*, and *vomer* (Fig. 14-2). The mastoid process, part of the temporal bone, has particular relevance during assessment of the ear, which is discussed in Chapter 16.

Clinical Significance 14-1

The major facial muscles are the *frontalis, temporalis, zygomaticus, masseter, buccinators, orbicularis oculi,* and *orbicularis oris.* These and other smaller muscles enable chewing, speaking, smiling, and frowning (Fig. 14-3).

Blood supply to the head is through the carotid artery, which then splits into the internal and external branches. The veins are the external and internal jugular. See Chapter 19. The temporal artery is a branch of the external carotid artery that supplies the face. Trigeminal nerve V supplies both motor and sensory innervations to the forehead, cheeks, and chin. See Chapter 24. The major neck muscles are the sternocleidomastoid and trapezius. The sternocleidomastoid muscle arises from the sternum and medial clavicle and extends to behind the ear. The trapezius arises from the occipital bone and vertebra and fans out to the clavicle and scapula.

Clinical Significance 14-2

These muscles are major accessory muscles used when the patient has difficulty breathing.

Three pairs of salivary glands are present. The parotid glands are in the cheek anterior to the bottom half of the ear. The submandibular glands are at the angle of the jaw below the mandible. The sublingual glands are in the mouth and under the tongue. See Chapter 17.

The Neck

The neck is supported by the cervical vertebrae, C1–7. A useful neck landmark is the *vertebral prominence*, which is the spinous process of C7, the longest cervical vertebrae (Ellis, 2002). Of the vertebrae of the neck, C7 and T1 are usually the most easily palpable, and the one that protrudes the furthest is C7 (Fig. 14-4). Locating C7 during assessment of the head, neck, and posterior thorax facilitates more accurate description of findings.

⚠ SAFETY ALERT 14.1

Falls or sudden jerking of the head and neck (whiplash) are particularly likely to result in dislocation of the cervical vertebrae. Fractures also may occur with head-first falls. Any history of falls or sudden jerks of the neck requires careful investigation.

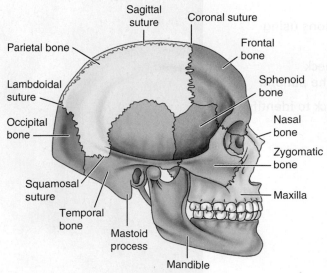

Figure 14.1 Bones and sutures of the cranium.

Sagittal suture
Coronal suture
Parietal bone
Frontal bone
Lambdoidal suture
Sphenoid bone
Occipital bone
Nasal bone
Zygomatic bone
Squamosal suture
Maxilla
Temporal bone
Mastoid process
Mandible

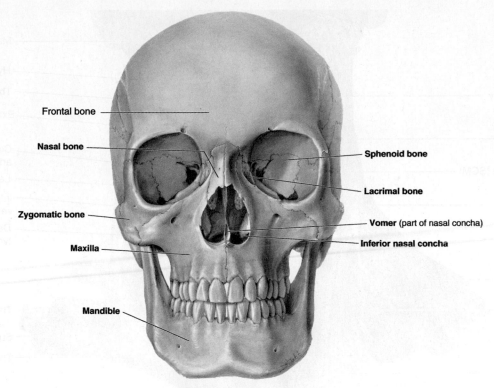

Figure 14.2 The facial bones.

Labels: Frontal bone, Nasal bone, Zygomatic bone, Maxilla, Mandible, Sphenoid bone, Lacrimal bone, Vomer (part of nasal concha), Inferior nasal concha

Trachea

The trachea passes down the midline of the neck and is part of the upper respiratory system (see Chapter 18). Important landmarks for the head and neck region also are in the tracheal area (Fig. 14-5). The usually palpable U-shaped *hyoid bone* is located midline just beneath the mandible. The large *thyroid cartilage* consists of two flat, plate-like structures joined together at an angle and with a small, sometimes palpable notch at the superior edge. This structure, usually more prominent in males, is also called the "Adam's apple."

The palpable *cricoid cartilage* is a ringed structure just inferior to the thyroid cartilage.

Clinical Significance 14-3

Palpation of the thyroid gland reveals important landmarks of the trachea. Such landmarks are noted when assessing for tracheal deviation, which accompanies a potentially life-threatening condition called *tension pneumothorax* (see Chapter 18).

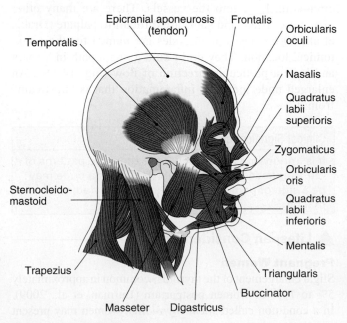

Figure 14.3 The facial muscles.

Labels: Temporalis, Epicranial aponeurosis (tendon), Frontalis, Orbicularis oculi, Nasalis, Quadratus labii superioris, Zygomaticus, Orbicularis oris, Quadratus labii inferioris, Mentalis, Triangularis, Buccinator, Digastricus, Masseter, Trapezius, Sternocleido-mastoid

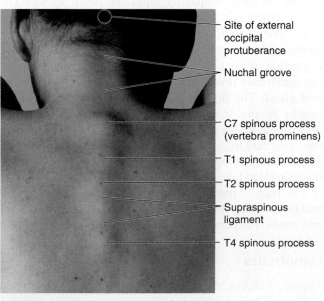

Figure 14.4 Posterior surface anatomy of the neck. Note the location of C7.

Labels: Site of external occipital protuberance, Nuchal groove, C7 spinous process (vertebra prominens), T1 spinous process, T2 spinous process, Supraspinous ligament, T4 spinous process

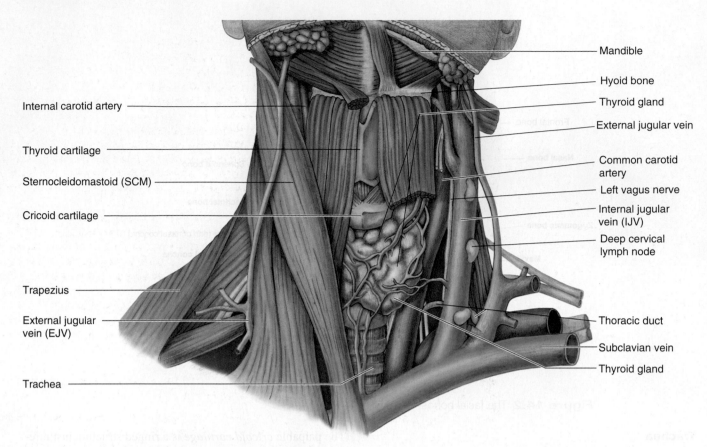

Internal carotid artery

Thyroid cartilage

Sternocleidomastoid (SCM)

Cricoid cartilage

Trapezius

External jugular
vein (EJV)

Trachea

Mandible

Hyoid bone

Thyroid gland

External jugular vein

Common carotid
artery

Left vagus nerve

Internal jugular
vein (IJV)

Deep cervical
lymph node

Thoracic duct

Subclavian vein

Thyroid gland

Figure 14.5 Key head and neck landmarks in the region of the trachea.

Thyroid and Parathyroid Glands

The butterfly-shaped *thyroid gland* consists of a band (the isthmus) that crosses the trachea and two symmetrical 3 to 4 cm lobes that lie on each side of the trachea. The *sternocleidomastoid muscle* largely covers the thyroid lobes (see Fig. 14-5). The thyroid gland produces thyroid hormones, the most frequently measured being T3 and T4, which control metabolic rates and can affect almost every body system. In all patients, the thyroid should be symmetric without discrete masses, nodularity, or tenderness. Inspection of the patient's neck while he or she swallows can sometimes reveal up and down movement of the thyroid gland. The thyroid gland is usually not palpable in healthy people. If only the posterior portion of the gland is enlarged, it also may not be palpable. Therefore, nurses must take care to gather thorough data in history taking that may identify symptoms of hypothyroid or hyperthyroid function (Haddow, et al, 2007).

Two pairs of parathyroid glands are imbedded in the thyroid lobes and produce calcitonin, which helps move calcium into bones. The parathyroids are usually not palpable.

Lymphatics

The major chains of lymph nodes in the neck are the *preauricular, posterior auricular, occipital, superficial cervical* (extending from the tonsillar to supraclavicular nodes), *deep cervical, posterior cervical, submental*, and *submandibular* (Fig. 14-6). Approximately 80 lymph nodes are in the head and neck region, serving as part of the immune system. These vessels filter potential pathogens from the body. They also drain fluid that has moved outside of the circulation back into the vessels. There are many other than those listed, and some are difficult to palpate (Drake, et al., 2005). The lymph nodes are named for their anatomical location. They drain fluid along a path in a chain and have a particular direction of flow (Fig. 14-6B). An enlarged node indicates inflammation that is "upstream" from it.

Clinical Significance 14-4

It is important to understand the drainage patterns of the lymphatics, because enlargement of a node may be a sign of pathology that is not directly adjacent to that node.

Lifespan Considerations

Pregnant Women

Slight enlargement of the thyroid is common in approximately 5% to 10% of women postpartum (Burman, et al., 2009). In a condition called *silent thyroiditis*, women may present

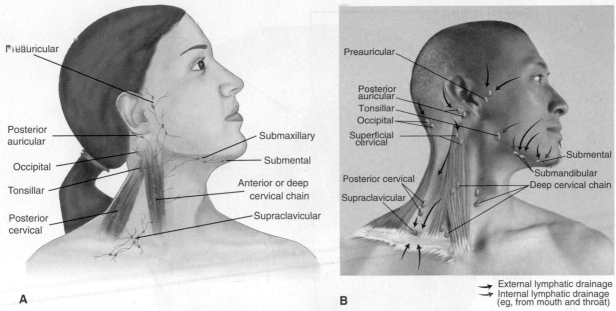

Figure 14.6 Lymphatics of the head and neck. **A.** Major chains of lymph nodes in the neck. **B.** Direction of lymphatic flow and drainage. See also Chapters 20 and 21.

with signs and symptoms of hyperthyroidism, followed by hypothyroid symptoms. It may be several months before usually returning to normal thyroid function (Uphold & Graham, 2003). Even though slight enlargement of the thyroid gland in pregnant or postpartum women may be normal, it still requires further investigation. A thrill may be palpable over the thyroid and a bruit may be auscultated; this is an abnormal condition.

Newborns, Infants, and Children

At birth, the newborn's head may be slightly asymmetrical, elongated, or both as a result of molding of the skull during passage through the birth canal. Head shape moves to normal usually within a few days or weeks after. Newborns have two *fontanels*, areas of the skull with a soft and nonossified matrix. Fontanels enable the head and underlying structures to grow as the child develops. Assessing the size of the anterior and posterior fontanels at each evaluation of the infant is important to determine if ossification is happening at the appropriate time (Fig. 14-7). The posterior fontanel closes by 3 months of age, while the anterior fontanel closes by 18 months of age (Ellis, 2002).

Fontanels should be flat—neither bulging nor retracted. A bulging fontanel may be normal when an infant cries but otherwise needs further evaluation as a sign of possible increased intracranial pressure. A depressed fontanel may indicate dehydration. An unusual head shape may be noted if fontanels close prematurely but may also be from prolonged positioning of the infant in one way. Parents are encouraged to change their infants' position regularly throughout the day while babies are awake to enhance normal physical development. Infants who spend nearly all

their time on their backs may develop significant flattening of the posterior skull.

In children 1 to 5 years, nurses may palpate small (<10 mm), nontender, movable nodes in the head and neck region (Kliegman, et al., 2007). These normal findings are sometimes referred to as "shotty," because they feel like BB gun pellets or shots. The thyroid gland and lymph nodes are usually nonpalpable in school-age children.

Older Adults

With aging, facial subcutaneous fat decreases, making the skeleton more pronounced. Skin may sag and wrinkle across the forehead, surrounding the eyes, at the tip of the nose, and on the cheeks, altering facial appearance. Skin lesions are more likely, and careful assessment for possible cancers, especially in commonly sun-exposed areas, is important (Ellis, 2002). See Chapter 13.

Cultural Considerations

The most noticeable difference among racial groups is skin color. Shape of the eyes, nose, and lips also varies based on background and genetics. Variations in skull or neck shape or size relate more to height and weight than to specific racial or cultural background.

Acute Assessment

Patients with acute head injuries and neurologic changes (see Chapter 24) must be quickly and accurately assessed by the health care team. Stabilization of the head and neck is essential to avoid further neurologic injury. Any history

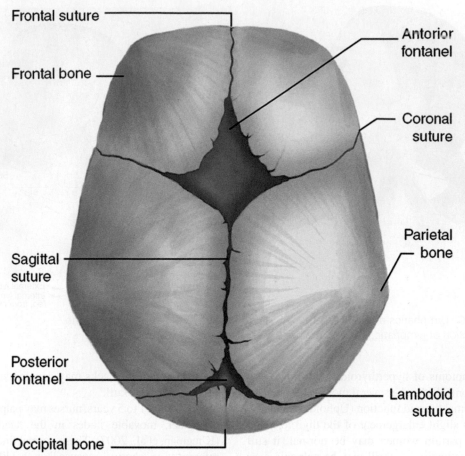

Figure 14.7 Anterior and posterior fontanels.

Labels on figure: Frontal suture, Frontal bone, Sagittal suture, Posterior fontanel, Occipital bone, Anterior fontanel, Coronal suture, Parietal bone, Lambdoid suture

of trauma to the head, neck, or both warrants a careful assessment of these structures for bleeding, swelling, loss of mobility or pain. Identifying the mechanism of injury helps the nurse to determine which anatomic regions require their focus. It is essential to keep the spine immobilized to prevent spinal cord injury, and immobilization devices should not be removed until the spine is cleared of injury. Patients with severe headaches may be unable to provide a complete history, but a focused history and physical examination looking for neurologic changes are critical nursing behaviors.

Neck pain, a common symptom, is most often related to muscle tension or spasm. Neck pain associated with fever and headache may signify serious illness such as meningitis and should be carefully evaluated (see Chapter 24 for meningeal signs). Patients experiencing a myocardial infarction may present with neck pain—so any patient with sudden onset of neck or jaw pain should be evaluated for possible cardiac etiologies (Swartz, 2006).

⚠ *SAFETY ALERT 14.2*

Patients may experience referred neck pain from myocardial infarction. If cardiac origin is suspected, the nurse focuses assessments on the heart and intervenes (see Chapter 19).

Lymphatics larger than 1 cm, fixed, irregular, or hard or rubbery require emergency investigation. Such signs raise the possibility of cancer.

Hyperthyroidism may present as an emergency, with symptoms of hypermetabolism in all systems. The most common sign is tachycardia, but other possibilities include diarrhea, anxiety, fever, weakness, and even psychosis, coma, or death. Nurses should recognize patients at greatest risk for this emergency state. Such patients include those with thyroid tumors and those who have undergone thyroid surgery (Nayak & Hodak, 2007).

Subjective Data Collection

Areas for Health Promotion/ *Healthy People*

Table 14-1 includes pertinent goals and education topics relevant to the head and neck regions based on the *Healthy People* goals.

Assessment of Risk Factors

When assessing for risk factors associated with head and neck pathology, nurses should remember that multiple systems may influence the structure or function of these regions.

Table 14.1 *Healthy People* Goals Related to Head and Neck Health

Goals	Patient Education Topics
Reduce the occurrence of developmental disabilities.	Teach rationale for assessing thyroid level and administering oral synthroid if needed.
Reduce activity limitation due to chronic back conditions.	Teach proper posture, bending, and lifting.
Increase the proportion of bicyclists and motorcyclists using helmets.	Encourage use of appropriate safety equipments to reduce risk of head or neck trauma.
Reduce deaths caused by motor vehicle crashes.	Encourage use of seatbelts to reduce risk of head or neck trauma, especially in populations at risk.

Source: *Healthy People 2010: What are its goals*? (n.d.). Retrieved May 10, 2010, from http://www.healthypeople.gov/About/goals.htm

Questions to Assess Risk Factors	Rationales
Have you ever had an accident that resulted in a loss of consciousness or head injury? Do you wear a seat belt? Bicycle helmet? Refer to Chapter 24 for more information.	Head injuries are a major cause of disability, which can be permanent. They may be preventable with appropriate use of protective gear, such as a helmet. Nurses can promote use of appropriate safety equipment for patients across the lifespan.
Were you ever treated with radiation to the neck, chest, or back?	Previously, acne on the neck and upper thorax was sometimes treated with radiation therapy. Patients who received such treatment are at significantly increased risk for thyroid and salivary-gland malignancies (Smith, 2008).
Have you had any surgeries involving your head or neck?	Because the head and neck have multiple structures, surgeries there may result in dysfunction of nerves, muscles, or vascular flow, or in endocrine changes. Nurses should understand the specific procedure and assess for any functional changes that could occur.
Do you have a family history of thyroid problems? • Who had the illness? • Was it hypothyroidism or hyperthyroidism? • When did the person have it? • How was it treated? • What were the outcomes?	*Graves' disease*, the most common type of *hyperthyroidism*, is autoimmune and may also be genetic. Some evidence supports that *medullary thyroid cancer* is genetically linked (Kim & Hatton, 2008).
Do you take any regular medications? How much alcohol do you drink? Do you take any herbal products?	Many medications (eg, bronchodilators, oral contraceptives) and alcohol can precipitate headaches. Some studies have found feverfew effective in relieving headaches (Evans & Taylor, 2006). While patients may use this and other herbal products for relief of symptoms such as headaches, these potentially potent chemicals could actually cause headache and other neurologic side effects.

Risk Assessment and Health-Related Patient Teaching

Teaching related to the head and neck involves reducing risk of injury to these areas, preventing complications from thyroid disorders, and promoting early detection of masses or lymph nodes that may be malignant. The *Healthy People* goals in Table 14-1 emphasize the wearing of helmets and use of seatbelts and child safety restraints to protect the head and neck. Other causes of injuries to these regions include motor vehicle collisions related to alcohol or drug use or sleepiness. Education for high-risk groups about not driving while under the influence or sleepy is critical. Another important education area, especially for older adults, is fall prevention.

A focus area for pregnant women is the need for regular examinations that include thyroid screening. Such prenatal care helps to ensure that thyroid levels remain within normal limits, protecting both mother and fetus.

Risk factors for cancers of the neck include male gender, age older than 50 years, tobacco use, and alcohol consumption (NCI, 2008). For patients with such risk factors, nurses should especially emphasize teaching related to smoking prevention or cessation (see Chapter 18).

Focused Health History Related to Common Symptoms

Common Head and Neck Symptoms

- Headache
- Neck pain
- Limited neck movement
- Facial pain
- Lumps or masses
- Hypothyroidism
- Hyperthyroidism

Questions to Assess Symptoms	Rationales/Abnormal Findings
Headache Have you had any unusually frequent or severe headaches? • Where is the headache? Does it radiate? Is it on one or both sides? • Describe the headache. What does it feel like? • How bad is it on a scale from 1 to 10, with 10 being the worst? • When did it start? How long has it lasted? How often do you get headaches? Do you ever have milder headaches? Is a pattern evident? • What makes it worse? What makes it better? What brings it on? Is there a relationship with food or alcohol? With activity? With menstrual cycle? • Do any other symptoms accompany the pain such as nausea, visual changes, or an aura? • Have you tried any treatments? How often do you take headache relievers or pain pills? Is it difficult to function without treatment? • Has there been any recent change in your headaches?	When taking history, pay attention to characteristics such as pain worse in the morning on awakening, precipitated or made worse by straining or sneezing (potentially *elevated intracranial pressure*) vs. worse as the day progresses (more likely *tension*). A throbbing, severe, unilateral headache that lasts 6–24 hours and is associated with photophobia, nausea, and vomiting suggests *migraine*, while a constant, unremitting, general headache that is described as a feeling of a tight band around the head and lasts for days, weeks, or even months is usually characteristic of a *tension muscle contraction headache*. Headaches may be categorized as primary or secondary. *Primary headaches* are benign, often recurring, and not associated with underlying pathology. *Secondary headaches* are associated with underlying pathology that ranges from mild (eg, common cold) to severe (eg, subarachnoid hemorrhage, brain tumor, meningitis). See Box 14-1 for concerning red flags.

BOX 14.1 LIST OF RED FLAGS FOR HEADACHES

- Onset of new or different headache
- Nausea or vomiting
- Worst headache ever experienced
- Progressive visual or neurological changes
- Paralysis
- Weakness, ataxia, or loss of coordination
- Drowsiness, confusion, memory impairment, or loss of consciousness
- Onset of headache after age of 50 years

- Papilledema
- Stiff neck
- Onset of headache with exertion, sexual activity, or coughing
- Systemic illness
- Numbness
- Asymmetry of papillary response
- Sensory loss
- Signs of meningeal irritation

Source: Sobri, M. S., Lamont, A. C., Alias, N. A., & Win, M. N. (2003). Red flags in patients presenting with headache: Clinical indications for neuroimaging. *British Journal of Radiololgy, 76*(908), 532–535.

Questions to Assess Symptoms	Rationales/Abnormal Findings

Neck Pain

- Where exactly is the pain?
- How long have you had it?
- On a scale of 1–10 how bad is it?
- Describe the pain.
- What makes it better? Worse?
- What is your pain goal?

Neck pain can be from musculoskeletal injury, tension, or pathologic changes (Piatt, 2005). Common causes include *trauma* at any age, muscle tension in adolescents or adults, and *arthritis* in older clients.

Limited Neck Movement

Are you having any difficulty turning or flexing/extending your neck?

Limitation of neck mobility may be from muscle tension/strain or cervical vertebral joint dysfunction.

Facial Pain

- Where exactly is the pain?
- How long have you had it?
- On a scale of 1–10 how bad is it?
- Describe the pain.
- What makes it better? Worse?
- What is your pain goal?

Trauma, infection, and neurologic disorders may result in facial pain, which also can be referred from another organ or system. Common causes of facial pain include the following:
- Muscle over-use
- Mouth/tooth infections
- Sinusitis
- Herpes zoster
- Trauma
- Migraine or cluster headaches
- Jaw pain, especially if associated with shoulder or arm pain (could be cardiac); this medical emergency requires immediate evaluation and treatment
- Skull pain, which may be related to tension headaches or tension of the neck muscles. Also consider skin lesions, trauma, and infection as possible causes.

Lumps or Masses

Have you noted any lumps or masses in your head or neck?
- How long have you had this?
- How many are there?
- How large are any?
- Are they changing?
- Are they tender or painful?

Nurses must differentiate the many structures in the neck by careful questioning of the characteristics of any neck lump, followed by careful physical examination grounded in knowledge of the anatomy of this region.

Hypothyroidism

Do you have any of these symptoms: fatigue; anorexia; cold intolerance; dry skin; brittle, coarse hair; menstrual irregularities; weight gain or difficulty losing weight; decreased libido?

Signs and symptoms of thyroid dysfunction are often nonspecific (Herrick, 2008). Nurses should consider that the patient has a thyroid problem when several symptoms are "clustered together." Metabolism is low.

Hyperthyroidism

Do you have any of these symptoms: fatigue; weight loss; anxiety; palpitations; rapid pulse; heat intolerance; fine, limp hair; diaphoresis; muscle weakness?

Similarly, hyperthyroidism usually presents with several of these signs or symptoms (Siraj, 2008). An overactive thyroid gland increases the metabolic rate.

Documentation of Normal Findings

Patient reports no unusual, severe, or frequent headaches. Denies loss of neck mobility or neck pain. Denies any lumps or masses in the neck. Reports no problems with fatigue, weight change, temperature discomfort, skin changes, sweating, or other unusual findings. *P. Rubin, RN*

Additional Questions	Rationales/Abnormal Findings
Pregnant Women Have you noticed any changes or swelling in your neck?	The thyroid gland enlarges slightly and symmetrically in pregnancy. Marked or unilateral enlargement is abnormal and requires further evaluation.
Do you have a headache or any sensory, motor, or visual changes?	*Migraines* are more common, possibly from increased hormones.
Newborns and Infants To caregiver, "Is the infant properly secured in an approved car seat every time he or she is in an automobile?"	Because infants' heads are disproportionately large, they are likely to sustain severe head injuries or death even in minor traffic accidents or sudden stops, if not positioned properly in a securely fastened car seat.
Was there any possible exposure of the infant to alcohol or drugs while the mother was pregnant?	Maternal use of alcohol or drugs can cause deformities of the fetal head and face, as well as other serious physical and mental disabilities. Thus, it is important to determine any and all in utero exposures.
Children and Adolescents Does the child wear a helmet for such actions as bicycling, scooter riding, or skateboarding? Does the child hold or bang his or her head?	Properly used helmets can reduce risk of significant head injury. Headache should be suspected in young children who hold or bang their heads but cannot describe their symptoms. In children older than 3 years, headache is significant, requiring thorough evaluation to rule out conditions related to increasing intracranial pressure.
Older Adult • Have you noticed any lumps/masses in your neck? • Do you have a new type of headache? • Do you have any pain in your neck? • Any weakness, numbness or tingling in your arms?	Cervical lymph nodes are usually *not* palpable, but submandibular glands may be more prominent from less subcutaneous fat. New headache in a patient older than 50 years requires thorough investigation to determine etiology. Arthritic changes in the cervical spine may present as neck pain or loss of sensation or strength in the upper extremities.

Cultural Considerations

Do you feel that you have a neck injury that has not been treated?	Diagnosis of a cervical spine injury is challenging and in many cases goes undiagnosed, especially in those lacking adequate health insurance (Rubenstein & van Tulder, 2008). Patients at risk include those following a fall or collision, and patients with osteoporosis, advanced arthritis, cancer, or degenerative bone disease (Harris, et al., 2008).

Objective Data Collection

Equipment

- Ambient lighting
- Penlight or flashlight for tangential lighting
- Gloves, if any lesions of the scalp or skin of head and neck are suspected
- Small cup of water

Preparation

If the patient is wearing a wig or hairpiece, ask him or her to remove it. Wash your hands. The patient is usually seated, facing the examiner. Instruct the patient that the head and neck will be inspected, palpated, and manipulated, but that the procedures should not be painful. Instruct the patient to tell you if any part of the head and neck examination causes discomfort.

Remember Faye Davis-Pierce, introduced at the beginning of this chapter. This 21-year-old college student has presented to the campus clinic with fatigue and weight gain. The nurse must use professional communication techniques to gather subjective data from the patient. The following conversations give two examples of interview styles used by different nurses. One style is more effective than the other.

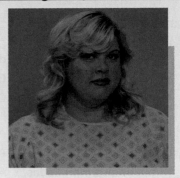

Less Effective	More Effective
Nurse: Hi, Ms. Davis-Pierce. My name is Brenda. Why are you here?	**Nurse:** Hi, I'm Brenda. What name do you prefer to be called?
Ms. Davis-Pierce: I've been feeling really tired.	**Faye:** Faye is fine. Thanks for asking.
Nurse: Many students are tired on college campuses. It's really stressful.	**Nurse:** Sure. So, how are you doing today?
Ms. Davis-Pierce: Yes. I've been under a lot of stress. It makes me hungry and I eat all the time.	**Faye:** I've just been feeling really tired.
Nurse: Have you gained any weight?	**Nurse:** Tell me a little about that.
Ms. Davis-Pierce: Yes—20 lb since the semester started! I guess it's the dorm food. It's full of fillers.	**Faye:** Well, I've been really stressed out and having trouble sleeping. It's hard to get out of bed sometimes in the morning.
Nurse: I know. We really should provide more nutritious food. I remember when I lived in the dorm and there was so much starch. We couldn't get anything fresh, and the desserts were wonderful. I gained 20 lb, too. Don't worry, you'll get it off.	**Nurse:** I see that you're in college, which can be stressful.
	Faye: Yes, it really can be.
Ms. Davis-Pierce: Yeah, I hope so.	**Nurse:** Have you noticed any other symptoms with your fatigue?
Nurse: I know that you will. All you have to do is eat more fruits and vegetables and get some exercise. Do you go to the gym?	**Faye:** Yeah, I've gained 20 lb. I think that it's the dorm food.
	Nurse: We can talk about some strategies for your nutrition later if you would like.
Ms. Davis-Pierce: I just haven't had the energy.	**Faye:** Yes, I would.
Nurse: Well, get somebody to go with you. It's more fun that way. You can keep each other on track.	**Nurse:** Have you noticed anything else, such as loss of appetite, dry skin, or hair?
	Faye: Well, yes, my skin and hair have been dry. You know my mother has been saying that she had a low thyroid when she was around my age. Could it be related?
	Nurse: It's possible. I'll make sure to report this information to the nurse practitioner when she sees you.

Critical Thinking Challenge

- What did the more effective nurse do to establish a therapeutic relationship?
- How did the more effective nurse use interview skills to collect pertinent data?
- What ineffective communication techniques did the less effective nurse demonstrate?

Common and Specialty or Advanced Techniques

The routine head-to-toe assessment includes the most important and common assessment techniques. Nurses may add specialty or advanced steps if concerns exist over a specific finding. Table 14-2 summarizes the most common techniques used in the comprehensive assessment of the head and neck, which are therefore essential to learn for use in clinical practice. Additional techniques may be added if the clinical situation warrants them.

Technique	Purpose	Screening or Registered Nurse Assessment	Focused or Advanced Practice Examination
Inspection of the head	Observe for symmetry, deformities	X	
Inspection of the hair	Observe for texture, color	X	
Inspection of the neck	Observe for lesions, limitations in movement	X	
Palpation of the scalp	Assess masses or lesions	X	
Palpation of the thyroid	Assess for enlargement		X
Palpation of lymph nodes	Assess for enlargement or tenderness		X
Auscultation of the thyroid	Listen for bruit		X

Comprehensive Physical Examination

Technique and Normal Findings	Abnormal Findings
Inspection	
Inspect the head (Fig. 14-8). *The head is centered, proportional to the body (1/7), erect, and without tremors, tics, or unusual movements. The skull is round without obvious deformities. The neck muscles are symmetric.*	Facial asymmetry may indicate damage to CN VII or a serious condition such as a *stroke*. Enlarged bones or tissues are associated with *acromegaly*. A puffy "moon" face is associated with *Cushing's syndrome*. Increased facial hair in females may be a sign of *Cushing's syndrome* or *endocrinopathy*. Periorbital edema is seen with *congestive heart failure* and *hypothyroidism (myxedema)*. See Tables 14-5 and 14-6 at the end of this chapter for visual examples.

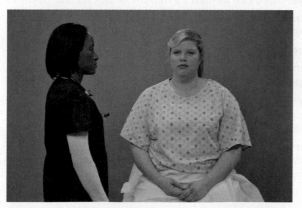

Figure 14.8 Inspecting the head.

Inspect facial features for symmetry and size. *Nasolabial folds are symmetric.*	If asymmetric, look for signs of trauma. Carefully assess any lesions for infection.
Inspect the hair (Fig. 14-9) for • Distribution and quantity • Texture • Cleanliness *Hair is evenly distributed across the scalp, extending from the superior aspect of the forehead to the base of the cranium and to the top of the ears bilaterally.*	Testosterone stimulates hair growth on the face, pubis, axilla, and chest but diminishes scalp hair growth. Male-pattern baldness occurs when there is both a genetic predisposition and increased testosterone or other male hormones (Kaufman, et al., 2008). Adult men may present with male-pattern baldness in either an "M" pattern on the scalp or, as hair loss continues, a "U" pattern with hair growth around the skull at the level of the temples.

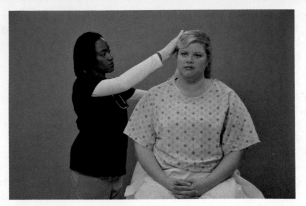

Figure 14.9 Examining the hair and scalp. The nurse wears gloves if there is any possibility of contact with an open sore or lesion.

Inspect the neck (Fig. 14-10). Look at the neck muscles, sternocleidomastoid, thyroid, and isthmus (may be visualized with tangential light and asking the patient to swallow a sip of water). *Trachea is midline. A slight symmetric elevation may be observed in the mid-neck.*

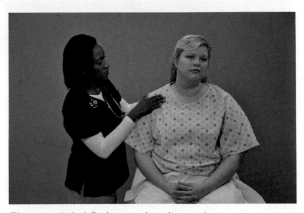

Figure 14.10 Inspecting the neck.

Palpation

Palpate the temporal artery in the space above the cheek bone near the scalp line.

The temporal artery pulse is 2–3 on a 4 point scale.

Palpate the scalp. Refer to Chapter 13. *The scalp is symmetric without tenderness, masses, lesions, or differences in firmness.*

Palpate the thyroid, either from the anterior or posterior approach.
• For the *anterior approach*, have the patient tilt the head slightly back. Locate the thyroid and cricoid cartilages. The thyroid cartilage is larger, shield-shaped, and in the mid-neck, sometimes referred to as the "Adam's apple" in males.

Such hair loss can occur any time after puberty but is usually more noticeable in middle and older adults (Guyton & Hall, 2006). Unusual distribution or patterns of hair growth on the face or skull are associated with endocrine abnormalities. Any nits (white to brown small 1 mm specks) attached to hair shafts may be signs of *pediculosis* (head lice). Usually, intense itching accompanies infestation. Traction alopecia may occur with tight braiding (Khumalo, et al., 2008) See also Chapter 13.

Thyroid enlargement or masses can be seen more easily when the patient swallows and while illuminating the neck with a tangential light.

Temporal arthritis is a painful inflammation of the temporal artery. A biopsy is necessary for diagnosis.

Bulging or depression of the bony structure of the scalp may result fro m trauma or tumor growth. Bulging fontanels in infants may be a clinical sign of *hydrocephalus*, or simply the result of lusty crying (see Table 14-5). Depressed fontanels are most often associated with dehydration.

• Unilateral bulging may be a thyroid goiter, cyst, or tumor.
• Neck masses may also originate from a lymph node or cyst.

(text continues on page 332)

Below is the ringed cricoid cartilage. Just below the cricoid cartilage the isthmus of the thyroid should be palpable as a smooth rubbery band that rises and falls with swallowing. With the pads of the fingers of one hand gently palpate the thyroid isthmus. Ask the patient to lower the head slightly and turn it slightly to one side. The sternocleidomastoid muscle will relax on the side to which the patient turns. Palpate behind the sternocleidomastoid muscle (Fig. 14-11).

- For the posterior approach, locate the thyroid and cricoid cartilages and the thyroid isthmus by palpation while standing behind the patient. Have the patient bend the head slightly forward and toward one side. Use your index finger to slightly retract the sternocleidomastoid muscle on the side toward which the patient has tilted the head. Use the middle two or three fingers to locate the lobe of the thyroid. The fingers of the other hand should gently displace the trachea and thyroid cartilage on the opposite side, which helps to move the thyroid gland slightly forward and prominent and allows for easier palpation. It is, however, not unusual for the thyroid lobes to also be nonpalpable with this approach (Fig. 14-12).

- Any new neck mass in a patient older than 35 years should be carefully evaluated to rule out cancer. It could be a lymph node enlarged by metastatic cancer, a primary lymphoma, or a tumor of structures of the neck.
- Unusual hardness is a dangerous finding, possibly associated with cancer (Kim & Hatton, 2008).
- A toxic goiter may feel softer than normal thyroid tissue.
- Tenderness is common with subacute infections, traumatic injury, and radiation thyroiditis (Burman, et al., 2009).
- The parathyroid gland is not independently palpated but may be noted when attempting to palpate the thyroid gland. Parathyroid carcinoma is a rare form of cancer. The tumors usually secrete parathyroid hormone, producing hyperparathyroidism, and increased calcium levels. Parathyroid carcinoma may be suspected, but it usually cannot be confirmed prior to surgery.

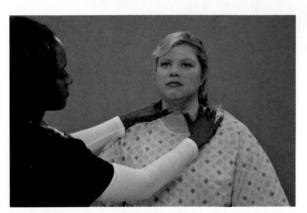

Figure 14.11 Palpating behind the sternocleidomastoid muscle for the anterior thyroid.

If palpable, the thyroid is smooth, rubbery, nontender, symmetrical, and barely palpable beneath the sternocleidomastoid.

Palpate for discernable lymph nodes in the head and neck following a systematic pattern (Fig. 14-13). The order of examination is usually preauricular, posterior auricular,

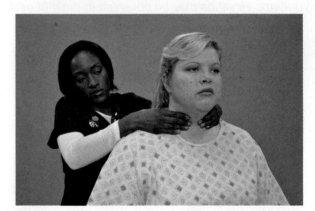

Figure 14.12 Palpating the thyroid from the posterior approach.

Palpable, tender, and warm lymph nodes usually indicate an infection in the area from which the lymph vessels drain to that node (Ellis, 2002):
- Anterior cervical nodes: *pharyngitis*
- Posterior cervical nodes: *mononucleosis*
- Posterior auricular nodes: *otitis media*
- Supraclavicular nodes: must be carefully evaluated as a possible sign of metastatic cancer. Virchow's node, the left supraclavicular, is associated with *lung and abdominal cancers.*

Hard, rubbery, irregular, fixed, and nontender lymph nodes are a possible sign of *lymphoma.*

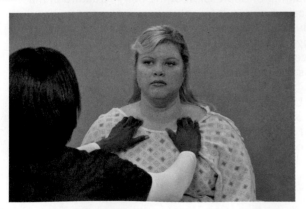

Figure 14.13 Palpating for any discernable lymph nodes.

occipital, submental, submandibular, tonsilar, anterior cervical chain, posterior cervical chain, and supraclavicular. Using the pads of the second, third, and fourth fingers, gently palpate with small circles, varying the amount of pressure over each lymphatic region. *Usually no lymph nodes are palpable in the adult.* If a node is palpable, it is important to describe the following characteristics:

* Location—which lymphatic chain and where along that chain is the node
* Size—in mm or cm
* Consistency—how hard or soft is the node? It should be smooth, slightly soft, and nontender.
* Mobility—it should be freely movable
* Delimitation—there should not be any matting together of lymph nodes

Auscultation

If the thyroid is enlarged, either unilaterally or bilaterally, auscultate over each lobe for a bruit using the bell of the stethoscope (Fig. 14-14). *No bruit or vascular sounds are audible.*

Bruits are most often found with a *toxic goiter, hyperthyroidism,* or *thyrotoxicosis.*

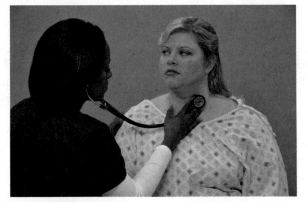

Figure 14.14 Auscultating the thyroid.

Documentation of Normal Findings

Thyroid gland palpable, symmetric, smooth, rubbery, and nontender. No bruit. *P Rubin, RN*

Documenting Abnormal Findings

The RN reports her findings and history to the APRN, who finishes conducting a physical examination of Faye Davis-Pierce, the 21 year old with fatigue and weight gain. Unlike the samples of normal documentation previously charted, Faye Davis-Pierce has abnormal findings. Review the following important findings revealed in each of the steps of objective data collection. Consider how the RN and APRN will collaborate related to these findings.

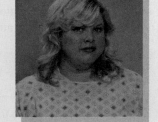

Inspection: Skull is normocephalic, atraumatic. Hair blondish and slightly dry. Skin dry and intact. Trachea midline. Skin color slightly pale, appears puffy.

Palpation: Thyroid gland palpable and enlarged, symmetric, smooth, rubbery, and nontender. No lumps or masses.

Auscultation: No bruit over thyroid.

R. Bustion, APRN

Lifespan Considerations

Pregnant Women

Chloasma may be present on the face. This blotchy and hyperpigmented patch appears on the cheeks and fades in the postpartum period. Detection of maternal (and fetal) hypothyroidism is of major importance because of potential damage to fetal neural development, an increased incidence of miscarriage, and preterm birth (Abalovich, et al., 2007). Autoimmune thyroid disease is associated with both increased rates of miscarriage and postpartum thyroiditis.

Infants and Children

Measure the infant's head circumference (see Chapter 6). Observe the head for shape and symmetry. Infants in one position for prolonged periods may have a flattening of one part of the head. Asymmetry may also result from premature closure of the sutures.

Note head control. The infant should be able to hold up the head by 4 months of age. Palpate the skull for patent sutures, fontanels, edema, fractures, or masses. Normally the posterior fontanel closes by 1–2 months; the anterior fontanel closes by 7 to 19 months. A caput succedaneum is a swollen and ecchymotic area caused from the birth process as the head is squeezed. It usually resolves in the first few days. A cephalahematoma is a hemorrhage defined over one cranial bone. It appears shortly after birth and increases in size. It also resolves on its own but the infant is more likely to develop jaundice because of the breakdown of the red blood cells.

Note any limitations in neck range of motion. If the child holds the head to one side with the chin pointing toward the opposite side, the sternocleidomastoid muscle may be injured. The neck is normally short in an infant. Skinfolds are present between head and shoulders in infancy.

To palpate the lymph nodes, tilt the child's head upward slightly but without tensing the sternocleidomastoid or trapezius muscles. Lymph nodes are not usually present in an infant but a child's may be palpable.

Observe the face or symmetry, movement and general appearance. Ask the child to make a face to assess for any paralysis. Note any unusual facial proportions that may be present with fetal alcohol syndrome or Down's syndrome.

Congenital hypothyroidism is rare, but if not identified early, it will result in cognitive delays (Lafranchi, 2008). All states screen all infants by measuring thyroid-stimulating hormone (TSH) levels shortly after birth (American Academy of Pediatrics, 2006). Early recognition and treatment (within 1 month of birth) can significantly mitigate associated developmental

delays. Hypothyroidism is more common in infants with Down's syndrome (Kliegman, et al., 2007).

Older Adult

The facial skin may appear more wrinkled and less elastic. Thinning of the hair is also a normal aging process. The neck may have reduced range of motion with chronic conditions such as arthritis. Additionally, there is an exaggerated concave curve of the spine.

Hypothyroidism in the older adult often lacks the classic symptoms seen in younger patients (Peeters, 2008). This is from a more subtle onset, chronic diseases, and the idea that typical signs and symptoms (fatigue, cold intolerance, constipation, or depression) may be attributed to aging. Additionally the older adult is more prone to hyperthyroidism (Brunk, 2008). Unexplained weight loss, diarrhea or constipation, nausea, and vomiting may be presenting symptoms. Depression and mania can be presenting symptoms of hyperthyroidism in the elderly.

Evidence-based Critical Thinking

Common Laboratory and Diagnostic Testing

Evaluation of headaches may indicate the need for several diagnostic tests, which would be determined by an APRN or other advanced health care professional. Examples of such tests include computed tomography (CT), magnetic resonance imaging (MRI), or lumbar puncture.

Musculoskeletal injury or disease can be confirmed with an X-ray, CT, or MRI (see Chapter 23). If test results are negative, the nurse should assess for complete range of motion of the neck, looking for any muscle tension, loss of mobility, or pain. The nurse should recall that cardiac disease may present with referred pain to the neck or jaw, making it important to assess for signs of cardiovascular disease.

Tests of thyroid function are commonly performed for patients at any age presenting with signs or symptoms of hyperthyroidism or hypothyroidism. Usually TSH, T3, and T4 are measured. Table 14-3 shows normal and abnormal values.

Diagnostic Reasoning

Nursing Diagnosis, Outcomes, and Interventions

Table 14-4 compares nursing diagnoses, abnormal findings, and interventions commonly related to assessment of the head and neck (NANDA-I, 2009). Nurses use assessment information to identify patient outcomes. Some outcomes related to head and neck problems include the following:

- Patient participates in physical activity with appropriate changes in vital signs.
- Patient verbalizes increased energy and well being.
- Pain goals are met (Moorhead, et al., 2007).

Once the outcomes area is established, nursing care is implemented to improve the status of the patient. The nurse uses

Table 14.3	Thyroid Hormone Levels			
Test	TSH	Free T4	Total T3	Total T4
Normal values	0.3–5.0 mU/L	0.8–2.3 ng/dL	80–200 ng/dL	5–12 μg/dL
Hypothyroidism	High	Low	Low	Low
Hyperthyroidism	Low	High	High	High

Table 14.4 Common Nursing Diagnoses Associated with the Head and Neck

Diagnosis and Related Factors	Point of Differentiation	Assessment Characteristics	Nursing Interventions
Activity intolerance related to hypothyroidism	Inability to complete or continue daily activities as a result of a lack of physical or mental energy, which is symptomatic of the thyroid problem	Verbal report of weakness, abnormal P or BP during activity, dyspnea, ECG changes	Determine cause.* If appropriate gradually increase activity. Monitor response to activity. Refer patient to physical therapy.
Fatigue related to low T3 and high TSH	A continual and overwhelming feeling of exhaustion or tiredness despite sleep that is normally sufficient for age, health, and lifestyle	Lack of energy, increased rest and sleep requirements, lethargy or listlessness, drowsiness	Assess severity. Evaluate sleep and nutritional status. Gather data to help determine if cause is physiological or psychological.
Chronic pain related to cervical spine injury	Pain lasting more than 6 months. Use pain scale to describe.	Report of pain, facial grimace, muscle tension, increased P, R, or BP, shifting or guarding	Assess characteristics. Work with pain team to determine appropriate medical treatment. Use nonpharmacologic interventions.

*Collaborative interventions.

critical thinking and evidence-based practice to develop the interventions. Some examples of nursing interventions for the head and neck are as follows:

• Allow for periods of rest before planned activities.

• Set small, achievable short term goals for activity that can be motivational.
• Treat pain before it becomes severe (Bulechek, et al., 2007).

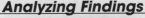

Analyzing Findings

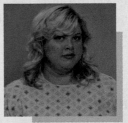

Remember Faye Davis-Pierce, whose problems have been outlined throughout this chapter. Initial subjective and objective data collection is complete. Tests of Faye's thyroid levels reveal an elevated TSH and low T3 and T4, indicating hypothyroidism. The following nursing note illustrates how the assessment data are analyzed and nursing interventions are developed.

Subjective: I've just been feeling really tired. I've had some weight gain and I've been really cold.

Objective: Hair blondish, slightly dry. Skin dry and intact. Skin color slightly pale, appears puffy and tired. TSH high and T3 and T4 are low. Skull is normocephalic, atraumatic. Trachea midline. Thyroid gland palpable and enlarged, symmetric, smooth, rubbery, and nontender. No lumps or masses. No bruit over thyroid.

Analysis: Symptoms are related to low thyroid. Need for teaching about new prescription for thyroid replacement.

Plan: Provide teaching about new thyroid replacement medication. Provide materials on nutrition for healthy food choices. Assess college stressors at next visit.

P. Rubin, RN

Critical Thinking Challenge

• How does the role of the RN and APRN differ in this case?
• What role and responsibility does the RN have for assessment of the laboratory values?
• How will the nurse approach teaching about diet and exercise given sensitivity in many patients about weight gain?
• Why did the RN decide to defer assessment of college stressors until the next visit?

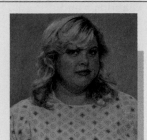

In many facilities, nurses initiate referrals based on needs related to teaching or interventions. Results that might trigger a pharmacy consult include questions about the drug dose, route, or time; drug interactions; appropriate therapies; discharge teaching; and patient education (Interdisciplinary Plan, 2007). Read the following dialogue below to see how the RN discusses with pharmacy personnel the new prescription for Faye Davis-Pierce.

Situation: Hi, I'm Patricia, an RN who saw Faye Davis-Pierce in the clinic today. She has been diagnosed with hypothyroidism. Her APRN has written a prescription for thyroid replacement for her.

Background: The patient is concerned about paying for the medication. I remember that there are some financial issues related to the generic versus trade name thyroid replacement drugs.

Assessment: We want to make sure that costs are controlled as much as possible so that she can obtain and take the medication correctly.

Recommendations: Can you tell me what her copayments will be between the generic and trade medications? She will need to be on this long term over the school year. It will be important for her to stay on the same medication without switching between brands.

Critical Thinking Challenge

- Is consideration of funding within the role of the RN, APRN, or pharmacist?
- What teaching will the RN provide compared to the pharmacist?
- What is the role of the RN and APRN in assessing for both the intended effects and also side effects of the new medication?

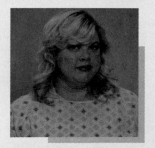

The nurse uses assessment data to formulate a nursing care plan with patient outcomes and interventions for Faye Davis-Pierce. After completion of interventions, the nurse reevaluates Ms. Davis-Pierce and documents findings in the chart to show progress toward goals. The nurse uses critical thinking and judgment to continue or revise the diagnosis, outcomes, or interventions. This is often in the form of a care plan or case note similar to below.

Nursing Diagnosis	Patient Outcomes	Nursing Interventions	Rationale	Evaluation
Knowledge deficit related to new diagnosis of hypothyroidism as evidenced by no knowledge of new medication	Patient will state intended effect and side effects of medication.	Teach patient not to take medication with food. Review effects and side effects of medication, including that it may take several weeks to notice a change. Provide written information. Give a phone number in case she has questions or experiences side effects.	Written instructions are a resource that the patient can access after leaving the clinic. Questions may not arise until the patient is home.	The patient stated the intended effect of resolution of her symptoms. She also stated the side effects of too high a level, including weight loss, anxiety, palpitations, rapid pulse, heat intolerance fine limp hair, and diaphoresis. The patient scheduled a follow-up appointment in 3 weeks.

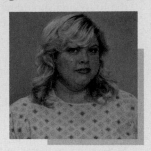

Using the previous steps of diagnostic reasoning, organizing, and prioritizing, consider all the case study findings woven throughout this chapter. When answering the following questions, begin drawing conclusions and see how the pieces of assessment must work together to create an environment for personalized, appropriate, and accurate care.

• How might Faye's physical issues relate to her psychosocial health, including potential issues related to her age and status as a college student?
• What other physical findings might be present, and what other body systems might be involved?
• What type of follow-up care and reassessment might the patient need at subsequent visits?

Key Points

• Structures of the head and neck also include the trachea, thyroid, and lymphatics.
• The anterior fontanel closes at 8 months of age, while the posterior fontanel closes at 3 months.
• Fontanels in the newborn should be flat, not bulging or retracted.
• Acute situations that need emergency assessment and intervention include head or neck injuries, neck pain (may be cardiac), enlarged hard nodes (which may indicate cancer), and thyrotoxicosis.
• Common symptoms of the head and neck include pain, limited neck movement, lumps or masses, hypothyroidism, and hyperthyroidism.
• The neck muscles, sternocleidomastoid muscle, thyroid, and isthmus are inspected in the neck.
• The thyroid is normally smooth, rubbery, and moveable. It is also common for the thyroid to be nonpalpable.
• A bruit may be present with hyperthyroidism or thyrotoxicosis.
• Common nursing diagnoses for the head and neck include activity intolerance, fatigue, chronic pain, and knowledge deficit.

Review Questions

1. While examining the patient's neck, the nurse finds the trachea midline but has difficulty palpating the thyroid. What action would the nurse take next?
   A. Document this finding as normal.
   B. Tell the patient that this finding is abnormal.
   C. Report to the physician a suspicion of a slow growing goiter.
   D. Look for signs of hypothyroidism.

2. The lymph nodes that lie superficial to the mastoid bone are the:
   A. Preauricular nodes
   B. Posterior auricular nodes
   C. Superficial cervical nodes
   D. Supraclavicular nodes

3. Which of the following descriptions is most consistent with a patient who has hypothyroidism?
   A. Slightly obese, perspiring female, who complains of feeling cold all the time and having diarrhea
   B. Slightly obese female with periorbital edema and a flat facial expression, who complains of constipation, deceased appetite, and fatigue
   C. Thin, anxious-appearing female with exophthalmos and a rapid pulse, and who complains of diarrhea
   D. Thin, perspiring male with a deep hoarse voice, facial edema, a thick tongue, and reports of diarrhea

4. Physical examination of a patient reveals an enlarged tonsilar node. Acutely infected nodes would be
   A. Hard and nontender
   B. Fixed and soft
   C. Firm but movable and tender
   D. Irregular and hard

5. While assessing the skin of a 24-year-old patient, the nurse notes decreased skin turgor. The nurse should further assess for signs and symptoms of
   A. hyperthyroidism
   B. hypothyroidism
   C. malnutrition
   D. dehydration

6. The nurse can best evaluate the strength of the sternocleidomastoid muscle by having the patient
   A. clench his or her teeth during muscle palpation
   B. bring his or her head to the chest
   C. turn his or her head against resistance
   D. extend his or her arms against resistance

7. Which of the following best describes the instructions the nurse should give a patient when assessing the thyroid from the posterior approach?
   A. Please tilt your head back as far as possible.
   B. Please turn your head as far to the right as you can.
   C. Please bring your chin down toward your neck.
   D. Please look straight ahead and tilt your head slightly down and to one side.

8. While assessing a patient, the nurse finds a palpable lymph node in the left supraclavicular region. Which of the following should be the next action?

A. Recognize that it is common to palpate lymph nodes in this region and they are usually not pathologic.

B. Recognize that a palpable node in this region is a dangerous indication of metastatic cancer that requires further evaluation.

C. Recognize that this is a common area for lymph nodes to be enlarged with minor infections.

D. Recognize that a palpable lymph node in this region is always indicative of malignancy.

9. While reviewing laboratory values for thyroid function on an adult patient, the nurse sees that the TSH is elevated, and the T3 and T4 are decreased. The nurse recognizes that these findings are indicative of

A. normal thyroid function

B. hypothyroidism

C. hyperthyroidism

D. thyroid cancer

10. A patient presents with a complaint of drooping of his eyes, cheeks, and mouth on one side. This finding is most likely associated with pathology of which cranial nerve?

A. Cranial nerve III

B. Cranial nerve VI

C. Cranial nerve VII

D. Cranial nerve IX

References

Abalovich, M., Amino, N., Barbour, L. A., Cobin, R. H., De Groot, L. J., Glinoer, D., et al. (2007). Management of thyroid dysfunction during pregnancy and postpartum: An Endocrine Society Clinical Practice Guideline. *Thyroid, 17*(11), 1159–1167.

American Academy of Pediatrics. (2006). Update of newborn screening and therapy for congenital hypothyroidism. *Pediatrics, 117*(6), 2290–2303.

Brunk, B. (2008). Elders are at risk for thyroid dysfunction. *Caring for the Ages, 9*(5), 23.

Bulechek, G. B., & Butcher, H. K., McCloskey Dochterman (2007). *Nursing Interventions Classification (NIC)* (4th ed.) St. Louis, MO: Mosby.

Burman, K. D., Ross, D., S., & Martin, K. A. (2009). *Overview of thyroiditis.* Retrieved December 14, 2009, from http://www.uptodateonline.com.proxy.seattleu.edu/online/content/topic.do?topicKey=thyroid/12274&selectedTitle=2%7E20&source=search_result

Drake, R. L., Vogl, W., & Mitchell A. W. M. (2005). *Gray's anatomy for students.* Philadelphia: Elsevier.

Ellis, H. (2002). *Clinical anatomy: A revision and applied anatomy for clinical students* (10th ed.). Oxford, UK: Blackwell Science.

Evans, R. W., & Taylor, F. R. (2006). Natural or alternative medications for migraine prevention. *Headache, 46*(6), 1012–1018.

Guyton, A. C., & Hall, J. E. (2006). *Textbook of medical physiology* (11th ed.). Philadelphia: Elsevier Saunders.

Haddow, J. E., McClain, M. R., Palomaki, G. E., & Hollowell, J. G. (2007). Urine iodine measurements, creatinine adjustment, and thyroid deficiency in an adult United States population. *Clinical Endocrinology and Metabolism, 92*(3), 1019–1022.

Harris, B. A., Blackmore, C. C., Mirza, S., & Jurkovich, J. (2008). Clearing the cervical spine in obtunded patients. *Spine, 33*(14), 1547–1553

Healthy People 2010: What are its goals? (n.d.). Retrieved December 5, 2009, from http://www.healthypeople.gov/About/goals.htm

Herrick, B. (2008). Cochrane for clinicians: Subclinical hypothyroidism. *American Family Physician, 77*(7), 953–955.

Interdisciplinary Plan. (2007). *Interdisciplinary plan for assessment/ reassessment and care planning.* Retrieved August 26, 2007, from https://hmcweb.washington.edu/ADMIN/APOP/Administration/5.20.htm

Kaufman, K. D., Girman, C. J., Round, E. M., Johnson-Levonas, A. O., Shah, A. K., & Rotonda, J. (2008). Progression of hair loss in men with androgenetic alopecia (male pattern hair loss): Long-term (5-year) controlled observational data in placebo-treated patients. *European Journal of Dermatology, 18*(4), 407–411.

Khumalo, N. P., Jessop, S., Gumedze, F., & Ehrlich, R. (2008). Determinants of marginal traction alopecia in African girls and women. *Journal of the American Academy of Dermatology, 59*(3), 432–438.

Kim, N., & Hatton, M. P. (2008). The role of genetics in Graves disease and thyroid orbitopathy. *Seminars in Ophthalmology, 23*(1), 67–72.

Kliegman, R. M, Behrman, R. E., Jenson, H. B., & Stanton, B. M. D. (2007). *Nelson Textbook of Pediatrics* (18th ed.). Philadelphia: Elsevier Saunders.

Lafranchi, S. (2008). Clinical features and detection of congenital hypothyroidism. Retrieved October 1, 2008, from http://www.uptodateonline.com.proxy.seattleu.edu/online/content/topic.do?topicKey=pediendo/2832&selectedTitle=4~150&source=search_result

Moorhead, S., Johnson, M., & Mass, M. (2007). *Nursing Outcomes Classification (NOC)* (4th ed.). Philadelphia: Mosby.

Mosby's medical nursing, and allied health dictionary (6th ed.). (2002). St. Louis, MO: Mosby.

National Cancer Institute. (2008). *Head and neck cancers: Questions and answers.* Retrieved October 2, 2008, from http://www.cancer.gov/cancertopics/factsheet/Sites-Types/head-and-neck

Nayak, P., & Hodak, S. P. (2007). Hyperthyroidism. *Endocrinology and Metabolism Clinics of North America, 36*(3), 617–656.

North American Nursing Diagnosis Association. (2009). *Nursing diagnoses, 2009–2011 Edition: Definitions and classifications (NANDA NURSING DIAGNOSIS).* West Sussex UK: John Wiley & Sons.

Peeters, R. P. (2008). Thyroid hormones and aging. *Hormones, 7*(1), 28–35.

Piatt, J. H. (2005). Detected and overlooked cervical spine injury among comatose trauma patients: From the Pennsylvania Trauma Outcomes Study. *Neurosurgery Focus, 19*(4), E6.

Rubenstein, S. M., & van Tulder, M. (2008). A best-evidence review of diagnostic procedures for neck and low-back pain. *Best Practice and Research: Clinical Rheumatolology, 22*(3), 471–482.

Siraj, E. S. (2008). Update on the diagnosis and treatment of hyperthyroidism. *Journal of Clinical Outcomes Management, 15*(6), 298–307.

Smith, R.V. (2008). *Tumors of the head and neck.* Retrieved May 23, 2010, from http://www.merck.com/mmpe/sec08/ch093/ch093a.htm

Sobri, M. S., Lamont, A. C., Alias, N. A., & Win, M. N. (2003). Red flags in patients presenting with headache: Clinical indications for neuroimaging. *British Journal of Radiololgy, 76*(908), 532–535.

Swartz, M. H. (2006). *Textbook of physical diagnosis: History and examination* (5th ed.). Philadelphia: Elsevier Saunders.

Uphold, C. R., & Graham, M. V. (2003). *Clinical guidelines in family practice* (4th ed.). Gainesville, FL: Barmarrae Books.

The Jensen suite offers these additional resources to enhance learning and facilitate understanding of this chapter:

- thePoint on line resource, http//thepoint.lww.com/Jensen1E
- Student CD-ROM included with the book
- *Laboratory Manual for Nursing Health Assessment: A Best Practice Approach*
- *Pocket Guide for Nursing Health Assessment: A Best Practice Approach*

Table 14.5   Head and Neck Problems More Common in Childhood

Hydrocephalus

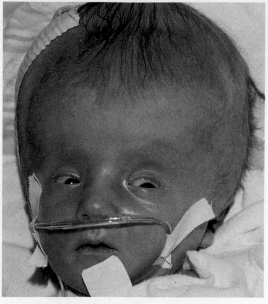

An abnormal collection of cerebrospinal fluid in the ventricles of the brain causes enlargement of the cranium. Infants with hydrocephalus may have separation of the cranial sutures, bulging fontanels, and dilated veins across the scalp.

Fetal Alcohol Syndrome (FAS)

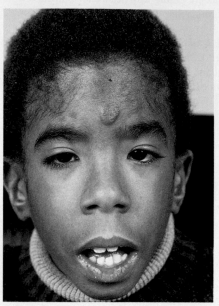

Developmental delays and congenital abnormalities are associated with maternal intake of alcohol during pregnancy. Physical manifestations include microcephaly, flattened cheekbones, small eyes, and a flattened upper lip. Children with FAS have multiple developmental and learning disabilities.

Down's Syndrome (Trisomy 21)

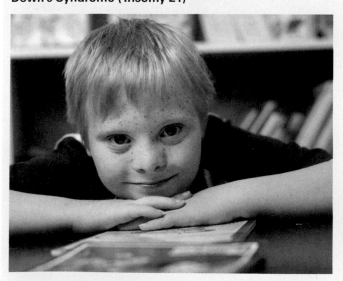

This congenital condition results from either an extra chromosome 21 or translocation of chromosome 14 or 15 with 21 or 22. Manifestations in the head and neck region include microcephaly, a flattened occipital bone, slanted small eyes, a depressed nasal bridge, low-set ears, and a protruding tongue.

Cretinism (Congenital Hypothyroidism)

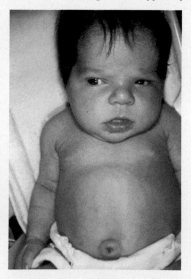

Affected infants have puffy facial features and often a larger than normal tongue. This syndrome is more common in parts of the world where diets are deficient in iodine.

Craniocytosis

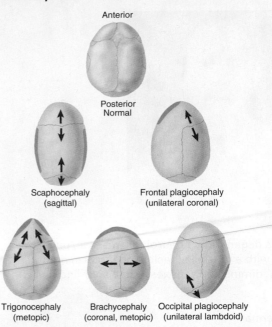

Premature closure and ossification of the fontanels results in skull deformities and microcephaly. Early diagnosis and surgical correction minimize malformations.

Torticollis

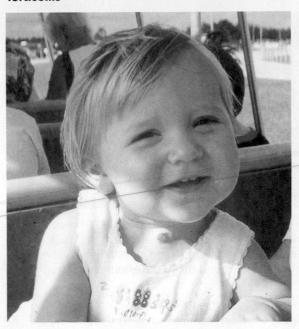

Congenital or acquired contraction of the sternocleidomastoid muscle causes the patient to incline the head to one side. Range of motion of the head and neck is decreased.

⚠ **Table 14.6   Head and Neck Problems More Common in Adults**

Acromegaly

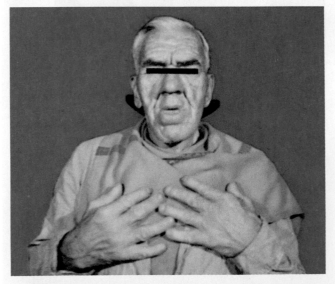

Overproduction of growth hormone in adults results in thickening of the skin, subcutaneous tissue, and facial bones and coarsening of facial features (see also Chapter 6).

Bell's Palsy

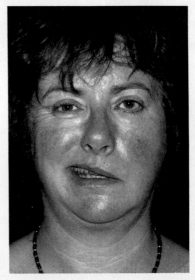

Paralysis, usually unilateral, of the facial nerve (CN VII) can be transient or permanent. Causes include trauma, compression, and infection.

(table continues on page 342)

Table 14.6   Head and Neck Problems More Common in Adults (continued)

Cushing's Syndrome

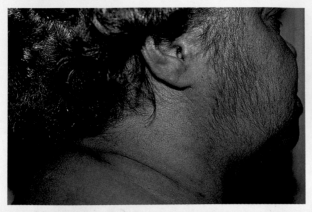

Excessive production of exogenous ACTH results in a round "moon" facies, fat deposits at the nape of the neck, "buffalo hump," and sometimes a velvety discoloration around the neck (*acanthosis nigra*).

Parkinson's Disease

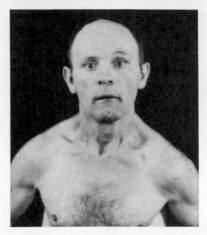

With this degenerative neurologic disease, patients present with a mask-like facial appearance, rigid muscles, diminished reflexes, and a shuffling gait.

Cerebral Vascular Accident (CVA/Stroke)

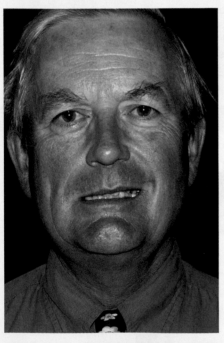

Also know as a "brain attack." Embolism, hemorrhage, or vasospasm in the brain results in ischemia of surrounding tissue and neurologic damage. Symptoms depend on the part of the brain affected.

Scleroderma

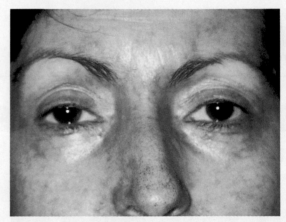

Hardening of the skin usually is noted first in the hands and face. Skin becomes firm and loses mobility, seemingly fixed to underlying tissues. Facial scleroderma presents with shiny taut immobile skin, which may make it difficult for patients to speak, chew, or even swallow. It can affect other organs and tissues.

Table 14.6　Head and Neck Problems More Common in Adults (continued)

Goiter

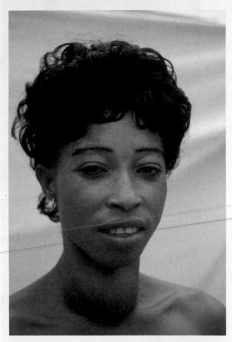

Enlarged thyroid gland can be associated with hyperthyroidism, hypothyroidism, or normal thyroid function. Enlargement can compress other structures in the neck, making surgical removal necessary. After thyroidectomy patients must be treated with exogenous thyroid hormone for the rest of their lives.

Myxedema

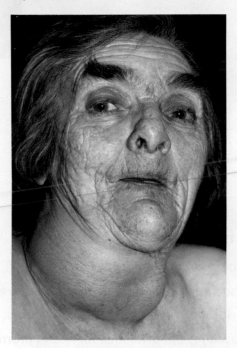

With severe hypothyroidism, patients present with periorbital swelling and edema of the face, hands, and feet. These patients must be identified and treated quickly and chronically with exogenous thyroid hormone.

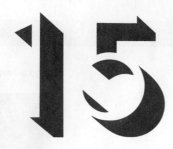

Eyes Assessment

Learning Objectives

1 Identify common landmarks of the eye.

2 Identify the structures and functions of the eye.

3 Relate periorbital landmarks to eye structures.

4 Identify teaching opportunities for health promotion and risk reduction related to the eye and vision.

5 Differentiate subjective data collected for visual changes.

6 Collect objective data on eye shape, ocular movements, vision, and retinal changes.

7 Identify normal ocular movements and vision.

8 Identify abnormal visual changes and ocular movements.

9 Identify normal and abnormal findings in the inspection and palpation of the eye.

10 Individualize ocular health assessment considering the condition, age, gender, and culture of the patient.

11 Use subjective and objective data to analyze ocular findings and plan interventions.

12 Document and communicate ocular data using appropriate medical terminology.

*M*r. Harris, a 61-year-old African American man, is in the adult medicine clinic for a routine physical examination. His temperature is 37°C, pulse 86 beats/min, respirations 16 breaths/min, and blood pressure 118/68. Upon reviewing documentation from his last annual assessment, the nurse notes that Mr. Harris takes a blood pressure medication and cholesterol-lowering agent. The patient previously worked as a janitor for the school system and now is a school bus driver. He has a 5-year history of glaucoma, for which he uses eye drops. Today, he states that his vision seems worse than usual.

You will gain more information about Mr. Harris as you progress through this chapter. As you study the content and features, consider Mr. Harris's case and the importance of patients seeking care for primary prevention. Begin thinking about the following points:

- What routine assessments should the nurse make related to the patient's eye health?
- What additional assessments should the nurse make based on the patient's reports of decreased vision?
- How can the nurse encourage Mr. Harris's desire for improved health?

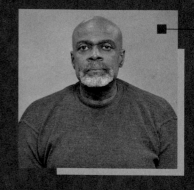

This chapter reviews anatomy and physiology pertinent to ocular and visual function, along with key variations in eye assessment related to lifespan and culture. It explores subjective data collection for eye health, including assessment of risk factors and focused history related to common symptoms. Content on objective data collection includes correct techniques for assessing vision, ocular movements, the external eye, and exterior and interior ocular structures; normal and unexpected visual and ocular findings; and appropriate documentation. Tests of visual acuity are part of screening during the complete physical examination and ongoing assessments for patients with identified ocular and visual problems or diseases. Although challenging, ocular and retinal assessments provide information that can assist with accurate diagnosis and related early interventions.

Structure and Function Overview

The *eye* (commonly referred to as the eyeball) is the sensory organ of sight. The orbital socket of the skull protects the complex internal structures of the eye (see Chapter 14); only the anterior portion of the eyeball is visible.

The eye is small, with an approximate diameter of 1 in (2.5 cm). It takes in information in the form of light, which internal structures then analyze and interpret to produce shapes, colors, and objects.

Extraocular Structures

The external (extraocular) structures of the eye support and protect it (Fig. 15-1). The **eyelids** are loose mobile folds of skin that cover the eye, protect it from foreign bodies, regulate light entrance, and distribute tears. The **palpebral fissure** is the almond-shaped open space between the eyelids. The lid margins normally approximate completely when the palpebral fissure is closed. The upper eyelid normally covers the upper portion of the iris. The lower eyelid's margin is at the **limbus**, which is the border between the cornea and sclera.

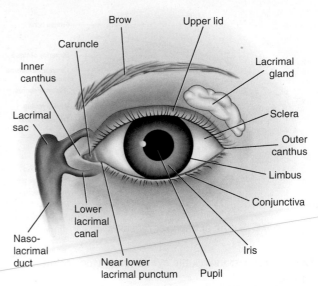

Figure 15.2 Structures of the eye and lacrimal apparatus.

The **conjunctiva** is a thin mucous membrane that lines the inner eyelid (palpebral conjunctivae) and also covers the sclera (bulbar conjunctivae). The **lacrimal apparatus**, which consists of the lacrimal gland, punctum, lacramal sac, and nasolacrimal duct, protects and lubricates the cornea and conjunctiva by producing and draining tears (Fig. 15-2).

Extraocular Muscle Function

The six extraocular muscles control eye movement and hold the eye in place in the socket. These muscles coordinate their actions to produce vision within both eyes (Fig. 15-3). Proper functioning of these muscles determines normal alignment or position of the eye. The muscles and their functions are as follows:

- **Superior rectus:** elevates the eye upward and adducts (toward the nose) and rotates the eye medially (inward)
- **Inferior rectus:** rotates the eye downward and adducts and rotates the eye medially

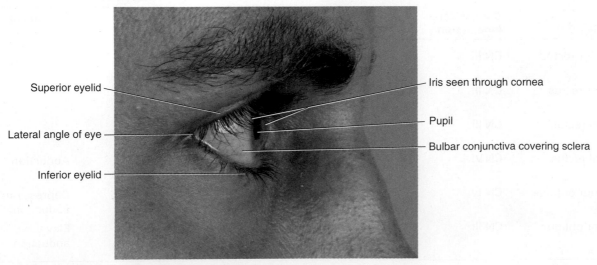

Figure 15.1 Surface anatomy of the eye in profile.

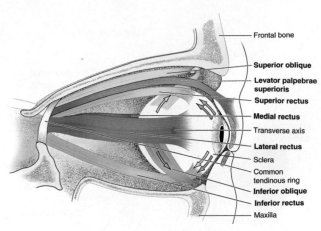

Figure 15.3 The extraocular muscles.

- **Lateral rectus:** moves the eye laterally (toward the temple)
- **Medial rectus:** moves the eye medially
- **Superior oblique:** turns the eye downward and abducts (toward the temple) and rotates the eye laterally
- **Inferior oblique:** turns the eye upward and abducts and turns the eye laterally.

The oculomotor (CN III), trochlear (CN IV), and abducens (CN VI) nerves innervate and control the motor nerve activities of the eye (Table 15-1).

The extraocular muscles oppose one another, much like the muscles surrounding joints of the skeleton. One muscle's contraction causes a relaxation of the corresponding muscle.

Intraocular Structures

The internal (intraocular) structures are involved in vision directly. The eye itself contains three layers of tissue:

1. An outer fibrous layer contains the sclera and cornea.

2. A vascular middle layer is composed of the iris, ciliary body, and choroids.
3. An inner neural layer is the retina.

The white **sclera** helps to maintain the size and shape of the eye. The transparent and avascular **cornea** allows light rays to enter the eye. It is highly sensitive to touch. The **iris** regulates the amount of light that enters the **pupil**. The color of the eye depends on the type and amount of pigment in the smooth muscles of the iris. The **pupil** opens and closes to permit light to enter the eye. Pupil size can range from 3 to 5 mm. The **lens**, which sits directly behind the pupil, refracts and focuses light on to the retina. The **ciliary body** produces aqueous humor and contains the muscle that controls the shape of the lens. The **choroids,** which cover the recessed portion of the eye, are a network of blood vessels to the eye (Fig. 15-4).

The interior eye has three chambers: anterior, posterior, and vitreous. The **anterior chamber** is the space between the cornea in the front and iris and lens in the back. It contains aqueous humor, produced by the ciliary body; the amount varies to maintain pressure in the eye. The **posterior chamber** starts behind the iris and goes to the lens. It is also filled with aqueous humor that helps to nourish the cornea and lens. The largest **vitreous chamber** is adjacent to the inner retinal layer and lens. This chamber is filled with vitreous humor, which is gel-like, holds the retina in place, and maintains the shape of the eyeball.

The **retina**, which is the innermost layer of the eye, receives and transmits visual stimuli to the brain for processing. The retinal structures are best viewed using an ophthalmoscope. The retina contains photoreceptors (rods and cones) that make vision possible. The rods on the outer edge of the retina are primarily responsible for vision in low light and produce images of varying shades of black and white. The cones, concentrated centrally, are adapted to bright light and produce color images and sharp, fine details.

Table 15.1	**Eye Muscles**				
			Action	
Muscle	**Cranial Nerve Innervation**	**Insertion**	*Medial (Toward Nose)*	*Lateral (Toward Temple)*
Superior rectus	CN III	Anterior, superior surface	Elevation, adduction	
Inferior rectus	CN III	Anterior, inferior surface	Depression, abduction	
Medial rectus	CN III	Anterior, medial surface	Adduction	
Lateral rectus	CN VI	Anterior, lateral surface		Abduction
Superior oblique	CN IV	Posterior, superior, lateral surface		Depression, abduction
Inferior oblique	CN III	Posterior, inferior, lateral surface		Elevation, abduction

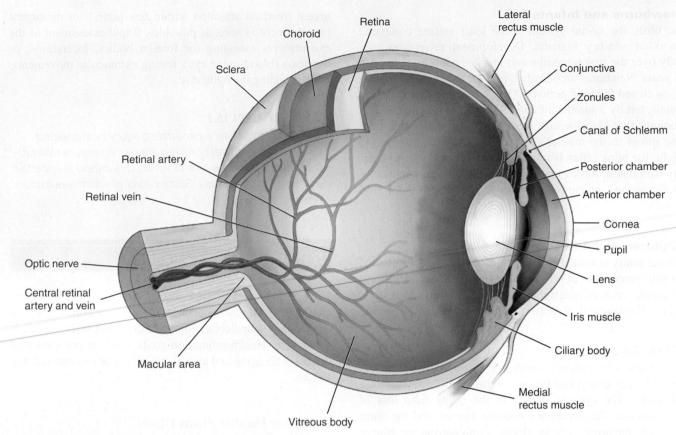

Figure 15.4 Intraocular structures.

The **optic disc**, a well-defined round or oval area, is the opening for the optic nerve head. The **macula**, lateral to the optic disc, is the area with the greatest concentration of cones.

Vision

The light rays from a viewed object enter the cornea and are refracted on to the central fovea (an area on the macula). The stimulus is then inverted, reversed, and focused on the retina, which sends the stimulus through the visual pathway to the brain where the image returns to its original form. The **neural pathway** consists of the optic nerves, optic chiasm, and optic tracts that continue into the optic region of the cerebral cortex. The neural pathway is part of the central nervous system (Fig. 15-5).

🔺 Lifespan Considerations

Pregnant Women

The most common eye problem during pregnancy is dry eyes, which result from decreased conjuctival capillaries. The cornea can thicken, making use of contact lenses uncomfortable. The corneal curvature also increases in some women, with subsequent loss of accommodation. Visual field changes may occur, possibly related to the pituitary gland affecting the optic nerve. Decreased intraocular pressure is significant

if the woman has glaucoma; adjustment of medications may be necessary. Chloasma, or increased pigmentation around the eyes, may result from increased progesterone levels (Somami, et al., 2008).

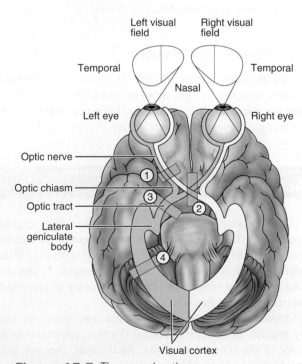

Figure 15.5 The neural pathway.

Newborns and Infants

At birth, the visual system is the least mature compared to other sensory systems. Development progresses rapidly over the first 6 months and reaches adult level by 4 to 5 years. Newborns are sensitive to light and often keep their eyes closed for long periods. They have a limited ability to focus, but by 3 months of age they can follow objects. It is thought that visual acuity is sharpest at the distance from the infant to the mother's face. The pupils are reactive to light, the blink reflex is intact, and the corneal reflex is easily stimulated. Reflex tearing is present at birth, while emotional tearing develops by 3 months (Lowdermilk & Perry, 2007).

Children and Adolescents

Visual acuity in toddlers ranges from 20/20 to 20/40 normally. Depth perception develops throughout childhood. Vision changes, such as nearsightedness, are common in adolescents (Hockenberry & Wilson, 2007).

Older Adults

Older adults have changes both in eye structures and vision. Eyelids may droop and become wrinkled from loss of skin elasticity. The eyes sit deeper in the orbits from loss of subcutaneous fat. Eyebrows become thinner, and the outer thirds of the brows may be absent. Conjunctivae are thinner and may appear yellowish from decreased perfusion. The iris may have an irregular pigmentation. Tearing decreases as a result of loss of fatty tissue in the lacrimal apparatus. Vision may decline. Because the pupil is smaller, there is loss of accommodation, decreased night vision, and decreased depth perception. The lens enlarges and transparency decreases, making vision less acute (Mackin, 2003).

Cultural Considerations

Eye color differs among people of various genetic backgrounds, with lighter eyes more prevalent in more Northern countries. Genetic background also influences the diameters of eyelids and eyebrows (Price, 2009).

Acute Assessment

Eye injuries account for 3% of all visits to U.S. emergency departments (Duffy, 2008). Acute assessment of the eye first involves identifying the problem and then determining if that problem requires immediate medical attention. In the case of emergent eye trauma or injury, time delay is potentially threatening to eye function.

Gradual vision loss, while significant, does not usually require an emergent referral. Further, ascertaining the source of the trauma/injury (eg, mechanical, thermal, radiant, chemical, electrical, or kinetic) helps determine whether the problem is emergent (immediate medical attention),

urgent (medical attention within few hours), or nonurgent (appointment as soon as possible). Rapid assessment of the eye involves assessing for foreign bodies, lacerations, or hyphema (blood in the eye), testing extraocular movements, and examining the optic disc.

⚠ SAFETY ALERT 15.1

Trauma that involves a penetrating injury or suspected fracture of the orbital bone requires an emergent referral. If a patient describes loss of vision, it is critical to ascertain a timeline of vision loss. Sudden loss of vision requires an emergent referral.

Subjective Data Collection

Subjective data collection begins with the health history, continues with questions about specific eye conditions, and ends with detailed collection of information involving areas of concern. Health-promotion goals focus on prevention of disease with aging and also occupational or recreational risk factors.

Areas for Health Promotion/ *Healthy People*

The goal of health promotion is to improve visual health through prevention, early detection, treatment, and rehabilitation (Healthy People, 2010). Table 15-2 details patient teaching related to *Healthy People* goals.

Assessment of Risk Factors

Eye and vision problems are common; 80 million Americans have some ocular abnormality, and 25% of all Americans have refractive errors (Lang & Hensrud, 2004). Some facts about eye problems include the following:

- Every 7 minutes someone in America loses his or her sight permanently.
- Leading causes of new cases of blindness are, in order, age-related macular degeneration (AMD), glaucoma, diabetic retinopathy, cataracts, and optic nerve atrophy.
- 88% of all computer users develop eye problems during, and related to, computer use.
- One in four children has an undetected vision problem that can interfere with learning.
- Tens of millions of Americans have uncorrected eye and vision problems.
- Vision problems are the second most prevalent health problem, affecting more than 120 million people (Lang & Hensrud, 2004).

The nurse needs to assess for risk factors related to eye problems, including family history, trauma, illnesses, and occupational hazards.

Table 15.2 Healthy People Goals Related to Eye Health and Education

Goals	Patient Education Topics
Increase the proportion of adults with diabetes who have an annual dilated eye examination.	Assess adults with diabetes for their last dilated eye examinations. Discuss with them the purpose and need for a dilated eye examination to establish the health of the retina.
Increase the proportion of public and private schools that require use of appropriate head, face, eye, and mouth protection for students participating in school-sponsored physical activities.	Assess with each patient the use of safety equipment when playing sports. Proper eye protection can prevent many sports-related eye injuries.
Increase the proportion of preschool children 5 years and younger who receive vision screening.	Assess history of last vision screening for preschoolers. Discuss with parents the negative effects of visual impairment on development and learning if not discovered early.
Reduce uncorrected visual impairment due to refractive errors.	Discuss with patients the need for vision screens. Discuss the sometimes dangerous consequences of uncorrected refractive errors (eg, driving).
Reduce blindness and visual impairment in children and teens 17 years and younger.	Assess history of last vision screening for children and adolescents. Assess for family history of blindness or visual impairment. Discuss with children, adolescents, and parents the signs and symptoms of visual loss.
Reduce visual impairment due to diabetic retinopathy, glaucoma, and cataracts.	Assess adults with diabetes for their last dilated eye examination. Discuss with them the purpose and need for such an examination to establish the health of the retina. Review the importance of maintaining blood glucose levels in the normal range to reduce eye damage.
Reduce occupational eye injury and increase the use of appropriate personal protective eyewear in recreational activities and hazardous situations around the home.	Assess with each client the use of safety equipment when playing sports. Discuss types of eye protective devices pertinent to the recreation or leisure activity involved. Proper eye protection can prevent many occupational eye injuries.

Source: U.S. Department of Health and Human Services (n.d.). *Healthy People 2010:* Retrieved May 20, 2010, from http://www.healthypeople.gov/About/goals.htm

Questions to Assess History and Risk	Rationales
Current Problems Are you having any eye problems now?	This general question opens discussion.
Family History Do any family members have myopia, hyperopia, strabismus, color blindness, cataracts, glaucoma, retinitis pigmatosa, or retinoblastoma?	Certain conditions and diseases that affect vision have a genetic link, which increases risk for patients. *Glaucoma* in a first-degree relative increases the patient's risk for the same problem two to three times (Jacobs, et al., 2009).
Personal History *Eye Conditions* • Do you have a history of cataracts, glaucoma, high blood pressure, diabetes, or thyroid disease? • Do you have any history of eye injury? • Have you ever had injuries or accidents, foreign bodies, or trauma to your eyes?	The focus is conditions that could affect vision and eye function.
Eye Surgery • Have you ever had any surgery on your eye(s)? • Have you ever had any facial surgery? • Have you ever had cataract removal, lens implant, or LASIK?	The focus is eye or facial surgeries, which can change the landscape of eye structures.

(text continues on page 350)

Questions to Assess History and Risk	Rationales
Medications Do you use artificial tears, decongestants, corticosteroids, antibiotics, antihistamines, or any prescribed eye drops?	Certain medications affect the eye and its functioning. Careful assessment is necessary.
Risk Factors *Allergies* • Do you have any allergies? • Are they seasonal? • Are you sensitive to pollen or animal dander, which can cause watery and itchy eyes? • How do you react to insect stings/bites: any swelling around the eyes?	The body's response to allergens affects not only the respiratory system, but also the eyes through excessive tearing, allergic conjunctivitis, and itching. Insect stings/bites to the eye often lead to periorbital edema and erythema. Previous occurrences increase risk of an angioedema-type allergic response with repeat exposure.
Exposure to Viruses. Has anyone ever told you that you were exposed to rubella in the womb? Were you diagnosed with congenital syphilis?	Maternal exposure to rubella can lead to congenital eye problems in the fetus. Fetal exposure to rubella can cause neonatal blindness secondary to cataracts. Congenital syphilis can also cause neonatal blindness.
Environmental Exposure • Are you exposed to toxins, chemicals, infections, or allergens at work? • How would you relate your current stress level: low, moderate, or high?	Many activities can increase risk for eye injury, infections, or trauma. Stress has been linked with decreased vision.
Eye Health • When was your last eye examination? • Were you screened for glaucoma?	The nurse needs to determine how the patient cares for the health of the eyes.
Corrective Prescriptions • Do you wear glasses and/or contacts? • Do you wear contacts for the recommended time frame only? • How do you care for your contacts? • How often do you change your contacts?	These questions address risks based on *Healthy People* goals to reduce the number of people with uncorrected refractive errors. The nurse can discuss the reason for not wearing prescribed glasses or contacts and care of contacts to prevent injuries to the eye.
Eye Protection • Are you exposed to any hazards that could affect your eyes? • Do you wear goggles or a face shield when you play sports or do home projects? • Do you wear your protective eyewear 100% of the time?	Questions address *Healthy People* goals to reduce injuries to the eyes of people whose occupation or leisure activities put them at risk.
Nutritional Status. Do you generally eat a well-balanced diet?	Assess the diet for any vitamin deficiencies that could affect the eyes.

Risk Assessment and Health-Related Patient Teaching

Diabetes mellitus increases risks for eye problems, including diabetic retinopathy, cataracts, and glaucoma. Sunlight exposure also increases risks, so use of sunglasses is important, especially if the patient lives in a sunny climate. Poor diet has been linked to eye problems. Foods that promote eye health include deep-water fish, fruits, and vegetables (eg, carrots, spinach). Because the lens has no blood supply, staying well hydrated keeps the lens supple and moist.

Focused Health History Related to Common Symptoms

In assessing the patient's health history, it is important to immediately determine if an eye problem results from trauma, is related to changes in vision, or involves visual symptoms. Failure to obtain an accurate and complete history can lead to loss of sight.

<table>
<tr><td colspan="2">Common Symptoms</td></tr>
<tr><td>• Pain
• Trauma or surgery
• Visual change
• Blind spots, floaters, or halos</td><td>• Discharge
• Change in activities of daily living (ADLs)</td></tr>
</table>

Questions for Common Symptoms	Rationale/Abnormal Findings
Pain Do you have any eye pain or discomfort? (Ask about location, intensity, duration, description, aggravating factors, alleviating factors, functional impairment, and pain goal.)	Pain in the eye is never normal and should always be further explored. See Chapter 7.
Trauma or Surgery Is the problem you are having related to trauma or an injury? If so: • How was the injury/trauma sustained? • Was this a high-velocity injury? • Was this a blunt force trauma?	High-velocity injuries are typically penetrating. Blunt-force trauma often results in fracture of the orbit.
Visual Change Have you noticed any recent changes to your vision? • What is the nature of the visual change? • When did the change begin? • Was onset sudden or gradual? • Have you noticed any double vision or halos/rainbows around objects?	If the patient describes loss of vision, it is critical to ascertain a timeline. Sudden vision loss requires an emergent referral.
Blind Spots, Floaters, or Halos • Have you noticed any blind spots in your vision • Any difficulty seeing at night? • Do you see any spots (floaters)? • Do you have any associated symptoms (eg, flashing lights, floaters, halos around lights)?	Loss of night vision is associated with *optiatrophy*, *glaucoma*, and *vitamin A deficiency*. Floaters (translucent specks that drift across the visual field) are common in people older than 40 years and nearsighted patients. No additional follow-up is needed.
Discharge • Are you having any eye discharge? • Is there any pain or grittiness, redness, or discharge associated? • Are one or both eyes affected? • Have you noticed any excessive tearing, dryness, or itching?	Discharge is associated with inflammation or infection.
Change in ADLs How has your eye problem (eg, diplopia, dry eyes) affected your ability to perform ADLs?	Assess functional limitations.

Documentation of Normal Findings

Denies pain, trauma, visual changes, blind spots, floaters, halos, and discharge. No changes in ability to perform ADLs.
B Ryan, RN

Lifespan Considerations

Additional Questions	Rationales/Abnormal Findings
Pregnant Women	
Have you noticed any changes in your visual acuity?	Hormonal fluctuations can cause refractive changes, which are typically minor, but should be discussed with a health professional.
Have you noticed that your eyes feel dry?	Dry eyes during pregnancy are usually temporary and resolve after childbirth.
Newborns, Infants, and Children	
Ask the parents of infants: Have you noticed tears when your infant cries?	Infants begin making tears at approximately 2 weeks old. Lack of tear production is a sign of a blocked lacrimal apparatus.
Does your infant have red, dry, or irritated eyes?	Such findings may indicate lacrimal apparatus blockage or *conjunctivitis* (ophthalmia neonatorum).
Do you think your child has something wrong with his or her eye/vision? What worries you?	Parents and immediate family members often notice things that do not seem to fit within the range of normal.
Have you noticed any problems or changes in the white of the eye, pupil, iris, or lashes?	Parents and immediate family often notice things that do not seem to fit the range of the normal.
Have you noticed that your child is sensitive to light? If yes, is it accompanied by nausea/vomiting, dizziness, or signs/complaints of headache?	These may be symptoms of other visual or eye problems.
Have you noticed your child exhibiting any of the following: • Poking at eyes or rubbing frequently? • Poor eye contact? • Turning of one eye? • Inaccuracy in reaching for an item of interest?	These could be symptoms of allergies, *blepharitis*, dry eyes, or visual field issues. Visual impairment could cause poor eye contact (eg, amblyopia, strabismus). This may indicate a visual refractive error.
Has your child been diagnosed with hearing problems?	Hearing-impaired infants are at increased risk for visual impairments.
Older Adults	
Do you have a history of diabetes, glaucoma, or high blood pressure?	Aging increases risks for visual complications related to other chronic diseases that affect blood vessels in the retina and fluid in the eye (Miller, 2008).
Have you noticed any tunneling of your visual field?	This is a symptom of *macular degeneration*.
Have you ever had your eyes checked for glaucoma, cataracts, or other eye conditions?	This provides the nurse with an opportunity to promote eye health.
Do you have any trouble managing your usual activities because of vision changes? Have you stopped doing any activities because of vision changes?	It is important to focus on any visual impairment and how the patient functions with it.
When did you last have a test for glaucoma (tonometery)?	Older adults are at increased risk; glaucoma screening should be done every 1–2 years (National Institutes of Health, 2005).
Have you ever tripped or fallen because of changes in your vision?	This question assesses awareness and presence of visual impairments.

Therapeutic Dialogue: Collecting Subjective Data

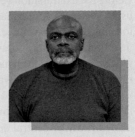

Mr. Harris, introduced at the beginning of this chapter, is in the clinic for follow-up care related to high blood pressure, high cholesterol, and glaucoma. The following conversations give two examples of interview styles used by different nurses. One style is more effective than the other.

Less Effective

Nurse: It looks like you have been diagnosed with high blood pressure, high cholesterol, and glaucoma, is that correct?

Mr. Harris: Yeah.

Nurse: What do you think caused these?

Mr. Harris: I don't know.

Nurse: Does anyone in your family have these problems?

Mr. Harris: Not that I know of.

Nurse: Well, glaucoma is more common in people with high blood pressure and cholesterol. And you're African American so that puts you more at risk, too.

Mr. Harris: (nods head)

Nurse: So, it looks like you're on medication for blood pressure and cholesterol and use eye drops for your glaucoma. Is that correct?

Mr. Harris: Yes.

Nurse: Did you bring them in so that I can double-check them?

Mr. Harris: No. I have a list in my wallet.

Nurse: That's great. Can I see it?

Mr. Harris: Sure.

More Effective

Nurse: I'm glad that you came back for your visit today. It's good to see you.

Mr. Harris: Thanks. I am really trying to take better care of myself.

Nurse: I noticed that your blood pressure is under good control.

Mr. Harris: Yes, I'm really trying to make sure to eat right, get some exercise, and take my medicine. I have two beautiful grandkids that I'm helping to raise. (pauses) I'm worried about my eyesight. I have glaucoma, and I can't see as well. I'm worried that I'll go blind and won't be able to help with my grandkids.

Nurse: You've had glaucoma for about 5 years now, is that correct?

Mr. Harris: Yes. The doctor gave me some drops for it.

Nurse: Can you take them as prescribed?

Mr. Harris: Well, I ran out a bit ago and had to wait a few days until the first of the month, but I have them now.

Critical Thinking Challenge

- What made the first nurse less effective?
- What did the more effective nurse do to establish a positive relationship?
- Compare the potential interventions between the less and more effective dialogues.

Objective Data Collection

A comprehensive physical examination of the eye involves assessment of visual acuity, the external eye, eye muscle function, external ocular structures (including pupil reflexes), and internal ocular structures. The external eyes and external ocular structures are examined through inspection and palpation. The interior ocular structures are inspected with an instrument called an *ophthalmoscope* (see Chapter 4). Identifying anatomical landmarks of the external eye assists nurses to document findings.

Equipment

Assemble the following equipments:

- Penlight
- Cotton wisps and cotton-tipped applicators
- Ophthalmoscope
- Snellen's chart for far-vision testing
- Jaeger's chart for near-vision testing
- Occlusive covers for individual eye testing
- Ishihara plates (optional for testing color vision)

Preparation

Before the examination begins, perform hand hygiene. If you are using hand gel, be sure that your hands are completely dry before touching the patient's eye. If there is a complaint or signs of an infection, make sure to avoid cross-contamination by wearing gloves, washing your hands, and cleaning all equipment before examining each eye. Always examine the infected eye last.

Assessment of visual acuity, visual fields, and the retina helps you evaluate not only the function of the eye itself, but also part of the central nervous system.

As you proceed with inspection and palpation of the eye you will assess for function of the sensory and motor function of four cranial nerves (Table 15-3). As you progress through the assessment, remember not only the sensory aspects of vision but also the motor function of the eyes. Thorough examination can make the difference in identifying risks and preventing blindness.

Common and Specialty or Advanced Techniques

Routine eye assessment includes the most important and common assessment techniques performed to screen for problems. Nurses may add specialty or advanced assessment techniques if concerns exist over a specific finding. Table 15-4 summarizes the most common and advanced techniques used in the comprehensive assessment of the eye.

Table 15.3 Cranial Nerves Associated with the Eyes

Cranial Nerve	Name of Cranial Nerve	Assessment of Cranial Nerve
II	Optic nerve	• Visual acuity • Visual fields • Fundoscopic examination
III	Occulomotor	• Cardinal fields of gaze • Eyelid inspection • Pupil reaction (direct/consensual/accommodation)
IV	Trochlear	• Cardinal fields of gaze
VI	Abducens	• Cardinal fields of gaze

Assessment of Visual Acuity

Visual acuity tests include testing for distance vision, near vision, peripheral vision, and color vision. This first step in an eye assessment is important to perform before any type of solution is used to dilate the pupil.

Table 15.4 Common Versus Specialty/Advanced Techniques Related to Eye Assessment

Technique	Purpose	Screening or Registered Nurse Assessment	Focused or Advanced Practice Examination
Inspect external eyes	To evaluate for symmetry, redness, and obvious deformities	X	
Test distance vision	To evaluate ability to see far, drive	X	
Test near vision	To evaluate ability to read	X	
Assess color vision	To evaluate ability to differentiate color		X
Test static confrontation	To screen for differences in the visual field from side-to-side and inferior and superior		X
Test kinetic confrontation	To assess the gross peripheral boundaries		X
Test corneal light reflex	To test for strabismus		X
Perform cover test	To assess the presence and amount of ocular deviation		X
Test cardinal fields of gaze	To assess for movement of the eye in several planes of movement	X	
Inspect and palpate lacrimal apparatus and conjunctiva	To evaluate swelling, tenderness	X	
Test pupillary reflex	To evaluate the pupil's response to direct and consensual light source	X	
Inspect cornea and lens	To assess for glaucoma and cataracts		X
Inspect posterior eye	To evaluate disk, vessels, macula, and periphery		X

Distance Vision

Assess distance visual acuity by having the patient read the Snellen's or Allen's Chart (based on developmental age or reading ability). With the Snellen's test, measure and place a mark or piece of masking tape on the floor 20 ft from the chart (Fig. 15-6). With the Allen's test, place the mark or piece of masking tape on the floor 15 ft from the chart. The area should be well lit, and the test should be at the patient's eye level.

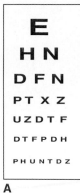 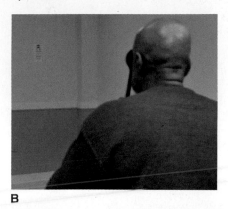

A   **B**

Figure 15.6 Assessing distance vision. **A.** The Snellen's chart. **B.** The patient reads the letters of the Snellen's chart from 20 ft away.

Give the patient an opaque card or eye occluder so that he or she can cover one eye at a time during assessment. Stand by the chart and request that the patient read through it to the smallest letters (pictures if using the Allen's chart) possible, occluding one eye at a time. Then request that the patient read the next smallest line. If the patient wears glasses/contacts they should remain on; only reading glasses should be removed for the assessment.

Abnormal findings include leaning forward, squinting, hesitation, misidentification of more than three of seven objects, or more than a two-line difference between eyes. Refer to Table 15-6, at the end of the chapter.

Acuity for distance vision is documented in two numbers, with reference to what a person with normal vision sees 20 ft from the test. Someone with "20/20" (normal) vision can read at 20 ft what the normal eye can read at 20 ft. On top, mark the distance in feet the patient was from the test (eg, 20). On bottom, mark the number under the smallest line of letters the patient correctly identified (eg, 40, 200). Also document the number of letters missed and if the patient wore corrective lenses (eg, right eye: 20/30 -2, with glasses). The larger the bottom number, the worse the visual acuity. *Refractive index (emmetropia) of the eye is 20/20 bilaterally.*

A larger number on the bottom (eg, 20/60) indicates diminished distance vision.

⚠ *SAFETY ALERT 15.2*

The abbreviations OD (oculus dexter-right eye), OS (oculus sinster-left eye), and OU (oculus uterque-each eye) are no longer used to document eye findings because of the potential for medical-order and medication errors. Instead it is recommended to use right eye, left eye, or both eyes to document findings.

Near Vision

Near vision is usually assessed in patients older than 40 years or younger patients who report difficulty reading. When no Jaeger test (pocket screener) is available, ask the patient to read newsprint (eg, newspaper, magazine).

Patients older than 40 years often have a decreased ability to accommodate; therefore, they move the card further away to read it.

(text continues on page 356)

Instruct the patient to hold the Jaeger chart 14 in (35 cm) from the eye. Request that the person read through the chart to the smallest letters possible, occluding one eye at a time (with corrective lenses on) (Fig. 15-7). *Visual acuity for near vision is 14/14 bilaterally.*

A patient who incorrectly identifies the embedded figures or color bars may have color blindness.

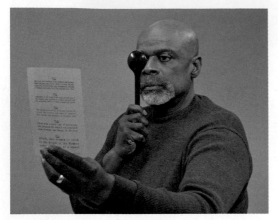

Figure 15.7 Assessing near vision with the Jaeger chart.

Color Vision

Color vision is assessed using Ishihara cards (Fig. 15-8) or by having the patient identify color bars on the Snellen's chart. *The patient correctly identifies the embedded figures in the Ishihara cards or the colors bars on the Snellen's chart.*

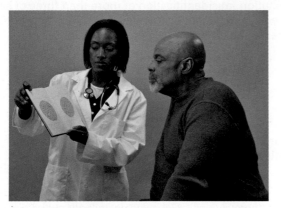

Figure 15.8 Testing color vision.

Assessment of Visual Fields

The *visual field* refers to what in the environment is visible when the eye fixates on a stationary object. Visual injury or disease usually causes defects in the normal full visual field. The confrontation test is used to screen for visual field defects, which may not be apparent to the nurse. When evaluating for visual field defects, the visual field is divided into four quadrants—inferior, superior, left, and right.

Visual field testing in the clinic setting can be performed without computerized automated perimetry; it is a gross screening of peripheral vision. The nurse can use either static or kinetic techniques.

The static test can help the nurse detect gross differences in all four quadrants of the visual field. The nurse does not move the fingers but presents one to four fingers in each quadrant. The static test effectively screens for differences from side-to-side (hemianopias) and inferior and superior (attitudinal).

The kinetic test assesses the gross peripheral boundaries of the patient's visual field. Kinetic technique is performed when the nurse moves an object or fingers from the periphery toward fixation at the point that the patient first becomes aware of the target (Dubois, 2005).

Static Confrontation

Stand approximately 2–3 ft (an arm's length) directly in front of the patient. Your eyes and the patient's eyes should be on the same level. Ask the patient to cover the left eye with the palm of the left hand (without putting pressure on the eye). Close your right eye and instruct the patient to look only at your open eye at all times. Present one to four fingers midway between yourself and the patient in each of the four quadrants of the visual field (Fig. 15-9). Ask the patient to report the number of fingers, without looking directly at them. Repeat the test with the other eye. *Patient accurately reports the number of fingers presented in all four quadrants.*

This screening test assumes that the nurse's visual field is normal and serves as the comparison for the patient's test. Reports of an incorrect number of fingers indicate a visual field defect.

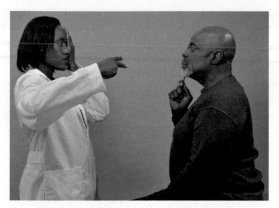

Figure 15.9 Performing the static confrontation test.

Kinetic Confrontation

As with static confrontation, your eyes and the patient's eyes must be on the same level. Instruct the patient to say "now" when the fingers first come into view. Wiggle your fingers from a far distal point and move them toward the center of each quadrant (Fig. 15-10). Your fingers should not be immediately visible (except in the inferotemporal quadrant). *Patient sees the fingers at about the same time as the nurse if the peripheral visual field is normal in that quadrant.*

A patient who sees fingers presented on either side only on one side may have a hemianopic defect. If the patient sees only from an inferior or superior position, an attitudinal defect is suspected.

⚠ *SAFETY ALERT 15.3*
Defects in any quadrant in either the static or kinetic confrontation test require referral to an optometrist or ophthalmologist for more precise testing.

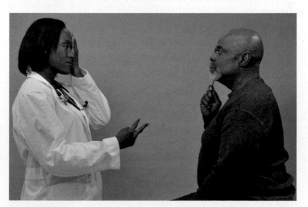

Figure 15.10 Performing the kinetic confrontation test.

Documentation of Normal Findings

Visual acuity 20/20. Accurately reads newsprint. Identifies color bars on Snellen's chart correctly. Patient sees finger at about 50 degrees superior, 90 degrees temporal, 90 degrees inferior, and 60 degrees nasal. *B. Ryan, RN*

Assessment of Extraocular Muscle Movements

Three basic tests allow examiners to assess the movement of the extraocular muscles: (1) the corneal light reflex (Hirschberg) test, (2) the cover test, and (3) the cardinal fields of gaze. They assess movements of the eye in several planes: up and down, side-to-side, diagonally from right superior to left inferior, and diagonally from left superior to right inferior (Fig. 15-11). The **corneal light reflex** tests for strabismus. The **cover test** is for presence and amount of ocular deviation. A low light level with no direct light sources shining in the patient's eyes is ideal. At rest the extraocular muscles have very little activity. The assessment referred to as **cardinal fields of gaze** allows

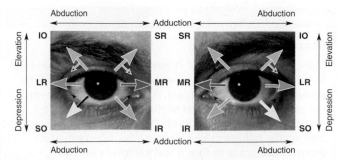

Figure 15.11 Extraocular movements.

nurses to detect muscle defects that cause misalignment or uncoordinated eye movements.

Technique and Normal Findings	Abnormal Findings
Corneal Light Reflex Instruct the patient to stare straight ahead at the bridge of your nose. Stand in front of the patient and shine a penlight at the bridge of the patient's nose. Note where the light reflects on the cornea of each eye (Fig. 15-12). *Light reflection is in exactly the same spot in both eyes.*	Abormal findings indicate improper alignment and appear as asymmetric reflections. Document abnormal findings using the face of the clock as a guide.

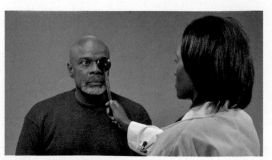

Figure 15.12 Testing the corneal light reflex.

Cover Test The cover test, most typically performed on children, helps with assessment of ocular alignment. Stand in front of the patient and ask the patient to focus on a near object (bridge of your nose). Place an opaque card or occluder over the eye; inspect for any movement of the uncovered eye that may indicate refixation of the gaze (Fig. 15-13). Remove the cover and observe the previously covered eye for refixation. Repeat the procedure for the other eye. *Gaze is steady and fixed.*	Any refixation is from muscle weakness in the covered eye (ie, while covered the eye drifted into a relaxed position).

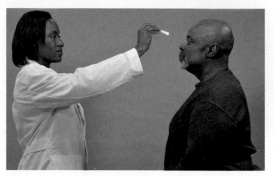

Figure 15.13 Performing the cover test.

Technique and Normal Findings (continued)	Abnormal Findings (continued)
Cardinal Fields of Gaze Further testing of the extraocular muscles assesses for symmetrical movements of the eyes in all nine cardinal fields of gaze. Instruct the patient to hold the head steady and to follow the movement of your finger or pen with the eyes. Hold your finger or pen approximately 12–14 in from the patient's face. Move slowly through position 2–9, stopping momentarily in each, and then back to center (Fig. 15-14). Proceed clockwise. *Patient's eyes move smoothly and symmetrically in all nine cardinal fields of gaze.* 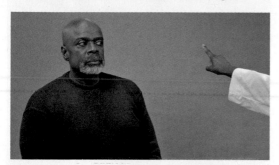 **Figure 15.14** Assessing the cardinal fields of gaze.	Document a deficit by noting in which field there is an abnormality. Mild nystagmus at the extreme lateral angles is normal; in any other position it is not. See Table 15-7 at the end of the chapter.

Documentation of Normal Response

Alignment symmetrical/corneal light reflex. Gaze fixed and steady. Extraocular movements intact (EOMI). *B. Ryan, RN*

Assessment of External Eyes

Ensure good lighting. Wash your hands before touching the eyelids or face of the patient.

Technique and Normal Findings	Abnormal Findings
Stand directly in front of and facing the patient (who is sitting on the examination table or bed). Inspect eyebrows, lashes, and eyelids; note eye shape and symmetry. *Eyebrows vary based on genetic background but show no unexplained hair loss. Lashes curve outward away from the eyes and are distributed evenly along the lid margins. Eyelids open and close completely, with spontaneous blinking every few seconds. Eye shape varies from round to almond but is symmetrical.* Note general appearance of the eyes. *Eyes are in parallel alignment.*	**Eyebrows:** unexplained hair loss; with normal aging, the outer third of the eyebrow thins **Eyelashes:** curved inward away toward the eye, distributed unevenly along lid margin, or both **Eyelids:** incomplete opening or closing; no spontaneous blinking; improper positioning with respect to iris and limbus **Eye shape:** asymmetry Eyes not in parallel alignment require further assessment. **Ptosis**, drooping of the eyelids, is a common finding with *stroke* (Fig. 15-15). 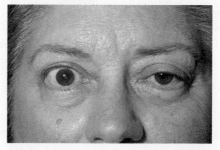 **Figure 15.15** Ptosis in a patient following stroke.

(text continues on page 360)

Lacrimal Apparatus

Inspect and palpate the lacrimal apparatus (if the patient reports eye fatigue or dry eyes). Identify the punctual opening of the lacrimal apparatus at the inner canthus. Gently stretch the bottom eyelids with your thumb downward to better expose the puncta. Gently press your index finger against the patient's nasolacrimal sac just inside the orbital ring (Fig. 15-16). *Lacrimal apparatus is not enlarged or tender.*

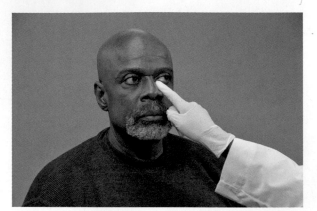

Figure 15.16 Palpating the lacrimal apparatus.

Bulbar Conjunctiva

Gently lift the upper eyelid. Instruct the patient to look down and then to the right and left. Note the surface for color, injection (redness), swelling, exudates, or foreign bodies. Gently stretch down the lower lid (Fig. 15-18). Instruct the patient to look up and to the right and left. Again note the surface for color, injection (redness), swelling, exudates, or foreign bodies. *Bulbar conjunctiva is normally transparent with small blood vessels visible.*

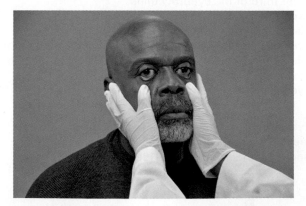

Figure 15.18 Inspecting the bulbar conjunctiva.

An enlarged lacrimal apparatus is rare. If you palpate an enlarged lacrimal apparatus, evert the eyelid and inspect the gland. Suspect conditions such as *sarcoid disease* and *Sjögren's syndrome* (Fig. 15-17).

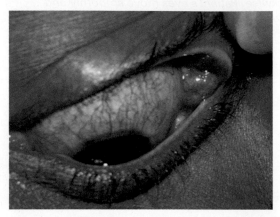

Figure 15.17 Sjögren's syndrome.

Erythema, cobblestone appearance, or both may indicate allergy or infection. Sharply defined bright red blood indicates a *subconjunctival hemorrhage* (Fig. 15-19).

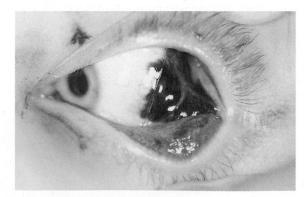

Figure 15.19 Subconjunctival hemorrhage.

An abnormal thickening of the conjunctiva from the limbus over the cornea is known as a *pterygium*. Pterygium is most common on the nasal side. Risk for development is heavy exposure to ultraviolet light, most commonly in equatorial areas. If pterygium advances over the pupil, it can interfere with vision (Fig. 15-20)

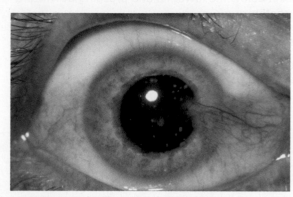

Figure 15.20 Pterygium.

Sclera

During inspection of the bulbar conjunctiva you can also inspect the sclera for color, exudates, lesions, and foreign bodies. *Sclera is clear, smooth, white, and without exudate, lesions, or foreign bodies.*

Scleral abnormalities include jaundice, bluing, and drainage. Refer to Table 15-8 at the end of the chapter for abnormalities of the external eye.

Eversion of the Eyelid

Eversion of the eyelid is an advanced practice skill used in specialized situations.

1. Grasp the lashes and lid margin gently between your thumb and forefinger.
2. Ask the patient to look down.
3. Pull the eyelid gently down and away from the eye.
4. Place a cotton tip applicator in the indentation between orbit and globe (Fig. 15-21).

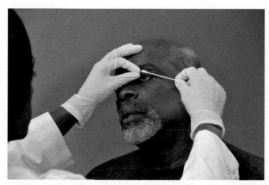

Figure 15.21 Placement of the applicator during eyelid eversion.

5. Pull the lashes and lid margin out and upward.
6. Fold the lid back over the cotton-tipped applicator, exposing the underside of the upper eyelid.
7. Hold the eyelid in this position while you remove the applicator.
8. Assess the underside of the eyelid, inspecting for any foreign bodies, chalazions, and so on.
9. Ask the patient to blink. The eyelid will return to its normal position.

(text continues on page 362)

10. Assess the inside of the lower lid by placing your thumb or a cotton-tipped applicator on the skin below the lower lid and pressing downward gently.
11. Ask the patient to look upward, to the right, and then to the left.

There are no foreign bodies, chalazions, redness, or injuries. Tissue is pink and smooth.

When examining the eye for a foreign body, it is important to examine the cornea, sclera, and palpebral conjunctiva. Eversion of the eyelid is essential in the assessment of an injured or red eye. Everting the upper eyelid allows for easy identification of foreign bodies.

⚠ SAFETY ALERT 15.4
Eversion of the eyelid should never be performed if a penetrating eye injury is suspected.

Documentation of Normal Findings

Eyebrows full and appropriate to age. Eyelashes evenly distributed. Blinking every 2–3 seconds. Eyes round, symmetrical, and in parallel alignment. Lacrimal apparatus not enlarged or tender. Conjunctiva with small vessels visible. Sclera clear and white.
B. Ryan, RN

Assessment of Exterior Ocular Structures

Cornea and Lens

Stand in front of the patient. Use a penlight or ophthalmoscope split light to inspect the cornea. Shine the light directly on the cornea. Move the light laterally toward the bridge of the nose. Repeat on the other eye. Observe the angle of the anterior space and the clarity and translucence of the lens. *A normal angle allows full illumination of the iris. Lens is transparent.*

A narrow angle indicates *glaucoma.*

Cloudiness of the lens can indicate a *cataract,* which is associated with increased age, smoking, alcohol intake, and sunlight exposure. Risk factors for cataracts are primarily environmental. See also Table 15-8.

Fluorescein Examination of Cornea. The advanced practitioner uses this technique to determine any abrasions or lacerations to the cornea. Fluorescein is a dye taken up by the damaged corneal epithelium. Under blue ultraviolet light it fluoresces, allowing assessment of the nature and extent of corneal injury.

Corneal fluorescence reveals the extent of the injury to the corneal epithelium.

⚠ SAFETY ALERT 15.5
Fluorescein is never used if a penetrating eye injury is suspected.

Remove a fluorescein strip, wet it with a drop of normal saline, and apply it to the lower conjunctival sac (fluorescein drops are also available). Ask the patient to blink several times to distribute the fluorescein over the cornea. Remove excess fluorescein with a gentle irrigation of normal saline. Darken the room and expose the eye to blue filtered, cobalt, or "black" light.

Iris

Inspect the iris for color, nodules, and vascularity. Brown is the most common eye color in the world. *Color is evenly distributed, smooth, and without apparent vascularity. A normal variation is mosaic variant.*

See Table 15-8.

Pupils

Examine the pupil using a direct method. Stand in front of the patient and use your light to observe the shape and size (mm) of the pupil. *Pupil is black, round, and equal with a diameter of 2–6 mm.* Gently place your open hand along the patient's nose. Shine the light into

See Table 15-9 at the end of the chapter for abnormal pupils. Also see Chapter 24 for more information on neurological findings related to altered pupils.

the right eyes as you observe the pupillary constriction (direct) (CN III) (Fig. 15-22). Repeat, except observe the left eye for pupillary constriction (consensual) (CN III). Repeat these two procedures in the left eye. *Pupils constrict directly and consensually.*

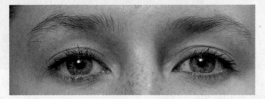

Figure 15.22 Pupillary constriction.

To test for accommodation (CN III), instruct the patient to stare at a distant object for 30 seconds. Hold an index finger, penlight, or other safe object (eg, pencil) about 14 in (10 cm) in front of the nose. Ask the patient to focus on your finger as you move it toward the patient's nose (Fig. 15-23). *Pupils constrict (accommodation) and eyes cross (converge). Accommodation is necessary for far-to-near focus. Documentation of this sequence of assessments is easily accomplished with the following acronym: PERRLA, which stands for Pupils Equal, Round, Reactive to Light, and Accommodation.*

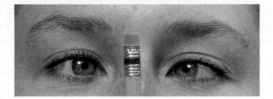

Figure 15.23 Accommodation.

Several abnormalities can be seen in the pupil during assessment. See Table 15-9.

Documentation of Normal Findings

Lens is transparent. Iris is brown, smooth, and without vascularity. PERRLA. *B. Ryan, RN*

Assessment of Internal Ocular Structures

Examination of internal ocular structures is in the domain of the APRN. The ophthalmoscope has some basic features that make inspecting the interior ocular structures easier: (1) a light source; (2) viewing aperture; and (3) a lens refraction adjustment (Fig. 15-24). These features allow nurses to direct the light source toward the pupil by looking through the viewing aperture.

The *aperture*, which has a lens selector wheel, allows for adjustment of refraction to bring the internal ocular structures into sharp focus, compensating for refractive errors of the patient or nurse. The aperture is set on large for the dilated pupil or small for the constricted pupil. The slit aperture is used to examine the anterior portion of the eye and evaluate lesions at the fundal level. The grid feature is used to locate and describe fundal-level lesions. The green beam (red-free filter) is often used to evaluate retinal hemorrhaging (which appears black with this filter) or melanin spots (which appear gray).

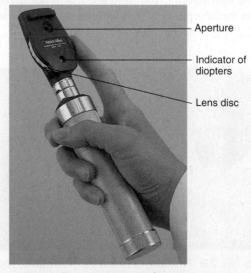

Aperture

Indicator of diopters

Lens disc

Figure 15.24 The ophthalmoscope.

Proper inspection of the posterior ocular structures with an ophthalmoscope requires that the pupils be slightly dilated. The optometrist or ophthalmologist will often use mydriatic eye drops, which are short-acting ciliary muscle paralytics that dilate the pupil. However, accommodation reflexes may be lost with the use of eye drops. Mydriatic drops are not used if a neurological assessment is necessary, because they may obscure pupil size and reactivity parameters used to determine neurological status.

⚠ SAFETY ALERT 15.6

Midriatic drops may precipitate acute angle closure glaucoma. Those at risk include patients with a history of glaucoma and extremely farsighted patients. Additionally, the patient should be warned about blurring of vision and sensitivity to light. The patient should not drive for 1 to 2 hours following pupil dilation.

In the nonophthalmic setting, partial dilation of the pupil is accomplished by darkening the room. The skill of assessing the fundus of the eye is advanced and requires much practice. For the nurse to be able to assess the fundus through a partially dilated pupil, his or her technique must be very proficient.

Examination of the fundus is conducted in a darkened room to increase pupillary dilation without medications. First set the ophthalmoscope on the 0 lens and aperture on small round light. When examining the right eye, grasp the ophthalmoscope in your right hand and then turn on the light source. When examining the left eye, grasp the ophthalmoscope in the left hand. This helps you to avoid bumping noses with the patient.

Ask the patient to focus on a distant object across the room. Start by placing your hand on the patient's head; this puts you about 2 ft from the patient. From an angle of about 15 degrees lateral to the patient's line of vision, shine the ophthalmoscope toward the pupil of the right eye (Fig. 15-25).

Look through the ophthalmoscope's viewing hole. Note the red reflex. Continue to look through the viewing hole and focus on the red reflex. Now, move toward the patient until you are about 10 in (25 cm) away from the patient's forehead. Move the lens selector from 0 to the + or black numbers to focus on the anterior ocular structures. Inspect the anterior

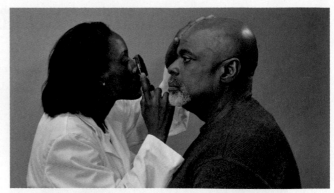

Figure 15.26 Using the ophthalmoscope to inspect the anterior ocular structures.

structures for transparency (Fig. 15-26). Now move the lens selector from the + black numbers to the – or red numbers to focus on structures progressively more posterior.

If the retinal structures are not in focus, adjust the focus with an index finger on the lens focus until the retina comes into focus. Look toward the nasal side of the retina. If you are having difficulty, ask the patient to look toward the right. Inspect the optic disc, which is the most prominent structure. The direct ophthalmoscope technique is difficult to master, and takes months of practice. The easiest way to find the optic disc is to find a blood vessel and then follow this vessel back to its origin at the optic disc. Inspect the shape (round or oval), color (creamy yellow-orange to pink), disc margins (distinct and sharply demarcated), and size of the disc cupping (brighter yellow-white than rest of disc) (Fig. 15-27). Cup-disc ratio is genetically determined and normally equal in both eyes. You may be able to pick up AV nicking from high blood pressure and retinal hemorrhages in the form of dot-blot spots or flame hemorrhages (Fig. 15-28).

The blood vessels can be directly observed in the retina. Systemic diseases of the body are often reflected in the blood vessels and can be directly observed in the eye. When examining the vascularity of the eye make note of the number, color, artery-to-vein ratio, tortuousity, and arteriovenous crossing. Also make note of the ratio of arteries to veins width, which is normally 2:3 or 4:5.

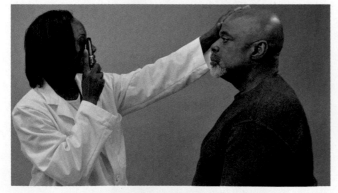

Figure 15.25 Positioning of the patient, nurse, and ophthalmoscope.

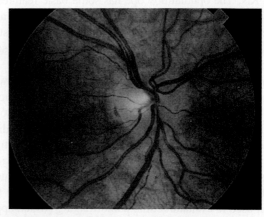

Figure 15.27 A normal optic disc.

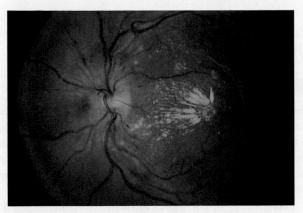

Figure 15.28 Flame hemorrhage in a patient with hypertensive retinopathy.

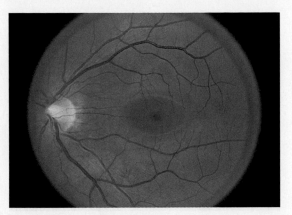

Figure 15.29 Normal macula.

The final retinal structure to be assessed is the macula. Move the ophthalmoscope approximately two disc diameters (2DD) temporally to view the macula. You can also ask the patient to look at the light. It can be difficult to find because the macula is light-sensitive. You may find that turning the aperture to green light (red-light filter) may make it easier to assess. The macula is a darker, avascular area with an ophthalmoscope light reflective center known as the fovea centralis. The color of the macula varies with ethnicity and age (Fig. 15-29).

Review the structures and what you are looking for

- **Disc:** What is the cup-to-disc ratio? Do the rims look pink and healthy?
- **Vessels:** Any signs of AV nicking?
- **Macula:** Does it look flat? Is there a good light reflex off the surface?
- **Periphery:** Any lattice or tears?

See Table 15-10 at the end of the chapter.

△ **SAFETY ALERT 15.7**

*A lack of **red reflex** may need urgent follow-up. If a white pupil reflex (leukokoria) is elicited, then an urgent ophthalmologic referral is required. Disease or trauma (eg, retinoblastoma, hyphema, toxocariasis, retinal detachment) often causes a white pupil reflex.*

🔺 **Lifespan Considerations**

Infants, Children, and Adolescents

Usually the iris has little color at birth, but by 3 months of age it attains its permanent color. Ability to follow objects is usually present by 3 months. Binocular vision develops between 3 and 7 months (Coats, et al., 2009).

Assess distance vision in children using a screening test based on developmental stage. Assess vision in infants through testing for pupillary light reflex and observing behavior. Assess a toddler's visual acuity through the Allen's test, which uses picture cards of common objects (Fig. 15-30). Normal findings in toddlers are 20/200 bilaterally. In preschool children (3 to 5 years old), assess visual acuity with the Snellen's E chart (Fig. 15-31). Normal visual acuity in a preschool child is 20/40, improving to 20/30 or better by 4 years. The Snellen's E chart is used to assess visual acuity in school-age children until the child acquires reading skills. By 5 to 6 years of age, normal visual acuity should approximate that of adults or 20/20 in both eyes. Children should be screened for color blindness between 4 and 8 years old.

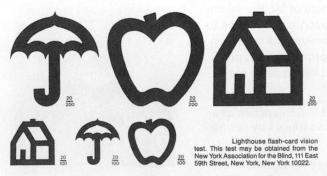

Lighthouse flash-card vision test. This test may be obtained from the New York Association for the Blind, 111 East 59th Street, New York, New York 10022.

Figure 15.30 Picture cards similar to those used in the Allen's test.

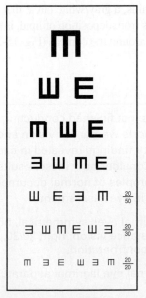

Figure 15.31 The Snellen's E chart.

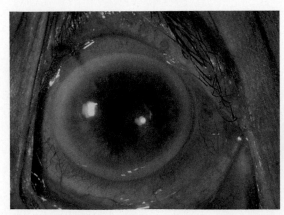

Figure 15.32 Arcus senilis.

Older Adults

Age-related visual changes and negative functional consequences occur slowly over time and are often overlooked. Visual impairments can begin to affect the older adult's functional capacity, decreasing ability to drive and perform usual activities. It is important to assess visual changes and how they affect lifestyle.

With aging, ability of the lens to accommodate decreases. Near vision is subsequently impaired, and thus older adults need reading glasses. *Presbyopia* is considered a normal part of aging.

Cataracts and AMD are the two leading causes of loss of vision and blindness in the United States. Approximately 22 million Americans suffer from cataracts and AMD. In the United States these diseases are primarily seen in the elderly (though there are congenital forms of cataracts). Glaucoma is also more common with increased age.

Loss of acuity of central vision may decrease, especially after 70 years of age. Loss of visual acuity puts the older adult at increased risk for falls and associated hip fractures (Friedman, et al., 2002). Additional findings related to aging include loss of adipose tissue in the orbit, decreased tear production, and decreased papillary response. Diabetic retinopathy is also increased in the elderly. Arcus senilis, a gray/white circle that circumscribes the limbus and results from deposition of lipid, is a common cloudiness that appears around the corneas (Fig. 15-32).

Keep in mind that testing visual acuity in the older adult with dementia can be challenging. Provide simple, one-step directions for these patients.

⊕ Cultural Considerations

The Snellen's E chart can be used for people who cannot read or speak English (see Fig. 15-31). Ethnic variations are found in the ocular sclera, depending on skin tone. In light-skinned people, the sclera appears white with some superficial vessels. In dark-skinned people, the sclera often has tiny brown patches (patches of melanin) or is grayish-blue.

Four-to-five times more African Americans develop glaucoma compared to other races. In fact, 11% of African Americans older than 80 years have glaucoma. Rate of blindness from glaucoma in African Americans is seven times that of Caucasians; blindness begins 10 years earlier in African Americans (Jacobs, et al., 2009).

Evidence-based Critical Thinking

Diagnostic Reasoning

When formulating nursing diagnoses, nurses use critical thinking to cluster data and identify patterns that fit together. The nurse compares these data clusters with defining characteristics (abnormal findings) for the diagnosis to ensure the most accurate labeling and appropriate interventions. A nursing diagnosis is a clinical judgment about responses to health problems or life processes. Table 15-5 provides a comparison of nursing diagnoses, abnormal findings, and interventions commonly related to the eye assessment (NANDA-I, 2009).

Nurses use assessment information to identify patient outcomes. Some outcomes related to eye problems include the following:

- Patient will plan to modify lifestyle to accommodate vision disturbance.
- Patient will remain safe in home environment.
- Patient will state measures to reduce risk of visual loss (Bulechek, et al., 2007).

Documenting Abnormal Findings

The nurse has just finished conducting a beginning assessment of Mr. Harris, the patient who reports worsening vision and has a history of glaucoma. Review the following important findings revealed in each of the steps of objective data collection for Mr. Harris. Consider how these results compare with the normal findings presented in the samples of normal documentation. Note that inspection is the major technique used in eye assessment.

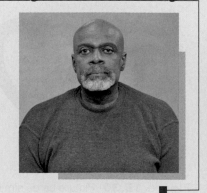

Inspection: External eyes symmetrical, no ptosis. PERRLA. EOMI. Conjunctiva clear, sclera white. Distance vision: right 20/30, left 20/50. Visual fields reduced by approximately 20% by confrontation.

Palpation: External eye lacrimal apparatus without swelling or redness, nontender.

B. Ryan, RN

Table 15.5   Common Nursing Diagnoses Associated with the Eyes

Diagnosis and Related Factors	Point of Differentiation	Assessment Characteristics	Nursing Interventions
Disturbed sensory perception related to vision disturbance	Alterations in the way the patient takes in, processes, uses, or otherwise deals with sensory (especially visual) stimuli	Wears eyeglasses, uses contacts, uses computer assistive devices	Converse with and touch patient frequently. Use lighting for reading. Use a magnifying glass for shaving or to apply makeup.
Risk for injury related to impaired vision	At risk for physical harm and damage as a result of environmental limitations imposed by impaired vision	Near or far vision impaired, difficulty seeing in low lighting, difficulty seeing at night	Refer to optometrist for corrective lenses. Ensure that patient wears lenses and that eyeglasses are clean. Make sure that objects are out of the path. Remove hazards from room, such as razors and matches.

Once outcomes are established, nursing care is implemented to improve the status of the patient. The nurse uses critical thinking and evidence-based practice to develop nursing interventions. Some examples of nursing interventions for the eye are as follows:

- Identify name and purpose of visit when entering patient's personal space.
- Keep furniture out of pathways and keep cords against walls.
- Ensure access to eyeglasses or magnifiers as needed (Moorhead, et al., 2007).

Analyzing Findings

The APRN has seen Mr. Harris, performed an ophthalmoscopic examination, and is concerned about Mr. Harris's worsening vision. The following nursing note illustrates how subjective and objective data are collected and analyzed and nursing interventions are developed.

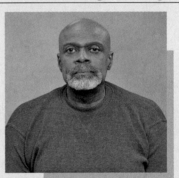

Subjective: "I'm here for my checkup to make sure that my medicines are doing what they're supposed to." Personal history of high blood pressure, high cholesterol, and glaucoma.

Objective: A 61-year-old African American man, alert and oriented, appears stated age. External eyes symmetrical, no ptosis. Conjunctiva clear, sclera white. Distance vision: right 20/30 left 20/50. Reads newsprint but says it is somewhat blurred compared to 1 year ago. Visual fields reduced by approximately 20% by confrontation.

Analysis: Disturbed visual sensory perception related to loss of visual field and visual acuity.

Plan: Make referral to ophthalmologist for further testing. Additionally refer to social work to assist with getting funding for new eyeglasses and medication. Teach about safety issues related to impaired vision, especially risk for falling. Encourage him to use magnifying devices for reading until he can get his new glasses.

B. Ryan, RN

Critical Thinking Challenge

- What other assessment data might the nurse collect?
- What other nursing diagnoses might be appropriate for Mr. Harris?
- How does the role of the APRN differ from the RN role?

Collaboration with Other Health Care Professionals

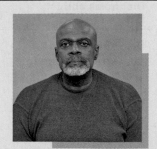

Because of Mr. Harris's abnormal findings, he needs referral to an ophthalmologist. The role of specialists is important in eye care, because they have more advanced assessment skills and techniques. Examples include more accurate testing of the visual fields with a machine and tonometry to measure pressure inside the eye. The following conversation illustrates how the RN might organize data and make recommendations about the patient's situation to an ophthalmologist.

Situation: Hi, I'm Bev Ryan, a nurse referring a patient for a consult.

Background: The name is Mr. Edward Harris. Date of birth is 10–31–1949. He's a 61-year-old man with a history of high blood pressure, high cholesterol, and glaucoma. We saw him for his annual visit and found some abnormalities on his eye examination. Both his near and far vision have worsened, and he says that his vision is blurrier compared to 1 year ago. His visual fields are also reduced by about 20%. Unfortunately, he also has some financial restrictions, and he had a few months where he couldn't afford to buy his eye drops. We have a social work consult in to work on that issue.

Assessment: Because he has symptoms of worsening glaucoma, he'll need further evaluation.

Recommendations: If possible, would you have time to work him into your schedule in the next week? He also will most likely need new glasses. We can also have social work help to get funding for his glasses.

Critical Thinking Challenge

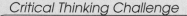

- What might the nurse further assess related to Mr. Harris's medication management?
- What additional information might the ophthalmologist request?
- How will the team collaborate to promote Mr. Harris's health?

Pulling It All Together: Reflection and Critical Thinking

The nurse uses assessment data to formulate a nursing care plan with patient outcomes and interventions. Outcomes are specific to the patient, realistic to achieve, measurable, and have a time frame for meeting the outcome. The interventions are actions that the nurse performs, based on evidence and practice guidelines. After these interventions are completed, the nurse reevaluates and documents findings to show progress toward the patient outcome. The nurse uses critical thinking and judgment to continue or revise the diagnosis, outcomes, or interventions. This is often in the form of a care plan or case note similar to the one below.

Nursing Diagnosis	Patient Outcomes	Nursing Interventions	Rationale	Evaluation
Disturbed visual sensory perception	Patient will remain free from harm resulting from a loss of vision.	Refer to ophthalmologist for further testing. Refer to social work to assist with funding for eyeglasses. Teach patient to clear cords and furniture from pathways, and use good lighting.	Referral to the ophthalmologist will correct the low vision. Furniture and cords are environmental hazards that increase risk of falling. Good lighting increases visibility.	Referral made to ophthalmologist. Patient will be seen in 2 days. Patient states that his home environment is uncluttered and all furniture and cords are out of the way. He plans to get lamp for the hallway at night.

U sing the previous steps of diagnostic reasoning, organizing, and prioritizing, consider all of the case study findings woven throughout this chapter. When answering the following questions, see how the pieces of assessment work together to create an environment for personalized, appropriate, and accurate care. As you study the content and features, consider Mr. Harris's case and how it is important to seek care for primary prevention. Begin thinking about the following points:

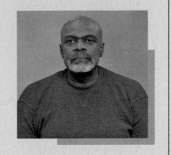

- What routine assessments should the nurse make related to the patient's eye health?
- What additional assessments should the nurse make based on the patient's reports of decreased vision?
- How can the nurse encourage Mr. Harris's desire for improved health?

Key Points

- Cranial nerves involved with the eyes include CN II (optic nerve), III (occulomotor), IV (trochlear), and VI (abducens).
- An important health promotion activity is the use of protective eyewear for contact sports and occupational exposure.
- Sudden visual loss is an emergency.
- Common symptoms related to the eye and vision include pain, trauma, visual change, blind spots, floaters, halos, discharge, and a related change in ADLs.
- The Snellen's chart is used to assess far vision; the Jaeger test is used for near vision. A patient with 20/20 vision can read at 20 ft what the normal person can read at 20 ft. A higher number on the bottom indicates worse vision.
- Patients older than 40 years often have a decreased ability to accommodate, moving the object further away to read.
- Static and kinetic confrontation tests measure peripheral vision.
- The cardinal fields of gaze allow the nurse to detect muscle defects that cause misalignment or uncoordinated movement of the eyes.
- PERRLA is documented when the pupils are equal, round, reactive to light, and accommodation.
- Assessment of the eye with an ophthalmoscope is considered an advanced skill.
- Cloudiness in the lens can indicate a cataract.
- Common abnormalities include being nearsighted or farsighted, astigmatism, pstosis, and nystagmus.
- Cataracts, glaucoma, and macular degeneration are more common in older adults.

Review Questions

1. Which of the following patients would require the most emergent nursing care?
   A. An 8-year-old girl with pink conjunctiva and drainage
   B. A 20-year-old man with sudden visual loss after playing football
   C. A 52-year-old woman with clouding of vision
   D. A 77-year-old man with loss of vision in his peripheral fields

2. Which of the following teaching points would the nurse emphasize related to eye health?
   A. Always wear eye protection for occupational exposures.
   B. Eat a diet high in animal protein and dairy.
   C. Exercise five times a week for at least 20 minutes.
   D. Get at least 7 hours of sleep each night.

3. Which of the following symptoms would the nurse expect the patient to report as translucent specks that drift across the visual field?
   A. Blind spot
   B. Ptosis
   C. Halo
   D. Floater

4. When working with an older adult, what would the nurse emphasize as increased risks for the patient?
   A. Myopia and strabismus
   B. Blepharitis and chalazion
   C. Glaucoma and cataracts
   D. Exophthalmos and presbyopia

5. A school nurse is performing annual vision screening for seventh grade students. Which of the following charts would the nurse most likely be using?
   A. Allen's chart
   B. Snellen's chart
   C. Ishihara cards
   D. Confrontation cards

6. Which of the following scores for distance vision indicates the patient with the poorest vision?
   A. 200/20
   B. 18/20
   C. 24/20
   D. 20/100

7. The nurse recognizes that the 60-year-old patient may have difficulty reading fine print because of the loss in the ability of the eye to
   A. accommodate
   B. aniscoria
   C. amblyopia
   D. asthenopia

8. Peripheral vision is evaluated by the nurse using
   A. corneal light test
   B. cover test
   C. confrontation test
   D. cardinal fields of gaze

9. The cranial nerves involved with eye movement include
   A. II, V, and VII
   B. III, IV, and VI
   C. IV, V, and VIII
   D. V, VI, and VII

10. The nurse assesses the response of the eye to light and documents normal findings as
    A. PEERLA
    B. PERRLA
    C. PERLLA
    D. PERLAA

References

Bulechek, G. B., Butcher, H. K., & McCloskey Dochterman, J. (2007). *Nursing Interventions Classification (NIC)* (4th ed.) St. Louis, MO: Mosby.

Centers for Disease Control and Prevention. (2006). Visual impairment and eye care among older adults—Five States, 2005. *Morbidity and Mortality Weekly Report, 55*(49), 1321–1325.

Childstats.gov. (2009). *America's children: Key indicators of national well being, 2009*. Retrieved July 12, 2009, from http://www.childstats.gov/americaschildren/index.asp

Coats, D. K., Paysse, E. A., & Torchia, M. M. (2009). Visual development and vision assessment in infants and children. Retrieved June 15, 2009, from http://www.uptodateonline.com.proxy.seattleu.edu/online/content/topic.do?topicKey=ped_opth/4522&selectedTitle=1~150&source=search_result

Dubois, L. (2005). Informal visual fields. In *Clinical Skills for ophthalmic examination: Basic Procedures* (2nd ed., pp. 37–45). Thorofare, NJ: Slack Inc.

Duffy, B. (2008). Managing chemical eye injuries. *Emergency Nurse, 16*(1), 25–29.

Friedman, D. S., Munoz, B., Massof, R. W., Bandeen-Roche, K., & West, S. K. (2002). Grading visual acuity using the preferential-looking method in elderly nursing home residents. *Investigative Ophthalmology and Visual Science, 43*(8), 2572–2578.

Healthy People 2010: What are its goals? (n.d.). Retrieved June 15, 2009, from http://www.healthypeople.gov/About/goals.htm

Hockenberry, M. J., & Wilson, D. (2007). *Wong's nursing care of infants and children* (8th ed.) St. Louis MO: Mosby Elsevier.

Jacobs, D. S., Trobe, J., & Sokol, H. N. (2009). *Primary open-angle glaucoma*. Retrieved June 4, 2009, from http://www.uptodateonline.com.proxy.seattleu.edu/online/content/topic.do?topicKey=priophth/7711&linkTitle=Risk%20factors&source=preview&selectedTitle=1~150&anchor=3#3

Javitt, J. C., Wang, F., & West, S. K. (1996). Blindness due to cataract: Epidemiology and prevention. *Annual Review of Public Health, 17*, 159–177.

Knowing, D., & Kester, K. (2007). Keep an eye out for glaucoma. *Nurse Practitioner, 32*(7), 18–23.

Lang, R. S., & Hensrud, D. D. (Eds.). (2004). *Clinical preventative medicine* (2nd ed.). Chicago, IL: American Medicine.

Lowdermilk, D., & Perry, S. (2007). *Maternity & women's health care* (9th ed.). St. Louis, MO: Mosby Elsevier.

Mackin, L. A., Mangin, E. J., Park, R., et al. (2003). *Handbook of geriatric nursing care* (2nd ed.). Philadelphia: Lippincott.

Miller, C. A. (2008). *Nursing for wellness in older adults* (5th ed.). Philadelphia: Lippincott Williams & Wilkins.

Moorhead, S., Johnson, M., & Maas, M. (2007). *Nursing outcomes classification (NOC)* (4th ed.). St. Louis, MO: Mosby.

Mozaffariehm, M., Greishaber, M. C., & Flammer, J. (2008). Oxygen and blood flow players in the pathogenesis of glaucoma. *Molecular Vision, 14*(Jan), 224–233.

National Eye Institute, National Institutes of Health. (2005). Eye health needs of older adults literature review. *National Eye Health Education Program Five-Year Agenda*. Retrieved June 3, 2009, from http://www.nei.nih.gov/nehep/research/The_Eye_Health_needs_of_Older_Adults_Literature_Review.pdf

North American Nursing Diagnosis Association. (2009). *Nursing diagnoses, 2009–2011 Edition: Definitions and classifications (NANDA NURSING DIAGNOSIS)*. West Sussex UK: John Wiley & Sons.

Price, K. M., Gupta, P. K., Woodward, J. A., et al. (2009). Eyebrow and eyelid dimensions: An anthropometric analysis of African Americans and Caucasians. *Plastic and Reconstructive Surgery, 124*(2), 615–623.

Somami, S., Bhatti, A., & Iqbal, I. K. (2008). *Pregnancy, special considerations*. Retrieved October 29, 2009, from http://emedicine.medscape.com/article/1229740-overview

Sperduto, R. D., Clemons, T. E., Lindblad, A. S., & Ferris, F. L. (2008). Age-related eye disease study research group: Cataract classification using serial examinations in the Age-Related Eye Disease Study: AREDS Report No. 24. *Archives in Ophthalmology, 145*, 504–508.

The Jensen suite offers these additional resources to enhance learning and facilitate understanding of this chapter:

- thePoint on line resource, http//thepoint.lww.com/Jensen1E
- Student CD-ROM included with the book
- *Laboratory Manual for Nursing Health Assessment: A Best Practice Approach*
- *Pocket Guide for Nursing Health Assessment: A Best Practice Approach*

Tables of Abnormal Findings

Table 15.6   Refractive Errors

Finding	Description
Asthenopia (eye strain)	Eye strain develops after reading, computer work, or other visually tedious tasks from tightening of the eye muscles after maintaining a constant focal distance. Symptoms include fatigue, red eyes, eyestrain, pain in or around the eyes, blurred vision, headaches, and, rarely, double vision.
Astigmatism 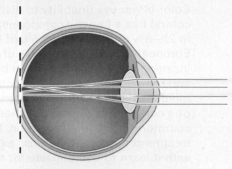 **Focal point of light rays:** multiple areas of the retina	Abnormal (football-shaped) curvature of the cornea prevents light from focusing on the retina. Images appear blurred because not all optical planes are focused. This condition is corrected with a cylindrical lens that has more focusing power in one access than the other.
Myopia (nearsightedness) 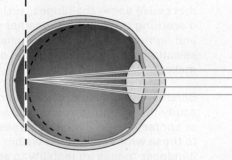 **Focal point of light rays:** in front of the retina	Images of distant objects focus in front of, instead of on, the retina from an imperfection in the shape of the eye or lens. Myopia occurs in approximately 25% of the U.S. population (Sperduto, et al., 2008). It is found in 2% of children entering first grade and 15% of those entering high school (Childstats, 2009). People with myopia can see clearly objects up close, but have difficulty seeing distant objects. Myopia is corrected with a concave lens that moves the focus back to the retina.
Hyperopia (farsightedness) 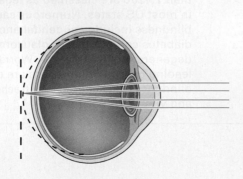 **Focal point of light rays:** behind the retina	Images of near objects focus behind, instead of on, the retina from an imperfection in the shape of the eye or lens. Approximately 25% of the U.S. population has hyperopia. People with it can see distant objects clearly but have difficulty seeing objects up close. A convex lens is used to treat hyperopia, moving the focus forward onto the retina.

(table continues on page 372)

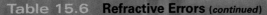
Table 15.6 **Refractive Errors** (*continued*)

Finding	Description
Presbyopia  **Focal point of light rays:** behind the retina 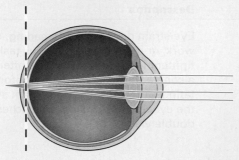	This symptom, considered a natural part of aging, is believed to result from loss of elasticity of the crystalline lens. As this happens, the ciliary muscles that bend and straighten the lens lose their power to accommodate. This condition affects near vision and therefore is corrected with a convex lens in front of the eye in the form of half-glass or as bottom of a bifocal or multifocal lens if other correction is needed for distance viewing.
Color blindness	Color blindness (inability to distinguish colors) has a genetic component. It occurs in 2%–8% of males and 0.5% of females of European descent. The cones of the eye, located in the macula, contain blue, green, and red pigments that allow color sight. Color blindness results with damage to the cones or a cone that is missing pigment. The most common form is the red/green. No effective treatment for color blindness exists. Many with it learn to compensate for the deficit and at times can discern details that a normal-sighted person would miss. Most people are not totally color blind but have deficiencies that cause some challenges, such as with discerning traffic lights, weather forecasts, and light-emitting diodes; purchasing clothes; selecting crayons; cooking; and applying makeup.
Blindness	Blindness means loss of vision or visual acuity that cannot be corrected with glasses or contact lenses. Partial blindness refers to those with very limited vision; complete blindness means an inability to see anything, including light. People with vision worse than 20/200 are classified as legally blind in most US states. Numerous causes of blindness include congenital anomalies, diabetes complications, glaucoma, macular degeneration, and trauma. Worldwide, the leading causes of blindness are cataracts, river blindness (onchocerciasis), trachoma, leprosy, and vitamin A deficiency.

Table 15.7 Abnormalities of Eye Movement

Finding	Description
Nystagmus 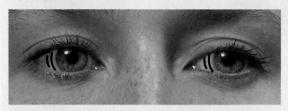	Involuntary rhythmic wobbling of the eyes; degree and direction of the movement can impair vision, with impairment varying greatly among patients
Strabismus (cross- or wall-eyed) 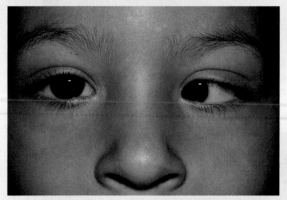 Crossed eye (esotropia) 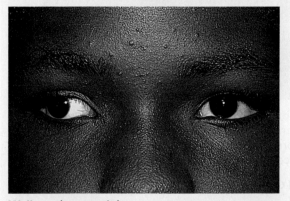 Wall eye (exotropia) 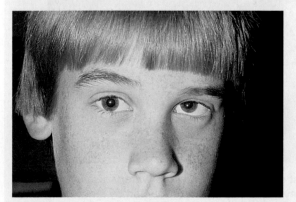 One eye pointing upward or downward (vertical deviation)	Different forms of strabismus; appropriate evaluation and treatment required for this condition in which a person cannot align both eyes simultaneously under normal conditions. To a certain degree strabismus occurs in 5% of all children. Strabismus is not the same as amblyopia. Children do not outgrow strabismus. Strabismus can be constant (eye turns out all the time) or intermittent (turning out only some of the time).

Table 15.8 External Eye Abnormalities

Jaundice

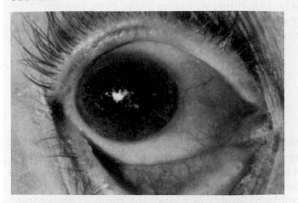

Yellowing of the sclera, which indicates liver disease

Hyphema

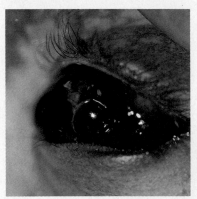

Blood in the anterior chamber of the eye, usually caused by blunt trauma

Chalazion

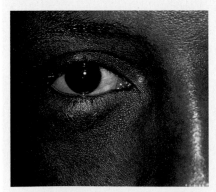

A cyst (meibomian gland lipogranuloma) in the eyelid resulting from inflammation of the meibomian gland. Most often on the upper eyelid and are sometimes confused with a hordelum (sty); they can be differentiated because they are usually painless and tend to be larger. Rarely resolves spontaneously; usually requires treatment

Iris Nevus

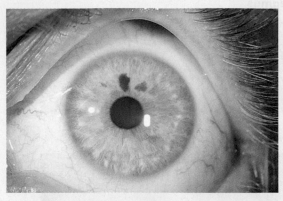

Rare condition affecting one eye, with abnormalities in appearance of the iris, pain, and decreased vision; patients may also have glaucoma on the same side

Blepharitis

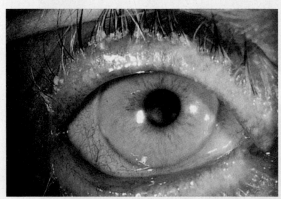

Inflammation of the margin of the eyelid; two types are anterior and posterior. Most common type is seborrheic, followed by staphylococcal, and then rosacea-associated

Viral Conjunctivitis

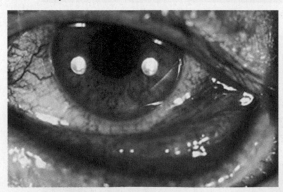

Most often associated with a watery discharge from the eye that may be accompanied by sinus congestion and rhinorhea (runny nose), slightly injected (diffusely pink), and numerous follicles on the inferior conjunctiva

Table 15.8 **External Eye Abnormalities** (*continued*)

Bacterial Conjunctivitis

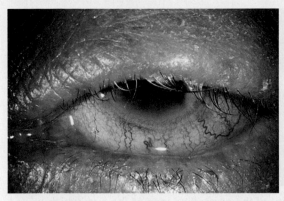

Should be suspected if there is purulent discharge (yellow or green), injected (red), and numerous follicles. Occasional blurring is common; should not be painful, constant blurring, or photophobia

Allergic Conjunctivitis

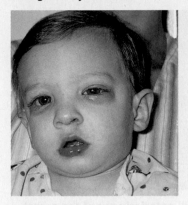

Usually bilateral and common in people with ectopic (allergic) conditions; associated with slight watery discharge and itching of the eyes

Glaucoma

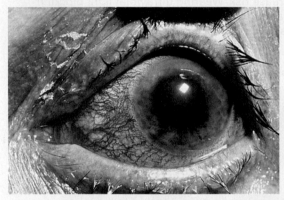

The leading cause of irreversible blindness and most common chronic optic neuropathy. Disease of the optic nerve that involves loss of retinal ganglion cells. A significant risk factor is increased intraocular pressure. Impaired flow of aqueous humor leads to increased intraocular pressure. In open-angle glaucoma, aqueous humor flows in the trabecular meshwork (Mozaffariehm, et al., 2008). In closed-angle glaucoma, the anteriorly displaced iris pushes against the trabecular meshwork, blocking fluid flow. Glaucoma has three main types: primary (primary open-angle or closed-angle); secondary (inflammatory, phacogenic, related to intraocular hemorrhage); and developmental (primary congenital, infantile). The most common type is primary open-angle glaucoma (POAG), affecting 2.2 million US citizens (Knowing & Kester, 2007). POAG has a genetic link. Rarer are congenital eye malformations that develop in the third trimester of gestation, which cause early-angle closure and ocular hypertension, leading to optic neuropathies. Those at risk for glaucoma need an annual dilated eye examination (CDC, 2006).

Amblyopia (Lazy Eye)

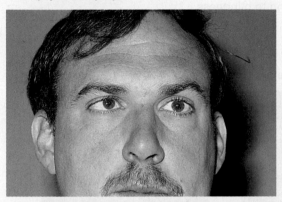

Condition in which the vision in one eye is reduced because the eye and brain are not working together. It is the most common cause of visual impairment in children (2–3:100). The eye upon examination looks normal, but vision is not normal because the brain is favoring the other eye. If amblyopia is not properly treated, it persists into adulthood, leading to monocular visual impairment. Amblyopia can be caused by strabismus, visual field discrepancies, and occasionally cataracts. The direction that the lazy eye moves is described as esotropia (medial), exotropia (lateral), hypertropia (superior), or hypotropia (inferior).

(table continues on page 376)

Table 15.8 **External Eye Abnormalities** (*continued*)

Exophthalmos

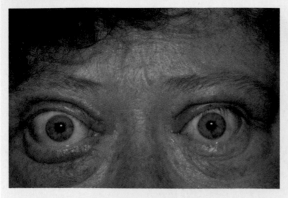

Protrusion of the eyeball anteriorly out of the socket. The most common cause is a thyroid disorder known as Graves' disease. Untreated exopthalmos can impair the ability of the eyelid to close properly, especially during sleep, which increases dryness of the corneal epithelium. The process and displacement of the eye can lead to compression of the optic nerve or artery, leading to blindness.

Cataracts

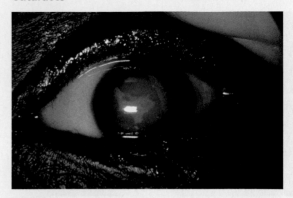

Opacity of the crystalline lens of the eye, which obstructs the passage of light. The most common causes are long-term exposure to ultraviolet light, radiation, diabetes, hypertension, and advanced age. Opacity develops from a change in the lens protein (denatured). Genetics plays a role in congenital cataracts; positive family history of cataracts seems to increase risk. Wearing ultraviolet light blocking sunglasses is believed to slow the development of cataracts (Javitt, et al., 1996).

Hordelum (Stye)

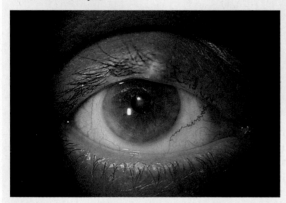

Caused by a blockage and infection of the sebaceous gland at the base of the eyelashes. While painful and unsightly, there is generally no lasting damage.

Osteogenesis Imperfecta

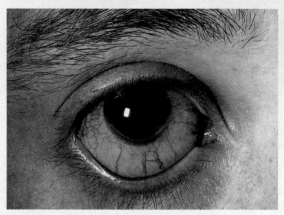

A blue sclera is due to a thinning of the sclera and is indicative of osteogenesis imperfecta.

Anisocoria (Unequal Pupils)

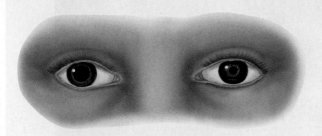

These usually result from a defect in the efferent nervous pathways controlling the oculomotor nerve. Deformities of the iris or eye must be ruled out.

Horner's Syndrome

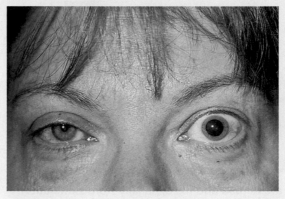

Pupillary miosis (constricted pupil) and dilation lag on the affected side. Also often present is ptosis.

Argyle Robertson

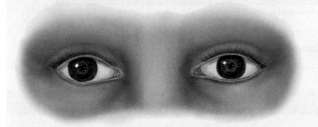

Bilateral pupils accommodate but do not dilate when exposed to bright light. Direct and consensual pupil reflexes are absent.

Adie's Pupil

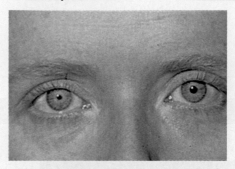

Pupils are fixed, dilated, and tonic. Direct and consensual pupil reactions are weak or absent.

Key Hole Pupil (Coloboma)

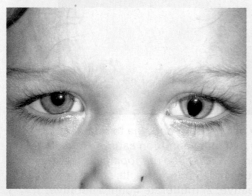

A gap appears in the iris. It can be congenital or caused during cataract or glaucoma surgery.

Miosis (Small Fixed Pupil)

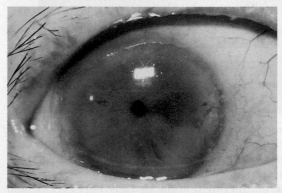

Pupils are constricted and fixed. Miosis occurs with eye drops for glaucoma, iritis, brain damage to pons, and narcotic drug use.

(table continues on page 378)

Table 15.9 Abnormal Findings in the Pupil *(continued)*

Mydriasis (Dilated Fixed Pupil)

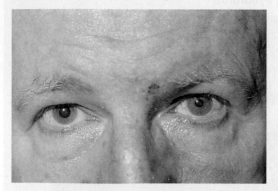

Pupils are dilated and fixed, usually from stimulation of sympathetic nerves as a consequence of CNS injury, circulatory arrest, deep anesthesia, acute glaucoma, or recent trauma. This may also follow administration of sympathomimetic eye drops.

Oculomotor (CN III) Nerve Damage

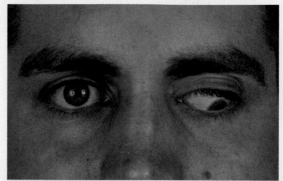

(A) Oculomotor paralysis

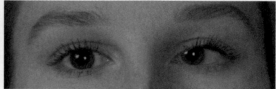

(B) Abducent paralysis

A unilateral dilated pupil has no reaction to light or accommodation.

 Table 15.10 Retinal Abnormalities

AMD

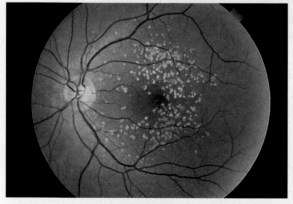

AMD gradually causes loss of sharp central vision, needed for common daily tasks (eg, driving, reading). The macula degenerates (dry) or abnormal blood vessels behind the retina grow under the macula (wet). The more common dry AMD occurs slowly in stages: early, intermediate, and advanced. Wet AMD develops quickly without stages. The main risk factor for AMD is age, with those older than 60 years mostly affected. Other risks are smoking, obesity, European ancestry, family history, and female gender. Health education for at-risk patients includes review of a healthy diet high in leafy green vegetables and fish, smoking cessation, blood-pressure and weight control, and exercise. Management options include ocular injections, laser surgery, and photodynamic therapy. None of these cure AMD, but they may slow vision loss.

Retinopathy

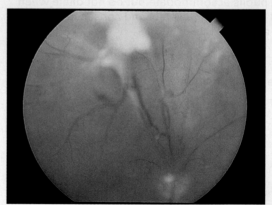

Retinopathy occurs from damage to retinal blood vessels. The two most common causes are diabetes and hypertension. *Diabetic retinopathy* is the most common cause of US blindness. Its stages are 1) mild nonprolifereative; 2) moderate nonproliferative; 3) severe nonproliferative; and 4) proliferative (most advanced). *Hypertensive retinopathy* presents with a dry retina (few hemorrhages, rare edema or exudate, multiple cotton wool spots), while diabetic retinopathy presents with a wet retina (multiple hemorrhages and exudate, extensive edema, few cotton wool spots).

Table 15.10 Retinal Abnormalities (*continued*)

Copper Wiring

Notching of vein by artery ——

Retinal artery with "copper wire" effect

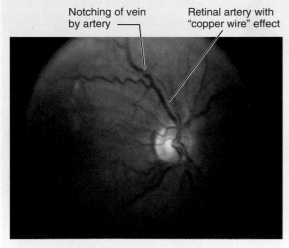

Chronic hypertension causes the retinal arterioles to thicken. The name *copper wiring* comes from the initial bronze appearance of the retina light reflection. As uncontrolled hypertension continues, the retina takes on a silvery or whitish appearance. The change comes from thickening of the retinal arterioles.

Retinitis Pigmentosa

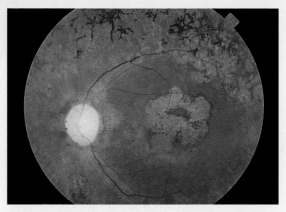

In this genetically transmitted disease, the retinas in both eyes progressively degenerate. It starts with loss of night vision, then loss of peripheral vision, progressing to tunnel vision, and finally no vision.

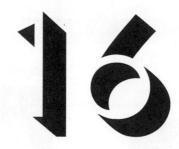

Ears Assessment

Learning Objectives

1 Identify the structures and functions of the ear.

2 Identify the common landmarks of the tympanic membrane.

3 Differentiate subjective data for otalgia, otorrhea, vertigo, and changes in hearing.

4 Identify teaching opportunities for health promotion and risk reduction related to the ear and hearing acuity.

5 Collect objective data on physical structures of the ear.

6 Identify normal and unexpected findings in the inspection and palpation of the ear.

7 Identify proper techniques for otoscope use.

8 Use subjective and objective data to analyze findings of and plan interventions for the ear and hearing acuity.

9 Document and communicate data from ear assessment using appropriate medical terminology.

10 Individualize health assessment considering the condition, age, gender, and culture of the patient.

*M*rs. Petino is a 25-year-old immigrant from El Salvador. She comes to the clinic today with concerns of ear pain, "buzzing" in her ears, and hearing loss. Mrs. Petino has been to the clinic five times in the last 4 months for ear concerns. She was treated once for bilateral otitis media. She currently works in a tuna-packing plant as a line custodian. Her immunizations are current. Temperature is 37.4°C orally, pulse 86 beats/min, respirations 16 breaths/min, and blood pressure 126/78 mm Hg. Current medications include 500 mg acetaminophen taken 2 hours ago.

You will gain more information about Mrs. Petino as you progress through the chapter. As you study the content and features, consider Mrs. Petino's case and its relationship to what you are learning. Begin thinking about the following points:

- How will the nurse assess and document the patient's pain?
- How will the nurse assess and document the patient's hearing loss?
- What information will the nurse need to collect to assess the patient's risk for hearing loss?
- When will the nurse make a referral to the audiologist?

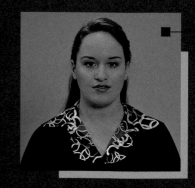

This chapter explores ear assessment. It reviews anatomy of the ear and physiology related to hearing and equilibrium, including key variations associated with lifespan, culture, and the environment. The section on subjective data collection covers family history, personal history, medications, and risk factors contributing to otitis media, loss of hearing, and vertigo. Information on collecting objective data describes methods for assessing anatomy, auditory perception, and equilibrium. A hearing screen is an essential portion of a complete physical examination. Early intervention for hearing deficit helps patients interact socially and decreases risk of injury.

Structure and Function Overview

The *ear* is divided into three distinct portions: (1) the *external ear*, most of which is visualized easily without tools; (2) the *middle ear*, a small space behind the tympanic membrane (TM) extending to the eustachian tube; and (3) the inner ear, the vestibular portion. All three portions contribute to the process of hearing. An important additional structure is the *mastoid process*, a bony protrusion of the skull present behind the lobule (see Fig. 14-1). The eustachian tube, though not part of the ear, affects its function. This small tube connects the anterior middle ear to the nasopharynx. The ear has two separate functions: hearing and sustaining equilibrium.

External Ear

The external ear (also called the auricle or pinna) starts to develop in the 6th week of gestation and is identifiable by the 12th week of gestation (Isaacson, 2009). It is made up of flexible cartilage and skin (Fig. 16-1). Its design guides sound waves into the meatus of the *external auditory canal*, which is a chamber that transitions from firm cartilage to bone and ends at the **TM**.

In adults, a thin, sensitive layer of skin covers the external auditory canal, which is shaped similar to an S. Lining the canal are hairs and glands that secrete **cerumen**, a waxy substance. The slight S curve, hair, and cerumen help protect the canal and TM from foreign objects (see Figure 16-2).

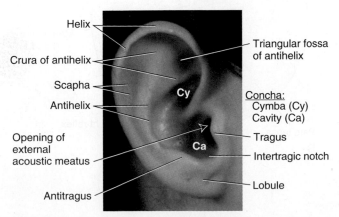

Figure 16.1 Surface anatomy of the external ear.

The TM is the oblique, multilayered, translucent, and pearly grey barrier between the external auditory canal and middle ear. There is a first layer of epidermis uninterrupted from the external auditory canal, a center layer, and a final mucosal layer consistent with the mucosa of the middle ear (Cummings, et al., 1998). The TM adheres through its concave shape to the malleus near the center. Some auditory ossicles in the middle ear can be distinguished on visualization of the translucent TM, as can portions of the malleus, umbo, manubrium, and short process (Fig. 16-3). A well-aerated middle ear allows visualization of part of the incus as well.

In the anterior quadrant of the TM, a distinct cone of light is visible, which is caused by the light of the otoscope reflecting-off the posterior wall of the middle ear. The outer rim of the TM, the *annulus*, is thicker and more fibrous than the rest. Most of the TM, *pars tensa*, is stretched tightly and easy to see through. *Pars flaccida*, a small portion of the TM above the short process of the malleus, is more relaxed and opaque.

Middle Ear

The air-filled space behind the TM contains the **malleus, incus**, and **stapes**—tiny bones responsible for conducting sound waves to the inner ear. The middle ear acts as a volume dampener to protect the inner ear. There are four openings to the middle ear chamber.

1. The TM, the largest, leading to the external ear
2. The *cochlear window*, also known as the round window, which connects the middle and inner ear
3. The *oval window*, on which the stapes rests to complete connection to the cochlea
4. The **eustachian tube**, a conduit that connects the middle ear to the nasopharynx and allows for pressure regulation of the middle ear. See Figures 16-2 and 16-6.

Clinical Significance 16-1

Ability to equalize pressure keeps the TM intact with atmospheric variances. The eustachian tube opens briefly with swallowing and yawning; otherwise, this conduit remains closed.

Inner Ear

The inner ear is responsible for the translation of sound to cranial nerve VIII (auditory nerve; see Chapter 24), which transmits it to the brainstem. While the external ear, middle ear, and inner ear all play roles in hearing, the inner ear is the only section responsible for vestibular function. The conduits of the inner ear are known collectively as the *bony labyrinth*, which consists of the **semicircular canals**, **vestibule**, and **chochlea**. The cochlea includes the portions of the inner ear responsible for hearing. Vestibular function is maintained in the semicircular canals and vestibule.

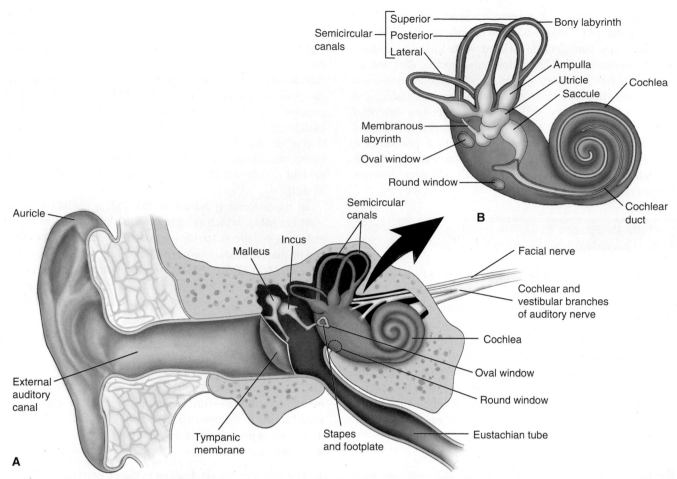

Figure 16.2 **A.** Anatomy of the external and middle ear. **B.** Anatomy of the inner ear.

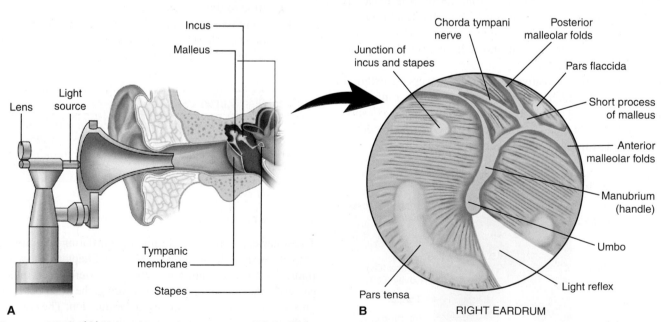

Figure 16.3 **(A)** Using the otoscope to view **(B)** the TM.

Hearing

Hearing is a complex experience. The external ear channels sound waves into the external auditory canal through the TM, to ossicles in the inner ear via the oval window, then to the cochlea. The basal membrane in the cochlea vibrates the receptor hair cells of the **organ of Corti**, which transfer the signal into electrical impulses for the auditory nerve. The auditory nerve then delivers those impulses to the auditory cortex in the temporal lobe of the brain (see Chapter 24), which interprets them as and assigns meaning to the sound. The brainstem detects origination of the sound and can distinguish from which ear the electrical impulses originated, even though there may be only a slight delay of sound from one ear to the other.

The cochlea interprets two components of sound: amplitude (volume) and frequency (pitch). *Amplitude* is the change in atmospheric pressure against the TM and is directly related to the intensity of a sound. Decibels (dB) are the measurement units of amplitude. *Frequency,* the number of cycles per second the sound waves make, is measured in units of hertz (Hz). Normal conversation occurs between 10 to 60 dB and 200 to 5,000 Hz. A jet engine is approximately 140 dB; a whisper is approximately thirty dB (Fig. 16-4).

Air and Bone Conduction

Sound is perceived two ways: air conduction (AC) and bone conduction (BC) (Fig. 16-5). **AC**, the most efficient method, is the normal pathway for sounds to travel to the inner ear. BC uses a different pathway, bypassing the external ear and delivering sound waves/vibrations directly to the inner ear via the skull. A compromise in either pathway causes hearing loss.

Hearing Problems

Conductive hearing loss occurs when sound wave transmission through the external or middle ear is disrupted. It may result with either blockage of the external auditory canal by cerumen or fluid in the middle ear. The health care provider can easily remedy external auditory blockage by clearing the obstruction. Fluid in the middle ear requires further investigation for pathology. Increasing the amplitude of sound will overcome conductive hearing loss.

⚠ *SAFETY ALERT 16.1*

The most common cause of conductive hearing loss in adults is auditory trauma related to excessive noise exposure. This problem is increasing among younger people as well. Twenty-five percent of the US workforce is exposed regularly to potentially damaging noise (Suter & von Gierke, 1987). Because of occupational risk of noise-induced hearing loss, government standards regulate allowable noise exposure.

Sensorineural hearing loss results from a problem somewhere beyond the middle ear, from inner ear to auditory cortex. Sites of dysfunction include the cochlea, organ of Corti, auditory nerve, or auditory cortex. **Presbycusis**, a common form of sensorineural loss, results from gradual degeneration of nerves and sensory hair cells of the organ of Corti. Such degeneration may be related to either aging or use of ototoxic drugs (eg, gentamicin).

Tinnitus is a perception of buzzing or ringing in one ear or both ears that does not correspond with an external sound. It is fairly common, affecting up to 15% of the population (Berry, et al., 2002). The perceived sound of tinnitus may be quiet and a minor annoyance or so loud that it makes hearing normal conversation or restful sleep impossible. Little is known about what causes tinnitus, though some degree of hearing loss often accompanies it. Tinnitus may be the perception of normal sounds within the body that external noise normally blocks. Currently very few treatments for tinnitus are available (Davis, et al., 2007).

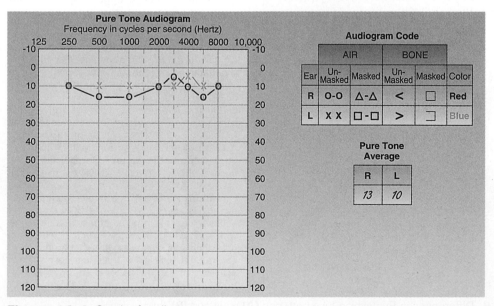

Figure 16.4 Graph of audiogram.

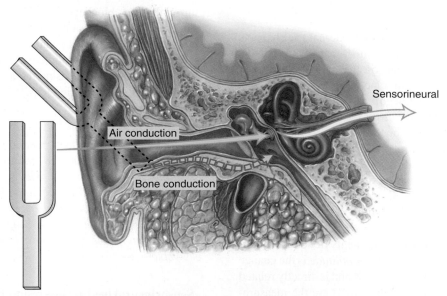

Figure 16.5 Pathways of hearing: air conduction and bone conduction.

Vestibular Function

The semicircular canals and vestibule (utricle and saccule) provide the body with proprioception and equilibrium. Each organ contains specialized epithelium for sensing position. With illness the labyrinth can become inflamed and cause loss of equilibrium, which leads to a sense of vertigo. Symptoms of Meniere's disease include vertigo along with severe nausea and vomiting. This illness has a pattern of exacerbations that often last for 24 hours followed by periods of remission (Rubin & Strayer, 2008).

Lifespan Considerations

Pregnant Women

During pregnancy estrogen levels stimulate the expansion of blood flow throughout the body. Increased blood flow and subsequent vessel changes in the middle ear may cause a sensation of fullness in the ear or intermittent otalgia. Vertigo in pregnant women can result from increased vascularity and edema.

Newborns, Infants, and Children

Infants and children are susceptible to otitis media, largely because of the size and shape of their eustachian tubes, which are shorter, wider, and more horizontal compared to those of adults (Fig. 16-6). Infants with Trisomy 21 or cleft palate have increased incidence of otitis media. Because of the frequent number of upper respiratory infections that infants and children have and their immature anatomy, bacteria and

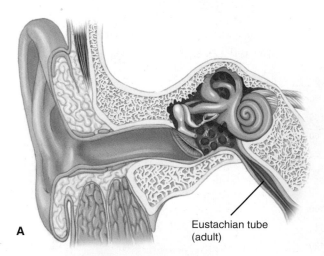
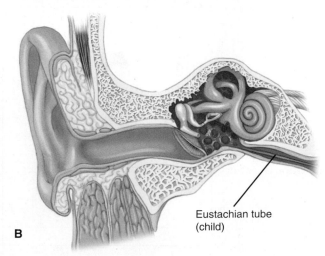

A Eustachian tube (adult)

B Eustachian tube (child)

Figure 16.6 Differences in Eustachian tube between **(A)** adult and **(B)** child.

viruses have more opportunity to reflux into the middle ear via the eustachian tube. The middle ear also acts as a perfect reservoir for pathogens because it is dark, warm, and moist. Both bacteria and viruses thrive in this environment.

> ## Clinical Significance 16-3
>
> Enlarged adenoids related to nasal allergies often obstruct the outlets for the eustachian tube to drain in children (see Chapter 17).

While otitis media can cause severe discomfort, including difficulty feeding, sleeping, and general fussiness, it rarely causes permanent hearing loss. Following an episode, it is normal for fluid to remain in the middle ear for up to 3 months. Repeated infections or persistent middle ear effusion (fluid) does cause temporary conductive hearing loss, which may delay onset or advancement of speech (because the child cannot hear the full range of spoken sounds). Hearing will become normal once the effusion is gone. Otitis media may also contribute to temporary attention difficulty from conductive hearing loss accompanied by persistent middle ear fluid.

The surgical placement of small tubes through the TM to treat otitis media is the most common US surgery. This intervention reduces the overall number of cases of otitis media. Any otitis media can now be treated with topical antibiotic drops instead of oral antibiotics. Drops have the advantage of treating bacteria directly without side effects associated with oral antibiotics, such as diarrhea.

Adolescents

Recreational exposure to loud tones or noises may cause temporary or permanent hearing loss. With increased use of portable MP3 players and headphones designed to fit into the external ear canal, hearing loss in school-age and adolescent populations has escalated dramatically. For this reason, Apple (manufacturer of the iPod) has created software that limits the maximum volume possible. Unfortunately, this option exists for newer iPods only—it is not currently available for other MP3 players.

Older Adults

Cartilage formation continues over the lifespan, which may make ears seem more prominent in older adults. Though it may seem that extra cartilage would help to funnel sound to the external auditory meatus, it does not. In fact, it can lead to loss of rigidity and potential collapse of the external auditory canal. In addition, fine hairs lining the ear canal become coarser and stiffer, often protruding from the external auditory meatus. The coarse hair can interfere with sound waves as they move toward the TM, decreasing hearing. With decreased hair mobility, cerumen accumulates more readily in the ear canal. This is compounded by cerumen itself becoming drier. This combination of factors can lead to impaction and decreased hearing in older adults. Removing mechanical blockage can restore hearing and enhance socialization. It also helps to prevent injury by preserving the sense of hearing.

Otosclerosis is another common conductive hearing loss in this age group, resulting from the slow fusion of any combination of the ossicles in the middle ear. The fusion leads to obstruction of the transmission of sound waves from the TM to the oval window and inner ear (American Hearing Research Foundation, 2007).

> ## Clinical Significance 16-4
>
> While hearing aids can help many people with hearing loss, 80% of those who would benefit do not use them. Many factors limit use such as cost, ill-fitting devices, and failure to follow-up.

Over time some people experience a natural sensorineural loss called *presbycusis*. It happens regardless of exposure to excessive noise. Just as the hair in the external auditory canal becomes less flexible, so do the hair cells in the cochlea. Difficulty distinguishing sounds increases, especially in noisy environments. Presbycusis includes loss of higher-pitched sounds such as the spoken "s" or "th." Garbled or mumbled speech is a symptom. Amplification of sound, such as with simple hearing aids, does little to alleviate presbycusis. Some hearing aids are designed with noise cancellation to help manage this problem.

Adults older than 70 years face greater delays in the electrical responses in the brain; thus, it takes longer for the brain to interpret input. This is one factor that contributes to the increased auditory reaction time for those in the oldest age groups.

Cultural Considerations

Caucasian men older than 70 years have the highest incidence of hearing loss; the next highest prevalence is in Caucasian women (Pratt, et al., 2009), followed by African American men and women. Incidence of hearing loss declines with increases in socioeconomic status, regardless of ethnicity.

Incidence rates of otitis media are highest among Native Americans, Alaskan and Canadian Eskimos, and indigenous Australian children, compared to children of Caucasian descent (Klein, et al., 2009). Forty percent of these high-risk populations may have chronic perforation by 18 months of age. Socioeconomic status and environmental exposure are also indicators of risk for otitis media. Lower socioeconomic status corresponds to higher rates of otitis media (Klein, et al., 2009). Exposure to cigarette smoke, propping bottles for babies to feed, and bottle feeding in a supine position are all environmental factors that increase risk for otitis media.

Color and consistency of cerumen differs according to cultural background. Most commonly cerumen is yellow to dark brown, varying from liquid to firm paste (known as *wet cerumen*). Wet cerumen is most common in Caucasians and African Americans (Hosford-Dunn, et al., 2008). Grey to white cerumen is often flaky and misdiagnosed as eczema. This type of cerumen, called dry cerumen, is most prevalent in Asians and Native Americans (Pawson & Milan, 2005).

Acute Assessment

If inspection of the outer ear canal reveals a foreign object, it is best to refer the patient to an otolaryngologist for removal of the object. If the object appears to be a button battery, the patient must be referred to the emergency department for immediate object removal. Button batteries can quickly erode the ear canal and extensively damage the tissues and middle ear.

Foul-smelling drainage from the ear demands immediate attention. When possible wick the fluid from the external ear canal with either a wisp of cotton or cotton wick. Sending a culture of the fluid removed will identify the pathogen and help determine the proper antibiotic treatment. A patient with a chronically draining ear that is unresponsive to treatment requires referral to an otolaryngologist. The greatest concern with chronically draining ears is *cholesteatoma*, an abnormal accumulation of squamous epithelium within the middle ear. The growth can erode the auditory ossicles and cause great damage to the patient's hearing.

Patients with ear trauma also need evaluation for injury to nearby structures, including brain injury, basilar skull fracture, and neck injury. Hemotympanum, otorrhea, or TM rupture may indicate barotrauma from pressure changes or a basilar skull fracture. Sudden hearing loss also can be an acute situation; the cause must be found so that appropriate treatment can be initiated.

Subjective Data Collection

Subjective data is gathered by performing a complete and thorough health history, which begins with obtaining general information regarding the ear and its function. During the interview process it is important for the nurse to observe for any signs that the patient is having difficulty hearing. Some nonverbal cues of hearing loss include leaning forward, positioning the head or "good ear" to hear better, concentrating on lip or face movement instead of making eye contact, mumbling answers or giving answers not congruent with the question asked, asking the nurse to repeat questions frequently, responding with a loud voice, or using a monotone conversational voice. If any of these signs is present, the nurse needs to adjust the interview and environment to facilitate communication and gather accurate data.

Areas of Health Promotion/*Healthy People*

While gathering the patient's health history, the nurse needs to think critically about the data being gathered. The patient will reveal information about level of knowledge, health, and lifestyle. It is the nurse's role and responsibility to analyze these data for an overall sense of the patient's wellness and to give feedback about how the patient is meeting current evidence-based health guidelines. The nurse also needs to follow-up on any deficits with patient teaching (see Table 16-1).

Assessment of Risk Factors

Risk factors play an important part in determining a patient's health status and degree of wellness related to the ear and its functions. Risk factors that cannot be controlled include age, gender, heredity, and family history. Risk factors that can be influenced are lifestyle choices and environmental risks. For example, as people age, so do the ears—like the rest of the body, the ears change with time. Nevertheless, people can influence the extent to which hearing changes or loss occurs by taking precautions to guard ears from loud noises. It is the nurse's role and responsibility to assess for risk factors such as listening to loud music or working with construction equipment. Once these factors have been thoroughly assessed, patient education can take place during the conversational interview. The nurse can give educational materials on how to prevent hearing loss to the patient to reinforce content covered.

Table 16.1 *Healthy People* Goals Related to Ear Health	
Goals	**Patient Education Topics**
Increase the proportion of newborns who are screened for hearing loss by age 1 month, have audiologic evaluations by age 3 months, and are enrolled in appropriate intervention services by age 6 months.	Emphasize to parents that early detection of hearing deficits allows for early intervention and increased ability to communicate with the child.
Reduce otitis media in children and adolescents.	Teach parents who bottle-feed infants to do so with their babies in an upright position.
Reduce new cases of work-related, noise-induced hearing loss.	Emphasize the importance of using ear-protective devices and practices with exposure to industrial noise.
Reduce noise-induced hearing loss in children and adolescents aged 17 years and under and adults.	Teach proper use of volume control on personal entertainment equipment.
Increase access by persons who have hearing impairments to hearing rehabilitation services and adaptive devices including hearing aids, cochlear implants, or tactile or other assistive or augmentative devices.	Advocate and get involved politically to establish assistance for economically challenged people for access to assistive hearing devices.
Increase the proportion of persons who have had a hearing examination on schedule.	Recommend primary prevention and screening.

Source: *Healthy People 2010: What are its goals?* (n.d.). Retrieved May 21, 2010, from http://www.healthypeople.gov/About/goals.htm

Questions on History and Risk	Rationales

Family History

Tell me about your family's history of ear or hearing problems, if any.
- Who had the illness?
- What was the illness?
- When did the person have it?
- How was the illness treated?
- What were the outcomes?

Identifying a family history of possible inherited and chronic disorders (eg, *Meniere's disease, otosclerosis*) is important in determining the patient's risk and providing anticipatory guidance (American Hearing Research Foundation, 2008).

Personal History

How do you protect your skin from the sun?
- How often do you wear a hat?
- How often do you apply sunscreen?
- What SPF is the sunscreen you use?
- When are you usually in the sun?
- How long do you usually stay in the sun?

The ear is commonly forgotten when it comes to sun protection. For this reason, 20% of all melanomas are found in the head and neck region. Of melanomas in this area, 7%–15% affect the external ear, most commonly the helix (Mondin, et al., 2005).

What ear problems have you been diagnosed with—ear infections, hearing loss, tinnitus, vertigo?
- What was the illness?
- When did you have it?
- How was the illness treated?
- What were the outcomes?

In children, ear infections are extremely prevalent. As many as 75% of children have at least one episode by their third birthday; 50% of these have three or more episodes in their first 3 years (National Institute on Deafness, 2009). These children are at risk for TM rupture, scarring, and hearing loss.

What surgeries have you had?
- What was the surgery?
- When did you have it?
- What were the outcomes?
- What complications or lasting effects (sequela) did you encounter?

Surgeries may be performed for artificial eustachian tube placement, TM repair, and cochlear implants. Cochlear implants for the hearing impaired are performed frequently (Watson, et al., 2007). Ear surgery increases the likelihood of being exposed to ototoxic medications (eg, aminoglycoside antibiotics).

Medications

What prescription and over-the-counter medications are you currently taking?
- How often do you take them?
- What dosage?
- What route?

Several drugs have possible adverse effects (eg, hearing loss, tinnitus, vertigo) on the ears. Examples of ototoxic agents include all aminoglycosides, antiinflammatory agents (eg, Ibuprofen), antimalarials (eg, quinine), diuretics (eg, furosemide), nonnarcotic analgesics containing salicylates, antipyretics containing salicylates, erythromycin, quinidine sulfate, and antineoplastic drugs.

What immunizations have you received?
- What was the date of your last vaccinations?
- Have you received all required doses?

Mumps (a vaccine-preventable disease and part of the Measles, Mumps, Rubella [MMR] shot) can cause sensorineural deafness in those who have not been vaccinated, did not develop immunity with vaccination, or had decreased immunity over time. Maternal exposure to rubella (a vaccine-preventable disease and part of the MMR shot) causes deafness in almost 90% of affected fetuses (Banatvala & Brown, 2004).

Risk Factors

What type of loud noises have you been exposed to over your lifetime?
- When were you exposed to them?
- How long were you exposed to them?
- What protective ear equipment did you use?
- How did you monitor your exposure?

Hearing loss from loud noises is a major worldwide health issue (Hong & Samo, 2007). Approximately 29 million Americans suffer from hearing loss, with risks 5.5 times higher for males than females (Agrawal, et al., 2008). Workers at high risk for harmful noise exposure are farmers, fire fighters, police, emergency medical technicians, heavy machinery operators (eg, construction workers), military personnel, and members of the music industry.

(text continues on page 388)

Questions on History and Risk	Rationales
What exposure to cigarette, pipe, or cigar smoke have you had over your lifetime? • When were you exposed to it? • How long were you exposed to it?	Those exposed to smoke show an increased prevalence of early-onset hearing loss (Agrawal, et al., 2008).
What allergies have you had? • To what are you allergic? • When did you have this problem? • What were the symptoms? • How were these treated? • What were the outcomes?	Allergy symptoms such as runny nose and stuffy sinuses may lead to eustachian tube dysfunction in some patients.
How often do you travel by airplane? What related ear problems have you experienced, if any?	Air-pressure changes with altitude. Those who travel by plane commonly experience some middle-ear discomfort during the aircraft's descent. The eustachian tubes help equalize pressure on either side of the TM. Those whose eustachian tubes may malfunction include those with colds, sinus infections, other upper respiratory infections, and other ear conditions. If the eustachian tubes cannot equalize pressure, intense middle ear and sinus pain can occur. In severe cases the TM may rupture (Keystone, et al., 2004).
What experience with diving do you have? • How often do you dive? • What ear problems have you experienced, if any?	Air pressure changes with altitude; those who dive are risk for middle-ear trauma. Those at highest risk suffer from eustachian tube malfunction (as discussed under air travel).
How do you clean your ears?	Inserting cotton-tipped applicators into the external ear canal may lead to impaction of cerumen, which can contribute to hearing loss.

Risk Assessment and Health-Related Patient Teaching

The most significant topic for patient teaching based on thorough risk assessment of the ears is general hearing loss. Although ability to hear decreases somewhat with age, much hearing loss is preventable. Patients need to be asked about their exposure to noise and what protective equipment they use. Educating patients on the types, effectiveness, and instructions for use of protective ear equipment allows them to make decisions based on their needs. Education becomes even more important if a patient cannot make changes to the environment. For example, a construction worker who works daily surrounded by large, loud equipment may not be able to change the amount of machinery in close proximity to the work site.

Another important topic to address is skin cancer prevention. Many melanomas are found near or on the helix of the ear. Teaching patients how to protect themselves from unnecessary sun exposure increases the likelihood of preventative behaviors. See Chapter 13.

In addition, it is important to address how the patient cleans the ears. Many people associate cerumen in the ear canal with lack of hygiene and therefore clean their ears routinely. Often patients think cotton-tipped applicators are for this purpose. This self-care behavior is unsafe, placing patients at risk for cerumen impaction. Nurses should reinforce proper cleaning techniques.

Focused Health History Related to Common Symptoms

While taking the health history it is important for the nurse to ask about common symptoms of the ear. Questions about common symptoms will aid in identifying any concerns and possible problem areas related to the chief complaint or a chronic diagnosis.

Common Ear Symptoms

• Hearing loss
• Vertigo
• Tinnitus
• Otalgia

Questions to Assess Symptoms

Rationales/Abnormal Findings

Hearing Loss
Describe your hearing. What changes, if any, have you noticed?
- When did this start?
- Did it start suddenly or gradually?
- In what situations do you find it hardest to hear?
- What have you done for it?
- What were the outcomes?
- Do you have a family history of hearing loss?
- Have you been exposed to loud noises such as machinery or gunshots?

Determining onset of hearing loss may help uncover cause and if it can be reversed, such as with a cerumen or foreign-body obstruction. Sudden hearing loss indicates trauma or obstruction. Family history of hearing loss indicates *presbycusis*. Environmental damage to hearing may involve consistent or one-time exposure to loud noise.

Vertigo
Have you ever felt dizzy or had problems with balance?
- Under what circumstances has this happened?
- How long does this continue?
- Does it feel like you are, or the room is, spinning?
- How have you treated the problem?
- What were the outcomes?

Transient vertigo and persistent vertigo have different etiologies and thus necessitate different treatments. *Vertigo*, the sensation of the room spinning, indicates dysfunction of the bony labyrinth in the inner ear.

Tinnitus
Do you ever have a sensation of a buzzing or ringing that no one else can hear?
- Is there any time that this seems louder?
- Are you currently taking any medications, vitamins, or herbal supplements?

Tinnitus is thought to be an inability to filter internal noise from the external input of sound. Ototoxic agents can cause tinnitus. Stopping their use may resolve tinnitus, although some ototoxic agents cause lasting damage.

Otalgia
Do you experience pain in either ear?
- Is it in both ears or just in one ear?
- Have you ever had this pain before?
- If so what was the cause?
- Do you feel the pain deep inside or more on the outside of the ear?
- Does it hurt to touch your ear?
- Describe the pain—is it persistent or intermittent?
- What makes the pain better or worse?
- Have you had any drainage from your ears?
- What color was the drainage?
- Did it have an odor?
- Have you had any surgeries or illnesses recently?
- How do you clean your ears?

Otalgia usually indicates ear dysfunction, most commonly *otitis media* or *otitis externa*. Pain in the ear can be referred from the pharynx. It is not uncommon for a patient recovering from tonsil surgery to complain of ear pain. Severe pain followed by relief and drainage indicates a *ruptured TM*. External ear sensitivity indicates *otitis externa*, which may result from self-induced trauma, such as inserting bobby pins, keys, or fingernails into the external ear canal.

Documentation of Normal Findings

Patient alert and following conversation with no evidence of hearing loss. Denies hearing difficulty, vertigo, tinnitus, and otalgia.
C. Borundi, RN

▲ Lifespan Considerations

Additional Questions

Rationales/Abnormal Findings

Newborns, Infants, and Children
Otitis Media
- When was the last case of otitis media?
- How was it treated?
- How many cases of otitis media has your child had?
- Did your child have otitis media over the summer months?
- Has your child ever had surgery for otitis media?
- Is your child exposed to cigarette smoke?
- Does your child attend daycare?

Repeat or persistent infections may require surgery if conductive hearing loss causes great discomfort or speech delays. Incidence of otitis media is highest in winter months (Klein, et al., 2009). Exposures to passive smoke or cigarette residue on clothes are risk factors for otitis media. Daycare attendance is also a risk factor and increases the risk of antibiotic-resistant otitis media.

(text continues on page 390)

Hearing

- Did your child pass his or her newborn hearing screen?
- Do you have concerns regarding your child's hearing?
- Do you have concerns about your child's speech development?
- Was your child born full term?
- How long did your child stay in the hospital following birth?

Routine newborn hearing screening enhances early intervention for hearing loss. Speech development is delayed in children with a hearing deficit. Premature infants are at increased risk for hearing deficits. Incidence of hearing deficits increases greatly with prolonged hospital stays and exposure to ototoxic drugs.

Therapeutic Dialogue: Collecting Subjective Data

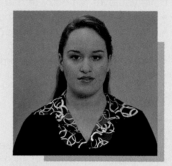

Remember Mrs. Petino, introduced at the beginning of the chapter. She was admitted to the clinic today with concerns of ear pain. The nurse uses professional communication techniques to gather subjective data. The following conversations give two examples of interview styles used by different nurses. One is more effective than the other.

Less Effective

Nurse: Hi, Mrs. Petino. I'm Lee and I'm going to be your nurse today. How are you feeling?

Mrs. Petino: Fine.

Nurse: How are your ears doing?

Mrs. Petino: Fine.

Nurse: Your chart says that you have an infection in your ears. Is that right?

Mrs. Petino: Yes. It's fine.

Nurse: But you have an infection in your ears, so you need to get it treated, right?

Mrs. Petino: Yes.

Nurse: Your chart also says you can't hear very well.

Mrs. Petino: I could if people just talked louder.

Nurse: I bet that would help you a lot. Just tell them that they have to speak louder. They need to realize that you have a hearing problem.

Mrs. Petino: But you know I can hear really well.

Nurse: So why did you come to the clinic then?

More Effective

Nurse: Hello, Mrs. Petino. I'm going to be your nurse today. My name is Lee. (smiles, pauses) How are you feeling?

Mrs. Petino: Fine.

Nurse: Your chart says that you came in because of your ears. Is that right?

Mrs. Petino: Yes, I have had problems with pain. But the pain gets better with medicine and a warm cloth.

Nurse: Are you having other problems with your ears?

Mrs. Petino: Yes, I have a buzzing noise in my ears. My husband says I can't hear well. My kids say I am yelling when I'm just talking. I can't understand them anymore.

Nurse: It sounds like your family is worried about you. (pauses)

Mrs. Petino: My mom had problems hearing when she was my age, and it was hard for the family.

Nurse: This must bring back some of those memories for you. Let's talk about how your hearing has changed (smiles).

Critical Thinking Challenge

- How might the more effective nurse's nonverbal communication promote a therapeutic relationship?
- How might the patient's experience and culture influence her perceptions, values, and beliefs about her diagnosis and healing?
- What is the role of the nurse in giving advice versus listening to the patient's perspective?

Objective Data Collection

Equipment Needed (for Advanced Practice Assessment)

- Otoscope
- High-pitched tuning fork

Preparation

To obtain objective data about the ears, it is best to make sure the patient is comfortable and the room is quiet. It is ideal for the patient's ears to be at the nurse's eye level to be able to inspect them without discomfort to the patient. For adults and older children the examination can be performed with the patient sitting on the examination table.

Begin the examination by first washing your hands in warm water. Hand sanitizer is effective for bacteria control but leaves the hands cold and may cause discomfort for the patient.

When meeting with patients you will be able to move forward with the examination and intervention when you address the problem that is most important to them first. Often this may not be the issue of greatest clinical significance. Once you address this you will find your patient is more receptive to issues of greater significance such as hearing loss or cholesteatoma. Patient education is the primary tool to engage your patient in greater heath care and address issues that unaddressed may cause the patient harm or impair quality of life.

Common and Specialty or Advanced Techniques

Routine head-to-toe assessment includes the most important and common assessment techniques. The nurse may add specialty or advanced steps if concerns exist over a specific finding. Table 16-2 summarizes the most common techniques used in the comprehensive ear assessment, which are therefore essential to learn for use in clinical practice. Additional techniques may be added if indicated by the clinical situation or used in advanced practice for diagnosis.

Table 16.2 Common Versus Specialty or Advanced Techniques Related to Ear Assessment

Comprehensive Assessment Technique	Purpose	Screening or Registered Nurse Assessment	Focused or Advanced Practice Examination
Observe behavioral responses to speech	To identify cues that might indicate hearing loss	X	
Inspect the external ear position	To evaluate for congenital problems	X	
Inspect the size, shape, and condition of skin on external ear	To evaluate for skin breakdown or lesions, edema, erythema, discharge	X	
Palpate external ear	To note lumps, masses, tenderness	X	
Perform whisper test	To evaluate for high-pitched hearing loss		X
Perform Weber's test	To evaluate air and BC		X
Perform Rinne's test	To evaluate unilateral hearing loss		X
Inspect external canal with otoscope	To evaluate cerumen, discharge, foreign bodies, erythema, lesions		X
Inspect TM	To note color, characteristics, position, integrity		X

Inspection

Inspect the ears (Fig. 16-7). *Ears are symmetrical, equal size, and fully formed*

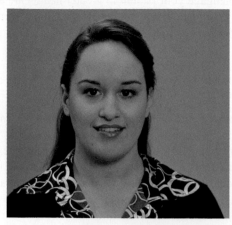

Figure 16.7 Normal surface anatomy of the ears.

Inspect the face. *Facial tone is uniform with the ears. Skin is intact. Small painless nodules on the helix are a variation of normal anatomy known as Darwin's tubercle* (Fig. 16-8).

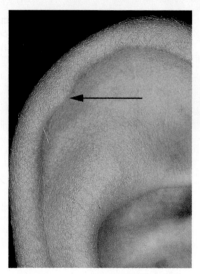

Figure 16.8 Darwin's tubercle, a normal anatomical variation.

Palpation

Palpate the auricle. *Ears are firm without lumps, lymph tissue is not palpable, ears are nontender, and no pain is elicited with palpation or manipulation of the auricle. No pain occurs with palpation of the mastoid process.*

Whisper Test

The **whisper test** evaluates for loss of high-frequency sounds. Instruct the patient to plug (or plug for the patient) the ear opposite to the one you are testing. With your head approximately 18 in from the patient's ear and your mouth not visible to the patient, whisper a simple sentence

Microtia, macrotia, edematous ears, cartilage *Pseudomonas* infection, carcinoma on auricle, cyst, and frostbite are abnormal findings. See Table 16-4 at the end of this chapter.

Enlarged lymph nodes indicate pathology or inflammation.

Pain with auricle movement or tragus palpation indicates otitis externa or furuncle.

Not being able to repeat the sentence clearly or missing components may indicate hearing loss of higher frequencies and requires follow-up with formal testing.

of words and numbers (Fig. 16-9). Have the patient repeat what you have said. Repeat on the opposite side. *Patient repeats the entire sentence to you without errors.*

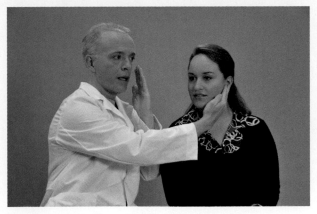

Figure 16.9 The whisper test.

Rinne's Test

A tuning fork is a U-shaped piece of metal with a handle attached at the apex of the U. When struck lightly against an object, it will vibrate at a specific frequency. Use of a tuning fork helps the nurse determine if hearing is equal in both ears and if there is either a conductive or sensorineural hearing loss by allowing the nurse to compare the difference in BC versus AC. Remember AC has less resistance than BC.

The Rinne's test examines the differentiation between BC and AC.

BC that is longer or the same as AC is evidence of conductive hearing loss. Conductive hearing loss on one side may indicate external or middle ear disease. Patients with conductive hearing loss should have an assessment of the auricle and external auditory canal to look for blockage. The TM should be assessed to ensure that there is no middle ear abnormality, such as fluid or a TM perforation.

1. To begin, grasp and tap the handle of the tuning fork against the back or heel of your hand (Fig. 16-10).

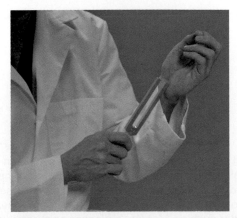

Figure 16.10 Striking the tuning fork against the back of the hand.

(text continues on page 394)

2. Place the base of the handle on the patient's mastoid process (Fig. 16-11). Note the time on the second hand of your watch.

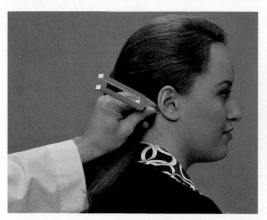

Figure 16.11 Rinne's test: placing the tuning fork on the mastoid process.

3. Instruct the patient to tell you when he or she no longer hears the sound of the fork. Note the number of seconds.

4. Once the patient no longer hears the sound through the mastoid process, move the tip of the tuning fork to the front of the external auditory meatus (Fig. 16-12). Again note the time on the second hand of your watch.

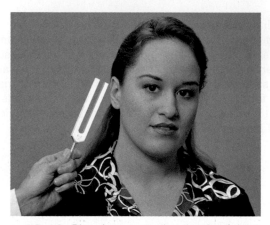

Figure 16.12 Rinne's test: moving the tip of the tuning fork to the front of the external auditory meatus.

5. Instruct the patient to inform you when he or she no longer hears the sound.
AC is twice as long as BC.

Weber's Test

The Weber's test helps to differentiate the cause of unilateral hearing loss. After activating the fork, place its handle on the midline of the parietal bone in line with both ears (Fig. 16-13). *The patient hears the sound in both ears and at equal intensity.*

Unilateral identification of the sound indicates sensorineural loss in the ear that the patient did not hear or had reduced perception of the sound. Sensorineural hearing loss on one side may be related to an inner ear disorder such as *Meniere's disease* or a *vestibular schwannoma* (*acoustic neuroma*).

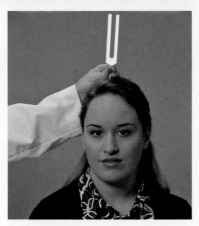

Figure 16.13 Weber's test: placing the tuning fork on the midline of the parietal bone.

Otoscopic Evaluation

The RN rarely uses an otoscope to inspect the ear. An APRN completes the otoscopic examination. Inspect the external meatus and canal. Several sizes of speculum can be used for the otoscope. Choose one that fits into the external canal without discomfort.
The canal has fine hairs; some cerumen lining the wall skin is intact, with no discharge.

Redness, swelling of the external auditory canal, and discharge are signs of external otitis. Either a foreign body or cerumen can obstruct the canal.

Hold the otoscope so that your thumb is by the window and you are bracing the shaft with your fingers along the patient's cheek. This allows you to stabilize the otoscope and decreases risk of scraping the external auditory canal with the speculum. Hold the patient's ear at the helix and lift up and back to align the canal for best visualization of the TM (Fig. 16-14). After visualization of the canal you will rotate the otoscope slightly to be able to visualize the entire TM. Visualize portions of the malleus, umbo, manubrium, and short process through the translucent membrane (Fig. 16-15).

Swelling or budging of the TM indicates acute otitis media (see Table 16-5). A diffuse cone of light indicates *otitis media with effusion*. Air bubbles caused by a functioning eustachian tube allow drainage of effusion and aeration of the middle ear. A perforated TM may allow for direct visualization into the middle ear.

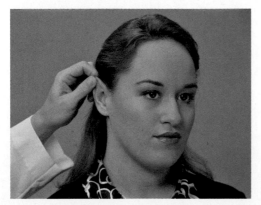

Figure 16.14 Otoscopic examination: holding the patient's ear at the helix and lifting up and back to align the canal for best visualization of the TM.

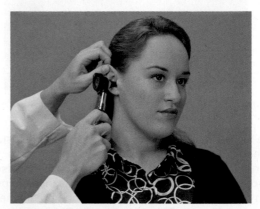

Figure 16.15 Correct placement of the otoscope.

(text continues on page 396)

A well-aerated middle ear allows visualization of part of the incus as well (Fig. 16-16). *TM is intact and translucent and allows visualization of the short process of the malleus. The cone of light is visible in the anterior inferior quadrant.*

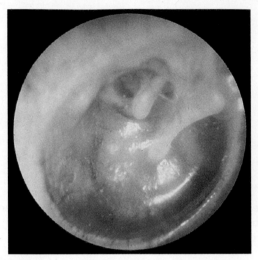

Figure 16.16 Normal TM.

A variation of normal is a TM with white areas (sclerosis). These white areas are visible scars from repeated ear infections. This scarring may make the TM less flexible (Fig. 16-17).

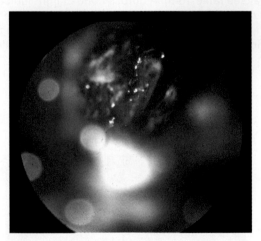

Figure 16.17 TM with tympanosclerosis.

Once the TM is visualized you may use the bulb insufflator attached to the head of the otoscope (Fig. 16-18) to observe TM movement. First perform positive pressure that forces air into the external auditory canal and pushes down the TM. Then release pressure and note the negative pressure pulling the TM outwards. *The TM moves inward when inflated and outward with release.*

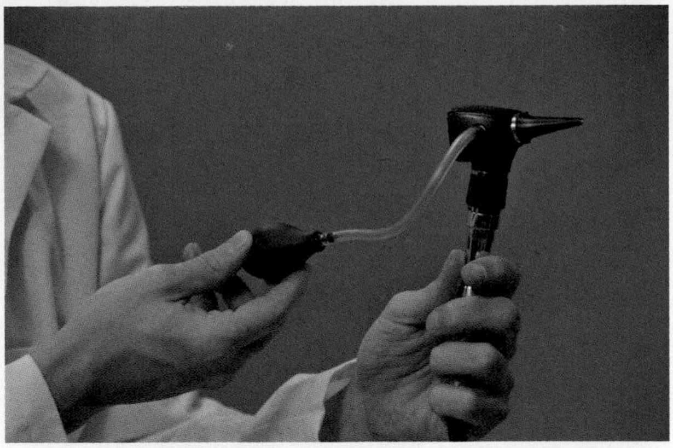

Technique and Normal Findings (continued)	Abnormal Findings (continued)
Figure 16.18 Otoscope with bulb insufflator attached.	
Auditory Acuity The most accurate way to evaluate hearing is by an audiologist performing an **audiogram** in a soundproof room. An audiogram gives exact information about absent or diminished frequencies for the patient. It also distinguishes sensorineural from conductive loss. Including tympanometry with the audiogram will show the compliance of the TM and if there is a pinhole rupture by providing the volume of the external ear canal. The primary provider in an advanced practice role orders this test. Though an audiogram is the most accurate test, most clinics are not supplied with it.	
Equilibrium Equilibrium can be assessed by using the Romberg's test as described in Chapter 24.	Failure of the Romberg's test may indicate dysfunction in the vestibular portion of the inner ear, semicircular canals, and vestibule.

Documentation of Objective Findings

Right pinna normal, canal well aerated, TM translucent with visible bony prominence of the malleus and sharp cone of light. Left pinna normal, canal well aerated, TM translucent with visible bony prominence of the malleus and sharp cone of light. Hearing intact bilateral with whisper test. Rinne's test normal. Weber's test normal. *C. Borundi, RN*

Lifespan Considerations

Infants and Children

Assessing ears for children can be challenging and fun. When working with them, addressing parents' concerns helps you gain their trust and will encourage them to assist with examination. Ensure that you approach children in a playful manner and involve them in conversation as developmentally appropriate. They will often be more compliant with examination once they are involved in the process (eg, holding the otoscope, helping explain their history).

While you are introducing and acclimatizing a child to the equipment, note the placement of the external ear on the skull. The superior portion of the pinna should be congruent with the outer canthus of the eye. There should be no more than a 10-degree deviation from the medial fold of the lobe to attachment of the superior portion of the helix. More than 10-degree deviation from requires further investigation—it can signify a genetic defect in the renal system. It can also indicate neurodevelopmental challenges.

Older children can sit for the examination on the examination table. Children tend to be active, and you need to be creative with gaining cooperation for the otoscopic examination. Have them touch the light to see that it does not hurt or help you place the speculum on the head of the otoscope. Ask playful questions, such as "What do you think I will find in here?" Some children are distracted by coming up with answers. Younger children and infants may need to be held safely to reduce the risk of injury to the external auditory

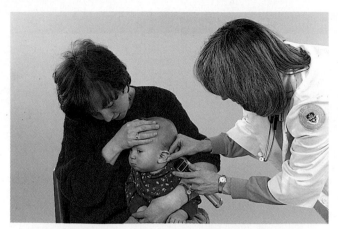

Figure 16.19 Adult holding infant for ear examination.

canal during the otoscopic examination. Parents may use one arm to hold infants firmly against the chest while using the other arm to stabilize the baby's head (Fig. 16-19). For the right ear have the parent hold the child on the left side and position the head so the infant faces away from the parent. Reverse for the left side.

Toddlers are best examined by sitting on the parent's lap facing forward while the parent "hugs" them with one arm and holds the head steady with the opposite arm. Preschoolers often need to be held down on an examination table. It is best to have the older children to be supine with the head turned toward the parent (Fig. 16-20). Once you examine the exposed ear, trade sides of the table with the parent and examine the opposite ear.

To insert the otoscope tip into a child's ear canal, the pinna must be manipulated differently than with an adult. Gently grasp the child's lobe and pull downward. A child's ear canal is narrower and positioned in a more posterior angle than an adults' (see Fig. 16-6).

If a child has had tympanostomy tubes placed because of recurrent or persistent otitis media, the tube should be in the inferior portion of the TM with the lumen of the tube patent.

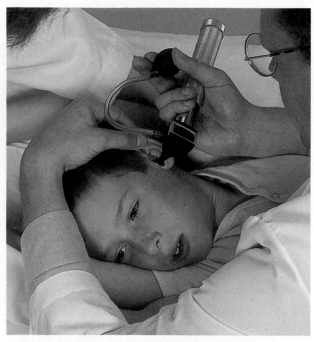

Figure 16.20 Older child on the examination table to facilitate ear examination.

Screening for hearing acuity in infants and young children includes evaluation of developmental milestones, such as the Moro reflex in neonates. If there is a developmental lag or concern by caregivers, a pediatric audiologist should perform a formal pediatric evaluation. Abnormal findings include lack of Moro reflex, inability to localize sound, or lack of understandable language by 24 months.

Older Adults

The cartilage and skin around the external ear may be less pliable in older adults. The stiff hairs in the canal may require a smaller otoscope tip to separate them and increase visualization of the TM. The membrane itself may seem more opaque and less mobile.

Documenting Abnormal Findings

The nurse has just finished a beginning ear examination of Mrs. Petino, who has abnormal findings. Review the following important findings revealed in each of the steps of objective data collection for Mrs. Petino. Consider how these results compare with the normal findings presented in the samples of normal documentation. Note that inspection is the major technique used in ear assessment.

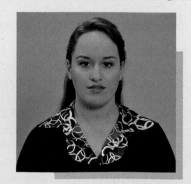

Inspection: Right ear is pink, skin is intact, external auditory canal appears clear. Left ear is pink, skin is intact, purulent drainage is noted in the external auditory canal.

Palpation: Right ear warm, no pain with palpation. Left ear is warm, painful with manipulation of the external ear and pain with pressure on the tragus.

L. Sang, RN

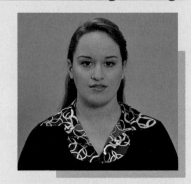

The APRN has seen the patient and performed further assessments including the otoscopic examination. The patient is diagnosed with an ear infection. The following nursing note illustrates how subjective and objective data are collected and analyzed and nursing interventions are developed.

Subjective: States 5/10 pain that is constant. Increased to 8/10 when she touches her left ear.

Objective: Withdrawing from touch applied to left ear during assessment. Purulent drainage noted at the meatus of the external ear canal.

Analysis: Pain related to otitis externa of left ear.

Plan: Apply heat or cold for comfort. Encourage administration of ordered oral pain medication and adherence to antibiotic schedule to promote healing. Assess if Mrs. Petino has sufficient resources to obtain necessary medications. Work with the patient's family and encourage them to speak more clearly and make eye contact.

L. Sang, RN

Critical Thinking Challenge

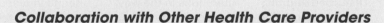

- How is the role of the RN different from that of the APRN?
- What type of ongoing assessment would you predict?
- How would you address the issue of pain assessment and management?
- What teaching should be performed related to Mrs. Petino's otitis externa, loss of hearing, and treatment plan?

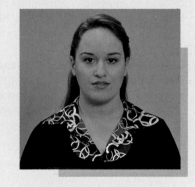

An audiology consult is indicated for evaluation of hearing loss. Audiologists are available in many specialty clinics to ensure proper evaluation. The APRN has recommended an audiology consult; the RN will make the referral. The following conversation illustrates how the RN might organize data and make recommendations about Mrs. Petino to the audiologist.

Situation: Hello. I'm taking care of Mrs. Petino in the clinic today. She's a 25-year-old woman with ear pain, tinnitus, and possible hearing loss.

Background: Her mother had hearing loss at a young age. Mrs. Petino also works in a tuna factory with many loud noises and uses ear protection. Her hearing was stable until 6 months ago when she noticed a buzzing sound in her ears. Around that time she also required the television to be turned up to hear it clearly.

Assessment: Her right ear is clear. She is having some drainage from her left ear and the APRN diagnosed otitis externa. He would like her to have an audiogram to evaluate her hearing loss.

Recommendations: When you perform your audiogram would you please perform a tympanogram as well to check for a ruptured TM? What times do you have available for her? Thanks so much.

Critical Thinking Challenge

- What assessments might be performed on other body systems related to the patient's findings?
- What health promotion and teaching needs would be related to the patient's history and risk factors?
- What further assessment information might the nurse want to collect in preparation for the end of the appointment?

Clinical Significance 16-5

For patients who wear hearing aids, accumulated cerumen and otitis externa can be ongoing challenges. It is important for this population to have frequent examination of their ear canals to ensure patency and health, and to receive maximum benefits from their hearing aids.

Evidence-based Critical Thinking

Common Laboratory and Diagnostic Testing

Most common hearing tests in primary-care offices and schools are done with a device called an *audiometer*. This simple screening device consists of headphones and a box that delivers tones to each ear at variable frequencies and volumes. The purpose is to identify those patients who require further testing and examination by an audiologist. Audiologists perform various hearing tests, such as an audiogram, which is conducted in a sound-proof booth. This test differentiates conductive from sensorineural hearing loss. Audiologists also use tympanograms and tests to reveal oto-acoustic emissions, which provide information about the function of the outer hair cells of the cochlea. The oto-acoustic emissions test helps determine suspected hearing loss from ototoxic drugs. If a patient complains of otalgia and drainage is present in the ear canal, this fluid may be cultured to determine the best topical treatment for either otitis externa or otitis media with TM perforation.

Diagnostic Reasoning

Nursing Diagnosis, Outcomes, and Interventions

When formulating a nursing diagnosis, it is important to use critical thinking to cluster data and identify patterns that fit together. The nurse compares these clusters of data with the defining characteristics (abnormal findings) for the diagnosis to ensure the most accurate labeling and appropriate interventions. Table 16-3 compares nursing diagnoses, abnormal findings, and interventions commonly related to the ear assessment (NANDA-I, 2009).

Table 16.3 Common Nursing Diagnoses Associated with the Ear

Diagnosis and Related Factors	Point of Differentiation	Assessment Characteristics	Nursing Interventions
Disturbed auditory sensory perception related to hearing loss	Alterations in the way the person interprets, uses, or organizes sensory (especially hearing-related) stimuli	Change in responses to environment, impaired communication, difficulty with concentration	Minimize background noise. Sit directly in front of patient. Allow patient to see your face. Do not overenunciate or shout at patient.
Pain related to inflammation of ear canal	Unpleasant sensory and emotional experience from skin or tissue damage	Self report of pain is subjective. Expressions are variable and include facial grimace, guarding, muscle tension, tachycardia, tachypnea, and nausea.	Use pain scale to identify current pain intensity and effectiveness of medication. Develop pain goal collaboratively with patient. Provide pain medications as ordered.* Provide alternatives such as distraction, breathing, and relaxation.
Risk for infection	At risk for pathogenic organisms due to break in the skin or tissue, the body's primary defense	Break in skin integrity, tubes and procedures, exposure to pathogens, malnutrition, inadequate immunity, chronic disease	Follow frequent handwashing, universal precautions. Protect wound with dressing. Monitor for fever, WBC, wound drainage, or erythema. Discontinue tubes as soon as possible. Encourage adequate nutrition.

*Collaborative interventions.

The nurse uses assessment data to formulate a nursing care plan with patient outcomes and interventions. This is often in the form of a care plan or case note similar to the one below.

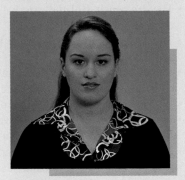

Nursing Diagnosis	Patient Outcomes	Nursing Interventions	Rationales	Evaluation
Pain related to ear infection as evidenced by stating pain 5/10 scale	Patient rates ear pain at zero.	Provide warm or cool pack for comfort. Provide analgesics as prescribed.	Pain is subjective and treatment is aimed at controlling the symptoms until the cause can be resolved.	Patient states that ear pain is now 2/10 scale. Continue to provide analgesic every 4 hours.*

*Collaborative interventions.

Nurses use assessment information to identify patient outcomes. Some outcomes related to ear problems include the following:

• Patient is free from ear pain.
• Patient demonstrates understanding with a verbal response.
• Patient explains plan to accommodate hearing impairment (Moorhead, et al., 2007).

Once the outcomes area is established, nursing care is implemented to improve the status of the patient. The nurse uses critical thinking and evidence-based practice to develop the interventions. Some examples of nursing interventions for the ear and hearing are as follows:

• Turn-off television and radio when communicating.
• Close the door if hallway noise is loud.
• Provide a communication board and visual aids for detailed discussions (Bulechek, et al., 2007).

The nurse then evaluates the care according to the patient outcomes that were developed, therefore reassessing the patient and continuing or modifying the interventions as appropriate.

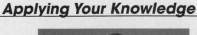
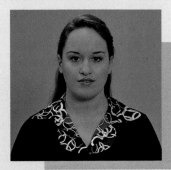

Using the previous steps of diagnostic reasoning, organizing, and prioritizing, consider all the case study findings woven throughout this chapter. When answering the following questions, begin drawing conclusions and see how the pieces of assessment must work together to create an environment for personalized, appropriate, and accurate care.

• How will the nurse assess and document the patient's pain?
• How will the nurse assess and document her hearing loss?
• What information will need to be collected to assess the patient's risk for hearing loss?
• When will the nurse make a referral to the audiologist?
• What type of follow-up will the patient need?

Key Points

- The ear consists of the external ear, middle ear, and inner ear.
- The TM is the barrier between the external auditory canal and the middle ear.
- The middle ear contains the malleus, incus, and stapes that conduct sound waves to the inner ear.
- The inner ear translates sound to the nerves and brainstem.
- The semicircular canals and vestibule provide the body with proprioception and equilibrium.
- The functions of the ear are hearing and equilibrium.
- Clues of hearing loss include leaning forward to hear, positioning the head with the "good ear" forward, concentrating on lip movement, asking to repeat questions, and using a loud or monotone voice.
- Risk factors for hearing loss include family history, frequent ear infections, use of some medications, lack of immunizations, exposure to loud noises, exposure to smoke, allergies, airplane travel, diving, inappropriate cleaning of ears, and increased age.
- Common disorders of the ear include hearing loss, vertigo, tinnitus, and otalgia.
- Otitis media is more common in children.
- Routine screening of newborn hearing leads to early intervention for hearing loss.
- The RN assessment includes inspection and palpation of the external ear.
- The APRN inspects the auditory meatus, canal, and TM with the otoscope.
- The most accurate evaluation of hearing is with an audiogram.
- The whisper test evaluates loss of high-frequency sounds.
- During the Rinne's test, AC should be twice as long as BC. If BC is equal to or greater than AC, this is evidence of conductive hearing loss.
- The Weber's test differentiates unilateral hearing loss.
- A child's ear canal is narrower and more posterior than an adult's.

Review Questions

1. The function of the ear is for
  A. hearing and equilibrium
  B. equilibrium and perforations
  C. perforations and balance
  D. balance and equilibrium

2. The inner ear
  A. contains the malleus, incus, and stapes
  B. conducts sound waves to the external ear
  C. translates sound to the nerves and brainstem
  D. provides the body with proprioception

3. Cues of hearing loss include which of the following? Choose all that are correct.
  A. Using a loud or monotonous voice
  B. Asking to repeat questions
  C. Concentrating on lip movement
  D. Leaning forward to hear

4. Risk factors for hearing loss include which of the following? Choose all that are correct.
  A. Frequent ear infections
  B. Being current on immunizations
  C. Exposure to smoke
  D. Decreased age

5. Tinnitus is described as
  A. inability to hear well
  B. dizziness
  C. ringing in the ear
  D. ear pain

6. Which of the following patients is most likely to have hearing loss?
  A. Caucasian man older than 70 years
  B. Hispanic woman older than 50 years
  C. Asian man younger than 30 years
  D. African girl younger than 10 years

7. Which of the following differentiates the RN assessment from the APRN assessment?
  A. History and risk factors
  B. Symptom analysis
  C. Inspection and palpation
  D. Otoscopic assessment

8. A nursing diagnosis appropriate for a patient with ear problems includes
  A. kinesthetic disturbed perception
  B. disturbed sensory perception
  C. sensory perception, gustatory
  D. olfactory sensory perception

9. An outcome that is appropriate for a patient with hearing impairment is
  A. Provide a communication board or picture to assist teaching.
  B. Minimize background noise and close door.
  C. Stand in front of patient and explain procedure.
  D. Patient explains plan to accommodate hearing impairment.

10. Which of the following are appropriate interventions for the patient who is at risk for ear infection? Select all that apply.
  A. Be current on immunizations.
  B. Avoid second hand smoke.
  C. Clean only external ear.
  D. Have audiogram yearly.

References

Agrawal, Y., Platz, E. A., & Niparko, J. K. (2008). Prevalence of hearing loss and differences by demographic characteristics among US adults. *Archives of Internal Medicine, 168*(14), 1522–1530.

American Hearing Research Foundation. (2007). *Otosclerosis*. Retrieved December 18, 2008, from http://www.american-hearing.org/disorders/hearing/otosclerosis2.html

American Hearing Research Foundation. (2008). *Meniere's disease*. Retrieved December 18, 2008, from http://www.american-hearing.org/disorders/menieres/menieres.html

Banatvala, J. E., & Brown, D. W. G. (2004). *The Lancet, 363*(9415), 1127–1137.

Berry, J. A., Gold, S., Frederick, E. A., et al. (2002) Patient-based outcomes in patients with primary tinnitus undergoing tinnitus retraining therapy. *Archives of Otolaryngology Head and Neck Surgery, 128*(10), 1153–1157.

Bulechek, G. B. & Butcher, H. K., McCloskey Dochterman, J. (2007). *Nursing Interventions Classification (NIC)* (4th ed.) St. Louis, MO: Mosby.

Cummings, C., Fredrickson, J., Harker, L., et al. (1998). *Otolaryngology in head and neck surgery*. St. Louis, MO: Mosby.

Davis, P. B., Paki, B., & Hanley, P. J. (2007). On tinnitus neuromonics tinnitus treatment: Third clinical trial. *Ear Hear, 2*, 242–259.

Healthy People 2010: What are its goals? (n.d.). Retrieved August 3, 2009, from http://www.healthypeople.gov/About/goals.htm

Hong, H. K. B., & Samo, J. (2007). Hazardous decibels: Hearing health of firefighters. *American Association of Occupational Health Nurses, 55*(8), 313–319.

Hosford-Dunn, H., Roeser, R. J., Valete, M. (2008). *Cerumen management in Audiology: Practice Management* (2nd ed.). New York: Thieme Medical Publishers Inc.

Isaacson, G. (2009). *Congenital anomalies of the ear*. Retrieved July 27, 2009, from UpToDate database.

Keystone, J. S., Kozarsky, P. E., Freedman, D. O., et al. (2004). *Travel medicine*. Expert Consult Elsevier.

Klein, J. O., Pelton, S., Kaplan, S. L., et al. (2009). *Acute otitis media in children: Epidemiology, pathogenesis, clinical manifestations, and complications*. Retrieved August 1, 2009, from http://www.uptodateonline.com.proxy.seattleu.edu/online/content/topic.do?topicKey=pedi_id/2870&selectedTitle=2~150&source=search_result

Mondin, A., Rinaldo, A., Shaha, A. R., et al. (2005). Malignant melanoma of the auricle. *Acta Otolaryngology, 125*(11), 1140–1144.

Moorhead, S., Johnson, M., & Mass, M. (2007). *Nursing Outcomes Classification (NOC)* (4th ed.). Philadelphia: Mosby.

National Institution on Deafness and Other Communication Disorders (2009). *Otitis media (ear infection)*. Retrieved January 2, 2009, from http://www.nidcd.nih.gov/health/hearing/otitism.asp

North American Nursing Diagnosis Association. (2009). *Nursing diagnoses, 2009–2011 Edition: Definitions and classifications (NANDA NURSING DIAGNOSIS)*. West Sussex UK: John Wiley & Sons.

Pawson, S., & Milan, F. A. (2005). Cerumen types in two Eskimo communities. *American Journal of Physical Anthropology, 41*(3), 431–432.

Pratt, S. R., Kuller, L., Talbott, E. O., et al. (2009). Prevalence of hearing loss in black and white elders: Results of the cardiovascular health study. *Journal of Speech Language and Hearing Research, 52*(4), 973–989.

Rubin, R. & Strayer, D. S. (2008). *Rubin's pathology: Clinicpathologic foundations of medicine*. Philadelphia: Lippincott Williams & Wilkins.

Suter, A. H., & von Gierke, H. E. (1987) Noise and public policy. *Ear Hear, 8*(4), 188–191.

Watson, L. M., Hardie, T., Archbold, S. M., et al. (2007). Oxford journals parents' views on changing communication after cochlear implantation. Retrieved December 10, 2009, from http://jdsde.oxfordjournals.org/cgi/content/full/enm036v1

The Jensen suite offers these additional resources to enhance learning and facilitate understanding of this chapter:

- thePoint on line resource, http//thepoint.lww.com/Jensen1E
- Student CD-ROM included with the book
- *Laboratory Manual for Nursing Health Assessment: A Best Practice Approach*
- *Pocket Guide for Nursing Health Assessment: A Best Practice Approach*

Table 16.4   Abnormalities of the External Ear

Microtia

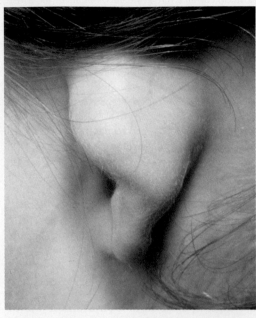

Small or deformed auricle that may be associated with a blind or absent auditory canal

Macrotia

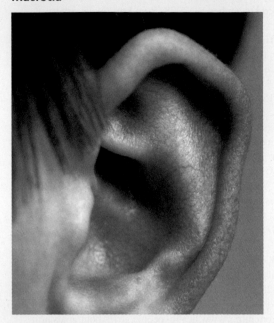

Excessive enlargement of the auricle; usually congenital

Edematous Ears

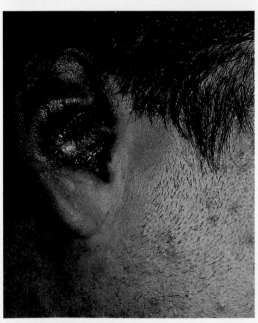

An external ear canal that is swollen with inflammation or infection

Cartilage *Staphylococcus or Pseudomonas* Infection

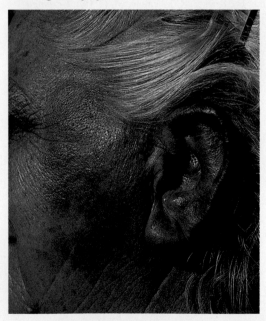

Painful, reddened ear usually surrounding incisions, ear piercing, or an area of traumatic injury

Table 16.4   Abalities of the External Ear (continued)

Carcinoma on Auricle

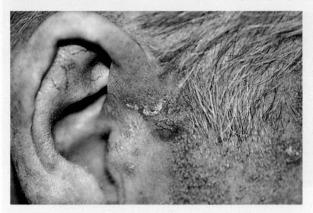

Common site of carcinoma related to sun exposure; either basal cell or squamous cell tumors may be present

Cyst

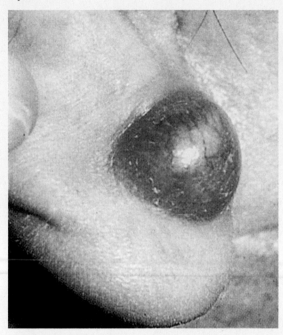

A sac or pouch with a membranous lining filled with fluid or solid material

Tophi

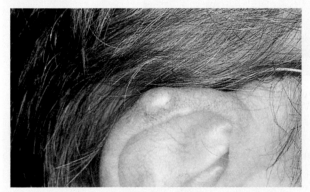

Uric acid crystals associated with gout; may appear as hard nodules on the ear surface

External Otitis

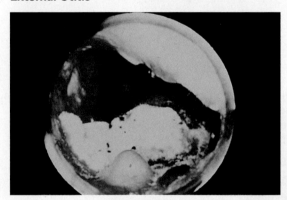

Inflammatory and infectious discharge in the external canal; associated with pain, itching, fullness, and reduced hearing

Table 16.5 **Abnormal Findings in the Internal Ear**

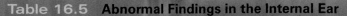

TM Rupture

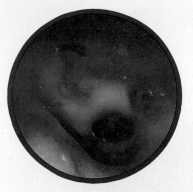

A nonintact TM; associated symptoms include clear, purulent, or bloody discharge; hearing loss in the affected ear; buzzing in the ear; and ear pain

Otitis Media with Effusion

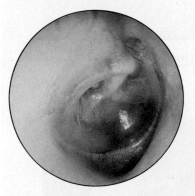

Purulent discharge associated with a bacterial infection. Redness and bulging on the eardrum. Onset can be sudden or gradual with increasing pain, fever, and hearing loss.

Foreign Body

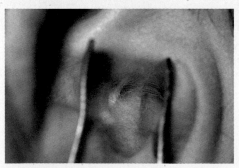

Most commonly these are found in the canal of a child who puts a bean or bead in the ear. If the object has been in the ear for several days, the patient may present with purulent discharge, pain, or hearing loss. If an insect is in the ear, the patient may hear a bug flying around in the ear.

Acute Otitis Media

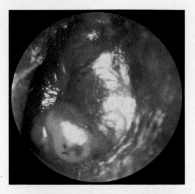

Acute infection in the middle ear. Onset is usually sudden and sometimes accompanied by fever and pain. Fluid may be in the middle ear, with signs or symptoms of middle ear inflammation. Causes may be viral or bacterial.

Scarred TM

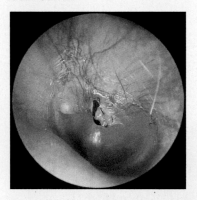

Caused by frequent ear infections with perforation of the TM. Scars are seen as dense white patches on the TM.

Tympanostomy Tube

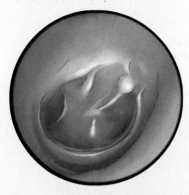

Tympanostomy tubes are indicated for chronic otitis media and its complications, recurrent acute otitis media, and antibiotic failure in children. The tubes are usually made of plastics such as silicone or Teflon. After 2–5 years, the tubes spontaneously fall out and the membrane most often closes.

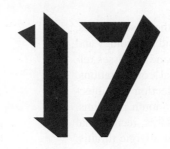

Nose, Sinuses, Mouth, and Throat Assessment

Learning Objectives

1 Identify the structures of the nose, sinuses, mouth, and throat.

2 Understand the anatomy and physiology involved in common symptoms of the nose, sinuses, mouth, and throat.

3 Identify key focus areas for health promotion and risk reduction related to the nose, sinuses, mouth, and throat.

4 Identify common subjective and objective findings in the upper respiratory area and mouth.

5 Differentiate normal from unexpected findings in the physical assessment of the upper respiratory system and mouth.

6 Document and communicate upper respiratory findings pertinent to risk reduction as well as to directing the patient's care.

7 Provide an individualized health assessment with sensitivity to the patient's age, gender, and culture.

8 Use assessment findings of the nose, sinuses, mouth, and throat to identify pertinent nursing diagnoses and initiate a patient care plan.

Mrs. Davis, an 89-year-old Caucasian woman, was admitted to the hospital 13 days ago with pneumonia. She had complications during her stay, was transferred to intensive care, and is now on the rehabilitation unit in preparation for her return home. Her temperature is 37°C orally, pulse 88 beats/min, respirations 20 breaths/min, and blood pressure 138/72 mm Hg. Current medications include a mild diuretic and beta blocker for blood pressure, an inhaler to open her airways, and an antibiotic for the pneumonia. Her assessment was documented on the previous shift.

You will gain more information about Mrs. Davis as you progress through this chapter. As you study the content and features, consider Mrs. Davis's case and its relationship to what you are learning. Begin thinking about the following points:

- The mucous membranes reflect the health of other body systems. What body systems are affecting the health of Mrs. Davis' oral mucous membranes?
- Why is it especially important for nurses to inspect the mouths of hospitalized patients?
- How might improvement in the patient's mouth affect her rehabilitation and functional abilities?

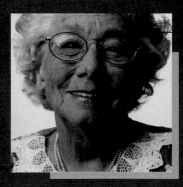

This chapter focuses on assessment of the nose, sinuses, mouth, and throat. It reviews anatomy and physiology and common variations from normal findings, and discusses relevant lifespan, cultural, and environmental considerations. The chapter serves as a guide to the collection of subjective data related to upper respiratory and mouth problems, which can result from occupational exposures, recreational activities (e.g., smoking), family history of allergic rhinitis, systemic disorders, and head and neck cancer. It reviews common signs and symptoms such as nasal discharge, congestion, and obstruction; snoring; sore throat; and facial pain and pressure. Presentation of objective data collection includes examination techniques and correct documentation of normal and abnormal findings. The emphasis is a systematic, uncomplicated approach to this rather complex anatomical area.

Structure and Function Overview

The upper respiratory system and mouth function as the entry point for air and food into the body. These organs serve as a common channel until air reaches the lungs and food reaches the esophagus. The upper respiratory tract warms, filters, humidifies, and transports air to the lower respiratory tract (see Chapter 18). The nose is the sensory organ for smell, while the mouth is the sensory organ for taste. An explanation of the anatomy of organs along this transport passageway promotes understanding of why structural deviations may interfere with function.

Nose

The external nose allows air to enter the respiratory tract (Fig. 17-1). The anterior slope of the nose is the *dorsum*, which ends inferiorly at the tip and laterally at the *ala*. Bone in the upper third and cartilage in the lower two thirds of the nose support its triangular shape. The nasal bone attaches superiorly at the bridge to the frontal bone and laterally to the lacrimal and maxillary bones. The floor of the nose rests on the superior portion of the hard palate, separating it from the mouth. The ethmoid bone forms and separates the roof of the

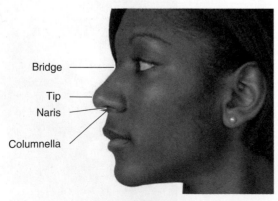

Figure 17.1 The external nose.

Bridge
Tip
Naris
Columnella

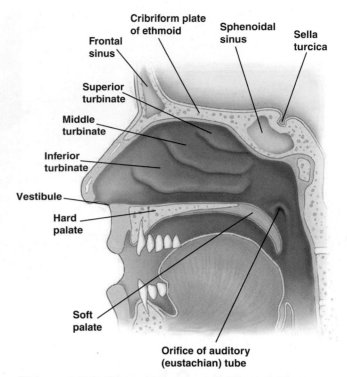

Figure 17.2 The nasal septum, left lateral wall.

Cribriform plate of ethmoid
Frontal sinus
Sphenoidal sinus
Sella turcica
Superior turbinate
Middle turbinate
Inferior turbinate
Vestibule
Hard palate
Soft palate
Orifice of auditory (eustachian) tube

nose from the brain. The midline **columella** divides the oval nares (nostrils), which are openings that lead into the internal nose and are lined with skin and ciliated mucosa. That lining is known as the **vestibule**.

Clinical Significance 17-1

The ciliated mucosa inside the nose warm, filter, and humidify inspired air at nearly 100% and expend more than 1 L/day of water (Andresen, et al., 2008).

The nasal septum is the center wall of bone and cartilage covered with mucosal membrane that divides the right and left nasal cavities (Fig. 17-2). Projecting from the lateral walls of the nose are three scroll-like bones covered with erectile mucous membranes: the inferior, middle, and superior turbinates. The inferior turbinates, which are most anterior, are usually the first internal structures seen on nasal examination. Lateral to each turbinate is an air space: the inferior meatus, middle meatus, and superior meatus. Cilia that trap particulates and sweep them posterior to the nasopharynx promote mucus drainage. The nasolacrimal duct drains into the inferior meatus (see Chapter 15). The middle turbinate and middle meatus area are known collectively as the **osteomeatal complex**.

Clinical Significance 17-2

The osteomeatal complex is the most anatomically significant area involved in chronic sinusitis (Yian, 2003).

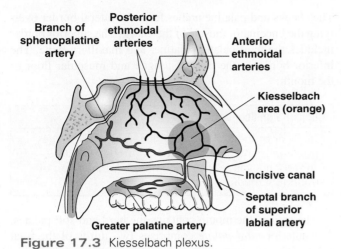

Figure 17.3 Kiesselbach plexus.

The nose is the primary organ for smell. Air within the nasal roof stimulates the olfactory receptors of cranial nerve (CN) I. Mucosal swelling from upper respiratory infections (colds) may obstruct olfactory sensory preceptors, compromising the sense of smell.

⚠ SAFETY ALERT 17.1

Patients with diminished smell are at risk for decreased detection of spoiled food, smoke, or gas fumes.

Nerve and Blood Supply

The maxillary and ophthalmic divisions of the trigeminal nerve (CN V) produce pain sensations. External movement of the nose, vasodilatation, and mucus production arise from the facial nerve (CN VII). The rhino-sino-brachial (sneeze) reflex results from the complex relationship of the medulla of the brain with CNs V, VII, IX (glossopharyngeal), and X (vagus).

Branches of the internal and external carotid arteries supply blood to the nose. The anterior portion of the nasal septum has a rich vascular supply known as *Kiesselbach plexus* (Fig. 17-3).

Clinical Significance 17-3

Kiesselbach plexus is the most common site of nosebleeds (Andresen, et al., 2008).

Lymph Drainage

Lymphatic drainage from the anterior nose leads to the preauricular and submandibular nodes. The deep cervical and retropharyngeal nodes drain the posterior nasal cavity.

Sinuses

The sinuses are hollow, bony, air-filled cavities within the forehead and facial cavities (Fig. 17-4). They lighten the weight of the skull and provide timbre and resonance to the voice. The sinuses also produce mucus that empties into the

Anterior view

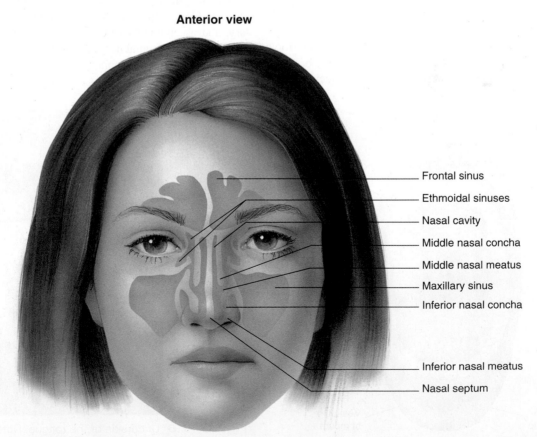

- Frontal sinus
- Ethmoidal sinuses
- Nasal cavity
- Middle nasal concha
- Middle nasal meatus
- Maxillary sinus
- Inferior nasal concha
- Inferior nasal meatus
- Nasal septum

Figure 17.4 The paranasal sinuses.

nasal cavity. Three major factors are related to normal function of the nose and sinuses: patency of the sinus ostia, normal cilia function, and normal quality and quantity of mucus.

The *frontal sinus* is above the eyebrows, the *ethmoid sinuses* are between the eyes, and the *maxillary sinuses* are below the eyes and above the teeth in each cheek. Sensory innervation of the sinuses is from CN V (trigeminal). Lymphatic drainage from the sinuses is to the lateral and retropharyngeal nodes.

The nasopharynx contributes to nasal resonance and assists with equilibration of middle-ear pressure (see Chapter 16). Air and nasal-sinus mucus passes through the posterior **choana** (opening) of the nose into the nasopharynx. The nasal end of the eustachian tube communicates with the middle ear by opening during swallowing and yawning. Just posterior to the eustachian tube opening is a mound of tissue known as the *torus tubarius.*

Clinical Significance 17-4

Posterior to the torus region is the pharyngeal recess or *Rosenmüller fossa*, which is a common site of occult nasopharyngeal malignancies (Andresen, et al., 2008).

The *adenoids* are lymphoid tissue located in the roof of the nasopharynx and laterally in the eustachian tube orifice. They have a rich blood supply from branches of the facial and internal maxillary arteries.

Mouth

The *mouth (oral cavity)* is the structure for taste, mastication, and speech articulation. It extends from the lips to the anterior pillars of the tonsils (Fig. 17-5). Anteriorly, the cavity begins at the vermillion border, or junction of the lip and facial skin.

The cheeks and palatine arches form the lateral border overlying the buccinator muscle of the cheek. The superior border includes the hard palate, palatine, and maxillary bone. The inferior border is the base of tongue and muscular floor of the mouth.

Clinical Significance 17-5

The floor of the mouth is highly vascular, with the largest percentage in the area at the base of the tongue. This vascularity allows rapid absorption of sublingual medication.

The roof of the mouth contains the hard and soft palates. The anterior *hard palate* comprises two thirds of the total palate. The adjacent, posterior *soft palate* forms the uvula and separates the mouth from the pharynx. The *uvula* is midline at the inferior border of the soft palate.

Tongue

The tongue is muscle tissue that covers the floor of the mouth, with posterior–inferior extension into the pharynx. The median fold, also known as the **lingula frenulum**, connects the base of the tongue to the floor of the mouth (Fig. 17-6). The tongue manipulates solids and liquids in mastication and deglutition. It is also involved in speech production and taste. The anterior two thirds of the tongue surface contain taste buds known as *vallate papillae*, which identify sweet, sour, salty, and bitter (Fig. 17-7).

The tongue is one of the body's most vascular muscles; its blood supply includes the lingual, exterior maxillary, and ascending pharyngeal arteries. Innervation of the tongue includes lingual nerve fibers from CN V, (trigeminal), VII (facial), IX (glossopharyngeal), X (vagus), and XII (hypoglossal).

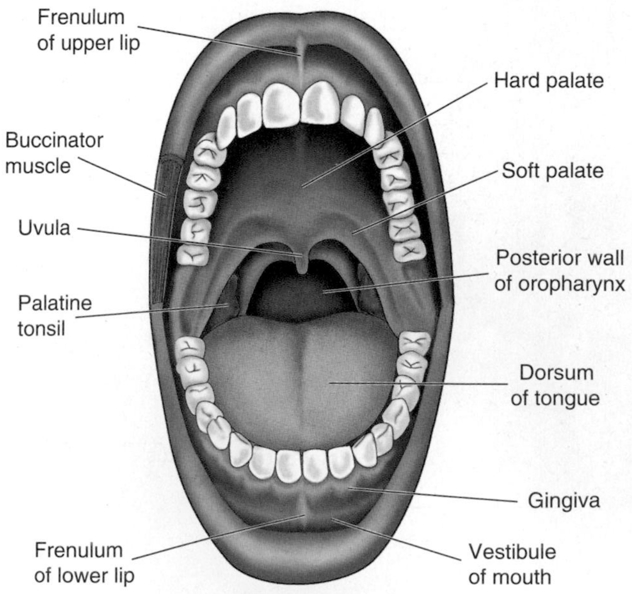

Figure 17.5 The oral cavity.

Frenulum of upper lip
Buccinator muscle
Uvula
Palatine tonsil
Frenulum of lower lip
Hard palate
Soft palate
Posterior wall of oropharynx
Dorsum of tongue
Gingiva
Vestibule of mouth

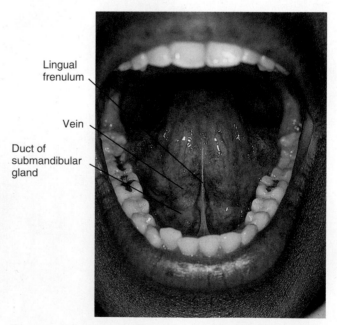

Lingual frenulum
Vein
Duct of submandibular gland

Figure 17.6 Underside of the tongue. Note the lingual frenulum.

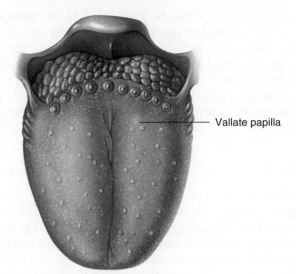

Figure 17.7 Vallate papillae.

microscopic minor salivary glands are scattered throughout the oral mucosa.

Saliva begins the digestive process by releasing enzymes upon contact with food. Saliva protects the oral mucosa from heat, chemicals, and irritants. Saliva also transmits taste information, rinses the oral cavity to maintain pH, and provides lubrication for the movement of food. Salivary production increases with smelling and seeing food, tasting, chewing, swallowing, and cigarette smoking. Decreased salivary flow, **xerostomia**, is related to emotional response, aging, disorders such as Sjögren syndrome, and damage to the glands (eg, radiation therapy, obstruction, infection).

Salivary Glands

The mouth also contains drainage ducts from three major salivary glands (Fig. 17-8). The largest, the *parotid gland*, is within the cheek anterior to the ear and extends from the zygomatic arch inferior to the angle of the jaw. The *parotid (Stensen's) duct* opens into the mouth in the buccal mucosa just opposite the upper second molar. The *submandibular gland* is beneath the body of the mandible. Its *Wharton ducts* run deep to the floor of the mouth and open on both sides of the frenulum. The small *sublingual salivary gland* lies within the floor of the mouth under the tongue with many openings along the submandibular duct. Many

The autonomic nervous system and CN VII (facial) and IX (glossopharyngeal) innervate secretions of the major and minor salivary ducts. CN XII (hypoglossal) innervates the submandibular glands.

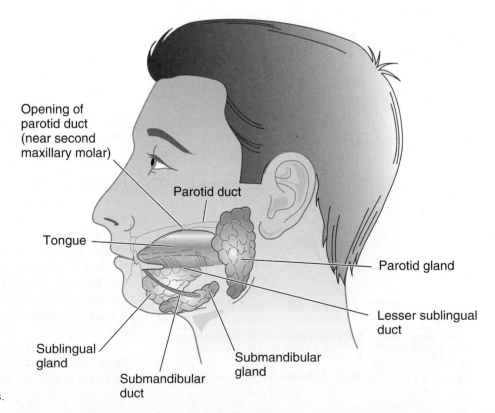

Figure 17.8 The salivary glands.

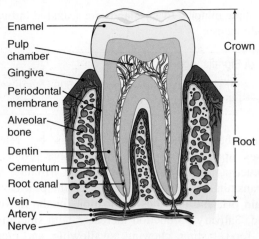

Figure 17.9 Anatomy of the tooth.

Teeth and Gums

The teeth contribute to the grinding and mastication of food to prepare for swallowing. They are composed of three layers: *crown*, *neck*, and *root* (Fig. 17-9). The crown, visible within the oral cavity, is the superior surface and also consists of three layers: enamel, dentin, and pulp. The outer *enamel* is an avascular surface with no pain receptors. It needs saliva to maintain its hard surface. Erosion of enamel may occur without pain. Regular dental follow-up is important in detecting early dental caries. The second layer, *dentin*, has tubules that connect to nerve fibers. Pain is experienced if damage to the dentin occurs by trauma or erosion. The innermost layer is the *pulp*, which has blood vessels and lymphatics, nerve tissue, and odontoblasts (dentin-forming cells). Increased pressure secondary to inflammation within the pulp may cause necrosis of the tooth.

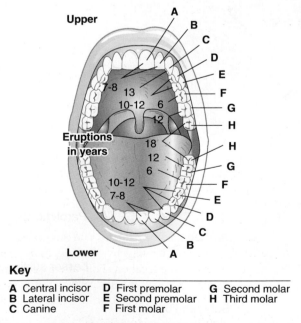

Key

A Central incisor	**D** First premolar	**G** Second molar
B Lateral incisor	**E** Second premolar	**H** Third molar
C Canine	**F** First molar	

Figure 17.10 Numbers and position of the adult teeth.

There are 32 permanent teeth (Fig. 17-10; Andresen, et al., 2008). The eight anterior incisors have flat surfaces for biting food. The most posterior teeth, the 12 molars, perform the grinding and final chewing process before swallowing. The maxillary bone supports the tissues of the upper jaw, while the mandibular bones support the tissues of the lower jaw. The periodontium is the gingival or gum tissue that supports the teeth.

Throat

The *throat (oropharynx)* is the common channel for the respiratory and digestive systems. It begins at the inferior border of the soft palate and uvula (see Fig. 17-5). The throat includes the base of the tongue, pharyngoepiglottic and glossoepiglottic folds, anterior and posterior pillars, and palatine tonsils. The *tonsils* are in the back of the throat between the anterior and posterior pillars. The tissue appears more granular and less smooth than the surrounding mucous membranes. Lymphatic tissue of the tonsils and adenoids provide immunologic defense. With chronic infections they may hypertrophy and produce chronic airway obstruction. **Tonsillitis** is inflammation of the tonsils. Hypertrophy of the tonsils and adenoids may develop secondary to sinusitis or otitis (middle-ear infection).

Clinical Significance 17-8
Removal of tonsils and adenoids does not increase risks of infection (Andresen, et al., 2008).

🔺 Lifespan Considerations

Pregnant Women

Rhinitis during pregnancy results from the increased vascularity of the respiratory tract as well as hormonal effects on the mucosal lining. Increased complaints of nasal congestion or obstruction are common in pregnant women. Increased sinus infections, epistaxis (nosebleeds), or both may occur. The gums also may become hyperemic and softened, leading to bleeding with tooth-brushing.

Infants and Children

Infants are obligatory nose breathers. Ability to smell is fully developed at birth, but the cilia that line the adult nose are lacking. Odors reach the olfactory receptor cells readily and provide a clear sense of smell in newborns. This heightened olfactory ability is key to infant–parent bonding. The maxillary and ethmoid sinuses are present at birth but small. The frontal and sphenoid sinuses appear by age 3 years and continue to develop through adolescence (Yian, 2003).

The sense of taste is present at birth, and salivation begins at 3 months. The taste buds for sweets are more abundant during the early years of life. Tactile sensation, particularly of the lips and tongue, is well developed at birth. Drooling may become noticeable at around 4 months of age. The development of teeth, temporary (deciduous) and permanent, begins in utero. Teeth erupt in infants and toddlers between 5 and 27 months of age, with primary dentition at about 6 months. Typically, by age 2½ years all deciduous teeth are present. Around age 6 years, children begin to loose their deciduous teeth, which are replaced by the permanent teeth. By age 12 to 13 years permanent teeth are present.

Older Adults

Gustatory rhinitis, clear rhinorrhea stimulated by the smell and taste of food, occurs most frequently in older adults. A decrease in olfactory sensory fibers occurs after age 60 years. In the oral cavity a thinning of the soft tissue of the cheeks and tongue results in an increased risk of ulcerations, infections, and oral cancers.

With advancing age, production of saliva and number of taste buds decrease. Resorption occurs in gum tissue, surrounding teeth, and the mandible bone. Natural tooth loss accompanies the breakdown of the tooth surface and receding gums. Malocclusion may occur with tooth loss and aggravate temporomandibular joint function (see Chapter 23). The number of older adults without teeth is declining because of more reconstructive dental practices. Nevertheless, incidence of dental caries is rising related to retention of the teeth (Mungia, et al., 2008).

Cultural and Environmental Considerations

Incidence of dental caries varies with sociodemographic groups. While spending trends for dental care have increased, an increase in dental insurance is lacking. Only 44% of people in the United States have some form of private insurance (many plans have limited coverage and high co–payments), 9% have public dental insurance (Medicaid and Children's Heath Insurance Program), 2% have other dental insurance, and 45% have no dental coverage (*Healthy People 2010*, 2008). The percentage of untreated dental carries is 36% in African American children, 43% in Hispanic children, and 26% in Caucasian children (*Healthy People 2010*, 2008).

Gingivitis, or inflammation with bleeding of the gums, is high among Hispanics, American Indians, Alaskan Natives, and adults of low socio-economic classes. It may progress to periodontal disease with a loss of connective tissue and bone (*Healthy People* 2010, 2008).

Cleft lip and cleft palate occur in 1 in 1,000 births with an increased incidence in Native Americans and Asian Americans (Newland, 2003). **Bifid uvula** is a minor cleft of the posterior soft palate and occurs in about 1 in 250 people (Langlais & Miller, 2002). Torus palatinus, a bony ridge running in the middle of the hard palate, is more common in Native Americans, Inunits, and Asians (Barnes, 2000).

Oral and pharyngeal cancers vary by race and ethnicity, most likely related to tobacco use. African Americans and Caucasians have 12.5 and 10.0 new cases per 100,000 per year; respectively Hispanics and American Indians and Alaskan Natives have only 6.5 and 8.8 new cases per year (Landis, et al., 1999). The 5-year survival rate for oral and pharyngeal cancers is lower among African Americans than Caucasians (34% versus 56%, respectively; NIH, SEER, 1999). An increased risk of nasopharyngeal cancer is noted with Chinese or Asian ancestry.

Acute Assessment

Severe nosebleeds need to be treated immediately. Infection in the floor of mouth may produce *Ludwig angina*, which is swelling that pushes the tongue up and back and results in eventual airway obstruction. Assessing risk for aspiration begins in the upper respiratory tract, focusing on laryngeal airway competency as well as the presence of dental prostheses or loose teeth, which may be accidentally swallowed and aspirated.

⚠ SAFETY ALERT 17.2
Acute airway obstruction such as in anaphylaxis, Ludwig angina, and epiglottis may limit the opportunity for data collection other than specifics related to presentation of the patient.

Abrupt loss of smell may indicate a brain tumor and warrants further evaluation with an MRI scan of the brain. Hard fixed nodes should be further evaluated by biopsy or radiologic films for cancer.

Subjective Data Collection

Subjective data collection for this body region involves taking a detailed health history. Investigation creates an environment in which the nurse can suggest strategies to manage symptoms, avoid exposures that may exacerbate symptoms, and suggest health-promotion measures. Examples include discussions of allergen/irritant exposure and smoking, which cause upper respiratory inflammation. Further education includes teaching patients to avoid environmental exposures to irritants and chemicals and suggesting the use of personal protective equipment when exposures may be toxic. Opportunities for education about allergy exposure and smoking cessation fall well within the scope of nursing practice (Table 17-1). Such health education may help the patient to avoid upper respiratory disease and exacerbation of current illnesses.

Table 17.1   Controlling Allergens in the Home Setting

Allergens	Precautions in the Home
Housedust Mites. Mites (microscopic bugs) live and feed in carpets, upholstery, and bedding. They produce droppings, which in humans cause allergic symptoms. Concentrate cleaning efforts in the bedroom to control dust mite allergies.	• Damp dust and vacuum weekly. • Change or clean furnace filter monthly. • Avoid feather pillows and down comforters. • Wash sheets and blankets weekly in hot water. • Avoid "dust catchers" (e.g., stuffed animals). • Consider using high efficiency particulate air filters in the bedroom and vacuum cleaner. • Use hardwood floors in the bedroom.
Mold Spores. Mold spores are found in damp, dark areas of the home.	Discourage and eliminate mold growth by: • Repairing leaks • Using dehumidifiers in damp basements • Cleaning shower grouting weekly • Decreasing houseplants, removing them from bedrooms, placing fungicide in soil • Cleaning refrigerator drip pan • Meticulously cleaning or avoiding portable humidifiers • Adjusting whole house humidity to 40% or less • Avoiding wool fabrics • Avoiding foods that contain mold: fermented beverages, especially wine and beer; vinegar; cheese; foods with yeast; breads and bakery products; canned tomato products; pizza; canned, smoked, and pickled meats; mushrooms
Foods. Any food can trigger an allergic reaction.	Eliminate forever foods suspected of producing acute life-threatening symptoms. Common culprits are shellfish and peanuts. Eliminate for 6 months foods that cause or contribute to chronic allergies, despite cravings for them. Then reintroduce the foods in a rotating manner. Common culprits are milk, egg, wheat, corn, soy, and yeast.
Pet Dander. Cat dander is light and highly allergic; dog dander is heavier.	Decrease pet dander by: • Having only outdoor pets • Removing pets from the bedroom • Grooming or bathing pets regularly (not by the allergic person) • Washing hands after touching pets
Pollens. Airborne pollens, present during blooming seasons, trigger allergic symptoms.	Decrease exposure to pollens by: • Keeping windows closed • Grooming pets, which can carry pollens into the home • Avoiding attic fans

Source: Adapted from *Patient Education: Allergy Precautions in the Home* by Margaret A. Kramper, RN, FNP, CORLN.

Areas for Health Promotion/ *Healthy People*

Consideration of *Healthy People* goals is essential in health assessment and patient education to increase the quality and quantity of healthy life and to eliminate health disparities. Major concerns for assessment of the nose, sinuses, mouth, and throat related to *Healthy People* include tobacco use, obstructive sleep apnea, oral heath, and cancer (see Table 17-2).

Assessment of Risk Factors

When exploring risk factors the intention is to determine how likely a person is to develop upper respiratory disease. Questions open discussion for educational opportunities as well as for identifying areas that may require emphasis and follow-up. Teaching and interviewing can be blended.

Table 17.2 *Healthy People* Goals Related to the Nose, Sinuses, Mouth, and Throat

Goals	Patient Education Topics
Reduce the oropharyngeal cancer death rate.	Offer smoking cessation programs and reduce exposure to second-hand smoke. Avoid use of smokeless tobacco, snuff, or chew.
Reduce the proportion of children and adolescents who have dental caries in their primary or permanent teeth.	Avoid leaving bottle in the baby's mouth. Encourage early dental care.
Reduce periodontal disease.	Encourage brushing and flossing.
Increase the proportion of local health departments and community-based health centers, including community, migrant, and homeless health centers, that have an oral health component.	Advocate for underserved populations as dental care is often undefended and not available to patients who can not pay.

Source: *Healthy People 2010: What are its goals? (n.d.)*. Retrieved June 2, 2010, from http://www.healthypeople.gov/About goals.htm.

Questions to Assess History and Risk	Rationales
Family History Do you have a family history of mouth or upper respiratory illness? • What family member had the illness? • What was the specific illness? • What management was implemented? • What was the outcome?	*Atopy* (allergic disease) occurs in 25% of the US population, or an estimated 18 million Americans (Lloyd & Naclerio, 2008). Hereditary prevalence is strong: if one parent has allergies, a child also has a 50% chance of developing them. Family history of *cancer* increases the patient's risk. Positive family history of genetic disorders such as *cystic fibrosis*, autoimmune disease such as *Wegener granulomatosis*, *Churg Strauss*, and *Sjögren syndrome* increases risk.
Personal History Have you ever been diagnosed with a mouth or upper respiratory condition? • What was the specific condition? • When did it occur? • How was the condition treated? • What where the outcomes?	Positive history of frequent *upper respiratory infections* suggests underlying allergy, chronic hypertrophy of the adenoids and tonsils, or *chronic sinusitis*.
Did you have a history of chronic upper respiratory infections as a child?	Frequent upper respiratory infections in childhood raise suspicion of *allergy*. Chronic inflammation of the respiratory tract may lead to mucosal damage with resultant chronic infections (eg, *sinusitis*).
Current Health Status Do you have any known sensitivities to inhalant allergens such as dust mites, mold, pollens, or animal dander? Have you had specific allergy testing? • What were the test results? • What were your symptoms? • When did you experience symptoms? • What treatment measures were taken? • What was the outcome of treatment?	Allergy can affect any target organ in the body. The nose and respiratory mucosa are the entry port for inhalant allergens. Thus, the nose and respiratory tract are common targets for inflammatory responses from allergen exposure.
Medications and Supplements What medications are you currently taking? • What are the names of all your current medications? • What dose and how frequently are they taken?	It is helpful to know the patient's complete medication list, because all medications have potential side effects, which may affect the mouth, nose, and sinuses. Blood-pressure drugs (eg, ACE inhibitors) may produce cough (Table 17-3). Anticoagulants may predispose patients to nosebleeds or exacerbate bleeding. Medication that dries the mouth may affect tooth and gum health.

(text continues on page 416)

Table 17.3 Medications That May Produce Symptoms in the Nose, Sinus, Mouth, and Throat

Drug Class	Possible Adverse Reaction
Antihypertensives	Cough, nasal congestion
Hormones	Nasal congestion
Anticoagulants	Epistaxis
Antihistamines	Dry mucous membranes, epistaxis
Herbal supplements	Epistaxis
Analgesics	Nasal congestion
CNS agents	Nasal congestion
Topical decongestants	Rebound nasal congestion
Antidepressants	Dry mucous membranes

Source: Lloyd, K. B., & Naclerio, R. M. (2008). Strategies for managing nasal congestion. *Post graduate healthcare education,* LLC. Philadelphia: GlaxoSmith Kline.

Questions to Assess History and Risk	Rationales
Are you taking any over-the-counter (OTC), natural, or herbal supplements. • What specific products? • How frequently are you taking them?	Patients sometimes have a false sense of safety with OTC medications. Potentially unsafe OTC medications include topical decongestant sprays. Used appropriately for a short time, they provide effective nasal decongestion. These sprays also facilitate quick vasoconstriction and are beneficial in treating nosebleeds. With persistent use, however, they produce rebound congestion and are addictive. Natural agents (eg, gingko biloba, garlic) may have undesirable effects on the respiratory lining, causing increased clotting times. They are thus contraindicated in patients with frequent nosebleeds (Bent, 2008). Other herbs may cross-react with pollen and stimulate *allergic rhinitis*. For example, echinacea taken to strengthen the immune system can cross-react with ragweed, increasing symptoms in sensitive patients (NCCAM, 2008).
Dental Health • How regularly do you brush and floss? • When were your teeth last cleaned? • Do you have any problems with your teeth or gums?	Regular dental cleanings are important to keeping teeth and gums healthy and identifying problems early.
Psychosocial History Do you currently smoke cigarettes, pipes, or cigars? • How many packs per day do you smoke? • How many years have you smoked? • Have you ever tried to stop smoking? • Are you currently interested in stopping smoking? • Do you currently or have you ever chewed tobacco?	Smoking increases respiratory inflammation, exacerbating *allergic rhinitis* and *chronic sinusitis*. It also increases risks for *head and neck carcinoma* (*Healthy People 2010,* 2008). Chewing tobacco increases risk for *oral cancer* (Mayo, 2007). See Chapter 18 for risks to the lower respiratory system related to smoking and tobacco use.
Are you frequently around others who smoke? What avoidance measures do you take to avoid smoke exposure?	Second-hand smoke increases risks for *head and neck cancer* and exacerbates *allergic rhinitis, pharyngitis,* and *sinusitis.* Researchers have identified more than 4,000 chemicals in tobacco smoke; of these at least 43 cause cancer in humans and animals (*Healthy People 2010,* 2008).
Do you inhale or have you ever inhaled marijuana, cocaine, methamphetamine, heroin, glue, or spray paint? If yes, are you interested in information to reduce associated risks or to help you quit?	Inhaling these substances can irritate the lining of the upper airway. Regular marijuana use may damage the cilia, leading to airway injury and potential infection, and increases the risk of *head and neck cancer.* Use of cocaine may permanently damage the nasal mucosa, resulting in nasal septal perforations. Use of methamphetamines may severely damage the teeth (Padilla & Ritter, 2008).

Questions to Assess History and Risk	Rationales

Environment Exposure

Are you currently or have you ever been exposed to chemical substances or irritants at work?
- Do you wear a mask or take other precautions to protect the respiratory tract?
- Do you monitor your exposures to chemicals?

Irritating chemicals may cause inflammation of the upper airway, which predisposes patients to chronic infections. Chemical exposures may damage the cilia, affecting the natural self-cleaning ability of the mucosal lining. Repeat exposures may produce allergic reactions in atopic patients. Chemicals may also be toxic.

Do you have hobbies that increase risk for upper-respiratory problems: farming; care of or frequent exposure to animals; exposure to paint, chemical fumes, or wood dust; airplane flying; scuba diving; or swimming?

Farming may expose patients to excessive pollen, animal dander, mold, or grain smuts. Atopic patients may experience adverse reactions with persistent allergen exposure. Chemical fumes from paints and solvents may irritate or damage the respiratory mucosa. Scuba diving and flying may produce negative pressure in the ear or sinuses, leading to barotrauma. Swimming may produce or aggravate *sinusitis* from chronic chlorine exposure. Chlorine may act as an allergen or irritant.

Risk Assessment and Health-related Patient Teaching

In assessing for risk factors, nurses can identify areas to focus efforts for patient teaching and related behavior changes. As discussed in Chapter 18, smoking is a major risk to the respiratory tract and the leading cause of preventable death (Risk Factors, 2005). At every encounter, patients should be questioned about smoking and their interest in stopping. Nurses should document this discussion each visit. Offering multiple choices for discontinuing smoking as well as providing resources, such as support groups or individual counseling, are helpful. Clinician interest can be an effective motivator in stimulating clients to quit smoking.

Visits to dental care providers are an excellent opportunity to improve oral health. Reduction of dental caries through daily oral hygiene, good dietary nutrition, community water fluoridation, and application of dental sealants after the eruption of permanent teeth are all examples of opportunities to improve oral health. Daily teeth brushing and flossing are essential to decreasing dental carries as well as reducing gingivitis and periodontal disease.

Focused Health History Related to Common Symptoms

Common Mouth and Upper Respiratory Symptoms

- Facial pressure/pain/headache
- Snoring/sleep apnea
- Obstructive breathing
- Nasal congestion
- Epistaxis (nosebleeds)
- Halitosis (bad breath)
- Anosmia (decreased smell)
- Cough
- Pharyngitis/sore throat
- Dysphagia (difficulty swallowing)
- Dental aching/pain
- Hoarseness/voice changes
- Oral lesions

Questions to Assess Symptoms	Rationale/Abnormal Findings

Describe your upper respiratory (nasal) breathing.

This question is an initial opportunity for patients to offer unbiased descriptions of how they feel their upper airway performs.

Facial Pressure, Pain, Headache

Do you have any pain, pressure, or a headache?

Sinus pain or pressure is common with *colds, influenza,* and *sinusitis.* See also Chapters 14 and 24.

Snoring and Sleep Apnea
- Do you snore?
- Are you a restless sleeper?
- Does anyone observe your sleep?
- Do you stop breathing during sleep?
- Are you rested in the morning? Do you experience daytime drowsiness?
- Do you drool at night?

Snoring can be a nuisance or complicated by sleep apnea. All patients with *sleep apnea* snore, but not all who snore have sleep apnea. Patients with sleep apnea are typically unaware of night-time arousals and at increased risk for hypertension, stroke, heart attack, and motor vehicle accidents. Hypertrophy of the tonsils or adenoids may cause airway obstruction or sleep apnea. Children with large tonsils and adenoids may be at risk.

(text continues on page 418)

Questions to Assess Symptoms	Rationale/Abnormal Findings

Obstructive Breathing

Do you experience decreased nasal breathing?
- Is this unilateral or bilateral?
- Is it related to any facial trauma?
- Does the congestion alternate from side to side?
- Does anything aggravate or improve your nasal breathing?

Inflammation of the nose and sinuses from allergen or irritant exposure may decrease nasal breathing. Structural abnormalities such as a *deviated nasal septum, nasal polyp*, or tumor may cause nasal obstruction. Trauma may result in a *deviated nasal septum* or *hematoma*, obstructing the nasal airway. The normal diurnal nasal cycle involves a cyclical alternating pattern of congestion and decongestion from side to side (Derebery & Berliner, 2002). With inflammation, this cycle may become exaggerated.

Nasal Congestion

Do you experience excessive nasal discharge?
- Is the discharge clear or cloudy?
- What color is it?
- Is it bilateral, from both sides, or unilateral, from one nostril?

Excessive clear rhinorrhea may represent *allergic* or *non-allergic rhinitis*. Unilateral clear discharge unresponsive to treatment may represent a rare *cerebrospinal fluid leak*. It can be determined by collection and laboratory examination of fluid for beta-2-transferrin (Nandapalan et al., 1996). Cloudy or discolored discharge indicates inflammation. Persistent inflammation may result in infection.

Epistaxis

Do you have difficulty with nosebleeds?

Do you habitually pick or remove crusts from the nose?

Nasal inflammation causes dilatation of its blood vessels. The most common site of nasal bleeding is Kiesselbach plexus on the anterior septum (Andresen, et al., 2008). Digital manipulation or nose picking may aggravate nasal bleeding.

Halitosis

Have you ever been told that your breath smells bad?

Foul breath suggests infection.

Anosmia

Do you have a decreased sense of smell? Is this a long-term or sudden problem?

Anosmia (decreased smell) may accompany chronic inflammation of the nose and sinus. A CT scan may reveal obstruction of one or more paranasal sinuses.

Cough

Do you have difficulty with cough?
- Does it feel like the cough comes from your chest or upper airway?
- Is your cough wet or dry?
- Is the cough productive or nonproductive?
- What makes the cough worse?
- What makes the cough better?

Sinus drainage, allergen or irritant exposure, or *chronic sinusitis* may produce cough. Persistent productive cough warrants a chest x-ray to determine lung pathology (see Chapter 18). Reactive airway in *asthma* may produce cough. Cough may be secondary to *gastro-esophageal reflux disease (GERD)*.

Pharyngitis

Do you experience sore throats?

Chronic hypertrophy or enlargement of the tonsils may produce sore throats. Typically hypertrophy of the tonsils is also associated with hypertrophy of the adenoids. Recurrent strep infections may occur with *chronic tonsillitis*.

Dysphagia

Do you have difficulty with swallowing?

Dysphagia (difficulty swallowing) may accompany a growth or lesion in the respiratory tract or result from inflammation of the upper respiratory tract secondary to *GERD*.

Dental Pain

Do you experience dental aching or pain?

Are your teeth sensitive to cold or heat?

Sinusitis may produce dental aching, particularly of the upper teeth. *Dental carries* or *abscess* may produce tooth pain.

Voice Changes

Have you experienced hoarseness or voice changes?

Common causes include sinus postnasal drainage, inflammation of the upper respiratory tract secondary to *GERD*, lesions of the upper respiratory tract, and inflammation from allergen or irritant exposure (eg, chemicals, cigarette smoke).

Oral Lesions

Do you have any sores in your mouth?

If so, has there been any change in the size or appearance of the sore?

Smoking or chewing tobacco increases risk for *oral cancer*. Persistent or changing lesions may indicate *oral cancer*. Biopsy is warranted for persistent lesions.

Documentation of Normal Findings

Patient states breathing is comfortable and quiet. Denies facial pressure, pain, headache, snoring, sleep apnea, obstructive breathing, or nasal congestion. Reports no epistaxis, halitosis, anosmia, or cough. States no pharyngitis, dysphagia, dental pain, hoarseness, or oral lesions. *C. Bond, RN*

Lifespan Considerations

Additional Questions	Rationale/Abnormal Findings
Pregnant Women Have you experienced increased nasal congestion or nosebleeds with pregnancy?	Hormonal fluctuations often result in increased nasal congestion and may exacerbate allergies. Epistaxis may be secondary to engorged nasal vessels.
Infants and Children How many upper respiratory infections has your child had in the past year?	Recurrent infections suggest underlying *allergy*. They may result in enlarged tonsils and adenoids, which in turn may be responsible for frequent *sinus infections*. Recurrent strep infections are an indication for consideration of removal of the tonsils and adenoids because of the risk of rheumatic fever with resultant heart or kidney disease.
Does your child have obstruction of the nasal airway? Is the obstruction unilateral or bilateral? Is your child a good eater? Does your child snore?	Decreased nasal breathing may be secondary to hypertrophy of the adenoids, which may result in mouth breathing. Mouth breathers are typically poor eaters because eating interferes with breathing. Hypertrophy of tonsils and adenoids may produce sleep apnea in children. Unilateral nasal obstruction in children may represent **choanal atresia** (restriction of the bucconasal membrane).
Does your child have persistent nasal discharge? Is it clear or cloudy? Is the discharge unilateral or bilateral?	Clear rhinorrhea suggests allergic disease. Thick discolored discharge may represent chronic infection. With unilateral purulent discharge in children a foreign body of the nose should be suspected.
Is your child exposed to cigarette smoke in the home?	Second-hand cigarette smoke is an irritant and increases risk for upper respiratory infections in children (U.S. Department of Health & Human Services, 2007).
Does your child have epistaxis or bloody nose? Is the bleeding unilateral or bilateral?	Suspicion for **hemangioma** or a benign mass of blood vessels should be considered. They are present at birth and may expand with crying (Newland, 2003). **Angiofibroma** of the nasopharynx should be suspected with epistaxis and nasal obstruction in adolescent boys (Woodson, 2001).
Does your child suck his or her thumb? Does the child use a bottle for feeding?	Thumb sucking past 6–7 years may cause malocclusion of the teeth. Prolonged use of baby bottles increases risk for dental decay.
Older Adults Do you experience decreased smell and taste? Do you experience increased nasal drainage at meal time?	Diminished smell and taste may produce safety risks. Gustatory rhinitis may occur in older adults with increased clear rhinorrhea at meal time.

Cultural and Environmental Considerations

Additional Questions	Rationale/Abnormal Findings
Have you recently immigrated to the United States?	Incidence of *tuberculosis* is approximately nine times higher among US immigrants (Burzynski & Schluger, 2008).
What type of heat do you use at home? Are you aware of any mold in your home?	Recent immigrants may use wood or kerosene heat, which may exacerbate allergies or produce inflammation of the upper respiratory tract leading to secondary infections. Mold may exacerbate allergies or, in the case of black mold, act as a toxin.
Note the patient's identified ethnicity and gender in relationship to known congenital and assessed health risks.	As discussed earlier, cleft lip and palate have increased incidence in Native and Asian Americans (Newland, 2003). African Americans and Caucasians are at higher risk for oral and pharyngeal cancers than are American Indians and Alaskan Natives (Landis, et al., 1999). The 5-year survival rate for oral and pharyngeal cancers is lower among African Americans than Caucasians (NIH, SEER, 1999).

Therapeutic Dialogue: Collecting Subjective Data

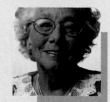

Remember Mrs. Davis, introduced at the beginning of this chapter. This elderly woman has been in the hospital 13 days with pneumonia and now is on the rehabilitation unit preparing to go home. The nurse uses professional communication techniques to gather subjective data from Mrs. Davis. The following conversations give two examples of interview styles used by different nurses. One style is more effective than the other.

Less Effective

Nurse: Hi, Mrs. Davis. How are you today?

Mrs. Davis: I'm fine.

Nurse: How did you do today?

Mrs. Davis: (swallows with difficulty). Just fine.

Nurse: Well, I'm glad to hear about that. How's your pneumonia?

Mrs. Davis: They tell me it's getting better (lips stick together).

Nurse: That's good.

Mrs. Davis: You nurses are taking such good care of me.

Nurse: Well, thanks. We always like to hear that.

Mrs. Davis: Can you get me a little water? My mouth seems so dry.

Nurse: (checks to see that there are no swallowing restrictions) Sure, here you go.

Mrs. Davis: (lips crusted and dry) Thanks. That tastes so good.

More Effective

Nurse: Hi, Mrs. Davis. I'm Jen and I'm going to be your nurse today.

Mrs. Davis: Nice to meet you.

Nurse: And you, too. How are you feeling?

Mrs. Davis: (swallows with difficulty). Just fine.

Nurse: It looks like you're having a little trouble swallowing ... (pauses)

Mrs. Davis: Well, my mouth seems so dry.

Nurse: I can see that. Let's wash your mouth out a little. Has it been awhile since you've brushed your teeth? (checks to see that there are no swallowing restrictions)

Mrs. Davis: It was yesterday. That would be so nice of you, honey.

Nurse: That's what we're here for. I'll get out your toothbrush and then we can clean things up and put on some lubricant to keep things moist. You'll feel a lot better.

Mrs. Davis: You're such a good nurse.

Critical Thinking Challenge

- Why did the more effective nurse discuss the dry mouth instead of the pneumonia?
- Why did both nurses check for swallowing restrictions?
- How did the assessment of the more effective nurse lead to a more effective ntervention?

Objective Data Collection

Much of the physical examination of the nose, sinuses, mouth, and oropharpharynx is performed by inspecting the area. Palpation for masses or tenderness is performed if abnormal findings are suspected. It is common to perform assessments in this region as focused examinations for symptoms, such as with nasal stuffiness or a sore throat.

Equipment Needed

- Hand-held otoscope
- Nasal speculum
- Tongue blades
- Cotton gauze 4 × 4
- Gloves
- Penlight
- Scratch or sniff test card
- Nasopharyngeal-laryngeal mirror

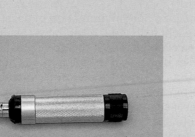

Preparation

Preparation involves good handwashing technique before beginning the examination. Gloves are used for the oral examination or with anticipated contact with mucous membranes. The patient is seated comfortably with the head at the examiner's eye level. If the patient wears dentures, offer a 4 × 4 gauze and ask the patient to remove them.

Common Specialty or Advanced Techniques

Table 17-4 summarizes common and specialized techniques used to assess the nose, sinuses, mouth, and throat. The registered nurse (RN) primarily performs inspection of these organs. Inspection of the mouth is especially important in patients taking antibiotics who are at risk for oral candidiasis. The hospital RN also assesses the patient's nares for patency when inserting a tube into the nose for feeding. A deviated septum or obstructed nares may make insertion difficult. The advanced practice nurse (APRN) uses the otoscope to visualize the nares.

Table 17.4	Common Versus Specialty/Advanced Techniques in Nose, Mouth, Sinus, and Throat Assessment		
Technique	**Purpose**	**Screening or RN Assessment**	**Focused or APRN Assessment**
Inspect the nose.	To provide information regarding the integrity of the nose	X	
Inspect the nose with otoscope and nasal speculum.	To gather information about inflammation, infection, structure		X
Palpate the nose.	To assess for inflammation, lesions, or fractures		X
Inspect the sinuses.	Transillumination results variable; typically assessed by CT scan; flexible fiberoptic examination allows visualization		X
Palpate/percuss the sinuses.	To look for signs of infection or inflammation		X
Inspect the mouth.	To gather information regarding the integrity of the oral cavity	X	
Palpate the mouth.	To look for lesions or salivary stones		X
Inspect the throat.	To gather information regarding the integrity of the throat	X	
Inspect/evaluate swallowing.	To investigate causes of complaints of dysphagia		X

Technique and Normal Findings	Abnormal Findings

External Nose

Inspection. Inspect the nose. *It appears symmetrical, midline, and proportionally shaped to facial features. Skin surface is smooth without lesions; coloration is consistent with other facial complexion.*

Asymmetry, swelling, or bruising may result from *trauma* or accompany lesions or growths.

Palpation. Generally the RN does not palpate the nose or sinuses unless there is a specific problem. For the APRN, gently palpate with the thumb and forefinger. *There is no pain, tenderness, or break in contour.*

Tenderness on palpation and crepitus suggest *fracture.*

Internal Nose

The APRN generally inspects the internal nose with an otoscope, nasal speculum, or both (Fig. 17-11). Insert a wide-tipped speculum gently into the nasal vestibule or naris and open vertically while gently lifting up on the tip of the nose. The nasal speculum may be inserted but should never be opened horizontally, because this puts uncomfortable pressure on the septum. Observe the color of the mucous membranes. Inspect any mucus. Note the color and character of the nose. The inferior turbinate is the first structure visualized. The middle turbinate can be noted superior and lateral. Assess nasal airflow by asking the patient to breathe out while holding the mouth closed. Gently manipulate the external nose to assess how these changes affect airflow. *Septum is midline; its mucosa is pink and moist with no prominent blood vessels or crusts. A small amount of drainage is clear. Airflow around the normal nasal structures is adequate.*

Infection and inflammation of nasal mucosa may be present with viral, bacterial, or allergic rhinitis. Excessive clear watery drainage suggests allergic rhinitis. Thick discolored mucus or gross pus may accompany infection. Absence of normal structures, such as the turbinates, suggests previous surgery. Deviation of the nasal septum may be congenital or acquired in trauma. Note any crusting or prominence of nasal vessels with special attention to the anterior septum. A septal perforation is a hole in the midline septum. It may be secondary to trauma, surgery, or illicit drug use. **Polyps**, grape-like swollen nasal membranes, may appear white and glistening. See Table 17-7 at the end of this chapter.

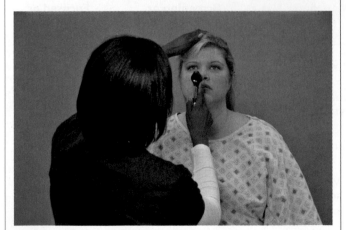

Figure 17.11 Inspecting the nasal mucosa.

If the patient notices a loss of smell, ask him or her to identify common scents. Smell testing may be performed with the use of a sniff test card. *The patient correctly identifies scents.*

Anosomia may occur with *trauma*, congestion, *polyps*, or *sinus infection*. Sudden loss of smell warrants consideration of radiological testing to rule out *intracranial masses*.

Sinuses

Inspection. Inspect the sinus areas (forehead, between the eyes, and both cheeks) for redness or swelling. *Findings are symmetrical with no redness or swelling.*

A historical method by which APRNs assess sinus cavities is transillumination (Fig. 17-12). This method has limited clinical significance and provides inconsistent results. The gold standard diagnostic technique in evaluating sinus disease is a CT scan.

Redness and swelling over the sinuses may represent acute *infection, abscess,* or *mucocele.*

Positive findings in inspection of the sinuses warrant radiological imaging to assess involvement.

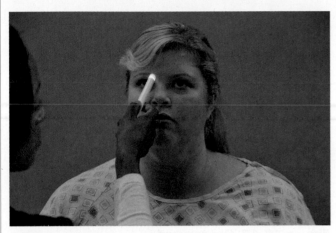

Figure 17.12 Transillumination of the sinuses.

Palpation and Percussion. Palpate and percuss the maxillary, ethmoid, and frontal sinus areas (Fig. 17-13). *No tenderness or fullness is present.*

Tenderness or fullness on palpation suggests infection. Positive findings on palpation may warrant radiological imaging.

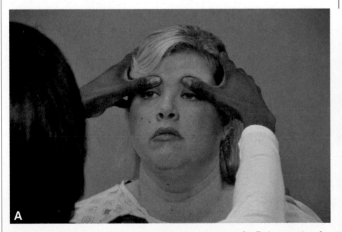
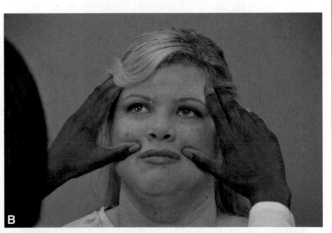

Figure 17.13 Palpating the sinus area. **A.** Palpate the frontal sinus. **B.** Palpate the maxillary sinus.

Mouth

External Inspection. Inspect lips, noting color, moisture, lesions, and oral competence. *Lips are pink and moist with no lesions.*

Dryness or cracking may indicate inadequate hydration. Lesions or aphthous ulcers may represent a *viral infection.* Swelling or edema of lips suggests *allergy.* Oral incompetence may occur in cleft lip or with inadequate repair. See Table 17-8 at the end of this chapter.

(text continues on page 424)

Internal Inspection

Buccal Mucosa. Holding a light in the nondominant hand and a tongue blade in the dominant one, gently separate areas to fully inspect the buccal mucosa, noting color and pigmentation (Fig. 17-14). Inspect the entire U-shaped area in the floor of mouth. Note the parotid (Stensen) duct appearing as a small dimple just opposite the second upper molar (Fig. 17-15). Small isolated white or yellow papules (**Fordyce granules**) may be noted on the cheeks, tongue, and lips (Fig. 17-16). These sebaceous cysts or salivary tissues are insignificant.

Poor oral hygiene has been linked to *pneumonia*. Inflamed buccal mucosa suggests *infection*. White patches (leukoplakia) may suggest a growth or lesion. Ulceration may represent viral infection or tumor. Petechiae or small red spots resulting from blood, which escapes the capillaries, may occur with trauma, infection, or decreased platelet counts (Fig. 17-17). Redness or swelling of Stensen duct may represent infection or blockage of the parotid gland.

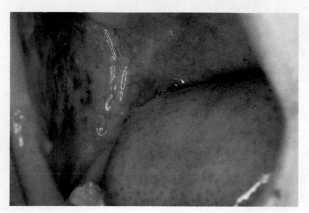

Figure 17.17 Oral petechiae.

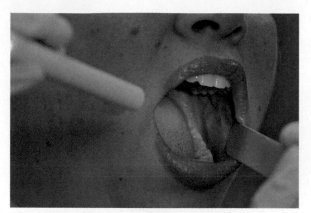

Figure 17.14 Inspecting the buccal mucosa.

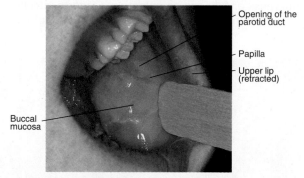

- Opening of the parotid duct
- Papilla
- Upper lip (retracted)
- Buccal mucosa

Figure 17.15 Examination of the parotid (Stensen) duct.

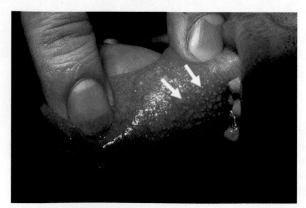

Figure 17.16 Fordyce granules.

Teeth and Gums. Inspect the teeth and gums. Note numbers and position of teeth. Note general appearance and signs of decay. Note alignment. Note the odor of the patient's breath.

Uvula. Note the position of the uvula (Fig. 17-18). Have the patient say "ah," noting the rise of the uvula and function of the vagus (CN X).

Teeth may be stained or have *decay*. Swollen or red gums with bleeding may indicate *gingivitis*. Foul breath may suggest infection. See Table 17-9 at the end of this chapter.

Uvula may be swollen with allergic reactions. It may be bifid or have a notch or cleft.

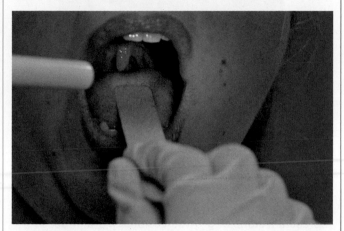

Figure 17.18 Observing the uvula.

Hard and Soft Palate. Inspect the color and surface of the hard and soft palate.

With *cleft palate*, nasopharyngeal incompetence may be present along with resultant nasal air leak during speech.

Tongue. Inspect the tongue, including the dorsum (top surface), sides, and underneath. Note papillae on the dorsum, small anterior, and large posterior. Ask the patient to stick out the tongue (Fig. 17-19). Although generally not done during a screening assessment, the gag reflex may be tested. Gently place a tongue blade on the posterior dorsum to produce the gag reflex, which ensures function of the hypoglossal nerve (CN XII).

Tongue may have lesions or ulcers. *Geographic tongue* (Fig. 17-20) tends to occur in people with allergic disease, but has no significant pathology. A white coating of the tongue may be oral candidiasis. This condition is very common in patients taking antibiotics. See Table 17-10 at the end of this chapter.

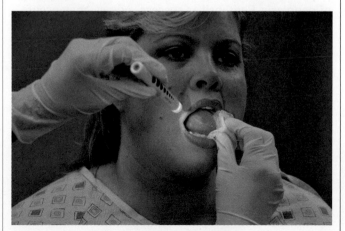

Figure 17.19 Sticking out the tongue.

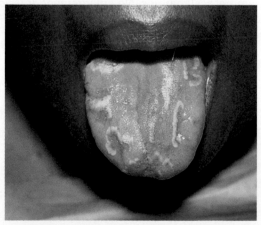

Figure 17.20 Geographic tongue.

(text continues on page 426)

Wharton Ducts and Salivary Flow. Inspect Wharton ducts in the floor of the mouth. Evaluate salivary flow from the submandibular salivary gland. *Buccal mucosa and soft and hard palates are pink with no lesions. Gingiva is pink and moist without inflammation. Breath has no foul odor. Tongue is smooth and midline. Teeth are well aligned with no evidence of decay. Uvula rises symmetrically with "ah." Ducts are smooth without inflammation.*

Swelling or redness of Wharton duct suggests inflammation of the submandibular gland (Fig. 17-21). No upward movement of the uvula when the patient says "ah" indicates dysfunction of CN X. Infection in the floor of the mouth may produce *Ludwig angina* (Wax, 2004).

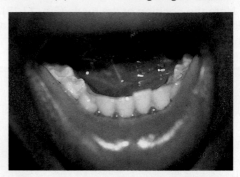

Figure 17.21 Swollen and red Wharton's ducts.

Swelling may occur with mumps, blockage of a duct, abscess, or tumor. Duct obstruction can occur as a result of aging, dehydration, or use of anticholinergics.

Palpation. Palpate the parotid, submandibular, and sublingual glands for swelling or tenderness (see Chapter 14). *There is no swelling or tenderness.*

Palpation of the mouth is usually completed as part of a specialty assessment. If performed, place a gloved hand inside the cheek to assess Stensen duct in the buccal mucosa opposite the second molars and Wharton duct. Assess these areas for a stone or growth. Palpate for any lesions. *Ducts are soft and nontender without lesions.*

A firm area at either Stensen or Wharton duct may represent a stone or growth. Lesions of oral mucosa may indicate a growth. Examination with biopsy or radiological films may be recommended for oral lesions. When palpating masses, hard fixed lesions have a higher incidence of cancer. Soft, mobile lesions are more often cysts or benign disease.

Throat

Inspection. Pressing down slightly with the tongue blade on the midpoint of the tongue, visualize the pharynx, tonsils, soft palate, and anterior and posterior tonsillar pillars. Note color, symmetry, enlargement, and any lesions. The tonsils are in the back of the oropharynx between the anterior and posterior pillars. The tissue appears more granular and less smooth than the surrounding mucous membranes. *Tissue is pink and moist with symmetrical margins. No enlargement or lesions are noted.* Grade the tonsils using the scale in Box 17-1. *Tonsils are absent or 1+.*

Mucosal inflammation may indicate *infection* or allergy. Hypertrophy of tonsils occurs with persistent recurrent infection. Frequent infections may leave superficial scars or crypts (Fig. 17-22). These crypts may collect food and oral debris, appearing as white curd-like material embedded in the tonsil mucosa. Generally, with chronic tonsillitis and hypertrophy, findings are symmetrical. Asymmetrical tonsillar enlargement raises suspicion of *neoplasia*. Peritonsillar abscess, *quinsy*, may occur with collection of fluid in the anterior tonsillar pillar

---

BOX 17.1 TONSILLAR GRADING SCALE

- 1+ tonsil obstructs 0%–25% to midline
- 2+ tonsil obstructs 25%–50% to midline
- 3+ tonsil obstructs 50%–75% to midline
- 4+ tonsil obstructs 75%–100% to midline

Source: Newland, D. (2003). Pediatric otolaryngology. In M. Layland & T. Lin (Eds.), *The Washington manual survival guide series. Otolaryngology survival guide* (pp. 153–166). Philadelphia: Lippincott Williams & Wilkins.

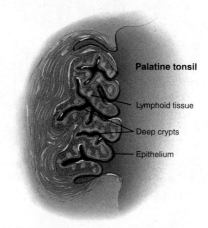

Palatine tonsil

Lymphoid tissue

Deep crypts

Epithelium

Figure 17.22 Tonsillar crypts with debris.

(Fig. 17-23). This presents as a sore throat with increasing unilateral pain, deviated uvula, hot potato voice, dysphagia, and trismus (inability to open jaw; Wax, 2004). Sleep apnea should be suspected with a squeezed appearance of the general proportion of the throat. Strep throat presents with red and white patches in the throat, difficulty swallowing, tender or swollen glands (lymph nodes) in the neck, or red and enlarged tonsils.

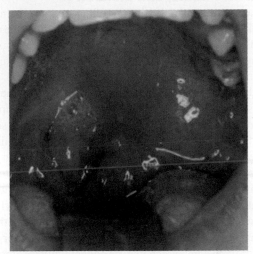

Figure 17.23 Peritonsillar abscess.

Palpation. An APRN will find palpation of the neck helpful to assess inflammatory and other changes that may occur in the throat. Anterior and posterior cervical chain lymph nodes and submental areas are palpated as part of a normal neck examination (see Chapter 14). *Nodes are symmetrical, soft, and nontender.*

Lymph nodes are quick to respond to inflammation and slow to resolve. Inflammation causes enlargement of the anterior, posterior, or submental lymph nodes of the neck. Soft and tender enlargement may accompany minor inflammation. Hard fixed nodes should be further evaluated by biopsy or radiologic films for cancer.

Swallowing Evaluation

Evaluation of swallowing is a technique typically performed by a speech therapist, APRN, or physician. Assess ability to swallow by positioning the thumbs and index finger on the patient's laryngeal protuberance. Ask the patient to swallow; feel the larynx elevate. Ask the patient to cough. Patients can aspirate even if they have an intact gag reflex (Nettina, 2006). Observe for signs associated with swallowing problems: coughing; choking; spitting of food; drooling; difficulty handling oral secretions; double or major delay in swallowing; watering eyes; nasal discharge; wet or gurgly voice; decreased ability to move tongue and lips, chew food, or move food to the back of mouth; pocketing of food; and slow or scanning speech (Nettina, 2006). *Swallowing takes <1 second with no sign of aspiration.*

Patients with *stroke*, *head injury*, or other neuromuscular disorders are at risk for dysphagia. Swallowing problems are common in hospitalized patients and may prolong length of stay because of an inability to obtain adequate nutrition for healing. Dysphagia may be from a growth in the airway or enlargement of surrounding glands or tissue. Dysphagia may be secondary to *GERD*, which should be suspected when inflammation of the larynx is visualized on indirect or direct view. Aspiration into the larynx may be observed with incomplete closure of vocal cords or impeded movement of the epiglottis.

Documentation of Normal Findings

Nose appears symmetrical, midline, and proportionally shaped to facial features. Skin surface is smooth without lesions; coloration is consistent with other facial complexion. Sinus areas are symmetrical with no redness or swelling. Lips are pink and moist with no lesions. Buccal mucosa, soft and hard palates are pink with no lesions. Gingiva is pink and moist without inflammation. Breath has no foul odor. Tongue is smooth and midline. Teeth are well aligned with no evidence of decay. Uvula rises symmetrically with "ah." Ducts are smooth without inflammation. Mouth is pink and moist with symmetrical margins. Tonsils are absent. *C. Bond, RN*

Lifespan Considerations

Pregnant Women
Increased nasal congestion may occur in response to hormonal fluctuations. Increased nosebleeds may be secondary to increased congestion. Gum hypertrophy may also occur. Localized gingival enlargement may lead to a tumor-like mass known as **epulis** forming on the gums (Fig. 17-24).

Newborns, Infants, and Children
The nasal and oral examination in infants and small children can be difficult; the APRN commonly performs it in the clinic setting. Having the parent hold the child may calm him or her. Coaching the parent to hold the child's head and restrain the arms can be helpful and less threatening to the child. With the child sitting on the parent's lap facing the examiner, the parent uses one hand to hold the child's head, while using the other arm to restrain the child's arms and one leg to secure the child's legs (see Chapter 14). If the child is unwilling to open the mouth, gently closing the nostrils will result in an open mouth for air within seconds. Use of flavored tongue blades may encourage small children to cooperate with the examination. Examiners can encourage children to growl "like a lion" to afford a thorough view of the oral cavity and throat.

Special pediatric considerations include checking for competency of the palate, which may be congenitally incompetent in the case of a cleft palate. Infants may have small white bumps or **milia** across the bridge of the nose (Fig 17-25). These self-limiting superficial cysts contain keratinous material and exfoliate on their own. Older children with allergies may develop a traverse ridge across the bridge of the nose from habitually performing the "**allergic salute**," (Fig. 17-26) an upward rubbing of the external nose induced by itching.

Examining the nose of children is best accomplished by gently pressing upward on the tip of the nose and visualizing the interior nares with the bright light from an otoscope. Assessing nasal breathing should include feeling for symmetrical airflow from each nostril. Holding a laryngeal mirror beneath the nose should demonstrate fogging from both nostrils. Congenital **choanal atresia** may be present when one nostril is not patent. This condition can present early in infancy as an emergency or may go undetected into adolescence. When suspected, a

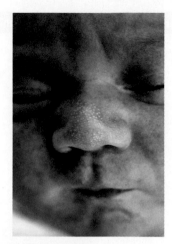

Figure 17.25 Milia.

small red rubber catheter can be passed through each nostril. Inability to pass the catheter suggests choanal atresia. Nasal flaring or narrowing of the nose with inspiration is an indicator of respiratory distress. Foul odor or unilateral thick nasal mucus suggests a foreign body in the nose. A normal finding in infants is the formation of a small pad of tissue in the middle of the upper lip known as the **sucking tubercle**.

Note age-appropriate eruption of teeth. For children younger than 2 years, the child's age in months minus the number 6 should equal the number of deciduous teeth (Hockenberry & Wilson, 2007). After 2½ years, all 20 deciduous teeth should be present. Tetracycline ingestion by the child or maternal ingestion in the last trimester of pregnancy may result in discoloration of an infant's teeth. Ingestion of excessive iron may cause a green or black discoloration of the teeth (Newland, 2003). Discoloration of the tooth enamel with plaque is a sign of poor dental hygiene. Brown spots in the crevices of the tooth may be caries (cavities).

Mobility of the tongue should extend to the alveolar ridge. **Ankyloglossia** (short lingual frenulum) may be congenital, restricting movement of the tongue and subsequently speech. An extremely narrow, flat roof or a high-arched palate affects placement of the tongue and can cause speech and feeding problems (Hockenberry & Wilson, 2007). A high arch may

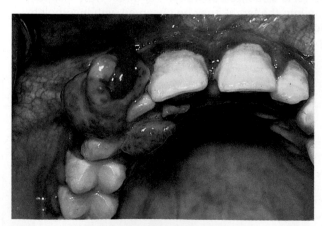

Figure 17.24 Epulis in pregnancy.

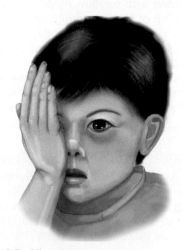

Figure 17.26 Allergic salute.

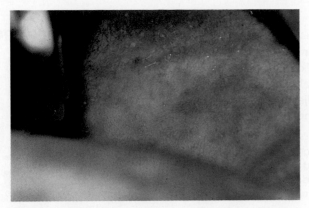

Figure 17.27 Koplik spots.

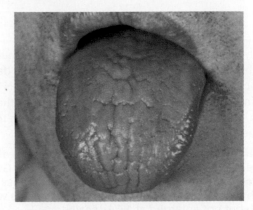

Figure 17.29 Smooth glossy tongue.

also develop in chronic mouth breathers with hypertrophy of adenoids or allergic disorders.

Bednar aphthae are ulcerative abrasions on the posterior hard palate that result from hard sucking. **Epstein pearls**, appearing as small, white, glistening, pearly papules along the median border of the hard palate and gums, are a normal finding in newborns. They represent small retention cysts that dissipate in the first few weeks of life. A maculopapular rash on the buccal mucosa that occurs within 24 hours of fever, inflammation of the nasal mucous membrane accompanied by nasal discharge (coryza), and cough are symptoms of **rubeola measles** The rash, known as **Koplik spots**, appears as grains of salt on an erythematous base on the buccal mucosa opposite the first and second molars (Fig. 17-27) (Bickley, 2009).

Tonsils are not visible in newborns but gradually enlarge in toddlers. Tonsils remain proportionally large in small children and decrease in size as they mature. After puberty the tonsils proportionally decrease in size and are typically small in adults (see Box 17-1).

Chromosomal disorders may result in major multisystem problems, some affecting the mouth, nose, and throat. Trisomy 21, **Down syndrome**, occurs in 1 in 800 to 1,000 live births with multiple-system involvement (Burns, 2000). Mouth, nose, and throat involvement in Down syndrome includes a protruding tongue and flat nasal bridge.

Older Adult

Loss of subcutaneous fat may cause the nose to appear more prominent in older adults. **Edentulous** (without any teeth)

older adults may develop a pursed-lip appearance as mouth and cheeks fold inward. Overclosure of the mouth may lead to maceration of the skin at the corners of the mouth; this condition is called **angular cheilitis** (Fig. 17-28) (Bickley, 2008). Teeth may appear yellow as worn enamel reveals the dentin layer. They also may appear larger as the gums recede. Teeth may loosen with bone resorption and move with palpation.

The tongue and buccal mucosa may appear smoother and shiny from papillary atrophy and thinning of the buccal mucosa. This condition is called **smooth, glossy tongue** (Fig. 17-29) and may result from deficiencies of riboflavin, folic acid, and vitamin B_{12} (Bickley, 2008). **Fissures** may appear in the tongue with increasing age. This condition, called **scrotal tongue** (Fig. 17-30), can become inflamed with the accumulation of food or debris in the fissures. An oral health screening tool is available that includes assessment of the lymph nodes, tissue inside the cheek, floor, and roof of the mouth, gums between the teeth or under dentures, saliva, condition of teeth, and oral cleanliness (Chalmers, et al., 2005).

🌐 Cultural Considerations

The nasal bridge may be flat in African American and Asians. In dark-skinned patients the gums are more deeply colored and a brownish ridge is often found along the gumline (Hockenberry & Wilson, 2007). An increased risk of nasopharyngeal cancer is noted with Chinese or Asian ancestry.

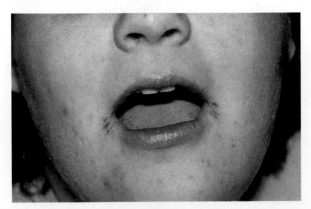

Figure 17.28 Angular cheilitis.

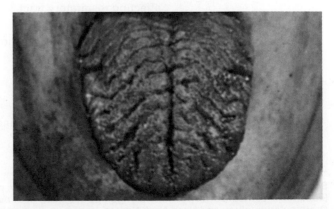

Figure 17.30 Scrotal tongue.

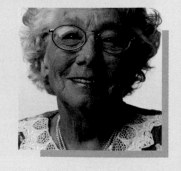

Ihe nurse has just finished conducting a physical examination of Mrs. Davis, the 89-year-old woman admitted with pneumonia 13 days ago. Unlike the samples of normal documentation previously charted, Mrs. Davis has abnormal findings. Review the following important findings revealed in each of the steps of objective data collection for her. Consider how these results compare with the normal findings presented in the samples of normal documentation.

Inspection: Lips pale and dry with large amounts of crusting. No ulcers or lesions. Teeth yellowed and slightly crusted. Correct occlusion. Gums pale and intact. Tongue and buccal mucosa with cheesy, white coating that scrapes off. Area under tongue is dry but smooth without lesions. Posterior palate also has white cheesy coating. Tonsils pink and smooth but not enlarged at 1+/4+ scale.

Palpation: No masses, lesions, or tenderness.

J. Tsang, RN

Evidence-based Critical Thinking

Common Laboratory and Diagnostic Testing—

Laboratory studies of blood or other body fluids can give measures that are helpful in constructing a diagnosis. An elevated white blood count suggests infection, such as sinusitis. Nasalsinus cultures can help with identification of bacteria type. Biopsies provide tissue to determine if cancer is present. Examination of clear nasal discharge for beta-2-transferrin can identify cerebrospinal fluid in the nose. Throat culture can identify the type of bacteria producing tonsillitis or pharyngitis. Nasal and oral findings also may be evidence of systemic disease (Table 17-5).

Table 17.5	Nasal and Oral Findings in Systemic Disease	
Disease	**Etiology**	**Nasal Findings**
Churg-Strauss syndrome	Vasculitis	Nasal crusting and polyps
Sjögren syndrome	Chronic inflammatory disorder characterized by decreased lacrimal and salivary gland secretion	Atrophy and drying of oral and nasal mucosa; may lead to epistaxis
Pemphigus-pemphigoid	Autoimmune disorder	Blister formation on external nose or anterior septum
Scleroderma	Systemic sclerosis from abnormal collagen synthesis	**Telangiectasias** of nasal mucosa with no cilia
Bechet disease	Chronic inflammatory disorder	Oral ulceration, rhinorrhea, rhinalgia, apthous ulceration of nose or nasopharynx that heals without scarring
Sarcoidosis	Noncaseating inflammatory disorder	Engorgement of turbinates with papules or nodules on septum
Wegner granulomatosis	Necrotizing granulomatous vasculitis affecting respiratory tract, kidneys, and peripheral vessels	Nasal crusting, ulcerations, epistaxis, chronic rhinosinusitis, septal perforations
Syphilis	Sexually transmitted infection	Primary 3–4 weeks after contact, ulceration in vestibule of nose or septum; secondary lesions after primary fades; tertiary nasal septal swelling may develop into perforation
Tuberculosis	Mycobacterial infection	Nasal crusting, mucosal ulcerations
Cystic fibrosis	Inherited absence of exocrine glands	Copious, thick, viscous mucus that blocks airways; chronic rhinosinusitis; nasal polyps
AIDS	HIV	Nasal ulcerations, lesions, Kaposi sarcoma

Source: Higgins, T., LeGrand, M., & Rudy, S. (2008). Nasal cavity, paranasal sinuses and nasopharynx. In L. Harris & M. Huntoon (Eds.), *Core curriculum for otorhinolaryngology and head-neck nursing* (2nd ed., p. 183). New Smyrna Beach, FL: Society of Otorhinolaryngology and Head-Neck Nurses, Inc.

Diagnostic testing for allergic sensitivity is helpful in managing persistent upper-respiratory inflammation. Allergy testing may be performed via skin or blood. Various approaches to allergy skin testing include percutaneous or prick testing and intradermal testing. A blending of both types of skin testing is performed typically when evaluating upper-respiratory conditions. Radioallergosorbent testing (RAST) is a blood test that measures allergen-specific IgE antibody, which is elevated in reaction to allergens to which the patient is sensitive (Emanuel, 2002).

Radiographic studies are helpful in diagnosing chronic sinusitis. Plain film x-rays may be used in acute sinusitis. The gold standard radiological film in evaluating chronic sinusitis is CT scan. Note the detail provided by the sinus CT scan over plain x-ray views. CT scans or MRI films are helpful is evaluating masses and lesions of the upper-respiratory tract. Routine dental x-rays improve early detection of dental carries.

Biopsy is performed on lesions of uncertain behavior for tissue diagnosis. This can be accomplished by fine-needle aspiration in some situations. Other lesions may warrant an incisional biopsy.

Sleep studies are available to assess sleep apnea. Patients spend the night in a sleep laboratory and are monitored for breathing, heart monitoring, oxygen saturation, and excessive leg movements.

Diagnostic Reasoning

Nursing Diagnosis, Outcomes, and Interventions

When formulating a nursing diagnosis, it is important to use critical thinking to cluster data and identify patterns that fit together. The nurse compares these data clusters with defining characteristics (abnormal findings) for the diagnosis to ensure the most accurate labeling and appropriate interventions. Table 17-6 provides a comparison of nursing diagnoses, abnormal findings, and interventions commonly related to nose, mouth, sinus, and throat assessment (NANDA-I, 2009).

Some outcomes commonly related to nose, mouth, sinus, and throat problems include the following:

- The patient's oral mucous membranes are pink and intact.
- Patient swallows with evidence of aspiration.
- Patient states breathing is more comfortable and less congested (Moorhead, et al., 2007).

Once outcomes are established, nursing care is implemented to improve the status of the patient. The nurse uses critical thinking and evidence-based practice to develop the interventions. Some examples of nursing interventions for the nose, mouth, sinuses, and throat are as follows:

- Provide oral hygiene every 8 hours.
- Consult with a speech therapist to evaluate swallowing.
- Push fluids to 2 L to liquefy secretions (Bulechek, et al., 2007).

Table 17.6	Common Nursing Diagnoses Associated with the Nose, Sinuses, Mouth, and Throat		
Diagnosis and Related Factors	**Point of Differentiation**	**Assessment Characteristics**	**Nursing Interventions**
Impaired dentition	Disease, disruption, trauma, or other factors that cause problems in development, eruption, or structural integrity of teeth	Malocclusion, tooth pain, caries, plaque, halitosis, premature loss of teeth, tooth fracture	Teach toothbrusing and flossing. Provide assistance as needed. Perform mouth care if patient is unable to do so independently.
Altered oral mucous membrane	Break in the integrity of the tissues of the lips, soft tissues of the oral cavity, or both	Dry mouth, oral lesions, aphthous ulcers, coated tongue, vesicles, nodules, patches	Provide fluids and mouth care. Moisturize mucous membranes. Treat infections.*
Impaired swallowing	Associated with oral, pharyngeal, or esophageal structure or function	Delayed swallowing, gurgly voice, frequent coughing, choking or gagging, inability to clear oral cavity, food falling from mouth	Evaluate swallowing ability. Provide sips of fluids before giving dry foods. Elevate head of bed. Thicken liquids if needed.
Altered breathing pattern	Respirations that fail to produce significant ventilation	Nasal flaring, dyspnea, orthopnea	Use tissues to clear upper airway. Elevate head of bed. Give frequent fluids to liquefy secretions.

*Collaborative interventions.

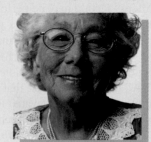

Remember Mrs. Davis, whose problems have been outlined throughout this chapter. Initial subjective and objective data collection is complete, and the nurse has spent time reviewing the findings and other results. The following nursing note illustrates how subjective and objective data are collected and analyzed and nursing interventions are developed.

Subjective: "My mouth is dry."

Objective: Lips pale and dry with large amounts of crusting. No ulcers or lesions. Teeth yellowed and slightly crusted. Correct occlusion. Gums pale and intact. Tongue and buccal mucosa with cheesy, white coating that scrapes off. Area under tongue is dry, but smooth without lesions. Posterior palate also has white cheesy coating. Tonsils pink and smooth but not enlarged at 1+/4+ scale. No masses, lesions, or tenderness palpated.

Analysis: Altered oral mucous membranes related to xerostoma, infrequent oral care, and possible infection.

Plan: Performed oral hygiene with positive results. Large reduction in crusting and mucous membranes now pink. White coating remains on tongue and buccal mucosa. Contact primary health care provider to evaluate for a possible infection. Continue oral hygiene every shift.

J. Tsang, RN

Critical Thinking Challenge

- Why did the RN decide to focus the SOAP on the status of the patient's mucous membranes rather than on the patient's diagnosis of pneumonia?
- What other effects might poor oral hygiene have on the patient's body systems?
- What data made the nurse suspect that there might be an associated infection?

Collaboration with Other Health Care Providers

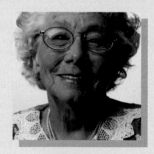

The nurse suspects that Mrs. Davis has a yeast infection (*Candida albicans*) in her mouth. Treatment requires a prescription medication. Therefore, the nurse will need to notify the primary care provider. The following conversation illustrates how the nurse might organize the data and make recommendations about the patient's situation to the provider.

Situation: I'm Jen Tsang, and I've been caring for Mrs. Davis today. She is an 89-year-old woman admitted 13 days ago with pneumonia.

Background: She's been on antibiotics for most of her stay here, which has been complicated with multiple infections and a 4-day stay in the ICU.

Assessment: When I performed oral care on her today, I noticed a white coating on her tongue. I was able to clean off most of the crusts and moisturize her lips, but the white coating remains. She doesn't have any lesions but she said that her tongue is quite tender and it got quite red when I tried to scrape off the coating.

Recommendations: I was thinking that she might have a fungal infection from the antibiotics and wonder if you could order a medication to swish and swallow in her mouth. Thanks so much.

J. Tsang, RN

Critical Thinking Challenge

- What information did the nurse decide not to include in the conversation and why?
- What risk factors does Mrs. Davis have for *C. albicans*?
- How can the nurse ensure that oral hygiene becomes one of the priorities in care?

Pulling It All Together: Reflection and Critical Thinking

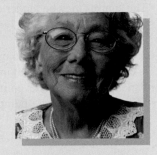

The nurse uses assessment data to formulate a nursing care plan with patient outcomes and interventions for Mrs. Davis. The nurse uses critical thinking and judgment to continue or revise the diagnosis, outcomes, or interventions. This is often in the form of a care plan or case note similar to the one below.

Nursing Diagnosis	Patient Outcomes	Nursing Interventions	Rationale	Evaluation
Altered oral mucous membrane	Oral mucous membranes pink, moist, and without coating, lesions, or masses	Encourage fluids. Provide oral care every shift. Obtain order for medication. After oral care, have patient swish and swallow medication.*	Fluids will keep the membranes moist. Provide fluids, then oral care, and then medication last to allow the medication time in the oral cavity to work.	Patient with no crusts or dryness in mouth. States oral cavity and lips are more comfortable. Approximately half of coating on tongue is present. Continue with care.

*Collaborative intervention.

Applying Your Knowledge

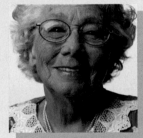

Using the previous steps of diagnostic reasoning, organizing, and prioritizing, consider all the case study findings woven throughout this chapter. When answering the following questions, begin drawing conclusions and see how the pieces of assessment must work together to create an environment for personalized, appropriate, and accurate care.

- The mucous membranes reflect the health of other body systems. What body systems are affecting the health of Mrs. Davis's oral mucous membranes?
- Why is it especially important for nurses to inspect the mouths of hospitalized patients?
- How might improvement in the patient's mouth affect her rehabilitation and functional abilities?

Key Points

- The nose, sinuses, and throat are parts of the upper airway.
- The mouth and throat are parts of the upper gastrointestinal tract.
- The nose is the primary organ of smell.
- The mouth is the primary organ of taste.
- Kiesselbach plexus is the most common site of expistaxis.
- The pharyngeal fossa is the most common site of oral cancer.
- The highly vascular floor of the mouth is a good location for absorption of sublingual medications.

- Tonsillitis is inflammation of the tonsils; their removal does not increase risk for infection.
- Dental care is lacking in vulnerable groups.
- Acute airway obstruction requires immediate intervention.
- Risk factors for nose, mouth, sinus, and throat problems include topical decongestant use, smoking, inhaling substances and chemicals, allergies, and dust exposure.
- Common symptoms in the nose, sinuses, mouth, and throat include facial pain, sleep apnea, obstructive breathing, nasal congestion, epistaxis, halitosis, anosmia, cough, pharyngitis, dental pain, dysphagia, hoarseness, and oral lesions.

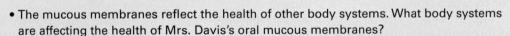

- The nose is normally symmetrical, midline, and proportional to facial features.
- The sinuses may be tender or full with infection.
- Fordyce granules are insignificant sebaceous cysts or salivary tissue.
- A white coating of the tongue may be oral candidiasis and is common in patients taking antibiotics.
- Patients can aspirate even if they have an intact gag reflex.
- Milia are small white bumps across the bridge of the nose in infants.
- After age 2½ years, all 20 deciduous teeth should be present.
- Epstein pearls are small white glistening pearly papules normally found in newborns.
- Fissures may appear in the tongue with increased age.

Review Questions

1. Which of the following is part of the upper gastrointestinal tract?
   A. Nasal septum
   B. Sinuses
   C. Throat
   D. Adenoids

2. The nurse is assessing the nares to evaluate the site of epistaxis. The most common site of bleeding is which of the following?
   A. Osteomeatal complex
   B. Nasal septum
   C. Kesselbach plexus
   D. Woodruff plexus

3. The nurse knows that the floor of the mouth is highly vascular so it is a good location for which of the following?
   A. Absorption of sublingual medications
   B. Identification of malignancy in the pharyngeal fossa
   C. Considering an infection with streptococcus
   D. Aspiration even if the gag reflex is present

4. Acute airway obstruction is a situation that should be
   A. reassessed during the next visit
   B. evaluated within 8 hours
   C. further assessed thoroughly
   D. quickly assessed and treated

5. Risk factors for nose, sinus, mouth, and throat problems include
   A. topical decongestant use, smoking, and allergies
   B. smoking, allergies, and high blood cholesterol
   C. allergies, high blood cholesterol, and topical decongestant use
   D. high blood cholesterol, topical decongestant use, and smoking

6. The nurse has assessed the nose and documents normal findings as
   A. nose asymmetrical with clear drainage
   B. nose symmetrical and midline
   C. nose asymmetrical and proportional to facial features
   D. nose symmetrical with yellow drainage

7. The nurse is assessing a patient who has been taking antibiotics for 10 days. Oral assessment is important because of the increased risk for which of the following?
   A. Fordyce granules
   B. Pharyngitis
   C. Anosmia
   D. *C. albicans*

8. An adolescent male presents with complaints of nosebleeds. The nurse would further assess for
   A. hemangioma
   B. nasal trauma
   C. angiofibroma
   D. cystic fibrosis

9. The nurse assesses the child with purulent unilateral nasal discharge. The nurse knows that the most likely causative factor is
   A. allergic rhinitis
   B. choanal atresia
   C. foreign body in nose
   D. cystic fibrosis

10. During routine physical examination of a 20-year-old woman, the nurse notes a septal perforation. This finding may be significant for which of the following causes?
    A. Illicit drug use
    B. Nose picking
    C. Nasal trauma
    D. Bifid uvula

References

Andresen, H., Hickey, M., Higgins, T., et al. (2008). Normal anatomy and physiology. In L. Harris & M. Huntoon (Eds.), *Core curriculum for otorhinolaryngology and head-neck nursing* (2nd ed., pp. 41–77). New Smyrna Beach, Florida: Society of Otorhinolaryngology and Head-Neck Nurses, Inc.

Barnes, L. (2000). *Surgical pathology of the head and neck* (2nd ed.). Revised

Bent, S. (2008). Herbal medicine in the United States: Review of efficacy, safety, and regulation: Grand rounds at University of California, San Francisco Medical Center. *Journal of General Internal Medicine, 23*(6), 854–859.

Bickley, L. S. (2009). *Bates' guide to physical examination and history taking* (10th ed.). Philadelphia: Lippincott Williams & Wilkins.

Bulechek, G. B., Butcher, H. K., & McCloskey Dochterman, J. (2007). *Nursing Interventions Classification (NIC)* (4th ed.) St. Louis: Mosby.

Burns, C. (2000). Genetic disorders. In C. Burns, M. Brady, A. Dunn, & N. Starr (Eds.), *Pediatric primary care: A handbook for nurse practitioners* (2nd ed., pp. 1260–1282). Philadelphia: W. B. Saunders.

Burzynski, J., & Schluger, N. W. (2008). The epidemiology of tuberculosis in the United States. *Seminars in Respiratory Critical Care Medicine, 29*(5), 492–498. Epub 2008 Sep 22.

Chalmers, J. M., King, P. L., Spencer, A. J., et al. (2005). The oral health assessment tool – Validity and reliability. *Australian Dental Journal, 50*(3), 191–199.

Derebery, J., & Berliner, K. (2002). Allergic disease and the middle ear. In J. Krouse, S. Chadwick, S. Gordon, & J. Dereberry (Eds.), *Allergy and immunology: An otolaryngic approach*. Philadelphia, PA: Lippincott Williams & Wilkins.

Emanuel, I. (2002). In vitro testing for allergens. In J. Krouse, S. Chadwick, S. Gordon, & J. Dereberry (Eds.), *Allergy and immunology: An otolaryngic approach* (pp. 124–133). Philadelphia: Lippincott Williams & Wilkins.

Epstein, J. (2007–2008). Oral malignancies associated with HIV, JCDA,www.cda-adc.ca/jcda December 2007-January 2008, Vol73, no10. Retrieved April 2008.

Healthy People 2010: What are its goals? (n.d.). Retrieved February 15, 2008, from http://www.healthypeople.gov/About goals.htm.

Higgins, T., LeGrand, M., & Rudy, S. (2008). Nasal cavity, paranasal sinuses and nasopharynx. In L. Harris & M. Huntoon (Eds.), *Core curriculum for otorhinolaryngology and head-neck nursing* (2nd ed., p. 183). New Smyrna Beach, FL: Society of Otorhinolaryngology and Head-Neck Nurses, Inc.

Hockenberry, M. J., & Wilson, D. (2007). *Wong's nursing care of infants and children*. St. Louis: Elsevier.

Landis, S. H., Murray, T., Bolden, S., et al. (1999). Cancer statistics, 1999. *CA: A Cancer Journal for Clinicians, 49*, 8–31.

Langlais, R. P., & Miller, C. S. (2002). *Color atlas of common oral diseases*. Philadelphia: Lippincott Williams & Wilkins.

Lloyd, K. B., & Naclerio, R. M. (2008). Strategies for managing nasal congestion. *Post graduate healthcare education*, LLC. Philadelphia: GlaxoSmith Kline.

Mayo Clinic.com. (2007). *Chewing tobacco: Not a risk-free alternative to cigarettes*. Retrieved May 25, 2008, from http://www.nim.nih.gov/medicineplus/smokelesstobacco.hmtl.

Moorhead, S., Johnson, M., & Mass, M. (2007). *Nursing Outcomes Classification (NOC)* (4th ed.). Philadelphia: Mosby.

Mungia, R., Cano, S. M., Johnson, D. A., Dang, H., & Brown, J. P. (2008). Interaction of age and specific saliva component output on caries. *Aging Clinical and Experimental Research, 20*(6), 503–508.

Nandapalan, V., Watson, I. D., & Swift, A. C. (1996). Beta-2-transferrin and cerebrospinal fluid rhinorrhea. *Clinical Otolaryngology Allied Science, 3*, 259–264.

NCCAM. (2008). *Herbs at a glance. National center for complimentary and alternative medicine*. Washington, DC: National Institute of Health.

Nettina, S. M. (2006). *Lippincott manual of nursing practice* (8th ed.). Philadelphia: Lippincott Williams & Wilkins.

NIH, SEER. (1999). *Cancer statistics review 1973–1996*. Retrieved April 6, 2009, from http://www.seer.ims.nci.nih.gov/Publications/CSR1973_1996>June.

Newland, D. (2003). Pediatric otolaryngology. In M. Layland & T. Lin (Eds.), *The Washington manual survival guide series. Otolaryngology survival guide* (pp. 153–166). Philadelphia: Lippincott Williams & Wilkins.

North American Nursing Diagnosis Association. (2009). *Nursing diagnoses, 2009–2011 Edition: Definitions and classifications (NANDA NURSING DIAGNOSIS)*. West Sussex UK: John Wiley & Sons.

Padilla, R., & Ritter, A. (2008). *Talking with patients about meth mouth: Methamphetamine and oral health*. Chapel Hill, NC: Department of Diagnostic Services & General Dentistry, University of North Carolina at Chapel Hill School of Dentistry.

Risk factors and use of preventative services, United States. (2005). Retrieved January 5, 2007, from www.cdc.gov.

U.S. Department of Health & Human Services. (2007). *The health consequences of involuntary exposure to tobacco smoke: A report of the Surgeon General*. Retrieved April 15, 2008, from http://www.sureongeneral.gov/library/secondhandsmoke/factsheets/factsheet2.html.

Wax, M., et al. (2004). *Primary care otolaryngology* (2nd ed.). Washington, DC: American Academy of Otolaryngology—Head and Neck Surgery Foundation.

Woodson, G. (2001). *Ear, nose and throat disorders in primary care*. Philadelphia: W.B. Saunders Company.

Yian, C. (2003). Rhinosinusitis. In M. Layland & T. Lin (Eds.), *The Washington Manual survival guide series. Otolaryngology survival guide*. Philadelphia: Lippincott Willliams & Wilkins.

The Jensen suite offers these additional resources to enhance learning and facilitate understanding of this chapter:

- thePoint on line resource, http//thepoint.lww.com/Jensen1E
- Student CD-ROM included with the book
- *Laboratory Manual for Nursing Health Assessment: A Best Practice Approach*
- *Pocket Guide for Nursing Health Assessment: A Best Practice Approach*

Tables of Abnormal Findings

 Table 17.7   Common Assessment Findings: Nose and Sinuses

Condition	Description and Risk Factors	Findings and Diagnostic Testing
Epistaxis (Nosebleed) 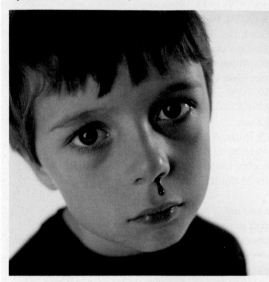 Most commonly involve Kiesselbach plexus in the anterior septum (Little area), which is vulnerable to trauma; also Woodruff plexus under the posterior portion of the inferior turbinate	Increased nasal congestion; dry mucosa; digital manipulation or nose picking; trauma; anticoagulants; foreign bodies; tumors; infection; inflammation; blood or coagulation disorders	*Subjective:* Dry sensation or crusting in nose *Objective:* Prominent vessels, scabs, or crusts on anterior septum; blood in nasal vestibule *Testing:* Consider hemoglobin and hematocrit levels with recurrent nose bleeds. Balloon angiography may locate posterior bleeds; intravascular embolization can occlude vessels.
Rhinitis 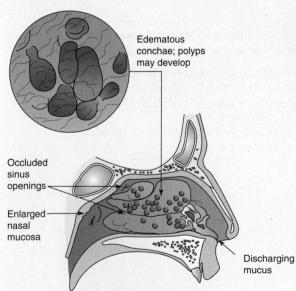 Inflammation of the nasal mucosa; may be subdivided as allergic and nonallergic	Familial or personal atopic disease; exposure to allergens (eg, pollens, dust, mold, animal dander, food) or chemical irritants (eg, smoke); use of illicit drugs; overuse of topical decongestant sprays	*Subjective:* Watery, itchy nose with frequent sneezing and congestion *Objective:* Excessive clear watery nasal drainage; pale blue, boggy, mucosa, or redness and inflammation *Testing:* Specific skin or blood testing known as RAST measures IgE antibody, which is elevated in atopic disease (Emanuel, 2002).

Labels on rhinitis illustration: Edematous conchae; polyps may develop · Occluded sinus openings · Enlarged nasal mucosa · Discharging mucus

Table 17.7   Common Assessment Findings: Nose and Sinuses *(continued)*

Condition	Description and Risk Factors	Findings and Diagnostic Testing
Sinusitis 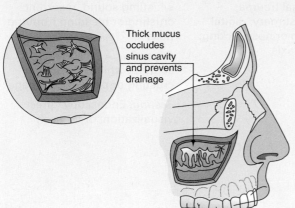 Thick mucus occludes sinus cavity and prevents drainage	Chronic mucosal swelling from allergy, irritants, or chemicals; inflammation secondary to GERD	*Subjective:* Facial pain or pressure, thick nasal discharge, fever, cough, halitosis. *Objective:* Redness and inflammation of nasal mucosa; thick purulent drainage *Testing:* Endoscopic examination of nose; CT scan (gold-standard radiographic tool)
Infection of one or more paranasal sinuses; may be acute or chronic; chronic sinusitis may result in fungal pathology		
Nasal Polyps 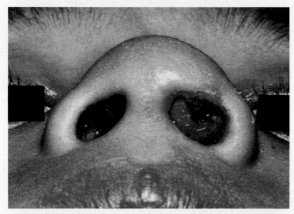	Chronic inflammation of the nose and paranasal sinuses, allergic or chronic rhinitis, asthma, cystic fibrosis, and chronic sinusitis.	*Subjective:* Nasal obstruction and congestion, facial pain and pressure *Objective:* White glistening grape-like structures in the nose that may also fill the sinus cavities *Testing:* Nasal/sinus endoscopy; CT scan
Grapelike swelling of the nasal and sinus mucosa leading to nasal obstruction; often associated with other inflammatory conditions of the nasal mucosa		
Deviated Septum 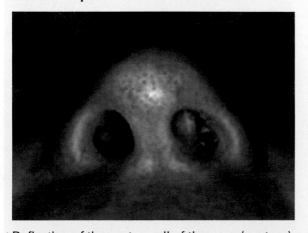	May be congenital or occur with trauma to the nose	*Subjective:* A unilateral decreased ability to breathe through the nose, pressure or headache *Objective:* Narrowing of the nasal chamber *Testing:* Endoscopy of the nose; x-ray or CT scan
Deflection of the center wall of the nose (septum)		

(table continues on page 438)

Table 17.7   Common Assessment Findings: Nose and Sinuses *(continued)*

Condition	Description and Risk Factors	Findings and Diagnostic Testing
Perforated Septum 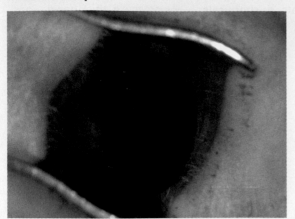 A hole in the nasal septum	Illicit drug use (eg, snorting cocaine); nasal trauma; nasal septal surgery; digital manipulation or nose picking; chronic epistaxis	*Subjective:* Foul odor, whistling sound, recurrent crusting or bleeding from the nose *Objective:* A hole in the septum, which may have crusting or purulent drainage *Testing:* Endoscopy, direct visualization, or CT scan
Foreign Body 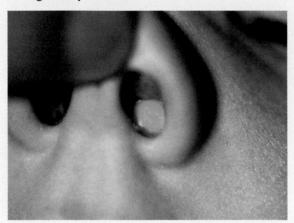 Any object not commonly found in the upper aerodigestive tract	Nasal piercing; deliberately placed objects in nose (as with small children); postsurgical remnant of cotton or gauze	*Subjective:* Unilateral nasal congestion or obstruction *Objective:* Unilateral purulence or thick nasal drainage *Testing:* Endoscopic examination; x-ray of the nose—in small children examination under anesthesia is typically performed with removal of the foreign body

Table 17.8   **Common Assessment Findings: Palate and Throat**

Condition	Risk Factors	Findings and Diagnostic Testing
Cleft Lip/Palate 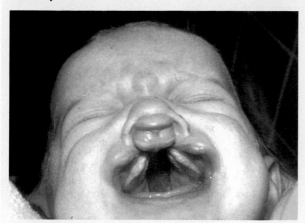 Most common congenital malformation of oral cavity (1 in 1,000 births); an opening or fissure of the lip/alveolus and palate; represents a fusion abnormality of the midfacial skeleton and soft tissues	Native American and Asians ancestry; maternal exposure to phenytoin, methotrexate, cigarette smoke, and alcohol abuse	*Subjective:* Recurrent middle ear and sinus infections; feeding difficulties *Objective:* Lip cleft apparent at birth; notch or full opening on hard palate, soft palate, or both *Testing:* Oral/facial examination
Bifid Uvula 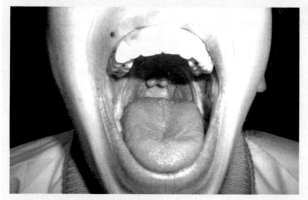 Congenital complete or partial split of uvula; adenoidectomy may be contraindicated	Submucosal cleft palate	*Subjective:* Usually asympyomatic *Objective:* A split or fork visible in uvula *Testing:* Oral examination
Kaposi Sarcoma 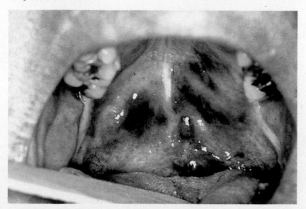 Rapidly proliferating malignancy of the skin or mucous membranes; oral involvement includes the tongue, gingiva, and palate	HIV; 5–10 times greater in male homosexuals infected with HIV than others with the illness (Epstein, 2007–2008)	*Subjective:* Non-healing oral lesions; may complain of facial lymphedema. *Objective:* Bruise-like lesions that form plaques and progress into nodular, red-purple, nonblanching firm lesions. *Testing:* Endoscopic examination of nose; Chest x-ray, CT scan, or MRI for disease surveillance

(table continues on page 440)

Table 17.8   Common Assessment Findings: Palate and Throat *(continued)*

Condition	Risk Factors	Findings and Diagnostic Testing
Acute Tonsillitis or Pharyngitis 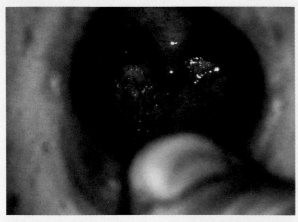 *Pharyngitis:* inflammation of the pharyngeal walls—may include tonsils, palate, uvula *Tonsillitis:* inflammation in lymphoid tissue of oropharynx including Waldeyer ring, palatine or lingual tonsils, pharyngeal bands, nasopharynx, adenoids	Beta-hemolytic streptococcus; may be viral; smoking; mouth breathing	*Subjective:* Sore throat, malaise, anorexia, headache, dysphagia, increased postnasal secretions *Objective:* Infection, redness of pharyngeal walls, exudate, fever, rash; in severe cases, airway obstruction *Testing:* Throat culture; complete blood count (CBC) with differential to determine viral or bacterial
Strep Throat 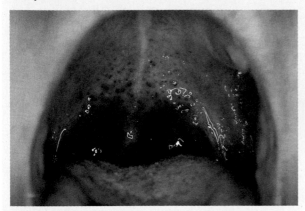 Infection of the tonsils involving streptococcus bacterium	Exposure to infected individuals; smoking	*Subjective:* Sore throat, chills, difficult painful swallowing, headache, laryngitis *Objective:* Infection and enlargement of tonsils; enlargement of jaw and neck lymph nodes *Testing:* Rapid strep swab, throat culture, monospot test, CBC with differential to determine viral or bacterial
Torus Palatinus 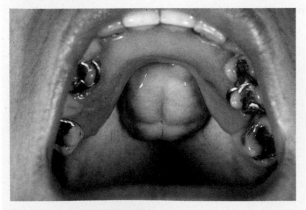 A bony prominence in the middle of the hard palate	Congenital; no clinical significance	*Subjective:* Foul odor, whistling sound, recurrent crusting, or bleeding from the nose *Objective:* A hole in the septum, which may have crusting or purulent drainage *Testing:* Endoscopy, direct visualization, or CT scan

Table 17.9 Common Assessment Findings: Lips and Tongue

Condition	Risk Factors	Findings and Diagnostic Testing
Herpes Simplex Virus 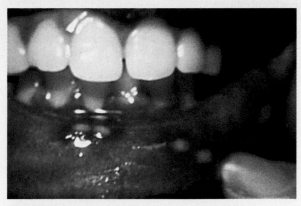 Clear vesicular lesions with indurated base caused by herpes simplex 1 virus	Direct contact with infected person, fever, colds, allergies; may be precipitated by sunlight exposure	*Subjective:* Painful oral lesions; frequently appears at lip–skin juncture *Objective:* Lesions evolve into pustules that rupture, weep, and crust; typical course is 4–10 days *Testing:* Typically none recommended, but may culture with persistent lesions
Aphthous Ulcers (Canker Sores) 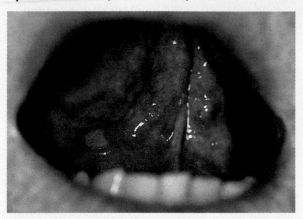 Vesicular oral lesion that evolves into a white ulceration with a red margin	Stress, fatigue, allergies, autoimmune disorders	*Subjective:* Pain at and around site *Objective:* Visible oral lesion(s) *Testing:* Typically not recommended, but may culture in persistent lesions
Candidiasis 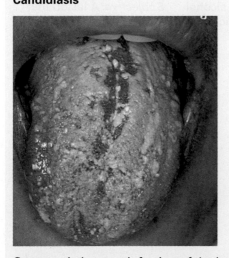 Opportunistic yeast infection of the buccal mucosa and tongue	May occur in newborns; antibiotic or corticosteroid therapy; immunosuppression	*Subjective:* White sticky mucus on tongue or oral mucosa *Objective:* White, cheesy mucus on tongue or buccal mucosa; may scrape mucus off yet tissue is raw and vascular beneath *Testing:* No specific recommendation; consider immune compromise work-up in recurrent infections

(table continues on page 442)

Table 17.9   Common Assessment Findings: Lips and Tongue (continued)

Condition	Risk Factors	Findings and Diagnostic Testing
Leukoplakia 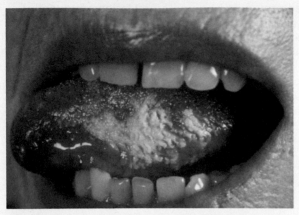 White patchy lesions with well-defined borders	Chronic irritation, smoking, excessive alcohol use	*Subjective:* Persistent oral lesion *Objective:* White lesion firmly attached to mucosal surface; does not scrape off *Testing:* May require biopsy
Black Hairy Tongue 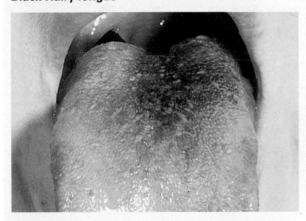 Fungal infection of the tongue involving elongation of the papillae	May follow antibiotic therap; immunocompromised status	*Subjective:* Brown/black hairy coating on tongue *Objective:* Black/brown hairy appearance from elongation of papillae with a painless overgrowth of fungus *Testing:* None reco-mmended
Carcinoma 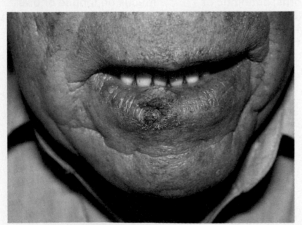 An initially indurated lesion with rolled irregular edges; later may crust or scab but does not heal	Tobacco use, heavy alcohol consumption, chemical exposure	*Subjective:* A lesion that may be painful or limit mobility of the tongue *Objective:* Initially indurated lesion with rolled irregular edges; later appears crusty; possible swelling in adjacent lymph nodes *Testing:* Biopsy

Table 17.10   Common Assessment Findings: Gums and Teeth

Condition	Risk Factors	Findings and Diagnostic Testing
Baby Bottle Tooth Decay 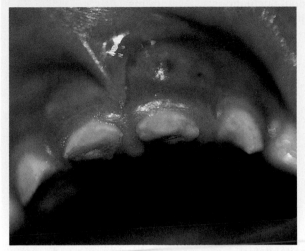Decay of deciduous teeth in older infants and toddlers from pooling of liquid carbohydrate around front teeth; as mouth bacteria act on the carbohydrate, liquid metabolic acid forms that breaks down tooth enamel	Infants taking milk or sweet juice to bed; bottle feeding past 1 year of age	Decay and destruction of upper front teeth *Testing:* Dental x-ray with extensive involvement
Dental Caries 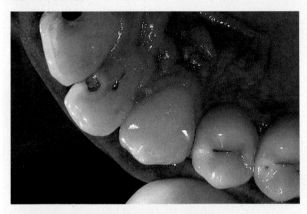Progressive destruction of tooth	Poor oral hygiene	*Subjective:* Early no complaints; with further destruction, pain with hot and cold substances *Objective:* Early may appear chalky white; later becomes brown or black and forms a cavity *Testing:* Dental x-ray
Gingival Hyperplasia 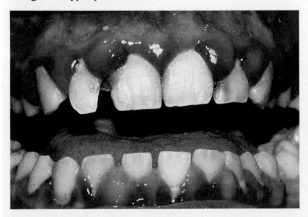Painless enlargement of the gums	May accompany states of hormonal fluctuation (eg, puberty, pregnancy); leukemia; side effect of drugs (eg, phenytoin [Dilantin])	*Subjective:* Swelling of gums *Objective:* Enlargement of gum tissue; may over-reach the teeth *Testing:* Dental x-ray

(table continues on page 444)

Table 17.10 Common Assessment Findings: Gums and Teeth (*continued*)

Condition	Risk Factors	Findings and Diagnostic Testing
Gingivitis 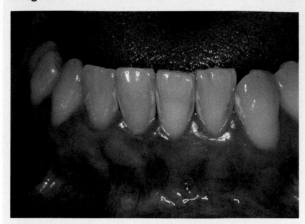 Painful, red, swollen gums	Poor oral hygiene; hormonal fluctuations; vitamin B deficiency	*Subjective:* Sore, bleeding gums *Objective:* Red, swollen, possibly bleeding gums; may involve desquamation of gingival tissue *Testing:* Dental x-ray
Ankyloglossia (Tongue-tie) 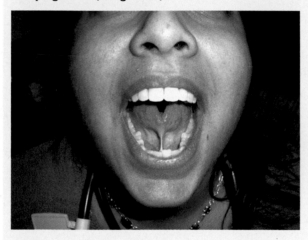 A shortened lingual frenulum	Congenital defect	*Subjective:* Limited movement of tongue; speech disruption, particularly with a, d, and n sounds *Objective:* A tight frenulum fixing the tongue to the floor of mouth *Testing:* None recommended

18

Thorax and Lungs Assessment

Learning Objectives

1 Identify common landmarks on the thorax.

2 Identify the structures and functions of the upper and lower airways.

3 Relate thoracic landmarks to the underlying lung position.

4 Identify teaching opportunities for health promotion and risk reduction related to the thorax and lungs.

5 Differentiate subjective data collected for chest pain, dyspnea, cough, sputum, and wheezing.

6 Collect objective data on skin color, respiratory pattern, chest expansion, and chest shape.

7 Identify normal and abnormal findings in the general survey, inspection, palpation, and percussion of the thorax.

8 Identify normal breath sounds and abnormal sounds including crackles, wheezes, gurgles, and stridor.

9 Use subjective and objective data to analyze respiratory findings and plan interventions.

10 Document and communicate respiratory data using appropriate medical terminology.

11 Individualize respiratory health assessment considering the condition, age, gender, and culture of the patient.

12 Use respiratory assessment findings to identify diagnoses and to initiate a plan of care.

*M*r. Jin, a 65-year-old Chinese man, has come to the clinic today reporting shortness of breath and fatigue. Mandarin is his first language, and he speaks English with a slight accent, well-developed vocabulary, and fluent pacing. He has smoked cigarettes for 49 years. Mr. Jin has a history of congestive heart failure (CHF) and high blood pressure, for which he takes a thiazide diuretic. He states that he uses prescribed albuterol and ipratropium inhalers to improve his breathing.

You will gain more information about Mr. Jin as you progress through this chapter. As you study the content and features, consider Mr. Jin's case and its relationship to what you are learning. Begin thinking about the following points:

- Is Mr. Jin's condition stable, urgent, or an emergency?
- What health promotion and teaching needs are identified? Which two areas are highest priorities?
- How will the nurse focus, organize, and prioritize subjective and objective data collection?
- What nursing diagnosis is the highest priority? Provide rationale.
- How will the nurse individualize assessment to Mr. Jin's specific needs, considering his condition, age, and culture?

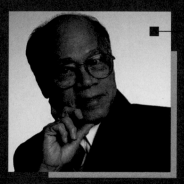

This chapter explores assessment of the thorax and lungs. It reviews pertinent anatomy and physiology related to respiratory and pulmonary function, as well as key variations based on lifespan, culture, and environment. The chapter explores methods for collecting subjective data about risks for pulmonary disease, such as smoking and family history of similar problems. It reviews specific respiratory signs and symptoms, such as shortness of breath and coughing. Content about objective data explains the correct techniques for assessing respiratory patterns, identifying normal and abnormal breath sounds, and labeling findings. Lung auscultation is performed as a screening during the complete physical examination, as well as in ongoing assessments for patients with identified pulmonary problems or diseases. Although challenging, lung auscultation provides information that can assist with accurate diagnosis and related early interventions.

Structure and Function Overview

The respiratory system is separated into the upper and lower divisions. The upper airway warms, moisturizes, and transports air to the lower airway, where oxygenation and ventilation occur.

Understanding the anatomy of the thoracic cage and how to use its landmarks to reference underlying structures when conducting examinations and reporting findings is essential. Knowledge of the placement and divisions of the lungs, other vital organs within the respiratory system, and physiology of respiration enhances the potential for accurate assessments of the thoracic and lung regions.

The Thorax

The thorax is one of the most dynamic regions of the body because it is constantly moving (Moore & Agur, 2007).

See Figure 18-1 for the surface anatomy of the thorax in men and women.

The bony **thoracic cage** includes the sternum and clavicle anteriorly, scapulae and 12 vertebrae posteriorly, and 12 pairs of ribs. The **thoracic cavity** contains the heart, lungs, thymus, distal part of the trachea, and most of the esophagus. The thoracic nerves in the chest (T1–T12) supply a surrounding area of skin horizontally, following the dermatomes (see Chapter 24). The phrenic nerve innervates the diaphragm, and the intercostals nerves innervate the intercostals muscles. The thoracic muscles include the intercostals, transverse thoracic, subcostal, levator costarum, and serratus posterior (Moore & Agur, 2007). Arterial blood supply to the chest is through the thoracic aorta, subclavian artery, brachial artery, and axillary artery; numerous veins return blood to the heart. Each lung has a pulmonary artery that supplies deoxygenated blood for gas exchange, while two pulmonary veins return oxygenated blood to the left side of the heart for circulation to the rest of the body.

To label findings on the thorax, locations must be identified both vertically (up and down) and horizontally (side to side). The ribs provide vertical reference points, while a series of lines provide horizontal reference marks.

Anterior Thoracic Landmarks

The anterior vertical landmarks involve the ribs and their associated interspaces. The easiest place to start is at the **suprasternal (jugular) notch** (Fig. 18-2). This U-shaped depression lies just above the **sternum** and between the clavicles. Place your fingers on your sternum and walk them up to the notch; alternatively, you can lightly feel the trachea and move your fingers down. From the suprasternal notch, walk your fingers down approximately 5 cm to the bony ridge that joins the **manubrium** to the sternum. This ridge, called the **sternal angle** (also known as the **Angle of**

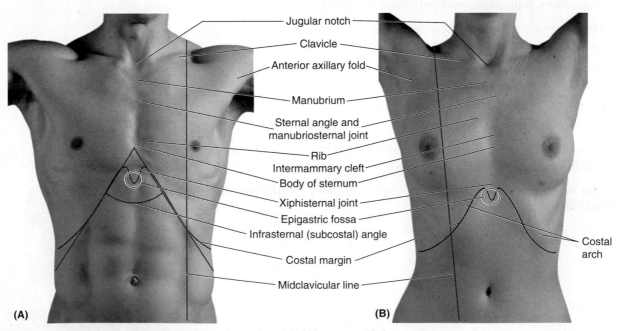

Figure 18.1 Surface anatomy of the thorax in adult **(A)** men and **(B)** women.

Labels: Jugular notch, Clavicle, Anterior axillary fold, Manubrium, Sternal angle and manubriosternal joint, Rib, Intermammary cleft, Body of sternum, Xiphisternal joint, Epigastric fossa, Infrasternal (subcostal) angle, Costal margin, Midclavicular line, Costal arch

(A) (B)

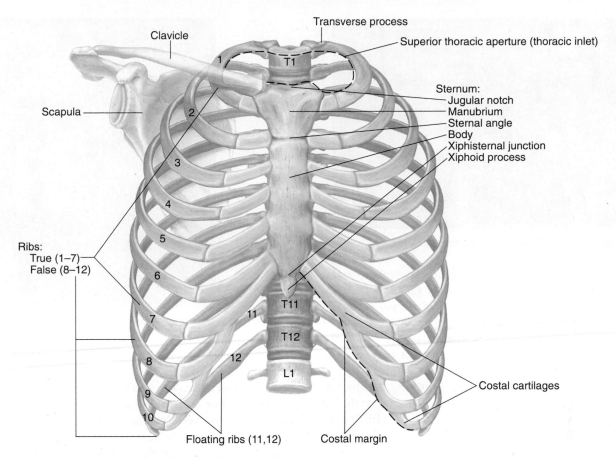

Figure 18.2 Landmarks of the thoracic cage, anterior view.

Louis or **manubriosternal angle**), varies in prominence and is usually easier to locate in thinner people. The sternal angle is continuous with the 2nd rib (Moore & Agur, 2007). It also marks the site of the apex of the heart and the bifurcation of the right and left mainstem bronchi.

Clinical Significance 18-1

The carina, found at the sternal angle, is also the site of the cough reflex. Patients who need nasotracheal suctioning will cough when the nasotracheal tube reaches the carina (approximately the 2nd rib space).

Landmarks are identified on the rib cage by the **intercostal space** (ICS) below each rib. Slide your fingers from the sternal angle over to the 2nd rib, and then down into the indentation that is the 2nd ICS. Take a moment to make sure that you can identify the bony raised rib and sunken rib space. From the 2nd ICS, walk another finger approximately 3 cm down the chest wall to the 3rd ICS. Continue to "walk" your fingers down, keeping one finger in the rib space and using a second to locate the next rib space (see Fig. 18-2). In women, it may be necessary to displace the breast laterally or stay closer to the sternum to avoid breast tissue. Also, avoid pressing too hard on tender breast tissue.

The ribs become too close together to count easily once you reach the 6th rib, which is usually at the bottom of the breast tissue (where underwire in a bra would lie). Also, the costal cartilages of the 8th, 9th, and 10th ribs articulate with the ribs above them, not the sternum. Thus, if you palpate more laterally in the locations, shown in Figure 18-2, you can palpate more easily down to the 10th rib anteriorly. From the 6th to 7th rib space, walk your fingers in the rib space to approximately the middle of the chest and then laterally and down to the 9th ICS. The 11th and 12th ribs do not join anteriorly.

The angle between the ribs at the costal margins forms the **costal angle**, found at the bottom of the sternum at the **xyphoid process**. It is usually 90 degrees or less.

Clinical Significance 18-2

During cardiopulmonary resuscitation (CPR), hands are placed above the xyphoid process to avoid breaking it off from the sternum and causing complications, such as pneumothorax, hemothorax, or liver laceration.

Posterior Thoracic Landmarks

The muscles in the back make it difficult to locate ribs and ICSs using the same technique as on the front. Specific posterior landmarks usually are less important, because most of the relevant organs are located anteriorly. Thus, rib spaces on the back are identified indirectly, and spinous processes of the vertebrae are used to identify rib location.

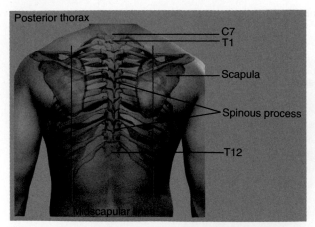

Figure 18.3 Posterior thoracic landmarks.

Flex your neck forward and feel the vertebral processes, the most protruding of which is usually C7 (Fig. 18-3; see also Chapter 14). If two are protruding, the upper one is C7, and the lower one is T1 (Moore & Agur, 2007). The spinous process of T1 usually correlates with the 1st rib. Posteriorly, the spinous processes correlate down to T4 only, because they start to angle down and overlie the vertebral body and underlying rib. A second method for identifying the ribs posteriorly is to locate the lower tip of the scapula; it is at the 7th to 8th rib (Moore & Agur, 2007). The tip of the 11th floating rib can be palpated laterally; the tip of the 12th floating rib can be palpated posteriorly.

Reference Lines

To label findings horizontally on the chest, a series of reference lines is used. On the anterior chest are the midsternal, midclavicular, and anterior axillary lines, named for the structures that they describe (Fig. 18-4). The **midsternal line** is in the center of the sternum. The **midclavicular line** (MCL) extends down

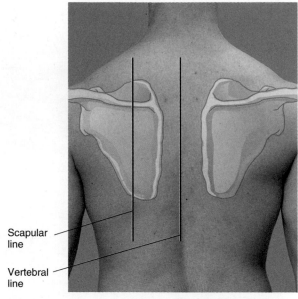

Figure 18.5 Reference lines of the chest, posterior.

from the clavicle halfway between the sternoclavicular and acromioclavicular joints. The **anterior axillary line** extends from the top of the axillary fold when the arms are at the sides.

The posterior chest wall lines are vertebral and scapular (Fig. 18-5). The **vertebral line** lies over the center of the spinous processes of the vertebrae. The **scapular line** originates from the inferior angle of the scapula and is parallel to the vertebral line.

In addition to the previously mentioned anterior axillary line, other lines from a side view are based on their relation to the axilla. The **posterior axillary line** drops from the apex of the axilla (Moore & Agur, 2007). The **midaxillary line** also drops from the apex of the axilla and is parallel to the anterior axillary line (see Fig. 18-6).

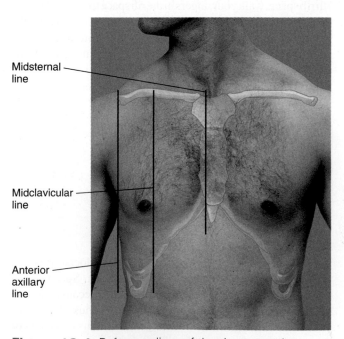

Figure 18.4 Reference lines of the chest, anterior.

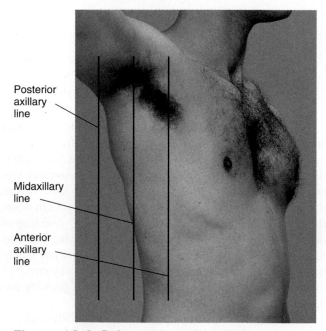

Figure 18.6 Reference lines of the chest, side.

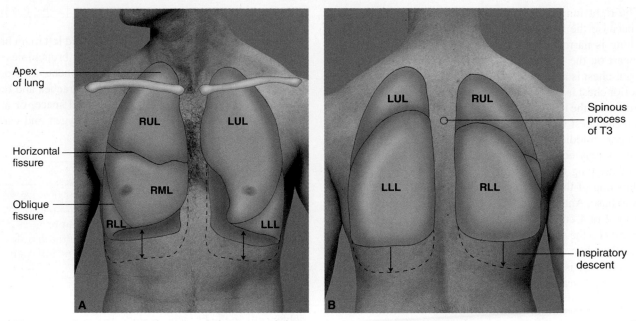

Figure 18.7 Views of the lungs. **(A)** Anterior. **(B)** Posterior.

Other areas that may be referenced when identifying findings include supraclavicular (above the clavicle), above or below the scapula, or medial or lateral to the reference lines.

Lobes of the Lungs

The previously described landmarks help pinpoint the approximate location of the lobes of the lungs on the chest wall. Each rib is divided almost in half by an **oblique fissure** that runs from the 6th rib MCL anteriorly to the T3 spinous process posteriorly (Figs. 18-7A & B). The left lung has two lobes, while the right lung has three. The **horizontal (minor) fissure** divides the right upper and middle lobes of the lung.

The right upper lobe (RUL) and right middle lobe (RML) are approximately the size of the left upper lobe (LUL). The RML extends from the 4th rib at the sternal border to the 5th rib at the midaxillary line (Fig. 18-8) (Moore & Agur, 2007). The right lower lobe (RLL) and left lower lobe (LLL) are approximately the same size.

Clinical Significance 18-3

The RML can be auscultated anteriorly only. It often is found under the breast, making it challenging to hear in women.

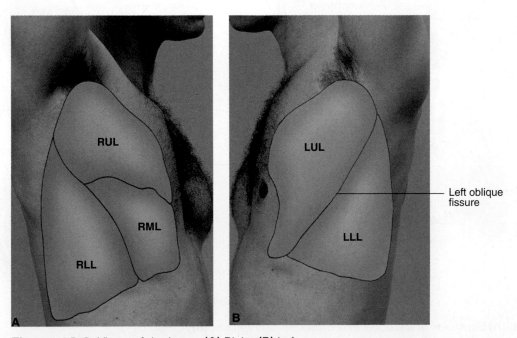

Figure 18.8 Views of the lungs. **(A)** Right. **(B)** Left.

The right lung is approximately 2.5 cm higher than the left because the liver displaces the lung tissue upward. The left lung is narrower than the right because the location of the heart on the left displaces the lung tissue. Note that the anterior chest is almost all middle and upper lobes, while the posterior chest is almost all lower lobe. These landmarks only approximate the lung lobes, so it is more accurate to label findings using chest wall landmarks instead of the lung lobes.

Upper, middle, and lower lung fields are divided into approximately equal thirds. The **base** refers to the very bottom of the lung fields; the **apex** is the very top (opposite of the labeling of the heart). Lungs should be auscultated from apex to base. Anteriorly, the apex of the lung extends approximately 2 to 4 cm above the inner third of the clavicle. The base rests on the diaphragm at the 6th rib MCL and the 8th rib midaxillary line. Posteriorly, the apex of the lung is near C7, while the base is near T10 (three rib spaces below the inferior tip of the scapula). With deep inspiration, the base may extend another two rib spaces to T12 (Moore & Agur, 2007).

Clinical Significance 18-4

The apex of the lung extends above the clavicle, where lung sounds may be audible. When primary health practitioners place a central line into the chest, they may accidentally nick the lung apex, causing a pneumothorax. The apex must be carefully auscultated following this procedure.

Lower Respiratory Tract

The trachea bifurcates into the right main and left main bronchi and then further branches into terminal bronchioles and then alveoli (Fig. 18-9). The right main bronchus is shorter, wider, and more vertical than the left. The trachea and bronchi contain approximately 150 mL of dead space, or areas that transport gas but do not exchange oxygen and carbon dioxide (Moore & Agur, 2007).

Clinical Significance 18-5

The structure of the right bronchus makes it more susceptible to aspiration and intubation if an endotracheal tube is inserted too far. If the right bronchus is intubated, breath sounds will be auscultated only on the right because the tube will block the left main bronchus.

Narrowed **bronchioles** may lead to wheezing. If the goblet cells in the bronchi produce excessive mucus or if the cilia that transport mucus are slowed, crackling or gurgling breath sounds may result. Breath sounds differ in the trachea and bronchi because the trachea is much larger and thus has wider airways. As the airways narrow, sounds become softer, finer, and more difficult to auscultate.

The **alveoli** are the primary units in the lungs that absorb oxygen and excrete carbon dioxide. When fluid

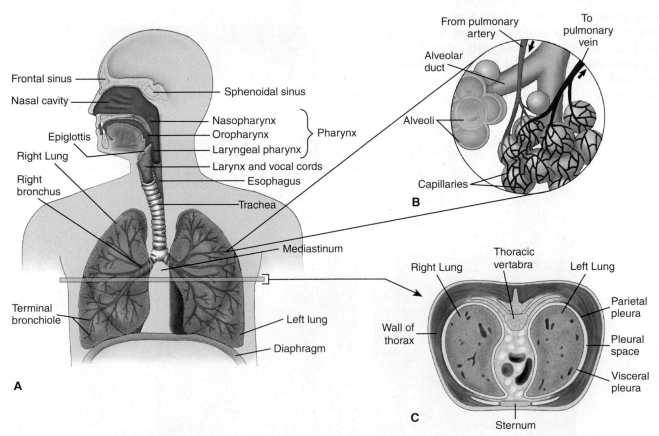

Figure 18.9 (A) Structures of the upper and lower respiratory tracts. **(B)** Alveoli. **(C)** Horizontal cross-section of the lungs.

fills the alveoli, fine crackles may be audible on auscultation. Excessive fluid in the alveoli may lead to airway collapse and decreased breath sounds. Pulmonary arterioles take oxygen from the alveoli to the cells, while pulmonary veins return carbon dioxide to the alveoli for excretion. Obstruction of a pulmonary artery by a blood clot or pulmonary thromboembolism can lead to decreased blood oxygenation.

The pleurae are two overlapping membranes. The **visceral pleura** lines the lungs, including the surfaces within the fissures, while the **parietal pleura** lines the thoracic wall, mediastinum, and diaphragm. The pleural space lubricates the two surfaces. Although called a "space," it really is a very thin (less than a few milliliters) coating of fluid that seals the lungs open with negative pressure. In cases of trauma to the chest wall, the seal may be broken, leading to separation of the visceral pleura and, subsequently, a collapsed lung (pneumothorax).

The **mediastinum** extends from sternum to vertebrae, containing the organs and tissues between the right and left lungs. These structures include the trachea, pulmonary vasculature, heart, great vessels, esophagus, and lymph vessels. The other two cavities in the thorax are the pulmonary cavities that contain the lungs.

Upper Respiratory Tract

The upper respiratory tract is responsible for moisturizing inhaled air and filtering noxious particles. It is covered in depth in Chapter 17.

Mechanics of Respiration

Respiration is primarily an automatic process triggered in the respiratory center of the brainstem (pons and medulla) based on cellular demands (Benditt, 2006). The main trigger for breathing is increased carbon dioxide in the blood. Decreased oxygen or increased acidity also may trigger breathing. Some medications (eg, opiates) or an overdose of drugs may reduce the ability of the brain to trigger breathing, causing hypoventilation (slow breathing). Anxiety or brain injury may stimulate breathing, causing hyperventilation (fast breathing).

When breathing is triggered, the **diaphragm** contracts and flattens, pulling the lungs down. The thorax and lungs elongate, increasing the vertical diameter. The external intercostals muscles open the ribs and lift the sternum, and the anteroposterior diameter of the thorax increases. With increased thoracic size, pressure in the lungs is less than pressure in the atmosphere. As a result, approximately 500 to 800 mL of air enters the lungs with each breath in adults (Moore & Agur, 2007).

Expiration is primarily passive. As the diaphragm, internal intercostals muscles, and abdominal muscles relax, pressure in the lungs is greater than in the atmosphere. Subsequently, air is pushed out, and the chest and abdomen return to their relaxed position.

Sufficient innervation, muscle excursion, and strength are needed for effective breathing. Patients with diseases or problems of the spinal cord, especially injuries above C3–C5, may require ventilatory support. Extreme obesity can limit chest wall expansion (and thus compromise breathing), and progressive loss of muscle function (eg, muscular dystrophy) can limit ability to ventilate and cough (Benditt, 2006).

Lifespan Considerations

Pregnant Women
In late pregnancy, the lower ribs flare as the fetus and uterus grow. The costal angle increases, and the diaphragm rises approximately 4 cm above its usual position. Tidal volume increases because the diaphragm moves more, although respiratory rate remains approximately the same. Increased tidal volume meets the increased demands that the growing fetus places on the mother.

Infants and Children
The respiratory system does not function until birth. The fetus depends on the placenta for exchange of oxygen. Prenatal lungs contain no air, and the alveoli are collapsed. Passive air movements prepare the fetus to respond to chemical and neurological stimuli that will trigger breathing after birth. Surfactant production begins at 32 weeks of gestation to keep the alveoli open.

After the umbilical cord is cut at birth, the newborn's lungs fill with air as he or she takes the first breath. Blood perfuses the lungs quickly. The pulmonary arteries offer less resistance than the systemic circulation, so the lungs get more of the blood supply. The foramen ovale closes between the right and left atria of the heart. The ductus arteriosus, which shunts blood from the pulmonary artery to the aorta, closes; right to left blood flow in the heart is established (Woods, et al., 2005).

The chest in the newborn is round and consistent with the size of the head until approximately 2 years of age. The thin chest wall makes the ribs more prominent in newborns. Increased cartilage makes the chest wall also more compliant and flexible than in adults. Respiratory function continues to develop throughout childhood with increases in the size of the airways and in the size and number of alveoli.

Older Adults
With aging, respiratory strength declines. Lungs lose elasticity, cartilage in the ribs loses flexibility, and bones lose density. These changes result in smaller breaths (decreased inspiratory volumes) and more air remaining in the lungs after exhalation (increased residual volume) (Hankinson, et al., 2003). The anterior to posterior depth of the chest widens, causing the thorax to become more rounded or barrel shaped. When the thorax is rounded, it is harder to inhale deeply. Costal cartilages are calcified, creating a less flexible thorax and more use of the upper lung fields, which are less efficient than the bases. As breathing becomes shallower,

older adults inhale less air and may need to increase rate of breathing to maintain oxygenation.

More significantly, the alveoli are less elastic and more rigid, and the lungs may become "stiff." It takes more work to ventilate stiff lungs. Loss of alveoli renders less surface area available for gas exchange. The elderly are at increased risk for chronic obstructive pulmonary disease (COPD) (Crapo, et al., 2006). Their decreased reserves make it difficult to maintain ventilation during stress, such as exercise or illness. Additionally decreased function of the cilia leads to the pooling of secretions in the lungs. Weaker chest muscles also decrease the older person's ability to cough up secretions. Thick, pooled secretions increase risks for pneumonia.

🌐 Cultural and Environmental Considerations

Chest size influences how much a person can inhale and exhale. There is no significant difference in the chest volumes of Caucasians, African Americans, or Hispanics. Reference values for Caucasian adults are 5% to 19% higher than for Asian adults (Ip, et al., 2006). Variability is more closely linked to body size versus ethnicity. Women have a lower forced expiratory capacity than men (Hankinson, et al., 2003), and older adults have a lower forced expiratory capacity than younger adults (Ip, et al., 2006).

Genetic patterns of inheritance increase risks for respiratory problems such as cystic fibrosis and alpha-1 anti-trypsin deficiency (associated with COPD). Cystic fibrosis is characterized by high sodium and chloride levels in sweat, COPD, and pancreatic insufficiency. Ninety percent of people with cystic fibrosis die from pulmonary complications (Crapo, et al., 2006).

Before birth, the lecithin/sphigomyelin ratio can be calculated to help determine a preterm newborn's risk of fetal respiratory distress. Infants of African descent have a higher ratio and better outcomes than Caucasian infants because of accelerated lung maturation (Berman, et al., 1996).

Acute Assessment

Accurately prioritizing assessments and interventions in urgent or emergency respiratory situations is absolutely critical. If a patient has acute shortness of breath, immediate assessments include respiratory rate, pulse, blood pressure, and oxygen saturation. The lungs are auscultated. Simultaneously, oxygen is administered and inhalers may be given. If the patient is in bed, the head of the bed is elevated to reduce the effect of gravity. Because anxiety increases the work of breathing; the nurse's role is to stay with and to calm the patient. Conversations should be limited while the nurse implements interventions to improve oxygenation. As oxygen levels drop, patients become more dyspneic and cyanotic; they also may become confused. If the situation does not resolve, an emergency response team or personnel from respiratory therapy may be necessary for assistance.

In some cases, patients are stable, but fatigue limits collection of assessment data. In such instances, listen to the bases of the lungs first, and to the posterior lungs before the anterior lungs. Consider clustering care. Auscultate the lungs when turning the patient or getting the patient up in a chair. Positioning with the head of the bed at a 30- to 45-degree angle may be more comfortable than lying flat. Prioritize the subjective data collected; ask only those questions important to current care. Questions relating to the future can be deferred. Simple daily tasks such as eating may consume much energy, so it is important to cluster interventions and time assessments for when the patient is more rested.

Subjective Data Collection

Subjective data collection begins with the health history, continues with questions about specific respiratory conditions, and ends with detailed collection of information involving areas of concern. If patients are short of breath, the interview will need to be shortened. In such instances, ask only those questions pertinent to the current condition and necessary for current care.

△ SAFETY ALERT 18.1

If the patient is having extreme difficulty breathing, stop the assessment and get help. A decreased level of consciousness, respiratory rate above 30 breaths per minute, O_2 saturation less than 92%, cyanosis, retractions, and use of accessory muscles may indicate hypoxia (a medical emergency).

Areas for Health Promotion/ *Healthy People*

An important purpose of the health history is to gather information to promote health and provide health teaching. Health-promotion activities focus on preventing disease, identifying problems early, and reducing complications of existing or established diagnoses. They also serve to reinforce existing healthy habits and to encourage refinements to approaches patients already are practicing.

Patient education, health promotion, and risk reduction are some of the most important roles in nursing. Relevant topics should be woven into conversation during the collection of health history data and follow-up teaching sessions. Nurses can promote patient education and healthy behaviors as they apply the nursing process to care. Table 18-1 includes pertinent goals and education topics for respiratory health.

Table 18.1   *Healthy People* Goals Related to Respiratory Health

Goal	Patient Education Topics
Increase the proportion of adults vaccinated against influenza and pneumococcal disease.	Promote participation in influenza-shot clinics. Encourage patients at high risk to receive the pneumococcal vaccine.
Reduce the number of school or work days missed because of asthma, asthma emergency visits, asthma hospitalizations, and asthma deaths.	Provide instruction about the self-management of asthma symptoms.
Reduce the proportion of adults whose activity is limited because of chronic lung and breathing problems; reduce associated deaths.	Teach how to manage symptoms, pace activities, and use medications properly. Encourage exercise.
Reduce the proportion of nonsmokers exposed to environmental tobacco smoke.	Emphasize the importance of avoiding smoking in the home or car. Teach patients who smoke to do so at least 25 ft away from the entrance to enclosed spaces.
Increase smoking cessation attempts by adult and adolescent smokers and during pregnancy.	Investigate each patient's willingness to quit. Develop a plan for individual, group, or pharmacology resources that works at every visit.
Establish laws on smoke-free indoor air that prohibit smoking or limit it to separately ventilated areas in public places and worksites.	Advocate and get involved politically in professional organizations that encourage smoke-free indoor air.

U.S. Department of Health and Human Sevices. (n.d.). *Healthy People 2010: What are its goals?* Retrieved January 7, 2007, from http://www.healthypeople.gov/About/goals.htm

Assessment of Risk Factors

When questioning patients about risk factors, the intent is to identify how likely they are to develop or to already be experiencing consequences of respiratory diseases. Such investigation creates an environment in which health care providers can implement necessary interventions to control symptoms, direct education to prevent new problems or complications, and establish within the record areas needing ongoing follow-up and emphasis. For example, smoking contributes to COPD. Thus, the smoking history requires thorough assessment so that health care providers can give educational materials to patients willing to begin a smoking-cessation program. Teaching and questioning can be woven together.

Questions to Assess Risk Factors	Rationales
Family History Do you have any family history of respiratory problems? • Who had the illness? • What was the illness? • When did the person have it? • How was the illness treated? • What were the outcomes?	A positive family history, especially of genetic problems such as *cystic fibrosis*, increases the patient's risk for respiratory illness. Note any contagious diseases and the possibility for familial transmission. Also consider whether the condition is chronic (eg, *COPD*) or transient (eg, *common cold*). Family history of *lung cancer* increases risk by two to three times (Crapo, et al., 2006).
Past Medical History Have you ever been diagnosed with a respiratory problem such as asthma, bronchitis, emphysema, or pneumonia? • When was the illness? • How was the illness treated? • What were the outcomes?	History of respiratory disease increases risk for recurrence. Chronic diseases such as *COPD* often have long-term effects that result in a slow but progressive decline in function. *Asthma* symptoms may occur at any age and improve or worsen over time. *Pneumonia* usually has an acute course that improves with treatment.
Did you have frequent respiratory infections as a child?	Frequent childhood infections may lead to problems later in life (Stick, 2000).

(text continues on page 454)

Questions to Assess Risk Factors	Rationales
Do you now or have you ever had allergies? • What are the allergens? • When did you have allergies? • What were the symptoms? • How were the allergies treated? • What were the outcomes?	Allergies to foods or medications may precipitate bronchoconstriction. Common allergens include pollens, dust mites, grasses, molds, animal dander, and latex. Exercise also induces allergies in some people.
When was your last tuberculosis (TB) skin test or chest x-ray? • What was the result? • Do you receive any treatment?	Risk factors include close contact with an infected person, being foreign-born, low income, substance abuse, and infection with HIV (Taylor, 2005). Health care workers should be screened annually (Centers for Disease Control and Prevention [CDC], 2006a).
When did you receive your last influenza or pneumococcal vaccine? Are you interested in being immunized this year?	Influenza vaccine is recommended annually for people at high risk for influenza-related complications and severe disease. Pneumococcal vaccine is recommended every 5 years for immunocompetent adults, people older than 65 years, patients with AIDS, and children older than 2 years with chronic illnesses or HIV infection (CDC, 1997).

Medications

Are you taking any medications for respiratory problems? • What are they? • How often are you taking them? • How well are you following your prescribed medication regimen?	Many respiratory medications, such as inhalers, are used as needed. Trends of increased use may indicate a worsening condition. Steroids also may be used during times of increased inflammation, such as an *acute asthma attack*.
Are you taking any natural supplements or over-the-counter medications? • What are they? • How often are you taking them?	Over-the-counter medications that block beta 2 receptors may exacerbate bronchoconstriction. Sensitivity to nonsteroidal antiinflammatory agents (eg, Motrin, Indocin) may cause wheezing in patients with asthma.

Lifestyle and Personal Habits

Do you smoke or have you ever smoked cigarettes, pipes, or cigars? • How many packs per day do you smoke? • How many years have you smoked? • Have you ever tried to stop smoking? • Are you interested in quitting?	Smoking is described by the number of **pack years** (number of years × number of packs per day). For example, a patient who has smoked ½ pack per day for 30 years has a 15-pack-year history. Increased pack years increase the risk for respiratory problems including *lung cancer* and *COPD* (Tessier, et al., 2000).
Are you frequently around people who smoke in the home or car? What measures do you take to control this exposure?	Secondhand smoke increases risks for *emphysema* and *lung cancer* (Health Effects, 2006).
Do you use or have you ever inhaled recreational drugs such as marijuana, cocaine, methamphetamine, glue, or spray paint? Are you interested in information about how to quit or reduce your risk?	These inhaled substances can irritate the linings of the upper or lower airway. People with injection substance use disorders are at risk for *infectious pulmonary disease*, as well as *HIV* and its pulmonary manifestations (Wolff & O'Donnell, 2004.) Regular marijuana use can lead to extensive airway injury, potentially causing pulmonary infection and respiratory cancer. Crack cocaine use can lead to exacerbations of asthma and an acute lung injury syndrome ("*crack lung*"). Heroin inhalation can induce severe and sometimes fatal exacerbations of asthma (Tashkin, 2001).

Questions to Assess Risk Factors	Rationales
Do you have any hobbies that might increase your risk for respiratory problems, such as exposure to paint fumes or wood dust, bird breeding, mushroom growing, scuba diving, swimming, and high-altitude activities?	Such hobbies may cause lung injury. Exposure over time to bird droppings or feathers may cause *hypersensitivity pneumonitis* and *pulmonary fibrosis*. Risk of drowning is increased for those younger than 18 years, especially toddlers. Being male and ingesting alcohol also increases risk (Crapo, et al., 2006). With rapid ascent to high elevation, *acute mountain sickness* may develop, causing fluid retention, hypoventilation, and mechanical dysfunction (Crapo, et al., 2006).
Occupational History Have you ever been or are you now exposed to substances or irritants at work? • Do you wear a mask or take other precautions to protect your lungs? • What steps do you take to monitor your exposure?	Coal miners have an increased risk of *pneumoconiosis*, or black lung disease (McPhee, et al., 2007). *Silicosis* is increased in glassmakers, stonecutters, miners, cement workers, and semiconductor manufacturers (Singh, et al., 2006). *Occupational asthma* may develop in 2% to 5% of workers exposed to grain dust, wood dust, soldering flux, and dyes (McPhee, et al., 2007). *Industrial bronchitis* is found in textile workers. Shipyard and construction workers, pipefitters, and insulators may develop *asbestosis* (McPhee, et al., 2007).
Enviromental Exposures Have you ever been or are you now exposed to substances or irritants at home such as pollen, dust, pet dander, cockroaches, or cooking smoke particles? Is there any history of exposure to radon or asbestos from heating/cooling systems?	Common household irritants can contribute to *asthma*, as well as itchy eyes, sneezing, and runny nose. Radon and tobacco smoke can cause even more dangerous health effects, including *lung cancer* (American Lung Association, 2004).
Have you recently traveled to any high-risk areas for respiratory conditions such as Asia, southern Africa, Indonesia, or Turkey? • Where? • How long were you there? • Were you exposed to people with a cough, cold, or the flu?	*Histoplasmosis*, a fungal infection, is common in the Midwestern United States and endemic in Ohio, Missouri, and the Mississippi River valley (Rakel, 2006). Another fungal infection, *coccidioidomycosis*, is found in the southwestern United States and Central and South America (Rakel, 2006). *Avian flu* can be contracted through exposure to dead or infected birds in China, Indonesia, or Turkey (World Health Organization [WHO], 2006a). High-risk areas for TB include Asia and southern Africa (WHO, 2006b). *SARS*, although uncommon, may be contracted in China, Hong Kong, or Taiwan (CDC, 2005a). Quick identification and treatment of these contagions is essential.

Risk Assessment and Health-Related Patient Teaching

As mentioned, risk assessment helps identify potential problems so that health care providers can give patients information to influence behavioral choices. The most important focus area for the respiratory system involves smoking.

Smoking Cessation

All patients who smoke should be asked at every appointment about their readiness to stop. Smoking has been linked to *lung cancer, emphysema, bronchitis, cardiovascular disease,* and *oral cancer*; it is considered the leading cause of preventable death (CDC, 2005b). Studies have

shown that when health care providers ask patients about their willingness to quit, smoking cessation is more likely (Smoking Cessation Leadership Center, n.d.). Patients can be given several choices to assist with quitting, such as individual or group counseling, medical treatment, or nicotine replacement.

Prevention of Occupational Exposure

Another focal point is modification of the work environment to limit exposure to irritants. In some cases, consultation with employees at the work site may be recommended. Occupational health and safety guidelines should be followed. For example, people exposed to dust should have the opportunity to wear respirator masks.

Prevention of Asthma

Asthma triggers include tobacco smoke, dust, dust mites, molds, furred and feathered animals, and cockroaches and other pests. For patients with allergies, modification of the home environment may be recommended. Examples include covering the bed and pillows and ensuring that pets sleep separately (eg, outside the bedroom) from owners.

Immunizations

All adults should be counseled to obtain the influenza vaccine annually. This consideration is especially important for health care providers. In addition to being at increased risk for contracting influenza from patients, providers also need to consider that they may infect others at risk, including those with suppressed immune systems and older adults (CDC, 2006b).

Focused Health History Related to Common Symptoms

Some common symptoms should be assessed in all patients to screen for the early presence of respiratory disease. Nurses can use any special concerns from patients about respiratory problems to identify focal areas. A thorough history of symptoms assists with identifying a current problem or diagnosis.

Common Respiratory Symptoms

- Chest pain or discomfort
- Dyspnea
- Orthopnea or paroxysmal noctural dyspnea
- Cough
- Mucus or phlegm
- Wheezing or tightness in chest
- Change in functional ability

Questions to Assess Symptoms	Rationales/Abnormal Findings
Patient Perspective Describe your breathing.	This question allows patients to share an unbiased perspective.
Chest Pain Do you have chest pain or discomfort? • Where is it? Can you point to where it hurts? Does the pain go anywhere? Describe the discomfort. • When did it start? How long has it lasted? What brings it on? • How bad is it on a scale from 1 to10 with 10 being the worst? Do any other symptoms accompany the pain? • What does it feel like? • What makes it better? Have you tried any treatments? Did they help? What makes it worse? What brings it on? • What is your goal for the pain? What would you like to be able to do that you can't because of the pain?	**⚠ SAFETY ALERT 18.2** *Health care providers should assume that chest pain is heart pain from cardiac ischemia until proven otherwise. Chest pain is an emergency requiring immediate help (see Chapter 19).* Lung tissue has no pain fibers. Pleuritic chest pain (*pleurisy*) can follow inflammation of the parietal pleura. Patients usually describe such pain as sharp or stabbing, worsening with deep breathing or coughing, and often lateral or posterior in the lung. Antiinflammatory agents often relieve pleuritic pain. *Tracheobronchitis* can cause pain starting in the trachea and large bronchi. Patients usually describe this as burning and in the upper sternum. It is associated with a cough. Chest wall pain can be muscle strain secondary to frequent coughing. Patients may describe it as achy; muscles may be tender to palpation.
Dyspnea Have you had any difficulty breathing? • How bad is it on a scale from 1 to 10, with 10 being the worst? • When did it start? How long has it lasted? • What activities make it worse? What makes it better? • Do you have other symptoms? • How has this limited your activities? • Is the breathing difficulty associated with anxiety?	**Dyspnea** is a subjective term used when patients report labored breathing and breathlessness. This response to exercise or heavy activity is normal if it rapidly disappears upon return to rest. Patients with *lung disease*, however, may experience dyspnea with normal activities or even at rest. Note what causes dyspnea, such as climbing two stairs, walking one block, or walking uphill. Also note if onset was gradual (eg, *COPD*) or sudden (eg, *pneumonia*). *Anxiety* can precipitate dyspnea and hyperventilation. Anxious patients may describe dyspnea as smothering; they also may report tingling around the lips from a low carbon dioxide level. Patients with *COPD* or *CHF* may describe dyspnea as scary, hard to breathe, shortness of breath, cannot get enough air, or gasping (Caroci & Lareau, 2004).

Questions to Assess Symptoms	Rationales/Abnormal Findings

Orthopnea and Paroxysmal Nocturnal Dyspnea

Do you have difficulty breathing when you sleep?
- On how many pillows do you sleep?
- Do you have difficulty breathing when lying flat?
- Do you wake up suddenly at night short of breath?
- Do you snore or stop breathing when you sleep?
- Do you have night sweats?

Gravity increases work of breathing when lying flat. Patients with **orthopnea** (difficulty breathing when lying flat) often sleep on two or more pillows or even in recliners. Patients who waken at night with sudden shortness of breath have **paroxysmal nocturnal dyspnea**. The cause is fluid overload from elevation of the legs, which shifts fluid there to the body's core. The excess fluid cannot be pumped through the heart and suddenly accumulates in the lungs, causing dyspnea. *Sleep apnea* commonly interrupts sleep and can lead to pulmonary complications over time. Night sweats are associated with *TB*.

Cough

- Do you have a cough?
- Where does the cough come from—sinuses, throat, or lungs?
- What does it feel or sound like?
- How bad is it?
- How often do you cough? When is it worse?
- When did it start? How long has it lasted?
- Is it worse in any particular setting?
- What makes it worse? What makes it better?
- Do you have other accompanying symptoms?
- What do you think has caused the problem?

Cough can originate in the upper or lower airway. With *sinus congestion*, mucus can drip into the throat and cause coughing. A tickle in the throat also can trigger coughing. A cough that accompanies laryngeal irritation is croupy, barking, or brassy. Alternatively, lung irritation can trigger coughing, such as with a *cold, early heart failure, viral infection*, or *bronchitis*. These coughs are usually dry and hacking. With *pneumonia* or the *common cold*, mucus in the lungs may trigger coughing. Such coughs usually are productive (wet or moist). Coughs upon waking are associated with pooled secretions secondary to smoking or *bronchitis*. Coughs at night may be from *sinus drainage, heart failure*, or *asthma*. Coughs following a meal may be related to *GERD* or a *hernia* (Hancox, et al., 2006). Treatment for conditions underlying coughs are different, so accurate detection of the cause is important.

Sputum

Do you cough up any mucus or phlegm? How much? Has the amount increased or decreased?
- What color is it?
- Is it thick or thin?
- Do you notice an odor?
- Has the amount, consistency, or color changed?

Quantifying the amount of sputum (eg, teaspoon, tablespoon, quarter cup, half cup) may provide clues about the severity of the problem. Sputum color may differentiate the cause. The **mucoid** sputum of *bronchitis* is clear, white, or grey. **Purulent** yellow or green sputum indicates the presence of white cells and *bacterial infection*. Rust-colored sputum is found with *TB* and *pneumococcal pneumonia*. **Tenacious sputum** may be thick with *dehydration* or *cystic fibrosis*; sputum from *heart failure* is thin and frothy and may be slightly pink. Sputum may be bloody with *lung cancer* or *TB* (Crapo, et al., 2006). Examine such sputum carefully to see if blood is integrated or just coats the outside. An irritated throat or sinus may bleed and contact the sputum during expectoration. **Hemoptysis** is the term for frankly bloody sputum. Some patients may expectorate from the mouth; this is not considered sputum but instead oral secretions.

Wheezing

Do you have any wheezing or chest tightness?
- How severe is wheezing compared to your normal function?
- Do you use a peak flow meter? What are your usual/current values?
- When did the problem start? How long has it lasted?
- Is wheezing associated with allergies? If so, what are they? Do you notice that the problem is worse in a particular environment?

Wheezing is associated with *asthma*, *CHF*, and *bronchitis*. It occurs in response to narrowed bronchioles. Wheezing with asthma is worse in response to offending allergens, at night, and in the early morning (Crapo, et al., 2006). Patients with asthma are taught to use a peak flow meter to provide objective data about how much they can inhale with each breath. If airways are greatly constricted, breaths will be small, and patients may need to use their inhalers.

(text continues on page 458)

Questions to Assess Symptoms	Rationales/Abnormal Findings

- What makes it worse? What makes it better? How often do you use your inhalers?
- Do you have other symptoms?
- What do you think is causing this? What will make it better?

⚠ **SAFETY ALERT 18.3**
In an acute asthma attack, observe for wheezing that progresses to decreased lung sounds, which may indicate worsening status.

Functional Abilities
Have breathing difficulties changed any of your normal activities? How do you plan the day and pace activities? (in addition to eating, grooming, and dressing, also consider the patient's ability to perform home maintenance, such as vacuuming, bed making, cooking, cleaning, and buying groceries).

Patients with respiratory problems commonly have more energy in the morning and need frequent rest during the day. Some are short of breath even at rest, needing to pause after a few words. Others become breathless when eating, grooming, or dressing. Patients with declining health may need plans for assistance. Ask what they like to do and if they can do these things. Patients with respiratory problems may be able to engage in sexual activity and exercise if they plan to do so during high-energy times.

Documentation of Normal Findings

Patient denies chest pain or discomfort, dyspnea, orthopnea, paroxysmal noctural dyspnea, cough, mucus, wheezing or tightness in chest, and decrease in functional ability. *S. Garcia, RN*

 Lifespan Considerations

Additional Questions	Rationales/Abnormal Findings

Pregnant Women
How is your breathing? Are you having any difficulty sleeping because of breathing problems?

Dyspnea is common in late pregnancy as the uterus begins to compress the diaphragm. Assess the woman for sleep disturbances; teach that side lying may be more comfortable. Multiple fetuses contribute to increased size and associated maternal discomfort.

Newborns, Infants, and Children
How many colds has your child had over the past year? How serious were they?

Poor and limited independent hygiene places infants and children at risk for *respiratory infections*; thus, emphasize infection-reduction measures such as handwashing and proper use of tissues. Frequent childhood infections are linked to later COPD and asthma (Crapo, et al., 2006).

What measures are you taking to avoid allergies in your child? Is your baby breast or bottle fed? How are you introducing new foods?

Teach parents of young infants about the proper introduction of solid foods (one at a time for 1 week at a time) to help determine new possible allergens. High body mass index is associated with increased risk of *asthma* in childhood, while regular intake of seafood, fresh fruits, and vegetables is associated with a decreased risk (Hong, et al., 2006).

How have you safety-proofed your home and yard? Have you learned emergency techniques, such as first aid or CPR?

Accidental aspiration of toys, foods, and poisons is a risk for young children. Evaluate the family's knowledge about common problematic items; teach prevention measures.

Is your infant experiencing apneic episodes? Is there any family history of sudden infant death syndrome (SIDS)?

Teach parents the importance of placing all infants on the back to sleep to help prevent *SIDS*.

Did your child have any problems related to birth?

For low birth weight or premature infants, review the duration of ventilator support and any complications or chronic issues. Meconium aspiration may cause *pneumonia* in newborns.

Additional Questions	Rationales/Abnormal Findings
Has your child had frequent spitting up or difficulty swallowing?	Be aware of the risk of pulmonary complications related to *gastroesophageal reflux disease (GERD)*. Teach parents measures to prevent aspiration in children at high risk for GERD, such as elevating the head after meals. GERD in childhood is a risk factor for asthma in adulthood (Hancox, 2006).
Older Adults Have you noticed any shortness of breath or fatigue with your activities of daily living (ADLs)?	Older adults have less tolerance for ADLs than younger patients. Assess how any respiratory disease or problems are affecting ability to function. Assess energy level and activities that cause patients to tire more easily. Consider recommendations for pacing activities, allowing for rest, and performing higher energy tasks earlier in the day when well rested.
Have you had any recent pulmonary infections or worsening of your current condition?	Counsel high-risk patients to avoid exposure to infections and to plan modifications for weather variations, such as walking in a shopping mall instead of outside on a cold day. Educate about lifestyle changes to increase health and prevent chronic disease (eg, not smoking).

🌐 Cultural and Environmental Considerations

Additional Questions	Rationales/Abnormal Findings
Have you recently immigrated to the United States? Have you been immunized with the BCG vaccine?	Incidence of *TB* is approximately nine times higher among North American immigrants (Taylor, et al., 2005).
Do you have concerns about exposure to environmental pollution?	Children in urban environments are more likely to have *asthma* (Lee, et al., 2003). Air pollution contributes to *COPD* and *lung cancer* (Crapo, et al., 2006). Owning a home, a mark of socioeconomic status, is linked to less susceptibility to childhood *colds* (Cohen, et al., 2004).
Are there any concerns about exposure to dust, fumes, or mold in your home?	Recent immigrants may cook or heat with kerosene or wood. Make sure that there is proper ventilation to avoid *carbon monoxide poisoning*. Also consider quality of housing, including density of residents, ventilation systems, and black mold (Crapo, et al., 2006).
Note the patient's self-identified ethnic group and gender.	Pacific Islanders, Filipinos, Cubans, and Puerto Ricans are at risk for *asthma* (Davis, et al., 2006). Hispanics, Blacks, and Asians have *TB* rates 7–19 times higher than Caucasians (Taylor, et al., 2005). Cigarette smokers, African Americans, and Native Americans are more susceptible to *lung cancer* than are Caucasians (Haiman, et al., 2006). Women smokers also have increased susceptibility to adverse effects from tobacco and greater risk for *lung cancer* and *COPD* (Crapo, et al., 2006; Henschke, et al., 2006).

🔍 Objective Data Collection

Equipment

- Examination gown
- Stethoscope and alcohol swab
- Marking pen and small ruler for diaphragmatic excursion (optional)

Preparation

Make sure that the room is a comfortable temperature. Take measures to facilitate a private and quiet setting. Wash and warm your hands to avoid spreading infection and to facilitate patient comfort.

For inspection, expose only the area of the chest that you will be examining, especially for women. When visualization is required, gather the gown from the bottom to the shoulders so that the patient feels less exposed anteriorly. Cover the anterior

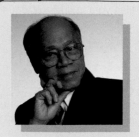

Therapeutic Dialogue: Collecting Subjective Data

The nurse's role relative to subjective data collection is to gather information to improve the patient's health status and to help determine the cause of current symptoms. Remember Mr. Jin, who was introduced at the beginning of this chapter. He has had COPD for 15 years. Today, he is visiting the clinic because of increasing dyspnea and fatigue. Because Mr. Jin is fatigued, efficient questioning is essential. Thus, questions must be prioritized, with the most important issues addressed first.

The following conversations give two examples of interview styles used by different nurses. One style is more effective than the other.

Less Effective

Nurse: I'm going to ask a few questions to get information on your health history, if that's OK with you.

Mr. Jin: Sure.

Nurse: Do you have any history of respiratory disease?

Mr. Jin: Yes, I have had COPD for 15 years.

Nurse: Do you smoke?

Mr. Jin: Yes, I've smoked since I was 16.

Nurse: Were you around any pollution or dust?

Mr. Jin: I used to work in the steel mill, so there was always some kind of fume.

Nurse: Did you have respiratory infections as a child?

Mr. Jin: Not that I remember. I was born in China and never had good records.

Nurse: Do you have any allergies?

Mr. Jin: Just to pollen.

Nurse: Does anyone in your family have lung problems?

Mr. Jin: Not that I know of.

Nurse: Do you have a cough?

Mr. Jin: Yes.

Nurse: How about mucus?

Mr. Jin: Yes.

More Effective

Nurse: (Before beginning, he reads the chart and notes that Mr. Jin has a 98 pack-year history of smoking and COPD for 15 years. The record states that Mr. Jin is allergic to pollen, with symptoms of red teary eyes and sinus congestion.) It looks like your last visit was 2 weeks ago, Mr. Jin. How do you feel now?

Mr. Jin: I'm still not feeling well. When I came in last time, they said I had bronchitis, but it feels like it's getting worse.

Nurse: It feels like it's getting worse... (pause)

Mr. Jin: Last time I felt wheezy. This time I'm coughing more.

Nurse: Are you coughing anything up?

Mr. Jin: Yes.

Nurse: What does it look like?

Mr. Jin: It's yellow.

Nurse: And is it thick or thin?

Mr. Jin: It's quite thick.

Nurse: How much would you say you're coughing up—a few teaspoons, a half cup, or a cup?

Mr. Jin: I probably cough something up three to four times an hour. Maybe a half cup.

Critical Thinking Challenge

- Compare and contrast the data collected in the two dialogues. What approaches made the second dialogue more effective?
- Could the "more effective" nurse have done anything differently to further improve data collection and communication with the patient?
- Does the patient's childhood and family history require further exploration? Provide rationale.
- Is this an appropriate time to discuss risk factor modification and smoking cessation? Provide rationale.

---

chest when inspecting posteriorly. Explain the rationale for the need to expose the chest to ease the patient's anxiety.

Lung auscultation is easiest to perform with the patient sitting. If sitting is not possible, the anterior lungs can be auscultated when the patient is lying, and the posterior lungs can be heard when the patient is turned from side to side. Alternatively, a second person may be able to assist the patient to sit.

Studies have shown that a stethoscope can be a source of bacterial transmission across patients (Marinella, et al., 1997). Thus, be sure to use an alcohol swab to clean the diaphragm of the stethoscope before bringing it into contact with the patient.

You also may warm the diaphragm of the stethoscope with your clean hands prior to placing it on the patient's chest.

Common and Specialty or Advanced Techniques

Routine assessment includes the most important and common techniques. Examiners may add specialty or advanced steps if concerns exist over a specific finding. Table 18-2 summarizes the most common techniques for thoracic and lung assessment, which are therefore essential to master in clinical practice.

Table 18.2 Comprehensive Versus Advanced Respiratory Assessment Techniques

Comprehensive Assessment Technique	Purpose	Screening or Registered Nurse Assessment	Focused or Advanced Practice Examination
Inspection of patient	Assists to determine the acuity of the situation	X	
Inspection of chest	Provides information on chest shape and breathing pattern	X	
Palpation of chest	Assessed when tenderness, masses, or lesions are present	X	
Chest expansion	Assessed in cases of physical or neuromuscular limitations		X
Tactile fremitus	Assessed when consolidation or hyperinflation is anticipated		X
Percussion of chest	Assessed when consolidation or hyperinflation is anticipated		X
Diaphragmatic excursion	Assessed in cases of physical or neuromuscular limitations		X
Auscultation	Performed to accurately identify breath and adventitious sounds	X	
Auscultation of voice sounds	Assessed when consolidation is anticipated		X

Initial Survey

Technique and Normal Findings	Abnormal Findings
Closely assess the position that the patient is using to breathe. *Posture is relaxed and upright with the arms at the sides.*	Patients in respiratory distress may assume a **tripod** position, leaning forward on a stationary object such as a table or with their elbows on their knees (Fig. 18-10). This relaxes their abdominal, intercostals, and neck muscles and allows for less work in breathing. 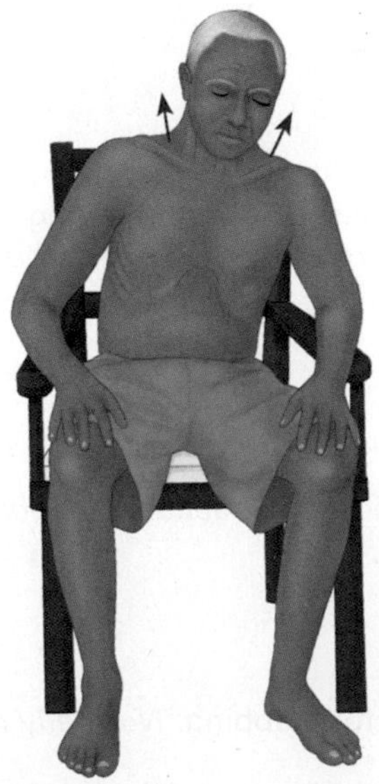 **Figure 18.10** A patient with COPD assuming the tripod position.
Observe for **pursed lips** and **nasal flaring**. *Facial expression is relaxed.*	Patients in *respiratory distress* may have an anxious expression. Patients with *COPD* may have pursed lips, providing some positive pressure in the bronchial tree to prevent airway collapse. Nasal flaring may accompany *respiratory distress*, especially in children.

(text continues on page 462)

Technique and Normal Findings (continued)	Abnormal Findings (continued)
Evaluate level of consciousness. *Patient is alert, cooperative, and normally oriented to time, place, and person.*	The patient with *hypoxemia* may be irritable, somnolent, restless, confused, combative, or disoriented.
Inspect skin color. Document the absence of cyanosis or pallor. *Skin color is an appropriate tone for the patient's racial background. Observe the undertone of the skin rather than the amount of melanin. Normal skin color is pink.*	With hypoxemia, **cyanosis** (bluish discoloration) may occur either centrally or around the mouth (circumoral). **Pallor** (pale whitish color) and grayish tones indicate poor oxygenation or *anemia*. Chronic respiratory disease may lead to **rubor** (reddish-purple color) or **erythema** (flushed appearance).
Observe respiratory movements. Note if the patient uses the upper or lower chest to breathe. *Normally expiration is twice as long as inspiration (inspiration:expiration = 1:2).*	Patients with disease that impedes outflow (eg, *COPD*) may have **forced expiration**. **Guarding** may accompany pleuritic or postoperative pain. **Work of breathing** is less efficient with use of upper chest muscles.
As you observe the patient's respiratory movements, also count the rate. Do not tell the patient that you are assessing rate, because he or she may subconsciously alter it. If it is difficult to see the chest moving, gently rest your hand on the patient's shoulder to feel the rate. *Rate of a normal respiratory pattern is 12–20 breaths/min for adults. Rhythm is regular, and breathing appears easy and quiet. This is labeled eupnea. An occasional sigh is normal.*	Wheezing may be audible in severe asthma or bronchitis. **Tachypnea** is breathing >24 breaths/min; **bradypnea** is <10 breaths/min. See Table 18-8 at the end of this chapter for other abnormal respiratory patterns. ⚠ SAFETY ALERT 18.4 *Stridor, a high-pitched crowing sound from the upper airway, results from tracheal or laryngeal spasm. In severe laryngospasm the larynx may completely close off. This life-threatening emergency requires immediate medical assistance.*
Assess oxygen saturation level (see Chapter 6). *Normal is 95% to 100%.*	*Pulmonary embolism* produces hypoxemia because of shunting of blood to atelectatic areas of the lung. ⚠ SAFETY ALERT 18.5 *Oxygen saturation <92% may require immediate intervention.*
Assess the muscles used for breathing. *The diaphragm and external intercostals do most of the work.*	Patients with *respiratory distress* may use accessory muscles. **Sternocleidomastoid, scalene, trapezius, latissimus dorsi**, and occasionally **pectoralis major and minor** and **platysma** muscles are used in severe breathing difficulties (Benditt, 2006). The rectus abdominis and internal intercostals are used to facilitate expiration, such as in *COPD*.
Note any retractions. *Retractions are absent.*	Supraclavicular or intercostals retractions accompany resistance to airflow such as in *severe asthma*. Retractions appear as an indentation in the spaces in an effort to "suck in" more air.
Observe fingers for clubbing. *Normally no clubbing is present.*	Clubbing of the fingers is noted with chronic lung disease (see Chapter 13).

Documentation of Normal Findings

Patient lying in bed with head of bed flat. Relaxed breathing, posture, and facial expression. Respirations 16 breaths/min without accessory muscle use or retractions. Skin pink without cyanosis or pallor. *S. Garcia, RN*

Technique and Normal Findings	Abnormal Findings

Posterior Chest

Inspection. Note the shape and configuration of the thoracic cage. Observe spontaneous chest expansion. *Spinous processes of the vertebrae are midline; scapulae are symmetric in each hemithorax. Chest wall is cone-shaped (narrower at the bottom than the top), symmetric, and oval (narrower from front to back than from side to side). The transverse (side to side):anterior-posterior (AP) ratio is between 1:2 and 5:7. Although ribs are not visible in most people, those that are slope at approximately 45 degrees. Chest expansion is symmetric.*

Skeletal **scoliosis** and **kyphosis** can limit respiratory excursion. In **barrel chest**, which can accompany *COPD*, the transverse:AP ratio approximates 1:1, giving the chest a round appearance. Also with COPD, the expanded ribs slope more horizontally, inverting the chest's normal cone shape. **Pectus excavatum** and **pectus carinatum** are sternal abnormalities that limit respiratory excursion. Asymmetry and paradoxical respirations occur in flail chest. See Table 18-9 at the end of the chapter.

Palpation. Palpate the chest for tender areas. Using the fingertips, start above the scapula over the lung apex and progress from side to side to compare findings bilaterally, ending at the base of the lung and moving laterally to the midaxillary line (Fig. 18-11). Note any lesions, lumps, or masses; use gloves if there are lesions or open areas. Palpate for crepitus if the patient has had rib fractures, recent chest surgery, or chest tubes. *Thorax is nontender without any lesions, lumps, masses, or crepitus.*

Tender areas may indicate *muscle strain*, *rib fracture*, or *soft tissue damage*. In chest trauma, air can enter the lungs to escape into subcutaneous tissue. This free air creates a crackling sensation similar to bubble wrap or crispy rice cereal under the skin (**crepitus**). Because air floats, *subcutaneous emphysema* migrates, so it may be found in the head and neck. If there is a large amount, mark the borders with a pen so that changes can be noted.

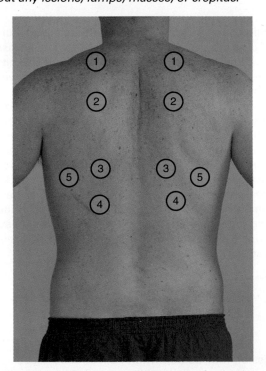

Figure 18.11 Sites for and sequence of palpation of the posterior thorax.

Test for symmetric chest expansion when there are concerns about reduced lung volumes. With the thumbs at T9–T10, wrap the palmar surface of the hands laterally and parallel to the rib cage (Fig. 18-12). Slide the thumbs and hands medially to pinch up a small fold of skin between the thumb and vertebra. Ask the patient to inhale deeply and observe the thumbs. *The thumbs move apart symmetrically, approximately 5–10 cm.*

Asymmetrical movements indicate collapse or blockage of a significant portion of the lung such as with *pneumothorax*, *rib fracture*, *severe pneumonia*, *pleural effusion*, or *atelectasis*. Patients with muscle weakness, respiratory disease, recent surgery, chest wall abnormalities, or obesity may have reduced chest expansion (Jones & Nzekwu, 2006).

(text continues on page 464)

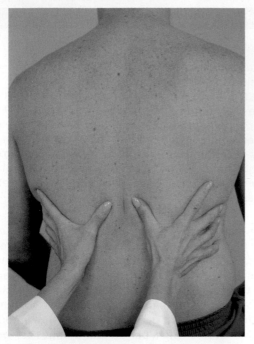

Figure 18.12 Testing for chest expansion.

Tactile fremitus is tested when concern exists about obstruction or consolidation of lung tissue. Following the sequence for palpation but avoiding the scapula, place the palmar base or ulnar surface of the hand on the patient's chest above the scapula. Ask the patient to say "ninety-nine." Vibrations of air in the bronchial tree are transmitted to the chest wall when the patient speaks. Assess for intensity and symmetry of fremitus. If fremitus is difficult to palpate, ask the patient to speak louder. As the technique is learned, fremitus may be palpated with a hand on each side simultaneously to further assess symmetry and gain efficiency. Because of the wide variation in findings, fremitus is usually interpreted in combination with other data. *Normal variations are wide-ranging, depending on voice intensity and pitch, position of the bronchi in relation to the chest wall, and chest size. Fremitus is normally more intense between the scapulae, where the bronchi bifurcate, and less intense at the bases, where more porous tissue reduces the transmission of vibrations.*

Percussion. Percussion is used when obstruction or consolidation of lung tissue is suspected (similar to testing of fremitus). This technique can help establish if underlying tissues contain air or fluid, or are solid. Use the percussion technique covered in Chapter 4. On the posterior chest, begin at the apex of the

Conditions that may obstruct lung tissue include an obstructed bronchus, *COPD, pleural effusion, fibrosis, tumor,* or *pneumothorax.* In these conditions fremitus is decreased or absent. Fremitus also is reduced with increased distance between the lung parenchyma and chest wall, as with obesity or an extremely large chest. Fremitus is increased in conditions of increased consolidation close to the chest wall, in which a bronchus is open. Examples include severe localized *pneumonia* or *lung tumor.* **Ronchal fremitus** is a coarse vibration produced by passage of air through or around thick exudates in the airways, such as in *pneumonia.* **Pleural friction fremitus** results from inflamed pleural surfaces rubbing together and causing a grating sensation synchronous with respirations and more commonly felt on inspiration.

Percussion may be dull when fluid or solid tissue replaces the normally air-filled spaces in the lungs, such as with lobar pneumonia, hemothorax, or tumor. If fluid is in the pleural space (eg, empyema, pleural effusion), the sound may also be dull. Generalized hyperresonance may be heard over the hyperinflated lungs found with COPD or emphysema. Unilateral hyperresonance may be found with a large pneumothorax.

lungs (C7 bilaterally) and percuss from side to side to compare symmetry (Fig. 18-13). Working toward the bases side to side in the ICSs, move fingers approximately 5-cm apart. When the fingers are below the level of lung tissue, the sound changes from resonant to dull (around T10); from this point move laterally to percuss near the anterior axillary line and the 7th and 8th ICSs. Avoid the area over the ribs and scapulae, because normal bone is flat. Percussion penetrates only 5–7 cm into the thorax, so abnormalities must be close to the surface and large enough (at least 2–3 cm) to be detected. Thus, percussion usually is combined with other tests (eg, chest x-ray). *Healthy lung tissue sounds resonant. In patients with extremely large chests, percussion sounds may become dull secondary to the increased tissue mass.*

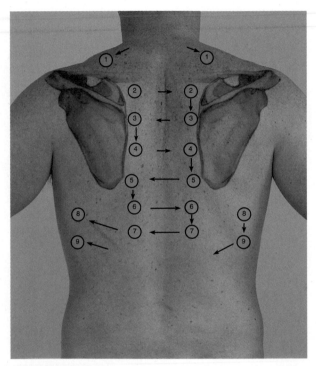

Figure 18.13 Sites and sequence for posterior chest percussion.

Test **diaphragmatic excursion** in cases of concern about chest expansion (eg, spinal cord injury). Diaphragmatic excursion helps estimate how much the diaphragm moves between inhalation and exhalation. Ask the patient to deeply exhale and hold it; then, percuss in the ICSs down the scapular line (Fig. 18-14). A helpful strategy is for the nurse to hold the breath at the same time as the patient to remember to let the patient breathe after a short time. When the sound changes from resonant to dull, go back to the previous resonant rib space. This marks the location of lung tissue on deep expiration (it may also be marked with a pen) (Fig 18-15). Allow the patient to breathe if needed or ask the patient to take in and hold a deep breath. Percuss in the previously resonant spot; *it should remain resonant.*

Diaphragmatic excursion may be reduced in *emphysema* (in which the diaphragm is already flat) or *atelectasis* (in which lung tissue is collapsed at the base). Extreme *ascites*, advanced pregnancy, and extreme obesity also limit diaphragmatic excursion. Neuromuscular paralysis or weakening of the diaphragm in *spinal cord injury, stroke, Guillian-Barré's syndrome*, or *muscular dystrophy* can also inhibit respiratory excursion. Lag in expansion may occur with *atelectasis, pneumonia*, or postoperative pain.

(text continues on page 466)

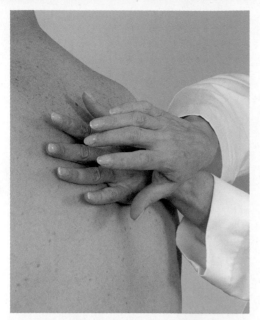

Figure 18.14 Assessing diaphragmatic excursion: percussing in the ICSs.

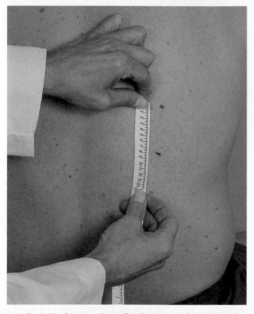

Figure 18.15 Assessing diaphragmatic excursion: marking the location of lung tissue.

Move down into the previously dull ICS; *it should now be resonant at deep inspiration because the lungs should have moved down with the diaphragm.* Move down one or two more rib spaces until the sound is dull again; *the difference should be one or two rib spaces, or 3–5 cm and 7–8 cm in well-conditioned adults (it may also be marked with a pen).* This estimates the amount of diaphragmatic movement between maximum inspiration and expiration, although this estimate does not correlate well with radiographic findings (Kleinman, 2002). As always, interpret these data within the context of other findings, such as strength of cough.

Technique and Normal Findings (continued)	Abnormal Findings (continued)

Technique and Normal Findings (continued)

Auscultation of Breath Sounds. Auscultation of the lung fields is the most important physical examination technique for assessing air flow through the respiratory passages and alveoli. In the larger airways, sounds are louder and coarser, while sounds in the smaller airways are softer and finer. Auscultate by listening from the top down alternating between left and right sides. It is very important to make sure that the stethoscope is in direct contact with the skin. If the patient is wearing a gown or clothing, the stethoscope can be placed underneath either from the top or bottom. Avoid listening through the gown, which can generate additional sounds that mimic adventitious sounds or that muffle existing sounds. Avoid allowing the tubing to rub against bed rails, patient, or nurse, which can create additional noise. Be careful not to interpret chest hair sounds as crackles; press more firmly or moisten the chest hair. Be sure to listen to the most important areas instead of only auscultating in convenient places. Additionally, listen for extra, abnormal sounds of breathing such as wheezes. Ask the patient to breathe through the mouth a bit deeper than normal. Place the flat side of the stethoscope diaphragm on the chest wall firmly to block extraneous noise. Listen to one full breath in each location, moving from side to side to compare symmetry.

Stand behind and beside the patient and listen from the lung apices to the bases and then laterally in the same sequence as percussion (see Fig. 18-11). If breath sounds are too soft, ask the patient to breathe deeper.

Identify the breath sounds by listening for their intensity, quality, pitch, and duration of inspiration versus expiration:

* ***Vesicular*** *sounds are soft, low-pitched, and found over fine airways near the site of air exchange.*
* ***Bronchovesicular*** *sounds are found over major bronchi that have fewer alveoli.*
* ***Bronchial*** *sounds are loud, high-pitched, and found over the trachea and larynx.*

Expiration is longer than inspiration, similar to normal breathing. As auscultation progresses down to the smaller airways, it takes time for air to move in, so inspiration is longer than expiration in vesicular sounds. See Table 18-3 for more complete descriptions of the sounds.

Abnormal Findings (continued)

⚠ *SAFETY ALERT 18.6*
Deep breathing can be especially exhausting for patients with respiratory disease; it also can cause some patients to hyperventilate and become dizzy. Instruct patients to tell you if they need a break.

Careful auscultation of the bases is important, because they often are the first area to collapse with atelectasis secondary to immobility. They are also often the first place to collect fluid in CHF or fluid overload.

Breath sounds are considered abnormal when heard outside their normal location, such as bronchial breath sounds in the bases. Bronchial or bronchovesicular sounds in the normal vesicular location indicate airway thickening. Decreased lung sounds are very common, especially in patients with *atelectasis* or *pleural effusion* (Greco, 2004). Auscultating sounds in patients with large chests may be difficult, because the lungs are at a greater distance from the chest wall. The breath sounds may be very soft, so a quiet room and a good seal with the skin are especially important. Absent lung sounds may be noted over areas where air transmission through the bronchioles is completely blocked, as with dense areas of atelectasis.

⚠ *SAFETY ALERT 18.7*
Absent sounds over a large portion of the lung, such as with a large mucus plug, may be an emergency. Get help immediately.

Breath sounds can increase when normal sounds are transmitted more easily over areas of consolidation or compression, such as in *lobar pneumonia or pleural effusion.*

(text continues on page 468)

Table 18.3 Characteristics of Normal Breath Sounds

	Intensity and Pitch	Quality	Duration	Locations
Bronchial	Loud and high	Coarse or tubular	Inspiration < expiration	Larynx and trachea
Bronchovesicular	Intermediate and intermediate	Intermediate	Inspiration = expiration	Anteriorly between first and second interspaces; between scapula
Vesicular	Soft and low	Whispering undertones	Inspiration > expiration	Over most of the lung fields

---

Technique and Normal Findings (continued)

Normal breath sounds are vesicular without crackles, wheezes or ronchii. In some people audible crackles with the first deep breath or before coughing are normal. These crackles are the sound of collapsed alveoli opening, which is a common consequence of immobility. It is important to note the absence of adventitious sounds when documenting.

Abnormal Findings (continued)

Adventitious (added) sounds are not normally heard. These extra sounds are layered on top of underlying breath sounds. If extra sounds are heard, listen for their loudness, pitch, duration, number, timing in the respiratory cycle (inspiration versus expiration), location on the chest wall, any variation from breath to breath, and any change after a cough or deep breath. It may be necessary to listen in the same area for a few cycles of breathing to differentiate the timing in the respiratory cycle and note changes that occur with breathing. If crackles or wheezes are audible, ask the patient to cough to hear if they clear.

- **Crackles** can result from fluid in the airways or alveoli or from the opening of a series of collapsed airways and alveoli that reinflate during deep breaths. They sound like hairs rubbing together near the ear or Velcro opening.
- **Wheezes** sound more musical, and are caused by the fluttering of narrowed airway walls (as with *asthma* or *bronchitis*). Note if wheezes occur on inspiration, expiration, or both.
- **Ronchi** (also called coarse wheezes or gurgles) are lower pitched and louder sounds resulting from secretions moving around during inhalation or exhalation. They commonly accompany *pneumonia*.

See Table 18-4 for a more complete comparison.

Technique and Normal Findings (continued)	Abnormal Findings (continued)
Auscultate voice sounds when an area of consolidation or compression is suspected. They may be assessed if other findings (eg, increased breath sounds) suggest these conditions.	Brochophony, egophony, and whispered pectoriloquy (described next) are all found with increased consolidation or compression, as with *lobar pneumonia, atelectasis,* or *tumor.*
Ask the patient to say "ninety-nine" as you auscultate the chest wall with a stethoscope, comparing sides. *Sounds are muffled and difficult to distinguish.*	The word "ninety-nine" is easily understood and louder over dense areas. It sounds as if the patient were directly talking into the stethoscope. This is called **brochophony**.
Ask the patient to say "ee" while listening to the chest, comparing sides. *This sound is also muffled and difficult to hear.*	In **egophony**, the "ee" sounds like a loud "A."
Ask the patient to whisper "one-two-three" while listening to the chest, comparing sides. *Normal sounds are faint, muffled, and difficult to hear.*	Sounds are louder and clearer than the whispered sounds, as if the patient is directly whispering into the stethoscope. This is called **whispered pectoriloquy**.

Documentation of Normal Findings

Symmetrical chest shape without kyphosis or scoliosis. Vesicular breath sounds over lung fields. Denies chest pain or tenderness. No crackles or wheezes. *S. Garcia, RN*

Table 18.4 Adventitious Breath Sounds

Abnormal Sound	Description	Mechanism	Associated Conditions
Fine crackles (rales)	High-pitched, soft, brief crackling sounds that can be simulated by rolling a strand of hair near the ear or stethoscope	Deflated small airways and alveoli will pop open during inspiration. In early CHF, small amounts of fluid in the alveoli may cause fine crackles.	Late inspiratory crackles are associated with restrictive disease (eg, fibrosis and heart failure). Early inspiratory crackles occur with obstructive diseases (eg, asthma and COPD).
Coarse crackles (rales)	Low-pitched, moist, longer sounds that are similar to Velcro slowly separating	Small air bubbles flow through secretions or narrowed airways.	Pulmonary fibrosis, pulmonary edema, COPD
Wheeze (high-pitched or sibilant)	High-pitched musical sounds heard primarily during inspiration	Air passes though narrowed airways and creates sound, similar to that of a vibrating reed. Note if inspiratory or expiratory.	Asthma, bronchitis, emphysema
Ronchi (gurgle, low-pitched wheeze, sonorous wheeze)	Low-pitched snoring or gurgling sound that may clear with coughing	Airflow passes around or through secretions or narrowed passages.	Pneumonia
Pleural friction rub	Loud, coarse, and low-pitched grating or creaking sound similar to a squeaky door during inspiration and expiration; more common in the lower anterolateral thorax	Inflamed pleural surfaces lose their normal lubrication and rub together during breathing.	Pleuritis
Stridor	Loud high-pitched crowing or honking sound louder in upper airway	Laryngeal or tracheal inflammation or spasm can cause stridor, as can aspiration of a foreign object.	Epiglottitis, croup, partially obstructed airway; can indicate an emergency requiring immediate attention

Anterior Chest

Inspection. Inspect the anterior chest using the same techniques as for the posterior chest. Look for any deformities or asymmetry, retraction of the supraclavicular or ICSs, or impaired respiratory movement. *Normal findings are similar as for the posterior chest.*

Palpation. Palpate the anterior chest for tenderness, masses, or lesions. Begin at the lung apices and move from side to side, ending below the costal angle and moving laterally to the midaxillary line. *Normally there is no tenderness.*

Assess anterior chest expansion by palpating with the thumbs along each costal margin near the sternum and with the palmar surface laterally on the rib cage (Fig. 18-16). Slide the thumbs medially so that they raise a small skin fold between them. Ask the patient to inhale deeply; observe the thumb movement. Feel for the extent of symmetric chest expansion. *Anterior chest expansion is greater than with posterior because the rib cage has more anterior mobility.*

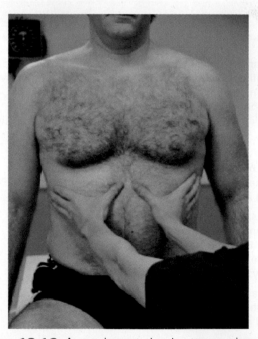

Figure 18.16 Assessing anterior chest expansion.

Assess for tactile fvremitus, beginning at the lung apices and continuing to the bases and laterally, comparing bilateral symmetry. It may be necessary to ask female patients to lift or to displace their breast to the side, because fremitus is decreased over this soft tissue. *Fremitus is decreased or absent over the precordium because of the heart. Fremitus is greatest over large airways in the 2nd and 3rd ICSs near the sternum.*

Abnormal findings are similar to those for the posterior chest. The costal margin is widened in hyper-inflation of the lungs. The chest may be barrel shaped in diseases that obstruct air outflow such as *COPD* and *asthma.* See Tables 18-10 and 18-11 at the end of the chapter.

Percussion. Percuss the anterior and lateral chest in the ICSs and laterally, comparing bilateral findings. Women may need to displace the breast to avoid percussion over breast tissue, which produces a dull sound. Avoid percussing over bone, which produces a flat tone. *The heart produces dullness from the 3rd to 5th ICS to the left of the sternum. The upper border of liver dullness is percussed in the 5th ICS in the right MCL. Tympany is percussed over the stomach in the 5th ICS in the left MCL.*

Auscultation. Auscultate the trachea and anterior and lateral lung fields, beginning at the trachea. Listen to the lung apices, moving the stethoscope from side to side to evaluate symmetry. Place the stethoscope around the breasts in female patients. Listen down to the 6th ICS bilaterally or when breath sounds become absent, signaling the end of the lung fields. *Breath sounds are usually louder in the upper chest, where the larger airways are closer to the chest wall. Bronchial breath sounds are audible over the trachea; bronchovesicular sounds are heard over the 2nd to 3rd ICSs to the right and left of the sternum over the bronchi. Vesicular sounds are heard in other areas of the lung fields. No adventitious sounds are heard (see Table 18-3).*

If indicated, auscultate for transmitted voice sounds using the same pattern and technique as for the anterior chest.

Documentation of Normal Findings

Symmetrical chest shape and expansion. Lungs clear, no crackles or wheezes. Denies chest pain or tenderness. *S. Garcia, RN*

Documenting Abnormal Findings

The nurse has just finished conducting a physical examination of Mr. Jin. Review the following important findings revealed in each step of objective data collection for this patient. Compare these results with the normal findings presented in the samples of normal documentation.

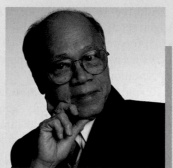

Inspection: T 38°C oral, P 102 beats/min, R 24 breaths/min, BP 156/78 mm Hg, SaO_2 90%. Alert and oriented. Patient sitting in chair with increased respiratory effort. Nasal flaring and pursed lip breathing. Needs to pause to breathe in the middle of sentences. Skin color pale, using neck muscles to breathe, no retractions. Clubbing present in fingers. Coughing up moderate amounts of thick-yellow sputum. Denies chest pain. Increased dyspnea and respirations 32 breaths/min when ambulating in hall.

Palpation: Tactile fremitus increased in right base.

Percussion: Right base dull to percussion.

Auscultation: Few wheezes scattered through lung fields. Decreased breath sounds noted in right base. Bronchophony, egophony, and whispered pectolioquy over right base.

J. Nguyen, RN

Table 18.5	Apgar Scoring System		
	0	1	2
Heart rate	Absent	Slow below 100 beats/min	>100 beats/min
Respiratory effort	Absent	Slow or irregular	Good crying
Muscle tone	Limp	Some flexion of extremities	Active motion
Reflex irritability (response to catheter in nostril)	No response	Grimace, frown	Cough or sneeze
Color	Blue or pale	Body pink, extremities blue	Completely pink

Lifespan Considerations

Pregnant Women

The woman's chest may appear wider and the costal angle larger in late pregnancy as the uterus pushes up on the diaphragm. Pregnant women may have strained or fractured ribs because of expansion of the thoracic cage.

Newborns, Infants, and Children

In newborns, Apgar scores are taken at 1 and 5 minutes after birth to determine health status and need for interventions (Table 18-5). In the respiratory component of the Apgar, the nurse evaluates respirations, using a sliding scale from absent to accompanied by strong crying.

The first breaths take great effort as the airways and alveoli are inflated. Sedatives given to the mother during labor, a compromised newborn blood supply, or airways obstructed by mucus may depress the baby's ventilation. All of these require interventions to correct the underlying cause. Premature infants are especially at risk for pulmonary problems, because their lungs may not produce enough surfactant, causing the alveoli to collapse.

Add the scores of the five observations to get the full Apgar score. Lower the score, the more likely that there is a problem. A score of 7–10 is desirable. A score of 0–2 is a severely depressed newborn in need of emergency resuscitation.

Respiratory patterns in infants vary based on feeding, sleep state, and body temperature. Because of this irregularity, respirations in infants should be counted for 1 minute. Respiratory rates are fastest in newborns; they decrease with age (Table 18-6). The more premature the newborn, the more irregular may be the respiration because of the lack of a well-developed nervous system (Bader, et al., 2004).

SAFETY ALERT 18.8

Apnea that lasts 10–15 is common; longer apneic periods or cyanosis in the baby are causes for concern.

Another criterion of the Apgar score is skin color (see Table 18-5). The lowest rating is blue or pale; the highest rating is completely pink. **Acrocynosis** (cyanosis of the hands and feet) is normal immediately after birth or if newborns are exposed to a cool environment. If poor peripheral circulation causes the acrocyanosis, the sole of the foot turns pink when it is vigorously rubbed; if it is true cyanosis, the foot stays blue.

Newborns are nose breathers, and nasal flaring is common because their noses are often congested. Suctioning immediately after birth is usual practice. Respiratory grunting indicates increased effort to expel air or fluid. Coughing in newborns raises concern over lung involvement. Newborns use the diaphragm and abdominal muscles for respiratory effort, movements that are noticeable in this age group. Crepitus around the clavicle requires assessment; a positive finding may indicate a pneumothorax, especially following forceps delivery. Newborns delivered by cesarean section have more apnea, especially during sleep (Bader, et al., 2004).

Table 18.6	Normal Range of Resting Values for Respiration
Age	Respirations (/min)
Newborn	30–60
6 months	24–38
1 year	22–30
3 years	22–30
5 years	20–24
10 years	16–22
12 years	16–22
14 years	14–20

Source: National Institutes of Health. (n.d.). *Age appropriate vital signs*. Retrieved March 11, 2007, from http://clinicalcenter.nih.gov/ccc/pedweb/pedsstaff/age.html

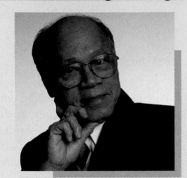

Remember Mr. Jin, whose problems have been outlined throughout this chapter. The initial subjective and objective data collection is complete, and the nurse has spent time reviewing the findings and other results. The following nursing note illustrates how subjective and objective data are analyzed and nursing interventions are developed as part of the nursing process described above. The subjective and objective data provide evidence for the analysis (the nursing diagnosis or problem). The plan includes interventions related to the diagnosis, previously described.

Subjective: "I'm still not feeling very well. When I came in last time, they said that I had bronchitis, but it feels like it's getting worse. Last time I felt wheezy; this time, I'm coughing more."

Objective: Alert and oriented. Sitting in chair with increased respiratory effort. T 38°C oral, P 102 beats/min, R 24 breaths/min, BP 156/78 mm Hg, SaO_2 90%. Skin color pale, using neck muscles to breathe, no retractions. Coughing up approximately ½ cup of thick-yellow sputum daily. Few wheezes scattered through lung fields. Decreased breath sounds noted in right base. No chest pain noted. Also complaining of increasing fatigue. Dyspnea and respirations 32 breaths/min when ambulating in hall.

Analysis: Increasing dyspnea, cough, sputum, and fatigue. Impaired gas exchange with reduced SaO_2. Risk for ineffective airway clearance with increasing sputum. Potential for infection in the lungs.

Plan: Contact primary health practitioner about findings. Further assess effect of problems on patient's sleep pattern and ADLs. Teach to drink 2 L of fluid to liquefy secretions. Teach patient about coughing and deep breathing techniques. Teach to pace activity and rest when dyspneic. Have patient take temperature three times daily and call if >38.5°C or 101.5°F. Contact respiratory therapy about administration of inhalers and interventions to reduce dyspnea. Contact primary health practitioner to discuss possibility of obtaining sputum culture and sensitivity, chest x-ray, and medical treatments. Discuss concerns with patient's wife.

J. Nguyen, RN

Critical Thinking Challenge

- Critique the objective data that were documented. How will the nursing data collection differ from that of the primary health care provider?
- What other data might be collected to identify problems affecting other body systems or functional status?
- How will the nurse work collaboratively with the primary health care provider to evaluate interventions?

Percussion is not useful in newborns because an adult's hands are too large for the small chest. When auscultating the lungs, make sure to use the pediatric diaphragm on the stethoscope appropriate for the newborn's size. If the baby is crying, wait for a quiet moment to auscultate. Also, take advantage of sleep in newborns to listen to breath sounds. If the baby is quiet, breath sounds are easier to hear in newborns than in adults because of their thinner and smaller chest wall. Breath sounds are also transmitted more easily, so they may be referred to areas where there are absent breath sounds; listen to fine differences in quality. Expect to auscultate crackles or gurgles because of small amounts of fluid that remain in the lungs.

If adventitious lung sounds are asymmetrical, meconium aspiration may have occurred in one section of the lung. If gastrointestinal gurgling sounds are heard in the chest, communicate these findings to a primary health practitioner, because the newborn may have a diaphragmatic hernia.

Parents may hold a hesitant child or a child may want to sit in a parent's lap. Children are curious about stethoscopes; gain trust by having them listen to their own breath sounds first. Detecting expiratory sounds in children with rapid respirations is difficult. Asking them to blow out the penlight will prolong expiratory sounds and wheezing may be detected. A child may also like to breathe like a hot or tired dog during auscultation. A child's breath sounds are louder and harsher; therefore, bronchovesicular breath sounds may normally be heard through the chest.

Children begin using their intercostals muscles to breathe by 6 to 7 years old. A round chest shape that persists past 5 to 6 years may indicate pulmonary disease. If the child is crying, auscultate the chest during the deep breath that follows a sob.

Older Adults

Immobility creates a risk for airway collapse (atelectasis), reduced air exchange, hypoxia, hypercapnia, and acidosis. Reduced gag and cough reflexes can place older people at risk for aspiration of secretions and, potentially, aspiration pneumonia. Postoperative pulmonary complications are another possibility because of impaired cough reflex, weaker muscles, and decreased inspiratory capacity.

Older adults are at increased risk for pulmonary complications during stress. Attention must be paid to maintaining effective ventilation, keeping lung volumes high, clearing secretions, and positioning to prevent aspiration. Respiratory assessment may be tiring for people of this age group, so allow frequent rest periods. Postpone those activities that can wait until strength has returned so that these patients can use energy for breathing.

Evidence-based Critical Thinking

Organizing and Prioritizing

Nurses must continuously think critically about the patient's condition to organize and prioritize assessments and patient care. Laboratory and diagnostic tests related to the respiratory system can add to the database of findings created after the health history and physical examination. The analysis of history, physical examination, and laboratory data helps to identify the underlying cause of signs and symptoms. Nurses use these data to identify the underlying functional problem, label the problem (sometimes in a nursing diagnosis format), and plan interventions based

on patient outcomes. At times nurses make referrals for a complex problem. They need to clearly communicate assessment findings and reasons for referrals to other health care providers. Nurses also work with primary health practitioners to gather information to make a diagnosis and to prescribe appropriate collaborative care. They reassess patients to evaluate the effectiveness of both nursing and collaborative care measures.

Laboratory and Diagnostic Testing

Laboratory data taken from samples of blood or other body fluids give indirect measures of disease. For example, an elevated white blood cell count may indicate infection (eg, pneumonia). Analysis of a sputum sample may help pinpoint the type of causative bacteria. Arterial blood gas sampling is a direct measure of blood levels of oxygen, carbon dioxide, and pH. Other diagnostic tests can help visualize the thorax and lungs in different ways to identify structures and densities.

Chest x-rays are commonly performed in patients with respiratory problems. Radiography can identify areas of consolidation, which accompanies pneumonia, TB, and cancer. When more accurate testing is needed to identify the size and shape of lesions, a CT scan or MRI may be indicated. These methods, however, are expensive.

A V/Q scan identifies differences in ventilation and perfusion and is commonly ordered in cases of suspected pulmonary embolism. If findings are abnormal, the patient's oxygen saturation level should be closely monitored; deep vein thrombosis prophylaxis may be indicated.

Pulmonary function tests provide information about the patient's ability to move air into and out of the lungs. Total vital capacity, inspiratory volume, and expiratory reserve are measured for patients at risk for disease or dyspneic symptoms. These tests may show whether a patient requires home oxygen therapy or assistance with ADLs at home.

Refer to table at the end of the chapter that compares assessment findings for common medical diagnoses related to the thorax, lung, and respiratory functioning.

Diagnostic Reasoning

Assessment findings are used as a basis for nursing care. An accurate and complete assessment provides a firm foundation for setting outcomes, providing individualized interventions, and evaluating progress.

Nursing Diagnoses, Outcomes, and Interventions

Difficulty breathing could be a manifestation of many different underlying problems. Alveolar exchange of oxygen and carbon dioxide might be impaired. The airway may have too many secretions. Breathing could be too shallow or slow. Interventions for each of these problems are very different.

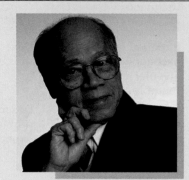

In many facilities, nurses initiate referrals for respiratory care based on assessment findings. Results that might trigger a respiratory therapy consult include an unexpected change in respiratory status; increased wheezing; absent breath sounds; gurgles; sudden decrease in oxygen saturation; accessory muscle use; respiratory rate greater than 30 breaths/min; change in pattern and rate of breathing; cyanosis; dyspnea; or an acute change in oxygen saturation or arterial blood gasses (Interdisciplinary Plan, 2005).

Mr. Jin has been experiencing many of the problems outlined above; therefore, a respiratory therapy consult might be indicated. In this case, the situation and background are the assessment information. The analysis is the nursing diagnosis or problem and the recommendations are the interventions. The following conversation illustrates how the nurse might organize data and make recommendations about the patient's care to the respiratory therapy department.

Situation: Hi, I'm June Nguyen, a nurse working with Mr. Jin. He is 65 years old with a history of COPD, CHF, and high blood pressure.

Background: He came in 2 weeks ago for bronchitis and returned to the clinic today with increasing cough, thick-yellow sputum production, and fatigue. His temperature is 38°C, respirations are 24 breaths/min, and pulse is 112 beats/min. His saturations usually are 92% to 94% but now are 90%. He is short of breath with even walking in the hall. He usually has scattered wheezes but now has new decreased breath sounds in the right base.

Analysis: I'm concerned about his low oxygen saturation and ability to handle his increased sputum.

Recommendations: He is continuing to use his inhalers, and he says that they help. I was wondering if you could come to assess his need for more inhalers and make sure that he is using them properly. Could you also listen to his lungs and see if you think that he might benefit from some chest physiotherapy to assist with mobilizing his secretions?

Critical Thinking Challenge

- How did the nurse prioritize which subjective information to share?
- Critique the objective data. Is the organization logical? Would it be clearer to add to or take out any of the information?
- Critique the analysis and recommendations. What is the nurse's role in coordinating collaborative care with respiratory therapy?

If the problem is with airway clearance, fluids are given to help liquefy secretions. If the problem is shallow breathing, deep breathing exercises are indicated. When formulating a nursing diagnosis, it is important to use critical thinking and to ensure the accuracy of assessment findings to increase the chances for arriving at correct diagnosis. Note that the diagnosis is supported by the abnormal assessment findings. The point of differentiation summarizes the major problem related to the diagnosis. See Table 18-7 for nursing diagnoses commonly related to thorax, lung, and respiratory assessment (Johnson, et al., 2005).

Nurses use assessment information to identify patient outcomes. Some outcomes related to respiratory problems include the following:

- Demonstrate improved ventilation and adequate oxygenation
- Maintain clear lung fields and remain free of signs of respiratory distress
- Demonstrate effective coughing
- Maintain a patent airway at all times (Moorhead, et al., 2008).

Table 18.7 Nursing Diagnoses for the Respiratory System

Diagnosis and RelatedFactors	Point of Differentiation	Assessment Characteristics	Nursing Interventions
Impaired gas exchange related to alveolar–capillary membrane changes	Describes changes at the capillary level	Low pO_2, confusion, cyanosis, fatigue, tachycardia, use of accessory muscles	Administer oxygen,* deep breathing, incentive spirometer, inhalers*
Ineffective airway clearance related to thick tracheobronchial secretions	Describes problems related to expectorating sputum	Cough, thick secretions, adventitious sounds, cyanosis, nasal flaring	Cough and deep breathe, increase fluids, expectorants,* postural drainage*
Ineffective breathing pattern related to fatigue	Describes changes in respiratory rate, rhythm, or depth	Decreased chest excursion, dyspnea, nasal flaring, increased rate, decreased depth, accessory muscles	Position to decrease workload of breathing, pace activity, provide rest, reduce fever
Excess fluid volume related to CHF	Describes peripheral edema and fluid accumulation in the lung	Low pO_2, frothy sputum, decreased breath sounds, pleural effusion, shortness of breath, orthopnea, paroxysmal nocturnal dyspnea	Elevate head of bed, administer diuretics,* intake and output, daily weights

*Collaborative interventions.

Pulling It All Together: Reflection and Critical Thinking

The nurse uses assessment data to formulate a nursing care plan for Mr. Jin. He or she may independently perform teaching on appropriate inhaler-use, teach cough and deep breathing techniques, and teach the need for increased fluids to liquefy secretions. The nurse also may initiate a referral to respiratory therapy about inhaler-use and possible chest physiotherapy and consulting with the primary health practitioner about his potential infection. The assessment data is included as the "as evidenced by" section of the care planning. Outcomes and interventions are established collaboratively with the patient. After the interventions are completed, the nurse will reevaluate (or reassess) Mr. Jin and document the findings in the chart to show the progress toward the patient outcomes. This is often in the form of a care plan or case note similar to the one below.

Nursing Diagnosis	Patient Outcomes	Nursing Interventions	Rationale	Evaluation
Ineffective Airway Clearance related to fatigue and inability to cough effectively as evidenced by RR, dyspnea	Breath sounds return to baseline wheezing with no gurgles in right base within 1 week.	Teach patient cough and deep breathing techniques to perform every 2 hours. Identify fluids that patient likes to reach goal of 2 L/day. Teach patient to call clinic for T > 38.5°C increased dyspnea, increasing sputum.	Increases force and depth of breath to clear secretions. Fluids liquefy secretions to make them easier to expel. Signs and symptoms of worsening status should be reevaluated.	Demonstrated accurate cough and deep breathing techniques. Drank 1 L/day. Stated when to call clinic. Lungs sounds with wheezing and gurgles in right base. Encourage fluids every 2 hours. Encourage cough and deep breathing every hour. Reassess in 4 hours.

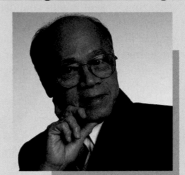

Thus, subjective and objective assessment data are used in developing a diagnosis, planning care and evaluating progress toward established outcomes. Using this nursing process and critical thinking, consider all the case study findings woven throughout this chapter. When answering the following questions, begin drawing conclusions and see how the pieces of assessment must work together to create an environment for personalized, appropriate, and accurate care.

• Is Mr. Jin's condition stable, urgent, or an emergency?
• What health promotion and teaching needs are identified? Which two areas are highest priorities?
• How will the nurse focus, organize, and prioritize subjective and objective data collection?
• Which nursing diagnosis is highest priority? Provide rationale.
• How will the nurse individualize assessment to Mr. Jin's specific needs, considering his condition, age, and culture?

Once outcomes are established, nursing care can be implemented to improve the patient's status. Nurses use critical thinking and evidence-based practice to develop the interventions. Some examples of nursing interventions for respiratory care are as follows:

• Monitory respiratory rate, depth, accessory muscle use, and breath sound every 1 to 4 hours.
• Monitor oxygen saturation using pulse oximetry.
• Position the patient with the head of the bed at 45 degrees; reposition every 2 hours.
• Obtain incentive spirometer and teach the patient to use it to prevent atelectasis and retained bronchial secretions (Bulechek, et al., 2008).

Nurses then evaluate care according to the patient outcomes that were developed, thereafter reassessing the patient and continuing or modifying interventions as appropriate.

An accurate and complete nursing assessment is an essential foundation for holistic nursing care. Even beginning nursing students can use the patient assessment to implement new interventions, evaluate the effectiveness of those interventions, and make a difference in the quality of patient care.

Key Points

• Anterior and posterior landmarks are used to identify the location of lung fields.
• Reference lines include the midsternal anterior axillary, mid-clavicular line, verbral line, posterior axillary line, and midaxillary line.
• Anteriorly, the apex of the lung extends approximately 2 to 4 cm above the inner third of the clavicle and posteriorly the base is near T10.

• With ageing, the lungs lose elasticity, respiratory strength decreases, cartilage loses flexibility, and bones lose density.
• Dyspnea, decreased level of consciousness, respirations > 30 breaths/min, oxygen saturation < 90, retractions, and acces-sory muscle use may indicate an acute or emergency situation.
• Health promotion includes avoidance of smoking, occupational exposure to irritants, recreational drugs, high risk travel and recommendation on influenza and pneumoncoccal vaccines.
• Common respiratory symptoms include chest pain, dyspnea, orthopnea, paroxysmal nocturnal dyspnea, cough, mucus, wheezing, and change in functional ability.
• The initial survey includes position, pursed lips, nasal flaring, level of consciousness, skin color, respiratory movement and rate, oxygen saturation, accessory muscle use, and retractions.
• Abnormal respiratory patterns include tachypnea, hyperventilation, bradypnea, hypoventilation, Cheynes-Stokes, biots, agonal, and apnea.
• Objective assessment includes inspection, palpation, chest expansion, tactile fremitus, percussion, and diaphragmatic excursion.
• Breath sounds are auscultated and labeled as vesicular, bronchial, or bronchovesicular.
• Adventitious lung sounds include fine and coarse crackles, wheezes, ronchi, pleural friction rub, and stridor.
• Ausculatate voice sounds for bronchophony, egophony, and whispered pectorilioquy.
• The Apgar scoring system is used to assess the newborn, including respiratory effort and skin color.
• Common nursing diagnoses include impaired gas exchange, ineffective airway clearance, ineffective breathing pattern, and excess fluid volume.

• A respiratory therapy consultation may be indicated with an unexpected change in respiratory status; increased wheezing; absent breath sounds; gurgles; sudden decrease in oxygen saturation; accessory muscle use; respiratory rate greater than 30 breaths/min; change in pattern and rate of breathing; cyanosis; dyspnea; or an acute change in oxygen saturation or arterial blood gasses.

Review Questions

1. When the nurse assesses a 78-year-old client with pneumonia, which finding should be evaluated first?
   A. Breath sounds
   B. Airway patency
   C. Respiratory rate
   D. Percussion sounds

2. A 45-year-old man has been admitted to the hospital with pulmonary embolism. Which of the following symptoms should the nurse report to the primary health practitioner immediately?
   A. Chest pain
   B. Shortness of breath
   C. Respirations 20 breaths/min
   D. Productive cough

3. A 62-year-old woman comes to the clinic with an exacerbation of asthma. Which of the following findings indicate worsening status of her asthma?
   A. Increased wheezing
   B. Bloody sputum
   C. Increased tympany
   D. Flushed red skin

4. A 3-year-old boy is in the emergency department with stridor, intercostal and supraclavicular retractions, and respiratory rate of 40. What type of situation is this?
   A. Stable
   B. Acute
   C. Urgent
   D. Emergency

5. A 92-year-old woman with a history of COPD presents with increasing shortness of breath, decreased lung sounds in the bases, increased edema, and weight gain. What is the most likely problem?
   A. Impaired gas exchange
   B. Ineffective airway clearance
   C. Activity intolerance
   D. Excess fluid volume

6. Which of the following factors is most likely to increase the risk of a patient developing COPD?
   A. Increased age
   B. Immune suppression
   C. Smoking
   D. Occupational exposure

7. When the nurse assesses the client with respiratory symptoms, which of the following complaints should be evaluated first?
   A. Chest pain
   B. Shortness of breath
   C. Cough
   D. Sputum

8. When assessing the client with atelectasis, what assessment findings are expected? Choose all that apply.
   A. Shortness of breath
   B. Decreased breath sounds
   C. Decreased oxygen saturation
   D. Increased tactile fremitus
   E. Hyper-resonance

9. Which assessments would indicate that the inhaled bronchodilators have their desired effect?
   A. Wheezing, O_2 saturation 94%, pallor
   B. Vesicular breath sounds, O_2 saturation 96%, pink
   C. Bronchial breath sounds, O_2 saturation 100%, erythema
   D. Crackles, O_2 saturation 90, cyanosis

10. The nurse auscultates bronchovesicular breath sounds in the 2nd ICS near the sternum. The nurse interprets this as
    A. a normal finding over the trachea
    B. a normal finding over the bronchi
    C. an abnormal finding over the lung
    D. an abnormal finding over the trachea

References

American Lung Association. (2004). *American Lung Association offers tips to improve indoor air quality during high pollution season*. Retrieved January 7, 2007, from http://www.lungusa.org/site/apps/s/content.asp?c=dvLUK9O0E&b=34706&ct=66959

Bader, D., Riskin, A., Paz, E., Kugelman, A., & Tirosh, E. (2004). Breathing patterns in term infants delivered by caesarean section. *Acta Paediatrica, 93*(9), 1216–1220.

Benditt, J. O. (2006). The neuromuscular respiratory system: Physiology, pathophysiology, and a respiratory care approach to patients. *Respiratory Care, 51*(8), 829–837.

Berman, S., Tanasijevic, M. J., Alvarex, J. G., Ludmir, J., Liberman, E., & Richardson, D. K. (1996). Racial differences in the predictive value of the TDx fetal lung maturity assay. *American Journal of Obstetrics and Gynecology, 175*(1), 73–77.

Caroci, A. S., & Lareau, S. C. (2004). Descriptors of dyspnea by patients with chronic obstructive pulmonary disease versus congestive heart failure. *Heart Lung, 33*(2), 102–110.

Centers for Disease Control and Prevention. (1997). *Prevention of pneumococcal disease: Recommendations of the Advisory Committee on Immunization Practices (ACIP)*. Retrieved February 17, 2007, from http://www.cdc.gov/MMWR/preview/MMWRhtml/00047135.htm

Centers for Disease Control and Prevention. (2005a). *Cinical guidance on the identification and evaluation of possible SARS-CoV disease among persons presenting with community-acquired illness.* Retrieved January 7, 2007, from http://www.cdc.gov/ncidod/sars/clinicalguidance.htm

Centers for Disease Control and Prevention. (2005b). *Risk factors and use of preventative services, United States.* Retrieved January 7, 2007, from http://www.cdc.gov/nccdphp/burdenbook2004/Section03/smokeadult.htm

Centers for Disease Control and Prevention. (2006a). Prevention and control of influenza: Recommendations of the Advisory Committee on Immunization Practices (ACIP). *Morbidity and Mortality Weekly Report, 55*(RR10):1–42.

Centers for Disease Control and Prevention. (2006b). *TB facts for health care workers 2006.* Retrieved January 7, 2007, from http://www.cdc.gov/nchstp/tb/pubs/TBfacts_HealthWorkers/populations.htm

Cohen, L., Doyle, W. J., Turner, R. B., Alper, C. M., & Skoner, D. P. (2004). Childhood socioeconomic status and host resistance to infectious illness in adulthood. *Psychosomatic Medicine, 66*(4), 553–558.

Crapo, J., Glassroth, J., Karlinsky, J. B., & Talmadge, E. K. (2006). *Baum's textbook of pulmonary disease* (7th ed.). Philadelphia: Lippincott Williams & Wilkins.

Davis, A. M., Kreutzer, R., Lipsett, M., King, G. M., & Shaikh, N. (2006). Asthma prevalence in Hispanic and Asian American ethnic subgroups: Results from the California healthy kids survey. *Pediatrics, 118*(2), e363–e370.

Bulechek, G., Butcher, H., Dochtermna, J. (2008). *Nursing Interventions Classification (NIC)* (5th ed.). St. Louis: Mosby.

Greco, F. A. (2004). Interpretation of breath sounds. *American Journal of Respiratory and Critical Care Medicine, 169,* 1260.

Haiman, C. A., Stram, D. O., Wilkens, L. R., Pike, M. C., Kolonel, L. N., Henderson, B. E., et al. (2006). Ethnic and racial differences in the smoking-related risk of lung cancer. *New England Journal of Medicine, 354*(4), 333–342.

Hancox, R. J., Poulto, R., Taylor, D. R., Greene, J. M., McLachlan, C. R., Cowan, J. O., et al. (2006). Associations between respiratory symptoms, lung function and gastro-oesophageal reflux symptoms in a population-based birth cohort. *Respiratory Research, 5*(7), 142.

Hankinson, J. L., Crapo, R. O., & Jensen, R. L. (2003). Spirometric reference values for the 6-s FVC maneuver. *Chest, 124,* 1805–1811.

Henschke, C. I., Yip, R., & Miettinen, O. S. (2006). Women's susceptibility to tobacco carcinogens and survival after diagnosis of lung cancer. *Journal of the American Medical Association, 296,* 180–184.

Health effects: hazards of second hand smoke (July 21, 2006). Retrieved January 7, 2007 from http://www.secondhandsmokesyou.com/health_effects/index.php

Hong, S. J., Lee, M. S., Lee, W. Y., Ahn, K. M., Oh, J. W., Kim, K. E., et al. (2006). High body mass index and dietary pattern assocated with childhood asthma. *Pediatric Pulmonology, 41*(12), 1118–1124.

Interdisciplinary plan for assessment/reassessment and care planning (2005). Retrieved February 19, 2007 from https://hmcweb.washington.edu/ADMIN/APOP/Administration/5.2.htm

Ip, M. S., Ko, F. W., Lau, A. C., Yu, W. C., Tang, K. S., Choo, K., et al. (2006). Updated spirometric reference values for adult Chinese in Hong Kong and implications on clinical utilization. *Chest, 129*(2), 384–392.

Johnson, M., Bulechek, G. M., McCloskey Dochterman, J, & Maas, M. L. (2005). *NANDA, NOC, and NIC linkages: Nursing diagnoses, outcomes, and interventions.* St. Louis: Mosby.

Jones, R. L., & Nzekwu, M. M. (2006). The effects of body mass index on lung volumes. *Chest, 130*(3), 827–833.

Kleinman, B. S., Frey, K., VanDrunen, M., Sheikh, T., DiPinto, D., Mason, R., et al. (2002). Motion of the diaphragm in patients with chronic obstructive pulmonary disease while spontaneously breathing versus during positive pressure breathing after anesthesia and neuromuscular blockade. *Anesthesiology, 97*(2), 298–305.

Lee, T., Brugge, D., Francis, C., & Fisher, O. (2003). Asthma prevalence among inner-city Asian-American schoolchildren. *Public Health Report, 118*(3), 215–220.

Marinella, M. A., Pierson, C., Chenoweth, C., Marinella, M. A., Pierson, C., & Chenoweth, C. (1997). The stethoscope. A potential source of nosocomial infection? *Archives of Internal Medicine, 157*(7), 786–790.

McPhee, S. J., Papadakis, M. A., & Tierney, L. M. (2007). *Current medical diagnosis and treatment* (46th ed.). McGraw Hill: New York.

Moore, K. L., & Agur, A. M. (2007). *Essential clinical anatomy* (2nd ed.). Philadelphia: Lippincott Williams & Wilkins.

Moorhead, S., Johnson, M., Maas, M., & Swanson (2008). *Nursing outcomes classification (NOC)* (4th ed.). Philadelphia: Mosby.

National Institutes of Health. (n.d.). *Age appropriate vital signs.* Retrieved March 11, 2007, from http://clinicalcenter.nih.gov/ccc/pedweb/pedsstaff/age.html

Rakel, R. E. (2006). *Conn's current therapy 2007.* Philadelphia: Elsevier.

Singh, S. K., Chowdhary, G. R., & Purohit, G. (2006). Assessment of impact of high particulate concentration on peak expiratory flow rate of lungs of sand stone quarry workers. *International Journal of Environmental Research in Public Health, 3*(4), 355–359.

Smoking Cessation Leadership Center (n.d.). *30 seconds to save a life.* Retrieved January 7, 2007, from http://smokingcessationleadership.ucsf.edu/30seconds.html

Stick, S. (2000). Paediatric origins of adult lung disease: The contribution of airway development to paediatric and adult lung disease. *Thorax, 55,* 587–594.

Tashkin, D. P. (2001). Airway effects of marijuana, cocaine and other inhaled illicit agents. *Current Opinion in Pulmonary Medicine, 7*(2), 43–61.

Taylor, Z., Nolan, C. M., Blumberg, H. M., American Thoracic Society, Centers for Disease Control and Prevention, & Infectious Diseases Society of America. (2005). Controlling tuberculosis in the United States. Recommendations from the American Thoracic Society, CDC, and the Infectious Diseases Society of America. *Morbidity and Mortality Weekly Report, 54*(RR–12), 1–81.

Tessier, J. F., Nejjari, C., Letenneur, L., Barberger-Gateau, P., Dartigues, J. F., & Salamon, R. (2000). Smoking and eight-year mortality in an elderly cohort. *International Journal Tuberculosis Lung Disease, 4*(8), 698–704.

U.S. Department of Health and Human Sevices. (n.d.). *Healthy People 2010: What are its goals?* Retrieved January 7, 2007, from http://www.healthypeople.gov/About/goals.htm

Woods, S. L., Sivarajan Froelicher, E., & Motzer-Underhill, S. (2005). *Cardiac nursing* (5th ed.). Philadelphia: Lippincott Williams & Wilkins.

Wolff, A. J., & O'Donnell, A. E. (2004). Pulmonary effects of illicit drug use. *Clinical Chest Medicine, 25*(1), 203–216.

World Health Organization. (2006a). *Avian influenza (bird flu) fact sheet*. Retrieved January 7, 2007, from http://www.who.int/mediacentre/factsheets/avian_influenza/en/index.html

World Health Organization. (2006b). *Tuberculosis fact sheet*. Retrieved February 18, 2007, from http://www.who.int/mediacentre/factsheets/fs104/en/#global

The Jensen suite offers these additional resources to enhance learning and facilitate understanding of this chapter:

- thePoint on line resource, http//thepoint.lww.com/Jensen1E
- Student CD-ROM included with the book
- *Laboratory Manual for Nursing Health Assessment: A Best Practice Approach*
- *Pocket Guide for Nursing Health Assessment: A Best Practice Approach*

Table 18.8 Abnormal Respiratory Patterns

Visual Pattern	Description	Associated Conditions
Normal Inspiration Expiration	Rate of 10–20 breaths/min Ratio of respiration:pulse is approximately 4:1 500–800 mL per breath Regular rhythm	Normal findings
Tachypnea	Rate >24 breaths/min <500 mL/breath, shallow Regular rhythm	Anxiety, fear, elevated metabolic rate, fever, exercise, respiratory diseases in which rate must be increased to maintain oxygenation
Hyperventilation	Rate >24 breaths/min >800 mL/breath, deep Regular rhythm	Extreme anxiety or fear, exercise, increased intracranial pressure Kussmaul respirations are seen with diabetic ketoacidosis, because the body is attempting to remove carbon dioxide to normalize pH.
Bradypnea	Rate <10 breaths/min 500–800 mL/breath, shallow Regular rhythm	Conditions in which the breathing center in the medulla is depressed, such as narcotic overdose; diabetic coma and increased intracranial pressure
Hypoventilation	Rate <10 breaths/min <500 mL/breath, shallow Irregular rhythm	Narcotic or anesthetic overdose, increased intracranial pressure
Cheyne-Stokes respiration Hyperpnea Apnea	Rate variable Depth variable Regular irregular rhythm that cycles from deep and fast to shallow and slow, with some periods of apnea	Normal in children and the elderly; also, terminal illness, renal failure, drug overdose, increased intracranial pressure, and heart failure. Count the rate for 1 full minute and record the length of apnea.
Biot's respiration	Rate variable Depth variable Irregular irregular rhythm	Severe brain damage, commonly at the level of the medulla. Count the rate for 1 full minute and record the length of apnea.
Agonal	Rate intermittent Depth variable Irregular rhythm	Finding in patients at end of life. Count the rate for 1 full minute and record the length of apnea.
Apnea	No breaths	Cardiac arrest and brain death

Table 18.9   Abnormal Thoracic Configurations

Normal Adult

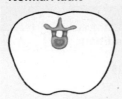

AP:lateral ratio is 1:2, wider than it is deep, oval shaped. Cone shaped from head to toe.

Kyphoscoliosis

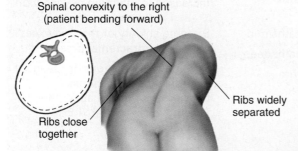

Spinal convexity to the right (patient bending forward)

Ribs widely separated

Ribs close together

With kyphosis, the thoracic spine curves forward, compressing the anterior chest and reducing inspiratory lung volumes. With scoliosis, a lateral S-shaped curvature of the spine causes unequal shoulders, scapulae, and hips. In severe cases, asymmetry may impede breathing.

Pectus carinatum (pigeon chest)

Depressed costal cartilages

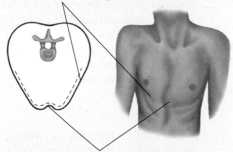

Anteriorly displaced sternum

Sternum is displaced anteriorly, depressing the adjacent costal cartilages. Congenital condition with increased anteroposterior diameter.

Pectus excavatum (funnel chest)

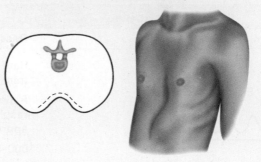

Depression in lower part of and adjacent to sternum. Congenital condition may compress the heart or great vessels and cause murmurs.

Barrel chest

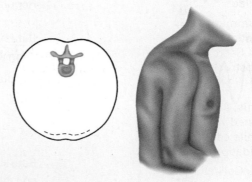

Anterior-posterior:lateral ratio near 1:1, round shaped. Ribs are more horizontal and costal margin is widened. Associated with COPD, chronic asthma, and normal aging.

Flail chest

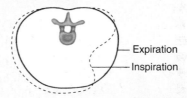

Expiration
Inspiration

When multiple ribs are fractured, paradoxical movements of the chest may occur. As the diaphragm pulls down during inspiration, negative pressure causes the injured area to cave inward; during expiration it moves out.

Table 18.10 Common Respiratory Conditions

Condition	Risk Factors	History and Subjective Data	Objective Data	Diagnostic Tests
Asthma: Allergic hypersensitivity to allergens that produces bronchospasm	Hyper-responsive airways Bronchospastic triggers	Cough worse at night and early morning	Wheezing, especially during exhalation Diminished lung sounds Clear sputum	Pulmonary function with short-acting bronchodilator
Atelectasis: Collapsed section of alveoli from immobility, obstruction, compression, or decreased surfactant	Immobility	Dyspnea Fever possible No sputum	Decreased or absent breath sounds over the atelectatic area, reduced inspiratory capacity	Chest x-ray
Emphysema: Destruction of pulmonary capillary bed and alveoli creating large air sacs and bullae	Smoking Occupational exposure	Shortness of breath Chronic cough	Cough, shortness of breath, decreased breath sounds, barrel chest	Pulmonary function tests
Bronchitis: Inflammation of bronchi that stimulate mucous glands. Secretions may partially obstruct the airways	Recent infection COPD presents with both bronchitis and emphysema	Chest tight or wheezy Clear sputum	Occasional wheezing or fine crackles	Chest x-ray
Lobar pneumonia: Alveoli become congested with bacteria and white cells causing consolidation	Elderly, immune compromised	Productive cough with yellow or green sputum	Ronchi or gurgles from secretions Fever	Sputum culture
Pleural effusion: Collection of fluid in the intrapleural space that compresses the lung tissue	CHF, fluid overload	Frothy white sputum	Decreased, bronchial or absent breath sounds over effusion	Chest x-ray
Pneumothorax or hemothorax: Collapsed or blood-filled lung	Trauma, central line placement	Dyspnea	Absent breath sounds over area of collapse or bleeding	Chest x-ray
CHF: Fluid overload and pulmonary congestion	High blood pressure, renal disease	Dypsnea, edema, weight gain	Decreased breath sounds, fine late inspiratory crackles	Chest x-ray
TB: Slow growing mycobacterium that may form lesions or cavities in the lung	Exposure to infected person	Night sweats	Cough productive of reddish sputum, decreased breath sounds or crackles	Acid fast bacilli sputum culture Chest x-ray
Pulmonary embolism: Blood clot in the lungs that causes shunting of blood to atelectatic area	Risk for deep vein thrombosis	Severe dyspnea, no sputum	Clear or if large may be decreased. Severe hypoxemia	V/Q scan or CT of lung
***P. carinii* pneumonia:** Protozoal infection that is common in the immune suppressed	HIV/ AIDS	Dry nonproductive cough	Decreased breath sounds	Chest x-ray Sputum culture

Condition	Auscultation	Sputum	Percussion
Asthma	Wheezes Diminished lung sounds	Clear	Occasional hyperresonance
Atelectasis	Diminished lung sounds in lower lobe	None	Dullness over affected lung
Bronchitis	Occasional wheezing or fine crackles	Clear	Resonance
COPD	Wheezes	Clear	Hyperresonance
Pneumothorax	Absent sounds	Absent	Hyperresonance over affected area
Hemothorax	Absent sounds	Bloody	Dull over affected area
Pneumonia	Wheezes, crackles, or gurgles	Purulent	Dull over affected area
CHF	Absent bases	Frothy	Dull bases
Pleural effusion	Absent over affected lung	None	Dull over affected lung
Pulmonary embolism	Clear or mild wheezes	None	Tympanic

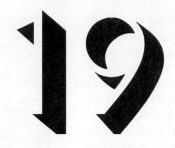

19

Heart and Neck Vessels Assessment

Learning Objectives

1 Identify the structures and functions of the heart.

2 Identify the location of the heart and common auscultatory areas on the precordium.

3 Identify teaching opportunities for cardiovascular health promotion and risk reduction.

4 Collect data about common cardiovascular symptoms: chest pain, dyspnea, orthopnea, cough, diaphoresis, fatigue, edema, and nocturia.

5 Collect objective data about the carotid artery, jugular veins, and heart.

6 Identify normal and abnormal findings from the inspection, palpation, and percussion of the precordium.

7 Auscultate normal and abnormal heart sounds, including S1, S2, split sounds, extra sounds, murmurs, and rubs.

8 Use subjective and objective data to analyze findings and plan interventions related to the cardiovascular system.

9 Document and communicate data about the cardiovascular system using appropriate medical terminology.

10 Individualize cardiovascular health assessment considering the condition, age, gender, and culture of the patient.

*M*rs. Lewis, a 77-year-old Caucasian woman, has been admitted to the hospital with chest pain and myocardial infarction (MI, heart attack). She has been on the cardiac unit for 4 hours. Nurses from the previous shift documented their admitting assessment data. The patient's vital signs are oral temperature 37°C, pulse 112 beats per minute (bpm), respirations 20 breaths/min, and blood pressure 148/78 mm Hg. Current medications include a thiazide diuretic and beta blocker for high blood pressure and a cholesterol-lowering drug. She has nitroglycerin tablets ordered as needed for chest pain.

You will gain more information about Mrs. Lewis as you progress through this chapter. As you study the content and features, consider Mrs. Lewis's case and its relationship to what you are learning. Begin thinking about the following points:

- Is Mrs. Lewis's condition stable, urgent, or an emergency?
- What immediate health promotion and teaching needs are evident?
- How will the nurse focus, organize, and prioritize subjective data collection?
- How will the nurse focus, organize, and prioritize objective data collection?
- How will the nurse individualize assessment to Mrs. Lewis's specific needs, considering her condition, age, and culture?

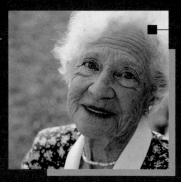

The complex cardiovascular system affects the entire body. Thus, it is important to understand the many factors that contribute to performing an accurate and complete assessment of this region for each patient. Thorough knowledge of pertinent anatomy and physiology, especially the cardiac cycle, is essential to conduct accurate assessment and understand normal and abnormal findings. Nurses and other health care providers assess cardiovascular risk factors and common symptoms as part of subjective data collection. During the interview and health history, they gather knowledge about risks such as a diet high in fat and cholesterol, high blood pressure, physical inactivity, and smoking. Auscultation of the heart helps examiners to check for the normal sounds heard upon closure of the heart valves and also for abnormal and extra sounds, including murmurs and gallops. Nurses document and communicate assessment information to appropriate health care providers. They also plan care to promote healthy heart habits, prevent cardiovascular disease, and treat identified problems.

Structure and Function Overview

The cardiovascular system includes the heart and blood vessels (great vessels and peripheral vascular system). It delivers oxygen and nutrients to the cells and tissues and returns waste products to the central circulation for excretion. This section concentrates on the heart and great vessels; see Chapter 20 for detailed discussion of the peripheral vascular system.

Anatomy

The heart and great vessels are located in the mediastinum between the lungs and above the diaphragm from the center to the left of the thorax (Fig. 19-1). The total

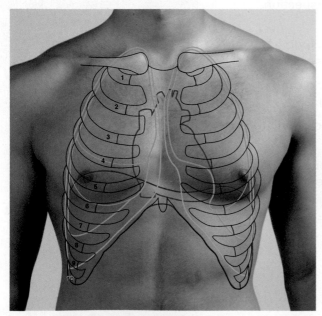

Figure 19.1 Surface anatomy of the thoracic contents. Note the outline of the heart's placement in relation to the thoracic cage.

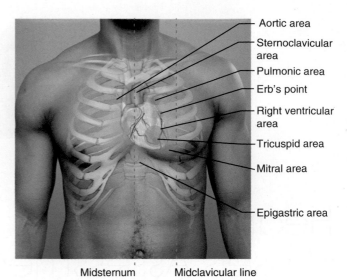

Midsternum   Midclavicular line

Figure 19.2 The anterior chest and cardiac landmarks.

size of the heart is approximately that of a clenched adult fist. The female heart is normally smaller and weighs less than the male heart across all age groups (Woods, et al., 2010).

The location for auscultating heart sounds is identified by landmarks on the anterior thoracic wall. The intercostals spaces (ICSs), sternal lines, and midclavicular line (MCL) are used to describe the location of heart sounds and impulses (see Chapter 18). The top of the heart is referred to as the base because it is broad; the bottom of the heart is referred to as the apex. This is opposite of the lungs, where the top is the apex and the bottom is the base. The base of the heart is at the right and left 2nd ICS at the sternal border, while the apex is in the 5th ICS 7 to 9 cm left of the midsternal line. The beating inferior tip of the heart may cause a pulsation in this area, referred to as the point of maximal impulse (PMI). The inferior border of the heart lies at the junction between the xyphoid process and the sternum to the left 5th ICS in the MCL laterally. The precordium on the anterior chest overlies the heart and great vessels, between the 2nd and 5th ICS at the right sternal border to approximately the 2nd and 5th ICS at the left MCL (see Fig. 19-2).

The *arterial great vessels* include the carotid arteries, aorta, and pulmonary veins. The *venous great vessels* are the jugular veins, superior vena cava, inferior vena cava, and pulmonary arteries. The great vessels are superior to the heart and then turn in the direction of the body part that they supply (Fig. 19-3).

Neck Vessels

The neck vessels include the carotid arteries and internal and external jugular veins (Fig. 19-4). The *carotid arteries* are located in the depression between the trachea and sternomastoid muscle in the anterior neck. They follow bilaterally along the trachea from clavicle to jaw. Palpation of the carotid arteries normally reveals a strong pulsation.

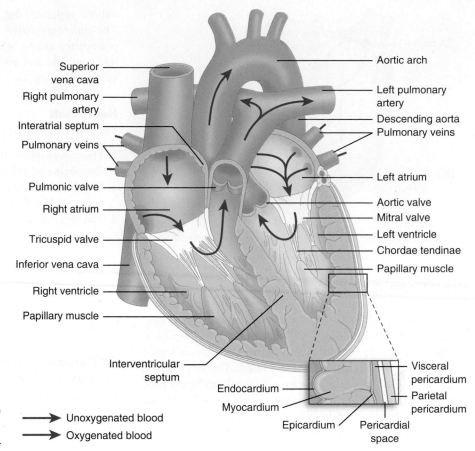

Superior vena cava

Right pulmonary artery

Interatrial septum

Pulmonary veins

Pulmonic valve

Right atrium

Tricuspid valve

Inferior vena cava

Right ventricle

Papillary muscle

Aortic arch

Left pulmonary artery

Descending aorta

Pulmonary veins

Left atrium

Aortic valve

Mitral valve

Left ventricle

Chordae tendinae

Papillary muscle

Interventricular septum

Visceral pericardium

Endocardium

Parietal pericardium

Myocardium

Epicardium

Pericardial space

Unoxygenated blood

Oxygenated blood

Figure 19.3 Interior anatomy of the heart. The arrows show the direction of blood flow through the heart chambers.

The internal and external jugular veins are named for their position in the neck. The *internal jugular vein* is deeper and near the carotid artery. Because of its location, it usually is not visible; because it is a vein, it is not palpable. The more superficial *external jugular vein* is visible in the depression above the middle of the clavicle. It is lateral instead of anterior to the sternomastoid muscle, and travels from the clavicle up to the jaw line.

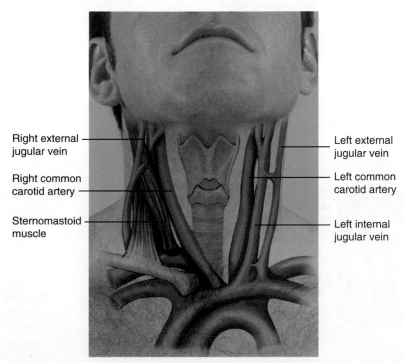

Right external jugular vein

Right common carotid artery

Sternomastoid muscle

Left external jugular vein

Left common carotid artery

Left internal jugular vein

Figure 19.4 Anatomy of the neck vessels.

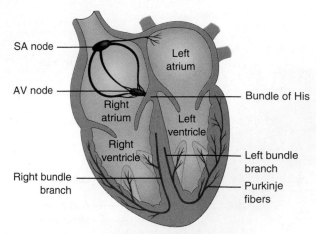

Figure 19.5 The heart wall, chambers, and valves.

Heart Chambers

Two main walls divide the heart into two upper and two lower chambers (Fig. 19-5). The upper chambers, or *atria*, collect and pump blood into the ventricles. The *ventricles* pump blood out to the lungs and body. The *septum* separates the left and right sides of the heart. The left side is larger and more muscular, because it circulates blood further and against a higher pressure (similar to the blood pressure). The right side circulates blood in the lower pressure pulmonary system, so it is thinner walled and smaller.

Valves

Two valves are located on each side of the heart (see Fig. 19-3). They open and close to permit blood to flow forward in one direction instead of going backward during contraction. The two atrioventricular (AV) valves separate the atria from the ventricles: the *tricuspid valve* separates the right atrium and ventricle, while the *mitral valve* separates the left atrium and ventricle. The two semilunar

valves separate the ventricles from the great vessels. The *pulmonic valve* lies between the right ventricle and pulmonary artery, while the *aortic valve* lies between the left ventricle and aorta. These valves are named after the vessel that they fill.

Heart Wall

The wall of the heart consists of three layers:

1. The thin *endocardium* lines the inside of the heart chambers and valves.
2. The thick muscular *myocardium* is the middle layer responsible for the pumping action of the heart.
3. The thin *epicardium* is a muscle layer on the outside of the heart.

The tough fibrous *pericardium* encloses and protects the heart. Its two layers contain a small amount of fluid for lubrication during pumping. The pericardium adheres to the great vessels, esophagus, sternum, and pleurae and is anchored to the diaphragm.

Coronary Arteries and Veins

The muscular heart needs its own blood supply. The coronary arteries arise from the base and branch out to the apex of the heart. The more muscular left side has a greater blood supply with two main arteries instead of one (Fig. 19-6). The left coronary and circumflex arteries supply the left side, and the right coronary artery supplies the right. The arteries fill when the heart relaxes. Cardiac veins empty deoxygenated blood into the coronary sinus at the base.

Clinical Significance 19-1

The coronary arteries may develop atherosclerotic plaques that narrow them, leading to an MI (heart attack) or angina.

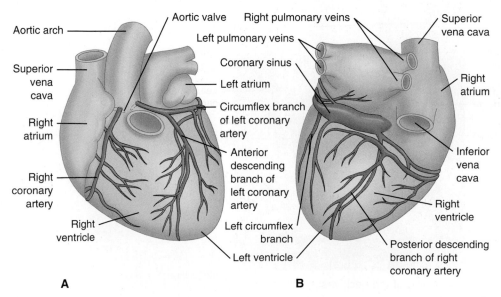

Figure 19.6 The coronary arteries adjust the flow of oxygenated blood to the heart muscle according to metabolic needs. **A.** Anterior view. **B.** Posterior view.

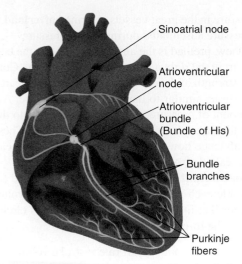

Figure 19.7 Outline of the path and involved structures of the cardiac conduction system.

Labels: Sinoatrial node; Atrioventricular node; Atrioventricular bundle (Bundle of His); Bundle branches; Purkinje fibers

Conduction System

A small electrical impulse that fires in the sinoatrial (SA) node in the right atrium generates the normal heartbeat. The SA node functions as the "pacemaker" of the heart (Fig. 19-7). The cells in the SA node are unique because they possess **automaticity** (property that enables the heart to generate its own impulses). After it has been generated, the impulse moves through an electrical "wiring" pathway through the left and right atria (via intra-atrial pathways). The electrical impulse causes the atrial muscle cells to contract. Then the impulse pauses briefly at the AV junction, travels through the electrical pathways in the bundle of His and bundle branches in the left and right ventricles, and finally moves to the Perkinge fibers (see Fig. 19-7). This impulse causes the ventricular muscle cells to contract. In healthy people, the rate of firing in the SA node determines ventricular contraction and pulse rate.

Physiology

Pulmonary and Systemic Circulation

The cardiovascular system is really a double pump system with two major divisions: the pulmonary and systemic circulation (see Fig. 19-6). Blood that enters the right side circulates to the lungs; blood that enters the left side circulates to the body.

The *pulmonary artery* carries deoxygenated blood to the lungs. At the lungs, the blood picks up oxygen and releases carbon dioxide. The *pulmonary vein* delivers oxygenated blood to the left atrium, which circulates the blood to the left ventricle and then out to the systemic circulation. Note that this process is the opposite of other body areas, where arteries carry oxygenated blood and veins carry deoxygenated blood.

The systemic circulation supplies the tissues with oxygen and nutrients and returns waste to the central circulation for excretion. The jugular veins and carotid arteries perfuse the brain, the superior vena cava and subclavian arteries perfuse the upper limbs, and the inferior vena cava and thoracic aorta perfuse the lower limbs.

Cardiac Cycle

The continuous rhythmic movement of blood during contraction and relaxation of the heart is the *cardiac cycle*. Squeezing of the heart during contraction is referred to as **systole**; relaxing of the heart is called **diastole** (Fig. 19-8).

Deoxygenated blood enters the right atrium from the superior and inferior vena cava. The right and left atria fill

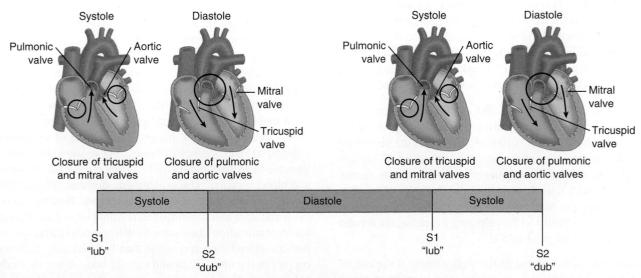

Figure 19.8 The cardiac cycle and normal heart sounds. Arrows represent the direction of blood flow. Closure of the mitral and tricuspid valves produces the first heart sound (S1, "lub"). Closure of the aortic and pulmonic valves produces the second heart sound (S2, "dub"). *Systole* is the phase between S1 and S2. *Diastole* is the phase between S2 and the next S1.

with blood until the SA node initiates atrial contraction by firing its pacemaker cells. When atrial contraction begins, the mitral and tricuspid valves open in response to the increased pressure. Blood moves from the atria into the ventricles.

As the impulse begins traveling down the bundle branches, it initiates ventricular contraction, leading to increased ventricular pressure. This increased pressure causes the mitral and tricuspid valves (between the atria and ventricles) to close. The closure of the valves is the *first heart sound (S1)*.

The aortic and pulmonic valves open to allow blood to flow to the lungs and body, producing the pulse. Opening of these valves is normally silent (ie, no sounds are heard). As the ventricles finish contracting and start relaxing, pressure in the ventricles drops, and the aortic and pulmonic valves close (between the ventricles and great vessels). This causes the *second heart sound (S2)*.

To summarize, S1, or "lub," results from closure of the mitral and tricuspid valves. S2, or "dub," results from closure of the aortic and pulmonic valves. Understanding this basic physiology is essential to understand normal and abnormal heart sounds. If the nurse hears an abnormal sound, he or she uses knowledge of normal physiology to determine where the pathophysiology may be.

Systole. During systole, the ventricles contract and eject blood to the lungs and body. The beginning of systole correlates with the pulse as blood is being circulated. During systole, the closed mitral and tricuspid valves prevent regurgitation (backflow) of blood into the atria. The aortic and pulmonic valves are open as blood moves forward.

Diastole. Diastole is twice as long as systole to allow time for the ventricles to fill. As the heart rate increases, however, length of diastole shortens and becomes approximately equal to systole.

During diastole the aortic and pulmonic valves are closed to prevent regurgitation of blood from the aorta and pulmonary artery into the ventricles. The open mitral and tricuspid valves allow filling from the atria to the ventricles. The three phases of ventricular filling are early filling, slow passive filling, and finally, during atrial systole, the "atrial kick." An additional 30% of blood is squeezed into the ventricles during the atrial kick.

Relation to Heart Sounds (S1 and S2). As mentioned, closure of the heart valves during the cardiac cycle causes healthy sounds. The "lub" sound of S1 signals the beginning of ventricular systole, while the "dub" sound of S2 signals the end of systole and beginning of diastole. Systole occurs between S1 and S2, while diastole occurs between S2 and the next S1. When the heart rate is faster than 100 bpm, it may be necessary to identify S1 by palpating the pulse; the carotid upstroke occurs just prior to S2.

Cardiac Output. Volume in the right atrium at the end of diastole is called **preload**, an indicator of how much blood will be forwarded to and ejected from the ventricles. With increased blood in the right ventricle, force of contraction will be stronger, called **contractility**. The heart has to pump against the high blood pressures in the arteries and arterioles.

This pressure in the great vessels is termed **afterload**, similar to the pressure auscultated during blood pressure.

To review, preload is the amount of blood at the beginning of the heart in the right atrium to be squeezed out. Contractility is the strength of the contraction in the actual heart muscle during systole, similar to having a strong muscle. Afterload is the amount of pressure after the heart, similar to the resistance in the arterioles with the blood pressure. These three factors influence how much blood is ejected with each beat or stroke, called **stroke volume**.

Cardiac output is the amount of blood ejected from the left ventricle each minute. In addition to stroke volume, the other factor that influences how much blood is circulated is heart rate. The formula is

$$\text{cardiac output} = \text{heart rate} \times \text{stroke volume}.$$

A normal cardiac output is 6 to 8 L/min, or approximately 80 bpm with 80 mL in each beat. Ways to increase circulating blood (cardiac output) are by increasing heart rate, stroke volume, or both. The stress hormones epinephrine and norepinephrine increase both heart rate and stroke volume during exercise, trauma, or anxiety. The heart is continually adjusting heart rate and stroke volume during daily activities to supply needed oxygen and nutrients to active tissues.

Clinical Significance 19-2

Reduced cardiac output is associated with the medical diagnosis of heart failure. In this condition, reduced contractility causes preload to increase. Blood backs up, causing congestion. Congestion on the left backs blood into the lungs, while congestion on the right backs blood into the body, especially the legs and feet. Signs and symptoms of heart failure are shortness of breath, weight gain, and swollen ankles with decreased cardiac output.

Control of Heart Rate. The sympathetic and parasympathetic divisions of the nervous system control heart rate in response to stress and other variables (see Chapter 24). Overstimulation of the sympathetic division can cause heart rates that are too fast, while overstimulation of the parasympathetic division can cause rates that are too slow.

Stimulation of the sympathetic nervous system, or "fight versus flight" reactions, triggers the release of epinephrine (adrenalin) and norepinephrine. These neurotransmitters increase heart rate, contractility (to increase cardiac output), and blood pressure. The sympathetic division acts indirectly through baroreceptors and chemoreceptors. Baroreceptors in the aortic arch and carotid sinus regulate heart rate. Reduced baroreceptor stimulation (as with dehydration) increases sympathetic stimulation and subsequently heart rate. Chemoreceptors in the aortic arch and carotid body sense the body's pH, carbon dioxide, and oxygen levels. Accumulated acid or depleted oxygen levels stimulate the chemoreceptors, increasing heart rate.

The parasympathetic division, or "rest and digest" reaction, triggers a decreased heart rate by stimulating the vagus nerve that innervates the SA node to slow the natural pacemaker. The vagus nerve also slows conduction through the AV junction, which in turn slows the heart rate.

Relation to Electrocardiogram. As previously described, the heart has a pacemaker (SA node) and electrical conduction system that transmits signals for the cardiac muscle cells to contract at 60 to 100 bpm. This specialized "wiring" is a pathway similar to an electrical cord, by which signals travel quickly and efficiently to muscle cells. Once the signal is delivered, the muscle cells depolarize, causing filaments within to slide over one another and contract. Depolarization occurs when there is an exchange of electrolytes, including sodium and calcium. This shift in electrolytes causes electrical changes that can be detected by the **electrocardiogram (ECG)**.

The ECG is measured through special patches placed in specific areas on the chest, arms, and legs. The ECG records cellular depolarization primarily when sodium is released from the inside to the outside of cells. The ECG also records when sodium shifts back into cells at the end of contraction. The ECG records the electrical changes of contraction (depolarization) and relaxation (repolarization) as specific waves and intervals (Fig. 19-9):

- *P wave:* the spread of depolarization in the atria to cause atrial contraction (note that atrial repolarization is not seen because it is hidden when the ventricles contract in the QRS complex)
- *PR interval:* the time from firing of the SA node to the beginning of depolarization in the ventricle (includes a slight pause at the AV junction)
- *QRS complex:* the spread of depolarization and sodium release in the ventricles to cause ventricular contraction
- *T wave:* relaxation of the ventricles and repolarization of the cells, with a return of sodium and restoration of the resting state

Reading the ECG is an advanced skill used by nurses on cardiac and intensive care units. It takes practice and repetition

to learn the normal variations and abnormal findings. Health care providers use information from the ECG to analyze assessment data and plan care (see later discussion).

Heart Rhythm. The heart rhythm is an important element to assess in addition to the heart rate. **Arrhythmias** are abnormal heart rhythms with early (premature), delayed, or irregular beats. They can arise from the atria, AV junction, or ventricles; however, the type of arrhythmia cannot be diagnosed from auscultation alone. Analysis of the ECG or rhythm strip that shows the electrical changes is necessary.

A type of rhythm common in older adults is called *atrial fibrillation*. In this situation, many sites in the atria send signals to the ventricles. The ventricles contract very irregularly, causing an irregular heart rhythm.

Many other types of heart arrhythmias can be diagnosed depending on where the impulse originates, how fast it is, and if it is continuous or intermittent. An irregular pulse indicates a need to test with an ECG or rhythm strip to diagnose the type of arrhythmia.

Jugular Pulsations
The venous neck vessels reflect the pressure in the right atrium because no valve exists between the right atrium and jugular veins. The jugular pulse has five pulsations resulting from the backward effects of activity in the heart. The waves reflect atrial contraction and relaxation, ventricular contraction, and passive atrial and ventricular filling. Refer to Figure 19-10.

Lifespan Considerations

Pregnant Women
Maternal blood volume increases throughout pregnancy, beginning in the first trimester and peaking at 40% to 50% (approximately 1,500 mL above normal) by the 32nd to 34th week (Cunningham, et al., 2005). Volume may increase as much as 70% with a multiple pregnancy (Malone & D'Alton, 2004).

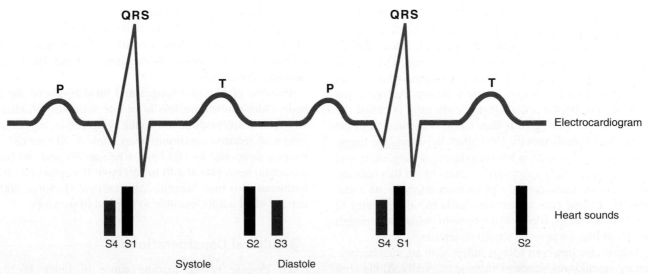

Figure 19.9 Correlation of the waves of the ECG with the cardiac cycle.

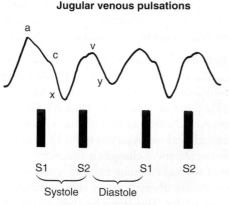

Jugular venous pulsations

S1   S2   S1   S2
└─Systole─┘ └─Diastole─┘

Jugular venous pressure curves

a = atrial contraction

c = carotid transmission not visible clinically

x = descent in right atrium following *a*

v = passive venous filling of atria from the vena cavae

y = descent during atrial resting phase before contraction

Figure 19.10 Jugular venous pressure curves.

Increased stroke volume and heart rate elevate cardiac output by 30% to 40% to keep up with the increased demands of supplying nutrients and oxygen to the developing fetus.

Cardiac output peaks at 30% to 50% greater than the nonpregnant state by approximately gestational week 32; it returns to prepregnancy levels about 2 weeks postpartum (Monga & Sanborn, 2004). Cardiac output is reduced when the mother is supine, because the uterus impedes venous return (Lowdermilk & Perry, 2007). This positioning may be significant enough to reduce blood pressure; thus, a side-lying position is recommended for pregnant women. The left ventricle increases both the wall thickness and muscle mass. Also the uterus enlarges and pushes the diaphragm upward, and the position of the heart shifts more horizontally. Many of the changes in pregnancy are related to the large increase in blood volume.

Newborns and Infants

Before birth, the fetus depends on the mother for blood circulation. The placenta supplies both nutrients and oxygen because the fetus is not using the lungs yet. The umbilical vein and artery connect the fetus to the placenta. The umbilical vein connects to the inferior vena cava, which empties nutrient-rich blood into the right atrium. An open flap in the septum between the left and right atria is called the *foramen ovale*. Through this flap, blood is shunted from the right atrium directly into the left atrium, bypassing the lungs. Additionally, a connection between the pulmonary artery and aorta, called the *ductus arteriosis*, shunts blood that remains in the right ventricle from the pulmonary artery to the aorta. Because of these two connections, little blood circulates to the uninflated lungs. Blood then returns to the mother through the descending aorta to the umbilical arteries.

At birth, the newborn's lungs inflate with air, causing pulmonary vascular resistance to increase markedly. Along with clamping of the umbilical cord, this forces the pulmonary

and systemic circuits to function separately. Within minutes to hours after birth, the atrial septum is pushed closed and right to left blood flow is established. Blood flow decreases in the ductus arteriosis, causing it to constrict and close within a few days, separating the pulmonary artery and aorta. In some congenital heart defects, the patent ductus arteriosis and foramen ovale remain open. If the openings are significant, they may need surgical repair.

The infant's blood pressure and arterial resistance increase when the umbilical cord is cut. Because of this increased work, the left ventricle hypertrophies and becomes more muscular than the right. By 1 year of age, the left ventricle is twice the size of the right, which is similar to adult size. The heart rate of the newborn is increased because the muscle has not yet developed and stroke volumes are lower. At birth the rate may be as high as 180 bpm in response to stress or crying and decrease to approximately 120 bpm at rest. The heart is positioned more horizontally in infants than in adults, which causes the apex to be in the 4th left ICS slightly lateral to the MCL (see Fig. 19-11).

Children and Adolescents

The heart grows and moves lower as the child's body changes. By 7 years of age, the child's heart is similar to an adult's. Both the left ventricular cavity size and wall thickness increase linearly with age. By 7 years, the apex is palpable in the 5th left ICS at the MCL.

Older Adults

With aging, the left ventricular wall thickens, most likely from the increased stress of pumping blood into stiffer vessels. The left atrium increases, and the mitral valve closes more slowly. The heart fills more slowly in early diastole but compensates by filling more quickly in late diastole during atrial contraction. In young hearts, approximately twice as much blood enters the ventricle during early diastolic filling compared to late diastole; in older hearts, blood flow is approximately equal during early and late diastole. Consequently, the volumes in the heart remain about the same as in younger people. During stress or exercise, younger people pump out more blood in the ventricle (ejection fraction); in older adults there are only slight increases in the ejection fraction, possibly causing exercise intolerance (Lakatta, 2002).

Because of fibrotic changes and fat deposits on the SA node, older adults have less heart rate variability. Additionally, their hearts respond less to the sympathetic nervous system, with reduced maximum heart rates. A 20 year old can increase heart rate to 180 bpm, while an 80 year old has a maximum heart rate of 140 to 150 bpm. Receptors for stress hormones also may become less sensitive (Lakatta, 2002), making older adults less able to respond to stressors.

Cultural Considerations

Heart disease is the leading cause of death in high-income countries, and coronary heart disease contributes to

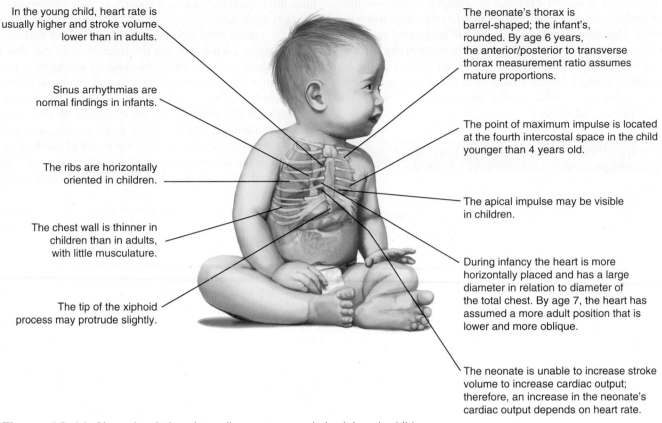

In the young child, heart rate is usually higher and stroke volume lower than in adults.

Sinus arrhythmias are normal findings in infants.

The ribs are horizontally oriented in children.

The chest wall is thinner in children than in adults, with little musculature.

The tip of the xiphoid process may protrude slightly.

The neonate's thorax is barrel-shaped; the infant's, rounded. By age 6 years, the anterior/posterior to transverse thorax measurement ratio assumes mature proportions.

The point of maximum impulse is located at the fourth intercostal space in the child younger than 4 years old.

The apical impulse may be visible in children.

During infancy the heart is more horizontally placed and has a large diameter in relation to diameter of the total chest. By age 7, the heart has assumed a more adult position that is lower and more oblique.

The neonate is unable to increase stroke volume to increase cardiac output; therefore, an increase in the neonate's cardiac output depends on heart rate.

Figure 19.11 Normal variations in cardiac anatomy and physiology in children.

approximately 50% of deaths from heart disease (NHLBI, 2007). Heart disease is the leading killer across most U.S. racial and ethnic minority communities, accounting for 27% of all deaths in 2004.

African American men are 30% more likely to die from heart disease than non-Hispanic white men, despite that 10% of African Americans have heart disease versus 13% of whites. The reasons for this disparity remain largely unknown, although some studies have indicated potential differences in knowledge of risk factors, physician–patient relationships, access to the health care system, and treatment beliefs (Woodard, et al., 2005). African Americans are 1.5 times more likely to have high blood pressure than Caucasians (32% to 21%). African American women are 1.6 times as likely as non-Hispanic white women to be obese (NHLBI, 2007). Although African American women have higher rates of heart disease with earlier onset and more severe consequences, they are less aware of their susceptibility to and the seriousness of the disease than other groups (Jones, et al., 2006).

Mexican Americans, who comprise the majority of the U.S. Hispanic population, suffer in greater percentages than Caucasians from overweight and obesity, two of the leading risk factors for heart disease. Premature death is higher for Hispanics (24%) than non-Hispanics (17%). Although Hispanic women believe that the best way to prevent heart disease is exercise, procrastination and culture-related issues are barriers to physical activity, as well as to regularly seeing a

doctor. Perceived self-efficacy, having a concern for own and family health, social support and norms for physical activity, serving as a role model to others, and perceived neighborhood resources are factors that promote health maintenance (Keller & Fleury, 2006).

In the Asian and Pacific Islander community, heart disease causes 25% of deaths, ranking as the overall leading contributor to mortality. Overall, Asian/Pacific Islander adults are less likely than non-Hispanic white adults to have and to die from heart disease.

The number of premature (younger than 65 years) deaths from heart disease is greatest among American Indians or Alaska Natives (36%) and lowest among Caucasians. American Indian/Alaska Native adults are 1.2 times as likely as Caucasians to have heart disease, and 1.4 times as likely to be current cigarette smokers. American Indian/Alaska Native adults are 1.6 times as likely as Caucasians to be obese and 1.3 times as likely as Caucasians to have high blood pressure (NHLBI, 2001).

Women and men present with heart disease differently (Pilote, et al., 2007). Women with diabetes have a significantly higher cardiovascular mortality rate than men with diabetes. Also women with atrial fibrillation are at greater risk for stroke than their male counterparts. Clinically significant heart failure is increasing in women. Women are also more likely to live with more cardiovascular disabilities and have a lower health-related quality of life than are men. Historically, women have been underrepresented in clinical trials.

The lack of complete evidence concerning gender-specific outcomes has led to assumptions about treatment in women, which may have resulted in inadequate diagnoses, suboptimal treatment, and reduced outcomes. Mortality rates in men have steadily declined, while mortality rates in women have remained stable over the past decade (Pilote, et al., 2007). The incidence of cardiovascular disease increases with age for both men and women.

Acute Assessment

⚠ SAFETY ALERT 19.1

If a patient is experiencing chest pain, dyspnea, cyanosis, diaphoresis, or dizziness, the nurse must focus assessment on collecting data to resolve the problem. The nurse should gather information while treatments, including administration of oxygen and nitroglycerine tablets sublingually as ordered, are performed. If chest pain continues, the nurse must ask for help, because more than one person may be necessary to collect data and to intervene appropriately.

Cardiac emergencies that necessitate rapid assessment and intervention include *acute coronary syndrome, acute severe heart failure, hypertensive crisis, cardiac tamponade, unstable cardiac arrhythmias, cardiogenic shock, systemic or pulmonary embolism,* and *aortic dissection.* Patients with these conditions may have chest pain, shortness of breath, abnormal (too high or too low) blood pressure, or inadequate tissue perfusion. Initial assessment includes a brief exploration of the presenting symptom (location, onset, intensity, alleviating and aggravating factors, associated symptoms); a focused physical examination of the cardiovascular and respiratory systems; an ECG; and a chest x-ray. Selected laboratory tests are done emergently to evaluate for cardiac muscle damage, embolism, or electrolyte imbalance. Team members perform interventions while gathering assessment data because prompt treatment is essential.

Accurate assessment of patients with cardiovascular problems is essential, because nurses are often the health care providers who first identify abnormal findings. Nurses play a key role in assessment of chest pain and assist in gathering data so that the source is quickly identified and treated. Differential diagnosis of chest pain is important, because ischemic cardiac pain involves loss of muscle cells that can cause further damage if left untreated. An accurate description of the pain and alleviating or aggravating factors is often pivotal to identify the source.

Other assessments that assume priority are related to arrhythmias. Nurses quickly assess the effects of the arrhythmia by evaluating level of consciousness and obtaining the blood pressure as an indicator of peripheral perfusion. If level of consciousness, blood pressure, or both are decreased, nurses page the rapid-response team. Nurses who work frequently with patients who have cardiac problems must think quickly, because the status of such patients often changes rapidly.

Fluid volume overload and severe heart failure that leads to pulmonary edema also are priorities. Nurses can evaluate the significance of volume overload by auscultating lung sounds, measuring respiratory rate, and obtaining an oxygen saturation level. Other infectious or inflammatory disorders (eg, endocarditis, pericarditis) are evaluated by assessment of related findings, such as fever, heart sounds, and pain. Patients with cardiac disease are often aware of subtle symptoms that indicate improving or worsening status; they can often provide valuable data that assists in accurate diagnosis and treatment.

Nurses organize data according to the clustering of signs and symptoms related to a specific problem. For example, if a nurse identifies a new murmur, he or she completes assessments that relate to fluid volume overload. Examples include weighing the patient, evaluating intake and output, auscultating lung sounds for fluid, and inspecting the extremities for edema. The nurse then analyzes findings to determine the effects of the murmur on the patient's physical and functional status.

Subjective Data Collection

Areas for Health Promotion/*Healthy People*

Health-promotion activities related to the cardiovascular system focus on preventing heart disease, identifying any problems related to the heart and blood vessels early, and reducing complications of existing or established diagnoses. Important healthy habits to emphasize include following a low-fat diet, regularly exercising, undergoing regular screening for diabetes and cholesterol, and quitting (or continuing not) smoking. See Table 19-1 relating to the cardiovascular system, which contains pertinent points for counseling when conducting the health history with patients.

Assessment of Risk Factors

When questioning patients about risk factors, the goal is to identify how likely they are to develop or to already be experiencing consequences of cardiovascular diseases. Such investigation creates an environment in which health care providers can implement necessary interventions to control symptoms, direct education to prevent new problems or complications, and establish within the record areas needing ongoing follow-up and emphasis. For example, smoking, high blood pressure, physical inactivity, and diabetes mellitus are major contributors to heart disease (EPIC-Potsdam, 2007). Nurses assess these risks in the interview. After assessment, nurses identify focused teaching areas and evaluate the patient's ongoing progress in controlling modifiable risks.

The following screening questions are important to establish the patient's risks for cardiovascular disease.

Table 19.1 *Healthy People* Goals Related to Cardiovascular Health

Goal	Patient Education Topics
Reduce coronary heart disease deaths.	Reduce risk factors.
Increase the proportion of adults aged 20 years and older who are aware of the early warning symptoms and signs of a heart attack and the importance of accessing rapid emergency care by calling 911.	Teach signs and symptoms of MI and to call 911 with chest pain that remains unrelieved after 20 minutes.
Increase the proportion of eligible patients with heart attacks who receive timely electrical shock and artery-opening therapy.	Advocate for automatic cardiac defibrillators in public buildings. Become involved in reducing time to treatment by reducing treatment delays.
Increase the proportion of adults with high blood pressure whose blood pressure is under control.	Participate in blood pressure screening; teach the importance of good control.
Reduce the mean total blood cholesterol levels and LDL cholesterol levels among adults.	Teach the importance of a low-fat, low-cholesterol diet.
Increase the proportion of physician office visits made by patients with a diagnosis of cardiovascular disease, diabetes, or hyperlipidemia that include counseling or education related to diet and nutrition.	Advocate for office visits that focus on health promotion, counseling, and education for healthy nutrition.
Increase the proportion of adults who engage in vigorous physical activity that promotes the development and maintenance of cardiorespiratory fitness 3 or more days per week for 20 or more minutes per occasion.	Teach the importance of physical activity in promoting health and reducing cardiovascular disease. Identify choices that the patient is willing to engage in and follow his or her progress.

Questions to Assess History and Risks	Rationales
Obtain the following information from the patient's chart: • Age • Heredity • Gender • Date and result of last blood pressure measurement • Date and result of last cholesterol level • Date and result of last C-reactive protein level • Date and result of B type natriuretic peptides (BNPs) • Thyroid levels	Increased age, male gender, and African American, Mexican-American, American-Indian, native Hawaiian, or Asian-American heritages are risk factors for *cardiovascular disease*. Risk of cardiovascular events more than doubles with elevated cholesterol and C-reactive protein levels (Ridker, et al., 2002). BNP is both sensitive and specific to *heart failure* (Chen & Burett, 2007). Hyperthyroidism has been linked to *atrial fibrillation* but not to cardiovascular disease or mortality (Cappola, et al., 2006).
Family History Do you have any family history of cardiovascular problems? • Who had the illness? • What was the illness? • When did the person have it? • How was the illness treated? • What were the outcomes?	*Premature coronary artery disease* in a first- or second-degree relatively increases the patient's risk for the same problem. Premature onset is before 55 years in men and before 65 years in women. Evidence suggests that premature coronary artery disease in siblings is a stronger risk than in parents or grandparents (Murabito, et al., 2005; Nasir, et al., 2004). Also assess family history for risk factors such as high blood pressure, high cholesterol, diabetes, heart disease, and obesity.
Past Medical History Have you ever been diagnosed with a cardiac problem such as chest pain, heart attack, heart failure, or irregular rhythm?	A history of past problems provides information that can assist with anticipating future needs.
Has anyone ever told you that you have high blood pressure? • What is the normal range? • Do you take anything for it?	In untreated hypertension, the risk of dying from cardiac disease is approximately twice as high as if the systolic pressure is normal (Benetos, et al., 2002).

(text continues on page 496)

CHAPTER 19   Heart and Neck Vessels Assessment   495

Questions to Assess History and Risks	Rationales
Has anyone ever told you that you have high blood cholesterol? • What is the usual level? • Do you take anything for it?	Patients with an elevated low-density lipoprotein (LDL) ("bad") cholesterol level are twice as likely to develop cardiovascular disease (Taubert, et al., 2003).
Do you have a history of diabetes mellitus? • What is your usual glucose level? • Do you take anything for it?	Patients with diabetes mellitus are approximately twice as likely to develop cardiovascular disease (Taubert, et al., 2003).
Medications Are you taking any medications for cardiac problems? • What are they? • How often are you taking them? • How well are you following your prescribed medication regimen?	Note the drug, dose, and frequency. Obtaining the reason for the medication is important, because some drugs have several purposes. Compliance with medications also is essential to review, because many cardiac medications have side effects that cause patients to stop taking them.
Are you taking any natural supplements or over-the-counter medications? • What are they? • How often do you take them?	Some supplements, such as ephedrine, may have cardiac side effects. Also note any potential drug interactions between prescribed and over-the-counter medications.
Lifestyle and Behavioral Issues Do you smoke cigarettes or use other tobacco products? • How long? • How many packs per day?	Smokers are two to four times more likely to develop *coronary heart disease* and are twice as likely to have sudden cardiac arrest (AHA, 2005).
What is your usual weight? What is your height?	Being overweight is not independently associated with an increased risk of dying from cardiovascular disease; associated variables such as diabetes, high blood pressure, and high cholesterol also may contribute (Romero-Corral, et al., 2006).
What is your usual level of physical activity? • Do you exercise? • What type? • How long and how often?	A low level of activity is associated with an increased risk for cardiovascular disease (AHA, 2005). Physical activity can help control blood cholesterol, diabetes, and obesity, as well as help lower blood pressure. Assess occupational activities, commuting patterns, and recreational exercise to determine how much these factors contribute to overall physical activity.
What is your typical diet?	A diet low in fruits and vegetables and high in fat and cholesterol is associated with an increased risk of cardiovascular disease (AHA, 2005).
How much alcohol do you usually drink per day? Week? Month? Do you use any recreational drugs such as cocaine?	Drinking more than two drinks of alcohol per day for men or one drink of alcohol per day for women can raise blood pressure and contribute to *heart failure*. It also can elevate triglyceride levels, contribute to obesity, and produce irregular heartbeats (AHA, 2005). Cocaine increases the risk of *MI* and *coronary vasospasm*.

Risk Assessment and Health-Related Patient Teaching

As mentioned, risk assessment helps to identify potential problems so that health care providers can give patients information to positively influence behavioral choices. Both primary prevention, in those without evidence of cardiovascular disease, and secondary prevention, to detect early disease through blood pressure and cholesterol screening, are priorities for public health. The most important cardiovascular focus areas are the modifiable risk factors of smoking, high blood pressure, and high cholesterol level. Additionally, a high-fat diet, overweight or obesity, and physical inactivity contribute to cardiovascular disease. Nurses work with patients over time to modify lifestyle choices that reflect healthy behaviors. The most important are stopping smoking, reducing high blood pressure, and reducing high cholesterol.

Smoking Cessation

Nurses should ask patients who smoke about their willingness to quit at every visit. Patients who quit reduce their risk of cardiac events by 50% after the first year (AHA, 2005). Nurses can give patients choices about tools to help them quit, such as referrals to behavioral therapy, information about support groups, or medication.

Control of Blood Pressure and Cholesterol Level

High blood pressure should be controlled with medication if diet, exercise, and weight reduction are unsuccessful. Patients may not adhere to prescribed medications because of side effects or difficulty following the schedule. Nurses might suggest a dosing regimen simplified to improve adherence (Schroeder, et al., 2004).

High cholesterol can also be modified by eating a low-cholesterol diet, with reduced animal fat. Lean cuts of grilled or roasted meat are better than deep-fried, fatty cuts. Nevertheless, dietary changes can usually lower cholesterol by only 5% to 10% (Pasternak, et al., 2002). If diet alone is unsuccessful, the physician may prescribe a statin, which reduces the risk of cardiovascular events by approximately 30% (Pasternak, et al., 2002).

Focused Health History Related to Common Symptoms

Nurses assess some common symptoms in all patients to screen for early signs of cardiac disease. If patients are concerned about cardiac problems, nurses can use these concerns to identify focused areas of assessment. A thorough history of cardiovascular symptoms assists with identifying the current problem or diagnosis.

Common Cardiovascular Symptoms

- Chest pain
- Dyspnea, orthopnea, and cough
- Diaphoresis
- Fatigue
- Edema
- Nocturia
- Palpitations

Questions to Assess Symptoms	Rationales/Abnormal Findings
⚠ SAFETY ALERT 19.2 *All health care providers should assume that a patient's chest pain is heart pain until another cause can be found. If chest pain is ischemic, rapid treatment is necessary to prevent the death of cardiac cells. If medication or angioplasty can open the artery, the size of the MI can be reduced.*	Heart pain indicates ischemic heart tissue and, if unrelieved after 20 minutes, can cause cell death and MI.
Chest Pain Do you have any chest pain or discomfort? • Where is the pain? Can you show me where it hurts? Does it go anywhere? • When did you first notice the pain? Is it constant or does it come and go? How long has it lasted? • How bad is it on a scale from 1 to 10, with 10 being the worst? • Describe the pain or discomfort. What does it feel like? • What makes it worse? What makes it better? Have you taken any nitroglycerin? How many tablets and how far apart? • What were you doing when you noticed it? Does anything consistently bring it on? • Do any other symptoms accompany the pain? • Have you tried any treatments for the pain? Did they help? • What is your goal for the pain? What would you like to be able to do that you are unable to do because of the pain?	The pain of *MI* typically is on the left side of the chest, radiates down the left arm or into the jaw, and is diffused rather than localized. Onset can be sudden or gradual. Patients often describe the pain as crushing or viselike. Others may not identify ischemia as pain but rather as pressure or discomfort, like "having an elephant on the chest." Some patients become nauseous and vomit; others describe indigestion resulting from cardiac ischemia. Associated symptoms include diaphoresis, pallor, anxiety, and fatigue. Palpitations, tachycardia, and dyspnea may also be present. Only one-third of women with acute MI report having this typical chest pain (McSweeney, et al., 2003). *Angina* is temporary heart pain, resolving in less than 20 minutes. It can be aggravated by physical activity and stress, or there may be no triggers (unstable angina). Chest pain may also be from pulmonary, musculoskeletal, or gastrointestinal origin. Factors that aggravate or alleviate the pain may help identify the cause. Nitroglycerin often relieves angina, while an antacid may relieve pain from reflux. Patients exhibit gestures such as a closed fist or palm on the chest in only approximately 50% of cases; so they are not particularly useful in diagnosing angina or MI (Marcus, et al., 2007). Refer to Table 19-2 for the differential diagnosis of chest pain.

(text continues on page 498)

Table 19.2   Differential Diagnosis of Chest Pain

Condition	Significant Findings in the History	Symptoms	Aggravating Factors	Alleviating Factors
MI	Cardiac risk factors	Chest pain or discomfort in men; fatigue and shortness of breath in women last more than 20 minutes Accompanied by nausea and diaphoresis	Anxiety, physical exertion	Nitroglycerin; thrombolytic medication or angioplasty are necessary to prevent damage
Stable angina	Cardiac risk factors	Discomfort lasting <20 minutes	Cold, fatigue, physical exertion	Nitroglycerin and rest
Unstable angina	Cardiac risk factors	Discomfort lasting <20 minutes	Occurs at rest	Nitroglycerin; no relation to activity
Gastrointestinal disease: esophageal, gastritis, biliary	History of ulcer, reflux, or gallbladder disease	Described as indigestion, difficulty swallowing, burning, acid stomach; biliary pain may be colicky or cramping	Food intolerances, large or fatty meals	Antacids
Pulmonary disease/pleural chest pain	History of lung disease, pneumonia	Stabbing or grating pain, typically at the bases of the lungs	Worse with deep inhalation or coughing	Splinting chest, nonsteroidal antiinflammatory medications
Musculoskeletal	History of trauma, such as CPR, musculoskeletal history	Muscle tenderness with palpation, located near joints or costochondral cartilages, chronic	Increased movement	Rest
Aortic dissection	Cardiovascular disease	Middle or upper abdominal pain, ischemic pain in legs	Not relieved until treated	Measures to increase perfusion
Pericardial pain	History of cardiac inflammation such as with MI	Described as stabbing	Position changes, such as leaning forward	Nonsteroidal antiinflammatory medications

Questions to Assess History and Risks	Rationales

Dyspnea

Have you had any shortness of breath?

- How bad is it on a scale from 1 to 10, with 10 being the worst?
- When did it start? How long has it lasted?
- What makes it worse? What makes it better?
- Do any other symptoms accompany the shortness of breath?
- Have you tried any treatments for the shortness of breath? Did they help?
- Is it better or worse when compared to 6 months ago?

Patients with *heart failure* may be short of breath from fluid accumulation in the pulmonary bed. Onset may be sudden with *acute or chronic pulmonary edema*. It is important to assess how much activity brings on dyspnea, such as rest, walking on a flat surface, or climbing. **Dyspnea on exertion** is common with physical activity. Note the amount of activity that elicits dyspnea, such as four stairs or one block. Fatigue, chest pain, or diaphoresis may accompany dyspnea. Typically, resting alleviates it; if not, there may be another cause such as worsening *heart failure*, *pulmonary embolism*, or *MI*. Women are more likely to have dyspnea than chest pain as an acute symptom of MI (McSweeney, et al., 2003).

Questions to Assess History and Risks	Rationales

Orthopnea and Paroxysmal Nocturnal Dyspnea

Have you had difficulty sleeping?
- How many pillows do you sleep on at night?
- Do you wake in the night short of breath?
- Have you had difficulty sleeping?

Patients with *heart failure* may have fluid in their lungs, making it difficult to breathe when lying flat (**orthopnea**). Fluid "backs up" into the pulmonary veins, the heart cannot keep up with the volume, and fluid leaks into the lungs. Patients also may wake up suddenly as the fluid is redistributed from edematous legs into the lungs (**paroxysmal nocturnal dyspnea or PND**), typically after a few hours of sleep. They may waken feeling tired, anxious, or restless. Approximately 50% of women report difficulty sleeping 1 month prior to an acute *MI* (McSweeney, et al., 2003).

Cough

Have you noticed a cough?
- When did it start? How long has it lasted?
- What makes it worse? What makes it better?
- What brings it on?
- Do any other symptoms accompany the cough?
- Have you tried any treatments for the cough? Did they help?
- Is it better or worse when compared to 6 months ago?

Coughing occurs for the same reason as dyspnea. The cough may produce white or pink blood-tinged mucus. Mild wheezing also may occur. Treatment with an angiotensin-converting enzyme inhibitor also can cause the side effect of a dry, hacking cough.

Diaphoresis

Have you noticed any excessive sweating?
- When? Is it during any particular activities?
- Are there any associated symptoms such as heart pounding or chest pain?

Night-time diaphoresis is associated with other diseases, such as *tuberculosis*. Diaphoresis in response to exercise or activity may be related to cardiac stress. Diaphoresis associated with chest pain or palpitations is an autonomic response of the body to stress.

Fatigue

Have you been especially fatigued or tired?
- When did it start? How long has it lasted?
- What makes it worse? What makes it better?
- Do any other symptoms accompany the fatigue?
- Have you tried any treatments for the fatigue? Did they help?

Fatigue occurs because the heart cannot pump enough blood to meet the needs of tissues. The body diverts blood away from less vital organs, particularly limb muscles, and distributes it to the heart and brain. Common activities that might cause fatigue include shopping, climbing stairs, carrying groceries, and walking. Seventy percent of women report unusual fatigue 1 month before *acute MI* (McSweeney, et al., 2003). It is the most common symptom of MI in women.

Edema

Have you noticed any swelling in your feet, legs, or hands?
- When did it start? How long has it lasted?
- What makes it worse? What makes it better?
- Do any other symptoms accompany the swelling?
- Have you tried any treatments for the swelling? Did they help?

When blood flow out of the heart is reduced, blood returning to the heart through the veins "backs up," causing fluid to accumulate in the organs and dependent areas of the body. Blood flow to the kidneys is also reduced, decreasing excretion of sodium and water and causing further fluid retention in the tissues. Usually, standing exacerbates leg edema, while elevating the legs above heart level reduces it. Patients who retain fluid may also notice weight gain.

Nocturia

Do you need to get up at night to use the bathroom?
- How often?
- Have you made any changes because of this?

Nocturia is a common symptom associated with redistribution of fluid from the legs to the core when lying. As the fluid shifts, the kidneys are better perfused, increasing urine production. Patients may avoid drinking water after dinner because of this.

(text continues on page 500)

Additional Questions	Rationales/Abnormal Findings

Palpitations

Do you notice that your heart is beating faster? Are you having skipped or extra beats?
- When did it start? How long has it lasted?
- What makes it worse? What makes it better?
- Do any other symptoms accompany the heartbeats?
- Have you tried any treatments? Did they help?

Patients with *cardiovascular disease* may have tachycardia from decreased contractile strength of the heart muscle. With reduced stroke volume, the pulse increases to maintain cardiac output. **Palpitations** experienced as a rapid throbbing or fluttering of the heart may be associated with *arrhythmias*. Patients tolerate these arrhythmias differently, ranging from a mild awareness of the sensation to more severe dizziness or loss of consciousness.

⚠ *SAFETY ALERT 19.3*
Patients with a history of loss of consciousness should have a complete workup to diagnose the cause. They are at risk for falling and require fall precautions.

Documentation of Normal Findings

No chest pain or discomfort. Denies dyspnea, orthopnea, PND, cough, fatigue, edema, nocturia, and palpitations. *G. Indigo, RN*

 Lifespan Considerations

Additional Questions	Rationales/Abnormal Findings

Pregnant Women
- Have you noticed your pulse or blood pressure changing during pregnancy?
- Have you had any swelling in your face or hands?

Typically, heart rate rises in pregnancy from increased blood volumes and demands. Swelling may indicate the beginning of *pregnancy-induced hypertension* and should be monitored.

Newborns and Infants
- Did you have any complications during the pregnancy or labor?
- What medications are you taking?
- Did you take alcohol or drugs during the pregnancy?
- Do you notice any shortness of breath, fast breathing, unusual skin color, or fatigue in your baby?
- How is your baby feeding?

Risk for *congenital anomalies* increases when the mother takes lithium, dilantin, thalidomide, or excessive alcohol during pregnancy. Additional risks include maternal rubella, lupus, or diabetes mellitus in pregnancy (Lowdermilk & Perry, 2007).

The baby may have symptoms of cyanosis or pallor, dyspnea, fatigue, and difficulty feeding or growing related to heart defects.

Children and Adolescents
- Do you or does anyone in your family have a congenital heart problem?
- Do you notice any shortness of breath, unusual skin color, or fatigue in your child?
- Do you notice that your child squats or sits down to rest?
- Can your child keep up with friends when active?
- Is your child gaining weight and growing as normal?

If one parent has a congenital anomaly, the risk of a child also having one may be as high as 10% (Lowdermilk & Perry, 2007).

Children with cardiac disorders that reduce blood flow may sit down to increase cardiac output. Defects that allow a left to right shunt result in increased pulmonary volumes and heart failure. Obstructive defects prevent blood from being pumped from the ventricles. Obstruction on the left results in backup into the lungs and periphery with symptoms of heart failure; obstruction on the right causes cyanosis and hypoxemia because blood does not move forward for oxygenation. Defects that reduce pulmonary blood flow also produce cyanosis.

Older Adults
- Have you noticed any changes in your ability to tolerate activity?
- Have you had any periods where you felt dizzy or faint, or actually passed out?
- Have you been short of breath or had trouble breathing at night?

Age-related changes may cause decreased activity tolerance. *Arrhythmias* and *heart failure* are common symptoms for nurses to assess with people of this age group.

🌐 Cultural Considerations

- What do you do to keep your heart healthy?
- How would you describe your general health?
- Do you ever worry about heart disease?

Asking general questions may identify areas in which people of various cultural groups have different perceptions of heart health and risk for disease. Such questions may also provide an opportunity to educate patients and clarify misperceptions. For example, although heart disease is the number one cause of mortality in African American women, studies have shown that they generally do not perceive this problem as a threat and are less likely to modify risk factors (Jones, et al., 2006).

Therapeutic Dialogue: Collecting Subjective Data

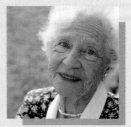

Remember Mrs. Lewis, introduced at the beginning of this chapter. She was admitted to the hospital 4 hours ago for chest pain and is experiencing some anxiety about a diagnosis of MI. The nurse is meeting Mrs. Lewis for the first time at the start of the shift. In addition to obtaining an assessment, the nurse must provide support and listen to the patient's responses to reduce anxiety. The following conversations give two examples of interview styles used by different nurses. One style is more effective than the other.

Less Effective

Nurse: You came to the hospital with chest pain. What did it feel like?

Mrs. Lewis: It felt like an elephant was sitting on my chest.

Nurse: How bad was it, on a 1–10 scale with 10 being the worst?

Mrs. Lewis: It was close to a 10. It was the worst pain that I've ever had.

Nurse: How long did it last?

Mrs. Lewis: Probably about 20 minutes.

Nurse: What took it away?

Mrs. Lewis: The paramedics gave me some nitroglycerin.

Nurse: Did you notice anything else with the pain, like nausea, sweating, or dizziness?

Mrs. Lewis: I was sweating and kind of dizzy, but that went away when the chest pain did.

Nurse: So what do you think the problem is?

Nurse: My doctor told me that I might be having a heart attack.

More Effective

Nurse: Tell me a little about what brought you to the hospital today.

Mrs. Lewis: I was taking a walk in my neighborhood and all of a sudden it felt like there was an elephant sitting on my chest. I couldn't breathe and had to stop. I was close to home, and when I got there my husband knew that something was wrong. He was the one who called 911.

Nurse: Tell me more about what you were feeling.

Mrs. Lewis: I've never felt anything like it before. It was right in the middle of my chest, and it didn't go away until the medics gave me a nitroglycerin tablet. It must have lasted about 20 minutes. I was so glad that they came fast. It was the worst pain that I've ever had. I felt all clammy and kind of dizzy.

Nurse: That must have been very scary for you.

Mrs. Lewis: I'm still scared. Do you think that I had a heart attack?

Critical Thinking Challenge

- Is this an appropriate time to perform a complete health history and review of systems? Provide rationale.
- What therapeutic communication techniques did the more effective nurse use?
- Compare and contrast the data collected in the two dialogues. Why is the more effective nurse more focused on Mrs. Lewis's experience versus assessment of her symptoms?
- How would the more effective nurse respond to Mrs. Lewis's question about the diagnosis of heart attack? Provide rationale.

Equipment

- Stethoscope with bell and diaphragm
- Watch with second hand
- Penlight or examination light for visualizing neck veins

Preparation

Evaluation of the neck vessels and heart requires contact with and exposure of the thorax. If possible, patients should wear a gown. Provide a drape to cover the patient when exposure of the chest is necessary. Ensure that the room is a comfortable temperature and take measures to facilitate a private and quiet setting. Wash and warm your hands to avoid spreading infection and to facilitate patient comfort.

For inspection, expose only the area of the chest that needs examination, especially for women. When visualization is required, gather the gown from the bottom to the shoulders so that the patient feels less exposed anteriorly. Cover the anterior chest when inspecting posteriorly. Explain the rationale for the need to expose the chest to ease the patient's anxiety.

If an abnormality is suspected, it may be necessary to listen to the heart in several different positions. Alert the patient that he or she will need to turn to the left or sit up to improve the volume and quality of the sounds. Also alert the patient that you will be listening for a longer period than usual and that doing so does not mean you have found abnormalities. Provide reassurance by saying, "I'm going to listen to your heart sounds carefully, but it doesn't mean that anything is wrong. I will let you know what I hear when I am finished."

Patient positioning is important for the cardiac examination. The patient may be sitting during auscultation of the carotid arteries. To evaluate the jugular pulses, lower the head of the bed to a 45-degree angle to allow for visualization of

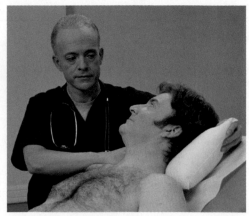

Figure 19.12 Lower the head of the bed to a 45-degree angle to better visualize the soft jugular venous pulses.

the softer impulses (Fig. 19-12). Most beds and examination tables have an indicator of the degree of elevation underneath to identify 45 degrees. The jugular pulse on the right side is usually easier to identify, so it may be most efficient and accurate for the examiner to stand on the patient's right. When auscultating the heart sounds, the patient may be sitting or lying (supine). Additionally, if there are concerns about cardiac problems, the heart can be auscultated with the patient supine, in the left lateral position, or leaning forward.

Studies have shown that a stethoscope can transmit bacteria among patients (Marinella, et al., 1997). Thus, be sure to clean the diaphragm of the stethoscope with the alcohol swab before bringing the diaphragm into contact with the patient. Also, warm the diaphragm of the stethoscope with your clean hands prior to placing it on the chest.

Common and Specialty/ Advanced Techniques

The focused examination mainly involves the neck vessels and precordium. A complete cardiovascular assessment incorporates additional data. The blood pressure, peripheral vascular

Table 19.3 Common Versus Specialty/Advanced Cardiovascular Techniques

Technique	Purpose	Screening or Registered Nurse Assessment	Focused or Advanced Practice Examination
Palpate the carotid arteries	Helps indicate the strength of the pulse		X
Auscultate the carotid artery	Enables the hearing of bruits		X
Inspect the jugular veins	Helps determine jugular venous pressure		X
Inspect the precordium	Identifies abnormalities	X	X
Palpate the PMI	Assesses for cardiac enlargement		X
Palpate the precordium	Assesses for masses, tenderness		X
Percuss the precordium	Evalutes heart size		X
Auscultate the pulse		X	X
Auscultate extra heart sounds	Determines rate, rhythm, and extra sounds	X	X

system, neck vessels, and heart sounds are all indicators of adequate circulation and tissue perfusion.

The routine head-to-toe assessment includes the most important and common cardiovascular assessment techniques. Nurses may add specialty or advanced steps if concerns exist over a specific finding. See Table 19-3, which summarizes the most common techniques that are essential to learn for use in clinical practice. Additional techniques may be necessary if indicated by the clinical situation or used more regularly in advanced practice.

◆ Comprehensive Physical Examination

Technique and Normal Findings	Abnormal Findings
Jugular Venous Pulses The jugular venous pulses are subtle, making their inspection challenging to learn. Accurate inspection requires practice and visualization with several patients, because chest size and shape and appearance of the jugular veins vary greatly. The jugular venous pulses have a waveform previously described. Rather than identify all the waves, nurses in clinical settings more commonly observe the pattern and rhythm.	If severe *heart failure* is suspected, invasive hemodynamic monitoring may be used. This waveform is often analyzed to identify the waves, pressures, and characteristics. These advanced techniques are used primarily in the intensive care setting.
Position the patient with the head of the bed at 30 to 45 degrees to promote visibility of the pulsation (see Fig. 19-12). Remove the pillow to avoid flexing the neck and to improve vein exposure. Move any long hair in patients away to enhance visibility. The right side is easiest to see; it may help the patient to turn the head away from the side being examined. Light the area to emphasize the shadows of the pulsations versus a bright light. Usually indirect lighting is best from a 45-degree angle. The external veins are lateral to the sternomastoid muscles, and the pulsations are best observed in the groove near the middle of the clavicle. The internal jugular veins can easily be confused with the carotid artery pulsation. The internal vein is not visible, but the pulsations are transmitted to the soft tissue and are usually most prominent in the suprasternal notch, the supraclavicular fossa, or just below the earlobe. If the pulsation is not visible, it may be necessary to lower the head of the bed. When learning to distinguish between the more subtle pulsations of the jugular veins, it may help to use a hand to shield the more prominent carotid pulsations and isolate the fluttery venous pulsations. *There are usually two pulsations with a prominent descent, compared to the carotid pulse, which has one pulsation and a prominent ascent with systole.*	If the patient is unusually dehydrated, it may be necessary to lower the head of the bed to visualize the vein, while the patient with fluid overload may need to have the head of the bed elevated. At times the neck veins are so distended that they extend all the way to the ear; in this case, raise the head of the bed until the pulsation is visible. Alternatively, patients with *dehydration* or *volume depletion* have barely visible neck veins, even when lying flat. These are described as flat neck veins.
Jugular Venous Pressure After locating the internal jugular vein in the sternal notch, identify the top height of the pulsation. If the internal vein is difficult to visualize, use the more prominent external vein (Techniques: Jugular, 2007). Locate the sternal angle in the 2nd ICS (see Chapter 18 for technique). Using a line parallel to the horizon, from the sternal angle estimate the difference between the parallel line and the top of the pulsation	Jugular venous distention (JVD) is associated with *heart failure* and *fluid volume overload*. The neck veins appear full, and the level of pulsation may be greater than 3 cm above the sternal angle.

(text continues on page 504)

in the external jugular vein (Fig. 19-13). Because of wide differences in chest shape and location of the sternal angle, exact measurement varies widely among patients (Van't Laar, 2002). Most commonly, nurses note whether neck veins appear distended, normal, or flat.

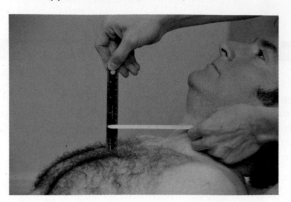

Figure 19.13 Estimate the jugular venous pressure.

Findings are up to 3-cm above the sternal angle, which is equivalent to a central venous pressure (CVP) of 8 mm Hg. If exact levels are not measured, document findings as "JVP normal," "JVP not elevated," "neck veins not distended," or "no JVD."

Hepatojugular Reflux

Pressing gently on the liver increases venous return (Fig. 19-14). Apply gentle pressure (30–40 mm Hg) over the right upper quadrant or middle abdomen for at least 10 seconds (some suggest to 1 minute) (Physical exam, 2007). *The pulsation increases for a few beats and then returns to normal less than 3-cm above the sternal angle.*

A positive result is when the highest level of pulsation stays above 3 cm for more than 15 seconds (Wiese, 2000). The pulsation remains elevated in disorders that cause a dilated and poorly compliant right ventricle or in obstruction of the right ventricular filling by tricuspid stenosis (Woods, et al., 2010). *Heart failure* is a common cause of hepatojugular reflux.

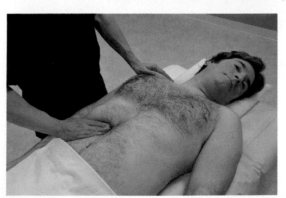

Figure 19.14 To assess hepatojugular reflux, press gently on the liver.

Carotid Arteries

Inspection. Inspect the carotid artery for a double stroke seen with S1 and S2. *The contour is smooth with a rapid upstroke and slower downstroke.*

The pulse may be bounding and prominent with hypertension, hypermetabolic states, and disorders with a rapid rise and fall of pressure (eg, patent ductus arteriosus) (Woods, et al., 2010). It may be low in amplitude and volume and have a delayed peak in aortic stenosis (from decreased cardiac output). If it is diminished unilaterally or bilaterally (often associated with a systolic bruit), the cause may be carotid stenosis from atherosclerosis (Woods, et al., 2010).

Palpation

⚠ SAFETY ALERT 19.4

Palpate the carotid arteries one at a time. Palpating them together poses a risk for obstructing both arteries, reducing blood flow to the brain and potentially causing dizziness or loss of consciousness.

Palpate the carotid artery medial to the sternomastoid muscle in the neck between the jaw and the clavicle (Fig. 19-15).

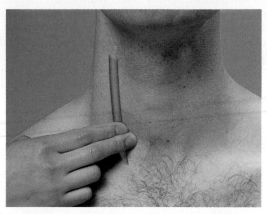

Figure 19.15 Palpate each carotid artery medial to the sternomastoid muscle in the neck.

⚠ SAFETY ALERT 19.5

Avoid compressing over the carotid sinus. Stimulation of the sinus also causes parasympathetic stimulation, which may lead to reduced pulse rate and bradycardia. Older adults and patients sensitive to this stimulation may develop periods of life-threatening asystole.

Palpate the strength of the pulse and grade it as with peripheral pulses (see Chapter 20). *Strength is 2+ or moderate. Pulses are equal bilaterally.*

Auscultation. Auscultation of the carotid arteries is performed in cases of suspected narrowing. Use the bell to hear the higher-pitched sound of the bruit.

Lightly apply the bell over the artery medial to the sternomastoid muscle at three locations: near the jaw, in the middle of the neck, and near the clavicle. Avoid compressing the artery, because doing so causes a bruit, similar to the compression from the cuff when taking blood pressure. *No sounds or bruits are heard.*

A diminished or thready pulse may accompany decreased stroke volume, found in *reduced fluid volume*. If the heart's ability to pump is decreased and cardiac output is low, as in *heart failure*, pulse strength may be reduced. Another cause of decreased pulse strength is a narrowed carotid artery from *atherosclerosis*. Pulse strength may increase during exercise or stress.

Bruits are swooshing sounds similar to the sound of the blood pressure. They result from turbulent blood flow related to *atherosclerosis*. A bruit is audible when the artery is partially obstructed. With complete obstruction, no bruit is audible, because no blood gets through. Bruits have been associated with an increased risk of stroke (Gillett, et al., 2003).

Distinguishing a murmur from a bruit can be challenging. Murmurs originate in the heart or great vessels and are usually louder over the upper precordium and quieter near the neck. Bruits are higher-pitched, more superficial, and heard only over the arteries (Woods, et al., 2010).

Documentation of Normal Findings

Without JVD, hepatojugular reflux negative. Carotid pulses 2+ bilaterally without bruits. *G. Indigo, RN*

Inspection of the Precordium

Inspect the anterior chest for any lesions, masses, or areas of tenderness (see Chapter 18). Observe for the PMI in the apex at the 4th–5th ICS at the left MCL. It is easier to observe in children, men, and adults with a thin chest wall. *Impulses are absent or located in the 4th–5th left ICS at the MCL with no lifts or heaves.*

The enlarged heart of *cardiomegaly* displaces the PMI laterally and inferiorly. Observe for a heave or lift, which appears as a forceful thrusting on the chest, and results from an enlarged left ventricle. A right ventricular heave is observed at the lower left sternal border; a left ventricular heave is observed at the apex.

Palpation of the Precordium

Palpate the anterior chest for any lesions, masses, or tender areas (see Chapter 18). When palpating for sensations related to the heart, use the palmar surface of the hand. Beginning at the apex of the heart, feel for the pulse in the location in which you observed it during inspection. To localize the impulse, it may help to use the fingerpads and depress in the left 5th ICS at the MCL (Fig. 19-16). If present, the PMI is usually felt as a light tap that lasts from S1 to halfway through systole and is less than 1–2 cm. It may or may not be palpable in adults. Also palpate in the sternoclavicular area, right and left upper sternal borders, right and left lower sternal borders, apical area, and epigastric area. Palpate all areas of the chest using the fingertips, heel, or ulnar surface of the hand. *The PMI is in the 5th left ICS at the MCL when present. No pulsations are palpated in other areas.*

An abnormal PMI is displaced left or downward, may raise a larger than normal area, and may be sustained throughout systole. It may result from *heart failure, MI, left ventricular hypertrophy*, or *valvular heart disease*. Abnormal sensations palpated on the chest include lifts and heaves. Thrills are vibrations detected on palpation. A palpable, rushing vibration (thrill) is caused from turbulent blood flow with *incompetent valves, pulmonary hypertension*, or *septal defects*. This vibration is usually in the location of the valve in which it is associated. With chest pain that increases with movement, palpation of the costochondral junction is performed to determine if the pain is of musculoskeletal origin.

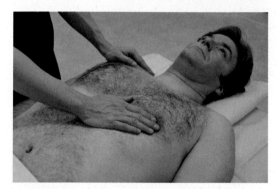

Figure 19.16 Location of the apical impulse.

Percussion of the Precordium

Chest x-ray has largely replaced chest percussion. Detecting percussion sounds over an obese or muscular chest or female breast tissue can be difficult. Without radiographic technology, percussion may be useful in identifying the left border if the heart is enlarged (as in cases of suspected heart failure). Identification of the right border is rarely useful. If heart failure or cardiomegaly is suspected, cardiac dullness may be percussed in the ICSs. Beginning at the anterior axillary line in the 4th ICS, percuss medially toward the sternum. Note the point at which the note changes from resonant (lung tissue) to dull (cardiac tissue). Repeat the procedure in the 5th and 6th ICSs. *The left border of the heart is percussed from the apex in the 4th–5th left ICS at the MCL.*

When the heart is enlarged, the left lateral border of the heart is percussed laterally and inferiorly to the normal location.

Documentation of Normal Findings

PMI observed and palpated in 5th left ICS at the MCL. No thrills, heaves, or lifts. *G. Indigo, RN*

Auscultation of the Precordium

Auscultation is the most important technique of cardiovascular examination. It is essential for the room to be quiet and for the stethoscope to be free of distracting noise. Chest hair, bumping of the stethoscope, or shivering may cause sounds that interfere with accuracy. Make sure that the patient is calm, warm, and draped as previously described.

Identify the locations for auscultation by accurately identifying the rib spaces and landmarks (Fig. 19-17). The most important landmark is the sternal angle at the 2nd rib space. There are two methods of identifying it. The first is to begin at the sternal notch and palpate to the right for the clavicle. Below the clavicle is the 1st rib; below the 1st rib is the 1st ICS. Feel the 2nd rib and then below it to the 2nd rib space. This is the first location for cardiac auscultation (*aortic area*). Recheck that this is the 2nd ICS by palpating the sternum for the indentation caused from the manubrium joining it (also called the sternal notch or Angle of Louis). The second method is to first locate the Angle of Louis on the sternum. A vertical motion is usually best for feeling this depression. Palpate directly across in the 2nd ICS at the left sternal border; this is the second location for auscultation (*pulmonic area*). The method used depends on the comfort of the nurse and the body structure of the patient; sometimes both methods are necessary to validate correct position. Walk the fingers one rib space at the left sternal border (approximately 1 in apart) to locate the 3rd left rib space; this is the third site for auscultation (*Erb's point*). Walk the fingers to the 4th ICS, this is the fourth site for auscultation (*tricuspid area*). Move the fingers to the 5th ICS, follow the ribs down and over to the MCL; this is the fifth location for auscultation (*mitral area*).

These auscultatory areas are near but not directly over the locations of the valves, because the sounds radiate in the direction in which blood flows. Note that although the pulmonic valve is on the right side of the heart, the valve is heard on the left sternal border. Not only does the sound radiate in this direction, but also the right side is more forward in the chest, so the pulmonic valve is turned more anteriorly and laterally. Also note that the aortic valve on the left side

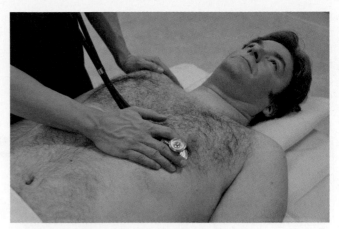

Figure 19.18 Auscultating the heart.

of the heart is heard best on the right side. It is more posterior in the chest, and the vessel branches to the right side before descending inferiorly. This flow of blood causes the aortic valve sound to radiate to the right. The tricuspid valve sound radiates to the left and is heard at the sternal border; the mitral sound is heard at the MCL. *Erb's point* is where the valves usually are equally audible; this site is especially effective for taking an apical pulse.

When listening to heart sounds, begin by hearing the rhythm of the beat and the characteristic "lub-dub." Usually the first heart sound is followed by the second with a pause before the next lub-dub. The lub, which correlates with the beginning of systole, is called S1 (see Fig. 19-7). The dub correlates with the end of systole and beginning of diastole (see Fig. 19-7). Each lub-dub is one pulse; when learning the heart sounds it may help to palpate and feel how the pulse (ventricular systole) occurs at the same time as S1.

First auscultate the heart rate and rhythm in one area (Fig. 19-18). Usually Erb's point is a good location to hear both S1 and S2 equally. Listen for a regular versus irregular rhythm. Count the heart rate for 30 seconds if regular and for 60 seconds if irregular (see Chapter 6). Then listen to each auscultatory area, usually beginning at the aortic area and proceeding laterally and inferiorly along the sternal border in each rib space. Listen first with the diaphragm and then with the bell to hear both high- and low-pitched sounds.

In all auscultatory areas:

1. Isolate the lub-dub rhythm, listening for a regular rhythmic cadence.
2. Listen first to S1 and then to S2 for a single sound or split sound. Identify if S1 or S2 is louder or softer, depending on the area being auscultated.
3. Listen for extra heart sounds (then identify if before or after S1 or S2).
4. Listen for murmurs (then identify if in systole or diastole).

Some normal variations in heart sounds include a split heart sound. When the valves close at the same time, one S2 is heard for both valves. If the valves close at slightly different times,

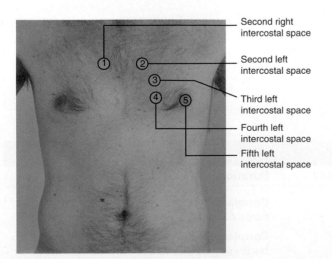

Figure 19.17 Sites for cardiac auscultation.

Second right intercostal space

Second left intercostal space

Third left intercostal space

Fourth left intercostal space

Fifth left intercostal space

however, two discernable components of the same sound are heard, a situation referred to as a **split heart sound**. The right-sided pressures are lower than the left, and with inspiration the intrathoracic pressures are even lower. The right heart can fill with more blood, which takes longer, and the closure of the pulmonic valve (on the right) is delayed. The split S2 is more commonly heard during inspiration and disappears during expiration. S1 can also be split because the tricuspid valve closes slightly after the mitral valve during systole. Splitting of S1 is usually constant and does not vary with respiration, because the AV valves are less sensitive to changes in intrathoracic pressures than are the semilunar valves. See Table 19-6 at the end of this chapter.

Technique and Normal Findings	Abnormal Findings
Identify Rate and Rhythm. Using the diaphragm, listen to Erb's point to identify S1, S2, heart rhythm, and heart rate as described. Rhythm may vary with respiration in some patients, especially children and young adults. Rate increases at the peak of inspiration and slows at the peak of expiration. This normal variation is referred to as a **sinus arrhythmia**. *Heart rate is 60–100 bpm and regular in adults.*	If the rhythm is irregular, identify if the irregularity has a pattern or is totally irregular. For example, every third beat missed would be described as a regular irregular rhythm. No detectable pattern is characteristic of atrial fibrillation, common in older adults. If the rhythm is irregular, take the radial pulse while listening to the apical pulse. Count the apical and radial heart rate at the same time. The easiest way to do so is to count the apical pulse while counting the number of missed beats; the difference is referred to as the **pulse deficit**. Refer to Chapter 6 for rate variations.
Identify S1 and S2. After identifying S1 as lub and S2 as dub, listen to each sound separately (Table 19-4). Normally they are each heard as one sound. S1 signals the beginning of systole as the mitral and tricuspid valves close. Because the right side of the heart may contract slightly slower than the right, the triscuspid valve may close slightly after the mitral, causing a split S1 as previously described. A split S1 is heard in the tricuspid area. S2 signals the end of systole and beginning of diastole as the aortic and pulmonic valves close. A split S2 may occur from the pulmonic valve closing slightly after the aortic; it may be heard in the pulmonic valve area during inspiration in children (see Table 19-6). Split sounds are very close together and difficult to auscultate. S1 is louder than S2 in the mitral and triscupid areas because those valves close at the beginning of systole (signaled by S1). S2 is louder than S1 in the aortic and pulmonic areas because those valves close at the beginning of diastole (signaled by S2). *S1 is greater than S2 in the mitral and tricuspid areas; S2 is greater than S1 in the aortic and pulmonic areas; S1 is equal to S2 at Erb's point.*	The rare split S1 is constant, does not vary with respiration, and thus is referred to as a fixed split. Wide splitting occurs when bundle branch block delays activation of the right ventricle or when *stenosis of the pulmonic valve* or *pulmonary hypertension* delays emptying of the right ventricle. A paradoxical split is the opposite of expected. When closure of the aortic valve is delayed (as in *left bundle branch block, right ventricular pacing, aortic stenosis,* or *left ventricular failure*), the pulmonic valve closes before the aortic. The split is heard during expiration and disappears with inspiration (Paradoxical split, 2007). See also Table 19-6 at the end of this chapter.

Table 19.4	Characteristics of Normal Sounds			
Visual Representation	Intensity and Pitch	Quality	Duration	Locations
S1	Louder at apex	Lub	Correlates with carotid pulse	Mitral tricuspid
S2	Louder at base	Dub	Correlates with beginning of diastole	Aortic pulmonic

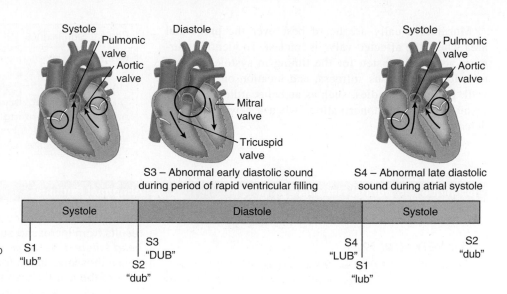

Figure 19.19 Extra heart sounds. Arrows represent the direction of blood flow. An S3 ("DUB") is an abnormal sound heard immediately following S2 (closure of the semilunar valves). S3 is generated very early in diastole as blood flowing into the right or left ventricle is met with resistance. S4 ("LUB") is an abnormal sound created during atrial systole as blood flowing into the right or left ventricle is met with resistance.

Extra Sounds. Extra heart sounds occur from vibrations during rapid ventricular filling. They include **S3 and S4** (Fig. 19-19). The third heart sound (S3) occurs during the early rapid diastolic filling phase immediately after S2. Blood rushes into ventricles abnormally resistant to filling, distending the ventricular walls and causing vibration. S3 is quiet, low pitched, and often difficult to hear. It usually is audible in patients with heart failure (Wang, et al., 2005). At the end of ventricular diastole, the atria contract and push an additional 25% to 30% of blood into the heart, called the "atrial kick." Abnormal resistance to filling during this phase also causes vibrations. S4 is heard late in diastole immediately before S1. Both S3 and S4 sound similar to S1 or S2. They are commonly referred to as ventricular "**gallops**." Presence of both S3 and S4 is referred to as a "summation gallop." S3 may be normal in children, young adults, or pregnant women in the third trimester. S3 is immediately after S2 early in diastole, and S4 is immediately before S1 late in diastole.

Systolic ejection **clicks** may occur early or in the middle of systole (see Table 19-6 at the end of this chapter). The early systolic sound occurs quickly after S1. Causes are either a sudden bulging of an abnormal aortic or pulmonic valve or the sudden distention of the associated great artery. *Aortic stenosis*, *pulmonic stenosis*, and a *bicuspid aortic valve* can all produce this sound, with or without a murmur. Pulmonic ejection sounds often decrease in intensity with inspiration and are best heard at the left sternal border. Aortic ejection sounds are best heard at the apex.

The midsystolic click is associated with *mitral valve prolapse* (see Table 19-7). There may or may not be an associated late systolic murmur, which is caused by mitral regurgitation. The click is produced by systolic prolapse of the mitral valve leaflets into the left atrium. If present, the Valsalva or squatting-to-standing maneuver should be performed to assess for increases in the click or murmur (Techniques: Heart sounds, 2007).

The opening **snap** is an early diastolic sound associated with *mitral stenosis* (see Table 19-7). It is audible shortly after S2 and may or may not be associated with a late diastolic murmur. It results from rapid opening of the anterior mitral valve leaflet during diastole with high left atrial pressures. The opening snap is challenging to differentiate from either S3 or split S2 (Techniques: Heart sounds, 2007).

The pericardial friction **rub** is the most important physical sign of *acute pericarditis*. It may have up to three components during the cardiac cycle and is high-pitched, scratching, and grating (see Table 19-7). It can best be heard with the diaphragm of the stethoscope at the left lower sternal border. The pericardial friction rub is heard most frequently during expiration and increases when the patient is upright and leaning forward (Strimel, et al., 2006).

Murmurs

Murmurs may result from intrinsic cardiovascular disease or circulatory disturbances (eg, anemia, pregnancy). Some murmurs have no underlying pathology (referred to as innocent murmurs). Fitting the clinical situation with the murmur is necessary to better determine if the murmur is insignificant or abnormal.

An innocent flow murmur may originate from higher blood flow velocities in the left ventricular outflow tract and aortic valve. The increased flow velocity results from a larger stroke volume passing through the relatively narrow left ventricle and aortic valve in children (Celebi & Onat, 2006). Innocent murmurs are usually systolic. Functional murmurs in pregnancy usually result from increased circulating fluid volumes.

Murmurs in adults usually indicate disease. If the heart valve fails to totally close, during systole the blood leaks back through the valve and causes a whooshing sound (similar to the Korotkoff's sounds heard during assessment of blood pressure). Similarly, a valve may fail to totally open, causing turbulence during diastole as the blood rushes against a partially closed valve to fill the heart. Therefore, these murmurs may occur during either systole or diastole. Murmurs also may result from vibration of tissue or excessive flow as in pregnancy. Additionally they may occur in any of the four valves.

Murmurs usually are heard best over the precordial area where the affected valve is loudest. To identify murmurs accurately, listen for the timing in systole or diastole, loudness versus softness, and location on the chest wall. Follow-up studies, such as an echocardiogram, will identify structural abnormalities when a new murmur is detected.

Technique and Normal Findings	Abnormal Findings
Listen for Extra Sounds ⚠ *SAFETY ALERT 19.6* *Auscultation of a new extra sound may indicate a change in the patient's condition or worsening heart failure. A new S3 or S4 requires investigation and may be the reason to consult with a physician for further diagnostic testing.* S3 and S4 are commonly called "gallops." When S3 exists, it follows S2 and sounds like "lub dub-dub." It usually is heard best in the apex with the patient lying on the left side. It may be normal in young patients. S4 in late diastole, right before S1, sounds like "lub-lub dub." It is usually abnormal.	S3 is abnormal in patients older than 40 years and results from increased atrial pressure related to *systolic heart failure* or *valvular regurgitation*. Using the bell of the stethoscope, listen for a left ventricular S3 over the apex of the heart. Listen for a right ventricular S3 over the lower left sternal border. Have the patient move to the left lateral position to bring the cardiac apex closer to the chest wall, making the left ventricular S3 easier to hear. S4 results from a noncompliant ventricle as a consequence of *hypertension, hypertrophy,* or *fibrosis* (Techniques: Heart sounds, 2007). A left ventricular S4 is heard best at the apex with the patient lying in the left lateral position; a right ventricular S4 is loudest over the left sternal border in the 5th ICS.
Also listen for the short scratching sound of the pericardial friction rub, high-pitched opening snaps, and ejection clicks as previously described. These sounds are difficult to differentiate between S3 and S4; referral to a cardiologist may be helpful in labeling them. *Normally no extra sounds are heard.*	Pericardial friction rubs can be differentiated from pleural friction rubs by having the patient hold the breath. If present without breathing, the rub is pericardial. An opening snap is associated with mitral stenosis. It is high-pitched, snapping, and best heard with the diaphragm of the stethoscope in the mitral area. In patients who have undergone cardiac surgery, related trauma may produce extra sounds. An audible respirophasic squeak may be related to mediastinal or pleural tubes. Air in the mediastinum produces a crunching sound (Hamman's sign) during auscultation of the precordium.
Listen to Murmurs In clinical practice, nurses are more concerned with recognizing changes in murmurs rather than in diagnosing and labeling them. Describe murmurs according to timing in the cardiac cycle, loudness, pitch, pattern, quality, location, radiation, and position. When learning murmurs it is helpful to identify how other health care professionals have labeled them and attempt to hear how they have been described (see Table 19-8 at the end of this chapter). *Normally no murmurs are heard.*	The most common systolic murmurs in adults are produced by aortic stenosis, mitral insufficiency, and ventricular septal defect. In older adults, the murmur of aortic sclerosis (thickening of aortic valve leaflets with age) is common. The most common diastolic murmurs are aortic insufficiency and mitral stenosis. Nurses are often the first to identify the onset of murmurs related to papillary muscle dysfunction associated with MI. This high-pitched, crescendo-decrescendo shaped, systolic murmur must be recognized immediately so that interventions can be instituted to prevent rupture, which poses a high mortality rate (see Table 19-9).

Documentation of Normal Findings

Heart rate and rhythm regular. Without gallops, murmurs, or rubs. *G. Indigo, RN*

Lifespan Considerations

Pregnant Women

Many changes in pregnancy relate to increased blood volume that accompanies gestation. Resting pulse rate increases, and blood pressure may rise slightly. Heart rate increases by 10 to 15 bpm between 14 and 20 weeks of pregnancy. In multiple gestation, heart rate increases significantly in the third trimester (Malone & D'Alton, 2004).

The woman's skin may be slightly redder than normal because of the increased volume and metabolic state. In late pregnancy, the uterus pushes up on the diaphragm. The PMI moves upward and laterally approximately 1 to 1.5 cm, depending on uterine size and position (Lowdermilk & Perry, 2007). Heart sounds may change because of the increased blood volume. S1 and S2 may be split after 20 weeks. Systolic and diastolic murmurs may be heard over the precordium, although systolic murmurs are more common.

A unique murmur in lactating women is referred to as a *mammary soufflé*. It results from increased blood flow through the internal mammary artery and is best heard in the 2nd to 4th ICS. Pressing on the artery can obliterate the mammary soufflé, unlike a murmur that originates in the heart.

Newborns and Infants

If possible, place the infant on the parent's lap during examination. Do not undress the baby until necessary, because exposure may be uncomfortable and cold, and assessing a restless baby with high respiratory and cardiac rates is difficult. If the baby is crying, a bottle or pacifier might help to calm him or her. During inspection, observe for associated chromosomal characteristics, such as found with Down's or Turner's syndrome. Up to 20% of infants with Down's syndrome may have an associated cardiac anomaly (Braunwald, et al., 2004).

Observe for cyanosis, especially with crying. Note that the infant's skin may normally be mottled if the examining environment is cool. Inspect for subcostal retractions, left-sided chest prominence, abnormal chest movement, and increased respiratory rates found with congenital heart disease (see Table 19-10 at the end of this chapter). Because infants have short necks, the jugular veins are not examined. Palpate the faint apical impulse to the left of the xyphoid, at the apex, and in the 2nd ICS left sternal border; a prominent pulse is abnormal. Percussion in infants and children is not performed, because related findings do not accurately reflect cardiac size or function. Use a pediatric stethoscope to auscultate the heart (Fig. 19-20). Innocent murmurs are less common in neonates than in children.

Children and Adolescents

If the child appears likely to cry, auscultate heart sounds before inspecting the precordium. By the time a child is 3 to 5 years old, complications from heart anomalies may manifest as cyanosis or heart failure. Angina is rare. Anomalies create diminished oxygenation, low cardiac output, or increased pulmonary pressure. Associated symptoms include fatigue, diaphoresis, and poor weight gain. Question older children about exercise, activities, edema, respiratory problems, chest pain, palpitations, fainting, and headaches.

If cardiac disease is suspected, auscultate the heart with the child in different positions, beginning with lying and standing (Fig. 19-21). During auscultation in the pulmonic area, S2 may be closely split in inspiration and single in expiration. Be aware that fixed splitting is an important finding that may indicate an atrial septal defect from a patent foramen ovale. In the tricuspid area, S1 may be closely split and S2 will be single; this does not vary with respiration.

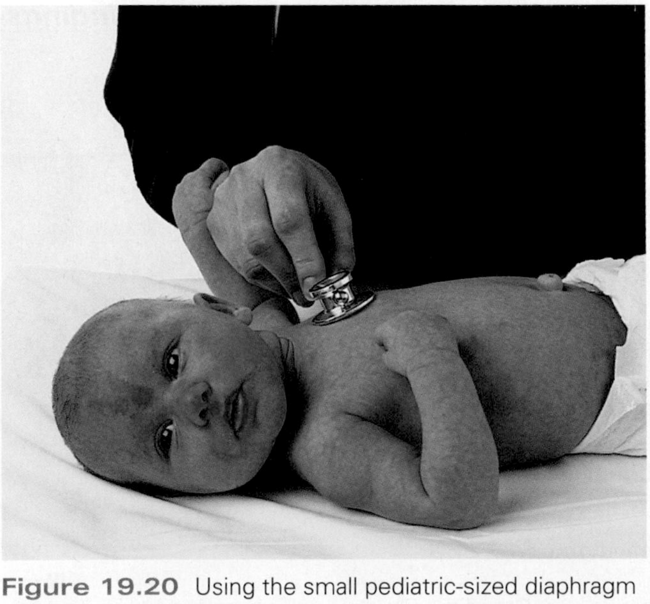

Figure 19.20 Using the small pediatric-sized diaphragm and bell.

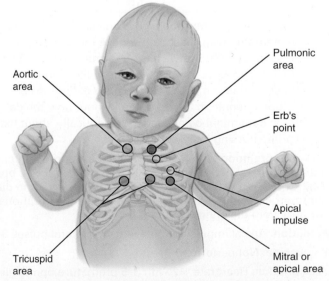

Figure 19.21 Palpate in the fourth interspace to the right of the MCL in children ages 7 years or younger.

At the apex, there is a single S1, single S2, and possibly an S3. S3 will be heard best with the bell; it is normal in children because of hyperdynamic circulation and a thin chest wall. If a murmur is heard, it may be innocent, functional, or pathologic. Listen carefully to determine the characteristics, and refer any patients with suspected problems to a physician if previously undiagnosed. Up to 50% of children have an innocent systolic murmur (Menasche, 2007). (See Chapter 28 for more information.)

Older Adults

Older adults develop changes in their hearts and blood pressures primarily from age-related stiffening of the vasculature and decreased responsiveness to stress hormones. Blood and pulse pressures increase from the stiff vessels. Additionally, BMI increases, causing the heart to work harder. Elevated late diastolic filling increases the volume of atrial contraction, which may be associated with the S4 gallop of late diastolic filling.

The ventricles hypertrophy, increasing the risk for heart failure and resultant atrial fibrillation. Approximately 17% of men and 6% of women live with this chronic problem, which causes an irregular heartbeat and increases the patient's risk for stroke (Lakatta & Levy, 2003). Assess older adults for symptoms of heart failure including weight gain, shortness of breath, and edema. Symptoms of atrial fibrillation include fatigue, palpitations, and heart failure with loss of the "atrial kick" that supports ventricular filling.

Older adults are also more likely to develop atherosclerosis and cardiovascular disease. The vasculature is undergoing constant remodeling, forming new capillaries and collateral circulation (Yang, 2007). Older adults, however, are more prone to atherosclerosis because they are more sensitive to the effects of lifestyle choices, such as smoking and high-fat diets (Lakatta, 2002). Assess these patients carefully for chest pain, fatigue, and dyspnea associated with symptoms. Ideally, counseling is effective in reducing risk factors and interventions are targeted toward primary prevention of disease.

Evidence-based Critical Thinking

Common Laboratory and Diagnostic Testing—

Laboratory and diagnostic testing helps confirm and expand information obtained through subjective and objective data collection. Some tests require explanation to the patient, some require special preparation (eg, a period of fasting), and some require special monitoring by nurses during and after the test (eg, exercise tolerance testing). Cardiac testing ranges from low-risk ECG to more invasive cardiac catheterization. Results from such tests help identify patterns of data that indicate areas for care planning and interventions.

Elevated levels of blood lipids are a risk factor for cardiovascular disease. A lipid profile includes total cholesterol, high-density lipoprotein (HDL), LDL, and triglyceride levels. For the general population, the guidelines designate a desirable cholesterol level less than 200, an optimal LDL level less than 100, an HDL level less than 40, and triglyceride level less than 150 (National Cholesterol Education Program Expert Panel, 2001).

The myocardium releases cardiac enzymes and proteins in response to cell damage. These enzymes and proteins

---

Documenting Abnormal Findings

The nurse has just finished a physical examination of Mrs. Lewis, the 77-year-old woman admitted with chest pain. Unlike the samples of normal documentation previously noted, Mrs. Lewis has abnormal findings. Review the following important findings that the steps of objective data collection for this patient revealed. Consider how these results compare with the normal findings presented in the samples of normal documentation. Begin to think about how the data cluster together and what additional data might be needed. Think critically about her problems, and anticipate appropriate nursing interventions.

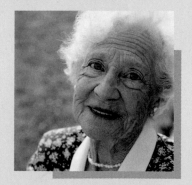

Inspection: Sitting with head of bed at 45-degree angle, appears comfortable but somewhat anxious. BP 122/62 mm Hg, P 112 bpm, R 16 breaths/min, T 37°C, oxygen saturation 94%. Skin color pale, some diaphoresis. Chest shape symmetrical without visible apical impulse. Respirations without dyspnea. No neck vein distention.

Palpation: Apical impulse not present. Peripheral pulses 3+ without edema.

Percussion: Not performed.

Auscultation: Heart rate 112 with 3–5 premature bpm. Pulse deficit of 5. S1 > S2 at apex and S2 > S1 at base. No murmurs, rubs, or gallops.

G. Indigo, RN

are measured in blood samples to diagnose or rule out MI. Creatine kinase-MB (CK-MB) and troponin-I are intracellular proteins specific to the myocardium; their values are elevated with MI.

The ECG discussed earlier, assists with diagnoses of myocardial ischemia, chamber hypertrophy, pericarditis, electrolyte imbalances, cardiac arrhythmias, and heart block. Electrodes are attached to the limbs and anterior chest wall using adhesive pads; the electrical changes in the heart are transferred onto a paper graph. Nurses with additional training may perform ECG testing. Home ECG monitoring can be conducted using an ambulatory ECG monitor or an event recorder.

A chest x-ray film helps determine the size, contour, and position of the heart; alterations in the pulmonary circulation; and acute or chronic lung disease. An echocardiogram uses high frequency sound waves and the Doppler effect to evaluate the size, shape, and motion of cardiac structures and the direction and velocity of blood flow through the heart. A gel (often cold) is placed on the patient's chest wall and the transducer is moved around the anterior chest wall. The echocardiogram may also be done with the transducer inserted through the mouth into the esophagus (transesophageal echocardiogram or TEE). Compared to the simple echocardiogram, this invasive procedure requires fasting and sedation, with potential complications such as a perforated esophagus or impaired swallowing.

Bedside hemodynamic monitoring includes measurement of central venous pressure, pulmonary artery pressures, and systemic interarterial pressures using a catheter placed in the heart. Systemic intra-arterial pressure monitoring provides access to direct and continuous blood pressures in critically ill patients; this catheter is usually placed in the radial artery. Hemodynamic monitoring requires advanced training and skill of nurses in critical care areas.

Stress testing compares cardiac function and perfusion at rest versus during stress. A simple exercise stress test consists of ECG monitoring for signs of ischemia or arrhythmia while the patient walks on a treadmill or rides a stationary bicycle. A radionuclide ventriculogram, also known as a *mu*ltiple-*g*ated *a*cquisition (MUGA) scan, is a test in which a small amount of a patient's blood is withdrawn, mixed with a radionuclide, and reinjected. This study is most commonly used to monitor the effects of potentially cardiotoxic chemotherapeutic agents. Both of these tests are performed in special settings.

Cardiac catheterization and coronary angiography are invasive diagnostic procedures that delineate coronary anatomy and coronary heart disease using fluoroscopy, usually in the radiology department. Right-sided heart catheterization is performed to measure right heart pressures and structures. Left-sided heart catheterization involves placing a catheter through the femoral artery to the coronary arteries where dye is used for visualization. Following the procedure, the patient is on bed rest and the puncture site and distal circulation must be monitored frequently. Nursing staff also monitor blood pressure and cardiac rhythm.

Cardiac electrophysiology studies are used in the diagnostic investigation of arrhythmias and syncope. Flexible catheters with multiple electrodes are placed within the heart to stimulate arrhythmias. The patient fasts for several hours before the study; usually, he or she is sedated during the procedure. Complications include the inability to induce arrhythmias, cardiac perforation and pericardial effusion, venous thrombosis or infection from the catheter site, and intractable ventricular fibrillation and death (Blancher, 2005). Patients are monitored closely following this procedure.

Diagnostic Reasoning

Nursing Diagnoses, Outcomes, and Interventions

Table 19-5 compares nursing diagnoses commonly related to cardiovascular assessment (NANDA-I, 2009). From the assessment information and established nursing diagnoses, nurses then work to identify patient outcomes. Some outcomes related to cardiovascular problems include the following:

• The patient demonstrates adequate circulation status with strong peripheral pulses, normal blood pressure, and adequate urinary output
• The patient demonstrates cardiac pump effectiveness with normal heart rate, negative JVD, no S3 or S4, and no arrhythmias
• The patient maintains fluid balance with no edema, clear lung sounds, stable body weight, and balanced intake and output (Moorhead, et al., 2007).

Once outcomes are established, nurses can implement care to improve the patient's status. Critical thinking and evidence-based practice are essential to develop effective interventions. Examples of nursing interventions for cardiovascular care are as follows:

• Teach the patient the signs of cardiac ischemia and when to call 911.
• Assess for chest pain, shortness of breath, and edema and document cardiac arrhythmias.
• Weigh the patient daily; monitor trends. Maintain accurate intake and output (Bulechek, et al., 2007).

Nurses then evaluate care according to the developed patient outcomes, thereafter reassessing the patient and continuing or modifying the interventions as appropriate. An accurate and complete nursing assessment is an essential foundation for holistic nursing care. Even beginning nursing students can use assessment data to implement new interventions, evaluate the effectiveness of those interventions, and make a difference in the quality of patient care.

Nurses also collect assessment data to assist physicians to identify medical diagnoses, so that appropriate treatment may be ordered. Nurses must understand the association of assessment findings to underlying problems to gather data to support or discount medical diagnoses. For example, chest pain may result from MI, pulmonary embolism, or musculoskeletal tenderness. Nurses assess the patient's history to determine if

Table 19.5 Common Nursing Diagnoses for Cardiovascular Conditions

Diagnosis and Related Factors	Point of Differentiation	Assessment Characteristics	Nursing Interventions
Decreased cardiac output related to MI, arrhythmia, sepsis, congenital heart defect	The heart pumps inadequate blood to meet the body's metabolic demands.	Arrhythmias, palpitations, ECG changes, increased fluid volume, decreased blood pressure, dyspnea, S3 or S4, murmur	Monitor for symptoms of heart failure. Observe for chest pain or discomfort. Place patient on cardiac monitor. Assess blood pressure carefully.
Impaired tissue perfusion, cardiac related to chest pain, shock, or dysrhythmia	Decreased oxygen results in failure to nourish tissues at the capillary level.	Chest pain, ECG changes, elevated CK-MB or troponin, diaphoresis, dyspnea, low oxygen saturation	Place patient on cardiac monitor. Administer nitroglycerin with MD order.* Place oxygen.* Ensure the IV is in place for emergency use.* Notify physician.
Excess fluid volume related to heart failure, excess fluid intake, excess sodium intake	Increased fluid retention and edema	Jugular vein distention, weight gain, dyspnea, orthopnea, PND, S3 or S4, edema	Monitor edema, intake and output. Weigh patient daily. Auscultate lung and heart sounds. Administer diuretic with order.* Elevate head of bed for dyspnea.

*Collaborative interventions.

Analyzing Findings

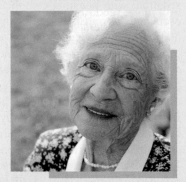

The problems of Mrs. Lewis have been outlined throughout this chapter. The initial collection of subjective and objective data is complete. Mrs. Lewis expressed concerns about her new diagnosis of MI; additionally, she developed an irregular rhythm with some pallor and diaphoresis.

Unfortunately, Mrs. Lewis also develops a new onset of chest pain, so the nurse must reassess her and document findings. The following nursing note illustrates how the nurse collects and analyzes subjective and objective data and begins to develop nursing interventions.

Subjective: "I'm having chest pain again." States chest pain 8/10 scale. Describes pain as a heavy weight in the center of her chest that radiates down her left arm. Started approximately 5 minutes ago and has been increasing. Is similar to the pain that she had earlier in the day, although this pain began at rest.

Objective: BP 100/66 mm Hg, P 122 with 3–5 premature bpm, R 28 breaths/min, O₂ saturation 94%. Increased diaphoresis, dizziness, and nausea. Skin pale, appears anxious. Peripheral pulses 2+ and thready.

Analysis: Impaired cardiac tissue perfusion related to possible myocardial ischemia.

Plan: Stay with patient and continue to monitor vital signs. Give nitroglycerin tablets as ordered by physician. Page rapid response team for assistance. Obtain 12-lead ECG and bedside monitor. Place oxygen as ordered and assess lung sounds. Elevate head of bed. Ensure that IV site is patent and suction is at bedside if needed. Provide calm reassurance that the patient will not be left alone and that treatment will be given for the chest pain. Use touch as appropriate. Inform family of new onset of chest pain.

G. Indigo, RN

Critical Thinking Challenge

- What type of assessment is this? Would you further investigate any subjective data?
- Critique the documented objective data. Is the organization logical? Would you add any data?
- Why did the nurse prioritize impaired cardiac tissue perfusion as the diagnosis to document?
- How is the nurse using assessment information to organize and plan nursing interventions?

the pain is acute (ie, MI, pulmonary embolism) or chronic (ie, chest wall tenderness). They assess heart sounds for S3, S4, or murmurs, which may accompany MI. Oxygen desaturation may be associated with pulmonary embolism, while tenderness to palpation is associated with chest wall tenderness. An ECG helps with diagnosis of MI. Therefore, nurses need to use critical thinking to know which data to collect, and then organize findings to assist physicians to arrive at a medical diagnosis.

Collaboration with Other Health Care Providers

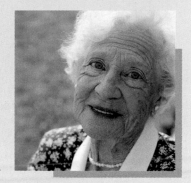

The Institute for Healthcare Improvement (Simmonds, 2005) has recommended the formation of rapid response teams to provide prompt assistance to patients with early warning signs of deterioration. Intervening before the patient's condition further declines has been proven to improve patient outcomes. The role of the team is to assess, stabilize, assist with communication, support, and assist with transfer if needed. Results that might trigger a page to the rapid response team are as follows:

- Any staff member is worried about the patient.
- The patient has an acute change in heart rate of less than 40 or more than 130 bpm.
- Systolic blood pressure changes acutely to less than 90 mm Hg.
- Respiratory rate changes acutely to less than 8 or more than 28 breaths/min.
- Saturation falls below 90% despite oxygen administration.
- Conscious state changes acutely.
- Urinary output falls below 50 mL in 4 hours (Grimes, et al., 2007).

Mrs. Lewis now has been admitted 6 hours ago with chest pain and is having new chest pain. Rapid response is indicated because the nurse is worried about the patient's new chest pain. The following conversation illustrates how to organize data and make recommendations about the patient's situation to team members when they arrive. Usually several people on the team come to assist with care at the bedside. Assessments and interventions occur simultaneously to resolve chest pain, which indicates cardiac ischemia and is an urgent issue.

Situation: I'm Galen Indigo and I'm the nurse for Mrs. Lewis. She was admitted with chest pain 6 hours ago and a diagnosis of MI. She has a new onset of chest pain that she rates as 8 out of 10.

Background: Her medical history includes hypertension. She is taking a beta blocker and a thiazide diuretic and also a statin to lower her cholesterol. Her blood pressure is 100/66 mm Hg, which is down from 148/78 mm Hg. Her pulse is 122 beats/min, respirations 28 breaths/min, and O_2 saturation is 94%. She's having 3–5 premature bpm and had a pulse deficit earlier. Her peripheral pulses are 2+ and thready. I have given her one nitroglycerin tablet, and she's still rating her pain as a 7 on a 1–10 scale.

Assessment: I called for you because I'm worried that she might be having some cardiac ischemia and can use some help in getting her treated.

Recommendations: (To a member of rapid response) It's time for her to have another nitroglycerin, so I can do that if you can get the ECG and then set up the bedside monitor. If someone else could hook up the oxygen, that would be great. She has an IV in place already. (To the charge nurse) Could you page the physician and let her know the situation? (To the Mrs. Lewis) I'll stay with you, because I know you're a little anxious. (To an assisting nurse) Her husband is in the waiting room—could you let him know that she's having chest pain? If he would like to come in that's OK. Let him know that we're working closely with her. (To the patient) "Mrs. Lewis, let me know if your pain is any better after this second nitroglycerin. How are you doing?"

Critical Thinking Challenge

- How will the nurse conduct assessments and nursing care while considering Mrs. Lewis's anxious state?
- Which part of the nursing process is highest priority during this time?
- What is the nurse's role in coordinating collaborative care with the rapid response team?
- What will be the frequency of assessment for Mrs. Lewis after this event? What items will be assessed?

Pulling It All Together: Reflection and Critical Thinking

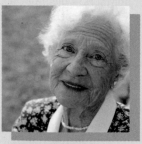

Nurses use assessment data to formulate a nursing care plan for Mrs. Lewis. After completing the outlined interventions, they reevaluate and document findings in the chart. This is often in the form of a care plan or case note similar to the one below.

Nursing Diagnosis	Patient Outcomes	Nursing Interventions	Rationale	Evaluation
Impaired Cardiac Tissue Perfusion related to possible cardiac ischemia	Blood pressure is stable within 30 minutes. Chest pain resolves within 5 minutes.	Monitor vital signs every 5 minutes until stable. Ensure IV access. Encourage patient to rest and reduce anxiety. Monitor for cardiac arrhythmias. Administer nitroglycerin and oxygen prn according to orders. Elevate head of bed.	IV access is essential in case the patient's condition deteriorates and IV medications are needed. Rest reduces the demand for oxygen. Arrhythmias may accompany ischemia. Nitroglycerin causes coronary arteries to dilate, relieving chest pain. Oxygen improves supply to the heart tissue.	Blood pressure has improved to 132/78. Chest pain has resolved with the third nitroglycerin. Patient is resting comfortably with head of bed elevated. Heart rate 102 and rhythm with no premature beats. Transfer to coronary intensive care for unstable chest pain.

Applying Your Knowledge

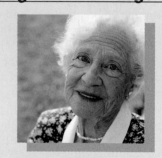

Using the previous steps of diagnostic reasoning, organizing, and prioritizing, consider all the case study findings woven throughout this chapter. When answering the following questions, begin drawing conclusions and see how the pieces of assessment must work together to create an environment for personalized, appropriate, and accurate care.

- Is Mrs. Lewis's condition stable, urgent, or an emergency?
- What immediate health promotion and teaching needs are evident?
- How will the nurse focus, organize, and prioritize subjective data collection?
- How will the nurse focus, organize, and prioritize objective data collection?
- How will the nurse individualize assessment to Mrs. Lewis's specific needs, considering her condition, age, and culture?

Key Points

- Knowledge of cardiac anatomy and physiology is essential to understanding cardiac assessment.
- The cardiovascular system is a double pump with pulmonary and systemic circulation.
- The cardiac cycle consists of rhythmic movements of systole (ventricular contraction) and diastole (relaxation).

- The S1 or first heart sound results from closure of the mitral and tricuspid valves; this sound signals the beginning of systole.
- The S2 or second heart sound results from closure of the aortic and pulmonic valves; this sound signals the beginning of diastole and end of systole.
- A newborn's cardiac function shifts dramatically at birth as the foramen ovale and ductus arteriosus close and the right heart pumps blood to the lungs.

- A pregnant female has increased blood volume, heart rate, stroke volume, and cardiac output by 30% to 40% above nonpregnant values.
- Health care providers assume that chest pain is heart pain until another diagnosis is established. Chest pain is an acute situation that requires intervention in addition to assessment.
- Risk factors for cardiovascular disease include increasing age, family history, male gender, high blood pressure, high blood cholesterol level, smoking, diabetes mellitus, overweight and obesity, decreased activity, high-fat diet, excessive alcohol intake, elevated C-reactive protein, and elevated B-naturetic peptide.
- Common symptoms of cardiovascular disease are chest pain, dyspnea, orthopnea, cough, diaphoresis, fatigue, edema, and nocturia.
- Inspection and palpation of the PMI should be at the 4th to 5th left ICS in the MCL.
- The nurse auscultates heart sounds in specific areas on the precordium: aortic, pulmonic, tricuspid, and mitral.
- A split heart sound is audible when the valves close at slightly different times: the S1 is split from the mitral and tricuspid, and the S2 is split from the aortic and pulmonic.
- Murmurs are identified by their location, intensity, quality, timing in the cardiac cycle, and radiation.
- S3 and S4 are extra sounds that result from ventricular filling; the S3 follows the S2 and the S4 precedes the S1.
- Cardiac anomalies in children cause symptoms of decreased oxygenation, low cardiac output, or increased pulmonary pressure.
- The nursing diagnoses most commonly associated with cardiac problems are decreased cardiac output, ineffective cardiac tissue perfusion and excess fluid volume.

Review Questions

1. Which of the following statements describes the cardiovascular system most accurately? The cardiovascular system
   A. is a double pump with pulmonary and systemic elements.
   B. has a heart with six chambers and valves.
   C. includes concepts of precontractility, after-contractility, and load.
   D. functions with a conduction system that starts in the ventricles.

2. In a healthy patient, the myocardial cells in the ventricle depolarize and contract during
   A. prediastole
   B. diastole
   C. systole
   D. postsystole

3. When the nurse listens to S1 in the mitral and tricuspid areas, the expected finding is
   A. S1 > S2
   B. S1 = S2
   C. S2 > S1
   D. No S1 is heard

4. The nurse assesses the neck vessels in the patient with heart failure to determine which of the following?
   A. The strength of the carotid pulse
   B. The presence of bruits
   C. The highest level of jugular venous pulsation
   D. The strength of the jugular veins

5. The nurse is caring for a patient with a sudden onset of chest pain. Which assessment is highest priority?
   A. Auscultate heart sounds.
   B. Inspect the precordium.
   C. Percuss the left border.
   D. Obtain a blood pressure.

6. A patient visits the clinic with the controllable risk factors of smoking, high-fat diet, overweight, decreased activity, and high blood pressure. What concept should the nurse use when performing patient teaching?
   A. Teach the patient the most serious information.
   B. Give the patient brochures to review upon the next visit.
   C. Discuss risk factors that the patient is interested in modifying.
   D. Describe consequences of risk factors to motivate the patient.

7. Which of the following clusters of symptoms are common in women preceding an MI?
   A. Chest pain, nausea, diaphoresis
   B. Weight gain, edema, nocturia
   C. Dizziness, palpitations, low pulse
   D. Fatigue, difficulty sleeping, dyspnea

8. The nurse auscultates a medium loud whooshing sound that softens between S1 and S2. The nurse documents this finding as which of the following?
   A. Grade III decrescendo systolic murmur
   B. Grade IV crescendo systolic murmur
   C. Grade II crescendo diastolic murmur
   D. Grade I decrescendo diastolic murmur

9. The nurse auscultates an extra sound on a patient 1 week following an MI. It is immediately after S3 and is heard best at the apex. Which of the following does the nurse suspect?
   A. S3 gallop
   B. S4 gallop
   C. Systolic ejection click
   D. Split S2

10. A patient has dyspnea, edema, weight gain, and intake greater than output. These symptoms are consistent with which nursing diagnosis?
    A. Ineffective cardiac tissue perfusion
    B. Decreased cardiac output
    C. Impaired gas exchange
    D. Excess fluid volume

References

American Heart Association. (2005). *Coronary heart disease, acute coronary syndrome, and angina pectoris.* Retrieved October 22, 2007, from http://www.americanheart.org/presenter.jhtml?identifier=3000090

Benetos, A., Thomas, F., Bean, K., Gautier, S., Smulyan, H., & Guize, L. (2002). Prognostic value of systolic and diastolic blood pressure in treated hypertensive men. *Archives of Internal Medicine, 162,* 577–581.

Blancher, S. (2005). Cardiac electrophysiology procedures. In S. L. Woods, E. S. Sivarajan Froelicher, S. U. Motzer, & E. J. Bridges (Eds.), *Cardiac nursing* (5th ed., pp. 425–438). Philadelphia: Lippincott Williams & Wilkins.

Braunwald, E., Zipes, D. P., & Libby, P. (2004). *Heart disease: A textbook of cardiovascular medicine* (7th ed.) Philadelphia: Saunders.

Bulechek, G. B., & Butcher, H. K., McCloskey Dochterman, J. (2007). *Nursing Interventions Classification (NIC)* (4th ed.) St. Louis, MO: Mosby.

Cappola, A. R., Fried, L. P., Arnold, A. M., Danese, M. D., Kuller, L. H., Burke, G. L., et al. (2006). Thyroid status, cardiovascular risk, and mortality in older adults. *Journal of American Medical Association, 295,* 1033–1041.

Celebi, A., & Onat, T. (2006). Echocardiographic study on the origin of the innocent flow murmurs. *Pediatric Cardiology, 27*(1), 19–24.

Chen, H. H. & Burett, J. C. (2007). Natriuretic peptides in the pathophysiology of congestive heart failure. *Current Cardiology Reports, 2*(3), 198–205.

Cunningham, F. M., Leveno, K., Bloom, S., Hauth, J., Gilstrap, L., & Wenstrom, K. (2005). *Williams' obstetrics* (22nd ed.). New York: McGraw-Hill.

EPIC-Potsdam. (2007). Potentially modifiable classic risk factors and their impact on incident myocardial infarction: Results from the EPIC-Potsdam study. *European Journal of Cardiovascular Prevention and Rehabilitation, 14*(1), 65–71.

Gillett, M., Davis, W. A., Jackson, D., et al. (2003). Prospective evaluation of carotid bruit as a predictor of first stroke in type 2 diabetes: The Fremantle diabetes study. *Stroke, 34,* 2145–2151.

Grimes, C., Thornell, B., Clark, A., & Viney, M. (2007). Developing rapid response teams: Best practices through collaboration. *Clinical Nurse Specialist, 21*(2), 85–92.

Jones, D. E., Weaver, M. T., Grimley, D., Appel, S. J., & Ard, J. (2006). Health belief model perceptions, knowledge of heart disease, and its risk factors in educated African-American women: An exploration of the relationships of socioeconomic status and age. *Journal of National Black Nurses Association, 17*(2), 13–23.

Keller, C., & Fleury, J. (2006). Factors related to physical activity in Hispanic women. *Journal of Cardiovascular Nursing, 21*(2), 142–145.

Lakatta, E. G. (2002). Age-associated cardiovascular changes in health: Impact on cardiovascular disease in older persons. *Heart Failure Review, 7*(1), 29–49.

Lakatta, E. G., & Levy, D. (2003). Arterial and cardiac aging: Major shareholders in cardiovascular disease enterprises: Part II: The aging heart in health: Links to heart disease. *Circulation, 107*(2), 346–354.

Lowdermilk, D., & Perry, S. (2007). *Maternity & women's health care* (9th ed.). St. Louis, MO: Mosby.

Malone, F., & D'Alton, M. (2004). Multiple gestation: Clinical characteristics and management. In R. Creasy, R. Resnik, & J. Iams (Eds.), *Maternal-fetal medicine: Principles and practice* (5th ed.) Philadelphia: Saunders.

Marcus, G. M., Cohen, J., Varosy, P. D., et al. (2007). The utility of gestures in patients with chest discomfort. *American Journal of Medicine, 120,* 83–89.

Marinella, M. A., Pierson, C., & Chenoweth, C. (1997). The stethoscope. A potential source of nosocomial infection? *Archives of Internal Medicine, 157*(7), 786–790.

McSweeney, J. C., Cody, M., O'Sullivan, P., Elberson, K., Moser, D. K., & Garvin, B. J. (2003). Women's early warning symptoms of acute myocardial infarction. *Circulation, 108,* 2619–2623.

Menasche, V. (2007). Heart murmurs. *Pediatrics in Review, 28,* 19–22.

Monga, M., & Sanborn, M. (2004). Biology and physiology of the reproductive tract and control of myometrial contraction. In R. Creasy, R. Resnik, & J. Iams (Eds.). *Maternal-fetal medicine: Principles and practice (5th ed.)* Philadelphia: Saunders.

Moorhead, S., Johnson, M., & Mass, M. (2007). *Nursing outcomes classification (NOC)* (4th ed.). Philadelphia: Mosby.

Murabito, J. M., Pencina, M. J., Nam, B., D'Agostino, R. B., Wang, T. J., Lloyd-Jones, C., et al. (2005). Sibling cardiovascular disease as a risk factor for cardiovascular disease in middle-aged adults. *Journal of the American Medical Association, 294,* 3117–3123.

Nasir, K., Michos, E. D., Rumberger, J. A., Braunstein, J. B., Post, W. S., Budoff, M. J., et al. (2004). Coronary artery calcification and family history of premature coronary heart disease: Sibling history is more strongly associated than parental history. *Circulation, 110*(15), 2074–2076.

National Cholesterol Education Program Expert Panel. (2001). Expert Panel on Detection, Evaluation and Treatment of High Blood Cholesterol in Adults. Executive summary of the 3rd report of the NCEP Expert Panel. *Journal of the American Medical Association, 285,* 2486–2490.

NHLBI (2001). Strong Heart Study Data Book. Retrieved June 1, 2010, from http://www.nhlbi.nih.gov/resources/docs/shs_db.pdf

NHLBI (2007). Disease statistics. Retrieved July 18, 2007, from http://www.nhlbi.nih.gov/about/factbook/chapter4.htm

North American Nursing Diagnosis Association. (2009). *Nursing diagnoses, 2009–2011 Edition: Definitions and classifications (NANDA NURSING DIAGNOSIS).* West Sussex UK: John Wiley & Sons.

Paradoxical split of the second sound (2007). Retrieved July 9, 2007, from http://sprojects.mmi.mcgill.ca/mvs/GLOSSARY/P.HTM

Pasternak, R. C., Sidney, C. S., Bairey-Merz, C. N., Grundy, S. M., Cleeman, J. I., & Lenfant, C. (2002). ACC/AHA/NHLBI clinical advisory on statins. *Journal of the American College of Cardiology, 40*(3), 567–572.

Physical exam: Neck veins. (2007). Retrieved July 9, 2007, from http://depts.washington.edu/physdx/neck/physical_hepa.html

Pilote, L., Dasgupta, K., Guru, V., Humphries, K. H., McGrath, J., Norris, C., et al. (2007). A comprehensive view of sex-specific issues related to cardiovascular disease. *Canadian Medical Association Journal, 176*(6), S1–S44.

Ridker, P., Rifai, N., Rose, L., et al. (2002). Comparison of C-reactive protein and low-density lipoprotein cholesterol levels in the prediction of first cardiovascular events. *New England Journal of Medicine, 347,* 1557–1565.

Romero-Corral, A., Montori, V. M., Somers, V. K., et al. (2006). Association of bodyweight with total mortality and with cardiovascular events in coronary artery disease: A systematic review of cohort studies. *Lancet, 368,* 666–678.

Schroeder, K., Fahey, T., & Ebrahim, S. (2004). How can we improve adherence to blood pressure-lowering medication in ambulatory care? Systematic review of randomized controlled trials. *Archives of Internal Medicine, 164,* 722–732.

Simmonds, T. (2005). Best-practice protocols: Implementing a rapid response system of care. *Nursing Management, 36*(7), 41–42, 58–59.

Strimel, W. J., Assadi, R., Sovari, A. A., Abraham, G., Kocheril, A. G., & Noe, S. (2006). *Pericardial effusion.* Retrieved July 16, 2007, from http://www.emedicine.com/MED/topic1786.htm on July 16, 2007

Taubert, G., Winkelmann, B. R., Schleiffer, T., et al. (2003). Prevalence, predictors, and consequences of unrecognized diabetes mellitus in 3266 patients scheduled for coronary angiography. *American Heart Journal, 145,* 285–291.

Techniques: Heart sounds and murmurs (2007). Retrieved July 16, 2007, from http://depts.washington.edu/physdx/heart/tech3.html

Techniques: Jugular venous pressure measurement (2007). Retrieved July 17, 2007, from http://depts.washington.edu/physdx/neck/tech1.html

Van't Laar, A. L. (2002). Why is the measurement of jugular venous pressure discredited? *Netherland Journal of Medicine, 61*(7), 268–272.

Wang, C. S., Fitzgerald, J. M., Schulzer, M., Mak, E., & Ayas, N. T. (2005). Does this dyspneic patient in the emergency department have congestive heart failure? *Journal of American Medical Association, 294,* 1944–1956.

Wiese, J. (2000). The abdominojugular reflux sign. *American Journal of Medicine, 109*(1), 59–61.

Woodard, L. D., Hernandez, M. T., Lees, E., & Peterse, L. A. (2005). Racial differences in attitudes regarding cardiovascular disease prevention and treatment: a qualitative study. *Patient Education and Counseling, 57*(2), 225–231.

Woods, S. L., Sivarajan Froelicher, E. S., Motzer, S. A., & Bridges, E. J. (2010). *Cardiac nursing* (6th ed.). Philadelphia: Lippincott Williams & Wilkins.

Yang, H. T. (2007). Effect of aging on angiogenesis and arteriogenesis. *Current Cardiology Reviews, 3*(1), 65–74.

The Jensen suite offers these additional resources to enhance learning and facilitate understanding of this chapter:

- thePoint on line resource, http//thepoint.lww.com/Jensen1E
- Student CD-ROM included with the book
- *Laboratory Manual for Nursing Health Assessment: A Best Practice Approach*
- *Pocket Guide for Nursing Health Assessment: A Best Practice Approach*

⚠ Table 19.6   Variations in S1 and S2

Heart Sound	Description
Accentuated S1 S1 S2 S1	S1 is louder when mitral valve leaflets are recessed into the ventricle, as with rapid heart rate, hyperkinetic states, short PR interval, atrial fibrillation, or mitral stenosis.
Diminished S1 S1 S2 S1	S1 is softer with long PR interval, depressed contractility, left bundle branch block, obesity, or a muscular chest.
Varying Intensity of S1 S1 S2 S1 S2	S1 varies in atrial fibrillation and complete heart block when the valve is in varying positions before closing.
Split S1 S1 S2 S1	The first component is heard at the base; the second component is heard at the lower left sternal border. Split S1 accompanies right bundle branch block.
Accentuated S2 S1 S2 S1	S2 is increased in systemic hypertension or when the aorta is close to the chest wall. Another cause is pulmonary hypertension.
Diminished S2 S1 S2 S1	S2 may be decreased from aortic calcification, pulmonic stenosis, and aging, with reduced mobility of the valves.

Table 19.6 Variations in S1 and S2 *(continued)*

Heart Sound	Description
Fixed Split 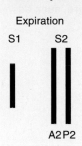 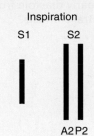	The two components are heard during both inspiration and expiration. The split is wide and results from right bundle branch block or early opening of the aortic valve.
Paradoxical Split 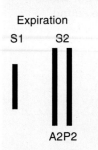 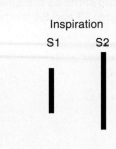	The pulmonic valve closes before the aortic from left bundle branch block, right ventricular pacemaker. The sounds usually fuse during inspiration.
Wide Split 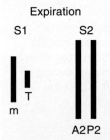 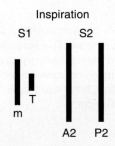	A wide split is found with right bundle branch block from delayed depolarization of the right ventricle.

Table 19.7 Identifying Extra Sounds

Heart Sound	Description
Ejection Click 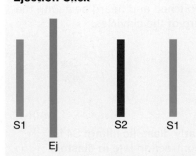	This sound results from an open valve that moves during the beginning of systole. It is heard best with the diaphragm of the stethoscope, and may be audible over aortic or pulmonic areas.

Heart Sound	Description
Opening Snap 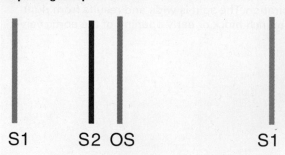	It indicates that the mitral valve is mobile and "snaps" during early diastole from high atrial pressure, such as with mitral stenosis.
Summation Gallop 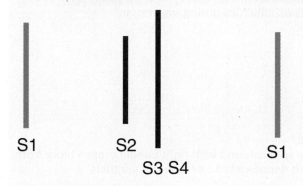	This is the same as the quadruple rhythm but with a faster rate. S3 and S4 merge to create one sound.
Pericardial Friction Rub 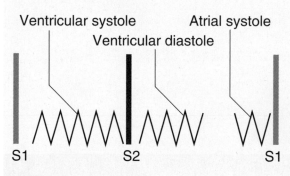	It is triple phased during mid-systole, mid-diastole, and pre-systole. The scratchy, leathery quality results from the parietal and visceral pleura rubbing together. The sound increases on leaning forward and during exhalation. It is heard best in the 3rd left ICS at the sternal border.
Venous Hum 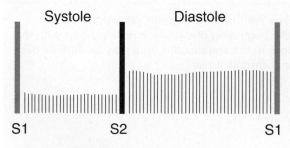	This continuous sound is normal in children and during pregnancy. It is rough, noisy, and occasionally accompanied by a high-pitched whine. It may be louder during diastole. It is low pitched and heard best with the bell above the medial third of the clavicles.
Quadruple Rhythm with S3 and S4	S3 is generated during early diastolic filling; S4 is generated during atrial contraction late in diastole. Both are present. It is heard best with the bell of the stethoscope over the apex of the heart.

Table 19.8   Description of Murmurs

Intensity: Loudness	**I.** Faint; heard only with special effort
	II. Soft but readily detected
	III. Prominent but not loud
	IV. Loud; accompanied by thrill
	V. Very loud
	VI. Loud enough to be heard with stethoscope just removed from contact with the chest wall (Braunwald, et al., 2004).
Timing: Point in the cardiac cycle	**Systolic:** Sounds like "swish-dub"; falls between S1 and S2
	Diastolic: Sounds like "dub-swish," falls after S2 and before the next S1
	More specifically murmurs may be labeled as early, mid, or late systolic and early, mid, or late diastolic.
	Holosystolic murmurs: Occur during all of systole
	Holodiastolic murmurs: Occur during all of diastole
	Continuous murmurs: Begin in systole and continue through S2 into part but not necessarily all of diastole
Pitch: High or low tone	**High:** Heard best with diaphragm
	Medium
	Low pitch: Heard best with bell
Pattern: Increasing or decreasing in volume	**Crescendo:** Increasing intensity
	Decrescendo: Decreasing intensity
	Plateau: Remain constant
Quality: Type of sounds	Harsh, blowing, raspy, musical, rumbling
Location: Site on the precordium	Area of maximum intensity using either the valvular areas or thoracic landmarks
Radiation: Direction it travels	Where the sound radiates, usually in the direction of blood flow in the vessel
Position: Changes with patient position	If the murmur changes depending on patient position. The patient may be turned to the left and right, lie down, sit up, and lean forward. Children may squat.

Table 19.9   Distinguishing Murmurs

Heart Sound	Description	Optimal Site for Auscultation
Physiologic Murmur 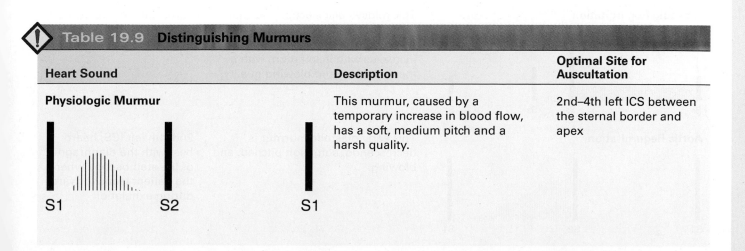 S1 .... S2 .... S1	This murmur, caused by a temporary increase in blood flow, has a soft, medium pitch and a harsh quality.	2nd–4th left ICS between the sternal border and apex

Heart Sound	Description	Optimal Site for Auscultation
Aortic Stenosis 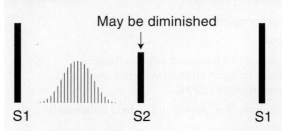	This midsystolic ejection murmur begins after S1, crescendos, and then decrescendos before S2. It radiates upward to the right 2nd ICS and into the neck. It is soft to loud, with a medium pitch and harsh quality. It is associated with ejection click, split S2.	2nd–3rd right ICS
Pulmonic Stenosis 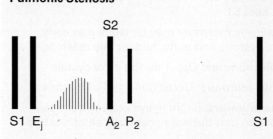	This midsystolic ejection murmur may radiate toward the left shoulder and neck. It is soft-loud, medium pitch, harsh quality, and associated with ejection click, split S2.	2nd–3rd left ICS
Mitral Stenosis 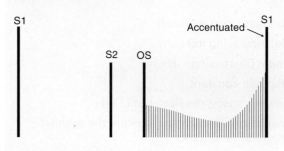	This mid-diastolic murmur is associated with an opening snap and has a low-pitched, rumbling quality.	Heard best with the bell over the apex with the patient turned to the left
Mitral Regurgitation 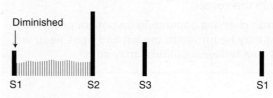	This midsystolic ejection murmur is soft to loud, medium to high pitch, with a blowing quality. It radiates to the left axilla and is associated with a thrill and lift at the apex.	Apex
Tricuspid Regurgitation 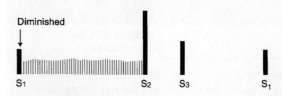	This midsystolic ejection murmur can be holosystolic with elevated right ventricular pressure. It increases with inspiration, with a medium pitch and blowing quality.	Lower left sternal border
Aortic Regurgitation 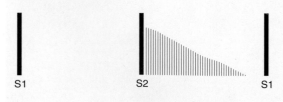	This early diastolic murmur is decrescendo, soft, high pitched, and blowing.	2nd–4th left ICS; heard best with the diaphragm of the stethoscope when the patient leans forward during exhalation

Table 19.9   Distinguishing Murmurs (continued)

Heart Sound	Description	Optimal Site for Auscultation
Pulmonic Regurgitation	This early diastolic murmur may begin with a loud S2. It is a high frequency blowing murmur with a crescendo-decrescendo pattern.	
Tricuspid Stenosis	The loudness of this mid-diastolic murmur increases with inspiration. It has a rumbling quality and is louder during inspiration.	Heard at the lower left sternal border

Table 19.10   Congenital Heart Disease

Heart Sound	Description	Optimal Site for Auscultation
Patent Ductus Arteriosus	The continuous murmur peaks just before and after S2. It has a rough, harsh, mechanical quality with a palpable thrill.	2nd left ICS
Atrial Septal Defect	This continuous murmur is altered by Valsalva's maneuver. It is a systolic ejection murmur with medium pitch.	Base in the 2nd left ICS

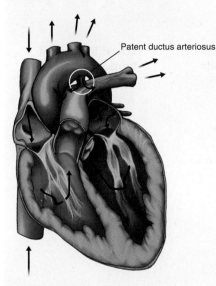

Patent ductus arteriosus

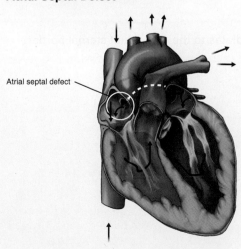

Atrial septal defect

(table continues on page 526)

Heart Sound	Description	Optimal Site for Auscultation
Ventricular Septal Defect 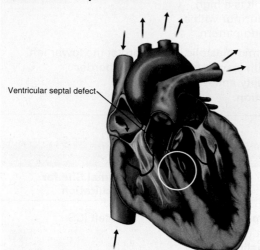 Ventricular septal defect	This murmur is holosystolic because left ventricular pressures exceed right ventricular pressures. It radiates, often loudly with a thrill. The quality is high-pitched and harsh.	3rd–5th left ICS
Tetralogy of Fallot 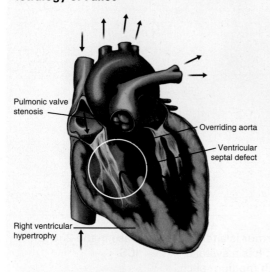 Pulmonic valve stenosis Overriding aorta Ventricular septal defect Right ventricular hypertrophy	This early diastolic murmur has a thrill. It is loud, with a crescendo-descrescendo pattern.	Lower left sternal border
Coarctation of the Aorta 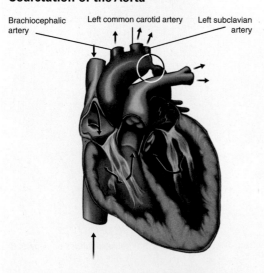 Brachiocephalic artery Left common carotid artery Left subclavian artery	This systolic murmur radiates to the back.	Left sternal border

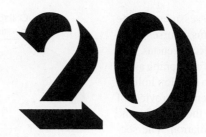

Peripheral Vascular and Lymphatic Assessment

Learning Objectives

1 Identify the structures and functions of the arterial, venous, and lymphatic systems.

2 Identify teaching opportunities for health promotion and risk reduction related to the arterial, venous, and lymphatic systems.

3 Collect subjective data related to peripheral vascular symptoms, including pain, numbness or tingling, skin changes, edema, cramps, and decreased functional ability.

4 Collect objective data about the peripheral vascular system, including color, temperature, pulses, capillary refill, and edema.

5 Identify normal and abnormal findings from the general survey, inspection, and palpation of the peripheral vascular and lymphatic systems.

6 Identify the locations of the peripheral pulses.

7 Use subjective and objective data to analyze findings of and plan interventions for the peripheral vascular and lymphatic systems.

8 Document and communicate data from peripheral vascular and lymphatic assessments using appropriate medical terminology.

9 Individualize peripheral vascular and lymphatic assessment considering the condition, age, gender, and culture of the patient.

10 Use assessment findings of the peripheral vascular and lymphatic systems to identify diagnoses and to initiate a plan of care.

*M*r. Tretski, an 88-year-old Caucasian man, lives in a long-term care facility. His medical diagnoses include a myocardial infarction 15 years ago, high blood pressure, high cholesterol level, chronic renal failure, and peripheral arterial disease (PAD). He is taking a statin for his cholesterol and an antiplatelet medication for the PAD. He also is slightly confused, with impaired recent memory.

You will gain more information about Mr. Tretski as you progress through this chapter. As you study the content and features, consider Mr. Tretski's case and its relationship to what you are learning. Begin thinking about the following points:

- How does the patient's health history relate to his current health status?
- What assessment findings might the nurse note if Mr. Tretski's PAD worsens?
- What assessment data will the nurse want to collect related to other body systems?
- How might the nurse modify history taking and physical examination based on the patient's age?

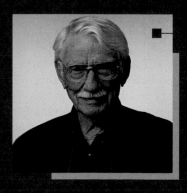

This chapter focuses on comprehensive assessment of the peripheral vascular and lymphatic systems. Nurses must understand the independent roles of the arterial, venous, and lymphatic systems, as well as their integrated functioning as the circulatory system. Doing so enables them to develop holistic plans for circulatory well-being in their patients. A review of pertinent anatomy and physiology provides the basis for the collection of subjective and objective information. The section on subjective data collection gives details to help nurses evaluate history, risk factors, and symptoms associated with peripheral vascular health. The content on objective assessment outlines a methodical approach to assessing peripheral pulses, extremity temperature, skin condition, perfusion, and fluid status, and describes alterations from normal. The chapter presents advanced assessment techniques as well.

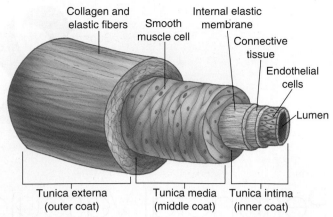

Figure 20.1 Structure of an artery.

Structure and Function Overview

The organs and tissues of the body depend on a healthy, intact peripheral vascular system, which consists of a complex network of arteries, veins, and lymphatic vessels. The vascular network transports oxygenated blood throughout the body and returns deoxygenated blood to the heart and lungs for reoxygenation. The lymphatic system supports the vascular system by returning excess fluid from the tissues to the vascular network. Disruption of the peripheral vascular or lymphatic system can have debilitating and, in some cases, fatal consequences. Thus, comprehensive and accurate assessment of the arterial, venous, and lymphatic systems provides an essential foundation for holistic and thorough nursing care. Such assessment depends on a solid understanding of the anatomy and physiology of these systems.

Arterial System

The arterial system consists of arteries, arterioles, and capillaries that deliver oxygenated blood from the heart to the rest of the body. The walls of the arteries and arterioles have three layers: the *tunica intima* or inner layer; the *tunica media*, which is the middle layer; and the *tunica externa (adventitia)* or outer layer (Fig. 20-1). Arteries have many elastic fibers, which allow them to constrict and recoil with systole and diastole.

> **Clinical Significance 20-1**
>
> Arterioles have more smooth muscle, and it is here that blood pressure is controlled (Porth, 2007).

The largest vessel of the arterial system is the *aorta*. The subclavian arteries come-off of the aorta to feed the vessels of the upper extremities. The largest arteries of the upper extremities are the *brachial arteries*. They bifurcate into the *radial* and *ulnar arteries*, which further divide into two arterial arches that supply the hand (Fahey, 2004).

The aorta bifurcates distally into the *iliac arteries*. The iliac arteries continue into the femoral arteries, which go to the

lower extremities. At the *popliteal fossa*, the femoral artery becomes the popliteal artery, which bifurcates into the *dorsalis pedis* and *posterior tibial arteries*. These arteries form a connecting arch at the foot (Fahey, 2004; see Fig. 20-2).

Smooth endothelial cells line the inner layer of all blood vessels and play a critical role in the prevention of platelet adhesion and thrombus formation. Injury to the endothelial layer thus contributes significantly to the pathogenesis of atherosclerosis (Porth, 2007). Interruption of arterial flow results from narrowing of the arteries, rupture or dissection of the layers of an artery, or thrombus formation.

Venous System

The venous system consists of veins, venules, and connecting veins called perforators, which collect unoxygenated blood from the body and return it to the heart (Fig. 20-3). In contrast to arteries, veins are thin walled. The venous system is a low-pressure system. Veins often are referred to as capacitance vessels, because they can stretch and accommodate large volumes of fluid (Fahey, 2004).

The veins of the upper extremities, upper torso, head, and neck drain into the superior vena cava and then the right atrium. Those of the lower extremities and lower torso drain into the inferior vena cava and right atrium. In the upper and lower extremities, veins are part of the superficial or deep systems. The superficial system includes the greater and lesser saphenous veins. The deep system includes the common femoral, femoral, profunda femoris, popliteal, and anterior, posterior, and peroneal tibial vessels (Fahey, 2004).

A pressure gradient created by respiration, skeletal muscle contraction, and intraluminal valves regulates blood flow in the venous system (Porth, 2007). During inspiration, the diaphragm drops and abdominal pressure increases. During expiration, abdominal pressure decreases, creating a suction effect that promotes venous return. Because veins do not have the same muscular walls that arteries do, they also rely on the calf muscle pump to combat the pull of gravity and promote venous return. For example, as a person walks, the contraction of the calf muscles promotes venous flow. Additionally, veins contain bicuspid valves that prevent the retrograde flow of venous blood, thus maintaining unidirectional flow.

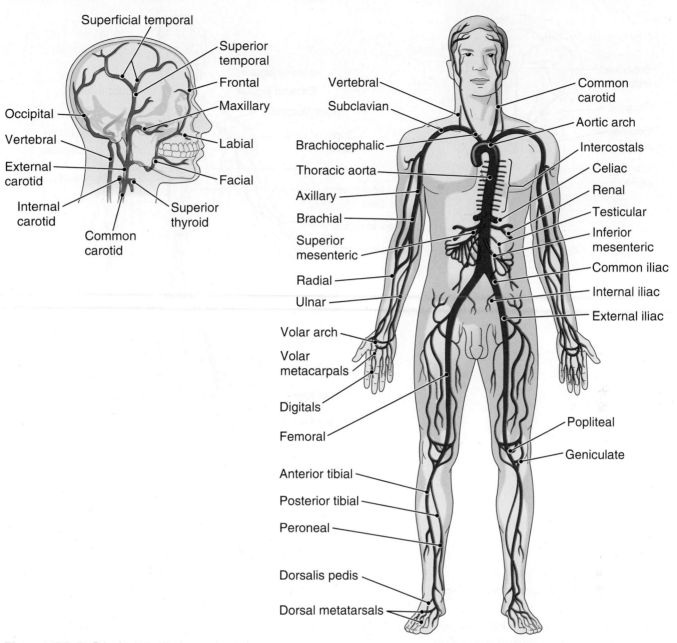

Figure 20.2 Principal systemic arteries.

The more distal a vein is, the greater the number of valves, because the pull of gravity is stronger (Porth, 2007). Interruption of venous flow results from obstruction, valve incompetence, or trauma.

Capillaries

The exchange of nutrients, gases, and metabolites between blood vessels and tissues occurs in the capillary beds

(Fig. 20-4). Oxygen-rich blood delivers nutrients from the arterioles to the capillaries. Venules then return metabolites from the capillary beds to the venous system.

Lymphatic System

The lymphatic system consists of the lymph nodes and lymphatic vessels (Fig. 20-4), as well as the spleen, tonsils, and thymus (Fig. 20-5). It maintains fluid and protein balance and functions with the immune system to fight infection. The lymphatic vessels carry lymph in the tissues back to the bloodstream. The pathways of these vessels often run parallel to the arteries and veins (Porth, 2007). The thoracic ducts at the junctions of the subclavian and internal jugular veins return the lymph fluid to the circulation (Fahey, 2004). The lymphatic vessels contain valves to maintain unidirectional

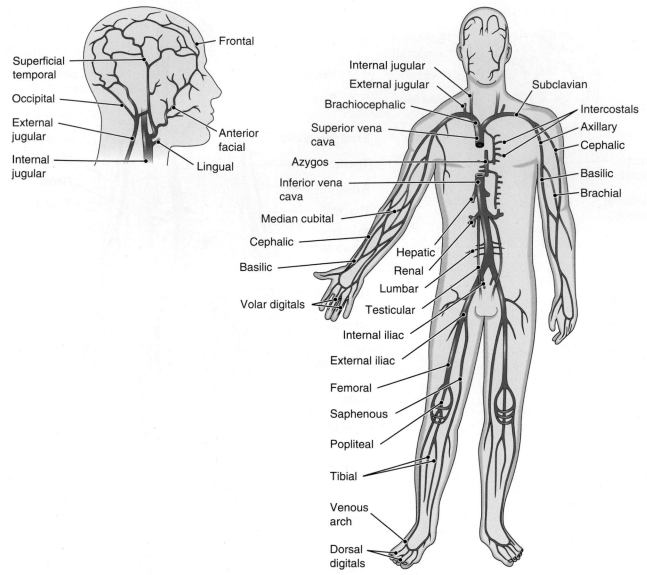

Figure 20.3 Principal systemic veins.

flow. Skeletal muscle contraction, passive movement, and increases in heart rate all support lymph flow.

Only the superficial lymph nodes are accessible for palpation. Lymphatic flow in the arms drains into the epitrochlear, axillary, and infraclavicular nodes. In the lower extremities, the lymph drains primarily into the inguinal nodes (Fahey, 2004).

When the amount of lymph in interstitial tissue exceeds the capacity of the lymphatic vessels, *lymphedema* occurs. Edema high in protein fills the tissue and is ultimately replaced by fibrous tissue and collagen. If untreated, the fibrosis may progress and result in irreversible tissue enlargement. Lymphedema may be congenital or result from scarring injury, removal of lymph nodes, radiation therapy, or chronic infection (Fahey, 2004).

🔺 Lifespan Considerations

Pregnant Women
Maternal blood volume nearly doubles during pregnancy. This volume, combined with obstruction of the iliac veins and inferior vena cava as a result of fetal growth, leads to increased venou s pressure. The result may be dependent edema, varicosities in the legs and vulva, and hemorrhoids (Porth, 2007). These findings are especially common in the last trimester.

Newborns, Infants, and Children
Intimal changes begin at birth. Atherosclerosis has been found in the arteries of children and adolescents, highly correlated with known familiar hypercholesterolemia (Noto, et al., 2006). Smoking, hypertension, elevated cholesterol level, obesity, physical inactivity, and high-fat diet are all risk factors that must be evaluated in children and adolescents (Kavey, et al., 2003). Obesity in children and adolescents increased two- to fourfold from 1980 to 2000; rates were highest among those of African American and Hispanic descent (Brunt, et al., 2008; Williams, et al., 2002). The association of obesity with other cardiovascular risk factors as well as other diseases makes its growing prevalence a great public-health concern (Williams, et al., 2002). Many cigarette smokers begin smoking in their

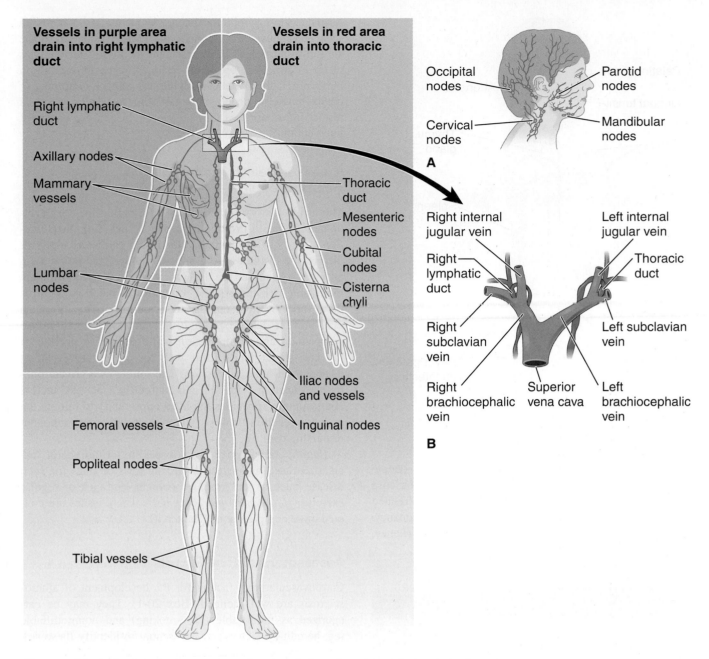

Figure 20.4 The lymphatic vessels and nodes. **A.** Lymph nodes and vessels in the head. **B.** The right lymphatic duct and thoracic duct drains into the subclavian veins.

preteen or teen years. Early education and intervention are key in this age group. The American Heart Association recommends that prevention of atherosclerosis begin in childhood (Williams, et al., 2002).

Older Adults

Calcification of the arteries, or *arteriosclerosis*, causes them to become more rigid in older adults. Less arterial compliance results in increased systolic blood pressure (Porth, 2007). This is often compounded by the coexistence of atherosclerotic disease in the arteries supplying the brain, heart, and other vital organs. The incidence of PAD increases dramatically in the seventh and eight decades of life (Porth, 2007). Prevalence of PAD in men and women is equal at this stage (Ostchega, et al., 2007).

🌐 Cultural Considerations

Incidence of PAD, the most prevalent vascular disease, is highest in African Americans of both sexes and Mexican-American women (Ostchega, et al., 2007; Porth, 2007). Hypertension, a significant risk factor for PAD, is increased in African Americans. Smoking, another primary risk factor, also may have environmental effects, such as in the case of secondary smoke inhalation. Genetics play a prominent role in atherosclerosis in addition to many of the cardiovascular risk factors. Hypertension, diabetes, and hyperlipidemia are cardiovascular risk factors with strong genetic components (Ostechega, et al., 2007; Porth, 2007).

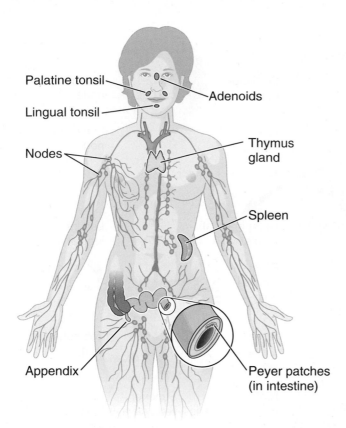

Figure 20.5 Lymphoid tissues.

Palatine tonsil

Lingual tonsil

Nodes

Adenoids

Thymus gland

Spleen

Appendix

Peyer patches (in intestine)

Primary varicose veins are seen more often in people older than 50 years and in those with obesity. Varicose veins are more common in women, which may be related to the increased venous stasis that accompanies pregnancy. Varicose veins and lymphedema may be familial (Fahey, 2004).

Acute Assessment

If the patient is experiencing symptoms of complete arterial occlusion such as pain, numbness, coolness, or color change of an extremity, stop the assessment and get help. This is a limb-threatening situation. If the patient is experiencing symptoms of deep vein thrombosis (DVT) such as pain, edema, and warmth of an extremity, stop the assessment and get help. Immediate intervention to start anticoagulants is necessary. A pulmonary embolism may result from a DVT. Be alert for any signs of a pulmonary embolism including acute dyspnea, chest pain, tachycardia, diaphoresis, and anxiety (see Chapter 15). This life-threatening emergency requires immediate intervention.

Subjective Data Collection

The subjective portion of the health assessment includes identification of cardiovascular risk factors and history

related to those symptoms that are frequently associated with arterial, venous, and lymphatic disorders. Evaluation of the subjective portion of the assessment should include analysis of the information for the development of health-promotion measures. If the patient is having any critical symptoms of complete arterial occlusion or DVT, nurses take only critical history information as they prepare the patient for emergent intervention.

Areas for Health Promotion/ *Healthy People*

The health history includes key information for the development of health-promotion measures including the educational needs of the patient. Identifying cardiovascular risk factors and evaluating the patient's understanding of them provides a basis for the development of a plan to eliminate modifiable risk factors and to control as much as possible the severity of those that cannot be changed. This approach may prevent disease through early intervention or lessen progression and complications. The subjective portion of the assessment lends itself well to incorporating patient education into the discussion. The setting of a private one-on-one meeting with the patient focusing on risk factors and symptoms provides the ideal opportunity to initiate the patient education process, which is an integral component of nursing care.

Healthy People goals are not specific for peripheral vascular disease, but instead focus on areas of risks for such disease, such as smoking, overweight, and lack of regular exercise (*Healthy People 2010*, n.d.). These issues are covered more completely in Chapter 19.

Assessment of Risk Factors

Cardiovascular risk factors for the development of atherosclerosis are well defined (Box 20-1). They may be categorized as modifiable (eg, smoking) and nonmodifiable (eg, hereditary factors). It is essential to identify these risk factors, the patient's understanding of them, and resources available to the patient and his or her support network. Exploring these areas yields the necessary information from which to formulate with the patient a comprehensive plan to improve his or her cardiovascular risk profile.

BOX 20.1 CARDIOVASCULAR RISK FACTORS

- Smoking
- Hypercholesterolemia
- Diet high in saturated fats
- Sedentary lifestyle
- Hypertension
- Diabetes
- Obesity
- Genetics

Questions to Assess Risk Factors	Rationales

Personal and Family History

Do you have a family history of cardiovascular problems?
• Who had the illness?
• Was the illness arterial, venous, or lymphatic?
• How was it treated?
• What was the outcome?

Cardiovascular disease has a well-established hereditary component (Fahey, 2004; Pei, 2006).

Do you have a family or personal history of diabetes?
• Who had/has the illness?
• How is it treated?
• How well is it controlled?
• Have there been any complications related to diabetes?

Family history of *diabetes* increases a person's risk of developing the same condition. Diabetes increases up to four times a patient's risk of lower-extremity PAD. Severity and duration of diabetes correlate with the likelihood of developing lower-extremity PAD (ACC/AHA, 2005; Chorzempa, 2006).

Do you have a family or personal history of hypertension?
• Who had/has the illness?
• How is it treated?
• How well is it controlled?
• Have there been any complications related to hypertension?

Patients with *hypertension* are at increased risk for cardiovascular disease, especially cerebrovascular and lower-extremity PAD and abdominal aneurysms (ACC/AHA, 2005).

Do you or does anyone in your family have an elevated cholesterol level?
• Who had/has the elevated cholesterol level?
• How is it treated?
• How well-controlled is it?

Increased levels of cholesterol are associated with the development of atherosclerosis and therefore lower-extremity PAD and abdominal aneurysms (ACC/AHA, 2005; Fahey, 2004).

Have you had any recent trauma to any of your extremities?
• If so, what was the trauma?
• What was the treatment?
• Have you had any long-term effects?

Thromboembolism should be monitored for as a possible side effect of trauma. Arterial damage can also result from trauma such as penetrating or blunt-force injuries (Fahey, 2004).

Do you have a family history of lymphedema?
• Who in your family had/has lymphedema?
• How was it treated?
• What was the outcome?
• Have you ever had any lymph nodes removed?
• Why were the lymph nodes removed?
• From what part of your body were they removed?
• When were they removed?
• Have you had any problems with swelling since they were removed?

Lymphedema may be familial (Fahey, 2004). It also may result from trauma or the excision of lymph nodes (Fahey, 2004).

Personal Behaviors and Lifestyle

Do you smoke cigarettes, pipes, or cigars?
• How many packs per day do you smoke?
• How many years have you smoked?
• Have you ever tried to stop smoking?
• Are you interested in quitting now?
• Does anyone living with you smoke cigarettes, pipes, or cigars?
• Are you frequently around people who smoke cigarettes, pipes, or cigars?
• What measures do you take to control your exposure to people who smoke cigarettes, cigars, or pipes?

Smoking is an extremely significant risk factor for lower-extremity PAD and abdominal aneurysms. The number of cigarettes smoked per day and the number of years the patient has smoked directly affect the degree of risk for developing lower-extremity PAD (ACC/AHA, 2005). Exposure to secondary smoke may affect risk as well (Fahey, 2004).

Do you exercise regularly?
• What type of exercise?
• How often and for how long do you exercise?
• Do you sit or stand for long periods?
• Do you have any problems with swelling in your legs because of this?

The American Heart Association recommends regular exercise, four to five times a week, to promote cardiovascular health and to decrease the risk of cardiovascular disease (Williams, 2002). Regular exercise also promotes the well-being of the venous system.

(text continues on page 534)

Questions to Assess Risk Factors	Rationales
Do you use oral contraceptives? • If so, for how long have you used them? • Have you experienced any side effects from them?	Oral contraceptives have the side effect of possible DVT formation.

Risk Assessment and Health-Related Patient Teaching

Risk assessment is essential for the health care provider to determine areas for focused teaching. Education provides the patient with the necessary information to make behavioral choices that may prevent future health concerns or improve the outcome of current health problems (Veazie, et al., 2005).

Atherosclerosis is a progressive, systemic disease. Initially it manifests in one area of the body, but it is likely to also be found in other vessels (Fahey, 2007). Risk assessment and patient education to modify risks are imperative.

Patients with Peripheral Arterial Disease

Identifying options for the modification of risk factors can significantly improve the outcome for patients with PAD. The most modifiable risk factors are smoking, high-fat diet, and limited activity level. Of these, smoking has been found one of the most devastating. Cessation of smoking can significantly delay the progression of atherosclerosis (Collins, et al., 2005). Nurses ask patients about their readiness to quit smoking. They offer various resources to assist patients with smoking cessation, including individual and group counseling, support groups, medical treatment, and nicotine-replacement therapy.

Diet modification includes weight management and decreasing the consumption of foods high in saturated fats. Monitoring of cholesterol and triglyceride levels is important for patients with PAD. They should have a thorough understanding of the relationship that diet, activity, and genetic factors have to cholesterol levels and the development of atherosclerosis (Aronow, 2007). Nurses also discuss with patients the preventative role of exercising four to five times a week as recommended by the American Heart Association.

Daily assessment of the feet is essential for these patients. With decreased arterial blood supply, minor cuts or areas with excessive pressure may quickly develop into arterial ulcers. Because of the decreased blood supply, these ulcers may be difficult to heal, leading to gangrene and limb amputation (Aronow, 2007).

Hypertension, diabetes, and heredity are also risk factors for PAD. Though they may not be eliminated, hypertension and diabetes are modifiable in terms of close monitoring and tight control (Aronow, 2007). Patients with diabetes are twice as likely to develop PAD as the general population (ACC/AHA, 2005). Maintaining glycemic control and blood pressure within the guidelines of the American College of Cardiology/American Heart Association (2005) is critical to slowing the progression of PAD (Mitka, 2006).

Patients with Venous Disease

Patients with venous disease should receive education on methods of decreasing venous pressure. Avoiding standing and sitting for long periods in addition to elevating the legs periodically help to combat the chronic edema that may accompany venous disease (Fahey, 2004). Compression stockings are recommended for some patients. Patients at risk for or with a history of DVT need thorough education on the signs and symptoms of DVT and, in some cases, anticoagulant therapy (AORN, 2007).

Patients with Lymphatic Disorders

Patients with lymphatic disorders have several issues that health care providers must address. Similar to venous disease, edema in the extremities is the primary symptom of lymphedema. Thus, management suggestions may include avoiding sitting or standing for long periods, periodically elevating the affected extremity, and applying compression wraps or stockings (Fahey, 2004). Patients with chronic lymphedema may experience disfigurement that affects their body image and self-esteem (Fahey, 2004). It is essential for nurses to address these areas that affect quality of life.

Focused Health History Related to Common Symptoms

Common symptoms of vascular disease should be part of the assessment of all adults. As discussed previously, the underdiagnosis of vascular problems and lack of aggressive treatment of risk factors have been identified as major areas of concern in primary care (Oka, 2006). Consistent evaluation of vascular and lymphatic wellness is necessary to better serve the adult population. Common symptoms are associated with various medical diagnoses (Box 20-2).

Common Peripheral Vascular and Lymphatic Symptoms

• Pain
• Numbness or tingling
• Cramping
• Skin changes
• Edema
• Decreased functional ability

BOX 20.2 COMMON SYMPTOMS OF VASCULAR DISORDERS

PAD

• Claudication
• Rest pain

Acute Arterial Occlusion

• The six Ps:
  • Pain
  • Poikilothermia
  • Paresthesia
  • Paralysis
  • Pallor
  • Pulselessness

Abdominal Aortic Aneurysm

• Bruit
• Laterally pulsating abdominal mass

Abdominal Aortic Aneurysm Dissection or Rupture

• Chest pain
• Abdominal pain
• Back pain
• Shortness of breath

Raynaud's Phenomenon and Disease

• Numbness
• Tingling

• Pain
• Coolness
• Extreme pallor

Chronic Venous Insufficiency

• Edema of the extremity

Deep Vein Thrombosis

• Unilateral edema
• Pain or achiness
• Erythema
• Warmth

Thrombophlebitis

• As with DVT
• Palpable mass or cord along the vein

Neuropathy

• Burning pain
• Numbness
• Paresthesias

Lymphedema

• Unilateral edema

Questions to Assess Symptoms	Rationales/Abnormal Findings

Pain

Do you have any pain in your arms or legs?

⚠ *SAFETY ALERT 20.1*
It is critical to determine if pain is acute or chronic before proceeding with the interview.

• Where is the pain?
• Can you point to where it hurts?
• Does it go anywhere?

The location of pain in PAD usually closely approximates the affected vessel.

• Describe it.
• What does it feel like?
• How bad is it on a scale from 0 to 10 scale, with 0 being no pain and 10 being the worst possible that you can imagine?
• What brings on the pain? How long does it last?
• What would you like to be able to do that you can't do because of the pain?

Chronic pain is described as dull or aching. Acute pain is often described as sharp and stabbing.

Pain brought on by exertion and relieved by rest is called *intermittent claudication*. It is important to quantify the claudication time as much as possible. An example would be "One block claudication."
The patient with PAD often describes feeling the need to hang the foot of the affected extremity over the side of the bed. Pain that awakens patients from sleep is termed *rest pain*.

• Do other symptoms accompany it?
• Does the pain wake you up at night?
• What do you think that the problem is?

Numbness or Tingling

Have you experienced any changes in sensation in your arms or legs?
• Do you experience any numbness or tingling in your hands or feet?
• What makes it worse?
• What makes it better?

Peripheral neuropathies often develop as a complication of diabetes. They may be very painful and also result in a loss of sensation, increasing the patient's risk for injuries. Subsequent damage to skin further increases risk for wounds that are difficult to heal (Smeltzer & Bare, 2009). Patients with *diabetes* often experience *peripheral neuropathy*, which may manifest as numbness and tingling or pain.

(text continues on page 536)

Cramping

Do you have any cramping in your legs?
- Do cramps come on suddenly or gradually?
- Are cramps associated with walking or activity?
- How many blocks can you walk without cramping?
- What makes the cramps better?

The area of cramping in arterial disease, termed *intermittent claudication*, closely approximates the level of arterial occlusion.

Skin Changes

Have you had any changes in your skin, hair or nails?
- Do you have hair loss in your hands or feet?
- Have your arms or legs become pale or cool?
- Have your nails changed? Have they become thicker?
- Have you had any color changes in your fingers or toes related to cold weather?

Decreased arterial blood supply may lead to changes on the lower extremities, such as loss of hair, pallor, or cool temperature. Another potential consequence is hypertrophic nail changes (Fahey, 2004). *Raynaud's disease* is characterized by color changes in cold weather (Smeltzer & Bare, 2009).

Edema

Have you experienced any swelling in your arms or legs?
- Does it go away when you put your legs up?
- Is it worse at night or in the morning?
- Have you experienced any swelling in your arms or legs that is accompanied by redness or tenderness?

Vascular causes of swelling in the arms or legs may result from venous occlusion or incompetence of the valves of the venous system (Fahey, 2004).

Functional Ability

Have difficulties with your arms or legs affected your daily life in any way? Can you continue activities without fatigue or pain in your arms or legs?

Decreased functional ability may result from arterial insufficiency (ACC/AHA, 2005). It is a symptom that may be overlooked.

Documentation of Normal Findings

Patient denies upper or lower extremity pain; no claudication, coldness, numbness, pallor, hair loss, or nail changes in the extremity; no color changes related to cold temperatures, swelling, or redness in fingers or toes. *A. Hukkanen, RN*

🔺 Lifespan Considerations

| Additional Questions | Rationales/Abnormal Findings |

Pregnant Women

Are you pregnant?
- If so, how many weeks' gestation is the pregnancy?
- Have you had prior pregnancies?
- Have you had any vascular changes related to them?

Venous valvular incompetence and *varicosities* may develop during pregnancy as a result of hormonal factors and increased venous pressure (Fahey, 2004).

Have you experienced any swelling in your feet or ankles? Is it worse after long periods of standing? Have you noticed any enlarged veins? Have you developed any hemorrhoids?

These symptoms are common in pregnancy.

Newborns, Infants, and Children

Is your child frequently exposed to secondary smoke? What measures are taken to avoid such exposure?

Secondary smoke is a cardiovascular risk factor.

Have you noticed any unusual swelling in your child's legs?

Primary lymphedema is congenital and may be seen as early as the first year of life (Fahey, 2004).

Older Adults

Have you experienced any fatigue, cramping, or aching in your legs? How have these symptoms affected your activities of daily living?

Many older adults have general, sometimes vague symptoms of arterial disease that primary care providers frequently overlook (Oka, 2006).

Have you noticed any swelling in your legs? Is it on one side, or both sides?

Because older adults often have multisystem problems, it is important for health care providers to clearly differentiate vascular disease from other sources.

Additional Questions	Rationales/Abnormal Findings
Note the patient's self-identified ethnic group and gender.	Non-Hispanic Blacks are approximately three times more likely than Caucasians to have *PAD* (Selvin & Erlinger, 2004).

Therapeutic Dialogue: Collecting Subjective Data

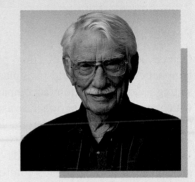

The nurse's role relative to subjective data collection is to gather information to improve the patient's health status and to help determine the cause of the patient's current symptoms. Remember Mr. Tretski, introduced at the beginning of this chapter. His long problem list includes PAD and confusion. His risk factors include 50 years of smoking a pack a day, high cholesterol level, and hypertension.

The long-term care nurse is working with Mr. Tretski today. Because the patient is confused; simple questioning is essential. Thus, the nurse must arrange questions with the simplest first, leading to more complex questions as the interview progresses. Cueing Mr. Tretski during the interview is another technique that can help keep him focused on the topic of the conversation.

The following conversations give two examples of two different interview styles. One style is more effective than the other.

Less Effective

Nurse: I would like to ask you a few questions about your arterial disease.

Mr. Tretski: What's that?

Nurse: That's the disease where your arteries are narrowed and the blood flow is reduced.

Mr. Tretski: Oh. OK. (Puzzled look on face)

Nurse: How is the circulation in your legs?

Mr. Tretski: Fine.

Nurse: Do you have any pain in your legs?

Mr. Tretski: Why are you asking me about my legs?

Nurse: I'm asking about your arterial disease.

Mr. Tretski: Oh. OK. (Puzzled look)

Nurse: So do you have any pain in your legs?

Mr. Tretski: Just when I walk. I like to walk a lot, but sometimes I can't feel my feet very well and I fall. The nurses don't like that when it happens, so they make me sit in this wheelchair.

Nurse: Do you have any tingling in your legs?

Mr. Tretski: No. Why are you asking so many questions about my legs?

More Effective

Nurse: Mr. Tretski, I'm your nurse and I want to ask some questions about the circulation in your legs. I want to talk about the circulation in your legs (pauses).

Mr. Tretski: You want to ask me some questions about my circulation. It's pretty bad.

Nurse: The circulation in your legs isn't very good. Do you have any pain in your legs or feet?

Mr. Tretski: Just when I walk. But I don't walk very much, because the nurses make me stay in this wheelchair. I fall sometimes.

Nurse: You fall because of your bad circulation in your legs. Sometimes people with bad circulation have tingling in their legs. Do you ever have tingling?

Mr. Tretski: No. You sure are asking me a lot of questions about my legs.

Nurse: I want to know how good the circulation is, and I think that you've helped me understand that. How's the feeling in your legs? (pauses 10 seconds) (touches him) How's the feeling in your legs?

Mr. Tretski: Sometimes I can't feel my feet and then I fall.

Critical Thinking Challenge

- What helpful therapeutic communication techniques did the more effective nurse use?
- What additional data about other body systems did the nurse gather during this interview?
- Is this an appropriate time to discuss risk for falling and safety issues? Provide rationale.

Objective Data Collection

Equipment Needed

- Examination gown
- Nonstretchable measuring tape
- Ultrasonic Doppler stethoscope
- Ultrasonic gel
- Sphygmomanometer
- Tourniquet

Preparation

Objective assessment of the peripheral vascular and lymphatic systems should take place in a quiet and private setting. Vasoconstriction accompanies cool temperatures, which may affect the peripheral vascular examination. Thus, the room should be at a comfortable temperature before the assessment begins.

Wash and warm your hands as an infection-control measure and for the patient's comfort. The patient will need to wear a gown for the examination. He or she may leave on undergarments. The arms and then legs must be accessible for inspection and palpation, because side-to-side visualization for comparison is essential.

The examination requires the patient to be sitting, supine, and standing. Take safety precautions while helping the patient to change positions. Pay attention to mobility constraints as well as the effects of position changes on respiratory effort as they apply to the patient.

Cleanse the ultrasonic Doppler stethoscope before and after use to prevent the spread of infection. Use soap and water, because alcohol is damaging to the transducer.

Common and Specialty or Advanced Techniques

The head-to-toe physical examination focuses on both the most common and most important assessment techniques. The examiner may incorporate advanced techniques to collect additional data for a special concern. Table 20-1 summarizes the most common techniques for peripheral vascular and lymphatic assessment, which are therefore essential to master in clinical practice.

Table 20.1	Common Versus Advanced Techniques in Peripheral Vascular and Lymphatic Assessment		
Comprehensive Assessment Technique	Purpose	Screening or Registered Nurse Assessment	Focused or Advanced Practice Examination
Inspect arms and legs	To identify symmetry, range of motion, color, hair, nails	X	
Palpate arms and legs	To identify tenderness, warmth, erythema	X	
Palpate peripheral pulses	To assess for effectiveness of peripheral circulation	X	
Perform Allen's test	To assess for blood flow in radial and ulnar arteries		X
Auscultate blood pressure	To compare circulation in both arms	X	
Auscultate Doppler stethoscope pulses	Performed when unable to palpate peripheral pulses		X
Assess for edema	To evaluate effectiveness of venous return	X	
Perform ABI	Performed if arterial insufficiency is suspected		X
Assess for color change	To assess for arterial insufficiency		X
Perform manual compression	To evaluate competence of valves in the patient with varicose veins		X
Perform Trendelenburg's test	To evaluate the saphenous vein valves and retrograde filling of the superficial veins		X

Technique and Normal Findings	**Abnormal Findings**

Arms

Inspection. Note the size and symmetry of the arms and hands as well as muscle atrophy or hypertrophy. *Arms and hands are symmetrical with full joint movement.*

PAD may result in muscle atrophy. Hypertrophy may result from activity in which the patient uses one arm more than the other, such as tennis.

Assess the color of the arms and hands; evaluate for venous pattern. *Color is pink, symmetrical, and consistent without prominent venous pattern.*

Pallor indicates arterial insufficiency. Erythema may accompany thrombophlebitis or DVT.

Evaluate the nail beds for color and angle. *Nail beds are pink. Nail-base angle is 180 degrees without clubbing.*

Capillary refill may be decreased with arterial disease.

Note any edema of the arms and hands. Evaluate for pitting by pressing the tissue with your fingers. *No indentation remains when you remove your fingers.*

Lymphedema results in unilateral edema. Use the scale in Box 20-3 to document degree of pitting edema.

BOX 20.3 PITTING EDEMA SCALE

+1: Slight pitting, 2-mm depression
+2: Increased pitting, 4-mm depression
+3: Deeper pitting, 6-mm depression; obvious edema of extremity
+4: Severe pitting, 8-mm depression; extremity appears very edematous

---

Evaluate for any ecchymoses or lesions of the upper extremities. *Ecchymoses and lesions are absent.*

Be alert for signs of abuse (see Chapter 12) or falls. Delayed wound healing occurs with arterial disease.

Palpation. Palpate the arms and hands for temperature. Use the dorsal aspect of the hands and assess the extremities simultaneously. *Arms and hands are warm and equal in temperature.*

⚠ *SAFETY ALERT 20.2*
Coolness of an extremity may indicate arterial occlusion. Assess quickly for the other 6 "Ps" (see Box 20-2) and determine emergent nature.

Assess skin texture and turgor by pinching the skin to evaluate elasticity and hydration. With aging, elasticity decreases. *Skin texture is firm, even, and elastic. Turgor is intact, as shown by rapid return of skin after pinching.*

Rough or dry texture and poor turgor may be noted with dehydration.

Assess capillary refill by depressing and blanching the nail bed, then releasing and noting the time it takes for the color to return (Fig. 20-6). *Capillary refill is <3 seconds.*

Capillary refill taking 3 seconds or longer may indicate vasoconstriction, decreased cardiac output, impaired circulation, significant edema, or anemia.

(text continues on page 540)

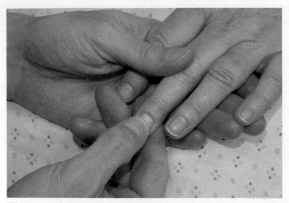

Figure 20.6 Testing capillary refill.

Palpate the brachial and radial pulses. Grade the pulses based on the scale in Box 20-4. The radial pulse site is used when assessing the pulse for vital signs (Fig. 20-7). The brachial pulses are located at approximately the inner third of the antecubital fossa when the palm is held up (Fig. 20-8). It is not usually necessary to palpate the ulnar pulse, which is difficult to locate. *A normal pulse is graded +3/4 on the scale shown. The denominator indicates the scale being used and should be indicated when documenting pulses, because two scale variations exist.*

BOX 20.4 GRADING OF PULSES

+1: Weak, thready
+2: Weak
+3: Normal
+4: Bounding
Document a normal pulse as +3/4.

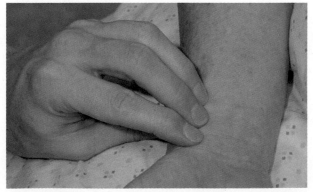

Figure 20.7 Assessing the radial pulse.

When indicated, perform the Allen's test to assess the patency of the collateral circulation of the hands (Fig. 20-9). Ask the patient to make a fist. Occlude the radial and ulnar arteries of one hand. Have the person open the hand; release pressure on the ulnar artery. *Color returns within 2–5 seconds, indicating adequate circulation.*

⚠ *SAFETY ALERT 20.3*
Evaluate any pulse that cannot be palpated with the Doppler stethoscope for an arterial signal. If pulselessness persists, quickly evaluate the remaining "Ps" to determine emergent nature (see Box 20-2).

See Table 20-3 at the end of the chapter.

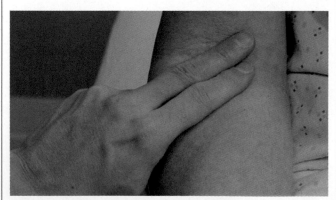

Figure 20.8 Assessing the brachial pulse.

⚠ *SAFETY ALERT 20.4*
The Allen's test is done prior to radial cannulation, such as for the drawing of arterial blood gases (ABGs) or the insertion of an arterial line. Lack of color return indicates inadequate collateral circulation. Do not draw ABGs or insert an arterial line in this hand—doing so will impede blood flow and ischemia may result.

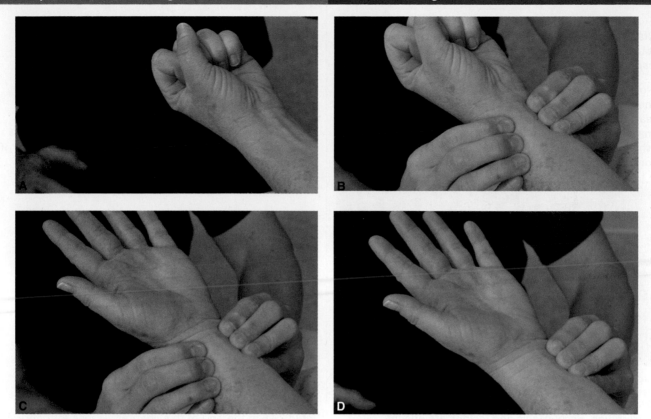

Figure 20.9 The Allen's test. **A.** Ask the patient to make a fist. **B.** Occlude the radial and ulnar arteries. **C.** Ask the patient to open the hand. **D.** Release pressure on the ulnar artery.

Palpate for the epitrochlear nodes. Flex the patient's arm and palpate in the groove between the biceps and triceps muscles just proximal from the medial epicondyle. *Normally the epitrochlear nodes are not palpable.* If palpated note size, consistency, mobility, and tenderness. *Normal palpable nodes are 2 cm or less.*

Auscultation. Evaluate the blood pressure in both arms. Document the arm with the higher pressure and take subsequent blood pressures in that arm. *A normal adult blood pressure is 100–120 mm Hg systolic and 60–80 mm Hg diastolic.*

Legs

Inspection. Note the size and symmetry of the legs as well as muscle atrophy or hypertrophy. *Legs are symmetrical with full joint movement.*

Assess the color of the legs; evaluate for venous pattern. *Color is symmetrical and consistent without predominant venous pattern.*

Enlarged nodes may be noted with regional inflammation, generalized lymphadenopathy, and some types of cancers such as *lymphomas*.

A difference >10 mm Hg may indicate arterial disease. A palpatory pressure should be taken first to avoid missing an auscultatory gap (see Chapter 6).

Atrophy may occur with arterial disease. See Table 20-4 at the end of the chapter.

⚠ *SAFETY ALERT 20.5*
Pallor may indicate arterial insufficiency. Evaluate the other five "Ps" to determine emergent nature. Erythema, edema, and tenderness may indicate DVT, also of an emergent nature.

Color change to white in the toes may indicate one of the Raynaud's syndromes. Venous insufficiency may result in dilated and tortuous veins. See Table 20-5 at the end of this chapter.

(text continues on page 542)

Evaluate the nail beds for color and capillary refill. Blanch the nail bed, release, and observe the time it takes for color to return. *Nail beds are pink, with capillary refill <3 seconds.*

Delayed capillary refill may be the result of arterial disease.

Note any edema of the legs. Evaluate for pitting by pressing the tissue with your fingers. Press firmly with thumb for at least 5 seconds over dorsum of each foot, over each medial malleolus, and over shins. No indentation should remain when you remove your thumbs (Fig. 20-10). See Table 20-2 for the grading scale for pitting edema. *No edema is found.*

Chronic venous insufficiency, DVT, and lymphedema result in edema. Asymmetry between the legs should be further investigated. Calf or leg swelling and unilateral pitting edema are associated with a DVT in 88% of patients. Localized pain or tenderness is noted in 56% of patients (Minichiello & Fogarty, 2008).

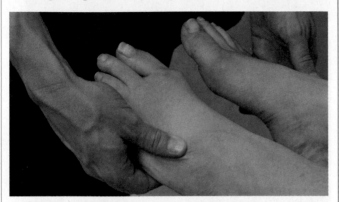

Figure 20.10 Assessing for pitting edema.

Evaluate for any ecchymosis or lesions of the lower extremities. *Ecchymosis and lesions are absent.*

Differentiate ulcers as arterial or venous in cause. See Table 20-6 at the end of this chapter. Assess for gangrene.

Palpation. Palpate the legs for temperature. Use the dorsal aspect of the hands and assess the extremities simultaneously. *Legs and feet are warm and equal in temperature.*

⚠ *SAFETY ALERT 20.6*
One extremity cooler than the other indicates arterial occlusion. Evaluate for the emergent nature of the condition. A warm, edematous, and tender extremity indicates DVT in 30%–40% of patients (Minichiello & Fogarty, 2008). This also is emergent.

Assess the texture and turgor of the skin by pinching the skin. *Texture is firm, even, and elastic. Turgor is intact when skin rapidly returns after pinching (indicating elasticity and hydration).*

Rough or dry texture and poor turgor are found in *dehydration.*

Palpate the femoral, popliteal, dorsalis pedis, and posterior tibial pulses. The femoral pulse is about halfway between the symphysis pubis and anterior iliac spine, just below the inguinal ligament (Fig. 20-11). The popliteal pulse is often difficult to locate. With your fingers braced on the knee, curl your hands around the back and press against the lower edge of the femur (Fig. 20-12). It may be felt immediately lateral to the medial tendon. The posterior tibial pulse is located in the groove between the medial maleolus and Achilles tendon (Fig. 20-13). A light touch is important to avoid obliterating the dorsalis pedis pulse. It is normally about halfway up the foot immediately lateral to the extensor tendon of the great toe (Fig. 20-14). Grade the pulses based on the scale in Box 20-3. *A normal pulse is +3/4 on the scale shown. The denominator indicates the scale being used and should be indicated when documenting pulses, because two scale variations exist. Evaluate any pulse that cannot be palpated with the Doppler stethoscope for an arterial signal.*

⚠ *SAFETY ALERT 20.7*
If pulselessness and no Doppler signal are present, quickly assess other 6 "Ps" to determine the emergent nature of the condition.

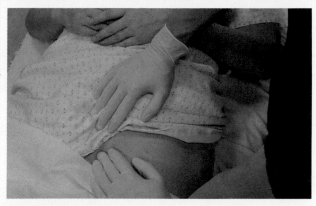

Figure 20.11 Assessing the femoral pulse.

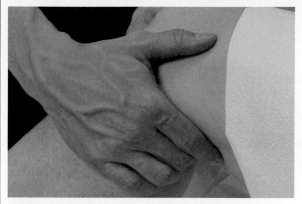

Figure 20.12 Assessing the popliteal pulse.

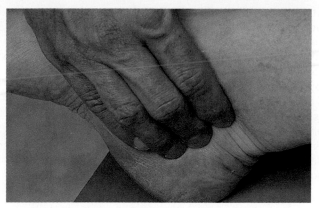

Figure 20.13 Assessing the posterior tibial pulse.

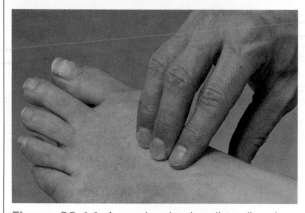

Figure 20.14 Assessing the dorsalis pedis pulse.

Palpate the upper and medial thigh for the superficial inguinal lymph nodes. *They may be palpable and up to 1–2 cm, movable, and nontender.*

Nodes >2 cm may be caused by either local or generalized conditions (Bickley, 2007). Local causes include inflammation from trauma or wounds. Generalized lymphadenopathy is noted if there are enlarged nodes in two or more noncontinuous lymph node regions.

The Homan's sign test is not recommended to test for DVT, because it not sensitive or specific. Additionally, palpating the calf may dislodge an existing DVT. With the patient supine, slightly support the knee and have the patient sharply dorsiflex the foot. *Pain or tenderness is a positive Homan's sign.*

False positive results are commonly related to muscle tenderness. Additionally, the Homan's sign is only present in 15% of patients with DVT (Minichiello & Fogarty, 2008).

Auscultation. The Doppler ultrasonic stethoscope can assess weak peripheral pulses (Fig. 20-15). It magnifies pulsatile sounds from the heart and blood vessels as an arterial signal. The arterial signal is a rhythmic whooshing sound. To use the Doppler, apply a drop of ultrasonic gel to the transducer, and then place the transducer slightly angled over the artery and turn on the volume.

(text continues on page 544)

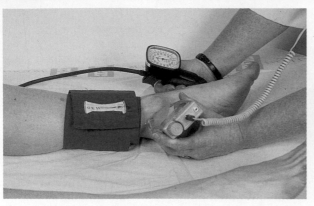

Figure 20.15 Doppler ultrasonic stethoscope.

To assess the ankle-brachial index (ABI), assist the patient to a supine position. Take the systolic pressure of the brachial artery. Then apply a blood pressure cuff to the ankle and obtain either a dorsalis pedis or posterior tibial artery systolic blood pressure. *The ankle pressure is slightly higher or equal to the brachial pressure.* Divide the ankle pressure by the highest brachial pressure.

$$\frac{134 \text{ systolic ankle pressure}}{128 \text{ systolic brachial pressure}} = 1.04 \text{ or } 104\%$$

The result is 1.0 (100%) or greater. Refer to Box 20-5 for a reference scale.

BOX 20.5 INTERPRETATION OF ABI VALUES

1.0–1.29: Normal
0.91–0.99: Borderline
0.41–0.90: Mild to moderate PAD
0.00–0.40: Severe PAD

Source: ACC/AHA. (2005). *Practice guidelines for the management of patients with peripheral arterial disease (lower extremity, renal, mesenteric, and abdominal aortic): A collaborative report from the American Association for Vascular Ssurgery/Society for Vascular Surgery, Society for Cardiovascular Angiography and Interventions, Society for Vascular Medicine and Biology, Society of Interventional Radiology, and the ACC/AHA Task Force on practice guideline (writing committee to develop guidelines for the management of patients with peripheral arterial disease).* Dallas, TX: Circulation.

Special Techniques

Color Change. This test is to check for arterial insufficiency. With the patient supine, elevate the legs 12 in above the level of the heart and have the patient pump their feet to drain off the venous blood (Fig. 20-16A). Have the client then sit up and dangle the legs over the side of the table (Fig. 20-16B). *Color returns to the feet and toes within 10 seconds. The superficial veins of the feet fill within 15 seconds.*

Arterial sounds should not be confused with the venous sound known as a "venous windstorm." Venous sounds are not rhythmic and should not be mistaken for an arterial signal. An ABI of 0.90 or less is considered to indicate arterial insufficiency. See Box 20-5 for delineation of approximate degree of occlusion based on ABI. Because of calcification of the arterial wall and subsequent arteries that are not compressible, patients with *diabetes, renal failure,* or both may have false high results. The same may be true for patients with prosthetic bypass grafts. The ABI is considered an essential assessment tool in evaluating for arterial insufficiency (Oka, 2006).

Return of color taking longer or persistent-dependent rubor indicates arterial insufficiency.

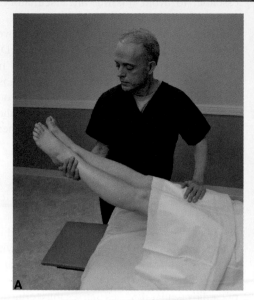
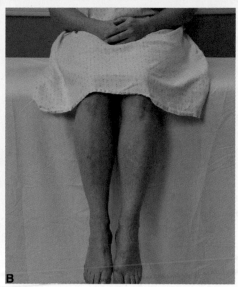

Figure 20.16 Testing for color change. **A.** Elevating the legs. **B.** Dangling the legs.

Manual Compression Test. This test evaluates the competence of the valves in the patient with varicose veins. Have the patient stand. Compress the lower portion of the vein with one hand and place your other hand 6–8 in higher (Fig. 20-17). If the valves are competent, a wave transmission is not palpable. This is considered a negative-negative result.

A transmission wave indicates that the valves are incompetent.

Figure 20.17 Manual compression test.

Trendelenburg's Test. For the patient with varicose veins, this test evaluates the saphenous vein valves and retrograde filling of the superficial veins. With the patient supine, elevate the leg 90 degrees for 15 seconds. Apply a tourniquet to the upper thigh. Assist the patient to stand and inspect for venous filling. After 30 seconds, release the tourniquet. *The saphenous veins fill from the bottom up while the tourniquet is on.*

Filling from above while the tourniquet is on or rapid retrograde filling when the tourniquet is removed indicates that the valves are incompetent.

Documentation of Normal Findings

The arms and legs are symmetrical with full joint movement. Arms and legs are pink and smooth with no ecchymosis or lesions. Skin is warm and dry, good turgor. Capillary refill in 2 seconds. Radial and posterior tibial pulses +3/4 bilaterally. No edema. No tenderness or pain. *A. Hukkanen, RN*

Lifespan Considerations

Pregnant Women

With the increased blood volume of pregnancy and the pressure of the growing fetus on vessels, some women may develop venous problems. An increased venous pattern over the breasts is common. Varicose veins and peripheral edema may develop, especially in the third trimester.

Newborns, Infants, and Children

Changes to the intimal layer of the arteries begin at birth. Significant atherosclerotic streaking that correlates with cardiovascular risk factors has been found on autopsy in children and adolescents. Cardiovascular disease does not typically manifest until later decades, but it may start histologically in childhood and adolescence (Williams, et al., 2002).

Venous disease is also uncommon in these developmental stages. With the increased use of venous access devices in children, however, it is becoming more common. Congenital lymphedema may be diagnosed in the first year of life (Fahey, 2004).

Older Adults

Arterial disease is common in older adults as a result of arteriosclerotic changes often coupled with atherosclerosis. The literature suggests that PAD is frequently underdiagnosed in the older population (Oka, 2003). Intimal changes in the arteries begin at birth and progress throughout life. The thickening of the arterial walls decreases nourishment of the tissue, often resulting in classic findings of trophic nail changes, thin shiny skin, and hair loss of the lower extremities. Decreased functional ability such as fatigue with walking may be an indication of PAD that providers often overlook or attribute to other factors (ACC/AHA, 2005; Oka, 2006). Evidence-based parameters suggest the integration of the ABI, a very simple and noninvasive tool, in the assessment of patients who have exertional leg pain, are older than 50 years with cardiovascular risk factors, have diabetes for more than 20 years, or are older than 70 years (ACC/AHA, 2005; Oka, 2006).

Systolic hypertension often increases with age as the arterial vessels become less compliant. Taking a palpatory blood pressure before taking the brachial blood pressure is essential to avoid missing an auscultatory gap caused by decreased compliance.

Older adults often become less active over time, increasing venous stasis and the development of DVTs. Decreased activity is also not beneficial to PAD and may be an overlooked symptom in patients with undiagnosed PAD (ACC/AHA, 2005). Venous insufficiency and chronic lymphedema may eventually decrease joint mobility (Fahey, 2004). Inclusion of the evaluation of joint mobility is therefore important to the peripheral vascular assessment.

Evidence-Based Critical Thinking

Research has shown that risk assessment and intervention have significant effects on outcomes for patients with cardiovascular disease. Modification of risk factors significantly slows disease progression (Aronow, 2007). Because of the systemic nature of cardiovascular diseases, nurses must critically investigate far beyond the initial reason for which the patient sought care. Once the nurse has analyzed the history, physical assessment, laboratory data, and diagnostic study results, he or she can develop a plan of care. Determining and prioritizing nursing diagnoses are the basis for the plan in collaboration with the patient and family. Patient education to facilitate modification of risk factors is paramount in this patient population. The nurse must educate the patient and family and coordinate support resources for effective care. A collaborative plan with the health care team is the most effective way to manage patient care.

Organizing and Prioritizing

Prioritizing assessment and interventions based on emergent rather than chronic situations is essential. The patient with PAD and symptoms of acute occlusion needs immediate intervention to avoid the threat of limb loss (ACC/AHA, 2005). Focused assessment on the six Ps (pain, pallor, poikilothermia, paresthesias, pulselessness, and paralysis) is critical. Nurses collect past cardiovascular history as physical

---

Documenting Abnormal Findings

The nurse has just finished conducting a physical examination of Mr. Tretski. Review the following important findings that each of the steps of objective data collection revealed for this patient. Consider how these results compare with the normal findings presented in the samples of normal documentation.

Inspection: Skin thin, shiny, and taut. Hair growth absent bilaterally. Toenails hard and thickened. Rubor on lower leg when limbs are dependent. Foot becomes pale when elevated. Able to wiggle toes slowly. Integument intact, no lesions.

Palpation: 1+ dorsalis pedis and posterior tibial pulses bilaterally. Feet cool. Capillary refill 7 seconds. No pedal edema. Unable to differentiate sharp versus dull sensations on feet and lower legs.

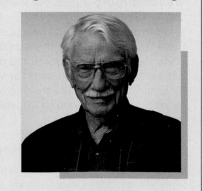

R. Renaldo, RN

assessment proceeds. They may then prepare the patient for interventional radiology, surgery, or both in emergent situations. The physical area may need to be shaved and cleansed, an intravenous access established, and consent forms signed. Patient education is done simultaneously with preparation.

In the patient with a DVT, the focus is initiation of intravenous anticoagulant therapy (AORN, 2007). Nurses document baseline assessment of calf size at the widest point in addition to any findings of pain, warmth, or tenderness. Past history of DVTs or other thrombus formation as well as family history are important to risk stratification. The possibility of PE is always a concern in the patient with a DVT. Ongoing assessments should include consideration of the signs and symptoms of a PE (see Chapter 15).

Common Laboratory and Diagnostic Testing

Accurate data collection is essential for the patient to receive the appropriate care. The physician relies on the accurate assessment of the nurse to determine the appropriate medical interventions. An example is the differentiation between problems that are arterial rather than venous. For example, an arterial ulcer has a deep necrotic base, whereas a venous ulcer is superficial and pale. The treatment for these ulcers is quite different (Sieggreen, 2006). An acute arterial occlusion will be painful with accompanying symptoms of pallor, pulselessness, poikilothermia, paresthesias, or paralysis. A venous occlusion will result in pain, edema, erythema, and warmth of the affected extremities (Fahey, 2004). The primary provider will order that the patient be prepared for an arteriogram for the arterial occlusion but venous duplex and anticoagulation for the venous occlusion. The nurse's critical thinking skills in assessment, prioritization, and organization will facilitate the arrival at a medical diagnosis.

Laboratory testing related to the peripheral vascular and lymphatic systems includes serum evaluation for known risk factors, as well as cholesterol and triglyceride levels. Patients with diabetes require monitoring of blood glucose level and hemoglobin A1C (Selvin, et al., 2006). Recently, research has led to the evaluation of C-reactive protein and homocysteine levels (Aronow, 2007). The d-dimer is indicated in the patient with a possible DVT (Porth, 2007).

Diagnostic ultrasonography is noninvasive and can evaluate anatomic and hemodynamic functions. At the bedside, the continuous wave Doppler is a common tool to evaluate arm and ankle pressures. In the vascular laboratory, an ultrasonic duplex imaging and plethysmography provide detailed anatomic and flow information. These diagnostics are used to evaluate the degree of venous obstruction and location and degree of arterial disease, as well as providing follow-up postoperatively. In the patient with arterial disease or aneurysm, the arteriogram remains the test for definitive diagnosis (Fahey, 2004).

Diagnosis of lymphedema may include magnetic resonance imaging and computerized tomography to identify features of lymphedema or obstruction. Lymphangiography has the drawback of possibly causing acute lymphangiitis. Lymphoscintography is a safe alternative (Fahey, 2004).

Diagnostic Reasoning

The different vascular systems have some separate and some shared nursing diagnoses. Tissue perfusion is altered in arterial disease, and interventions are specific to increasing arterial blood flow and preventing further progression of atherosclerosis through modification of risk factors and use of antiplatelet medications such as Clopidogrel and Aspirin (Oka, 2006). In patients with venous disorders, the focus is promotion of venous flow. With DVT, interventions seek to prevent increased thrombus size and PE with the use of anticoagulants (AORN). In chronic venous and lymphatic disease, interventions are similar. To promote venous and lymphatic return, use of compression devices, avoiding long periods of sitting or standing, increasing exercise and elevating the affected extremity are recommended (Sieggreen, 2006).

Nursing Diagnoses, Outcomes, and Interventions

When formulating a nursing diagnosis, it is important to use critical thinking to cluster data together and identify patterns that fit together. Table 20-2 provides a comparison of nursing diagnoses, abnormal findings and interventions commonly related to the peripheral vascular system assessment (NANDA-I, 2009). Additionally, pain, fatigue, impaired skin integrity, risk for infection, knowledge deficit, and a disturbance in body image may affect all vascular patients.

Critical assessment of the data gathered lead to a plan with the goal of achieving specific patient outcomes. Some outcomes that are related to vascular problems include the following:

- Peripheral pulses are strong and symmetrical.
- Capillary refill is <3 seconds.
- Patient states treatment regimen including exercise, medications and healthy behaviors.
- Patient senses sharp and dull accurately.
- Peripheral edema is decreased.
- Patient verbalizes an understanding or risk factors.
- Patient verbalizes a decrease in pain (Moorhead et al., 2008).

To achieve desired outcomes, evidence-based interventions are applied. Examples include the following:

- Monitor peripheral pulses every 4 hours.
- Assess and document degree of edema using scale every 4 hours.
- Evaluate pain on 10-point scale.
- Provide patient education on risk factors.
- Keep limbs warm and have patient wear skid free slippers
- Perform meticulous foot care once a day (Bulechek, et al., 2008).

Evaluation of the effectiveness of interventions is ongoing. The nurse modifies interventions as is appropriate. The continual process of reevaluation and modification to achieve desired outcomes requires a thorough knowledge of assessment and accurate application.

Table 20.2	Common Nursing Diagnoses Associated with the Peripheral Vascular System		
Diagnosis and Related Factors	**Point of Differentiation**	**Assessment Characteristics**	**Nursing Interventions**
Altered tissue perfusion, arterial related to reduced blood flow	Decrease in oxygen resulting in failure to nourish tissues at the capillary level	Reduced hair, thick nails, dry skin, weak or absent pulses, pale skin, cool, reduced sensation, long capillary refill	Assess dorsalis pedis and posterior tibial pulse bilaterally. If reduced or una ble to find them, assess with a Doppler and notify physician.
Risk for peripheral neurovascular dysfunction	Potential for one or more extremities to experience negative changes in circulation, sensation, or motion	Trauma, fractures, surgery, mechanical compression, burns, immobilization, obstruction	Perform assessment: pain, pulses, pallor, paresthesia, paralysis. Contact physician if present.
Activity intolerance related to pain and claudication with ambulation	Energy that is compromised and cannot facilitate endurance for completion of daily activities	Report of pain or claudication, fatigue, weakness	Gradually increase activity. Refer to physical therapy as indicated. Allow rest periods before and after activity.

Analyzing Findings

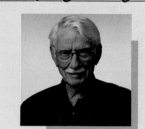

Remember Mr. Tretski, whose problems have been outlined throughout this chapter. The initial subjective and objective data collection is complete, and the nurse has spent time reviewing the findings and other results. The following nursing note illustrates how subjective and objective data are analyzed and nursing interventions are developed.

Subjective: "Sometimes I can't feel my feet and then I fall."

Objective: 1+ dorsalis pedis and posterior tibial pulses bilaterally. Rubor present on lower leg when limbs are dependent. Foot becomes pale when elevated. Feet cool. Capillary refill 7 seconds. Able to wiggle toes slowly. Cannot differentiate sharp versus dull sensations on feet and lower legs. Skin thin, shiny, and taut. Hair absent bilaterally. No pedal edema. Toenails hard and thickened. Integument intact, no lesions.

Analysis: Altered peripheral tissue perfusion related to PAD

Plan: Keep lower extremities in a dependent position. Keep socks and shoes or slippers on feet during the day and loose socks at night. Remind patient to change positions frequently and provide range of motion exercises twice daily. Assist with walking twice daily and stop when pain develops. Apply skin moisturizer to legs every morning. Inspect feet daily for injuries and pressure points. Consult with physical therapy to develop a daily walking program.

R. Renaldo, RN

Critical Thinking Challenge

- What might be included when writing another SOAP note focusing on Mr. Tretski's confusion?
- What overlap is present between the peripheral vascular assessment and other body systems?
- What assessments are highest priority based upon his health history and current problems?

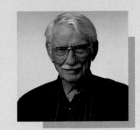

In many facilities, nurses initiate referrals for physical therapy based on assessment findings. Results that might trigger a consultation with physical therapy include musculoskeletal injury, reduced functional status, impaired balance, mobility issues, sensorimotor loss, assistance with techniques on seating or transfers, low endurance, impaired safety awareness, impaired strength or flexibility, use of adaptive equipment, and training for body mechanics.

Mr. Tretski has been experiencing many of the problems outlined above; therefore, a physical therapy consult might be indicated. The following conversation illustrates how the nurse might organize data and make recommendations about the patient's care to the physical therapy department.

Situation: I'm Ronald, the nurse who is taking care of Mr. Tretski, an 88-year-old man with multiple diagnoses, including arterial vascular disease in his legs.

Background: He has been falling because of reduced sensation in his feet and legs. He's also a bit confused.

Assessment: His peripheral pulses are decreased bilaterally. His feet are cool, and his capillary refill is prolonged. He has slower and reduced range of motion in his feet and legs also.

Recommendations: I think that a more structured walking program might help him improve his circulation and reduce his risk of falling. We are ambulating him twice daily, but it doesn't seem to be helping much. Could you come to evaluate if a program like this might be helpful for him? If you have other ideas about things that the nursing staff could do to reduce his pain and increase his circulation, that would be helpful, too.

Critical Thinking Challenge

- How will the nurse organize information before initiating the call for the consult?
- Comment on the reliability of the historian. How will the nurse collect assessment data based upon the patient's reliability?
- How will Mr. Tretski be reassessed to evaluate the effectiveness of therapy? How frequently?

Pulling It All Together: Reflection and Critical Thinking

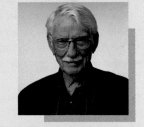

The nurse uses assessment data to formulate a nursing care plan for Mr. Tretski. He or she may independently perform teaching, give reminders to get assistance for transfers, and set up environmental cues for the patient to remember to call. Because Mr. Tretski is confused and his memory is poor, the nurse will need to take more initiative to remind him to keep his legs dependent and change position. The nurse also may initiate a referral to physical therapy about a daily walking program. After completing such interventions, the nurse will reevaluate Mr. Tretski and document the findings in the chart to show the nursing critical thinking. This is often in the form of a care plan or case note similar to the one below.

Nursing Diagnosis	Patient Outcomes	Nursing Interventions	Rationale	Evaluation
Altered Peripheral Tissue Perfusion related to PAD	Patient will state that pain, numbness, and reduced sensation are improved 1 month after starting walking program.	Keep lower extremities in a dependent position. Provide range-of-motion exercises twice daily. Assist with walking twice daily and stop when pain develops. Consult with physical therapy to develop a daily walking program.	Keeping legs in a dependent position uses gravity to flow toward the feet. Range of motion prevents loss of mobility. Walking programs stimulate improved oxygen extraction and prevent further loss of function.	Patient states that pain, numbness, and sensation remain about the same. He reports keeping his legs dependent except when in bed. Continue plan and reevaluate in another 2 weeks.

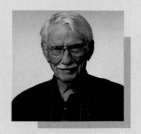

Using the previous steps of diagnostic reasoning, organizing, and prioritizing, consider all the case study findings woven throughout this chapter. When answering the following questions, begin drawing conclusions and see how the pieces of assessment must work together to create an environment for personalized, appropriate, and accurate care.

- How does the patient's health history relate to his current health status?
- What assessment findings might the nurse note if Mr. Tretski's PAD worsens?
- What assessment data will the nurse want to collect related to other body systems?
- How might the nurse modify history taking and physical examination based on the patient's age?

Key Points

- Arterioles have smooth muscle and are primarily responsible for blood pressure.
- Veins are thin-walled capacitance vessels that stretch and accommodate large volumes of fluid.
- The lymphatic system maintains fluid and protein balance and fights infection.
- Pain, numbness, coolness, and pallor are signs of acute arterial occlusion.
- Pain, edema, and erythema may be signs of a DVT.
- Risk factors for peripheral vascular disease include family history, diabetes mellitus, hypertension, elevated cholesterol level, smoking, lack of exercise, and oral contraceptives.
- Common symptoms of peripheral vascular disease include pain, numbness or tingling, cramping, skin changes, edema, and reduced functional ability.
- Edema is graded on a scale from 0 or absent to 4+ deep pitting.
- The six Ps to assess arterial obstruction are pain, pallor, poikilothermia, paresthesia, pulselessness, and paralysis.
- A normal pulse is 3+ on a 4-point scale.
- The Allen's test is performed prior to radial cannulation.
- A difference of more than 10 mm Hg in limbs may indicate arterial disease.
- Venous insufficiency may result in dilated and tortuous veins.
- Lymph nodes >2 cm may be caused by local or generalized conditions.
- The Homan's sign is not sensitive or specific for DVT.
- The Doppler ultrasound is used to locate pulses not palpable.
- An ABI of 0.90 or less indicates arterial insufficiency.

Review Questions

1. Which of the following is a normal ABI?
   A. 56
   B. 87
   C. 1.0
   D. 24

2. Which of the following peripheral vascular diseases is not known to have a hereditary component?
   A. Lymphadenopathy
   B. Raynaud's disease
   C. Abdominal aortic aneurysm
   D. PAD

3. When assessing the lower extremities, it is critical that the examiner
   A. starts at the feet
   B. compares side to side
   C. evaluates the venous system and then the arterial system
   D. starts at the femoral area

4. The six Ps of an acute arterial occlusion include
   A. polythermia
   B. popliteal edema
   C. pain
   D. polycythemia

5. A history of smoking has an extremely significant role in the development of which of the following?
   A. Venous insufficiency
   B. DVT
   C. PAD
   D. Raynaud's disease

6. A dorsalis pedis of +1/4 may indicate
   A. DVT
   B. PAD
   C. Raynaud's disease
   D. lymphadenopathy

7. During history taking, a patient reports cramping in his calf when walking a few blocks. He states that it goes away when he sits down for a few minutes. How would the nurse document this symptom?
   A. Intermittent claudication
   B. Rest pain
   C. Poikilothermia
   D. Venous stasis

8. A patient reports swelling in her ankles. How would the nurse proceed with physical examination?
   A. Have the patient elevate her feet to better visualize her ankles.
   B. Measure her ankles at their widest point.
   C. Evaluate further for the brown hyperpigmentation associated with venous insufficiency.
   D. Press the fingers in the edematous area evaluating for a remaining indentation after the nurse removes the fingers.

9. While evaluating the inguinal lymph nodes of a patient, the nurse palpates a 1-cm soft and freely movable node. What action should the nurse take next?
   A. Nothing—this finding is normal.
   B. Refer this patient to a specialist.
   C. Immediately check the patient's dorsalis pedis pulse.
   D. Refer the patient for immediate management of a life-threatening condition.

10. A patient with diabetes who closely monitors and controls her blood glucose level is very interested in preventing complications of her illness. The nurse would emphasize the following consideration in patient teaching:
    A. How to count calories
    B. How to assess her feet daily
    C. What are good carbohydrates
    D. The signs of venous insufficiency

References

American Operating Room Nurses. (2007). AORN guideline for prevention of venous stasis. *American Operating Room Nurses, 85*(3), 607–624.

ACC/AHA. (2005). *Practice guidelines for the management of patients with peripheral arterial disease (lower extremity, renal, mesenteric, and abdominal aortic): A collaborative report from the American Association for Vascular Ssurgery/ Society for Vascular Surgery, Society for Cardiovascular Angiography and Interventions, Society for Vascular Medicine and Biology, Society of Interventional Radiology, and the ACC/AHA Task Force on practice guideline (writing committee to develop guidelines for the management of patients with peripheral arterial disease).* Dallas, TX: Circulation.

Aronow, W. S. (2007). Management of peripheral arterial disease in the elderly. *Geriatrics, 62*(1), 19–25.

Bickley, L. S. (2007). *Bates' guide to physical examination and history taking* (9th ed.). Philadelphia: Lippincott Williams & Wilkins.

Brunt, H., Lester, N., Davies, G., & Williams, R. (2008). Childhood overweight and obesity: Is the gap closing the wrong way? *Journal of Public Health (Oxford).* Feb 29 [Epub ahead of print]

Bulechek, G. B., Butcher, H. K., & McCloskey Dochterman, J (2008). *Nursing interventions classification (NIC)* (5th ed.). St Louis: Mosby.

Chorzempa, A. (2006). Type 2 diabetes mellitus and its effect on vascular disease. *Journal of Cardiovascular Nursing, 21*(6), 485–492.

Collins, T. C., Peterson, N. J., Suarez-Almazor, M., & Ashton, C. M. (2005). Ethnicity and peripheral arterial disease. *Mayo Foundation for Medical Education and Research, 80*(1), 48–54.

Fahey, V. A. (2004). *Vascular nursing* (4th ed.). St. Louis, MO: Saunders.

Healthy People 2010: What are its goals? (n.d.). http://www.healthypeople.gov/About/goals.htm

Kavey, R., Daniels, S., Lauer, R., Atkins, D., Hayman, L., & Taubert, K. (2003). American Heart Association guidelines for primary prevention of atherosclerotic cardiovascular disease beginning in childhood. *Circulation, 107*, 1562.

Minichiello, T., & Fogarty, P. F. (2008). Diagnosis and management of venous thromboembolism. *Medical Clinics of North America, 92*(2), 443–465.

Mitka, M. (2006). Guidelines update: Aggressively target cardiovascular risk factors. *Journal of the American Medical Association, 296*(1), 30–31.

Moorehead, S., Johnson, M., Mass, M. L., & Swanson, E (2008). *Nursing outcomes classification (NOC)* (4th ed.). Philadelphia: Mosby.

NANDA International (2009). *Nursing diagnoses: Definitions and classification.* West Sussex, UK: Wiley-Blackwell.

Noto, N., Okada, T., Yoshino, Y., & Harada, K. (2006). B-flow sonographic demonstration for assessing carotid atherosclerosis in young patients with heterozygous familial hypercholesterolemia. *Journal of Clinical Ultrasound, 34*(2), 43–49.

Oka, R. H. (2006). Peripheral arterial disease in older adults: Management of cardiovascular disease risk factors. *The Journal of Cardiovascular Nursing, 21*(5), Suppl S15–S20.

Ostchega, Y., Paulose-Ram, R., Dillon, C. F., Gu, Q., & Hughes, J. P. (2007). Prevalence of peripheral arterial disease and risk factors in persons aged 60 and older: Data from the national health and nutrition examination survey 1999–2004. *Journal of the American Geriatric Society, 55*(4), 583–589.

Pei, H., Wang, Y., Miyoshi, T., Zhang, Z., Matsumoto, A. H., Helm, G. A., et al. (2006). Direct evidence for a crucial role of the arterial wall in control of atherosclerosis susceptibility. *Circulation, 114*, 2382–2389.

Porth, C. A. (2007). *Essentials of pathophysiology* (2nd ed.). Philadelphia: Lippincott Williams & Wilkins.

Selvin, E & Erlinger, T. P. (2004). Prevalence of and risk factors for peripheral arterial disease: Results from the National Health and Nutrition Examination Survey, 1999–2000. *Circulation, 110*(6), 738–743.

Selvin, E., Wattanakit, K., Steffes, M. W., Coresh, J., & Sharrett, A. R. (2006). HbAqc and peripheral arterial disease in diabetes: The atherosclerosis risk in communities study. *Diabetes Care, 29*(4), 877–882.

Sieggreen, M. (2006). A contemporary approach to peripheral arterial disease. *The Nurse Practitioner, 31*(7), 23–27.

Smeltzer, S., & Bare, B. (2009). *Brunner & Sudarth's textbook of medical-surgical nursing* (12th ed.). Philadelphia: Lippincott Williams & Wilkins.

Veazie, M., Galoway, J., Matson-Koffman, D., LaBarthe, D., Brownstein, J., Emr, M., et al. (2005). Taking the initiative: Implementing the American Heart Association Guide for Improving Cardiovascular Health at the Community Level:

Healthy People 2010 Heart Disease and Stroke Partnership Community Guideline Implementation and Best Practices Workgroup. *Circulation, 112*(16), 2538–2554.

Williams, C., Hayman, L., Daniels, S., Robinson, T., Steinberger, J., Paridon, S., et al. (2002). Cardiovascular health in childhood. *Circulation, 106*, 143–160.

The Jensen suite offers these additional resources to enhance learning and facilitate understanding of this chapter:

- thePoint on line resource, http//thepoint.lww.com/Jensen1E
- Student CD-ROM included with the book
- *Laboratory Manual for Nursing Health Assessment: A Best Practice Approach*
- *Pocket Guide for Nursing Health Assessment: A Best Practice Approach*

Tables of Abnormal Findings

Table 20.3   Variations in Arterial Pulses

Pulse	Characteristics	Causes
Weak Pulse	Decreased pulse pressure, weak on palpation and easily obliterated, slow upstroke with prolonged systolic peak	Decreased cardiac output, as with congestive heart failure, hypovolemia, and severe aortic stenosis; PAD
Bounding Pulse	Increased pulse pressure, strong and bounding, rapid rise and fall, brief systolic peak	Increased stroke volume such as with exercise and fever, hyperthyroidism, decreased aortic compliance as with atherosclerosis or aging
Pulsus Alternans	Alternating small and large amplitude, regular rate	Left ventricular failure, may be accompanied by S3
Pulsus Bigeminus *Premature contractions*	Alternating irregular beats; one normal beat and then one premature beat with alternating strong and weak amplitude	Premature ventricular or atrial contractions
Pulsus Bisferiens	Double systolic peak	Aortic regurgitation, combined aortic regurgitation and stenosis, less often hypertrophic cardiomyopathy
Pulsus Paradoxus *Expiration* — *Inspiration*	Palpable decrease in amplitude on quiet inspiration; with blood pressure cuff, systolic decreases of more than 10 mm Hg during inspiration	Pericardial tamponade, constrictive pericarditis, and obstructive lung disease

Peripheral Arterial Disease

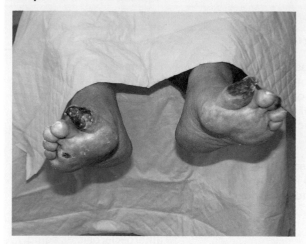

Chronic atherosclerotic occlusion may develop anywhere in the arterial system. As with coronary artery disease (CAD), peripheral arteries narrow from plaque, which limits oxygenated blood from reaching the tissues. Resulting ischemia causes cramping pain, which in the lower extremities is called *claudication*. It is usually exertional and occurs in relation to arterial blockage. Lower-arterial blockage may lead to calf claudication. Blockage at the sacroiliac bifurcation may cause hip claudication. As the disease progresses, rest pain may occur. Patients report being awakened by pain. At this point, dorsalis pedis and posterior tibial are decreased significantly compared to the opposite leg. Also, the diseased leg has a cool temperature and pale or blue color. ABI is decreased. Severe occlusion is chronically painful and may cause ulcers, which in turn may lead to gangrene and amputation. Total occlusion, often
from thrombus, is limb threatening. Any combination of the six Ps (see Box 20-2) constitutes a clinical emergency requiring immediate intervention.
Rest generally relieves claudication. Well-refined assessment skills are paramount. Modification of risk factors is critical. Smoking cessation is of utmost importance. Stringent control of unmodifiable risk factors (eg, blood glucose level in patients with diabetes) is essential. Pain assessment and management are other issues.

Acute Arterial Occlusion

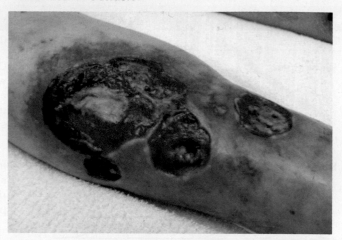

Acute arterial occlusion may result from progression of PAD (as discussed) or thrombus from another source (eg, cardiac catheterization puncture site). In the latter case, a thrombus may break-off and travel through the arterial system to a smaller vessel that is then occluded. The six Ps would again be assessment findings. As with PAD, this is a clinical emergency.

Table 20.4 Abnormal Arterial Findings (*continued*)

Abdominal Aortic Aneurysm

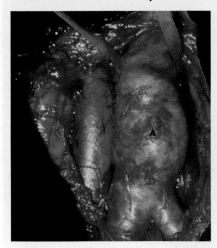

An aneurysm is an outpouching of an arterial wall which results from a weakened or damaged medial arterial layer. Aneurysms may occur in any artery but are most common in the aorta. Aortic aneurysms may be intracranial, below the renal arteries, or abdominal (thoracic). The predominant cause of aortic aneurysm is atherosclerosis. Hypertension may accelerate aneurysm development in an already damaged aortic wall. Aortic aneurysms are also seen with Marfan's syndrome, a congenital disorder. In addition to smoking and hypertension, family history of aortic aneurysm is a risk factor. Aortic aneurysms affect men nearly five times more than women. Aortic aneurysms may rupture or dissect, in which the layers of the artery separate and fill with blood. Either situation results in compromised blood supply to major arteries and therefore to organs and tissues. These critical emergencies are often fatal. Assessment findings include chest pain, abdominal pain, back pain, shortness of breath, laterally pulsatile mass on palpation, and a bruit. Patients with an abdominal aortic aneurysm are usually asymptomatic.

Raynaud's Phenomenon and Raynaud's Disease

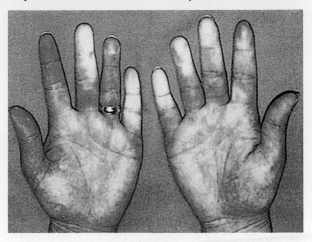

These vasospastic disorders primarily affect women. *Raynaud's phenomenon* is the term used when the cause is attributed to a connective tissue disorder (eg, lupus eryhtematosus, rheumatoid arthritis, scleroderma). When the etiology is unknown (most cases), it is called *Raynaud's disease*. Symptoms include numbness, tingling, sometimes pain, extreme pallor progressing to cyanosis, and coolness of the hands. They usually begin in the fingers and are symmetrical. When the ischemic episode is over, hyperemia, erythema, and burning pain may follow. Smoking, emotional stress, and exposure to cold often precipitate vasospasm. Management includes smoking cessation, avoiding cold temperatures, wearing thermal socks and gloves in cool temperatures, and stress management. In patients with Raynaud's phenomenon, treatment of the underlying cause may offer relief. Tissue injury is rare but with repeated ischemic episodes skin over the fingertips and even small ulcers may develop. The nails may become brittle. In rare cases gangrene of the fingers may occur.

Arterial diseases involve narrowing of the vessels, weakening of the vessel walls, and thrombus formation. Risk factors are the same as for CAD: smoking, diabetes, hypertension, hypercholesterolemia, and family history of arterial problems. Atherosclerosis is the most common cause.

Table 20.5 Abnormal Venous Findings

Chronic Venous Insufficiency

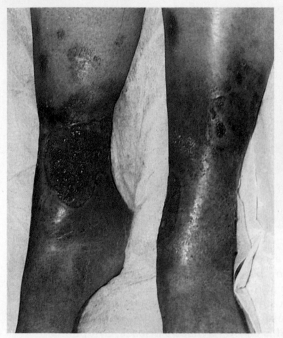

Deep Vein Thrombosis

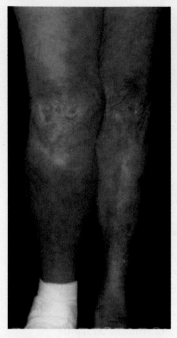

Malfunctioning of the unidirectional valves impairs venous blood return to the affected extremity. Causes are primary valvular incompetence (which may be from a congenital absence of valves), sequelae of DVT, or both. DVT permanently damages the valve leaflets, which cannot close. The veins then cannot empty, leading to edema. Venous insufficiency from dysfunctional valves causes tissue congestion, which eventually impairs nutrition to the tissue. Brown hyperpigmentation may develop from hemosidderrin deposits remaining after the breakdown of red blood cells. Lymphatic insufficiency follows venous insufficiency, compounding tissue congestion. Patients complain of edema and aching pain. As venous insufficiency progresses, stasis dermatitis (characterized by dry, scaling skin) may lead to superficial and relatively painless venous ulcers. Chronic pressure from edema makes these ulcers difficult to heal (see Table 20-6). Long periods of standing promote edema. Elevating the legs above the heart promotes venous return, providing some relief. Compression stockings are recommended to prevent increasing edema (Sieggreen, 2006).

DVT results from thrombus formation in the deep veins. They are more common in the lower extremities, but increasing use of venous access catheters is contributing to more upper-extremity DVTs. Virchow's triad identifies risk factors for venous thrombosis: blood stasis, vessel wall injury, and increased blood coagulability. Immobility and decreased mobility, both more common in older adults, pose risks for stasis. Trauma or surgery may damage vessel walls. Increased blood coagulability may stem from the prolonged sitting and dehydration associated with airplane travel, cancer, use of oral contraceptives, and inherited or acquired coagulation disorder. Treatment is anticoagulation; for some patients with chronic problems, anticoagulation may be long-term prophylaxis. Presenting symptoms of DVT are unilateral edema of the extremity, redness, pain or achiness, and warmth. The leg is measured daily at the same place throughout treatment. Unrecognized DVTs are responsible for most deaths from pulmonary emboli (PE). Acute-care patients often have at least one risk factor for venous thrombosis, so knowledge of the features of DVT and PE is critical.

Table 20.5   **Abnormal Venous Findings** (*continued*)

Thrombophlebitis

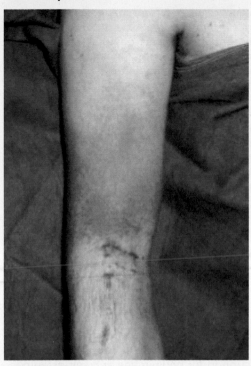

Superficial thrombophlebitis results from thrombus formation in the superficial veins. The same risk factors apply as with DVT. Assessment findings are unilateral localized pain or achiness, edema, warmth, and redness. In superficial veins, a palpable mass or cord may also be present along the vein.

Neuropathy

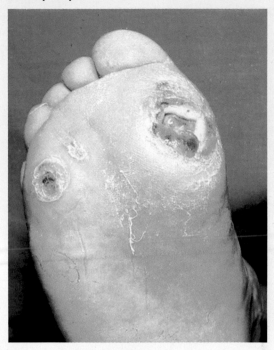

Peripheral neuropathies, most common in patients with diabetes and chronic hyperglycemia, are classified as somatic or autonomic. *Somatic neuropathies* typically affect lower extremities. Paresthesias, burning sensations, and numbness may occur, along with decreased senses of vibration, pain, temperature, and proprioception. These symptoms increase risks for tissue injury and falls. Daily foot assessment is critical, because these patients may not feel a break in the skin or burn and develop subsequent foot lesions, which are challenging to heal. For some patients, peripheral neuropathies cause chronic lower-extremity pain. Pain assessment and management are crucial to their quality of life. A pharmacologic approach to management is often employed.

(table continues on page 558)

Table 20.5 Abnormal Venous Findings (*continued*)

Lymphedema

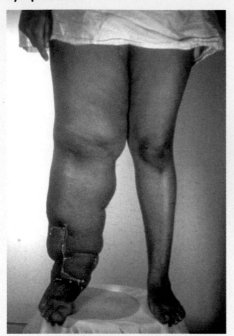

Lymphedema occurs when lymph channels or nodes are obstructed. *Primary lymphedema* is congenital. *Secondary lymphedema* results from injury, scarring, excision of lymph nodes, or, sometimes, trauma or chronic infection. Assessment initially reveals nonpainful pitting edema of the extremity. As lymphedema progresses, the skin may thicken, redden, and show nonpitting edema. Small vesicles with lymphatic fluid may develop in more advanced stages. Cellulitis is a frequent complication. Management begins with treating the cause. Bed rest with the leg elevated 45 degrees at night and frequently during the day for several days is usually very effective in reducing edema. Compression pumps and manual lymphatic drainage may also be used. Patients should wear elastic compression wraps or stockings when the extremity is dependent to combat gravity-related pooling. They apply these devices in the morning when edema is lowest. Exercise enhances treatment, as do weight control and decreased salt intake. Ongoing skin assessment is essential, because breaks in the skin occur more easily in edematous extremities and are difficult to treat. Diuretics may also promote fluid elimination. Chronic lymphedema can be disfiguring and limit joint mobility. Psychosocial support for body image and self-esteem is very important in care.

The structure of veins and their reliance on a unidirectional valve, the skeletal muscle pump, and changes in abdominal and intrathoracic pressures lend them to problems of stasis and insufficiency.

Table 20.6 Arterial Versus Venous Ulcers

	Arterial	Venous
Location	Toes, metatarsals, malleoli, heel	Ankle, medial malleolus, distal third of leg
Borders	Regular	Irregular
Ulcer base	Pale, yellow	Red, pink
Drainage	Minimal	Moderate to large amount
Gangrene	May be present	Not present
Pain	Painful; decreased with dependency	Aching pain, feeling of heaviness; decreased with elevation
Skin	Pale, inflamed, necrotic	Stasis dermatitis, pigmentation changes
Pulses	Decreased or absent	Normal, may be difficult to palpate because of edema

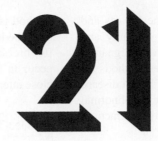

Breasts and Axillae Assessment

Learning Objectives

1   Identify the location of the internal and external breast structures.

2   Identify the structure and function of the lymphatics.

3   Identify teaching opportunities for health promotion and risk reduction related to breast health.

4   Collect subjective data related to conditions of the breast and axillae, including history of present illness, past medical history, family history, and personal and social history.

5   Use inspection and palpation to collect objective data related to pain, lumps, discharge, rashes, and swelling in the breasts and axillae.

6   Identify normal and abnormal findings of the breast and axillae during the general survey, and when performing inspection and palpation.

7   Use subjective and objective data from assessment of the breasts and axillae to analyze findings and plan interventions.

8   Document and communicate data about the breasts and axillae using appropriate medical terminology.

9   Individualize health assessment of the breasts and axillae considering the condition, age, gender, and culture of the patient.

10 Use findings from the assessment of the breasts and axillae to identify nursing diagnoses and to initiate a plan of care.

*M*rs. Randall, a 66-year-old African American woman, is receiving home care for the management of stage III breast cancer. She recently had preoperative chemotherapy and a mastectomy; she is currently undergoing radiation treatments. Medications include oxycodone for moderate to severe pain, acetaminophen (Tylenol) for mild to moderate pain, senna (Senokot) as a laxative, and metoclopramide (Reglan) for nausea. Mrs. Randall can get out of bed for meals, but she has not been eating much because of a lack of appetite and fatigue. The nurse performed and documented an assessment of Mrs. Randall last week. Temperature was 37°C (98.6°F) orally, pulse 78 beats/min, respirations 24 breaths/min, and blood pressure 138/70 mm Hg.

You will gain more information about Mrs. Randall as you progress through this chapter. As you study the content and features, consider Mrs. Randall's case and its relationship to what you are learning. Begin thinking about the following points:

- Are Mrs. Randall's psychosocial or physical needs in this case more important? Provide rationale.
- What health promotion and teaching needs are apparent? Which two areas are highest priorities?
- How should the nurse organize and prioritize data collection, considering Mrs. Randall's multiple problems?
- How should the nurse individualize assessment to Mrs. Randall's specific needs, considering the patient's condition, age, and culture?

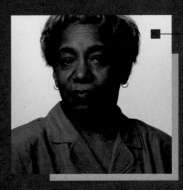

This chapter discusses the assessment of the breasts and regional lymphatics. It reviews pertinent anatomy and physiology, as well as key variations based on pregnancy, lifespan, sex, and culture. The chapter explores methods for collecting subjective data related to the risk of breast disease (cancerous and benign). It also presents specific abnormal findings, such as color changes, nipple discharge, retraction, heat, warmth or redness, and lumps.

Structure and Function Overview

Breasts are paired mammary glands found in both sexes. Male breasts, which remain rudimentary, have a thin layer of breast tissue with a centrally located small **nipple** and surrounding **areola**. Mature female breasts are accessory reproductive organs that respond to cyclical changes in sex hormones and provide nourishment for infants through milk production. Many cultures associate the breasts with female sexuality.

Landmarks

Female breasts are located on the anterior chest wall between the 3rd and 7th ribs. They extend from the sternal margin to the midaxillary line, with the tail of each breast extending into its respective axilla. The pectoral muscles and superficial fascia provide support.

To describe clinical findings, it is best to divide each breast into four quadrants by imagining horizontal and vertical lines that intersect at the nipple. The **tail of Spence**, which extends from the upper outer breast quadrant into the axilla, can be described separately (Fig. 21-1). An alternative

method is to compare the breast to the face of a clock and describe findings based on their distance from the nipple (eg, [R] breast at 8:00, 3 cm from nipple). Most breast cancers occur in the upper outer quadrant, so examiners must pay close attention to this area (Sohn, et al., 2008).

Breast Structures

On the surface, the breasts lie anterior to the serratus anterior and pectoralis major muscles (Fig. 21-2A). Each breast has a nipple with a surrounding areola, as well as Montgomery

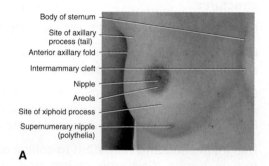

Body of sternum
Site of axillary process (tail)
Anterior axillary fold
Intermammary cleft
Nipple
Areola
Site of xiphoid process
Supernumerary nipple (polythelia)

A

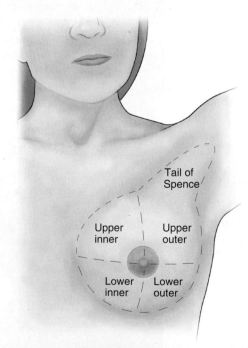

Figure 21.1 Breast with four quadrants and tail of Spence delineated.

Tail of Spence
Upper inner
Upper outer
Lower inner
Lower outer

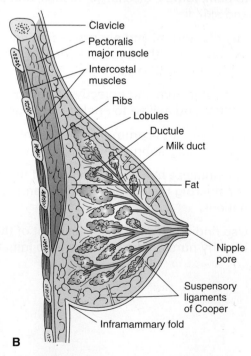

Clavicle
Pectoralis major muscle
Intercostal muscles
Ribs
Lobules
Ductule
Milk duct
Fat
Nipple pore
Suspensory ligaments of Cooper
Inframammary fold

B

Figure 21.2 A. Surface anatomy of the breast. **B.** Internal structures of the breast.

glands, fibrous tissue, glandular tissue, and lymph nodes (Fig. 21-2B). The **nipple** is in the center of the breast. It is darkly pigmented, round, rough, and usually protuberant; it is composed of smooth muscle fibers. Autonomic, sensory, or tactile stimulation produces nipple erection and emptying of lactiferous ducts during breastfeeding. Surrounding the nipple is a 1- to 2-cm **areola**, which is also darkly pigmented. Within the areola are small sebaceous glands called **Montgomery glands**. During lactation, these glands secrete a protective lubricant.

Breasts consist of two types of tissue, fibrous and glandular, and two types of fat, subcutaneous and retromammary. The fibrous tissue is supportive. **Cooper ligaments** (fibrous bands) extend from the connective tissue to the muscle fascia, providing additional support. The glandular tissue consists of 15 to 20 glandular lobes in each breast that extends from the nipple in a radial fashion. Within each lobe, 20 to 40 lobules contain milk-producing **acini** cells. When milk is produced, it drains into the **lactiferous ducts**; the milk from each lobe empties into one sinus that terminates at the nipple. Milk is stored in these sinuses until it is released. This ductal system may be noticeable in pregnant or lactating women.

Most of the breast consists of subcutaneous and retromammary fat surrounding the glandular tissue. Actual breast size and the proportions of each tissue component vary with age, genetic predisposition, pregnancy, lactation, and nutritional status.

Branches of the internal mammary and lateral thoracic arteries provide most of the blood supply to the deep breast tissues and nipple. The superficial tissues receive blood from the intercostal arteries.

Axillae and Lymph Nodes

Each breast has an extensive lymphatic network for drainage. Most lymph drains into the axillary lymph nodes on the same side (ipsilateral lymph nodes; Fig. 21-3). Axillary nodes are relatively superficial, so they are more accessible than deep lymph nodes and fairly easy to palpate when enlarged.

- The *lateral axillary (brachial) nodes* are located inside the upper arm along the humerus.
- The *central axillary (midaxillary) nodes* are palpable high up in the axilla at the top of the ribs. These nodes receive lymph from the lateral, posterior, and anterior axillary nodes.
- The *posterior axillary (subscapular) nodes* lie inside the posterior axillary fold along the lateral edge of the scapulae.
- The *anterior axillary (pectoral) nodes* are located inside the lateral axillary fold along the pectoralis major muscle.

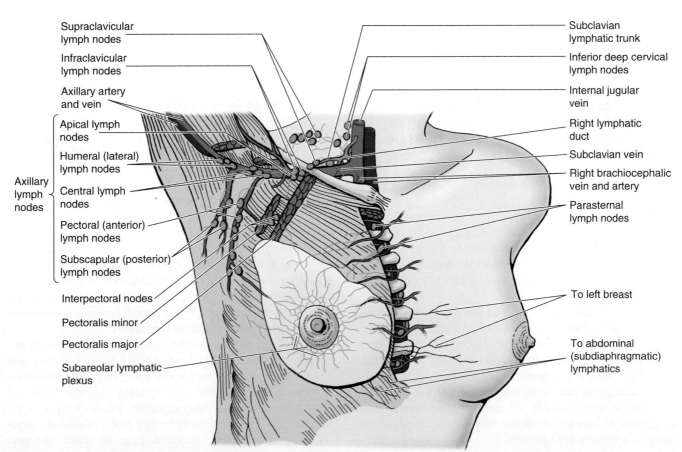

Figure 21.3 Location of lymph nodes in relation to breasts.

⚙ Lifespan Considerations

Pregnant Women

Women experience breast changes as early as the first 2 months of pregnancy. The ductal system expands, secretory alveoli develop, and breasts enlarge, often feeling nodular as the mammary alveoli hypertrophy. Placental hormones stimulate this growth. Breasts enlarge, often feeling tender and nodular. Nipples darken, enlarge, and become more erect. As pregnancy progresses, areolae also become larger, darker, and more prominent. Small, scattered Montgomery glands develop within the areolae. Because of increased blood flow, a bluish venous pattern is often evident on the breast tissue.

The breasts may begin to express *colostrum* (milk precursor) during the fourth month of pregnancy. Colostrum is rich in protein, carbohydrates, and antibodies and low in fat, which makes it easier for newborns to digest. For the first few days after they give birth, women continue to produce colostrum. Actual milk replaces colostrum if breastfeeding occurs.

After childbirth, decreased levels of placental hormones and prolactin secretion by the pituitary gland stimulate lactation (Singleton, et al., 2008). The alveolar cells produce breast milk, which is rich with antibodies that protect against infection in newborns. Breast milk is also high in protein and lactose. During breastfeeding, smooth muscle in the nipple and areola contracts to express milk from the sinuses. After completion of lactation, the breast glandular tissue shrinks.

Newborns and Infants

Development of breast tissue in utero is identical for both genders. During this time, the mammary ridge, or "milk line," extends from the axillae through the nipple and down to the inguinal ligament. Prior to birth, most of the ridge atrophies, leaving two bilateral breasts along the ridge over the thorax.

Enlarged breast tissue and white discharge (commonly called "witch's milk") in newborns of either gender may occur for the first few weeks of life, secondary to the effects of maternal estrogens. If breast enlargement, witch's milk, or both are present, it is important to reassure the newborn's parents/caregivers that nothing is wrong and the conditions will resolve spontaneously. At birth, the lactiferous ducts are present in females within the nipples, but alveoli do not develop in females until puberty.

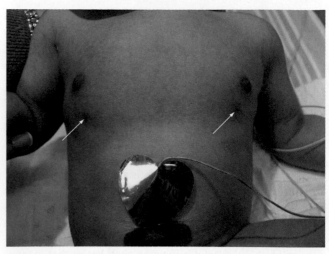

Figure 21.4 Supernumerary nipples in a newborn.

In a small percentage of males and females, a **supernumerary (accessory) nipple** persists. It often looks like a mole, but when inspected closely a tiny nipple and areola are evident. If an examiner finds a supernumerary nipple, he or she should also begin evaluation of the kidneys, because of the association between extra nipples and renal anomalies (Fig. 21-4; Laufer & Goldstein, 2005). Accessory breast tissue (polymastia) is most often seen in the axilla, also along the mammary ridge.

Children and Adolescents

Until puberty, breasts consist of only a few ducts without acini. During adolescence, breasts in females develop secondary to increased production of several hormones. Adipose tissue and the lactiferous ducts grow in response to estrogen. Progesterone stimulation results in lobular growth and alveolar budding (De Silva & Brandt, 2006).

In most girls, changes in the nipples and areolae and development of breast buds are the earliest signs of puberty. Fat deposits accumulate, and nipples and areolae grow and become more darkly pigmented and more protuberant. The breasts also may become tender.

Breast development begins at a mean age of 10 years for Caucasian girls and 9 years for African American girls (Smigal, et al., 2006). The average age has decreased over the past century as a result of improvements in nutrition, sanitation, and infection control; this decrease has not occurred in countries where children are malnourished or have high rates of disease (de'Onis, et al., 2004). Full breast development occurs on average over a 3-year period. Breast development is described by **Tanner staging** (Fig. 21-5).

Breast growth over this 3-year period is usually not steady or symmetrical. It may occur rapidly and then subside, changing with an uneven pace. It is not uncommon for one breast to grow more quickly than the other, but with time breast size may equalize. These changes in the breasts are linked to body image and self-esteem, especially during a developmental stage in which the peer

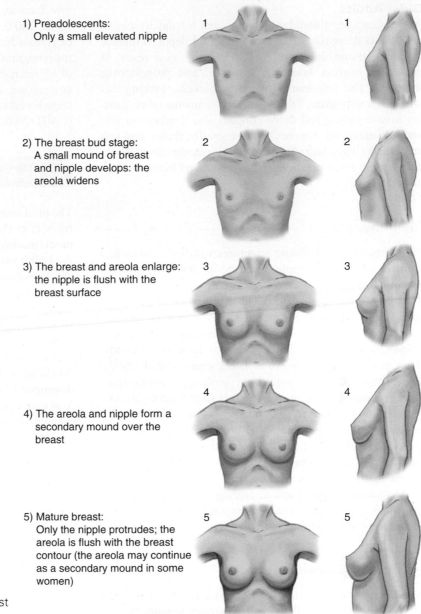

1) Preadolescents:
Only a small elevated nipple

2) The breast bud stage:
A small mound of breast
and nipple develops: the
areola widens

3) The breast and areola enlarge:
the nipple is flush with the
breast surface

4) The areola and nipple form a
secondary mound over the
breast

5) Mature breast:
Only the nipple protrudes; the
areola is flush with the breast
contour (the areola may continue
as a secondary mound in some
women)

Figure 21.5 Tanner staging of breast development.

group assumes increasing importance. Additionally, the breasts often symbolize the development of sexuality and reproductive capacity. The adolescent girl often will compare her growth to that of others. Early-maturing girls may experience more dissatisfaction with their physical appearance, because most of their peers have the slim body shape that cultural norms perpetuate. Late-maturing girls may worry that they will be "flat." Timing of breast development in girls has a social stigma; girls who mature either too early or too late may be concerned. The nurse reassures the adolescent that the rate of breast growth is uniquely individual, as are the size and shape of the mature breast.

Menarche (the beginning of menstruation) occurs during late puberty or Tanner stage 3 or 4, which coincides with the peak of the adolescent growth spurt (Kronenberg, et al., 2008). During menstruation, the glandular tissues of the breasts change in response to cyclical hormonal fluctuations. At the start of the cycle, the ductal cells grow, interstitial fluid increases, and the tissue may become slightly inflamed. These conditions peak just before menses and may lead to dilatation or hyperplasia of the ducts, hypertrophy of the surrounding connective tissue, and benign conditions referred to as fibrocystic changes (Singleton, et al., 2008).

Clinical Significance 21-3

In adult women, unilateral or bilateral breast tenderness and changes in size and nodularity (lumpiness) may accompany menses. Breasts often feel full, sore, or heavy just prior to menstruation and are smallest and least tender in the days following menstruation.

Older Adults

As women age, glandular, alveolar, and lobular tissues in the breasts decrease. After menopause, fat deposits replace glandular tissue that continues to atrophy as a result of decreased ovarian hormone, estrogen, and progesterone secretion. The inframammary ridge thickens, making this area easier to palpate. The suspensory ligaments relax, causing breasts to sag and droop. Breasts also decrease in size and lose elasticity. Nipples become smaller, flatter, and less erectile. Axillary hair may stop growing at this time. These changes are more apparent in the eighth and ninth decades of life.

Male Breasts

Male breasts are immature structures with well-developed areolae and small nipples. During midpuberty, one or both male breasts commonly and temporarily enlarge as a result of changing hormone levels, a condition referred to as **gynecomastia**. Pubescent males also may develop breast buds or tenderness, which also is usually temporary. Almost one-third of adolescent males have these conditions, which usually resolve in 1 to 2 years (Rakel, 2007). The breasts may also enlarge in adolescent males from adipose tissue related to obesity. It is important to investigate feelings related to body image and sexual identity in adolescent males with enlarged breasts. Gynecomastia is physically benign but can cause emotional distress. Reassurance that this is temporary and normal may help alleviate the distress.

As males age, gynecomastia (enlarged breasts) may recur from decreases in testosterone levels, causing the female hormones to predominate.

🌐 Cultural Considerations

Nurses are aware of variations in breast development related to ethnicity. For example, African American females mature earlier than Caucasians (Office of Minority Health [OMH], 2008). Variations in the color of the skin and nipple relate to ethnic background. Differences exist in the incidence and outcomes of breast cancer. Hispanic, Asian, and American Indian women have a lower risk for developing breast cancer. African American women experience a lower incidence but higher mortality rate from breast cancer than Caucasian women do. African American women 35 to 44 years have a breast cancer death rate more than twice that of Caucasian women in the same age group (OMH, 2008). This may be from breast cancer being diagnosed at a more advanced stage in the African American population, possibly from them having less access to breast health care. Breast cancer is the leading cause of death among Filipino women.

Overall factors that may impede access to health care include remote geographic location, lack of health insurance,

low income, and cultural, racial, and language barriers (ACS, 2007). Only approximately half of American Indian or Alaska Native women 40 years or older report having a mammogram within a 2-year period (OMH, 2008). Women of Mexican, South and Central American, and Puerto Rican descent are 20% more likely to be diagnosed with late-stage breast cancer when compared to non-Hispanic women (OMH, 2008).

Acute Assessment

The most common breast concerns that cause women to seek medical evaluation are a newly discovered lump, pain, and nipple discharge. In any of these situations, it is important for the health care provider to perform a focused health history and examination. The greatest fear a woman has related to these symptoms is that she has breast cancer, although often the cause is benign. Specific questions to ask depend on presenting symptoms.

Following the subjective health history, the examination includes inspection and palpation. When performing palpation in an acute situation, begin with the unaffected breast to determine what the patient's normal breast tissue feels like. You may even ask the patient to show you where she feels the lump or pain.

⚠ SAFETY ALERT 21.1

Conditions requiring further investigation to determine a need for tests to rule out cancer include the following:
- *A new breast lump*
- *A lump that has changed in size, shape, texture, or tenderness*
- *A lump in the axilla*
- *Bloody nipple discharge*

Nipple discharge alone is not a reliable sign of cancer; this symptom should be considered with other symptoms and the clinical presentation (Richards, et al., 2007). Ductal ectasia (expansion) may cause green, brown, or other colored discharge.

Subjective Data Collection

Subjective data collection begins with the current health history related to the breast (such as breast discomfort, masses or lumps, or nipple discharge), and continues with questions related to past history (previous breast disease; surgeries; menstrual, pregnancy, and lactation history; and past hormone replacement therapy), family history (of breast cancer or other breast disease), and personal history (breast trauma, surgery, and self-care behaviors). It is important to ask questions sensitively when obtaining data, because conditions related to the breast may be difficult or embarrassing for some women to discuss.

Areas for Health Promotion/ *Healthy People*

Gathering health history information related to the breast and lymphatic system identifies specific areas of patient needs or concerns, which aid nurses in providing education regarding health-promotion activities that focus on disease prevention, early identification of problems, and reduction of complications if problems exist. Health promotion also reinforces existing healthy habits. Nurses are often primary patient educators, and the promotion of healthy behaviors and risk reduction are very important nursing roles.

Educational level and financial situation influence ability to practice healthy behaviors. For example, the prevalence of women with less than a high school education reporting a recent mammogram is approximately 10% lower than the prevalence for all women. Even more striking is that the prevalence for women with no health insurance is approximately 25% lower than the prevalence for women with health insurance (ACS, 2007).

Table 21-1 includes pertinent goals and education topics for promoting healthy behaviors, based upon *Healthy People* criteria.

Assessment of Risk Factors

The most common cause of cancer in US women is breast cancer, accounting for an estimated 26% of cancer cases and 15% of cancer deaths in 2007 (ACS, 2008a,b). The probability of developing breast cancer increases with age, but breast cancer also occurs in young women and (rarely) in men. The National Cancer Institute (NCI, 2007) estimated that more than 178,000 women and 2,000 men would be diagnosed

with breast cancer in 2007. A woman's risk for breast cancer is as follows (NCI, Cancer Facts, 2007):

- From 30 to 39 years, 0.5% (often expressed as "1 in 229")
- From 40 to 49 years, 1.5% (often expressed as "1 in 68")
- From 50 to 59 years, 2.8% (often expressed as "1 in 37")
- From 60 to 69 years, 3.8% (often expressed as "1 in 26")

During the last half of the 20th century, incidence of breast cancer in the United States doubled, with early-stage and in situ discoveries being most prevalent. More diligent screening may be a factor in the increased cases; however, environmental factors, such as fewer pregnancies and improved nutrition (which increases life expectancy), may also be contributing factors (Fletcher, 2008).

The good news is that US cancer deaths have decreased from 30 per 100,000 to 25 per 100,000 since 1969, when national statistics began to be recorded. The greatest decline has been in Caucasian women, although African American women have also seen a decline (McCullough, et al., 2005). A possible reason for differences in deaths according to race is that more infrequent mammogram screenings for the African American population may lead to breast cancers being discovered at a more advanced stage (Gabram, 2008).

The purposes of assessing risk factors are to identify a patient's likelihood of developing breast cancer and to work with him or her to modify controllable factors. Breast cancer risk factors that nurses should review with patients are included in Table 21-2. These include increased age, prior history of breast cancer, family history, genetics, reproductive history, having children, and ethnicity.

If patients already have a breast condition, it is important to gather more information about its effects and how it is being treated (Bowen, et al., 2007). This information provides nurses with needed information to implement appropriate interventions that will control or improve symptoms and prevent complications. Additionally, these discussions illuminate areas in which patients need further follow-up or education. Questioning and education can occur simultaneously.

Table 21.1	*Healthy People* Goals Related to Breast and Axillary Health	
Goals	**Patient Education Topics**
Increase the proportion of mothers who breastfeed their babies.	Encourage pregnant women to breastfeed. Provide written and verbal information about the benefits.
Reduce the breast cancer death rate by 20%.	Teach SBE, and encourage monthly checks. Schedule mammograms according to guidelines.
Increase the proportion of cancer survivors who are living 5 years or longer after diagnosis.	Ensure that patients have access to culturally competent care. Teach the importance of early detection.

Source: Healthy people 2010: What are its goals? (n.d.). Retrieved June 4, 2010, from http://www.healthypeople.gov/About/goals.htm

Table 21.2   Risk Factors for Breast Cancer

Modifiable	Non-Modifiable	Controversial Possibilities
History of childbirth: Nulliparity or having first child after age 30 years slightly increases risk. **Oral contraceptive use:** Controversial; findings suggest that women currently using oral contraceptives have a slightly increased risk, which declines when they stop use. **Combined and estrogen-alone postmenopausal hormone therapy (PHT):** Long-term combined (estrogen and progesterone) PHT increases risks of breast cancer and death from it; risks return to that of the general population within 5 years of stopping use of combined PHT. Long-term estrogen alone (estrogen-replacement therapy [ERT]) increases risk of ovarian and breast cancer. **Breastfeeding:** Nursing children for 1.5–2 years may decrease risk. **Alcohol:** Risk is slightly higher for those who consume one alcoholic drink/day; risk increases to 1½ times that of non-drinkers in those who consume two to five drinks/day. **Overweight or obesity, especially after menopause:** Prior to menopause, the ovaries produce most of a woman's estrogen, and fat produces a small amount. After menopause, fat produces estrogen because the ovaries stop doing so. Estrogen levels can increase postmenopause with increased fat (which increases breast cancer risk). **Physical inactivity:** The ACS recommends 45–60 minutes of exercise at least 5 days/wk to reduce breast cancer risk.	**Gender:** Women are at a much greater risk of developing breast cancer than are men. **Aging:** Approximately two out of three diagnoses of invasive breast cancer occur in women older than 55 years, while one out of eight occurs in those younger than 45 years. **Genetic risk factors:** Women with BRCA1 or BRCA 2 genes have up to an 80% chance of developing breast cancer at some point in their lives. These mutations are most common in Jewish women of Ashkenazi origin, but they also occur in African American and Hispanic women. Other less common genes, such as ATM, CHEK2, p53, & PTEN, may also increase the risk of breast cancer. **Family history:** Having one or more first-degree relatives (i.e., mother, sister, daughter) with breast cancer doubles risk. Having two first-degree relatives with breast cancer increases risk five-fold. **Personal history of breast cancer:** Those with previous incidence have a 3- to 4-fold increased risk of developing breast cancer in another part of the same breast or in the other breast. **Race:** Caucasian women are slightly more likely to develop breast cancer, but African American women are slightly more likely to die from it. Risk is lowest in Asian, Native American, and Hispanic women. **Abnormal breast biopsy results:** Proliferative lesions (overgrowth of breast tissue) without atypia (abnormal cells) increase risk 1½ to 2 times that of normal; proliferative lesions with atypia increase risk four to five times that of normal. **Menstrual periods:** Women who begin menstruating before 12 years or stop after 55 years have a slightly increased risk. **Previous chest radiation:** Those who underwent such treatment for another cancer are at a significantly increased risk. **DES exposure:** Patients exposed to diehtylstilbestrol (DES) have a slightly increased risk of developing breast cancer.	High-fat diets Antiperspirants Bras Induced abortion Breast implants Environmental pollution Tobacco Night work

Adapted from ACS. (2007). *Detailed guide: Breast cancer. What are the risk factors for breast cancer?* Retrieved June 4, 2010, from http://www.cancer.org/docroot/CRI/content/CRI_2_4_2X_What_are_the_risk_factors_for_breast_cancer_5.asp

Questions to Assess Risk Factors	Rationales
Family History Do you have a family history of breast cancer? • If so, who had it? • What type of breast cancer was it? • How old was she (he) when it was diagnosed? • How was it treated?	The patient's risk for breast cancer increases if one or more first-degree blood relatives (eg, mother, sister, daughter) had breast cancer (especially if it was diagnosed before the affected person was 40 years old). Breast cancer in second-degree relatives (eg, grandmother, aunt) also may increase the patient's risk.
Past Medical History Have you ever been diagnosed with breast cancer? • If yes, what kind of breast cancer? • When was it diagnosed? • Any treatment? What and when? • At what age were you diagnosed? • How were you treated?	It is important to evaluate the patient's previous breast conditions, especially those that may increase risk for breast cancer (ie, personal history of previous breast cancer or cancer in situ; previous atypical epithelial hyperplasia found on biopsy; personal history of endometrial, colon, ovarian, or thyroid cancer; or family history of breast cancer) to encourage diligent breast examinations and medical follow-up. Previous history of breast cancer increases risk for a new mass being cancerous by three to four times (ACS, 2008a,b).
Have you ever been diagnosed with any breast conditions such as cysts or benign breast disease (BBD), fibroadenoma, or breast abscess?	*Cysts (BBD)* are common lumps that are usually elliptical or round, soft, and mobile. Size may vary, and they often occur in multiple numbers, usually in both breasts, and frequently in the upper outer quadrants (Katz, 2007). They occur during the childbearing years and are most tender just before menses. BBD with a positive biopsy for atypical hyperplasia (increased abnormal cells) or lobular carcinoma in situ carries an increased risk for breast cancer later in life (Katz, 2007). *Fibroadenoma* is a well-defined, usually single (can be multiple), nontender, firm or rubbery, round or lobular mass that is freely movable. It does not change in size with menses as BBD does and occurs most commonly in patients in their 20s–40s (Katz, 2007). *Breast abscess* (infection) may occur after *mastitis* (inflammation from a blocked duct that may develop with lactation), traumatic injury, or chest/breast surgery.
Have you ever had any breast surgery? • If yes, what kind (eg, breast biopsy, reduction, augmentation, mammoplasty, mastectomy)? • What was the result of the surgery?	Surgery of the breast is very personal; patients may have difficulty talking openly about it. A relaxed but professional demeanor is especially important when obtaining this information. A patient who has had breast augmentation (enlargement) could have the complication of a ruptured implant.
Have you been treated for a breast infection recently?	Recent breast infection may block ducts, causing a change in breast tissue.
When was your last period?	Breast tissue may be tender in the days before the onset of menses.
Lifestyle and Personal Habits Do you jog or run? If so, do you wear a sports bra?	Jogging or running increases breast movement, which may put strain on the shoulders or back. Sports bras can reduce movement by about 50% (Bryner, 2007).
Medications Are you taking any medications? • Medication/dose/schedule?	Some medications that can affect breasts include the following: • Androgens: female: decreased breast size; male: gynecomastia • Antidepressants: female: engorgement; male: gynecomastia • Antipsychotics: female: engorgement, mastalgia, galactorrhea; male: gynecomastia • Cardiac glycosides: male: gynecomastia • Oral contraceptives: female: breast secretions, enlargement, tenderness • Progestins: female: galactorrhea, breast tenderness

(text continues on page 568)

Questions to Assess Risk Factors	Rationales
Are you taking any natural supplements or over-the-counter medications? • Which ones/how often?	Although over-the-counter supplements are not known to affect breast lumps or pain, they may interfere with concurrent medications and contribute to side effects.
Breast Examination Have you ever been taught how to perform self-breast examinations (SBEs)? • If yes: How often do you perform them? Can you show me how you perform your SBEs? • If no: Would you like me to show you how to perform an SBE?	Monthly SBE coupled with yearly clinical breast examinations (CBE) by a medical professional increase the chances of detecting cancer in early stages. To optimize health maintenance, women should familiarize themselves at a young age with how their breasts normally feel to detect even slight changes. Women who perform BSE are more likely to discover cancer at an earlier stage (Katz, 2007). For this reason, it is important to guide patients through SBE that emphasizes timing, inspection, and palpation.
Have you ever had a mammogram or ultrasound? If yes, when was it done and what were the results?	Annual mammograms should begin at age 40 years; ultrasounds should begin at an earlier age if indicated (ACS, 2008a,b).

Risk Assessment and Health-Related Patient Teaching

As mentioned previously, risk assessment helps to identify potential problems so that health care providers can educate patients to influence their behavior choices. It is important for women to be aware of their specific risk factors for breast cancer. Although many factors are not modifiable, some are. When a patient is aware of her own specific risk factors, she may be more diligent in practicing healthy habits (monthly SBEs, yearly physical examinations, and mammograms if indicated) and adjust other personal behaviors (especially physical inactivity and obesity; see Table 21-2).

Nurses should teach patients how to perform SBEs and alert them to the importance of being diligent about performing them monthly beginning in their early 20s. Although breast cancer is more common in older women, recognizing what her normal breast tissue feels like alerts the patient to changes if they develop. Between 20 and 39 years, women should also have CBEs performed by a health professional every 3 years; from 40 years onward, patients should have CBEs yearly. They also should begin yearly (or every other year) mammograms at 40 years. Women at high risk should get a magnetic resonance imaging (MRI) and a mammogram every year. Women at moderately increased risk should talk with their care providers about the benefits and limitations of adding MRI screening to their yearly mammogram (ACS, 2008a,b). Refer to SBE instructions later in the chapter.

Focused Health History Related to Common Symptoms

Common Breast and Axillary Symptoms

• Breast pain	• Swelling
• Rash	• Discharge
• Lumps	• Trauma

Questions to Assess Symptoms	Rationales/Abnormal Findings
Pain Do you have any pain or discomfort in either or both breasts? • *Location*: Where is the pain? Can you point to where it hurts? Does it stay in the one spot or move around? • *Intensity:* Can you rate the pain using a 0–10 scale? • *Duration:* How long have you had the pain? When did the pain start? How long has it lasted? Does it fluctuate (or is it worse at certain times of the month)? Have you ever had this pain before? If so, when? Does the pain occur at the same time every month? • *Quality/Description:* Can you describe the pain (eg, sharp, dull, throbbing, shooting, burning, tingling)?	When asking questions about the symptom (pain in this case), it is important to gather all the relevant information. Severe pain (**mastalgia**) is more likely to result from trauma or infection. Breast pain is common at some point during a woman's life, especially during menstrual years. Pain may occur in one or both breasts and may be cyclical (same time each month). Cyclical pain is very common in women who take oral contraceptives or have BBD (Katz, 2007). Typically, cyclical pain is worst in the days preceding menstruation and spontaneously disappears during or immediately after a period. It is often generalized, whereas pain from trauma is usually localized to one spot. Patients may describe noncyclic pain as sharp or burning; they tend to describe cyclic pain as heaviness.

Questions to Assess Symptoms	Rationales/Abnormal Findings
• Do you have any other symptoms along with the pain (eg, warmth or redness, fever, muscle aches, nausea, vomiting)?	Pain associated with warmth or redness at the site, may indicate a localized infection; fever, muscle aches, nausea, and vomiting may indicate a systemic infection.
• *Aggravating factors*: Does anything make the pain worse? • *Alleviating factors*: Have you tried anything to make it feel better (eg, heat, ice, Tylenol or other medications)? If so, did it work?	Determining what treatments or remedies the patient has tried will help determine future treatments.
Rash Do you have a rash? If so, when/where did it start?	Rashes from *contact dermatitis* or *eczema* usually start on the breast tissue and move toward the nipple. *Paget's disease* produces scaly lesions that begin at the nipple and progress to a lump behind the nipple well. Axillary rashes may result from allergy to deodorant or soaps.
Lumps Have you noticed any lumps in your breasts or axillae? • Where is the lump? • When did you notice it? • Has it changed at all (in size, is it more painful)? • If you have had previous lumps, does this feel the same or different? • Do you have a history of cystic breast changes or "lumpy" breasts?	Lumps can have many causes (eg, *BBD, fibroadenoma, cancer*). It is important to investigate any lump, especially if it is new or if patients have noticed changes. Nurses must also include information about the axillae, because breast tissue and many lymph nodes extend to this area. Single breast masses can indicate benign conditions (eg, *cysts, fibroadenoma, fat necrosis, lipoma*), or more serious conditions (eg, *cancer*).
Swelling Do you notice any swelling of the breasts? • Is it cyclical (or are you breastfeeding)? • Is it in one area or does it involve your entire breast? • Has your bra size increased from the swelling?	Cyclical swelling and tenderness on a continuum corresponding with the menstrual cycle are common and benign. Patients experiencing them often complain of a "full" feeling in their breasts during menstruation, most often affecting both breasts.
Discharge Do you have any discharge from your nipple? • What is the color? • Could you be pregnant?	Nurses must evaluate spontaneous nipple discharge. Milky discharge in the absence of pregnancy or lactation (*nonpuerpera l galactorrhea*) may be from *hyperprolactinemia* (caused by a prolactin-secreting tumor) or adrenergic medications (methyldopa).
	⚠ *SAFETY ALERT 21.2* *Nipple discharge can be associated with a benign papilloma, ductal ectasia, and less commonly, cancer. Early diagnosis and treatment are needed (Hussain, et al., 2006).*
• What medications are you taking?	Clear discharge may rarely occur from ingestion of steroids, calcium-channel blockers, or oral contraceptives (Hussain, et al., 2006). Tranquilizers may also cause nipple discharge. When the medication is discontinued, the discharge will cease.
Trauma Have you had any injuries or trauma to your breasts? • When/how did it occur? • Did it cause any break in the skin (or any residual lumps, swelling, or discoloration)?	Injuries to the breast may cause a patient to feel a previously undetected lump or mass. A break in the skin could lead to an infection.

Documentation of Normal Findings

Patient states she is without breast pain, lumps, nipple discharge, rashes, swelling, or trauma. Negative history of breast disease or breast surgery. Reports performing monthly breast exams; routine mammogram 9/10/10, which was "normal." *T. Quist, RN*

Additional Questions | **Rationales/Abnormal Findings**

Pregnant Women

Do you feel that your breasts are getting larger or feel "full?"

Breast changes are expected during pregnancy. Providing reassurance and answering questions is beneficial.

Are you planning to breast or bottle feed your baby?

Breastfeeding provides antibodies that protect infants against illnesses and allergies, and promotes bonding between mother and child.

Are your nipples inverted (go inward) or everted (go outward)?

Reassure the pregnant woman that breastfeeding is possible with inverted nipples.

Adolescent Females

Have you noticed any changes in your breasts (eg, are they getting larger or are they tender)? If yes, when did you first notice any changes?

It is important to assess the adolescent girl's perception of her own development and to provide appropriate teaching and reassurance.

Many changes occur as you grow up. Have you noticed any other changes? If yes, how do you feel about them?

This is a time when girls often compare themselves to other girls their age, and body image is important to address.

Therapeutic Dialogue: Collecting Subjective Data

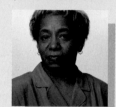

The nurse's role relative to subjective data collection is to gather information to improve the patient's health status and to help determine the cause of the patient's current symptoms. Remember Mrs. Randall, who was introduced at the beginning of this chapter. She was diagnosed with breast cancer 6 weeks ago, had a mastectomy, and is currently undergoing radiation. Some risk factors that the nurse assessed during subjective data collection were a family history of breast cancer in first-degree relatives (patient's mother and grandmother), early onset of menstruation (age 11 years), bottle feeding of her children, obesity, a high-fat diet, and lack of exercise. In addition to obtaining a health history and physical assessment, the nurse also assesses the patient's coping skills.

The following conversations give two examples of interview styles used by different nurses. One style is more effective than the other.

Less Effective

Nurse: Good morning, Mrs. Randall. How are you doing today?

Mrs. Randall: I'm feeling tired, real tired.

Nurse: I'm sorry. Well, I'm here to look at your breast and see how your wounds are healing.

Mrs. Randall: Yeah, that would be OK.

Nurse: How has your pain been?

Mrs. Randall: Not too bad.

Nurse: Have you been taking anything for it?

Mrs. Randall: Oh, just some Tylenol.

Nurse: How about any of the oxycodone?

Mrs. Randall: No, that stuff just makes me drowsy, and I don't like that.

Nurse: Can we take a look at your wound now?

More Effective

Nurse: Good morning, Mrs. Randall. How are you doing today?

Mrs. Randall: I'm feeling tired, real tired. (5-second pause) I can hardly get myself out of bed to eat. Why am I so tired?

Nurse: You sound a little discouraged.

Mrs. Randall: It's just been that after all of this happened, here I am feeling worse than when I started. (Begins to cry)

Nurse: (Silent. Touches Mrs. Randall on the arm, gives her a tissue.)

Mrs. Randall: I'm just tired of all of these treatments. And I'm worried that my breast won't heal. It's still all red and weepy (continues to cry).

Nurse: I'm sorry that you're not feeling well. Would this be a good time for me to look at it with you?

Critical Thinking Challenge

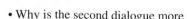

- Why is the second dialogue more effective, when the nurse's questions prompted Mrs. Randall to cry?
- How did the more effective nurse respond to Mrs. Randall's crying? Provide rationale.
- In addition to assessing her wound, what other things will the more effective nurse assess when examining the mastectomy incision?
- Is this an appropriate time to collect data on expected side effects from radiation, such as fatigue, anorexia, risk for infection, anemia, skin reactions, and coping? Provide rationale.

Table 21.3 Common Versus Specialty/Advanced Techniques for Breasts and Axillae

Technique	Purpose	Screening or RN Assessment	Focused or APRN Examination
Inspection of the breast	To assess healing following surgery	X	
Complete breast examination	A yearly examination by a health care professional (MD, NP, PA) as an adjunct to mammography to detect and evaluate breast abnormalities at an early stage		X
Transillumination of breast mass	Using a strong light to differentiate between a fluid-filled or solid mass		X

Objective Data Collection

Equipment

- Ruler marked in centimeters
- Small pillow
- Pamphlet or handout for BSE
- Gloves (if drainage is present)
- Adequate lighting

Preparation

The breast examination is an important part of a woman's health care. It provides an opportunity to identify breast disease, initiate early treatment, and demonstrate techniques for SBE. It is a good time to remind patients that mammography may not always detect breast cancer, and that they should perform SBE monthly. Variations in clinician technique and experience affect actual findings. As with any examination, the more breast examinations a nurse performs, the more likely he or she will be to identify abnormalities or variations. Additionally, using a standardized and systematic approach to palpate the breasts increases the likelihood of detecting breast changes and abnormalities. The following sections review actual techniques.

Keep in mind that hands-on palpation of the breasts may cause patients to feel apprehensive and embarrassed.

Adopting a professional, gentle, and reassuring approach is important. Before beginning, inform patients that you will be examining the breasts. Provide as much privacy as possible and answer any questions that patients may have. This is an opportune time to ask female patients if they perform monthly SBE. If not, instructing patients in it and watching return demonstrations can provide an opportunity to verify technique and provide helpful correction as indicated.

The breast examination involves inspection and palpation. It is important to expose both breasts fully initially during inspection to assess for symmetry, but then to cover or drape one breast while palpating the other. Patients should begin seated with the arms in different positions (first at the sides, then over the head, then against the hips while leaning forward). For palpation, patients should be supine. The best time to examine the breasts is when they are least congested and smallest (in adult women, days 4 to 7 of the menstrual cycle).

The comprehensive head-to-toe assessment includes the most important and common assessment techniques. Examiners may add focused or advanced techniques if concerns exist over a specific finding. Generally the registered nurse (RN) does not examine the breasts of patients unless a condition exists in the breast, such as recent breast surgery. The advanced practice nurse (APRN) includes a breast assessment with the comprehensive assessment, such as an annual physical examination (see Table 21-3).

Comprehensive Physical Assessment

Technique and Normal Findings	Abnormal Findings
Inspection Begin with the patient sitting with arms at the sides (Fig. 21-6). Inspect skin appearance for: • **Color and texture**: skin tone determines actual color. Pale, linear stretch marks (striae) may be evident after pregnancy or if a woman has gained then lost significant weight.	Redness (erythema) and heat can indicate infection or inflammation. Hyperpigmentation can signify *cancer*. A unilateral vascular appearance could indicate increased blood flow to a malignancy (produced by dilated superficial veins). *Peau d'orange* appearance is caused by

(text continues on page 572)

breast edema from blocked lymph drainage and indicates advanced cancer (Fig. 21-7). Rash or ulceration may occur in *Paget's disease of the breast*. See also Table 21-6 at the end of this chapter.

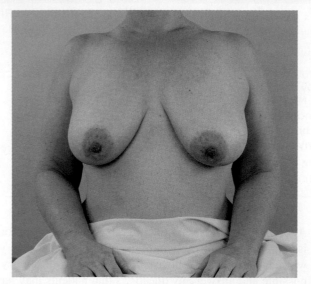

Figure 21.6 Patient sitting with arms at side as breast examination begins.

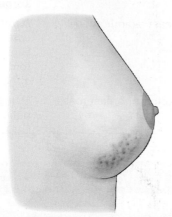

Figure 21.7 Peau d'orange.

- **Size and shape:** wide variation exists, from small to very large (pendulous).

- **Symmetry:** the left breast is often slightly larger than the right breast (Losken, 2007).

- **Contour:** should be uninterrupted

If a patient has pendulous breasts, it is easier to visualize irregularities if she leans forward with her arms on her hips.

Approximately 3% of women have one breast that is underdeveloped compared to the other (Losken, 2007).

Retractions or dimpling may occur with breast cancer (Fig. 21-8).

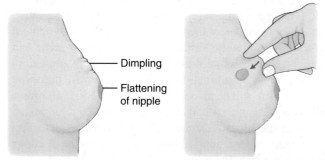

Retraction signs   Retraction with compression

Figure 21.8 Retraction signs.

- **Nipple and areola characteristics:** areola should be round or oval, and pink to dark brown or black. Most nipples are everted, but it may be normal for one or both nipples to be inverted.

Recent nipple changes from everted to inverted or in the angle the nipple points may indicate malignancy (caused from pulling of the malignant tissue; see Table 21-6.) Discharge (other than breast milk) can indicate cancer or infection and needs further evaluation; cracking or crusting can occur with breastfeeding.

An extra nipple (**supernumerary nipple**) along the embryonic nipple line (from axilla to groin bilaterally) is a common variation. If present, it is most often found 5–6 cm below the breast. On initial inspection it looks like a mole, but on careful inspection a tiny nipple and areola are present.

After inspecting with the arms at the side, re-inspect with the patient lifting the arms over head (Fig. 21-9A), pressed firmly on the hips (Fig. 21-9B), leaning forward from the waist (Fig. 21-9C), and then lying supine (Fig. 21-9D).

Any change in color, size (especially if unilateral), symmetry, or contour of the breast, or change in nipple characteristics requires further investigation. Lifting the arms over the head adds tension to the suspensory ligaments and accentuates any dimpling or retraction. Leaning forward may reveal breast or nipple asymmetry.

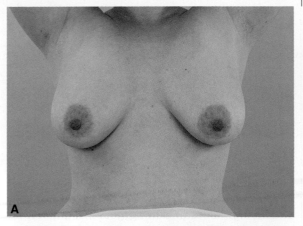
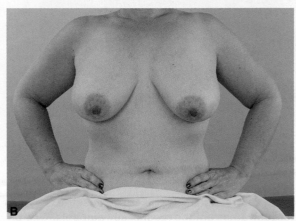
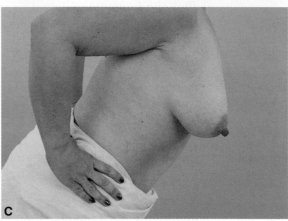
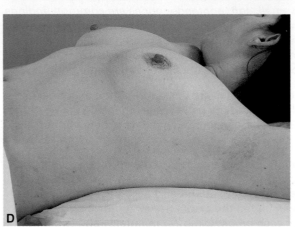

Figure 21.9 A. Arms over head. **B.** Arms pressed firmly on her hips. **C.** Leaning forward from the waist. **D.** Lying supine.

Also inspect the axillae while the patient is sitting, noting any rashes, infection, texture changes, or unusual pigmentation.

These signs suggest underlying cancer but may also be from benign lesions (eg, fat necrosis, mammary duct ectasia). Rashes or infection may occur from laundry detergent or deodorant. Velvety axillary skin or deep pigmentation is associated with malignancy.

Breasts are symmetrical; skin is smooth and even without redness, bulging, or dimpling. There is no rash, edema, or lesions. Nipples are symmetrical and protuberant. Nipples and areolae are the same color and smooth or wrinkled in appearance. There is no discharge (unless the woman is pregnant or lactating), cracking, or crusting.

Palpation

Palpating the axillae is best performed while the patient is sitting. Instruct the patient to gently raise the arm. Support the arm and wrist to aid in muscle relaxation. Use the right hand to palpate the left axilla and the left

(text continues on page 574)

hand to palpate the right axilla (Fig. 21-10). Point your fingers toward the midclavicle, directly behind the pectoral muscles.

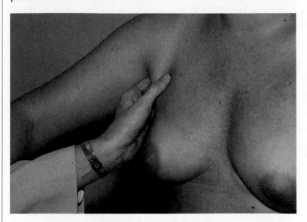

Figure 21.10 Palpation of the axilla.

Feel for the central nodes, which are against the chest wall, because these are the most easily palpable. *One or more small, soft, nontender nodes are common findings.* Also assess the other axillary lymph nodes, but these are more difficult to palpate. Pectoral nodes are located inside the border of the pectoral muscle. Lateral nodes are located along the upper humerus, high in the axilla.

Subscapular nodes are best felt with the examiner standing behind the patient, feeling inside the posterior axillary fold. Adjusting the patient's arm in various positions increases the surface area that can be assessed.

Palpating the breast tissue is best accomplished with the patient supine with her arm raised overhead and a small pillow or towel rolled under the side being examined. This will flatten the breast tissue. A thorough examination of each breast takes 2–3 minutes. Palpate the entire breast from the clavicle to the inframammary fold (bra line) and from midsternum to the posterior axillary line, making sure to examine the tail of Spence (Fig. 21-11).

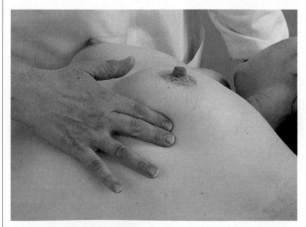

Figure 21.11 Palpation of the breasts with the patient supine.

Various techniques for palpation can be performed. The ACS currently recommends using the **vertical pattern**

Firm, hard, enlarged nodes (>1 cm) that are fixed to underlying tissues or skin suggest malignancy.

Tender, warm, enlarged nodes suggest infection of the breast, arm, or hand.

Enlarged axillary lymph nodes are sometimes mistaken for nodules in the tail of Spence and vice versa.

(Fig. 21-12A), because some evidence supports that this is the most effective means of examining the entire breast (Steiner, 2008). For this reason, this technique is described in detail. The circular (Fig. 21-12B) and wedge (Fig. 21-12C) patterns are also commonly used.

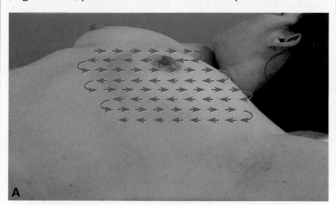

A

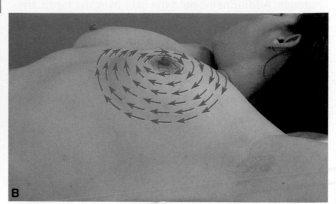

B

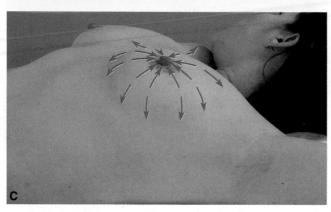

C

Figure 21.12 A. Vertical strip pattern. **B.** Circular pattern. **C.** Wedge pattern.

Vertical Pattern. Using the finger pads of the first three fingers, palpate in small, concentric circles beginning in the axilla and moving in a straight line down toward the bra line. Apply light, medium, and then deeper pressure at each examining point to reach the entire breast tissue. Continue in vertical overlapping lines until the sternal edge is met. Being systematic with the examination is important to always assess the entire breast for consistency, tenderness, and nodules.

Sliding the fingers along the breast to palpate each section increases the likelihood of palpating the entire breast.

Consistency. Breast tissue shows wide variations. Nodular masses may be present prior to menses, disappearing after menses has occurred. *The breast of a nulliparous woman feels smooth, elastic, and firm. Prior to menstruation, breasts are often engorged secondary to increased progesterone. The patient may notice nodules, a slight enlargement, and tenderness during this time. Upon examination, the lobes may be more prominent with distinct margins. After pregnancy, breasts feel softer and have less tone.*

Mammary duct ectasia (dilated, painful mammary ducts) should be suspected when a lump or thickening is palpable. This benign condition may result from hormonal changes, smoking, or lack of vitamin A. Additionally, an inverted nipple may block the mammary ducts, which can cause inflammation and mammary duct ectasia.

When assessing a pendulous breast, the examiner may feel the **inframammary ridge**, which is a firm transverse ridge of breast tissue. This finding is normal.

Do not rush through the examination of a pendulous breast, because lumps are harder to identify here from the increased size.

(text continues on page 576)

Tenderness. Breasts are often tender during the premenstrual period.

Nodules. If a lump is palpated, document the location, size, shape, consistency, mobility, tenderness, and distinctness. Additionally, note the skin over the lump, the nipple, and any lymphadenopathy.

- **Location:** Document by stating the quadrant or use clock measurements in centimeters from the nipple (eg, right upper outer quadrant or [R] breast, 10:00; 2 cm from nipple).
- **Size:** Measure or judge length × width × depth in centimeters using a ruler as a guide.
- **Shape:** oval, round, lobular, nodular, or indistinct?
- **Consistency:** smooth, soft, firm, or hard?
- **Mobility:** movable or immobile?
- **Tenderness:** tender or not?

- **Distinctness:** one lump or multiple nodules?

- **Skin:** dimpled, retracted, erythematous?
- **Nipple:** retracted or displaced?

- **Lymphadenopathy:** palpable lymph nodes?

Breast tissue is soft and homogeneous. No masses or tenderness. No lymphadenopathy.

Palpating the Nipple. Gently compress the nipple between your thumb and index finger to assess for discharge (Fig. 21-13). If discharge is evident, note the color, consistency, and amount. Massage around the areola if there is discharge to determine where it originates. *Nipple without discharge.*

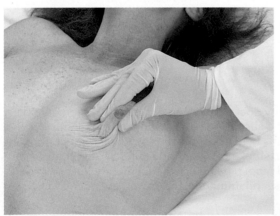

Figure 21.13 Palpating the nipple.

Bimanual Technique. If a patient has pendulous breasts, the bimanual technique may be more efficient in palpating lumps. With this technique, the patient should sit upright, leaning slightly forward. Place one hand underneath the breast (on the inferior surface) while palpating the breast tissue with the other hand (Fig. 21-14).

Tenderness or pain in the breast at other times may be from infection or trauma.

All breast masses require further evaluation and may require a mammogram, ultrasound, aspiration, or biopsy (discussed later).

The most common site for breast masses is in the upper outer quadrant, because this is where the most glandular tissue lies (Katz, 2007).

Indistinct lumps are more suspicious for breast cancer. Poorly circumscribed, fixed, hard, and irregular nodules strongly suggest cancer.

Tenderness indicates infection or inflammation. Some cancers may also be tender.

Cancer tends to be single; fibroadenoma or cysts may be single or multiple (see Table 21-7 at the end of the chapter).

Dimpling, retraction, or a retracted or displaced nipple can be signs of cancer. Erythema indicates inflammation.

Lymphadenopathy means swelling of the lymph nodes, which may occur postmastectomy, from blocked lymph nodes, or from infection.

If discharge is evident, it is important to obtain a cytological smear for examination.

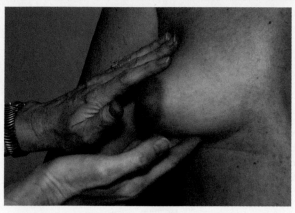

Figure 21.14 Palpating the breasts using bimanual technique.

Transillumination

Transillumination of a breast mass may be performed in a darkened room to differentiate between a solid and fluid-filled mass. When a strong light is pressed up against a mass filled with fluid, the rays will pass through, but when pressed up against a solid mass, they will not. This technique is rarely used, being largely replaced by mammography.

A solid mass is likely to be malignant, while a fluid-filled mass is more frequently a benign cyst (Katz, 2007).

Examining a Patient Postmastectomy

A woman who had had a mastectomy may be more self-conscious about being examined than one who has not undergone this procedure. The nurse must be empathetic and sensitive to her feelings. Malignancy can occur at the scar site or in other areas of the breast.

Masses, inflammation, color changes, and thickening may signify a recurrence of breast cancer.

Inspect the scar and axilla for signs of inflammation, rash, color changes, thickening, and irritation. Lymphedema may be evident in the axilla and arm secondary to impaired lymph drainage post-mastectomy. **Palpate** the surgical scar and chest wall with the pads of two fingers in a circular motion (as previously described) to assess for breast changes (lumps, tenderness, thickening, or swelling). Palpate the axilla and supraclavicular lymph nodes; assess for swelling and irritation.

If the patient has undergone breast reconstruction, lumpectomy, augmentation, or reduction, perform the breast examination as described, paying close attention to the scar tissue.

It is important to ask the patient to demonstrate SBE and to reiterate the importance of performing these monthly checks.

Male Breasts

Examining the male breast involves inspecting the nipple and areola for swelling, ulceration, or drainage. Additionally, palpate the areola and breast tissue for nodules or masses.

Firm, glandular tissue (**gynecomastia**) may occur when there is an imbalance of estrogen and androgen. An ulcer or hard, irregular mass suggests cancer. Obese men may have gynecomastia with increased fatty tissue. Gynecomastia also occurs with use of anabolic steroids, diseases, and as a side effect of some medications (see Table 21-6).

Documentation of Objective Findings

Inspection: (+) Symmetric breasts, everted nipples. Palpation (−) palpable masses in breast or axilla, nipple discharge, rashes, or dimpling. *T. Quist, RN*

Teaching the Self Breast Examination

After completion of CBE, it is appropriate to teach the patient how to perform an SBE. This practice is better than attempting to teach while performing the examination, because it allows nurses to concentrate on the examination separately from concentrating on teaching. See Box 21-1.

BOX 21.1 BREAST SBE TEACHING POINTS

*B*egin teaching the SBE by assisting the patient to establish a regular SBE schedule. As previously stated, the best time for an SBE is when the breasts are least congested (the fourth to seventh day of the menstrual cycle, which coincides with the end of the menstrual period). In postmenopausal patients, the time of the month for the SBE is irrelevant, because breast size remains stable. For them, discussing a day of the month that they will remember (eg, the first day of the month) may be a helpful suggestion.

Starting in their 20s, women should perform SBEs. Although most women will never get breast cancer, it is important for them to be aware of how their breasts feel and look so that they can immediately detect any changes. Emphasize to the patient that if she notices a significant change, such as dimpling or bulging of a section of the breast, a nipple that is inverted when it was previously outward, or a rash, soreness, swelling, or redness, then she should call her primary care provider for an appointment. Also inform the patient that many breast lumps are benign, but that if a lump is cancerous, the survival rate is very high if it is detected and treated before it becomes invasive.

Women with breast implants should still perform monthly SBEs. Help these patients identify the edges of the implants so they can determine what is normal for them. Implants actually push breast tissue outward and may make abnormalities easier to feel.

Instruct the patient to begin SBE by disrobing and lying down with one arm under the head and a pillow under the side she is going to examine first. (If her right arm is under her head, she should place a pillow under her right side.) The patient should use the pads of the middle three fingers to feel the entire breast in an up-and-down pattern (Fig. A). The patient should make sure she checks the entire breast. Using a soft pressure allows the patient to feel the breast surface, a medium pressure gets a little deeper, and a firm pressure allows her to feel the tissue closest to the ribs and chest. Teach her to use all three levels of pressure during her SBE. She should repeat all the previous steps on her other breast.

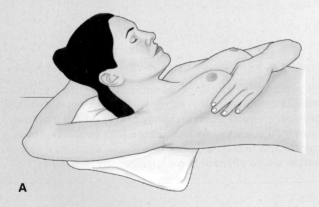

A

Next, she should look at her breasts in a mirror. Instruct her to keep her shoulders straight and her arms on her hips. Her breasts should be fairly equal in size, shape, and color (there may be

some variation), without any swelling, discoloration, dimpling, or drainage from the nipple.

Instruct the patient to raise her arms over her head to look for equal movement of the breasts. Sometimes, raising the arms accentuates dimpling or the lagging behind of a breast if either is present (Fig. B).

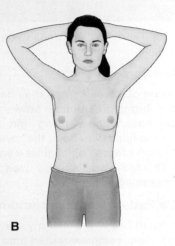

B

While the patient looks in the mirror, she should squeeze each nipple gently for any drainage. Generally, there is none (unless the woman is pregnant or breastfeeding, in which case there may be clear or milky white drainage).

From here, the patient should feel each breast in the same manner she did while supine (Fig. C). Often women like to perform SBE while in the shower, because the soap and water make the skin slippery.

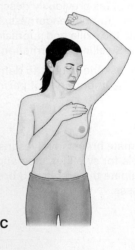

C

Instruct the patient to examine her underarm while she either stands or sits. It is easiest to feel the armpit with the arm only slightly raised, because the skin is loose. The skin tightens when the arm is fully raised and makes it difficult to examine.

Lifespan Considerations

Pregnant/Lactating Women

During pregnancy, breasts and nipples increase in size, which may cause mild discomfort. Linear stretch marks (**striae**) may be evident. Striae may disappear completely when breasts return to the pre-pregnant size. A blue, vascular pattern may also be visible from increased blood flow. Nipples and areolae darken and widen. Montgomery glands become more prominent. Breasts may feel nodular, and nipples may expel yellow colostrum (milk precursor) after the first trimester.

If the woman is breastfeeding, milk production occurs most often by the third postpartum day. Breasts may become larger, reddened, warm, and engorged, especially at this time. Frequent breastfeeding will stimulate milk production, drain the sinuses, and resolve the symptoms. If these symptoms occur at other times during lactation, they could indicate **mastitis**, which usually requires antibiotic therapy, as well as more frequent nursing to resolve. Nipples often become sore, but generally this resolves spontaneously. If they become cracked and irritated, bleeding may occur.

After pregnancy and lactation, breasts return to their pre-pregnant state, but often are less firm. The nipples and areolae usually remain darker than in the pre-pregnant state.

Newborns and Infants

As discussed previously, newborns may have enlarged breast tissue for the first few weeks of life from maternal estrogen. They also may secrete a clear white fluid from the nipples during this period. Should these findings occur, nurses reassure parents or other caregivers that they are normal and will resolve spontaneously.

Children and Adolescents

On inspection, the symmetrical nipples of prepubescent children lie between the 4th and 5th ribs just lateral to the midclavicular line. The nipples and areolae are flat and darker than the rest of the breast tissue.

During puberty females begin to develop breasts (usually between 8½ and 10 years). As previously mentioned, breast tissue may be asymmetric during growth. This temporary asymmetry may upset adolescents, who may need reassurance that this is normal and will resolve on its own. Breast tenderness may also occur. It is important to educate the adolescent female about expected body changes that will occur during this time period.

See Figure 21-5 for a review of Tanner staging. Breast development before 7 years in Caucasian girls or 6 years in African American girls is termed **precocious puberty** and may be secondary to either dysfunction of the thyroid gland or a tumor of the ovaries or adrenal gland. Isolated breast development in the absence of other hormone-dependent changes (eg, menses, pubic hair) in girls younger than 8 years is termed **premature thelarche** (Diamantopoulos, 2007). Delayed development may occur with anorexia nervosa, malnutrition, or hormonal imbalance. Girls may be considered to have a developmental delay if breast development has not

occurred by 13 years. Further evaluation is warranted if any of these conditions occur.

The breasts of an adolescent girl are uniform and firm. A mass at this age is most often benign (a cyst or fibroadenoma; see Table 21-6). Adolescence is a good time to introduce patients to what their breasts normally feel like, so that they will be more likely to perform SBE as they get older.

Older Adults

As a result of the relaxation of the suspensory ligaments and atrophy of the glandular tissue, the breasts of postmenopausal women sag, flatten, and look more pendulous. On palpation, they may feel more granular. Nipples become flatter and smaller, and the inframammary ridge is more prominent from thickening. As women age, care providers should remind them to continue monthly SBEs and yearly CBEs, because mature women are at increased risk for breast cancer. With the cessation of menses, hormonal changes will no longer affect their breasts. For this reason, patients can choose a convenient day of each month to perform SBEs (eg, first day of month).

Evidence-Based Critical Thinking

Organizing and Prioritizing

Nurses must continuously think critically about the patient's condition to organize and prioritize assessments and patient care. Laboratory and diagnostic tests related to the breasts and axillae can expand on findings from the health history and physical examination. Analysis of assessment and laboratory data help clinicians identify the underlying cause of signs and symptoms. Nurses use findings to identify the underlying functional problem, label it (sometimes in a nursing diagnosis format), and plan interventions based on patient outcomes. At times nurses need to communicate findings and reasons for referrals to other health care providers. Nurses also work with primary health practitioners to gather information to make a diagnosis and to prescribe appropriate collaborative care. They re-assess patients to evaluate the effectiveness of both nursing and collaborative care measures.

Laboratory and Diagnostic Testing

Mammography, ultrasound, MRI, and aspiration biopsy (fine-needle aspiration [FNA], coreneedle aspiration biopsy [CNB], or excisional biopsy) aid in accurately diagnosing breast cancer in 70% to 80% of cases (Dains, et al., 2007). A screening mammogram is suggested for patients at 40 years of age to detect nonpalpable breast masses (ACS, 2008a,b).

Mammography consists of two x-rays (digital or conventional film). If a palpable mass has been detected or if the woman has nipple discharge, magnification and additional views are necessary. A woman between 30 and 40 years may benefit from a mammogram if a mass is suspected, depending on breast density.

Table 21.4	Common Diagnostic Testing for Breasts
Technique	**Purpose**
Mammography	Low-dose x-ray of the breasts to aid in the diagnosis of breast disease; should be performed as a screening tool annually beginning at age 40 years
Ultrasound	Non-invasive test using high-frequency sound waves; differentiates between a solid and cystic mass; is used as a guide in needle aspirations
MRI	Uses a magnetic field (not x-ray), radio waves, and a computer to detect and stage breast cancer and other breast abnormalities
Excisional biopsy	An excision (cut) made into the breast to remove a portion of a suspicious lump and the surrounding tissue to examine for cancerous cells
Microscopy	Viewing cells under a microscope to enhance cellular features
Ductogram	Examination of the breast ducts to determine cause of unilateral, single-pore nipple discharge
Cytological smear	Smearing and staining a cell sample (obtained from breast discharge) to determine cause
TSH	Blood test drawn (thyroid stimulating hormone) to determine if nipple discharge is secondary to a thyroid problem

Ultrasound is used with women younger than 40 years, who tend to have denser breast tissue, those with silicone breast implants, pregnant women (so they are not exposed to x-ray), and as a guide when performing a CNB (Katz, 2007). This non-invasive test produces a picture through high-frequency sound waves of the internal breast structures to help practitioners differentiate between a solid and cystic mass.

FNA and CNB are types of biopsies in which a needle is inserted into the abnormal site to collect a sample of cells for analysis to determine if cancer exists. An excisional biopsy is similar to a lumpectomy, in which the lump or suspicious area and a portion of the surrounding tissue are removed and examined. It is the standard procedure for lumps that are smaller than 1 in in diameter and is performed on an outpatient basis.

MRI is a supplemental tool to mammography. This non-invasive, painless test uses a magnetic field (not x-ray), radio waves, and a computer to detect and stage breast cancer and other breast abnormalities. It may be used for women with dense breast tissue (as in those younger than 40 years), with breast implants, or with scar tissue from previous breast surgery. It also may provide more detailed information to help determine treatment choices for a woman with breast cancer.

The clinical situation may indicate a need for additional tests (see Table 21-4).

Diagnostic Reasoning

Nurses use assessment findings as the basis for ongoing care. An accurate and complete assessment provides a firm foundation for setting outcomes, providing individualized interventions, and evaluating progress.

Nursing Diagnoses, Outcomes, and Interventions

When formulating nursing diagnoses, it is important to use critical thinking to cluster data and identify patterns that fit together. Nurses compare clusters of data with the defining characteristics (abnormal findings) for the diagnosis to ensure the most accurate labeling and appropriate interventions. A nursing diagnosis is a clinical judgment about responses to health problems or life processes. See Table 21-5 for a comparison of nursing diagnoses, abnormal findings, and interventions commonly related to the breast assessment in a patient with cancer (NANDA-I, 2009).

Nurses use assessment information to identify patient outcomes. Some outcomes related to breast health include the following (Moorhead, et al., 2008):

- Patient looks at and touches changed or missing body part.
- Patient returns to previous social involvement.
- Patient verbalizes increased self-acceptance through positive self statements.
- Patient performs an SBE monthly.

Once the outcomes are established, nurses implement care to improve the status of the patient. They use critical thinking and evidence-based practice to develop the interventions. Some examples of nursing interventions for breast care are as follows (Bulechek, et al., 2008):

- Allow for privacy when examining breast tissue.
- Provide a mirror for the patient to visualize tissue and incisions.
- Teach SBE and encourage its monthly performance.

Table 21.5 Common Nursing Diagnoses Associated with Breast Cancer

Diagnosis and Related Factors	Point of Differentiation	Assessment Characteristics	Nursing Interventions
Disturbed Body Image related to surgery and treatment	Viewpoint or perspective of one's physical self that is significantly different from objective reality	Missing body part, avoiding looking at body part, behaviors of avoidance	Acknowledge feelings as normal when coping with change. Explore strengths. Encourage new clothes or wig in anticipation of changes.
Ineffective Coping related to changes in function	Failure to address stressors; using methods to handle stressors that worsen or fail to solve the problems	Substance abuse, complaining without acting, lack of resolution of the problem, over eating, sleeping too much, isolating oneself	Observe causes of ineffective coping. Help identify resources. Discuss changes and previous successful coping strategies. Evaluate suicide risk.
Ineffective Role Performance related to loss of ability to cook, clean for self	Behaviors that are out of the patient's usual context or character; failure to execute usual tasks	Inadequate resources to accomplish chores, change in normal responsibilities	Validate accomplishments. Locate community resources. Suggest physical accommodations.*
Grieving related to the loss of breast, functional ability and cancer diagnosis	Sadness related to loss of health, body part, function, or person	Sadness, crying, anger, depression, altered eating, and sleep patterns, reliving of past experiences	Encourage patient to express feelings and affirm that they part of the grief process. Refer to spiritual counseling if indicated.

*Collaborative interventions.

Analyzing Findings

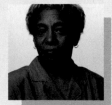

The initial subjective and objective data collection is complete, and the nurse has spent time reviewing the findings and other results. Mrs. Randall's skin is causing her discomfort and the radiation is causing anorexia and fatigue. The following nursing note illustrates how subjective and objective data are collected and analyzed and nursing interventions are developed.

Subjective: "I'm tired, real tired. And I'm worried that my breast won't heal." She also states that she has no appetite and is fatigued.

Objective: Appears tired, crying intermittently. Skin color pale, moving slowly. Right chest with 4-in curved scar extending from axilla to right sternal border 4th intercostal space. Bright red erythema present over 6 × 8 in area of anterior chest from radiation treatment. Dermis is exposed, small amount of serous-sanguineous drainage noted. Tenderness (3/10) over surgical site with palpation.

Analysis: Fatigue related to recent cancer diagnosis, surgery, radiation treatments, and situational grieving. **Impaired skin integrity** related to radiation treatments.

Plan: Allow time to talk and express thoughts. Validate her concerns and appropriateness of her feelings. Assess support systems and who might be available to assist with home maintenance and meal preparation while she is fatigued. Evaluate the need for supplements to provide nutrition for wound healing. Observe her caring for erythematous skin. Keep skin clean, avoid irritation and instruct on signs and symptoms of infection and when she should call physician.

T. Quist, RN

Critical Thinking Challenge

- How would the nurse transition from collecting data about coping to collecting physical assessment data?
- What additional assessment data might be gathered to evaluate side effects from the treatments?
- How do the coping, fatigue, treatment side effects, and ability to care for herself all fit together?

Collaborating with Other Health Care Providers

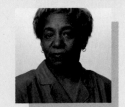

Homemaker and chore workers perform light household duties such as laundry, meal preparation, general housekeeping, and shopping. They direct services at maintaining patient households rather than providing hands-on assistance with personal care (National Association for Home Care, 2007). The following conversation illustrates how the nurse might organize data from Mrs. Randall and make recommendations about the patient's situation when making a referral to chore services.

Situation: Mrs. Randall is a 66-year-old woman who underwent a modified radical mastectomy for breast cancer 6 weeks ago and is currently receiving radiation therapy.

Background: She has been experiencing severe fatigue and anorexia and is a good candidate for chore services to assist with shopping, cooking, and cleaning. She has a decreased appetite and cannot cook her meals or do her housework..

Assessment: Increasing her food intake and rest will aid in healing, coping, and comfort. She seems very overwhelmed with all of the changes she has had to deal with in the last 6 weeks.

Recommendations: Please evaluate her mobility, strength, and home maintenance abilities. In particular, she may need an evaluation for housework and meals. Please let me know of your recommendations after your first visit. Your assessment in getting her some resources is greatly appreciated.

Critical Thinking Challenge

- What is the nurse's role in coordinating collaborative care with chore services?
- What family or community assessment information might be helpful?
- What other interventions might you recommend for Mrs. Randall?
- What information will the nurse gather when evaluating the effectiveness of the recommendations?

Pulling It All Together: Reflection and Critical Thinking

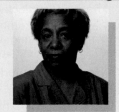

The nurse uses assessment data to formulate a nursing care plan for Mrs. Randall based on a complete and accurate assessment. After completing these interventions, the nurse will reassess Mrs. Randall and document the findings in the chart to show critical thinking. The plan of care integrates separate parts of the nursing process. This thinking is illustrated in a care plan or case note similar to the one below.

Nursing Diagnosis	Patient Outcomes	Nursing Interventions	Rationales	Evaluation
Fatigue related to disease state (breast cancer), recent modified radical mastectomy, radiation, decreased appetite, and life stress.	Patient will verbalize understanding of the effects of recent surgery and ra diation on her overall energy state. Additionally, she will verbalize feelings related to her emotional state (stress from diagnosis and current treatments). Also, she will identify personal strengths and accept support within the next 2 weeks.	Educate the patient about radiation treatments and the expected course. Allow her time to ask questions. Offer emotional support. Allow time to talk and express thoughts. Validate her concerns and appropriateness of her feelings. Assess support systems and who might be available to assist with home.	It is expected that a patient will experience fatigue at times with such recent surgery and while currently undergoing radiation. Confirming her feelings and assuring her that she will improve will aid in her recuperation. Effectiveness of coping is determined by the number, duration, and intensity of stressors. Her feelings are appropriate for the situation. Talking about her issues and finding support will help support her personal strengths during this difficult period.	Mrs. Randall is feeling less fatigued and more hopeful. She is looking forward to the end of her radiation treatments. Chore services have recommended a worker for the next 6 weeks to come once a week to shop and do housecleaning. Mrs. Randall appreciates the support. Continue to follow for her ability to perform household chores.

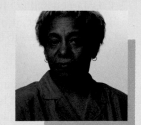

Using the previous steps of diagnostic reasoning, organizing, and prioritizing, consider all the case study findings woven throughout this chapter. When answering the following questions, begin drawing conclusions and see how the pieces of assessment must work together to create an environment for personalized, appropriate, and accurate care. Consider Mrs. Randall's case with her issues related to breast cancer, treatment, and side effects of treatment.

- Are Mrs. Randall's psychosocial or physical needs in this case more important? Provide rationale.
- What health promotion and teaching needs are apparent? Which two areas are highest priorities?
- How should the nurse organize and prioritize data collection, considering Mrs. Randall's multiple problems?
- How should the nurse individualize assessment to Mrs. Randall's specific needs, considering the patient's condition, age, and culture?

Key Points

- To describe clinical findings, nurses should divide the breast into four quadrants by imagining lines that intersect at the nipple.
- The lymphatic spread of breast cancer may cause enlarged lymph nodes, most commonly in the tail of Spence.
- Pregnant women experience breast changes and enlargement beginning in the first 2 months of pregnancy.
- Breast enlargement may occur in newborns as a result of the influence of maternal hormones.
- Breast development in adolescent females occurs over a 3-year period; the stage is identified by Tanner scale.
- Gynecomastia is common in approximately one-third of adolescent boys; it usually resolves in 1 to 2 years.
- A new breast lump, change in existing lump, or bloody discharge from the nipple needs further investigation to rule out breast cancer.
- The nurse teaches female patients how to perform an SBE as part of health-related patient teaching.
- Risks for breast cancer include history of childbirth, gender, oral contraceptive use, aging, combined and estrogen-alone postmenopausal hormone therapy (PHT), genetic risk factors, breastfeeding, family history, alcohol, personal history of breast cancer, overweight or obesity (especially after menopause), race, physical inactivity, abnormal breast biopsy results, menstrual periods, previous chest radiation, and DES exposure.
- Common signs and symptoms related to the breasts and axillae include breast pain, lumps, discharge, rash, swelling, and trauma.
- Palpation of the breasts may cause apprehension or embarrassment in patients; nurses provide reassurance and privacy.
- The best time to palpate the breasts is 4 to 7 days after the menstrual cycle begins.

- Size and shape of the breasts show wide variation.
- A supernumerary nipple is a normal variation.
- The sequence for inspecting the breasts is with the patient sitting with arms at the side, arms overhead, arms pressed on the hips, leaning forward at the waist, and lying supine.
- A vertical pattern of palpation is recommended.
- With pendulous breasts, a bimanual palpation technique is used.

Review Questions

1. When teaching the breast self-examination, which of the following times should nurses inform women that it is best to perform it? Select all that apply.
   A. Just before the menstrual period
   B. Just after the menstrual period
   C. On the fourth to seventh days of the menstrual cycle
   D. On the 10th day of the menstrual cycle

2. A male patient presents to the clinic with a complaint of a hard, irregular, nontender mass on his chest under the areola. Upon examination, the nurse notes that the mass is immobile and suspects
   A. gynecomastia
   B. benign lesion
   C. Paget's disease
   D. carcinoma

3. Gynecomastia may occur in an older male secondary to
   A. testosterone deficiency
   B. lymphatic engorgement
   C. trauma
   D. decreased activity level

4. When examining the breast of a 75-year-old woman, the nurse would expect to find which of the following?
A. Enlarged axillary lymph nodes
B. Multiple large, firm lumps
C. A granular feel to the breast tissue
D. Pale areola

5. It is important to examine the upper outer quadrant of the breast because it is
A. more prone to injury and calcifications
B. where most breast tumors develop
C. where most of the suspensory ligaments attach
D. the largest quadrant of the breast

6. A 23-year-old nulliparous woman is concerned that her breasts seem to change in size all month long and they are very tender around the time she has her period. The nurse should explain to her that
A. Nonpregnant women usually do not have these breast changes and this is cause for concern.
B. Breasts often change in response to stress so it is important to assess her life stressors.
C. Cyclic breast changes are normal.
D. Breast changes normally occur during pregnancy and she should have a pregnancy test.

7. A patient with BBD is likely to
A. develop breast cancer later in life
B. require hormone replacement therapy
C. be a teenager
D. resolve after menopause

8. The nurse palpates a fine, round, mobile, non-tender nodule and suspects that it is (a)
A. fibroadenoma
B. cyst
C. fibrocystic breast change
D. breast cancer

9. *Peau d'orange* appearance is highly suggestive of which of the following?
A. Breast cancer
B. Gynecomastia
C. Papillomas
D. Colostrum

10. The correct position to place the patient to palpate the breasts is
A. left lateral position with arm over head
B. sitting forward with hands on hips
C. supine with arm over head
D. supine with arms at side

References

American Cancer Society. (2007). *Risk factors for dying of breast cancer.* Retrieved December 13, 2007, from http://www.cancer.org/docroot/NWS/content/NWS_1_1x_Risk_Factors_for_Dying_of_Breast_Cancer_Similar_in_White_Black_Women.asp

American Cancer Society. (2008a). *Detailed guide: Breast cancer. What are the risk factors for breast cancer?* Retrieved February 20, 2008, from http://www.cancer.org/docroot/CRI/content/CRI_2_4_2X_What_are_the_risk_factors_for_breast_cancer_5.asp

American Cancer Society. (2008b). *Detailed guide: Breast cancer. Can breast cancer be found early?* Retrieved July 1, 2008, from http://www.cancer.org/docroot/CRI/content/CRI_2_4_3X_Can_breast_cancer_be_found_early_5.asp

Bowen, D. J., Alfano, C. M., McGregor, B. A., et al. (2007). Possible socioeconomic and ethnic disparities in quality of life in a cohort of breast cancer survivors. *Breast Cancer Research and Treatment,* Jan 27.

Bryner, J. (2007). *Bras don't support bouncing breasts.* Retrieved July 1, 2008, from http://www.livescience.com/health/070911_bounce_support.html

Bulechek, G. B., Butcher, J. K., & McCloskey Dochterman, J. (2008). *Nursing interventions classification (NIC)* (5th ed). St Louis: Mosby.

Dains, J., Baumann, L., & Scheibel, P. (2007). *Advanced health assessment and clinical diagnosis in primary care* (3rd ed.). St. Louis: Mosby.

de Onis, M., Garza, C., Victora, C. G., Bhan, M. K., Norum, K. R. (Guest Eds.) (2004). The WHO Multicentre Growh Reference Study (MGRS): Rationale, planning and implementation. *Food and Nutrition Bulletin,* 25(1, Suppl. 1), 1–89.

De Silva, N. K. & Brandt, M. L. (2006). Disorders of the breast in children and adolescents, Part 1: Disorders of growth and infection of the breast. *Journal of Pediatric and Adolescent Gynecology,* 19(5), 345–349.

Diamantopoulos, S. (2007). Gynecomastia and premature thelarche: A guide for practitioners. *Pediatrics in Review,* 28, e57–e67.

Fletcher, O., et al. (2008). Association of genetic variants at 8q24 with breast cancer risk. *Cancer Epidemiology Biomarkers & Prevention,* 17, 702–705.

Gabram, S. G. A. (2008). Effects of an outreach and internal navigation program on breast cancer diagnosis in an urban cancer center with a large African-American population. Retrieved July 1, 2008, from http://www.cancer.org/docroot/NWS/content/NWS_1_1x_Outreach_Programs_Help_African_American_Breast_Cancer_Patients.asp

Healthy people 2010: What are its goals? (n.d.). Retrieved January 7, 2007, from Healthy people 2010: http://www.healthypeople.gov/About/goals.htm

Hussain, A. N., Policarpio, C., & Vincent, M. T. (2006). Evaluating nipple discharge. *Obstetrical and Gynecological Survey,* 61(4), 278–283.

Katz, V. L., Lentz, G. M., Lobo, R. A., & Gershenson, D. M. (2007). Benign breast disease. In A. Katz (Ed.), *Comprehensive gynecology* (5th ed.). Philadelphia: Mosby Elsevier.

Kronenberg, H. M., et al. (2008). *Williams textbook of endocrinology* (11th ed.). Philadelphia: Saunders.

Laufer, M. R., & Goldstein, D. P. (2005). The breast: Examination and lesions. In A. Sydor (Ed.), *Pediatric & adolescent gynecology* (5th ed., pp. 729–759). Philadelphia: Lippincott Williams & Wilkins.

Losken, A., Fishman, I., Denson, D. D., et al. (2007). An objective evaluation of breast symmetry and shape differences using 3-dimensional images. Retrieved July 1, 2008, from http://cat.inist.fr/?aModele=afficheN&cpsidt=17314303

McCullough, M. L. Feigelson, H. S., Ryan Diver, W., et al. (2005). Risk factors for fatal breast cancer in African-American women and White women in a large U.S. prospective cohort. *American Journal of Epidemiology, 162*(8), 734–742.

Moorhead, S., Johnson, M., Maas, M., & Swanson, E. (2008). *Nursing outcomes classification (NOC)* (4th ed.). Philadelphia: Mosby.

NANDA International. (2009). Nursing diagnoses: *Definitions and classification*. West Sussex, UK: Wiley-Blackwell.

National Association for Home Care. (2007). *How to choose a home care provider*. Retrieved June 9, 2010, from http://www.nahc.org/consumer/coninfo.html

National Cancer Institute. (2007). *Fact sheet*. Retrieved January 24, 2008, from http://www.cancer.gov/cancertopics/factsheet/estimating-breast-risk/print?page=&keyword= (Estimating breast cancer risk: Questions & Answers)

National Cancer Institute. (2007). *What you need to know about breast cancer*. Retrieved January 24, 2007, from http://www.cancer.gov/cancertopics/wyntk/breast/page4

Office of Minority Health. (2008). Breast cancer: A guide for minority women. Retrieved May 6, 2008, from http://www.omhrc.gov/assets/pdf/checked/bcrg2005.pdf.

Rakel, R. E. (2007). *Textbook of family medicine* (7th ed.). Philadelphia: Elsevier.

Richards, T., Hunt, A., Courtney, S., & Umeh, H. (2007). Nipple discharge: A sign of breast cancer? *Annals of College Surgery England, 89*(2), 124–126.

Singleton, J. K., Sandowski, S. A., Horvath, T. V., et al. (2008). *Primary care*. Philadelphia: Lippincott.

Smigal, C., Jemal, A., Ward, E., et al. (2006). Trends in breast cancer by race and ethnicity: Update 2006. *American Cancer Journal Clinic, 56*(3), 168–183.

Steiner, E., Austin, D. F., & Prouser, N. C. (2008). Detection and description of small breast masses by residents trained using a standardized clinical breast exam curriculum. *Journal of General Internal Medicine, 23*(2), 129–134.

Sohn, V. Y., Arthurs, Z. M., Sebesta, J. A., & Brown, T. A. (2008). Primary tumor location impacts breast cancer survival. *American Journal of Surgery, 195*(5), 102–105.

The Jensen suite offers these additional resources to enhance learning and facilitate understanding of this chapter:

- thePoint on line resource, http//thepoint.lww.com/Jensen1E
- Student CD-ROM included with the book
- *Laboratory Manual for Nursing Health Assessment: A Best Practice Approach*
- *Pocket Guide for Nursing Health Assessment: A Best Practice Approach*

Table 21.6   Breast Abnormalities

Carcinoma (skin, areola, and nipple retraction)

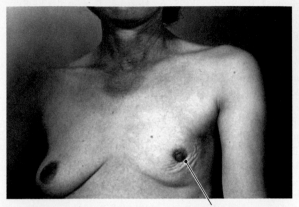

Skin, areola, and
nipple retraction

Carcinoma (bulging of breast and skin changes)

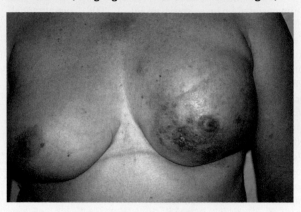

Paget's disease

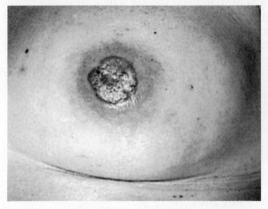

Follicular keratosis

Mastitis

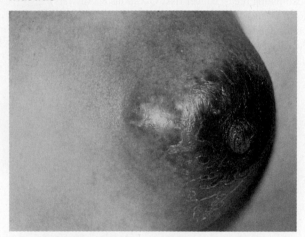

Mastectomy

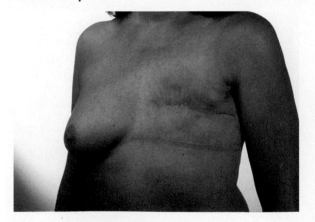

Gynecomastia

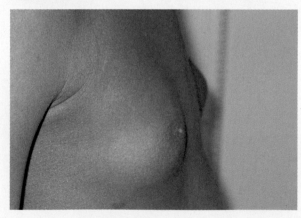

Characteristics	Fibroadenoma	Benign Breast Disease	Cancer
	Rubbery, circumscribed, freely movable benign tumor	Cyst Pectoralis muscles Fat Normal lobules	Skin dimpling Hard Irregularly shaped Immobile, fixed to chest wall Nipple retraction Blood or serous nipple discharge
Likely age	Appears most often before 30 years (15–39 years; some up to 55 years)	30–50 years; incidence decreases after menopause	30–80 years; risk increases after 50 years
Shape/size	Oval, round, lobular 1–5 cm	Round, lobular, variable size	Irregular, star-shaped, variable size
Consistency	Firm or rubbery	Firm to soft, rubbery	Firm to hard
Demarcation	Well demarcated, clear Margins	Well demarcated	Poorly defined
Number	Most often single; may be multiple	Most often multiple; may be single	Single
Mobility	Freely movable	Movable	Fixed
Tenderness	Painless	Painful; breast tenderness, which usually increases before menses, may be non-cyclic; breasts often swollen, usually bilateral	Nontender, can be tender
Suspicious signs	None	None	Dimpling, nipple inversion, spontaneous single-nipple bloody discharge, orange-peel texture (*peau d'orange*), axillary lymphadenopathy
Pattern of growth	Rapid growing during pregnancy, with HRT, or if immunosuppressed; approximately 10% disappear spontaneously	Size may increase or decrease rapidly	Continually increases in size (at varying rates)
Risk to health	None; they are benign—must diagnose by biopsy	Benign, although general lumpiness may mask other cancerous lump	Serious, needs early treatment

HRT, Hormone replacement therapy.

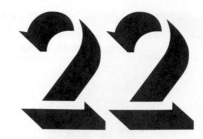

22

Abdominal Assessment

Learning Objectives

1 Identify anatomical landmarks that guide assessment of the abdomen and documentation of findings.

2 Explain the structure and functions of abdominal organs, muscles, and vascular structures.

3 Identify teaching opportunities for health promotion and risk prevention associated with organs found within the abdomen.

4 Collect subjective data including history, review of systems, and symptoms that affect the GI system.

5 Collect objective data on the inspection, auscultation, percussion, and palpation of the organs within the abdominal cavity.

6 Individualize the comprehensive health assessment by considering the condition, age, gender, and culture of the patient.

7 Identify normal, variations of normal and abnormal findings of the inspection, auscultation, percussion, and palpation of the organs located within the abdominal cavity.

8 Compare abnormal conditions that occur in the abdominal cavity.

9 Use subjective and objective assessment data to analyze findings, identify diagnoses, and plan interventions.

10 Document and communicate data using appropriate terminology.

*M*r. Chase, a 41-year-old Caucasian man, was admitted to the hospital with a gastrointestinal (GI) bleed. He has been on the acute care unit for 5 days following a 3-day stay in the intensive care unit (ICU). His temperature is 36.5°C tympanic, pulse 102 beats/min, respirations 20 breaths/min, and blood pressure 148/92 mm Hg. Current medications include a medication that blocks acid production and liquid antacid. He has had an assessment documented every shift.

You will gain more information about Mr. Chase as you progress through this chapter. As you study the content and features, consider Mr. Chase's case and its relationship to what you are learning. Begin thinking about the following points:

- How will the nurse prioritize health promotion and teaching needs?
- How does the nurse incorporate the different phases of the nursing process when performing the assessments?
- What information from other body systems might be useful to assess?
- How will the nurse organize the assessment during the shift?

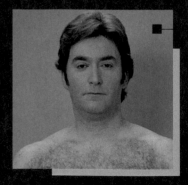

It is not possible to perform an assessment of the abdomen without realizing that every system (except respiratory) is found within the abdominal cavity. Awareness of this fact allows nurses to obtain valuable information about the functioning of the GI, cardiovascular, reproductive, neuromuscular, and genitourinary (GU) systems.

The focus of this chapter is abdominal assessment, and it primarily addresses issues within the GI system. The GI system is responsible for the ingestion and digestion of food, absorption of nutrients, and elimination of solid waste products from the body. Parts of the GI system also reside in the head, neck, and thoracic regions (see Chapters 14 and 18). Findings need to be evaluated based on the organ systems found in those regions as well.

GI symptoms are common and send people of all ages in search of relief. Diagnosis of abdominal diseases depends heavily on accurate and thorough history taking. During the health history, it is essential to delineate the sequence of the patient's symptoms. Additionally, it is important to master the abdominal assessment to provide quality health care.

Structure and Function Overview

Understanding the anatomy and physiology of GI structures is essential before beginning an assessment. The nurse must recognize normal GI structures and their functions before identifying abnormalities. Understanding the physiology associated with each organ and their interactions assists the nurse to accurately interpret findings from the assessment (Fig. 22-1; Tables 22-1 and 22-2).

Anatomical Landmarks

The abdomen is a large cavity extending from the xiphoid process of the sternum down to the superior margin of the pubic bone. It is bordered in the back by the vertebral column and paravertebral muscles and at the sides and front by the lower rib cage and abdominal muscles. Four layers of large, flat muscles form the ventral abdominal wall and are joined at the midline by a tendinous seam, the linea alba.

Reference Lines

For convenience in description, two methods are used to map the location of findings. The most common is the *quadrant method*, which divides the abdominal wall into four quadrants by imaginary vertical and horizontal lines bisecting the umbilicus. The quadrants are the right upper quadrant (RUQ), left upper quadrant (LUQ), right lower quadrant (RLQ), and left lower quadrant (LLQ) (Fig. 22-2). For most assessments and findings, this method is sufficient. A more specific method is to divide the abdomen into nine regions by drawing two vertical lines at the midclavicular lines (MCLs) and two horizontal lines, one beginning at the lower edge of the costal margin and the other beginning at the anterior-superior iliac spine of the iliac bones. The regions are named from right to left and top to bottom: right hypochondriac, epigastric, left hypochondriac,

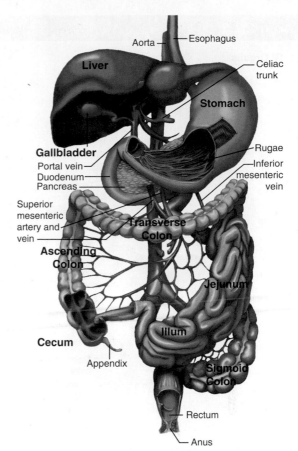

Figure 22.1 Overview of the GI system.

right lumbar, umbilical, left lumbar, right inguinal, hypogastric, and left inguinal. Findings that require a more specific location can be mapped to these regions (Fig. 22-3).

Abdominal Organs

GI Organs
The major GI organs found within the abdominal cavity include the stomach, small intestines, and colon (see Table 22-1). **Accessory organs** of the GI system within the abdomen include the liver, pancreas, and gall bladder (see Table 22-2).

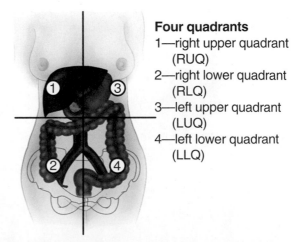

Four quadrants
1—right upper quadrant (RUQ)
2—right lower quadrant (RLQ)
3—left upper quadrant (LUQ)
4—left lower quadrant (LLQ)

Figure 22.2 Division of the abdomen into four quadrants.

Table 22.1   Major Organs of the GI/GU System

GI Organs

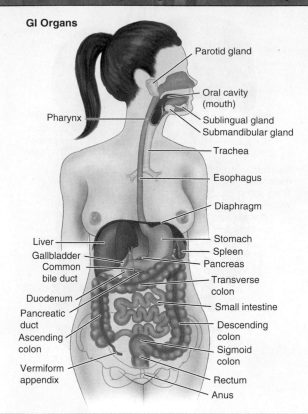

- Parotid gland
- Oral cavity (mouth)
- Pharynx
- Sublingual gland
- Submandibular gland
- Trachea
- Esophagus
- Diaphragm
- Liver
- Gallbladder
- Common bile duct
- Duodenum
- Pancreatic duct
- Ascending colon
- Vermiform appendix
- Stomach
- Spleen
- Pancreas
- Transverse colon
- Small intestine
- Descending colon
- Sigmoid colon
- Rectum
- Anus

GU Organs

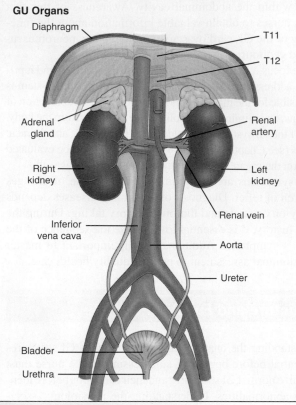

- Diaphragm
- T11
- T12
- Adrenal gland
- Renal artery
- Right kidney
- Left kidney
- Renal vein
- Inferior vena cava
- Aorta
- Ureter
- Bladder
- Urethra

Organ	Function
Esophagus	Propels food into the stomach, controlled by the cardiac sphincter—a one-way valve at the distal end
Stomach	Site for both mechanical and chemical digestion: Churns food into small particles that become liquid when mixed with gastric juices Stores food and slowly releases it into the small intestine Secretes hydrochloric acid to aid in digestion; mucus cells secrete substances to coat the stomach lining; chief cells secrete pepsinogen, which is converted to pepsin to aid in digestion of protein; secretes gastrin which stimulates secretion of acid and pepsinogen and increases gastric motility Secretes intrinsic factor that protects vitamin B_{12} from stomach acid and facilitates its absorption by the parietal cells in the small intestine Absorbs water, alcohol, and some medications Destroys some food-borne bacteria Allows emptying of stomach contents based on pressure gradient, a little at a time; gravity assists with emptying
Small intestine (18–20 ft in adults)	Propels contents by wormlike movements known as peristalsis Primarily responsible for absorption of nutrients

Table 22.1   Major Organs of the GI/GU System (*continued*)

Organ	Function
Duodenum (25 cm; 10 in)	Primary site for chemical digestion
	Enzymes, hormones, and bile from pancreas and liver enter and aid in absorption of nutrients:
	Peptidases help break down proteins.
	Enterokinase converts trypsinogen to active trypsin.
	Maltase, lactase, and sucrase break down carbohydrates.
	Cholecystokinin, secreted from duodenal wall, stimulates gallbladder to secrete bile.
	Gastric inhibitory peptide inhibits gastric motility.
	Secretin, secreted by duodenal wall, stimulates pancreatic secretions to neutralize gastric acid.
Jejunum (2.5 m or 8 ft) and ileum (3.5 m or 12 ft)	Absorb water, nutrients, and electrolytes for use in body
Large intestine (ascending and descending colon) (1.5–1.8 m or 5–6 ft)	Absorbs salt and water and excretes waste products of digestive process from the rectum (defecation)
	Aids in synthesis of vitamin B_{12} and K
Kidneys	Control blood pressure through the production of renin
	Stimulate red blood cell production by secreting erythropoietin
	Remove waste products filtered by the kidneys from the body
Bladder	Aids in the removal of waste products from the body in the form of urine
Aorta	Supplies oxygenated blood to the cells and organs of the lower half of the body

GU Organs

The organs of the GU system found within the abdominal cavity include the kidneys, ureters, and bladder; the spermatic cord in males; and the uterus and ovaries in females. Disease processes in these organs can produce abdominal symptoms.

The kidneys control blood pressure through the production of renin, stimulate red blood cell production by secreting erythropoietin, and remove waste products filtered by the kidneys

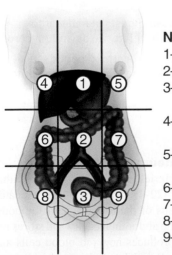

Nine regions
1—epigastric region
2—umbilical region
3—hypogastric or suprapubic region
4—right hypochondriac region
5—left hypochondriac region
6—right lumbar region
7—left lumbar region
8—right inguinal region
9—left inguinal region

Figure 22.3 Division of the abdomen into nine regions.

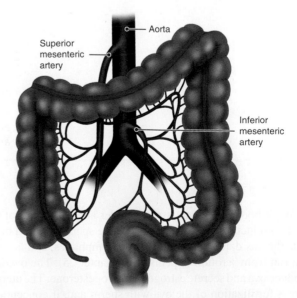

Figure 22.4 The aorta and branching arteries and veins within the abdominal cavity.

Table 22.2 Accessory Organs of the GI System

Accessory Organs	Function
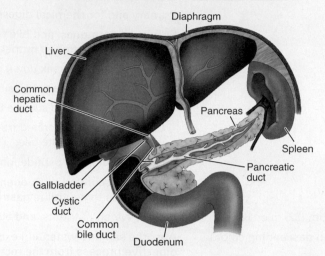	
Liver (located in RUQ)	Produces and secretes bile to emulsify fat
	Metabolizes protein, carbohydrates, and fats
	Converts glucose to glycogen and stores it
	Produces clotting factors, fibrinogen, and plasma proteins such as albumin
	Detoxifies drugs and alcohol
	Stores fat-soluble vitamins A, D, E, and K; vitamin B_{12}; and copper and iron
	Converts conjugated bilirubin from blood to unconjugated bilirubin
Gallbladder (located on back side of liver in RUQ)	Stores and concentrates bile
Pancreas (located in LUQ)	Endocrine functions:
	Secretes insulin and regulates blood glucose levels
	Secretes glucagons that store carbohydrates
	Inhibits insulin and glucagon secretion
	Secretes pancreatic polypeptide that regulates release of pancreatic enzymes
	Exocrine functions:
	Secretes digestive enzymes. Amylase digests starches into maltose. Lipase breaks down lipids into fatty acids and glycerol.
	Trypsinogen, chymotrypsinogen, and procarboxypeptidase are activated in the small intestine to break down proteins into amino acids.

from the body. The ureters and bladder aid with removal of waste products in the form of urine. The spermatic cord protects the vas deferens, blood vessels, lymphatics, and nerves that run from scrotum to penis (see Chapter 25). The ovaries produce ova and secrete estrogen and progesterone. The uterus allows fertilization of the ova with sperm and, if conception occurs, provides an environment for fetal development (see Chapters 26 and 27).

Blood Vessels, Peritoneum, and Muscles

The aorta and branching arteries and veins are found within the abdominal cavity (Fig. 22-4). They supply oxygenated blood to the cells and organs of the lower half of the body. The spleen also resides in the abdominal cavity and stores red blood cells and platelets, produces new red blood cells and macrophages, and activates B and T lymphocytes.

The **peritoneum**, mesentery, and muscles also make up the abdominal cavity. The peritoneum is a serous membrane that covers and holds the organs in place. It contains a parietal layer that lines the walls of the abdomen and a visceral layer that coats the outer surface of the organs. A small amount of fluid between these layers allows them to move smoothly within the cavity. The fan-like *mesentery* supplies blood vessels and nerves to the intestinal tract. The muscles protect and support the digestive system within the abdominal cavity. Muscles also assist with ingestion, mastication, and swallowing of food and with the voluntary defecation of its by-products.

Ingestion and Digestion

The digestive process consists of mechanical and chemical digestion. *Mechanical digestion* means the breakdown of food through chewing, peristalsis, and churning. *Chemical digestion* means the breakdown of food through a series of metabolic reactions with hydrochloric acid, enzymes, and hormones.

The digestive process begins in the mouth where food is ingested and mastication (chewing) begins. During this process, saliva mixes with the food and a bolus of food forms. The bolus passes into the oropharynx and esophagus, which propel the bolus via slow peristaltic movements into the stomach. In the stomach, the bolus is churned into a liquid, mixed with digestive juices and hydrochloric acid produced there. The liquid form is called chyme.

Absorption of Nutrients

Absorption of nutrients takes place almost exclusively in the small intestine. In the first portion of the small intestine, the *duodenum*, pancreatic juices and bile are secreted into the chyme, making it ready for absorption of nutrients by the many villi that line the walls of the *jejunum* and *ileum*. Each villus contains a blood vessel and a lymphatic vessel, which are responsible for nutrient absorption.

Elimination

Any food particles not absorbed by the small intestine pass into the large intestine, where a few electrolytes and water are further absorbed. Eventually, the remaining waste products are excreted as feces. On average, waste products of food ingested today are eliminated 48 hours later.

Lifespan Considerations

Pregnant Women
The abdomen changes dramatically in pregnancy. The abdominal muscles relax, allowing the uterus to protrude into the abdominal cavity to accommodate the growing fetus. The rectis abdominis muscles, which are located medially, become separated. As the fetus grows and takes up more room in the abdominal cavity, the stomach rises and may impinge on the diaphragm. Compression of the bowels by the uterus results in diminished bowel sounds. Thus, bowel activity decreases, which partly contributes to **constipation** in pregnant women.

Venous pressure in the lower abdomen increases, which may lead to hemorrhoids and further problems with elimination. During pregnancy, the appendix is displaced upward and laterally to the right, which can complicate the diagnosis of appendicitis in pregnant women. A darkly pigmented line, the linea nigra, appears in the midline of the anterior abdomen from pubis to umbilicus in many pregnant women. Near the end of pregnancy, the umbilicus may become everted, and **striae** (stretch marks) may develop on the skin of the abdomen. See also Chapter 27.

Newborns, Infants, and Children
Because of their small size, several anatomic differences related to the abdomen are found in infants. The newborn's bladder is located above the symphysis pubis. The liver takes up more space in the abdominal cavity and may extend 2 cm below the rib cage. The infant's abdominal muscles are not developed, so the abdomen of the infant usually protrudes. As the child grows, the abdominal protuberance becomes more obvious in toddlers and preschoolers because of the curvature of the back. It diminishes to adult proportions during adolescence. Because the abdominal muscles are underdeveloped, the organs are more easily palpated in children.

Older Adults
In older adults, production of saliva and stomach acid is reduced, and gastric motility and peristalsis slow. All these changes can lead to problems with swallowing, absorption, and digestion. Elderly people also have changes in dentition that may affect their ability to chew. Chewing difficulties, accompanied by limited financial resources, can dramatically alter dietary choices (less protein, more carbohydrates) and may result in painful mastication. All these factors along with generally reduced muscle mass and tone may contribute to constipation.

Fat accumulates in the lower abdomen in women and around the waist in men, making physical assessment more challenging. The liver decreases in size and liver function declines, making it harder for older adults to process medications.

Acute Assessment

If a patient has an acute abdominal problem, the history and physical examination will be focused on that problem and much of the history taking discussed next will be eliminated. Severe dehydration from nausea and vomiting, fever, and acute abdominal pain are potentially life-threatening symptoms that require prompt attention.

Subjective Data Collection

A comprehensive history normally precedes the physical assessment and involves asking the patient about his or her health status. It involves a broad range of questions to discern

Table 22.3   *Healthy People* Goals Related to Abdominal Health

Goals	Patient Education Topics
Increase the proportion of adults who receive a colorectal cancer screening examination.	Recommend assessments for health promotion including colonoscopy, sigmoidoscopy, and stool testing for occult blood.
Reduce the rate of new cases of end-stage renal disease.	Teach about risk factors for renal disease including control of high blood pressure.
Reduce cirrhosis deaths.	Perform CAGE screening for alcohol use at visits.

Source: *Healthy people 2010: What are its goals?* (n.d.). Retrieved June 7, 2010, from http://www.healthypeople.gov/About/goals.htm

possible problems associated with each organ and system within the abdomen. Approach the history from a head-to-toe direction and avoid skipping around with questioning. In many problems of the GI tract, a well-developed health history can point to a diagnosis 80% to 90% of the time. If time is an issue, a focused history on the abdomen will be sufficient.

Areas for Health Promotion/*Healthy People*

Healthy People (Chapter 1) describes focus areas that the U.S. government has identified for citizens to improve their health status. Three areas of focus involving the GI system include colorectal cancer, food-borne illness, and hepatitis (Table 22-3).

Colorectal cancer is the second leading cause of U.S. cancer deaths. The goal is to reduce death rates through educating patients about their risk factors and ensuring that every patient older than 50 years is appropriately screened for colorectal cancer (AHRQ, 2008).

Food-borne illnesses affect the very young, elderly, and immunocompromised patients most seriously. Risk of food-borne illness increases with emerging pathogenic organisms, improper food storage or preparation, an increasing global supply of foods, and inadequate training of food handlers. Food allergies, particularly to peanuts, are on the rise. Estimates are that food allergies affect almost 4% of children

younger than 6 years and 1% to 2% of adults (Eigenmann, et al., 2009). The goal for this risk factor is to reduce infections by food-borne pathogens and to reduce anaphylactic deaths from food allergies. Education about food handling in retail areas and at home as well as food labeling and proper preparation are the methods identified to achieve these goals.

Reducing the incidence of hepatitis A, B, and C is another *Healthy People* goal through screening, education, and immunization programs. Hepatitis C is the most common U.S. blood-borne viral infection. To date, no vaccine is available to prevent it. It is transmitted by contact with blood. Perinatal infection is the common mode of transmission of hepatitis B in infants. The infection rate among infants born to hepatitis B-positive mothers is 90% (Teo, et al., 2009). Identifying at-risk mothers and vaccinating them and their infants would reduce this transmission. In comparison, unprotected sexual intercourse and intravenous drug use are the major routes of hepatitis B spread in adults.

Assessment of Risk Factors

The nurse assesses current problems first, using symptom analysis. Then the nurse assesses personal and family history to assess genetic risk factors. After this initial history, the nurse assesses other risk factors and performs teaching about those that may be modified so that assessment is linked to health promotion and teaching.

Questions to Assess Risks	Rationales
Current Problems Are you having any abdominal problems now?	This question opens discussion with a general approach.
Have you had any unplanned changes in weight, either a loss or gain?	Unexplained weight changes may indicate undiagnosed *cancer, anorexia, bulimia, thyroid disorder*, psychosocial issues, or socioeconomic concerns.
Do you have any special dietary needs or concerns, or cultural or religious beliefs that affect your diet?	Special needs may indicate a nutrient imbalance or cause of symptoms. A 24-hour diet recall is helpful to determine what may be normal for the patient (see Chapter 8). If the patient has been sick for a prolonged period, ask what he or she "normally eats at each meal" rather than what was eaten in the previous 24 hours.

Questions to Assess Risks	Rationales
Have you had a fever or chills?	Fever may indicate an infection that could affect food or fluid intake.
Have you had any dizziness?	Dizziness may result from possible dehydration linked to inadequate fluid or caloric intake.
Family History Is there a family history of colorectal cancer in a first-degree relative?	Such a family history increases the patient's risk for this disease.
Do you have any family history of gastroesophageal reflux disease (GERD), peptic ulcer disease (PUD), inflammatory bowel disease (IBD), irritable bowel syndrome (IBS), anemia, thalassemia, or celiac disease?	Many of these conditions run in families.
Personal History How old are you?	Risk of colorectal cancer increases with age (Ahnen, et al., 2009). Colorectal cancer is the second leading cause of U.S. cancer deaths. It is often asymptomatic, but if caught early it is very curable.
Did you have a blood transfusion before the mid-1980s? Have you been vaccinated against hepatitis B?	Those who received blood transfusions prior to the mid-1980s (before the blood supply was tested for hepatitis B) may be at higher risk for the illness. Hepatitis B vaccine has been available to at-risk patients since the mid-1980s; since 1991, most U.S.-born infants have been vaccinated. Question patients about whether they received all three doses.
Do have a history of endometrial, ovarian, or breast cancer?	Personal history of endometrial, ovarian, or breast cancer also increases risk.
Have you ever had varicella?	Varicella, which always precedes herpes zoster (shingles), may appear along a dermatome on one side of the abdomen and back.
General GI Questions. Have you had any previous treatments or hospitalizations for GI problems such as GERD, PUD, IBD (either ulcerative colitis or Crohn's disease), IBS, anemia, thalassemia, or celiac disease?	The patient history may reveal an exacerbation of a previously diagnosed condition or a genetic predisposition or familial propensity for a particular disorder. Long-standing ulcerative colitis (more than 10 years) without remission increases the patient's risk for colorectal cancer. Crohn's disease may contribute to malnutrition or multiple surgical resections of the bowel, resulting in short gut syndrome.
Have you had any previous GI diagnostic tests such as stool for occult blood, colonscopy, upper GI series, barium enema, computerized tomography (CT) scan, or magnetic resonance imaging (MRI)?	
Do you have a history of previous abdominal or pelvic surgeries?	Previous surgeries increase risk for adhesions, infections, obstructions, and malabsorption. Appendicitis must be ruled out as the cause of the current problem.
Have you had any recent insertions of GI tubes?	GI tubes can be a source of infection.
Have you had any recent trauma, such as motor vehicle accident, occupational injury, or sports injury?	A history of trauma can provide insight into a previous surgery or injury, which may cause current symptoms.
Have you had any recent infection with mononucleosis?	Mononucleosis can cause hepatosplenomegaly.

(text continues on page 596)

Questions to Assess Risks	Rationales
Do you have a history of malabsorption disease?	This condition in self or family members may indicate lactose intolerance, food allergies, or celiac disease.
Do you have sickle cell anemia?	Abdominal pain is associated with *sickle cell crisis*.
Do you have history of eating disorders?	Eating disorders often begin in adolescence, with tendencies continuing into adulthood.
Have you ever had intestinal polyps?	History of intestinal polyps increases risk for colorectal cancer.
Chewing and Swallowing. Have you had any history of thyroid disease, neck masses, recent infection, vision changes, trouble swallowing, or sore throat?	Hypothyrodism or hyperthyroidism affects metabolism, weight, and elimination. Neck masses may indicate cancer or infection. Infections increase the caloric requirements. Visual changes may occur with nutritional imbalances. Difficulty swallowing may indicate an undiagnosed cancer or infection. Throat pain may impede swallowing. See also Chapter 14.
What is the date of your last dental assessment?	Poor dentition affects the intake of major food groups and nutritional status.
Breathing. Do you have a history of breathing problems, shortness of breath, or chronic obstructive pulmonary disease?	Respiratory problems diminish energy level and can decrease food intake. Some foods increase mucus in the throat. See also Chapter 18.
Weight Gain. Do you have a history of cardiovascular disease, high blood pressure, or congestive heart failure?	Weight gain and increased sodium in the diet can exacerbate these problems.
Genitourinary Issues. What is the color of your urine? Do you have any urinary burning, frequency, or urgency?	Dark urine can indicate inadequate fluid intake or blockage in the biliary system.
Do you have a history of sexually transmitted infections?	They may cause lower abdominal pain.
Females: What is the date of your last menstrual period?	Unplanned pregnancy is often a cause of nausea and vomiting.
Do you have any vaginal discharge?	Discharge may indicate an infection.
Males: Do you have a history of prostate problems?	An enlarged prostate may be a source of urinary difficulty and result in decreased intake of fluids.
Do you have any penile discharge?	Penile discharge may indicate a sexually transmitted infection.
Joint Pain. Do you have a history of fractures, joint pain, or weakness?	Joint pain may result in long-term use of nonsteroidal anti-inflammatory medications, which can cause GI bleeding. Joint issues may make food preparation difficult. Decreased mobility may result in constipation.
Neurological. How many alcoholic drinks do you have each day?	Excessive alcohol intake is the number one cause of liver disease. Excessive drinking may lead to decreased caloric intake.
Have you had any numbness, back problems, or loss of bowel/bladder control?	Numbness and changes in the bowel or bladder are symptoms of significant spinal injury.
Metabolism. Do you have a history of diabetes or thyroid problems?	Diabetes may cause polyphagia, polydipsia prior to diagnosis, improper carbohydrate metabolism, insulin resistance, and obesity.
	These are associated with an abnormal metabolism and weight changes.

Questions to Assess Risks	Rationales
Skin. Have you had any changes in your skin, hair, or nails?	Inadequate nutrition or imbalances in electrolytes or hormones may be exhibited in the skin, hair, or nails.
Have you had any rashes, itching, or lesions?	Rashes and itching suggest *liver disease* or malnutrition.
Lymphatic/Hematologic. Have you had any food allergies, infections, or sickle cell anemia?	Food allergies may cause belching, bloating, flatulence, diarrhea, or constipation. Sickle cell anemia may cause significant pain and anemia.
Medications Have you been taking any over-the-counter (OTC) or prescribed medications?	Patients will frequently take antacids that may interact with other medications.
Risk Factors **Alcohol or Substance Abuse.** Use the CAGE questionnaire if the patient has (or signs and symptoms lead you to suspect he or she has) a significant history of either alcohol or substance use (Gold, et al., 2009). See Chapter 10.	
Occupation • What is your profession? • Where do you work? • Are you vigilant about using personal protective equipment at work?	Health care workers are at high risk for hepatitis C, for which there is no vaccine.
Foreign Travel • Have you traveled to, or lived in, parts of the world where sanitation is less than optimal? • Have you eaten food prepared in places that are not sanitary? • Have you received the hepatitis A vaccine?	Hepatitis A is transmitted by the fecal-oral route, usually within 30 days of exposure. The disease is vaccine-preventable (Guerrant, et al., 2001).
Lifestyle • Do you use, or have you abused, IV drugs? • How many sexual partners have you had? • Have you ever had sex with sex workers?	Hepatitis B is transmitted through contact with bodily secretions (ie, blood, semen, saliva, and vaginal fluids) of infected people. Patients may not be aware of previous infection with it because symptoms may have felt like flu. Transmission time for hepatitis B is 6 weeks–6 months. Hepatitis C is the most commonly diagnosed form of hepatitis in the United States. It is transmitted through contact with the blood of infected people. IV drug users are at high risk for hepatitis C; 70% of patients with it develop serious liver complications of cirrhosis or hepatoma.

Risk Assessment and Health-Related Patient Teaching

Hepatitis A and B immunizations are recommended for all infants; people whose work may expose them to blood, body fluids, or unsanitary conditions (ie, health care, food services, sex workers); and those traveling to parts of the world where these illnesses are prevalent.

Risk of colorectal cancer increases with age. Initial screening for all people is recommended at 50 years, with serial fecal occult blood and colonoscopy for anyone whose results are positive. Follow-up screening is based on findings and risks, with colonoscopy repeated every 3 to 10 years.

Patient teaching concerning alcohol and substance abuse, and the possible effects on the organs in the abdomen, should be covered with all patients, especially those at high risk for abuse (see Chapter 10).

It is important to provide nutritional counseling to patients with food allergies, poor nutrition, and obesity at least annually, if not at every visit.

Focused Health History Related to Common Symptoms

The focused health history should address common symptoms of the abdomen: indigestion, anorexia, nausea, vomiting, hematemesis, abdominal pain, **dysphagia**, **odynophagia**, changes in bowel function, constipation, **diarrhea**, and jaundice. It should also include questions about the possibility of GU disorders. Additional questions can include suprapubic pain, dysuria, urgency, frequency of urination, hesitancy, decreased urine stream in males, polyuria, nocturia, urinary incontinence, kidney or flank pain, ureteral colic, pelvic pain, and vaginal discharge in females. Some common symptoms should be assessed in all patients to screen for the presence of GI disease. Nurses can use any special concerns from patients about GI problems to identify focal areas. A thorough history of symptoms assists with identifying a current problem or diagnosis.

Common Abdominal Symptoms

- Indigestion
- Anorexia
- Nausea, vomiting, hematemesis
- Abdominal pain
- Dysphagia, odynophagia
- Change in bowel function
  - Constipation
  - Diarrhea
- Jaundice/icterus
- Urinary/renal symptoms
  - Urinary incontinence
  - Kidney or flank pain
  - Ureteral colic

Questions to Assess Symptoms	Rationale/Abnormal Findings
Indigestion	
Have you had heartburn?	Heartburn suggests gastric acid reflux.
Do you have excessive gas, belching, abdominal bloating, or distention?	Increased intake of gas-forming foods, chewing gum, carbonated beverages, and motility problems can cause gas.
Have you noticed an unpleasant fullness after normal meals?	Gastric-emptying problems, outlet obstruction, and cancer can cause fullness.
Do you feel full shortly after eating? Are you unable to eat a full meal?	Early satiety can result from diabetic gastroparesis, anticholinergic drugs, or hepatitis.
Anorexia	
How is your appetite?	Loss of appetite can be related to stress, difficulty with ingestion, socioeconomic issues, age-related issues, or dementia.
Do you deliberately eat small meals?	With **anorexia nervosa**, food intake is intentionally limited.
Have you ever vomited after eating?	Bulimia is a disease in which the patient deliberately vomits after eating.
Nausea, Vomiting, Hematemesis	
Do you have nausea or vomiting? Have you ever vomited blood?	Nausea and vomiting may result from infections, food poisoning, or stress. Hematemesis may indicate gastric ulcer, gastritis, or esophageal varices from alcoholic cirrhosis.
Abdominal Pain	
Do you have any pain or discomfort?	Discerning pain characteristics can greatly assist in diagnosis of the problem by pinpointing the type of assessment and diagnostic procedures required:
• Location. Ask where the pain starts, and if it radiates or moves.	
• Intensity	• **Visceral pain** occurs when hollow organs are distended, stretched, or contract forcefully. It may be difficult to localize. The patient may describe it as gnawing, burning, cramping, or aching. If severe, it may be associated with sweating, pallor, nausea, vomiting, or restlessness.
• Duration	
• Description. Note if gnawing or sharp. Note if there is fever, chills, or pallor.	
• Aggravating factors	• **Parietal pain** results from inflammation of the peritoneum. It is usually severe and localized over the involved structure. Patients describe it as steady, aching, or sharp, especially with movement.
• Alleviating factors	
• Pain goal	• **Referred pain** occurs in more distant sites innervated at approximately the same spinal level as the disordered structure (see Chapter 7).
• Functional goal	

Questions to Assess Symptoms	Rationale/Abnormal Findings

Dysphagia/Odynophagia
- Do you have any difficulty swallowing or pain with swallowing?
- Does it feel like food gets stuck in your throat or esophagus?

Dysphagia may result from stress, esophageal stricture, GERD, or tumor.

Change in Bowel Function
What was your normal bowel pattern before symptoms developed?

The nurse needs to establish the patient's normal pattern, which may range from several times a day to once a week. This sets a basis for determining any current constipation or diarrhea.

Constipation. What is the change from your normal pattern? Are there any changes in your diet, medications, or physical activity?

Usually functional constipation results from inadequate fiber and fluids in the diet. It also can result from medications such as anticholinergics or narcotics.

Diarrhea
- What is change from your normal pattern?
- Is it associated with nausea/vomiting?
- Do you get diarrhea with a change in your diet, or only when you eat certain foods?
- Is there pain relieved with moving your bowels?

Diarrhea can result from an infection such as with *Clostridium difficile.* It also can be associated with food intolerances.

Jaundice/Icterus
Have you noticed a change in

- The color of your skin, sclera?
- The color of your urine or stool?

Jaundice can result from obstruction of the common bile duct by *gallstones* or *pancreatic cancer.*

Dark urine is from impaired excretion of bilirubin into the GI tract. Gray or light stool is common in obstructive jaundice.

Have you recently traveled to, or had meals in, areas of poor sanitation?

Recent travel may indicate exposure to hepatitis A.

Have you had any recent exposure to blood or body fluids of an infected partner, use of shared needles for IV drugs, or blood transfusion?

Exposure to blood or body fluids may indicate infection with hepatitis B or C.

Urinary/Renal Symptoms
Do you have

Many patients perceive these symptoms as abdominal in nature.

- Pain on urination or difficulty voiding (dysuria)

Pain may be from infection or irritation of either the bladder or urethra. Women often report internal urethral discomfort; men typically feel a burning proximal to the glans penis.

- Urgency or frequency of urination

Urgency may be from urinary tract or sexually transmitted infection.

- Suprapubic pain

Suprapubic pain is usually from *cystitis.*

- In males, hesitancy or decreased urine stream

Hesitancy may be from *benign prostatic hypertrophy (BPH).*

- Polyuria (how frequent?)

Polyuria is a common symptom of *diabetes.*

- Nocturia (how frequent)

Nocturia is usually from *BPH.*

- Hematuria, painful or not painful

Painful hematuria is usually the result of bladder infection in younger patients or renal calculi. Painless hematuria is common in older adults with urinary tract infections (UTIs) and patients with *bladder cancer.*

(text continues on page 600)

Questions to Assess Symptoms	Rationale/Abnormal Findings

Urinary Incontinence

- Do you ever leak urine, especially with coughing or sneezing?
- Have you had times where you could not make it to the bathroom fast enough?
- Have you ever lost urine before getting to the bathroom?

Patients need careful questioning on this topic, because they often do not volunteer this information from embarrassment. It may be the result of urinary sepsis, pelvic floor disorders, or multiparity.

Types of urinary incontinence are as follows:

- Stress: occurs with coughing, sneezing, or increasing intraabdominal pressure
- Urge: sudden urge and loss of continence with little warning
- Total: inability to retain urine, ask also about bowel incontinence

Kidney or Flank Pain. Do you have pain? Is it dull, achy, and steady? Did you have any burning, urgency, or bladder pain prior to its development?

Renal calculi and *pyelonephritis* can be causes of flank pain.

Ureteral Colic. Do you have severe, colicky pain in your flank? Is it associated with nausea or vomiting?

Ureteral obstruction of the ureters by blood clots or stones will cause a colicky cramping type of pain.

Documentation of Normal Findings

Patient reports normal appetite, no food intolerance, no excessive belching, no trouble swallowing, no heartburn, no nausea. Bowel movements are daily, brown in color, soft; denies changes in bowel habits, no pain with defecation, no rectal bleeding or black tarry stools. Denies hemorrhoids, passing of gas, constipation, or diarrhea. Denies abdominal pain. No jaundice, liver or gallbladder problems, no history of hepatitis. *D. Netter, RN*

 Lifespan Considerations

Additional Questions	Rationales/Abnormal Findings

Pregnant Women

Do you have heartburn, constipation, loss of urine, or hemorrhoids?

Heartburn occurs in 30%–50% of pregnant women. Bowel problems such as constipation, incontinence, and hemorrhoids are common during pregnancy and postpartum. Pregnant women commonly have abdominal bloating and constipation. Approximately, 30%–40% of them have hemorrhoids. Symptoms to assess include pruritus, discomfort, and bleeding (Bianco, 2009).

Newborns, Infants, and Children

Is the baby breast or bottle fed?

If bottle feeding, how does the baby tolerate the formula? What table foods have you introduced? How does the baby tolerate the food?

Consider formula or new foods possible allergens. Encourage parents to add only one new food at a time to help identify allergens.

How many wet diapers and bowel movements does your baby have in a day?

Early in life, feedings and diaper changes occur every 2–4 hours. As children grow and begin to eat solid foods, bowel movements decrease. Infants should have at least one bowel movement a day, more if breast fed.

How often does your toddler/child eat? Does he or she eat regular meals? How do you feel about your child's eating? Ask parent to describe previous day's eating, including meals and snacks.

Irregular eating patterns are common in young children and a source of great parental anxiety. As long as growth and development are normal and nutritious foods are offered, reassure parents.

Additional Questions	Rationales/Abnormal Findings
Does your child ever eat nonfoods: grass, dirt, paint chips?	*Pica* is the excessive ingestion of nonfoods. Most children attempt nonfoods at some time, but by 2 years, they should distinguish foods from nonfoods. Pica can be a source of *lead poisoning*.
Does your child have constipation? • If so, for how long? • What is the number of stools per day and week? • How much water and juice are in the child's diet? • Is constipation associated with attempts to toilet train? • What have you tried to treat the constipation?	Each child has his or her own "normal" bowel habits. Toilet training before a child is ready may result in the child withholding stool. Helping parents understand this to reassure them (van den Berg, et al., 2006).
Does your child have abdominal pain? Ask the parents to describe what they have noticed and when it started.	This symptom is difficult to assess in young children. Vague abdominal pain may be associated with unrelated organ systems, such as *otitis media* (see Chapter 16). It may also accompany inflammation of the bowel, constipation, UTI, and anxiety.
For the overweight child • How long has weight been a problem? • At what age, did it first appear? • Were there any changes in diet patterns at that time? • Describe the current diet pattern. • Do other family members have a weight problem? • How does the child feel about his or her own weight?	Reduced physical activity and food marketing practices contribute to the current obesity epidemic, as does intake of high fructose corn syrup in drinks and soda. Family history may contribute as well. Assess the child's body image.

Adolescents

What do you eat at regular meals? Do you eat breakfast? What do you eat for snacks? What do you like to drink? How many soft drinks/juice servings do you have per day?	Adolescents assume control of their eating and may reject family values. The only control parents may have is over what food is in the house, although they should still supply nutritional information to their children. Fast food is high in fat, calories, and salt and has little fiber.
What is your exercise pattern?	Boys need to eat an average of 3,000 cal/day to maintain weight and continue growth—the number of calories may be higher if boys participate in sports or regular exercise. Girls require 2,200 cal/day.
If weight is less than body requirements How much weight have you lost? Did you lose it by diet, exercise? How do you feel? Tired, hungry? How do you think your body looks? What is your activity pattern? Is the weight loss associated with any other body change (eg, menstrual irregularity)? What do your parents say about your eating? Your friends?	Screen any extremely thin adolescent (male or female) for *anorexia nervosa*. This serious psychosocial disorder involves loss of appetite, voluntary starvation, and excessive weight loss. People with anorexia may augment weight loss with purging (self-induced vomiting) and use of laxatives and diuretics. Denial of these feelings is common. Though these patients are thin, their distorted body image makes them think they are fat or disgusting. Patients with anorexia may have healthy activity patterns or exercise to the extreme. Amenorrhea is common in young women with anorexia. Eating disorders in teens constitute a family problem and warrant referral to a psychologist or an eating-disorder specialist.

Older Adults

How do you acquire your groceries and prepare meals?	Assess for risks for nutritional deficits: limited access to a grocery store, reduced income, compromised cooking facilities, physical disability (impaired vision, decreased mobility, decreased strength, neurological deficit).

(text continues on page 602)

Additional Questions	Rationales/Abnormal Findings
Do you eat alone or share meals with others?	Risks for nutritional deficit include living alone, not bothering or remembering to prepare meals, social isolation, and depression.
Ask for a 24-hour diet recall, starting with breakfast (see Chapter 8). • Do you have any trouble swallowing these foods? • What do you do right after eating—walk, take a nap?	A 24-hour recall may not provide sufficient information, because daily patterns may vary. Attempt to get a week-long diary of food intake. Food pattern may vary based on income.
How often do you move your bowels? Ask the patient to describe what is meant by constipation. • How much liquid and what types do you drink daily? • How much bulk, fiber, fresh fruits, and vegetables are in your diet? • Do you take anything for constipation? How often do you use it?	Many older adults have concerns about their bowel function. As the GI system changes with age, appetite may decrease, and constipation may result.
What medications do you take daily?	Consider GI side effects (eg, nausea, vomiting, anorexia, dry mouth) of all prescribed and OTC medications that the patient may take.

 ## Cultural Considerations

Additional Questions	Rationales/Abnormal Findings
African Americans Do you or your parents have sickle-cell disease or trait?	Sickle-cell anemia has an autosomal recessive inheritance pattern. Most states screen for the disease at birth. Symptoms begin to emerge in the second 6 months of life and include jaundice and splenomegaly.
Do you or does anyone in your family have Glucose-6-phosphate dehydrogenase (G6PD) deficiency?	G6PD is a drug-induced anemia caused by a genetic lack of the G6PD enzyme in the red blood cells. It is an X-linked recessive trait. Aspirin-containing medications, sulfonamides, antimalarials, and fava beans can trigger hemolysis.
Are you or is anyone in your family lactose intolerant?	Lactose intolerance tends to have a familial distribution and can develop at any age. Patients present with abdominal discomfort, bloating, belching, and diarrhea.
Asian Americans Do you have heartburn, indigestion, anorexia, or unplanned weight loss? Any family history of gastric cancer?	Incidence of gastric and primary liver cancers is increased in Asians. Because heartburn and indigestion are often treated with OTC preparations, patients may not report that they use them. Such medications may cover symptoms, leading to a delay in diagnosis until metastasis has occurred (Mandanick, et al., 2009).
Americans of Jewish Descent Is there any personal or family history of ulcerative colitis or Crohn's disease?	IBDs have a familial predisposition (Snapper, et al., 2009).
Is there any personal or family history of lactose intolerance?	Lactose intolerance may accompany the IBDs and cloud the history.
Americans of Mediterranean Descent Do you or does anyone in your family have lactose intolerance?	There is a familial predisposition as mentioned above.

Additional Questions	Rationales/Abnormal Findings
Do you or does anyone in your family have chronic anemia or thalassemia?	The thalassemias are a group of hereditary, hypochromic anemias. They are often confused with iron-deficiency anemia and lead poisoning but do not respond to iron supplementation. Minor pallor and splenomegaly may be present.
Native Americans • Do you drink alcohol? If so, how much and how often? • Have you ever had yellow skin or yellow eyes? • Have you had liver disease, gallbladder disease, or pancreatitis? • Do you have diabetes?	Alcoholism and diabetes are more prevalent in the Native American population.

Therapeutic Dialogue: Collecting Subjective Data

The nurse's role relative to subjective data collection is to gather information to improve the patient's health status and to help determine the cause of the patient's current symptoms. Remember Mr. Chase, introduced at the beginning of this chapter. This 41-year-old man was admitted to the hospital with a GI bleed that is related to his ongoing alcohol intake. In addition to obtaining an abdominal assessment, the nurse will assess Mr. Chase's needs to begin establishing a discharge plan.

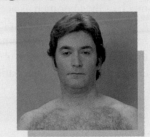

The following conversations give two examples of interview styles used by different nurses. One style is more effective than the other.

Less Effective

Nurse: Hi, Mr. Chase. We need to start thinking about where you're going after discharge. Do you have any plans?

Mr. Chase: No (pause).

Nurse: Where were you living before the hospital?

Mr. Chase: At the mission, why?

Nurse: We want to make sure that you have somewhere to go when you leave here. Are you homeless?

Mr. Chase: (pauses) I don't like living in that place. The people are too rough and dirty there. I'd rather live on the streets.

Nurse: Why are you living there?

Mr. Chase: Why do you think (irritated)?

Nurse: The chart said that you had a GI bleed and that you drink about nine shots a day.

Mr. Chase: I lost everything to alcohol—my wife, my family, my house. I just don't want to go back to that dirty mission.

Nurse: Why don't you stop drinking?

Mr. Chase: I've been through rehab twice. It doesn't help.

Nurse: Where else can you go?

More Effective

Nurse: Hi, Mr. Chase. We need to start thinking about where you're going after discharge. What are your thoughts?

Mr. Chase: I don't want to go back to that dirty mission. I would rather be on the streets than in there.

Nurse: Tell me more about that (pause).

Mr. Chase: The people are too rough, and I always get bedbugs there.

Nurse: It sounds like you don't like the mission, but we want you to have a safe place to go (pause).

Mr. Chase: I don't want to go there, but I've lost everything to alcohol—my wife, my kids, my house.

Nurse: Your drinking has created some problems for you. How are you feeling about quitting?

Mr. Chase: I've tried before, but it doesn't work.

Nurse: It's hard making a change. If you think that you're ready to try again, I could talk with a social worker about finding a rehab placement for you.

Critical Thinking Challenge

• Compare and contrast the questioning regarding alcohol use. Why is the second nurse more effective?
• How might your life experiences influence your attitude toward Mr. Chase?
• How does the more therapeutic nurse address the issue of homelessness?
• How might your values influence the patient assessment?

Objective Data Collection

Equipment

- Stethoscope
- Measuring tape
- Pen or marker
- Reflex hammer or tongue blade to ascertain abdominal reflexes
- Pillow placed under the knees to relax the abdominal musculature

Preparation

Make sure the environment is warm and private. Adequate lighting is essential. Have the patient empty the bladder before the assessment. He or she should lie supine with the arms at the sides. Using a sheet for draping, expose only as much of the abdomen as necessary as you proceed through the assessment. Be sure to explain what you are doing and to perform the assessment systematically, slowly, and without quick movements. Throughout, observe the patient's face for signs of discomfort. Distract the patient with questions or conversation to avoid tensing of the abdominal musculature, which will make the assessment more difficult and the findings obscure.

Clinical Significance 22-1

The order of assessment of the abdomen is different from previous systems. Inspection is followed by auscultation for bowel sounds *before* percussion and palpation. Failure to adhere to this order may result in the alteration of bowel sounds from either percussion or palpation, leading to inaccurate findings.

Common and Specialty or Advanced Techniques

The routine head-to-toe assessment includes the most important and common assessment techniques. Nurses may add specialty or advanced steps if concerns exist over a specific finding. Table 22-4 summarizes the most common techniques, which are therefore essential to learn for use in clinical practice. Additional techniques may be added if indicated by the clinical situation or used in advanced practice.

Table 22.4 Common Versus Specialty or Advanced Techniques for Abdomen

Technique	Purpose	Screening or Registered Nurse Assessment	Focused or Advanced Practice Examination
Inspect abdomen	To identify shape and contour	X	
Inspect urine	To identify if cloudy, clear, or with blood and to assess level of hydration	X	
Inspect emesis	To assess bleeding, hydration, acid-base balance	X	
Inspect stool	To assess for infection, *C. difficile*, need for drainage system	X	
Auscultate abdomen	To assess for sounds from peristalsis	X	
Percuss abdomen	To assess if normal, gas, or fluid filled		X
Percuss kidney	To assess for tenderness		X
Percuss liver	To measure size		X
Percuss spleen	To identify if enlargement is present		X
Percuss bladder	To evaluate if there is urine in the bladder		X
Perform bladder scan	To evaluate if there is urine in the bladder	X	
Lightly palpate abdomen	To assess overall impression	X	
Deeply palpate abdomen	To locate masses and organs		X
Palpate liver	To measure the size		X
Palpate spleen	To identify if enlargement is present		X
Palpate kidney	To assess for tenderness and enlargement		X
Test for fluid wave	To evaluate if gas or fluid		X
Test for shifting dullness	To evaluate if gas or fluid		X
Palpate abdominal aorta	To identify if there is enlargement		X
Palpate bladder	To evaluate if there is urine in the bladder		X
Palpate lymph nodes	To assess for inflammation and drainage		X
Assess abdominal reflex	To assess central neurological symptoms		X

Technique and Normal Findings	Abnormal Findings

Inspection

Inspect the abdomen. Look at the condition of the skin and umbilicus. Look at the abdomen for contour, peristaltic waves, and pulsations (Fig. 22-5). Inspect for size, shape, and symmetry. Note whether the umbilicus is inverted or everted and its position. Inspect from different angles to evaluate color, surface characteristics, contour, and surface movements. Note visible veins on the abdomen. Have the patient take a deep breath and bear down to determine any hernias or organomegaly.

Abnormal skin findings include scars, striae, and veins. The umbilicus may have a hernia or inflammation.

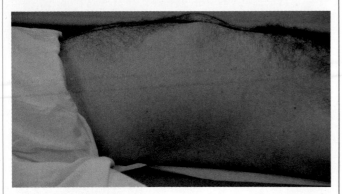

Figure 22.5 Inspecting the abdomen.

Assess for distention. If present, determine if it is generalized or only in one area. Ask the patient if the abdomen looks or feels different from normal. Inspect for any visible aortic pulsations, peristalsis, and respiratory pattern. Evaluate for ascites.

Several simultaneous conditions can cause distention. Consider all possible contributory factors. Abnormal contours include bulging flanks, suprapubic bulge of full bladder, enlarged liver or spleen, or a tumor. A peristaltic wave may indicate GI obstruction. It may be a normal finding in thin patients. Pulsation of the aorta may be increased and lateralized in an abdominal aortic aneurysm.

Urine. *Normal urine is clear and light yellow.*

Cloudy urine may indicate a UTI. Sediment may indicate kidney disease. Blood can be caused from renal injury, renal disease, or trauma to a catheter. Dark urine may be from dehydration.

Emesis. *There is no emesis.*

Medications or diseases may cause emesis. Green emesis usually results from reduced peristalsis with irritation. Coffee-ground emesis is digested blood; bloody emesis is an active bleed with undigested blood.

Stool. *Stool is soft and light brown.*

Foul-smelling stool may be from *Clostridium difficile*. This bacterial infection leads to very liquid and light brown stool. Dark stool can be from iron supplements or digested blood. Currant-jelly stool is noted with partially digested blood from GI bleeding.

Auscultation

Bowel Sounds. Auscultate all four quadrants for bowel sounds. Begin by placing the warmed diaphragm of

Bowel sounds increase and decrease and indicate GI motility. They may be hyperactive at a point above a

(text continues on page 606)

the stethoscope gently in one quadrant (Fig. 22-6). It is recommended to start at the point of the ileocecal valve, slightly right and below the umbilicus, and proceed clockwise. This is a very active area of bowel sounds. Bowel sounds are high-pitched gurgles or clicks that last from 1 to several seconds. *There are 5–30 clicks per minute or one sound every 5–15 seconds in the average adult. Sounds indicate bowel motility and peristalsis. If no sounds are audible, listen for up to 5 minutes.*

partial bowel obstruction and decreased or nonexistent below the point of obstruction. Increased bowel sounds occur with diarrhea and early intestinal obstruction. Decreased bowel sounds occur with *adynamic ileus* and *peritonitis*. High-pitched, tinkling bowel sounds indicate intestinal fluid, air under tension in a dilated bowel, and inadequate bowel sounds. High-pitched, rushing sounds indicate partial intestinal obstruction.

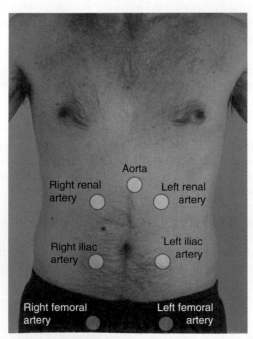

Figure 22.6 Auscultating the abdomen.

Vascular Sounds. Auscultate all four quadrants for vascular sounds. They are best heard with the bell of the stethoscope and include **bruits**, venous hums, and **friction rubs**.

Listen over the aorta in the epigastric region and over the renal and iliac arteries for bruits (Fig. 22-7).

Bruits sound like a swishing sound, which indicates turbulent blood flow from constriction or dilation of a tortuous vessel. Bruits in the hepatic area indicate *liver cancer* or alcoholic *hepatitis*. Bruits over the aorta or renal arteries indicate partial obstruction of the aorta or renal artery.

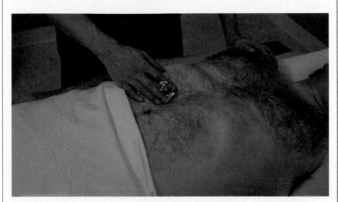

Aorta

Right renal artery

Left renal artery

Right iliac artery

Left iliac artery

Right femoral artery

Left femoral artery

Figure 22.7 Site for auscultating for bruits.

In the epigastric region, near the liver and over the umbilicus, venous hums are best heard (Fig. 22-8).

Venous hums are a soft-pitched humming noise with a systolic and diastolic component. They indicate partial obstruction of an artery and reduced blood flow to the organ.

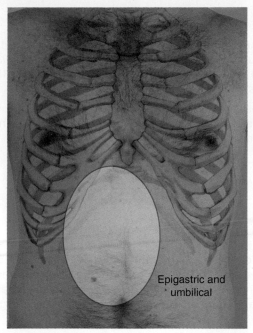

Epigastric and umbilical

Figure 22.8 Site for auscultating for venous hums.

Clinical Significance 22-2

Venous hums are a normal finding in children and pregnant women.

Lastly, auscultate over the liver and spleen for friction rubs (Fig. 22-9).

Friction rubs are grating sounds that increase with inspiration. They may indicate a *liver tumor*, *splenic infarction*, or *peritoneal inflammation*.

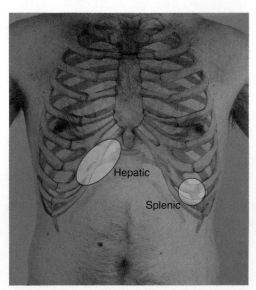

Hepatic

Splenic

Figure 22.9 Site for auscultating for friction rubs.

(text continues on page 608)

Percussion

Percussion is used to determine organ size and tenderness. It also detects any fluid, air, or masses in the abdominal cavity.

Percuss all four quadrants listening carefully for tympany or dullness. Ask the patient if there is abdominal pain. If an area is painful, percuss that area last. Ask the patient to point to the area of maximal tenderness and to suck in the abdomen. Place your hand 15 cm over the abdomen and ask the patient to push the stomach to your hand while coughing.

All these maneuvers move peritoneal surfaces without contact. Normal percussion findings include dullness over the liver in the RUQ and hollow tympanic notes in the LUQ over the gastric bubble. Over most of the abdomen, tympanic sounds should be heard and indicates the presence of gas.

Pain indicates peritoneal inflammation and can indicate a ruptured viscous in the area of the pain, *appendicitis* in RLQ, diverticulum in the LLQ, *cholecystitis* in the RUQ, or *cystitis* over the symphysis pubis.

Dullness may be heard over organs, masses, or fluid, such as ascites, GI obstruction, pregnant uterus, and an ovarian tumor.

Kidneys. Assessing kidney tenderness is accomplished by fist or blunt percussion at the costovertebral angle (CVA) posteriorly. (The CVA is where the rib cage meets the spine.) With the patient sitting, place the palm of your nondominant hand over the CVA and hit that hand with the fist of your dominant hand (Fig. 22-10). Repeat on the other side. *There is slight or no pain with fist percussion.*

Significant pain upon blunt percussion at the CVA is a positive sign and can be indicative of a kidney infection (pyelonephritis) or kidney stones, which cause stretching or inflammation of capsules surrounding these organs.

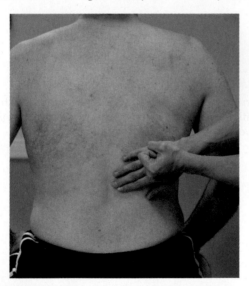

Figure 22.10 Percussing for kidney tenderness at the CVA.

Liver. A liver span test gives you an estimate of the size of the liver in the MCL. To assess the upper edge of the liver, start at the right MCL at the 3rd intercostal space (ICS) over lung tissue. Percuss down until you hear resonance change to dullness over the liver between the 5th and 7th ICS (Fig. 22-11). Place a mark where the dullness begins. To determine the lower border of the liver, start at the right MCL at the level of the umbilicus and percuss upward until tympany turns to dullness, usually at the sternal border, and mark this

Abnormal findings include hepatomegaly and the firm edge of *cirrhosis*.

area with a pen. Measure the distance between the two marks (Fig. 22-12).

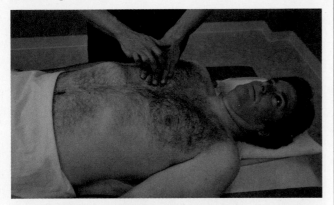

Figure 22.11 Percussing the liver.

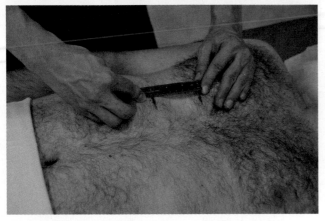

Figure 22.12 Measuring the liver border.

Liver span is 6–12 cm. If the liver span in the MCL is >12 cm, measure it in the midsternal line. Normal midsternal liver span is 4–8 cm (Fig. 22-13).

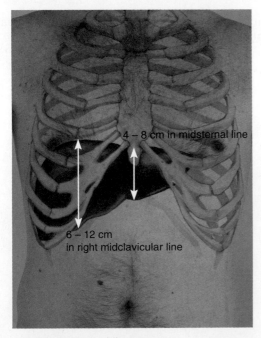

4 – 8 cm in midsternal line

6 – 12 cm
in right midclavicular line

Figure 22.13 Normal liver span.

(text continues on page 610)

Spleen. Three methods are used to assess the approximate size of the spleen:

1. Percuss from the left MCL along the costal margin to the left MAL. *If the nurse hears tympany, splenomegaly is unlikely.*
2. Percuss at the lowest ICS at the left MAL. Ask the patient to take a deep breath and hold it; percuss again. Tympany is normal, but with splenomegaly, tympany turns to dullness on inspiration.
3. Percuss from the 3rd–4th ICS slightly posterior to the left MAL, and percuss downward until dullness is heard. Dullness of the normal spleen is noted around the 9th–11th rib.

Bladder. Assessing bladder size is achieved by percussing for bladder distension. Begin at the symphysis pubis and percuss upward toward the umbilicus, noting any dullness. *An empty bladder does not rise above the symphysis pubis.*

Palpation

Light Palpation. Both light and deep palpations are used to assess the abdomen. Begin with light palpation in all four quadrants for a general survey of surface characteristics and to put the patient at ease. Press down 1–2 cm in a rotating motion, then lift your fingertips and move to the next location (Fig. 22-15). Observe for nonverbal signs of pain, such as grimacing and guarding. *No tenderness should be noted.* If guarding is present, place a pillow under the patient's knees and have him or her take a few deep breaths. While the patient is concentrating on breathing, lightly palpate the rectus abdominus muscles on expiration. The patient cannot voluntarily guard this muscle during expiration.

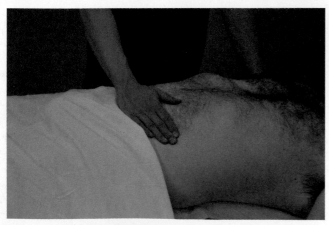

Figure 22.15 Lightly palpating the abdomen.

Dullness at the MAL is indicative of splenomegaly (Fig. 22-14).

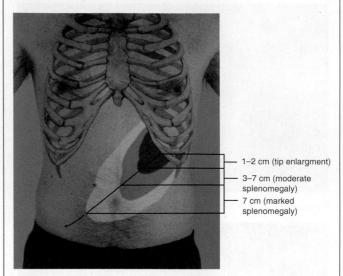

— 1–2 cm (tip enlargment)
— 3–7 cm (moderate splenomegaly)
— 7 cm (marked splenomegaly)

Figure 22.14 Indicators of splenomegaly.

Tenderness over the symphysis pubis may indicate a *UTI.*

⚠ *SAFETY ALERT 22.1*
Do not palpate the abdomen of patients who have had an organ transplant or of a child with suspected Wilms' tumor. Transplanted organs are often located in the anterior portion of the abdomen and not as well protected as the original placed organ. Palpating may cause the tumor to seed into the abdomen.

Involuntary guarding is a sign of possible peritoneal inflammation and should be carefully evaluated.

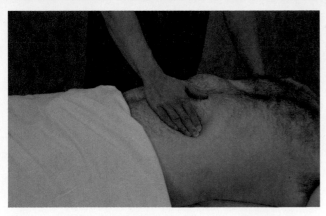

Figure 22.16 Single-handed deep palpation.

Deep Palpation. Deep palpation is used to assess organs, masses, and tenderness. To perform single-handed deep palpation, use the tips of your fingers and depress 4–6 cm in a dipping motion in all four quadrants (Fig. 22-16). *Tenderness may be noted in an adult near the xiphoid process, over the cecum, or over the sigmoid colon.* Bimanual deep palpation is necessary when palpating a large abdomen. Place your nondominant hand on your dominant hand and depress your hands 4–6 cm (Fig. 22-17).

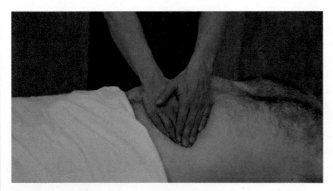

Figure 22.17 Bimanual deep palpation.

Liver. To palpate the liver, place your right hand at the patient's right MCL under the costal margin. Place your left hand on the patient's back at the 11th and 12th ribs; press upward to elevate the liver toward the abdominal wall (Fig. 22-18). Have the patient take a deep breath.

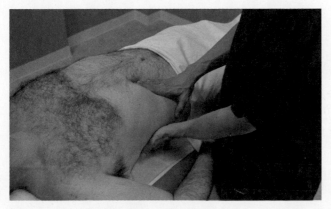

Figure 22.18 Pressing upward to elevate the liver.

If you find a mass, note its location, size, shape, consistency, tenderness, pulsation, mobility, and movement with respiration. Refer to Figure 22-1 for the location of abdominal and accessory organs. Size and changes over time offer insight into pathology and the extent of involvement.

An enlarged liver is palpable below the costal margin. Assess its size as described under "Percussion." An enlarged liver may indicate a *tumor* or *cirrhosis*.

(text continues on page 612)

Press your right hand gently but deeply in and up during inspiration. *The liver edge is palpable against your right hand during inspiration.*

The hooking technique is another method to palpate the liver. Place your hands over the right costal margin and hook your fingers over the edge. Have the patient take a deep breath and feel for the liver's edge as it drops down on inspiration, then rises up over your fingers on expiration (Fig. 22-19).

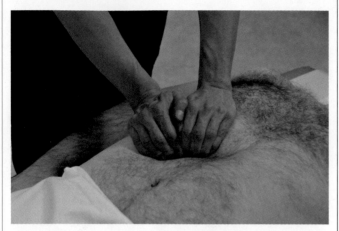

Figure 22.19 Using the hooking technique to assess the liver.

Spleen. To palpate the spleen, stand on the patient's right side. Place your left hand under the patient's left CVA and pull upward to move the spleen anteriorly (Fig. 22-20). Place your right hand under the left costal margin. Have the patient take a deep breath; during exhalation, press inward along the left costal margin and try to palpate the spleen. An alternative approach is to have the patient turn onto the right side to move the

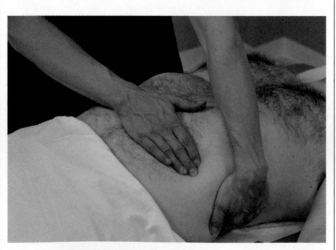

Figure 22.20 Placing the hand under the patient's left CVA to move the spleen.

In an enlarged spleen, you can palpate the spleen tip. Enlarged spleen occurs with *mononucleosis, HIV, cancers* of the blood and lymph, infectious *hepatitis,* and red blood cell abnormalities of *spherocytosis, sickle-cell anemia,* and thalassemia.

spleen more forward (Fig. 22-21). *A normal spleen is not palpable.*

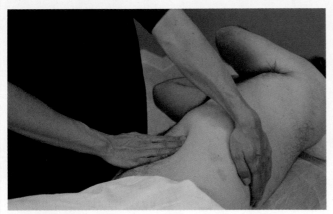

Figure 22.21 Palpating the spleen with the patient on the right side.

Kidneys. To assess the left kidney, stand on the patient's right side and place your left hand in the left CVA. Place your right hand at the left anterior costal margin. Have the patient take a deep breath; then press your hands together to "capture" the kidney. As the patient exhales, lift your left hand and palpate the kidney with your right hand (Fig. 22-22).

Kidneys enlarged from *hydronephrosis* or *tumors* may be palpable.

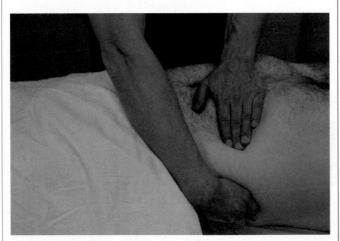

Figure 22.22 Palpating the left kidney.

To assess the right kidney (only palpable if enlarged), remain on the patient's right side, place your right hand on the right CVA, and your left hand on the right costal margin. When the patient exhales, palpate the right kidney (Fig. 22-23). *It is common to be unable to palpate the kidneys except in slender patients.*

(text continues on page 614)

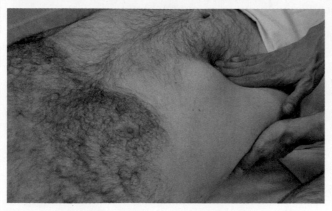

Figure 22.23 Palpating the right kidney.

Abdominal Aorta. To palpate the abdominal aorta, place your fingers in the epigastric region and slightly toward the left of the MCL. Palpate for aortic pulsations on either side of the aorta (Fig. 22-24). You can assess the width of the aorta by placing one hand on either side of the aorta. *Pulsations of the aorta are palpable; the aorta should measure 2 cm.*

An enlarged aorta (>3 cm) or one with lateral pulsations that are palpable can indicate an abdominal aortic aneurysm (*AAA*).

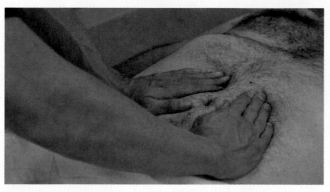

Figure 22.24 Palpating for aortic pulsations.

Bladder. Palpate the bladder using deep palpation in the hypogastric area. *The empty bladder is neither tender nor palpable.*

A palpable bladder is either full or enlarged from an underlying mass arising in the bladder or pelvis. A tender bladder usually indicates a *UTI*.

Lymph Nodes. Inguinal lymph nodes lie deep in the lower abdomen and can be palpated using the pads of your fingers just below the inguinal ligament for the superficial superior nodes and along the inner aspect of the upper thigh for the superficial inferior nodes. They drain the exterior iliac, pelvic, and paraaortic areas. *Inguinal lymph nodes are nontender and slightly palpable.*

If nodes are palpable, note size, shape, mobility, consistency, and tenderness. Enlarged nodes indicate an infection in the regions drained, such as *orchitis* in males, an infection of the lower extremities, or metastatic disease from the anus or vulva.

Assessing for Ascites

Assessing for *ascites*, which is detectable only after 500 mL of fluid has accumulated, is done in two ways: shifting dullness or fluid wave.

Ascites is found in patients with *cirrhosis* or primary or metastatic tumors of the liver.

Shifting Dullness. Shifting dullness can be detected by percussing dullness in the umbilical area when the

Dullness will move to the most dependent area.

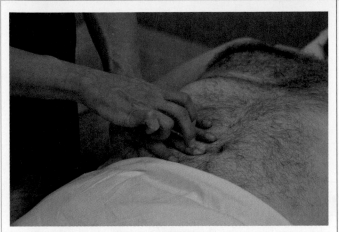

Figure 22.25 Percussing for dullness in the umbilical area with the patient supine.

patient is supine (Fig. 22-25), then having the patient lie on the right side and percussing again (Fig. 22-26). You can repeat this maneuver by having the patient turn to the left side.

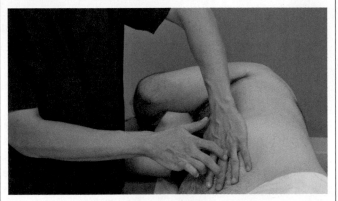

Figure 22.26 Percussing for dullness in the umbilical area with the patient turned to the side.

Fluid Wave. Have the patient place his or her hand vertically in the middle of the abdomen. Place your hands on both sides of the patient's abdomen and tap one side while palpating the other (Fig. 22-27).

If ascites is present, the tap will cause a fluid wave through the abdomen and you will feel the fluid with the other hand.

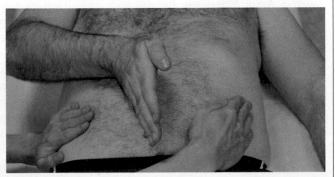

Figure 22.27 Assessing for a fluid wave to determine presence of ascites.

(text continues on page 616)

| **Technique and Normal Findings** (continued) | **Abnormal Findings** (continued) |

Eliciting the Abdominal Reflex

The abdominal reflex is a superficial cutaneous reflex measured by stroking the abdomen lightly with a tongue blade or the handle of a reflex hammer. The abdomen is stroked in all four quadrants toward the umbilicus. *The umbilicus moves toward the stimulus. This reflex may be masked and not determinable in obese patients.*

The abdominal reflex is absent in patients with upper and lower motor neuron diseases. See Chapter 24.

Documentation of Normal Findings

Abdomen is flat with active bowel sounds, soft, and nontender; no masses or hepatosplenomegaly. Liver span is 6 cm in the R MCL; liver edge is smooth and palpable 1 cm below the right costal margin. Spleen and kidneys not palpable. No CVA tenderness. *D. Netter. RN*

 ## Lifespan Considerations

Age-related changes that may be revealed during the physical assessment were discussed in the earlier sections on lifespan and cultural considerations. A brief review is presented here.

Pregnant Women

Assessing the abdomen of a pregnant woman can be very challenging. During pregnancy, abdominal muscles relax and the uterus protrudes into the abdominal cavity. The rectus muscles, which are normally aligned medially, separate, increasing the tendency for hernias later. The stomach rises from the increasing size of the uterus and may impinge on the diaphragm. Many women complain of increasing heartburn and indigestion as the pregnancy progresses. The uterus compresses the bowels, which may diminish bowel sounds. The enlarged uterus leads to increased venous pressure in the abdomen. The appendix is displaced upward and laterally to the right, making it more difficult for practitioners to diagnose appendicitis. A dark line, the linea nigra, may appear midline from the symphysis pubis to umbilicus. The umbilicus may evert. Stretch marks (striae) may appear as the abdominal wall and skin stretch to accommodate the enlarging uterus. See also Chapter 27.

Infants and Children

The abdominal musculature is less developed in infants and children who also have a much larger liver proportionately. The liver may protrude more than 2 cm below the ribcage. The less developed abdominal musculature makes the contents of the abdomen more palpable and results in a normally protuberant abdomen. The bladder is found above the symphysis pubis. This situation resolves in adolescence, when abdominal assessment findings become similar to those for normal adults.

Older Adults

Many elders are plagued with poor dentition, which may result in pain when chewing, dramatic changes in diet and weight, and long-term problems. Decreased production of saliva and stomach acid leads to changes in the digestive process. Motility and peristalsis decrease with age, which may result in more bloating, distention, and constipation. Also contributing is decreased muscle mass and tone. Fat accumulates in the lower abdomen of women and around the waist of men, making inspection more challenging and inaccurate. Liver size is smaller and the liver becomes less functional, resulting in less absorption of medications metabolized by the liver.

 ## Cultural Considerations

Certain health problems are more common in certain races and ethnic groups. African Americans more commonly present with sickle-cell anemia, G6PD deficiency, and lactose intolerance. Those with sickle-cell disease may have splenomegaly and jaundice on examination. In sickle-cell crisis, patients may present with complaints of acute abdominal pain and vomiting. Lactose intolerance may cause abdominal cramping and diarrhea. **Obesity**, defined as weight greater than 20% of ideal weight, is generally higher in racial and ethnic minorities than in Caucasians. It is highest in non-Hispanic black women. See also Chapter 8.

GI cancers, especially stomach cancer, are more often seen in Asian Americans. Patients with these illnesses present with long-standing complaints of heartburn, indigestion, anorexia, and weight loss. Asian Americans have a higher incidence of infection with *Helicobacter pylori*.

Lactose intolerance and IBD are more prevalent in Americans of Jewish ancestry. The most common presenting symptoms are abdominal cramping, diarrhea, and rectal bleeding. Ashkenazi Jews have a greater incidence of colon cancer than other groups and are believed to carry a gene linked to the development of familial colorectal cancer.

Americans of Greek and Italian descent more commonly present with lactose intolerance, thalassemia, and anemia. These illnesses cause abdominal cramping, **diarrhea**, jaundice, and splenomegaly.

Alcoholism, liver and gall bladder disease, pancreatitis, and diabetes are more common in Native Americans.

You have just finished conducting a physical assessment of Mr. Chase, the 41-year-old Caucasian man admitted to the hospital with a GI bleed. Review the following important findings revealed in each step of objective data collection for this patient. Consider how these results compare with the normal findings presented in the samples of normal documentation.

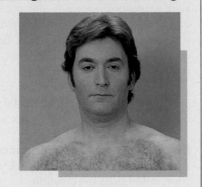

Inspection: Abdomen distended symmetrically. Umbilicus everted with significant ascites. Skin jaundiced with prominent venous network. Abdominal girth is 85 cm. Weight has decreased from 65 to 55 kg. Height 178 cm. Arms and legs lack muscle mass and tone.

Auscultation: Bowel sounds hyperactive in all four quadrants. No bruits present.

Palpation: Abdomen firm and slightly tender with muscle guarding. Lower border of the liver palpated 4 cm below the sternal border at the right MCL. Fluid wave and shifting dullness are present. No masses present, liver smooth.

Percussion: Lower border of the liver percussed 4 cm below the sternal border at the right MCL. Abdomen tympanic at the dome of the abdomen, flanks slightly dull.

K. Erickson, RN

GI symptoms in this group include jaundice, anorexia, ascites, abdominal pain, steatorrhea, weight loss, polyuria, polydipsia, polyphagia, and weakness.

Lactose intolerance is common among all cultural groups. In Europe and the United States, approximately, 7% to 20% of Caucasians are lactose intolerant. Approximately, 80% to 95% of Native Americans, 65% to 75% of Africans and African Americans, and 50% of Hispanics are intolerant. In eastern Asia, 90% may be intolerant (Montgomery, et al., 2009).

Evidence-Based Critical Thinking

The world of clinical decision making is uncertain. It is rare that the decision is absolutely positive or negative. Most situations involve a level of uncertainty for both health care providers and patients. The health care team will seek out additional clinical information such as laboratory studies or radiologic procedures only if these methods can change what is done for the patient. This form of decision making is called "wait and see" or "watchful waiting."

The nurse must be very clear to the patient as to what constitutes a change that requires further inquiry. Symptoms may evolve and a clearer clinical picture may emerge, or symptoms may resolve without intervention.

Nurse practitioners and other advanced health care providers construct a differential diagnosis by grouping symptoms that are present and absent and weighing the probability that a condition exists against the penalty for being wrong. Each provider compiles his or her own data and then constructs an argument for a particular disease based on the facts. The strength of the case depends on how information is gathered and analyzed.

Diagnostic decision making initially involves a search for the simplest possible explanation. The next step involves asking what other explanation exists. A differential diagnosis should be logical and listed from most to least likely. The list should highlight conditions that cannot afford to be missed— those that would result in significant morbidity and mortality. Strange symptoms and findings more likely represent an uncommon presentation of a common problem. The last step is asking what, if anything, can be done to rule out the "worst case scenarios" and how quickly.

Common Laboratory and Diagnostic Testing

Few specific laboratory tests focus on the abdomen and GI system. A complete blood count should be done to determine signs of anemia and infection. Iron-deficiency anemia in men, postmenopausal women, and elderly patients always warrants an endoscopy and colonoscopy to rule out GI cancer.

A basic metabolic panel (BMP) gives a good overview of various changes that can result from the malfunction of abdominal organs. Glucose level gives an indication of pancreatic endocrine function. The electrolytes Na, K, Cl, and CO_2 point to the state of the patient's hydration, which may be affected by vomiting or dehydration. The blood urea nitrogen (BUN) and creatinine are indicators of basic kidney function. Liver function tests (including ALT and AST) indicate the health of the liver. These levels remain normal until there is significant liver compromise. To determine the exocrine function of the pancreas, amylase and lipase levels indicate the status of these enzymes, which are necessary to digestion and absorption of nutrients. These studies would need to be added to the BMP.

If ulcer disease is suspected, a breath test for *H. pylori* is indicated. It is imperative that this test be done before any acid reducers (especially the proton pump inhibitors) are ordered to assist with pain relief (Malfertheiner, et al., 2007). If a patient has been taking OTC proton pump inhibitors, he or she must stop the medication for 2 weeks before the breath test will be accurate.

Several specialized tests are performed to identify specific problems along the alimentary canal and its accessory organs. These tests are briefly discussed below.

Esophagogastroduodenoscopy

Esophagogastroduodenoscopy (EGD), also called endoscopy, determines the condition of the mucosa of the esophagus, stomach, and duodenum. The patient is usually given conscious sedation, and the back of the throat is numbed with a spray anesthetic. The scope is passed, and the entire upper GI tract is assessed through pictures taken and biopsies of any abnormalities. EGD is usually ordered and performed in patients with suspected ulcer disease or cancer of the esophagus or stomach.

Barium Enema

Barium enema is a radiologic procedure in which the patient receives an enema of barium sulfate to outline the large intestine. This test helps determine if the patient has IBD or cancer of the colon. It can be done as single contrast with only the barium, or double contrast in which the barium is removed after the initial part of the assessment, air is inserted, and a closer look at the walls of the colon is possible.

⚠ SAFETY ALERT 22.2

A barium enema should not be performed on a patient suspected of having an acute inflammatory condition, such as appendicitis, diverticulitis, or ulcerative colitis, or a perforated hollow organ. The barium enema can cause an inflamed area of the bowel to rupture, and death can result.

Colonoscopy

Colonoscopy is done to determine the general condition of the colon and rectum and is used to determine polyps, ulcerations, and tumors of those entities. It is recommended as standard practice for patients older than 50 years as screening for colorectal cancer. The patient is given conscious sedation, the colonoscope is passed, and the entire length of the colon is visualized. Pictures of the walls of the colon are taken, and small polyps and tumors can be removed and biopsied as part of this test. This test requires preprocedure preparation of the bowel to remove all feces to enable the most accurate results.

Endoscopic Retrograde Cholangiopancreatography

Endoscopic retrograde cholangiopancreatography is performed to assess the ducts draining the liver and pancreas, to identify and remove gall stones in the common bile duct, and to diagnose pancreatic cancer. Similar but more extensive than the EGD, the patient receives conscious sedation, and the scope is passed through the mouth into the stomach and duodenum to the area of the ducts.

Computerized Tomography Scan

CT scan is a radiologic procedure performed with and without contrast to identify soft tissue problems that may arise in the abdominal cavity. Cysts, abscesses, infections, tumors, aneurysms, and enlarged organs such as the liver and gall bladder may be identified in this manner.

Magnetic Resonance Imaging

MRI is a radiologic procedure performed in a large magnetic tube. It is used to evaluate the condition of organs, ducts, and blood vessels. Patients with pacemakers, ventricular assist devices, and joint replacements cannot undergo MRI, because the magnetic force can cause problems with the metal components of their embedded life-sustaining equipment.

Diagnostic Reasoning

Table 22-5 provides a comparison of nursing diagnoses, abnormal findings, and interventions commonly related to the abdominal assessment (NANDA-I, 2009).

Nurses use assessment information to identify patient outcomes. Some outcomes that are related to system problems include:

- Diarrhea: Patient will defecate a formed soft stool every day to every third day.
- Constipation: Patient will maintain the passage of soft, formed stool every 1 to 2 days without straining.
- Patient will report relief from or decrease in the incidence and severity of incontinent episodes (Moorhead, et al., 2007).

Once the outcomes are established, nursing care is implemented to improve the status of the patient. The nurse uses critical thinking and evidence-based practice to develop the interventions. Some examples of nursing interventions for the GI system are as follows:

- Diarrhea: Consider inserting tube into rectum to drain stool and prevent skin breakdown.
- Constipation: Make sure to monitor last bowel movement and administer bulk, stool softeners, and laxatives as ordered.
- Incontinence: Teach patient to pace fluids and avoid fluids before bedtime (Bulechek, et al., 2007).

The nurse then evaluates care according to the patient outcomes that were developed, therefore reassessing the patient and continuing or modifying interventions as appropriate. An accurate and complete nursing assessment is an essential foundation for holistic nursing care. Even as a beginner, the nursing student can use the patient assessment to implement new interventions, evaluate the effectiveness of those interventions, and make a difference in the quality of patient care.

Table 22.5   Common Nursing Diagnoses Associated with the Abdomen

Diagnosis and Related Factors	Point of Differentiation	Assessment Characteristics	Potential Interventions
Imbalanced nutrition, less than body requirement related to nausea and vomiting	Dietary intake that is inadequate in quantity, quality, or both for metabolic needs	Body weight decreased, BMI less than normal	Provide nutritional supplements, eg, shakes. Administer antiemetics as ordered*
Diarrhea related to effects of bowel inflammation	At least 3 liquid stools per day	Passage of loose, unformed stools	Obtain stool specimens to determine infection, eg, *C. difficile* infection
Constipation related to immobility	Decrease in normal frequency of defecation with hard, dry stool	Abdominal distention, pain, tenderness, firm abdomen, no stool for days	Obtain order for stool softener if patient is on opioids, increase intake of fiber, assist with ambulation, assure adequate intake of fluids
Incontinence related to decreased level of consciousness	Involuntary passage of urine occurring with sudden desire to urinate (urge)	Voiding more than every 2 hours while awake, awakening at night to urinate, voiding more than eight times in a 24-hour period	Review medications that may contribute to incontinence, perform bladder scan to evaluate if residual is present, teach principles of bladder training.

*Collaborative interventions.

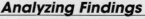

Analyzing Findings

Remember Mr. Chase, whose problems have been outlined throughout this chapter. The initial subjective and objective data collection is complete, and the nurse has spent time reviewing the findings and other results. Unfortunately, Mr. Chase vomits bright red blood, so it is necessary to reassess him and document the findings. The following nursing note illustrates how subjective and objective data are collected and analyzed and nursing interventions are developed.

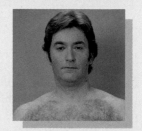

Subjective: I just felt it coming on fast. I knew I shouldn't have eaten that food. Am I going to have to go back to the ICU?

Objective: Vomited 250 mL of emesis with partially digested food and about 20% with bright red blood. Gastroccult tested positive for blood. T 37°C tympanic, P 124 beats/min, R 24 breaths/min, BP 100/62 mm Hg, oxygen saturation 93%. Sitting in bed with head of bed elevated. Abdomen slightly tender, firm, and distended with hyperactive bowel sounds. Tympany present over most of abdomen. Patient states feeling nauseous, fatigued, and anxious.

Analysis: Fluid volume deficit due to GI blood loss.

Plan: Saline lock intact. Notify primary provider about emesis. Inform patient about plans and assure that the nurse will be readily available if needed. Provide oral hygiene and hold food or fluids until discussed with provider. Administer medication for nausea according to physician orders.

K. Erickson, RN

Critical Thinking Challenge

- Why is information on the vital signs included as part of the nursing note?
- How has the nurse altered the assessment focus from the earlier conversation about discharge planning?
- What additional information might be documented on patient flow sheets?

Collaboration with Other Health Care Providers

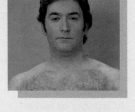

Mr. Chase, admitted 5 days ago with a GI bleed, is having a new onset of bleeding. The new bleeding, drop in blood pressure, and increase in pulse need collaborative interventions, so the physician needs to be contacted. The following conversation illustrates how the nurse might organize the data and make recommendations about the patient's situation to the physician.

Situation: Hi Dr. Plete. This is Kathy on 3 East. I'm taking care of Mr. Chase, a 41-year-old patient on your team.

Background: He was admitted 5 days ago with GI bleed and has been stable for the past few days.

Assessment: He just vomited 250 mL of emesis with partially digested food and about 50 mL of blood; the gastroccult was positive. His pulse is P 124 beats/min, R 24 breaths/min, BP 100/62 mm Hg, and oxygen saturation is 93%. Usually, his pulse is around 100, and the blood pressure is about 150/90 mm Hg. He has a saline lock in but no IV fluids, and I just gave him the as-needed antinausea medication.

Recommendations: I'll see if that works in a half hour. For now I've asked him to have nothing by mouth and was wondering if you wanted me to start IV fluids. I can also call lab to have them order a stat hemoglobin and hematocrit. He has three units of packed red blood cells on hold if they are needed. What would you like to do?

K. Erickson, RN

Critical Thinking Challenge

- Consider all the objective data that were collected. Why did the nurse omit some of the physical assessment findings previously documented in the SOAP note?
- Which of the assessments are within the nursing domain and which are within collaborative practice with the physician?
- What further assessments will you perform, and how frequently?

Pulling It All Together: Reflection and Critical Thinking

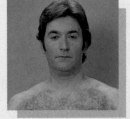

The nurse uses assessment data to formulate a nursing care plan for Mr. Chase. After completing interventions, the nurse will reevaluate Mr. Chase and document findings in the chart to show critical thinking. This is often in the form of a care plan or case note similar to the one below.

Nursing Diagnosis	Patient Outcomes	Nursing Interventions	Rationale	Evaluation
Fluid volume deficit	Maintain blood pressure and pulse within normal limits	Monitor P and BP every 15 minutes until stable. Assess for signs of hypovolemia including postural hypotension, poor skin turgor, thirst, sunken eyeballs, and weakness. Also monitor intake and output and daily weights. Assess IV site for infection, inflammation, and infiltration.	Decreased intravascular volume results in decreased tissue oxygenation. Signs of hypovolemia may be noted with continued bleeding or insufficient replacement. The IV site may be a source of infection because the skin is broken.	IV fluids started with normal saline at 100 mL/h.* IV site without redness, tenderness, or swelling. Patient placed on nothing by mouth. No further episodes of vomiting, no stools. BP 122/66 mm Hg, P 110 beats/min, skin turgor poor, eyeballs sunken, states feeling better.

*Collaborative interventions.

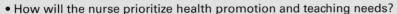

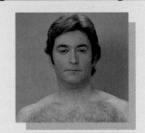

Using the previous steps of diagnostic reasoning, organizing, and prioritizing, consider all of the case study findings woven throughout this chapter. When answering the following questions, begin drawing conclusions and see how the pieces of assessment must work together to create an environment for personalized, appropriate, and accurate care.

- How will the nurse prioritize health promotion and teaching needs?
- How does the nurse incorporate the different phases of the nursing process when performing the assessments?
- What information from other body systems might be useful to assess?
- How will the nurse organize the assessment during the shift?

Key Points

- Auscultation of the abdomen is always performed before percussion and palpation, which can alter bowel motility and diminish the nurse's ability to hear bowel sounds.
- The nurse assesses tender areas last to avoid referred pain.
- The elderly are less likely to feel pain with abdominal conditions and do not always present with classic symptoms and laboratory findings. They are more likely to have vague, diffuse pain and tend to have a less acute presentation.
- Patients who present with fever, chills, leukocytosis, and rebound tenderness warrant a rapid assessment and referral to an acute care facility.
- Abdominal pain lasting more than 6 hours or pain that wakes a patient from sleep requires evaluation and possible referral.
- Hypoactive bowel sounds are common in patients with constipation and paralytic ileus.
- Hyperactive bowel sounds are common in patients with gastroenteritis and diarrhea.
- The location of the bruit sound can determine the cause of the bruit.
- Venous hums are continuous sounds found in the epigastric region and around the umbilicus and caused by portal hypertension.
- Eighty to ninety percent of GI diseases can be diagnosed by obtaining a thorough history.
- The liver takes up more space in the abdominal cavity of an infant and may extend 2 cm below the rib cage.
- As the fetus grows and the uterus enlarges into the abdominal cavity of a pregnant woman, the stomach rises up and may impinge on the diaphragm.
- Colorectal cancer is the second leading cause of U.S. cancer deaths.
- Food-borne illnesses affect the very young, the elderly, and immunocompromised patients more seriously.
- Hepatitis C is the most common blood-borne U.S. viral infection.

Review Questions

1. When performing an abdominal assessment, what is the correct sequence?
   A. Inspection, palpation, percussion, auscultation
   B. Palpation, percussion, inspection, auscultation
   C. Inspection, auscultation, percussion, palpation
   D. Auscultation, inspection, palpation, percussion

2. A patient reports a long history of changes in bowel pattern. Which is the BEST question to determine normal bowel habit?
   A. How often do you have a bowel movement?
   B. What was your bowel pattern before you noticed the change?
   C. Is there a family history of IBD?
   D. Have any of your parents or siblings had cancer of the colon?

3. When palpating the abdomen, the nurse notices a mass in the LUQ, lateral to the MCL. Which organ is involved?
   A. Liver
   B. Spleen
   C. Sigmoid colon
   D. Left kidney

4. What percussion sound is heard over most of the abdomen?
   A. Resonance
   B. Hyperresonance
   C. Dullness
   D. Tympany

5. A patient with a history of kidney stones presents with complaints of pain, hematuria, and nausea with vomiting. What assessment technique will illicit kidney pain?
A. Rosving's sign
B. Psoas sign
C. Fist percussion for CVA tenderness
D. Blumberg's sign

6. When auscultating the abdomen, the nurse hears a bruit to the right of the midline slightly below the umbilicus. The nurse documents this finding as a bruit of which of the following?
A. Right renal artery
B. Right femoral artery
C. Right iliac artery
D. Abdominal aorta

7. A patient with a history of cirrhosis tells the nurse that his or her abdomen seems to be getting larger and that he or she has gained 20 lb in the last 6 months. How will the nurse determine whether the abdominal enlargement is from accumulation of fluid or fat from the weight gain?
A. Listen for a fluid wave.
B. Percuss the abdomen with the patient in different positions.
C. Palpate lightly and note the movement on the surface.
D. Inspect the abdomen with the patient in different positions.

8. A patient with a protuberant abdomen complains of pain in the RUQ. Which sign would the nurse expect to be positive?
A. Murphy's sign
B. Psoas sign
C. Rosving's sign
D. Obturator sign

9. Which assessment technique would best confirm splenic enlargement?
A. Deep palpation under the left costal margin
B. Fist percussion of the spleen with the patient in a sitting position
C. Deep palpation over the RUQ with the patient lying on the right side
D. Percussion to estimate the size of the spleen and gentle palpation

10. When documenting a finding in the region over the stomach and above the umbilicus, the nurse would identify the region as
A. epigastric
B. hypogastric
C. RUQ
D. LUQ

References

Ahnen, D. J., Finlay A, Macrae, F. A., et al. (2009). *Epidemiology and risk factors for colorectal cancer*. Retrieved August 19, 2009, from http://www.uptodateonline.com.proxy.seattleu.edu/online/content/topic.do?topicKey=gi_dis/33858&selectedTitle=1~150&source=search_result

AHRQ. (2008). *Screening for colorectal cancer*. Retrieved August 19, 2009, from http://www.ahrq.gov/CLINIC/USPSTF/uspscolo.htm

Bianco, A., Lockwood, C. J., & Barss, V. A. (2009). *Maternal gastrointestinal tract adaptation to pregnancy*. Retrieved August 19, 2009, from http://www.uptodateonline.com.proxy.seattleu.edu/online/content/topic.do?topicKey=antenatl/10888&selectedTitle=2~150&source=search_result

Bulechek, G. B., Butcher, H. K., & McCloskey Dochterman, J. (2007). *Nursing Interventions Classification (NIC)* (4th ed.) St. Louis: Mosby.

Eigenmann, P. A, Scott, H., Sicherer, S. H., & TePas, E. (2009). *Pathogenesis of food allergy*. Retrieved August 19, 2009, from http://www.uptodateonline.com.proxy.seattleu.edu/online/content/topic.do?topicKey=food_al/7762&selectedTitle=2~100&source=search_result

Gold, M. S., Aronson, M. D., Schwenk, T. L., et al. (2009). *Screening for and diagnosis of alcohol problems*. Retrieved August 19, 2009, from http://www.uptodateonline.com.proxy.seattleu.edu/online/content/topic.do?topicKey=subabuse/8392&selectedTitle=17~112&source=search_result.

Guerrant, R. L., Van Gilder, T., Steiner, T. S., et al. (2001). Practice guidelines for the management of infectious diarrhea. *Clinics in Infectious Disease, 32,* 331.

Madanick, R. D., Shaheen, N. J., et al. (2009). *Early gastric cancer*. Retrieved August 19, 2009, from http://www.uptodateonline.com.proxy.seattleu.edu/online/content/topic.do?topicKey=gicancer/6577&selectedTitle=2~150&source=search_result

Malfertheiner, P., Megraud, F., O'Morain, C., et al. (2007). Current concepts in the management of *Helicobacter pylori* infection: The Maastricht III Consensus Report. *Gut, 56,* 772.

Montgomery, R. K., Grand, R. K., Büller, H. A., et al., (2009). *Lactose intolerance*. Retrieved August 19, 2009, from http://www.uptodateonline.com.proxy.seattleu.edu/online/content/topic.do?topicKey=gi_dis/13325&selectedTitle=1~77&source=search_result

Moorhead, S., Johnson, M., & Mass, M. (2007). *Nursing Outcomes Classification (NOC)* (4th ed.). Philadelphia: Mosby.

North American Nursing Diagnosis Association. (2009). *Nursing diagnoses, 2009–2011 Edition: Definitions and classifications (NANDA NURSING DIAGNOSIS)*. West Sussex UK: John Wiley & Sons.

Snapper, S. B., Podolsky, D, K., Rutgeerts, P., et al. (2009). *Epidemiology and genetic and environmental factors in inflammatory bowel disease*. Retrieved August 19, 2009, from http://www.uptodateonline.com.proxy.seattleu.edu/online/content/topic.do?topicKey=inflambd/8588&selectedTitle=1~150&source=search_result

Teo, E. K., Lok, A. S. F., Kaplan, S. L. (2009). *Epidemiology, transmission and prevention of hepatitis B virus infection.* Retrieved from http://www.uptodateonline.com.proxy.seattleu. edu/online/content/topic.do?topicKey=heptitis/11026&selected Title=2~150&source=search_result on August 19, 2009.

van den Berg, M. M., Benninga, M. A., & Di Lorenzo, C. (2006). Epidemiology of childhood constipation: A systematic review. *American Journal of Gastroenterology, 101,* 2401.

The Jensen suite offers these additional resources to enhance learning and facilitate understanding of this chapter:

• thePoint on line resource, http//thepoint.lww.com/Jensen1E
• Student CD-ROM included with the book
• *Laboratory Manual for Nursing Health Assessment: A Best Practice Approach*
• *Pocket Guide for Nursing Health Assessment: A Best Practice Approach*

Table 22.6   Abnormal Abdominal Findings

Common Sites of Referred Pain. Abdominal pain may present with pain directly over the organ involved or the pain may be referred to a site where the organ was located in fetal development because the human brain has no felt image for internal organs. During fetal development, the organs migrate to their final location, but the nerves persist in the former location, and the patient feels the referring sensation. Pain in referred areas without representative history or other physical findings may not have an abdominal origin.

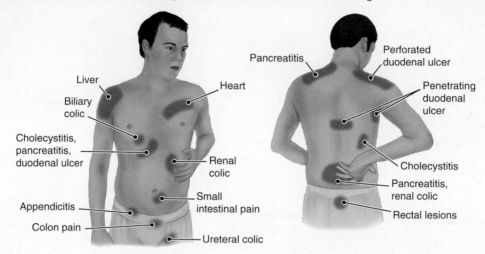

Abdominal Distention. Abdominal distention occurs for a variety of reasons including obesity, gaseous distention, tumors, and ascites.

Obesity

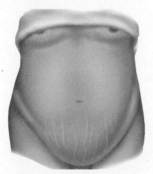

Obesity causes protuberance of the abdomen resulting in a thickened abdominal wall and fat deposits in the mesentery and omentum. Percussion sounds over an obese abdomen present as normal tympanic sounds.

Gaseous Distention

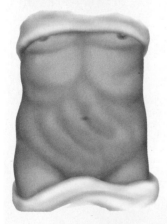

Gaseous distention is a result of increased production of gas in the intestines from the breakdown of certain foods and fluids. The average adult passes 500 mL of gas per rectum per day. It is also associated with altered peristalsis in which gas cannot move through the intestine. The altered peristalsis is seen in paralytic ileus and intestinal obstruction. Gaseous distention can be found in one area or generalized over the entire abdomen. Percussion sounds will be tympanic over the area of distention.

Table 22.6 **Abnormal Abdominal Findings** (*continued*)

Finding	Description

Abdominal Tumor

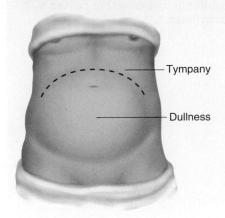

- Tympany
- Dullness

A large abdominal tumor also produces abdominal distention. The abdomen over a tumor is firm to palpation and dull to percussion. Ovarian and uterine tumors are common types of palpable tumors in the abdominal cavity, despite their pelvic origin. As the organs enlarge from the tumor, their mass protrudes into the abdominal cavity.

Ascites

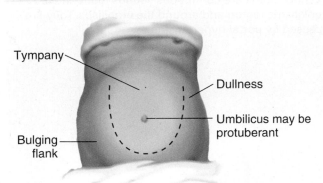

- Tympany
- Dullness
- Umbilicus may be protuberant
- Bulging flank

Ascites is the accumulation of fluid in the abdomen. The fluid descends with gravity resulting in dullness to percussion in the lowest point of the abdomen based on patient position. Changing the patient's position should move the fluid shift to the most dependent point. Ascites occurs in cirrhosis of the liver, CHF, nephrosis, peritonitis and metastatic neoplasms.

Abnormal Bowel Sounds. Auscultation of the abdomen results in bowel, vascular, and rubbing sounds. Bowel sounds may be hyperactive or hypoactive and occur in any quadrant of the abdomen. Hyperactive sounds are common in gastroenteritis and diarrhea. Hypoactive sounds are common in constipation and paralytic ileus. High-pitched bowel sounds with cramping are commonly heard in intestinal obstruction.

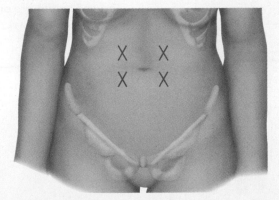

Abnormal Vascular Sounds. The most common abnormal vascular sound is a bruit. Its sound is blowing. Depending on location of the sound, the cause of the bruit can be determined. Bruits located in the midline below the xiphoid process are caused by aortic obstruction. Bruits located at the left and right costal borders at the MCL are caused by stenosis of the renal arteries. Other vascular sounds include venous hums and friction rubs.

(table continues on page 626)

Table 22.6 **Abnormal Abdominal Findings** (*continued*)

Finding	Description
Bruits 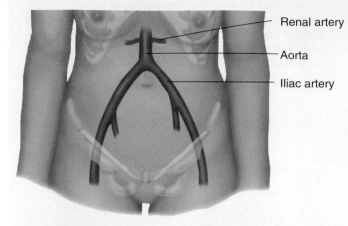	Bruits located at the left and right MCL between the umbilicus and the anterior iliac spine are caused by stenosis of the iliac arteries.

Renal artery

Aorta

Iliac artery

| **Venous Hums** 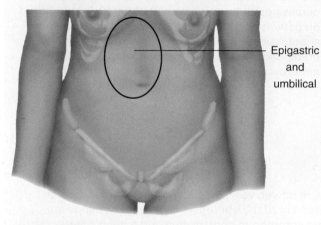 | Venous hums are continuous sounds found in the epigastric region and around the umbilicus. They are caused by portal hypertension. |

Epigastric
and
umbilical

| **Friction Rubs** 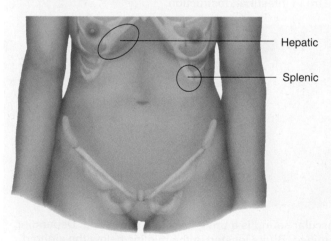 | Friction rubs are harsh, grating sounds found in the RUQ and LUQ, over the liver and spleen. They are caused by tumors or inflammation of the underlying organs. |

Hepatic

Splenic

Table 22.7 Common Tests for Abdominal Problems

Abdominal Problem	Special Techniques/Rationale
Acute Abdomen 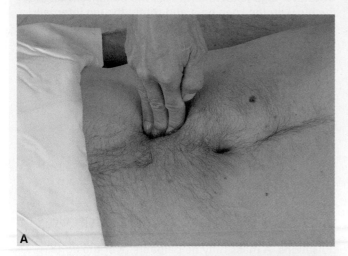 **A** 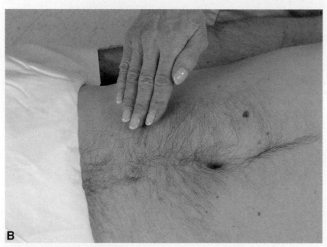 **B**	Apply light and deep palpation. A firm, board-like abdominal wall suggests *peritoneal inflammation.* Guarding occurs when the patient flinches, grimaces, or reports pain during palpation. Check for **rebound tenderness** (tenderness greater when you quickly withdraw your hand from the point of the pain [A] than when you press slowly on the tender area [B]), which also suggests *peritoneal inflammation.*
Appendicitis 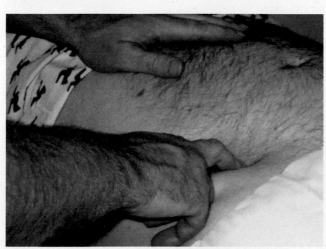	In classic appendicitis, the patient reports pain beginning at the umbilicus and moving to the RLQ. If you ask the patient to cough, he or she reports pain in the RLQ. The patient has local tenderness on palpation in the RLQ, at McBurney's point. A rectal examination, or in women, a pelvic examination, will reveal local tenderness, especially if the appendix is retrocecal. Other peritoneal findings include the following: **Rovsing's sign (shown left):** press deeply and evenly in the LLQ, and quickly withdraw your fingers. The patient reports pain in RLQ during LLQ pressure, suggesting appendicitis. **Psoas sign:** Place your hand just above the patient's R knee. Ask the patient to raise that thigh against your hand and turn to the left side. Extend the R leg at the hip to stretch to **iliopsoas** muscle. A positive sign is pain in the RLQ with this maneuver, suggesting appendicitis or peritoneal inflammation.

(table continues on page 628)

Abdominal Problem	Special Techniques/Rationale

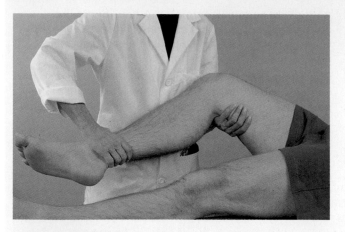

Obturator sign (shown left): Flex the patient's R thigh at the hip with the knee bent and rotate the leg internally at the hip, which stretches the internal obturator muscle. RLQ pain constitutes a positive obturator signs, suggesting an inflamed appendix or peritoneal inflammation.

Abdominal Aortic Aneurysm

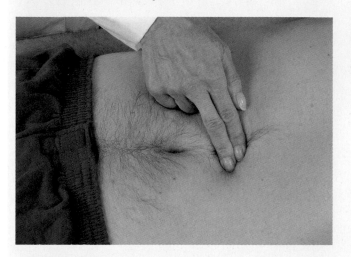

Patients complain of boring, tearing pain, and referred pain. Auscultation reveals bruits or exaggerated pulsations. A mass may be palpable over the aorta. Femoral pulses may be diminished or diffuse. Patients may seem in shock: hypotensive; tachycardic; tachypneic; pale, cool, clammy skin; cool extremities.

Acute Cholecystitis

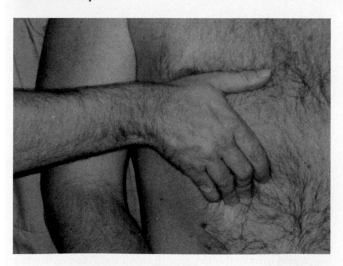

Auscultate, percuss, and palpate the abdomen for tenderness. Bowel sounds may be active or decreased. Tympany may increase with an ileus. There may be RUQ tenderness.

Assess for Murphy's sign by hooking your thumb under the right costal margin at the edge of the rectus muscle (as shown to the left); ask the patient to take a deep breath. Sharp tenderness and a sudden stop in inspiratory effort constitutes a positive Murphy's sign, suggesting cholecystitis.

Disease	Signs and Symptoms
Cancer of the stomach	This form of cancer, difficult to detect on physical examination, is associated with epigastric distress, abdominal fullness, anorexia, and weight loss. In late stages, patients may have ascites, a palpable liver mass, and lymph node enlargement.
Cancer of the colon	Colon cancer occurs most frequently in the descending and sigmoid colon and rectal areas. Patients report changes in bowel habits, blood in stool, and smaller diameter of bowel movement. Pain may accompany late stages of rectal cancer. A palpable mass may be found on rectal examination or on deep palpation of the LLQ.
Constipation	Results from slow, delayed movement of feces through the intestine. Bowel sounds may be diminished on auscultation. You may be able to palpate feces in the LLQ with deep palpation. Palpation in general may be uncomfortable depending on the amount of feces and the length of time it has been present.
Diverticulitis	Diverticula are common outpouchings of the walls of the intestine in which feces may get trapped, causing inflammation, possible infection, abscess, and perforation. Patients present with severe pain (usually LLQ), diminished bowel sounds on auscultation, nausea, vomiting, and a long history of constipation. Peritoneal signs (see appendicitis) may be present if the bowel perforates. The patient may report that he or she had "left-sided appendicitis."
Hernias	Hernias may be found in the inguinal area, umbilical area, or along an old incision. Inguinal hernias are more uncomfortable with long periods of standing and diminish with rest. Patients may complain of feeling full when straining to defecate.
	Umbilical hernias usually resolve in early life. Their protrusion worsens with crying. Incisional hernias become incarcerated or strangulated more frequently than other types. Incarceration involves the loop of intestine becoming "stuck" in the scar tissue of the incision. Strangulation is compromise of the blood supply to the loop of bowel, resulting in death of the tissue involved. It constitutes a surgical emergency.
	A hiatal hernia causes the stomach to move through the esophageal opening and rise above the diaphragm. Symptoms include acid reflux, esophageal constriction, and subsequent esophageal damage.
IBD	This inflammatory condition involves all layers of the GI tract and can occur anywhere from mouth to anus. Problems of malnutrition and vitamin absorption are common. Abdominal pain is not relieved with defecation. Diarrhea and steatorrhea are common.
Crohn's disease	Crohn's involves the mucosal and submucosal layers of the colon. It increases the risk for colon cancer if not in remission after 10 years; it can also cause bowel perforation and toxic megacolon.
Ulcerative colitis	Colitis presents with cramping pain in the lower abdomen, relieved with defecation. Watery diarrhea with mucus in the stool and rectal bleeding are common. Surgery that removes the colon can cure the problem.
IBS	Also known as spastic colon, this condition has symptoms of diarrhea, constipation, or both. It usually presents as intermittent constipation, with hard compacted stools, and abdominal pain relieved by defecation. Many patients have a range of stools from pebbles to liquid over several days.
Liver failure	Liver failure can develop within 2–8 weeks of onset of jaundice. It results from the acute onset of massive necrosis of liver cells, leading to sudden and severe impairment of liver function. Causes include acetaminophen toxicity, *viral hepatitis*, drug reaction, toxins (mushroom poisoning), *ischemic hepatitis*, *autoimmune hepatitis*, and the fatty liver of pregnancy.
Pancreatitis	This inflammation of the pancreas alters the flow of digestive enzymes to the small intestine. Symptoms include nausea, vomiting, weight loss, severe boring pain in LUQ, and referred pain to the back or shoulder.
Paralytic ileus	Lack of peristalsis, usually in the small intestine, may follow surgery, peritonitis, or spinal cord injury. The presentation is intermittent, colicky pain, with visible peristaltic waves on inspection and vomiting. Bowel sounds are absent. The abdomen is distended. Prompt attention is necessary to prevent bowel necrosis or perforation.

(table continues on page 630)

Disease	Signs and Symptoms
Peritonitis	This inflammation of the lining of the abdominal cavity presents with fever, nausea, and vomiting. Findings include abdominal pain of varying character, cutaneous hypersensitivity, abdominal rigidity, and guarding. Bowel sounds are diminished. Positive signs include psoas, obturator, Rovsing's, and Murphy's.
Pyelonephritis	Auscultate, percuss, and palpate the abdomen for tenderness. Bowel sounds may be active or decreased. Tympany may increase with an ileus; there may be tenderness anteriorly over the affected kidney on deep palpation. Check for CVA tenderness on the posterior thorax to be positive over the inflamed kidney.
Splenic rupture	This serious abdominal condition resulting in hemorrhage usually follows abdominal trauma, but can accompany mononucleosis from an enlarged spleen, which is subsequently traumatized. Presentation is severe LUQ pain, radiating to the left shoulder. Hemorrhagic shock can develop.
Ulcer	Ulcers form when gastric mucosa becomes permeable, protective mucus is reduced as a result of inflammation, or exposure to bile or other irritating substances (eg, medications, alcohol) is prolonged. *Gastric ulcers* present with gnawing pain, heartburn, anorexia, vomiting (possible hematemesis), eructations, and weight loss. *Duodenal ulcers* present with intermittent RUQ pain 2–3 hours after eating. Stools may be positive for occult blood.

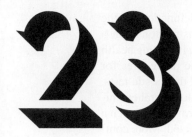

Musculoskeletal Assessment

Learning Objectives

1 Identify the structures and functions of the musculoskeletal system.

2 Identify teaching opportunities for health promotion and risk reduction related to the musculoskeletal system.

3 Collect subjective data related to the musculoskeletal system, including pain assessment and history of presenting symptoms.

4 Collect objective data on posture, gait, mobility, balance, and coordination.

5 Identify normal and abnormal joint range of motion (ROM) and muscle strength.

6 Use subjective and objective data from assessment of the musculoskeletal system to analyze findings and plan interventions.

7 Document and communicate data from musculoskeletal assessment using appropriate medical terminology.

8 Individualize musculoskeletal health assessment considering the condition, age, gender, and culture of the patient.

9 Use musculoskeletal assessment findings to identify diagnoses and initiate a plan of care.

*M*rs. Gladys Runningbird is an 82-year-old Native American who recently fell, requiring hospitalization. Twelve days ago, she was transferred from the hospital to a skilled nursing facility. Today, her temperature is 36.6°C orally, pulse 82 beats/min, respirations 18 breaths/min, and blood pressure 122/64 mm Hg. Current medications include alendrolate sodium (Fosamax) for osteoarthritis. Supplements are a multivitamin, vitamin D, calcium, and magnesium.

You will gain more information about Mrs. Runningbird as you progress through this chapter. As you study the content and features, consider Mrs. Runningbird's case and its relationship to what you are learning. Begin thinking about the following points:

- How are physiological and psychological data connected?
- What are some potential nursing diagnoses based on this patient's problem list? Provide rationale.
- What items will the nurse assess as part of a comprehensive musculoskeletal assessment? What other assessments should the nurse add?
- What are expected findings for Mrs. Runningbird based on her age? What findings would be associated with osteoarthritis?

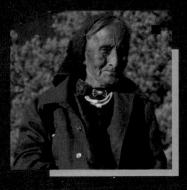

This his chapter discusses the structure and function of the musculoskeletal system. It provides instructions for a comprehensive musculoskeletal assessment, including health history, physical examination (with specific procedures for joint problems), and related laboratory and diagnostic tests. A patient would undergo a complete musculoskeletal examination during the first visit to a health care provider or when a condition that involves all the joints is suspected. More commonly, patients undergo focused assessments on a specific area with injury or pain, such as a shoulder, knee, or elbow.

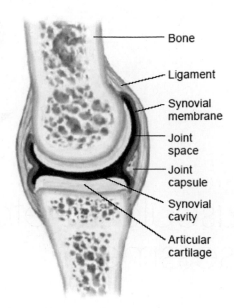

Figure 23.1 Example of a synovial joint.

Structure and Function Overview

The musculoskeletal system is composed of skeletal muscle and five types of connective tissues: bone, **cartilage**, **ligaments**, **tendons**, and **fascia**. Muscles and bones facilitate movement through the joints, or **articulations**. Connective tissues are located all around the muscles, bones, and joints and serve protective functions. The more elastic connective tissue found around a joint, the greater the ROM in that joint. The specialized forms of connective tissue in the musculoskeletal system are described in Table 23-1.

Bones

Bone is a living structure made up of a tough organic matrix strengthened by deposits of calcium phosphate. There are two types of bones: **compact bone**, which forms the shaft and outer layer, and spongy or **cancellous bone**, which makes up the ends and center. Bones are classified according to shape as short, flat, irregular, or long. Long bones are basically hollow tubes of compact bone with widened ends containing cancellous bone. Bones lengthen from the ends at areas called *epiphyses*.

Bones provide the framework for the body. They also protect vital tissues and are the primary site for storage and regulation of minerals, such as calcium and phosphate.

Their marrow cavities serve as sites of **hematopoiesis**, or the manufacturing of blood cells.

Muscles

The 600 skeletal muscles in the body make up 40% to 50% of its weight. Muscles may be cardiac, smooth, or skeletal. This chapter discusses only skeletal, or voluntary, muscles. Skeletal muscles consist of fibers bound together in bundles and attached to bone by tendons. They contract and relax to move joints. Muscles give the body shape and produce heat during movement.

Joints

A joint, or articulation, is the area where two bones come together. The function of joints is to provide mobility to the skeleton. Joints may be classified by the type of cartilage involved:

Table 23.1	Connective Tissues		
Type	**Functions**	**Example**
Cartilage	Allows bones to slide over one another, reduces friction, prevents damage, absorbs shock	Articular cartilage found on the ends of bones
Tendons	Connect muscles to bones	Biceps bronchii tendon in the shoulder, which connects the biceps muscle over the head of the humerus to the glenoid fossa
Ligaments	Connect bone to bone to stabilize joints and limit movement	Anterior cruciate ligament in the knee, which prevents lateral movement of the knee
Bursae	Fluid-filled sacs in areas of friction to cushion bones or ligaments that might rub against each other	Acromion bursa in shoulder to reduce friction during adduction
Meniscus	Cartilage disc between bones to absorb shock and cushion joints	The medial and lateral menisci in the knee, which cushion the tibia and femur
Fascia	Flat sheets that line and protect muscle fibers, attach muscle to bone, and provide structure for nerves, blood vessels, and lymphatics	The outer layer of fascia, which tapers at each end to form tendons

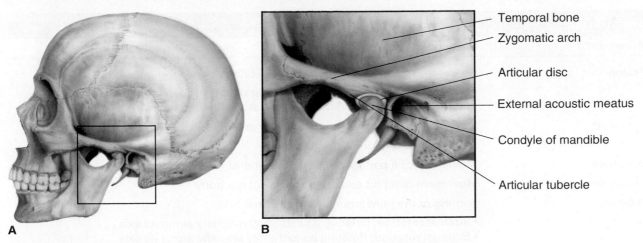

Figure 23.2 The temporomandibular joint (TMJ). **A.** Location of the TMJ within the skull. **B.** Close-up view of the TMJ.

- **Fibrous (synarthrotic) joints** are immovable, such as in the sutures in the skull.
- **Cartilaginous (amphiarthrotic) joints** are slightly moveable, such as the costal cartilage between the sternum and ribs and the symphysis pubis.
- **Synovial (diarthrotic) joints** are freely movable, the most common type, and named for their major type of movement: ball and socket (hip and shoulder), hinge (elbow and knee), pivot (atlas and axis), condyloid (wrist), saddle (thumb), and gliding (intravertebral).

Usually one of the bone ends is stable and serves as an axis for the motion of the other. The joint shape and ligaments determine the movement the joint can make (Fig. 23-1).

Temporomandibular Joint

The **temporomandibular joint** (TMJ) is where the mandible and temporal bone articulate (Fig. 23-2). The TMJ is palpable below and slightly anterior to the tragus of each ear. It permits three movements of the jaw for chewing and speaking: opening and closing, **protrusion** and **retraction**, and gliding from side to side.

Shoulder

The shoulder joint is where the humerus articulates with the glenoid fossa of the scapula (Fig. 23-3). Because it is a ball-and-socket joint, the shoulder permits many types of movement (Tables 23-2 and 23-3). Four strong muscles and their

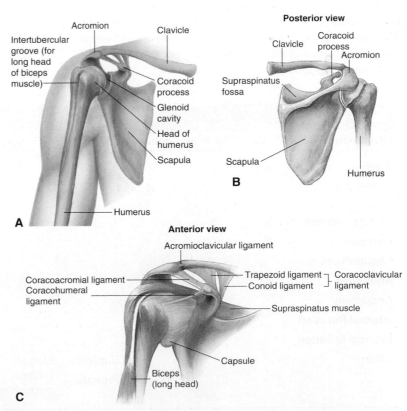

Figure 23.3 Shoulder. **A.** Anterior view. **B.** Posterior view. **C.** Ligaments.

Table 23.2   Terms for Joint Movement

Movement	Description
Flexion	Decreases the angle between bones or brings bones together
	• **Dorsiflexion:** Bending the ankle so that the toes move toward the head
	• **Plantar flexion:** Moving the foot so that the toes move away from the head
Extension	Increases the angle to a straight line or zero degrees
Hyperextension	Extension beyond the neutral position
Abduction	Movement of a part away from the center of the body
Adduction	Movement of a part toward the center of the body
Rotation	Turning of the joint around a longitudinal axis
	• **Internal rotation:** Rotating an extremity medially along its axis
	• **External rotation:** Rotating an extremity laterally along its axis
	• **Pronation:** Turning the forearm so the palm is down
	• **Supination:** Turning the forearm so the palm is up
Circumduction	A circular motion that combines flexion, extension, abduction, and adduction
Inversion	Turning the sole of the foot inward
Eversion	Turning the sole of the foot outward
Protraction	Moving a body part forward and parallel to the ground
Retraction	Moving a body part backward and parallel to the ground
Elevation	Moving a body part upward
Depression	Moving a body part downward
Opposition	Moving the thumb to touch the little finger

tendons, collectively known as the *rotator cuff*, surround the shoulder to support and stabilize it. A large bursa protects the bones and ligaments of the shoulder during movement. The scapula and clavicle connect to form the shoulder girdle. The **acromion process** of the scapula is at the top of the shoulder. The greater tubercle of the humerus is downward and lateral to the acromion, and the coracoid process of the scapula is a few centimeters medially.

Elbow

The **elbow** is the articulation of the humerus, radius, and ulna (Fig. 23-4). Its hinge action permits flexion and extension. A large bursa lies between the **olecranon process** and the skin. The olecranon process is centered between the medial and lateral **epicondyles** of the humerus. The sensitive ulnar nerve runs between the olecranon process and medial epicondyle. The radius and ulna articulate at two **radioulnar**

Table 23.3   Joints and their Movements

Movements	Neck	Shoulder	Elbow	Wrist	Fingers	Spine	Hip	Knee	Ankle	Toes
Flexion	X	X	X	X	X	X	X	X	Dorsi-flexion	X
Extension	X	X	X	X	X	X	X	X	Plantar flexion	X
Hyperextension	X	X		X	X	X	X			X
Rotation	X					X				
Circumduction		X					X			
Abduction	X	X			X	X	X			X
Adduction		X					X			
Internal Rotation		X					X			
External Rotation		X					X			
Other				Supinate Pronate	Finger-thumb-opposition				Inversion Eversion	

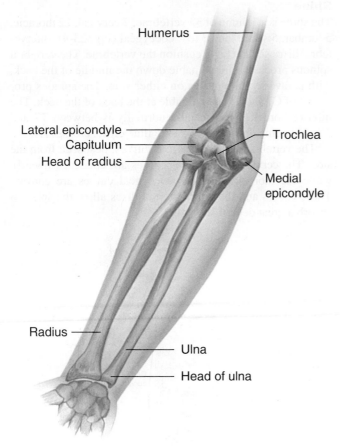

Figure 23.4 Bones of the elbow.

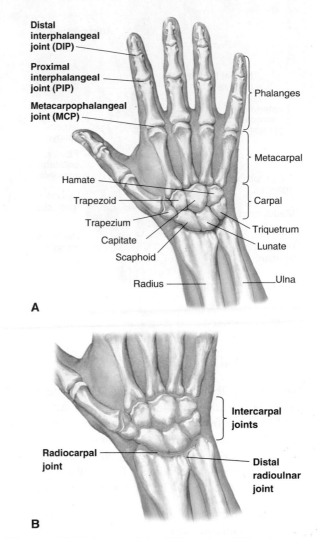

A

B

Figure 23.5 Bones of the **(A)** hand and **(B)** wrist.

joints, one at the elbow and one at the wrist. These bones move together to permit **pronation** and **supination** of the hand and forearm.

Wrist and Hand

The wrist, or **radiocarpal**, joint is the articulation of the radius (on the thumb side) and a row of carpal bones. Its condyloid action permits flexion, extension, and deviation (lateral movement of the hand). The **midcarpal joint** is the articulation between parallel rows of carpal bones. It allows flexion, extension, and some rotation. The **metacarpophylangeal** and **intraphalangeal** (proximal, medial, and distal) joints permit finger movement (see Table 23-2 and Fig. 23-5).

Hip

The hip joint is the articulation between the acetabulum and the head of the femur (Fig. 23-6). This ball-and-socket joint permits a wide ROM. Powerful muscles, strong ligaments, a fibrous capsule, and the insertion of the femur head into the acetabulum provide stability. Three bursae facilitate movement.

The iliac crest is palpable from the anterior superior iliac spine to the posterior. The ischial tuberosity is palpable when the hip is flexed. The greater trochanter of the femur is a depression on the upper lateral side of the thigh and is best palpated with the person standing.

Knee

The knee is the articulation of the femur, tibia, and patella (Fig. 23-7). The medial and lateral **menisci** cushion the tibia and femur. The **cruciate ligaments** cross within the knee to provide anterior and posterior stability and to control rotation. The **collateral ligaments** felt in the depressions on

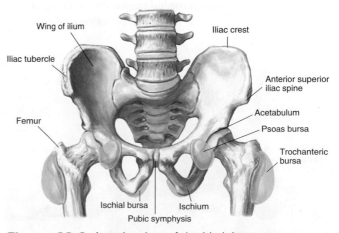

Figure 23.6 Anterior view of the hip joint.

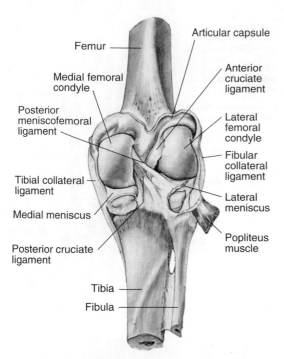

Figure 23.7 The right knee, posterior extended view.

both sides of the patella connect the joint at both sides to give medial and lateral stability and to prevent dislocation. Several bursae prevent friction. The tibial tuberosity is palpable on the midline of the tibia. The lateral and medial condyles of the tibia are to the sides and slightly above the tuberosity. The patella is above the condyles. The medial and lateral epicondyles of the femur can be felt above the patella.

Ankle and Foot
The ankle, or **tibiotalar joint**, is the articulation of the tibia, fibula, and talus (Fig. 23-8). It is a hinge joint limited to flexion and extension. The terms used to describe its movements are **dorsiflexion** and **plantar flexion**. The medial and lateral malleoli are palpable on either side of the ankle. Strong ligaments extend from each malleolus onto the foot to provide lateral stability of the ankle.

The subtalar joint in the foot permits **inversion** and **eversion**. Weight-bearing is distributed between the heads of the metatarsals and the **calcaneus** (heel) as a result of the longitudinal arch. The **metatarsophalangeal** and intraphalangeal joints permit flexion, extension, and abduction of the toes.

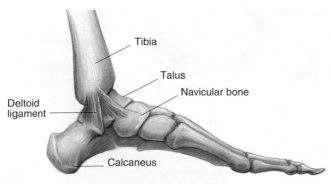

Figure 23.8 Bones of the ankle and foot.

Spine
The spine is a column of 33 vertebrae: 7 cervical, 12 thoracic, 5 lumbar, 5 sacral, and 3 to 4 coccygeal (Fig. 23-9). Intervertebral discs separate and cushion the vertebrae. The vertebral spinous processes are palpable down the middle of the back, with paravertebral muscles on either side. The spinous processes of C7 and T1 are palpable at the back of the neck. The inferior border of the scapula normally is between T7 and T8, and a line drawn between the iliac crests crosses L4.

The vertebral column has four curves, best seen from the side. The cervical and lumbar curves are concave (inward), while the thoracic and sacrococcygeal curves are convex. These curves and the intervertebral discs allow the spine to absorb a great deal of shock.

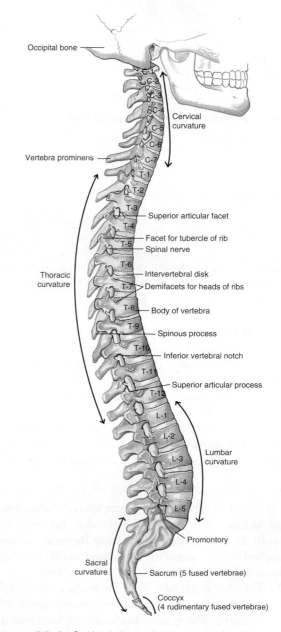

Figure 23.9 Sagittal view of the vertebral column (spine).

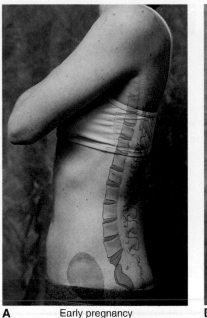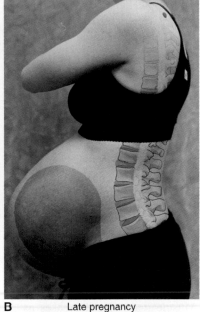

A Early pregnancy   **B** Late pregnancy

Figure 23.10 Note the change in spinal curvature from **(A)** early pregnancy to **(B)** late pregnancy.

Lifespan Considerations

While the human body is basically the same in all people, some changes occur with growth and development across the lifespan.

Pregnant Women

Pregnant women have increased joint mobility as a result of the hormones progesterone and relaxin. Increased mobility in the sacroiliac, sacrococcygeal, and symphysis pubis joints of the pelvis contribute to changes in maternal posture. **Lordosis**, increased lumbar curvature, compensates for the enlarging uterus (Fig. 23-10).

Infants and Children

The fetus forms a cartilaginous skeleton by 3 months, which calcifies and continues to grow into bone. Bones grow through infancy and childhood by depositing new bone around the shaft to increase width. They elongate by increasing the cartilage at epiphyses, or growth plates, at the ends of long bones. The cartilage later calcifies. This lengthening continues until approximately 21 years, when the epiphyses close. Any injury to the epiphyses before closure may result in bone deformity.

All muscle fibers are present at birth, but lengthen throughout childhood. During the adolescent growth spurt, muscle fibers grow following increased secretion of growth hormone, adrenal androgens, and, in boys, testosterone. Muscles vary in size and strength because of genetic factors, nutrition, and exercise. Throughout life, muscles strengthen with use and **atrophy** with disuse. Weight lifting can cause enlarged muscles, called **hypertrophy**.

Older Adults

Aging affects all components of the musculoskeletal system (Table 23-4). Bone resorption occurs more rapidly than deposition. This loss of bone density is termed **osteoporosis**.

Table 23.4	**Musculoskeletal Changes with Aging**
Physiological Change	**Nursing Implications**
Decreased bone density	Encourage weight-bearing exercise to decrease bone loss.
	Teach patients about hazards to prevent falls, because fragile bones break easily.
Increased bony prominences	Decrease pressure on bony prominences to prevent skin breakdown.
Cartilage degeneration	Encourage warm baths or showers prior to activity to increase blood flow and decrease joint stiffness.
Joint stiffness and lax ligaments	Encourage active ROM in all joints.
	Assess patient's ability to perform ADLs; provide assistive devices to help the patient perform self-care.
Muscle atrophy	Teach isometric exercises to maintain muscle strength.

Some osteoporosis occurs in all people, but it is most evident in women with small bone frames. Women experience rapid loss of bone density for the first 5 to 7 years after menopause. After the initial rapid phase, bone loss continues, but slows. Men also experience bone loss but at later ages and much slower rates than women. Bone mass is related to race, heredity, hormonal factors, physical activity, and calcium intake. Smoking, calcium deficiency, high salt intake, alcohol intake, and physical inactivity increase bone loss. Resistance exercise and soy isoflavones decrease bone resorption (Valachovicova, et al., 2004).

Postural changes and decreased height occur with aging. Loss of water content in the intervertebral discs contributes to height loss from 40 to 60 years. Shortening after 60 years results from osteoporosis, which compresses the vertebrae. **Kyphosis**, an exaggerated forward curvature of the spine, may occur in older adults.

With aging, joints become less flexible because of changes in cartilage. Tendons and ligaments shrink and harden, decreasing ROM. Muscle mass also decreases as a result of atrophy and loss in size. Muscle mass decreases 3% to 8% per decade after age 30 years, with even greater muscle loss after 60 years (Volpi, et al., 2004). This involuntary loss of muscle function increases the risk of falls and disability in older adults. Exercise training and adequate nutrition are successful in improving muscle mass and strength.

Subcutaneous fat distribution changes with aging. Men and women usually gain weight after 40 years, predominantly in the abdomen and hips. After 80 years, subcutaneous fat continues to decrease, causing bony prominences to be more obvious.

🌐 Cultural Considerations

Many changes related to ethnicity are visible in the musculoskeletal system. Bone density is most likely related to body weight rather than a particular genetic background (Finkelstein, et al., 2008). The curvature of long bones results from both ethnicity and body weight. African Americans have straight femurs, while Native Americans have anteriorly curved femurs. The femoral curve in Caucasians is intermediate. Thin people of all cultures have less curvature than obese people. Caucasians, Mexican Americans and African Americans have no difference in metabolism of vitamin D; however, conversion of active metabolites by sunlight is less efficient in African Americans (Tylavsky, 2005).

Gender also affects the skeletal system. Men have larger and stronger bones than women; therefore, men are less prone to problems related to osteoporosis. Caucasian women have the highest risk of developing problems from loss of bone density. Table 23-12 at the end of this chapter describes the relationship of age, ethnicity, and gender to certain musculoskeletal conditions.

Acute Assessment

Assessment of patients reporting musculoskeletal problems focuses on identifying the specific problem, alleviating pain, and preventing complications. Nurses look for alignment of limbs, joints, and the spine. They also observe for symmetry of size, shape, position, and movement of extremities. If a joint is swollen and tender following an injury, a strain or sprain is likely. If a bone is not aligned, it may be fractured, whereas if a joint is not aligned, it may be dislocated.

⚠ SAFETY ALERT 23.1
Nurses should not attempt to correct malalignment, because doing so can compound injury to muscle, nerves, or blood vessels. Rather, the extremity requires immobilization. Fractures require prompt care to prevent further injury or deformity. Efforts should focus on keeping the patient calm, quiet, still, and comfortable.

Damage to soft tissue often occurs at the same time as bone fracture. If there is soft-tissue injury and bleeding, nurses apply pressure to stop the bleeding and assess for swelling, pain, numbness, and guarding. Muscle contractions contribute to discomfort, so helping the patient to relax is essential. Nursing actions include taking vital signs, monitoring pulses, and assessing color, temperature, and capillary refill distal to the injury to evaluate tissue perfusion.

Subjective Data Collection

Areas for Health Promotion/ *Healthy People*

Nurses use the health history to gather information to discover areas requiring health teaching. *Healthy People* (see Chapter 1) describes focus areas that the US government has identified as ways for citizens to improve their health status. Table 23-5 organizes *Healthy People* foci related to the musculoskeletal system and pertinent health teaching.

Assessment of Risk Factors

Numerous factors affect the musculoskeletal system. The nurse asks the patient about family history, personal history, medications and supplements, sports and hobbies, and working conditions. In addition the nurse notes the patient's age, gender, and ethnicity. Knowledge of risk factors helps identify topics for health-promotion teaching.

Table 23.5 *Healthy People* Goals Related to Musculoskeletal Health

Goal	Patient Education Topics
Reduce the proportion of adults with chronic joint symptoms who experience a limitation in activity due to arthritis.	Encourage daily moderate exercise to maintain joint mobility. Promote self-management of arthritis symptoms.
Increase the proportion of adults who have seen a health care provider for their chronic joint symptoms.	Encourage adults to seek health care for joint discomfort.
Reduce the proportion of adults with osteoporosis and the number of adults who are hospitalized for vertebral fractures associated with osteoporosis.	Teach about calcium and vitamin D intake, weight-bearing exercise, effects of alcohol and tobacco on bone mineralization.
Reduce activity limitation due to chronic back conditions.	Teach patients how to manage symptoms, including core strengthening exercises.
Reduce hip fractures among older adults.	Encourage patients to correct environmental hazards such as slippery surfaces, uneven floors, poor lighting on stairs, loose rugs, unstable furniture, and objects on floors. Recommend installation of grab bars in restrooms for patients with poor balance. Encourage participation in physical therapy for patients with gait and balance problems.
Increase the proportion of adults who are at a healthy weight.	Teach safe weight reduction to decrease stress on joints.
Increase the proportion of persons aged 2 years and older who meet dietary recommendations for calcium.	Instruct patients about the recommendations for adequate daily calcium intakes: 500 mg for those 1–3 years, 800 mg for those 4–8 years, 1,300 mg for those 9–18 years, 1,000 mg for those 19–50 years, and 1,200 mg for those 51 years or older.
Reduce work-related injuries resulting in medical treatment, lost time from work, or restricted work activity.	Encourage participation in safety programs and use of protective equipment.
Reduce the rate of injury and illness cases involving days away from work due to overexertion or repetitive motion.	Instruct patients on correct positioning during lifting, ergonomics, and use of protective equipment.
Increase the proportion of adults who perform physical activities that enhance and maintain muscular strength and endurance.	Instruct the patient on correct performance of muscle strengthening and flexibility exercises.
Increase smoking cessation attempts by adult smokers.	Investigate the patient's willingness to quit. Assist the patient to develop a plan using social support, pharmacology, or complementary resources.

Source: *Healthy people 2010: What are its goals?* (n.d.). Retrieved July 7, 2010, from http://www.healthypeople.gov/About/goals.htm

Questions to Assess Risk Factors	Rationales
Demographic Data What is your age?	Table 23-12 at the end of the chapter reviews age-related musculoskeletal diseases. *Osteoporosis* affects 55% of people older than 50 years (National Osteoporosis Foundation [NOF], 2008). Failing eyesight and musculoskeletal changes increase older adults, risk for falls. Longer life expectancy has contributed to a growing number of people with disabilities. Young children are at risk for injury from impulsive actions, like running into the street after a ball. Adolescents are also at risk from impulsive actions, involvement in sports, and driving.
Note the patient's gender.	Incidence of many musculoskeletal diseases differs by gender (Table 23-12). Women are four times more likely than men to develop *arthritis*, and 50% of women will have an osteoporosis-related fracture in their lives (AHRQ, 2007). Female athletes have a four to six times higher incidence of ACL tears than males (Hewett, et al., 2006).

(text continues on page 640)

Questions to Assess Risk Factors	Rationales
What is your ethnic heritage or race?	Prevalence of some disorders varies by ethnicity. See Table 23-12.
Family History Do your parents or siblings have any muscle, joint, or bone problems? • Who had the problem? • When did it occur? • How was it treated? • What was the outcome?	Some musculoskeletal problems have a familial tendency. Examples include *osteoporosis*, *bone cancer*, and *rheumatoid arthritis*.
Past Medical History Have you ever had any musculoskeletal trauma or injury or been diagnosed with a musculoskeletal problem? Ask specifically about fractures, stroke, polio, infections of the bone or muscles, diabetes, and parathyroid problems. • When did it occur? • How was it treated? • What was the outcome?	Following hip replacement, hip dislocation can occur with hip flexion greater than 90 degrees or adduction of the joint past the midline. A person who has had a stroke is at increased risk of **subluxation**, or partial dislocation, of the shoulder from the weight of the arm and the lack of muscle tone to hold the joint together.
Nutrition and Medications How many servings of dairy products do you have per day?	Calcium is essential for bone growth and remodeling. Vitamin D is essential for calcium absorption.
What medications do you take? Ask women about current and past birth-control methods. Ask postmenopausal women about hormone replacement therapy (HRT). • Do you take calcium and vitamin D supplements? • Do you take any pain or antiinflammatory medications? Muscle relaxants? • Do you take any steroids? • Do you use complementary or alternative therapies (eg, chondroitin, glucosamine)?	Vitamin D deficiency has been linked to *osteoporosis* (van Schoor, et al., 2008). Oral contraceptive use in young adults may contribute to risk of *osteoporosis*, while HRT may help prevent it (Almstedt Shoepe & Snow, 2005; Dane, et al., 2007; MacLean, 2008). Pain or antiinflammatory medications and muscle relaxants can mask symptoms. Steroids can affect calcium absorption. Glucosamine and chondroitin have been found to improve joint pain resulting from *osteoarthritis* (Towheed, et al., 2005).
Occupation, Lifestyle, and Behaviors What type of work do you do? • Does your work involve any repetitive motion? Lifting or twisting? • How do you protect yourself from injury while working?	Some occupations increase risk of musculoskeletal injury through repetitive movements, twisting, frequent or heavy lifting, vibration, exposure to cold temperatures, and pushing or pulling heavy objects. Ergonomics and safety equipment can protect workers against injury.
What hobbies and sports do you enjoy? • How do you protect yourself from injury while exercising or participating in sports? • Do you consistently use car seats, helmets, and protective gear?	Sports such as basketball, baseball, football, and soccer contribute to knee injuries (Hewett, et al., 2006). Skiing increases risks for lower-extremity injuries, while skateboarding can lead to upper-extremity injuries. Stretching and warming up prior to strenuous exercise decreases injury. Car seats, helmets, and protective gear decrease the severity of injury during accidents.
What is your weekly or monthly income? How many people live on that income?	Women of lower socioeconomic status are more likely to report limitations in activity and *arthritis*, *obesity*, and *osteoporosis* (Women's Health Care, 2005).
Have you ever smoked cigarettes or cigars? • If yes, how many packs per day? • For how many years?	Smoking increases the risk of developing a vertebral fracture by 13% in women and 32% in men (Ward & Klesges, 2001). Smoking is an independent, dose-related risk factor. Smoking cessation may partially reverse the risk.
Have you ever consumed alcohol? • If yes, how many drinks per week? • What do you drink?	Alcohol use is associated with increased risk of *osteoporosis*. Alcohol raises parathyroid hormone levels, which causes calcium loss from bones. Regular consumption of 2–3 oz. of alcohol every day interferes with absorption and use of calcium and vitamin D (NOF, 2008).

Psychosocial History

Psychosocial assessment related to the musculoskeletal system is important, because problems that limit or compromise movement and mobility can have wide-ranging effects and consequences. For example, if a patient has a musculoskeletal injury, how will it affect his or her ability to work, participate in hobbies, or perform routine activities of daily living (ADLs) independently? If the patient does not have sick-leave benefits and cannot work, the financial strain may be immense. If the patient lives alone, can he or she perform self-care safely? Does the patient have pain that interferes with every aspect of living? Will immobility add stress or contribute to isolation and sensory deprivation? Are deformities altering sense of self or body image?

Scoliosis Screening

Scoliosis is the lateral curvature of the spine, usually affecting both the thoracic and lumbar parts, with a deviation in one direction in the thoracic and in the other direction in the lumbar spine. Scoliosis may be structural, caused by a defect in the spine, or functional, caused by habits (eg, consistently carrying a heavy backpack on one shoulder). If not corrected early, scoliosis can progressively worsen. Severe forms can interfere with breathing. The problem often develops in early adolescence, especially in girls. That is why school screening for scoliosis is so important.

To screen for scoliosis, inspect the patient's back. While the patient stands, look for symmetry of the hips, scapulae, shoulders, and any skin folds or creases (Fig. 23-11A and B). The patient then needs to bend forward with the arms hanging toward the floor. Look for any lateral curves or protrusions on one side. Then, the patient should slowly stand up while inspection of the spine continues. A **scoliometer** may be used to obtain a measurement of the number of degrees that the spine is deviated. A deviation in the thoracic area usually has a corresponding deviation on the other side in the lumbar area. During palpation of the spine, feel for any abnormal protrusions or deformities.

Today scoliosis screening is regularly done in schools, but older people likely did not undergo such screening. Thus, nurses may discover cases in the older population. Severe cases can interfere with normal functioning of the organs within the chest.

Risk Assessment and Health-Related Patient Teaching

Ask if the patient has any congenital bone, muscle, or joint problems. If responses are positive, ask if the congenital problem has any current effects. Knowledge of congenital problems can guide you to alter assessment and to anticipate findings during the physical examination. Assess how the patient is adapting to the deformity.

Ask about previous injuries or illnesses of muscles, joints, or bones. They can have long-lasting effects such as muscle weakness, decreased ROM, and impaired mobility. Specifically ask about fractures, sprains, strains, and dislocations, and also about childhood polio or **scoliosis**. If the patient reports previous injuries, ask about continuing effects.

Ask about surgery to the musculoskeletal system. Have the patient describe the procedure, when it occurred, and the results. Knowledge of previous surgeries provides additional information, allows the nurse to anticipate findings during the physical assessment, and enables the nurse to alter assessment procedures as needed to protect the patient.

A comprehensive method to determine the effects of previous or current problems in the musculoskeletal system is to perform a functional assessment. An example is the Short Musculoskeletal Function Assessment developed by Swiontkowski, et al. (1999).

People of all ages need to learn to maintain a healthy weight and perform weight-bearing exercise at least three times per week. Children should alternate the shoulders on which they carry back packs to help prevent functional

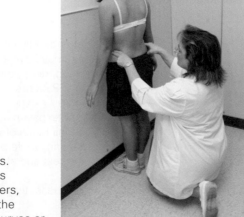 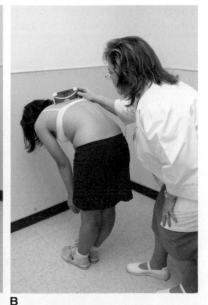

Figure 23.11 Screening for scoliosis. **A.** Standing behind the patient to assess symmetry of the hips, scapulae, shoulders, and any skin folds or creases. **B.** While the patient bends forward, looking for any curves or protrusions on one side.

A   B

scoliosis. Encourage all patients to use good body mechanics with lifting and pushing, to use protective equipment with sports and work, and to wear seat belts. Exercises to increase strength and flexibility and improve posture decrease the risk of falls. Exercise training and adequate nutrition are successful in improving muscle mass and strength in older adults (Volpi, et al., 2004).

Bone Density

Loss of bone density and muscle strength are major concerns of aging that lifestyle modification can help control. Calcium and vitamin D are important for people of all ages, as are weight-bearing exercises. Although there is treatment for osteoporosis, there is no cure. Prevention is very important, especially for women. Current treatment includes bisphosphonates calcitonin, estrogen and/or hormone therapy, raloxifene, and parathyroid hormone (NOF, 2008). HRT with estrogen may prevent bone loss but carries an increased risk of breast cancer and heart attacks.

The NOF (2008) recommends a comprehensive approach to prevent osteoporosis:

1. Consume the daily recommended amount of calcium and vitamin D. Limit caffeine, which increases excretion of calcium.
2. Perform at least 30 minutes of weight-bearing exercise three times per week.
3. Avoid smoking and excess alcohol consumption.
4. Discuss your risk for osteoporosis with your health care provider.

5. Have a bone density test and take medication when appropriate.

Clinical Significance 23-1

Because bone deposition begins to decrease after 30 years of age, women especially need to consume adequate calcium and perform weight-bearing exercises in the preceding decades. Weight-bearing exercise is required for older adults to prevent bone loss and muscle wasting. Walking, the most helpful form of exercise, is less detrimental to joints than other forms.

Focused Health History Related to Common Symptoms

Some common symptoms should be assessed in all patients to screen for the early presence of musculoskeletal disease. Nurses can use any special concerns from patients about joint problems to identify focal areas. A thorough history of symptoms assists with identifying a current problem or diagnosis.

Common Musculoskeletal Symptoms

- Pain or discomfort
- Weakness
- Stiffness or limited movement
- Deformity
- Lack of balance and coordination

Questions to Assess Symptoms	Rationales/Abnormal Findings
Pain or Discomfort Do you have any pain or discomfort in your muscles, bones, or joints?	Pain is a subjective experience.
Where is the pain located? Is it only in that area or does it radiate? Do you have pain in different areas at other times? If the pain is in more than one joint, is it symmetrical?	The location and timing of pain may help differentiate if it originates in muscle (**myalgia**), bone, or joint (**arthralgia**). Pain limited to one joint is described as **monoarticular**; pain in several joints is **polyarticular**.
How bad does it hurt? Use a scale to measure the intensity (see Chapter 7).	
What does the pain feel like?	Patients may describe it in many different terms. Burning pain may have a neurological cause. Bone pain may be aching, deep, and dull. Muscle pain is often cramping or sore. Patients often describe chronic pain as aching.
When do you feel pain? Is it constant or does it come and go? Does it start suddenly or gradually?	Arthritic pain may be worse during cold, damp weather. The joint pain of *rheumatoid arthritis* is often worse in the morning, while pain from *osteoarthritis* is usually worse after rest and at the end of the day.
Is there accompanying weakness, tingling, or numbness?	Weakness, tingling, and numbness indicate pressure on nerves.

Questions to Assess Symptoms	Rationales/Abnormal Findings
What makes the pain worse? What helps relieve it?	Bone pain does not increase with movement, unless there is a fracture. Muscle and joint pain increases with movement.
For patients with chronic pain, what level of pain would you like to achieve?	Patients with chronic pain may never experience its absence. The nurse and patient together need to determine what an acceptable level of pain is.
Does the pain limit your activities?	Pain can limit ability to perform usual activities (ambulating, bathing, dressing, preparing food, working, sitting, changing positions, climbing stairs, lifting, pushing, or pulling).

Weakness

Questions to Assess Symptoms	Rationales/Abnormal Findings
Do you have any muscle weakness?	Muscle weakness is associated with certain diseases.
Do all or just certain muscles feel weak?	Weakness may migrate from muscle to muscle or to groups of muscles. Knowing which muscles are involved helps with determining the disease process. Distal weakness is usually a neurologic problem, whereas proximal weakness is usually a muscle problem.
When does the weakness occur? How long does it last? What makes it worse? What helps the weakness? How bad is weakness on a scale of 1 to 10, with 10 being the worst?	Muscle weakness after prolonged activity may result from *dehydration* or electrolyte imbalances. Grading the degree of weakness can help patients see improvement or determine the time of day when they can perform better.
Does the weakness limit your activities?	

Stiffness or Limited Movement

Questions to Assess Symptoms	Rationales/Abnormal Findings
Do you have stiffness or limited movement in any part of your body?	Stiffness is one type of limited movement. It may result from pain in muscles or joints, swelling, or a disease process.
Is the stiffness in one or more joints?	Generalized body swelling from *renal failure* affects the entire body, while injury may involve one joint only.
Can you grade the stiffness on a scale of 0–10, with 10 being the inability to move?	
Is the stiffness constant or intermittent?	Early stages of *rheumatoid arthritis* may cause stiffness that is worse in the morning, while stiffness from *osteoarthritis* is usually worse at the end of the day.
Did the stiffness start after an injury or was onset gradual?	**Contracture,** shortening of tendons, fascia, or muscles, may result from injury or prolonged positioning. Once a contracture develops, it is difficult to stretch and may require surgery.
What makes the stiffness worse? What helps the stiffness? Does the stiffness limit your activities?	

Deformity

Questions to Assess Symptoms	Rationales/Abnormal Findings
Do you have a deformity? Was it present at birth or did it develop later?	Disuse, including wearing a cast, leads to some wasting or shrinking of the muscle (atrophy).
Does it affect the entire body or is it localized?	Deformities may be general (decreased overall body size) or localized (disruption in limb length and alignment from a fracture).
Does it affect your ability to perform ADLs?	

(text continues on page 644)

Questions to Assess Symptoms	Rationales/Abnormal Findings

Lack of Balance and Coordination

Do you have any problems maintaining balance?

Unusual gait or inability to perform ADLs may result from a balance or coordination problem, which may indicate a neurologic disorder.

Have you fallen recently?

Have you noticed your movements are uncoordinated?

Ataxia (irregular, uncoordinated movements) or losing balance may be from cerebellar disorders, *Parkinson's disease*, *multiple sclerosis*, strokes, brain tumors, inner ear problems, or medications.

Documentation of Normal Findings

Patient denies any discomfort, weakness, or stiffness in spine, bones, or joints. Patient reports no musculoskeletal difficulties with work, hobbies, or ADLs. *C. Chin, RN*

 Lifespan Considerations

Additional Questions	Rationales/Abnormal Findings

Pregnant Women

Have you noticed a change in your gait?

Hormones released during pregnancy cause ligaments to relax, which may contribute to a waddling gait in the last trimester.

Do you have back pain?

Lordosis frequently causes back pain during the last trimester of pregnancy.

Have you noticed numbness or tingling in your arms or hands?

Relaxation of the shoulder girdle and changes in neck curvature to counteract lordosis may cause pressure on nerves.

Newborns, Infants, and Children

Were you told about any trauma to the infant during labor and birth? Was the baby born head first? Was there a need for forceps?

Traumatic birth increases the risk for fractures of the clavicle or humerus (Pressler, 2008).

How much did the baby weigh at birth?

Large babies also have an increased risk for fractures of the clavicle or humerus (Pressler, 2008).

Did the baby require resuscitation?

Prolonged hypoxia can cause muscular hypotonia or hypertonia (spasticity).

Did the baby achieve motor milestones (eg, raising head, turning over) at about the same age as age-mates or siblings?

Failure to achieve motor milestones may be from muscular or neurological causes.

Have you noticed any bone deformity? Spinal curvature?

Scoliosis, lateral curvature of the spine, develops during growth spurts. Early stages may be treated with exercise and physical therapy. Advanced scoliosis may require braces or surgery.

Unusual shape of toes or feet? At what age? How were these treated?

Common foot deformities include **polydactyly** (extra toes), **syndactyly** (fused toes) and **talipes equinovarus** (club foot).

Has the child broken any bones? Had any dislocations? How were these treated?

Fractures of the arms or legs during childhood may injure the epiphyseal plate and prevent bone growth, resulting in a permanent deformity.

Questions to Assess Symptoms	Rationales/Abnormal Findings
Did you breastfeed the infant? Did you take vitamin D supplements while breastfeeding?	Mothers who breastfeed require vitamin D supplementation to prevent the development of *rickets*. This is especially important in lower socioeconomic areas (Gartner & Greer, 2003).
Does the 6- to 12-month-old child eat a variety of vegetables and citrus fruits (CACFP, 2008)?	Vitamin C deficiency is present in 14% of males and 10% of females (Goebel, 2007). Incidence of *scurvy* peaks in children 6 to 12 months whose diet is deficient in citrus fruits or vegetables. Incidence also peaks in elderly populations, who sometimes have diets deficient in vitamin C (Hampl, et al., 2004).
Is the child involved in any sports? How many times per week? How was the child trained for the sport? How does the child warm up for the sport?	Children involved in sports need good training and must warm up before every session to prevent injury.
What does the child do if injured?	Children may be reluctant to report injuries for fear of not being able to participate in the sport.
Does the child use any safety equipment during sports?	Properly fitted safety equipment is needed to minimize injuries.

Older Adults

Questions to Assess Symptoms	Rationales/Abnormal Findings
Have you noticed any decrease in strength in the last year?	Decreased muscle strength is common as people age, especially in those with sedentary lifestyles.
Have you noticed an increase in stumbling or falling in the last year?	Older adults have an increased rate of falls because of postural changes. Loss of balance may also result from sensory or motor disorders, ear infections, side effects of certain medicines, and other factors.
Do you use any aids to help you get around? Were you taught how to use the device?	Assistive aids help older adults ambulate but can cause falls if they do not use such devices correctly.
Postmenopausal women: Do you take bisphosphonates, calcitonin, estrogens and/or hormone therapy, raloxifene, or parathyroid hormone?	Calcium supplementation, HRT, and weight-bearing exercise decrease the development of osteoporosis (Dane, et al., 2007). Of the 10 million Americans estimated to have osteoporosis, 8 million are women, and 2 million are men (80% women, 20% men) (NOF, 2008).

Cultural Considerations

Questions to Assess Symptoms	Rationales/Abnormal Findings
What is your ethnicity? Where were you born?	Table 23-12 describes common musculoskeletal conditions based on ethnicity. Approximately 20% of Caucasian and Asian women 50 years or older are estimated to have osteoporosis compared to 7% of men (NOF, 2008). Additionally, 52% of Caucasian and Asian women 50 years or older have low bone mass, compared to 35% of men (NOF, 2008). Low bone mass increases the risk for osteoporosis. Estimates are that 10% of Hispanic women 50 years or older have osteoporosis, with 49% having low bone mass (NOF, 2008). In African American women older than 50 years, 5% have osteoporosis, with an additional 35% having low bone mass (NOF, 2008).

(text continues on page 646)

	People of Asian decent have lower fracture rates than Caucasians (Finkelstein, et al., 2008). Caucasian and Hispanic women have twice the risk for hip fracture as African Americans (AHRQ, 2007).
	Patients from countries with severe droughts or recent wars require assessment for signs of scurvy, including splinter hemorrhages in nails, ecchymosis, purpura, and hyperkeratotic papules on skin (Hampl, et al., 2004). These patients are also at risk for malnutrition, which increases the risk of osteoporosis.

Therapeutic Dialogue: Collecting Subjective Data

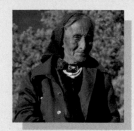

The nurse's role relative to subjective data collection is to gather information to improve the patient's health status and to help determine the cause of the patient's current symptoms. Remember Mrs. Runningbird, who was introduced at the beginning of this chapter. She is the 82-year-old Native American woman who has been in the skilled nursing facility for 12 days for rehabilitation. The nurse uses professional communication techniques to gather subjective data from Mrs. Runningbird. The following conversations give two examples of different interview styles. One style is more effective than the other.

Less Effective

Nurse: Hi, Gladys. How are you doing today?

Mrs. Runningbird: My joints feel kind of stiff today and I'm cold.

Nurse: Well let's just get you up and out of this room. Today's a great day to be alive.

Mrs. Runningbird: I feel like every day I'm losing ground. It's cold in here.

Nurse: It's not cold. It's 72 degrees in here. You just need to get up and moving.

Mrs. Runningbird: I don't know if I can do it. My hands don't work and my legs don't work and I just want to stay in bed.

Nurse: You need to get up and get something to eat. Once you get up you'll feel better.

Mrs. Runningbird: I don't think that I'm making any progress. I'm in here to get stronger and I feel like I'm getting weaker instead.

Nurse: You're doing fine. Here, let me help you with your clothing. You just relax and I'll put this on for you. We want to get you warmed up.

More Effective

Nurse: Good morning, Mrs. Runningbird. How are you doing today? (pauses)

Mrs. Runningbird: Not so good.

Nurse: I'm sorry to hear that. Do you think that you're more stiff and cold than you were yesterday?

Mrs. Runningbird: No, I don't think so honey. Thank you for asking.

Nurse: I know that it's been hard for you being away from your home. You're doing a great job participating in your therapies.

Mrs. Runningbird: Oh, thank you. My legs and hands don't work the way that they used to.

Nurse: That must be difficult for you. I'm glad that you're here so that we can help you get better.

Mrs. Runningbird: Yes, I'm really hoping that I can go home. I'll do whatever I can to get better.

Nurse: Let me help you get up and out of bed. I'll let you do what you can and help with the rest.

Critical Thinking Challenge

- What culturally appropriate behaviors did the more effective nurse use? Was any behavior or comment inappropriate in the less effective dialogue?
- What other assessments might the nurse make regarding Mrs. Runningbird's coldness, stiffness, and loss of function?
- What therapeutic communication techniques might be helpful to assess how Mrs. Runningbird is coping?

Objective Data Collection

Equipment

- **Goniometer** (Fig. 23-12) for measuring the angle at which a joint can flex or extend
- Tape measure to measure circumference of extremities or length of bones

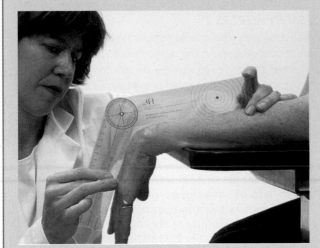

Figure 23.12 A goniometer is used to measure the angle at which a joint can extend or flex.

Preparation

Assemble needed supplies, as listed above. Make sure the room is warm and private. Wash and warm your hands. Help the patient to remove clothing so that the limbs and spine are visible. Drape the patient so that only the areas being currently observed are visible.

Weighing the patient is an important part of a comprehensive musculoskeletal examination. Obesity puts extra stress and strain on joints, increases the risk of degenerative joint disease, and decreases mobility. See Chapter 6.

Clinical Significance 23-2

Although nurses should compare each extremity to the other, they should examine last those areas that patients have identified as tender or painful.

Common and Specialty or Advanced Techniques

Inspection begins with the initial contact with the patient. Evaluate posture while the patient is sitting and standing and, if the patient is ambulatory, his or her gait and coordination. Assessment involves inspection and palpation. Advance practice nurses may use percussion to assess for joint injury (Table 23-6).

Table 23.6   Common Versus Specialty/Advanced Musculoskeletal Techniques

Technique	Purpose	Screening or Registered Nurse Assessment	Focused or Advanced Practice Examination
Assess posture.	Assess for kyphosis, scoliosis, or lordosis	X	
Observe gait, balance, and coordination.	Assess risk for falling and ease of movement	X	
Inspect extremities.	Observe for deformities	X	
Palpate extremities for swelling or tenderness.	Identify areas of inflammation	X	
Observe joint ROM.	Conduct a general overview of functional ability	X	
Assess muscle tone, strength, size, and symmetry.	Grade muscle bulk and function	X	
Inspect the spine.	Observe for symmetry and pressure areas	X	
Specifically inspect, palpate, and measure ROM in TMJ, cervical spine, shoulder, elbow, wrist, hand, hip, knee, ankle, foot, and thoracic and lumbar spine.	Perform if there is an area specifically affected, such as assessment of an ankle following a sprain.		X

Technique and Normal Findings	Abnormal Findings

Posture

Observe the patient's posture while he or she stands with feet together. Observe the relation of the head, trunk, pelvis, and extremities. Assess for symmetry in shoulder height, scapulae, and iliac crests. Also observe the patient's posture while sitting. *Posture is erect with the head midline above the spine. Shoulders are equal in height.*

Scoliosis or low back pain may cause the patient to lean forward or to the side when standing or sitting. **Acromegaly** may result in an enlarged skull and increased length to the hands, feet, and long bones.

> ⚠ *SAFETY ALERT 23.2*
>
> *When assessing the musculoskeletal system, prevent patient falls. Ask about the person's ability to transfer and to walk or stand. Encourage the patient to steady self by holding the examination table or wall when standing.*

Gait and Mobility

Watch the patient walk across the room while observing from the side and from behind. Gait can predict a person's risk of falling. The Gait Assessment Rating Scale is a useful tool for determining risk (www. ohcponline.com/tools/gars.html). *Walking is smooth and rhythmic with the arms swinging in opposition to the legs. The patient rises from sitting with ease.*

> ⚠ *SAFETY ALERT 23.3*
>
> *Before assessing gait, ask if the patient uses an assistive device, such as a cane or walker. Ensure that the patient has the equipment with him or her at the examination and knows how to correctly use it.*

Gait abnormalities include hesitancy, unsteadiness, staggering, reaching for external support, high stepping, foot scraping, inability to raise the foot completely off the floor, persistent toe or heel walking, excessive pointing of toes inward or outward, asymmetry of step height or length, limping, stooping, wavering, shuffling, waddling, excessive swinging of shoulders or pelvis, and slow or rapid speed. Table 23-13 at the end of this chapter describes some abnormal gait patterns; other gait patterns are in Table 24-10. Gait problems may result from muscle weakness, joint deterioration, malalignment of lower extremities, paralysis, poor coordination, poor balance, fatigue, or pain.

Balance

If the patient has a gait problem, you will not be able to assess balance. Ask the patient to walk on tiptoes, heels, heel-to-toe fashion (tandem walking), and backward. Ask the patient to step to each side, and to sit down and stand. Advanced assessment of balance includes the Romberg test, standing, and hopping on one foot.

To perform the Romberg, ask the patient to stand with feet together and eyes open; then have him or her close the eyes. If cerebral function is intact, the patient can do this without swaying (negative test). *Patient is balanced when standing and has a negative Romberg test.*

Balance is a function of the cerebellum; however, inner ear problems can also affect balance. Balance may be assessed with the musculoskeletal system, but also involves the neurological system.

Coordination

Ask the patient to rapidly pat the table or his or her thigh, alternating between the palm and dorsum of the hand. To assess fine motor coordination of the hand, ask the patient to perform finger to thumb opposition. Assess gross motor coordination in the legs by having the patient run the heel of one foot up the opposite leg from ankle to knee. *Patient performs rapid alternating movements of the arms and finger-thumb opposition and runs the heel of one foot down the opposite shin.*

The dominant side usually has slightly better coordination. Poor coordination may be from pain, injury, deformity, or cerebellar disorders. Coordination is often tested during assessment of the musculoskeletal system, but it is actually an assessment of the neurological system.

Inspection of Extremities

Look for any swelling, lacerations, lesions, deformity, length of long bones, size of muscles, and symmetry.

Asymmetry in bone length may be from injury. Asymmetry in muscle size may be from neurologic damage (eg, *polio*). Disuse, including while wearing a cast, leads to some wasting or shrinking of the muscle (atrophy).

Size and Shape of Extremities.
Assess both extremities at the same time to evaluate for symmetry. Bilateral assessment for muscle tone and strength is necessary for comparison. Note the size and shape of extremities and muscles, as well as alignment and any deformity or asymmetry. Are the limbs of equal length?

Limb Measurements.
Compare the circumference of the arms and legs. Compare the length of the radius by having the patient place the arms together from elbow to wrist. Observe the knee height with the patient sitting. Limb circumference may be measured on the forearms, upper arms, thighs, and calves. Measure circumference at the midpoint, so measure the length first. The dominant side may be 1 cm larger in circumference. Measure arm length from the acromion process to the tip of the middle finger. Measure true leg length from the anterior superior iliac crest to the medial malleolus (Fig. 23-13). Measure apparent leg length from the umbilicus to the medial malleolus.

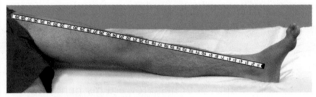

Figure 23.13 True leg length is measured from the anterior superior iliac crest to the medial malleolus.

Palpation

Joints are palpated for contour and size; muscles are palpated for tone. Feel for any bumps, nodules, or deformity. Ask if there is any tenderness during touch.

Joint ROM.
Assess both extremities at the same time to evaluate symmetry. Simultaneously observe and palpate each joint while the patient performs active ROM. If the patient cannot perform active ROM, carefully support the limb on either side of the joint and perform passive ROM. Ask the patient if there is any tenderness or discomfort. If there is limited ROM, use a goniometer to measure the angle of the joint at its maximum flexion and extension (see Fig. 23-12). Listen to and/or feel the joint while the patient moves. *A healthy joint moves smoothly and quietly.*

Muscle Tone and Strength.
When assessing muscle tone and strength, it is necessary to compare one side to the other. *Upper and lower extremity muscle strength is 5/5 bilaterally.*

Disuse, including while wearing a cast, will lead to some wasting or shrinking of the muscle (atrophy). Swelling or edema may be the result of trauma, inflammation, or lymph node resection.

Discrepancy in leg length of more than 1 cm may cause gait problems, hip and back pain, and apparent scoliosis. Unequal apparent leg length, but equal true leg length, is seen with hip and pelvic abnormalities. Unequal arm length does not cause as many problems as unequal leg length. Unequal circumference may be from disuse or neurologic disorders.

Asymmetry in muscle size and tone may be from disuse or neurological disease. Discomfort when touched may be because of inflammation or infection.

Limitation of movement, **crepitus** (cracking or popping), and nonverbal and verbal expressions of discomfort or pain are noted. With movement, ask the patient if there is any tenderness or discomfort. Do not apply force; rather, be gentle and stop if there is resistance or complaints of discomfort. Crepitus may be heard as a popping sound and may be felt as grating in the joint as it moves.

⚠ *SAFETY ALERT 23.4*
When performing passive ROM, do not force the joint. Stop if there is resistance or reports of discomfort.

Table 23-7 provides terms used when describing alterations in muscle tone, Table 23-8 describes the rating scale for muscle strength, and Table 23-9 provides instructions to give the patient when assessing muscle strength.

Documentation of Normal Findings

When standing, the trunk and head are erect with weight distributed equally on both feet. The head is midline and aligned with the spine. The shoulders, hips, scapulae, and iliac crests are level. The feet are under the hips and knees. The toes and knees point forward. The extremities are symmetrical and in proportion to the body. When full growth is reached, the arm span is equal to the height. When sitting, both feet are flat on the floor with toes pointed forward. The head and trunk are perpendicular to the floor. Walking is smooth and rhythmic with the patient erect. The arms swing freely at the sides and in the opposite direction that the leg is moving. The patient transfers from standing to sitting and sitting to standing with ease. The muscles are well formed, firm to touch, symmetrical. Joints have full active ROM. Patient denies any discomfort. *C. Chin, RN*

Table 23.7   Terms for Describing Alterations in Muscle Tone

Atony	Lack of normal muscle tone or strength
Hypotonicity	Diminished tone of skeletal muscles
Spasticity	Hypertonic, so the muscles are stiff and movements awkward
Spasm	Sudden violent involuntary contraction of a muscle
Fasciculation	Involuntary twitching of muscle fibers
Tremors	Involuntary contraction of muscles

Table 23.8   Rating Scale for Muscle Strength

5/5 (100%)	Normal	Complete ROM against gravity and full resistance
4/5 (75%)	Good	Complete ROM against gravity and moderate resistance
3/5 (50%)	Fair	Complete ROM against gravity
2/5 (25%)	Poor	Complete ROM with the joint supported; cannot perform ROM against gravity
1/5 (10%)	Trace	Muscle contraction detectable, but no movement of the joint
0/5 (0%)	Zero	No visible muscle contraction

Muscle strength can be described on a 0 to 5 scale, with 5 being the strongest, as percentage or by words.

Table 23.9   Instructions for Testing Muscle Strength

Muscle	Examiner Activity	Patient Instructions
Neck	Place hand on side of patient's head.	"Turn your head toward my hand."
Deltoid	Put hand on patient's upper arm and try to push arm down.	"Hold your arm straight out to the side. Try to prevent me from pushing down your arm."
Biceps	With elbow bent, place hand on patient's lower arm and have patient try to straighten arm.	"Push against my hand."
Triceps	With elbow bent, place hand on patient's lower arm and have patient try to flex the elbow.	"Prevent me from bending your arm."
Wrist	With wrist extended, place hand on dorsal surface of the patient's hand, and ask patient to try to flex the wrist. Place hand on palm, and ask patient to push to hyperextend wrist.	"Prevent me from pushing your hand downward." "Push against my hand."
Fingers	Push on dorsal surface of patient's fingers. Push on ventral surface of patient's fingers. Hold patient's fingers together. With patient's fingers spread apart, prevent patient from bringing fingers together.	"Do not let me bend your fingers." "Do not let me straighten your fingers." "Spread your fingers apart." "Bring your fingers together."
Hip	With patient supine, push down on his or her leg above the knee.	"Keeping your leg straight, raise your leg (do a leg lift)."
Quadriceps	Push down on patient's leg above the knee. Place your hand on the front of the patient's lower leg and prevent extension of knee.	"While sitting, raise your leg. Straighten your leg."
Hamstring	With patient's leg extended, place hand on back of the patient's lower leg and prevent flexion.	"Bend your knee."
Ankle	With patient's ankle flexed, push against sole of patient's foot. With patient's ankle flexed, push against dorsum of patient's foot.	"Bend your foot up." "Push against my hand."

Comprehensive Physical Examination

Clinical Significance 23-3

Handle the extremities of patients with fragile bones gently to prevent fractures.

Advanced practitioners use special assessment procedures for the musculoskeletal system. These tests are described in Table 23-10.

Table 23.10   Advanced Musculoskeletal Assessment Techniques

Phalen's Test

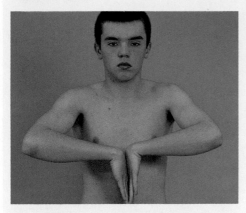

Evaluates for carpal tunnel syndrome. The patient flexes the wrists 90 degrees and holds the backs of the hands to each other for 60 seconds. Normal response is denial of any discomfort. Positive signs include numbness, burning, or pain.

Tinel's Test

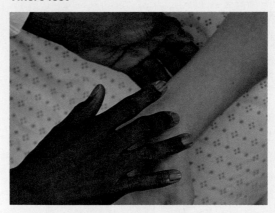

Evaluates for carpal tunnel syndrome. Percuss lightly over the median nerve located on the inner aspect of the wrist. Pain, numbness, or tingling is a positive (abnormal) finding.

Bulge Test

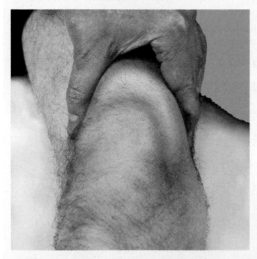

Differentiates soft tissue swelling from accumulation of excess fluid behind the patella. With the patient supine, milk upward along the medial aspect of the knee two, three, or four times. Then press on the lateral side of the knee and check for any bulging on the medial side. A bulge indicates mild joint effusion or liquid accumulation in the area, which is not a normal finding.

Ballottement

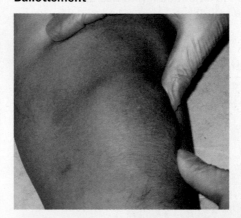

Evaluates presence of large accumulation of fluid behind the knee. With the patient supine and the knee extended, press on the quadriceps muscle just above the knee with one hand and keep that pressure there. This compresses the suprapatellar pouch. Palpate the patella with the other hand. If fluid is present, the patella will rebound or ballot against the fingers.

McMurray's Test

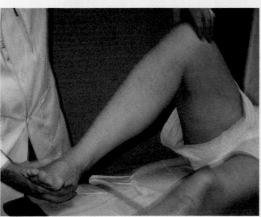

Checks for meniscus injury. The patient lies supine and flexes the hip and knee. The examiner supports the knee with one hand and holds the foot with the other, rotating the foot laterally. The examiner slowly extends the patient's knee, while assessing for the positive findings of pain or clicking. The examiner repeats the procedure, rotating the lower leg medially.

(table continues on page 652)

Table 23.10 Advanced Musculoskeletal Assessment Techniques (continued)

Thomas Test

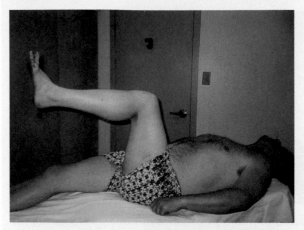

Assesses presence of a flexion contracture of the hip. Again, the patient is supine. Ask the patient to extend one leg, flex the hip and knee of the other leg, bringing the knee to the chest. A flexion contracture of the hip will cause the extended leg to rise up off the examination table.

Drawer Sign

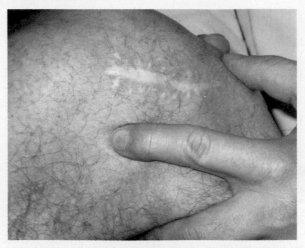

Checks for knee injury. The supine patient flexes the knee to a right angle. While standing at the patient's feet, grasp the leg just below the knee and see if you can move it toward and away from self. A normal finding is that the examiner cannot move the leg that way. A positive sign is the head of the tibia moves more than half an inch from the joint. May also be used for ankle injuries.

LeSegue's Test: Straight Leg Raising

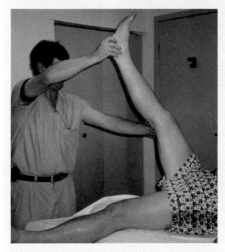

Checks for herniation of the lumbar disk and nerve irritation or pressure. With the patient supine and both legs extended, support and raise one leg. A positive response is the report of pain.

Trendelenburg Test

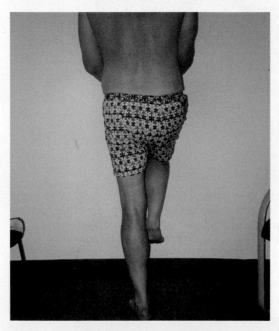

Assesses for hip disease with muscle weakness. Observe from behind the patient. Ask patient to stand first on one foot, then the other. Normally the pelvis remains level horizontally, which is a negative Trendelenburg sign. An abnormal or positive finding is that the other hip drops when the patient stands on the weak side.

Drop Arm Test

Assesses for rotator cuffv injury. Ask the patient to abduct the arm to shoulder level or 90 degrees. If the patient cannot fully abduct and remain there, the drop arm test is positive as the arm drops rapidly to the patient's side or the patient complains of severe shoulder pain.

TMJ

Inspection. Inspect the TMJ for symmetry, swelling, and redness. *The jaw is symmetrical bilaterally.*

Palpation. Place your fingerpads in front of the tragus of each of the patient's ears (Fig. 23-14). Ask the patient to open and close the jaw while you palpate the joints. You should feel a shallow depression, and the mandible motion should be smooth and painless. *The muscles are symmetrical, smooth, and nontender.*

Asymmetrical facial or joint musculature may indicate previous or current facial fractures or surgery.

Discomfort, swelling, limited movement, and grating or crackling sounds are unexpected and require further evaluation for dental or neurological problems or *TMJ syndrome.* TMJ dysfunction may present as ear pain or headache. Swelling or tenderness suggests *arthritis* or *myofascial pain syndrome* (inflammation of the fascia surrounding the muscle).

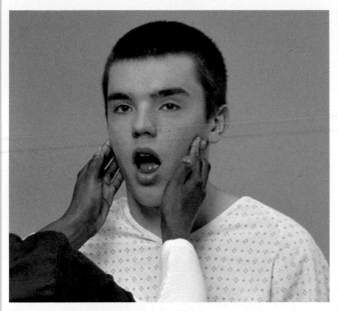

Figure 23.14 Palpating the TMJ.

ROM. Ask the patient to open the jaw as wide as possible, push the lower jaw forward (protrusion), return the jaw to neutral position (retraction), and move the jaw from side to side 1–2 cm. *The joint may have an audible or palpable click when opened. The mouth opens with 3–6 cm between the upper and lower teeth. The jaw moves with ease.*

Difficulty opening the mouth may be because of injury or arthritic changes. Pain in the TMJ may indicate misalignment of the teeth or arthritic changes.

Muscle Strength. Ask the patient to repeat the above movements while you provide opposing force. This tests cranial nerve V. *The strength of the muscles is equal on both sides of the jaw; the patient can perform the movements against resistance. Muscle strength is 5/5, with no pain, spasms, or contractions.*

Decreased muscle strength may be because of muscle or joint disease.

Documentation of Normal Findings

The TMJ is symmetrical bilaterally. The muscles are smooth with normal strength of 5/5. The joint moves smoothly through all ROM without pain. A slight popping sound is heard when the jaw is widely opened. The teeth align correctly. *C. Chin, RN*

Cervical Spine

Inspection. With the patient standing, inspect the cervical spine from all sides. It should position the head above the trunk (Fig. 23-15). Observing from the side, check for the concave curve of the cervical spine. *As viewed from behind, the patient holds the head erect, and the cervical spine is in straight alignment. From the side, the neck has a concave curve.*

Degenerative joint disease of the cervical vertebrae may cause lateral tilting of the head and neck. Lateral deviation of the neck (**torticollis**) may be because of acute muscle spasms, congenital problems, or incorrect head posture to correct vision problems. Weight lifting will cause hypertrophy of the neck muscles, resulting in a thickened appearance of the neck.

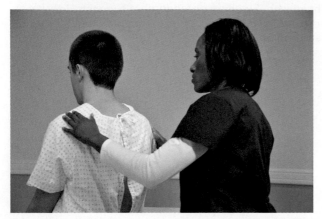

Figure 23.15 Inspecting the cervical spine from behind the patient.

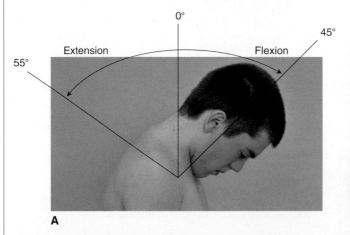

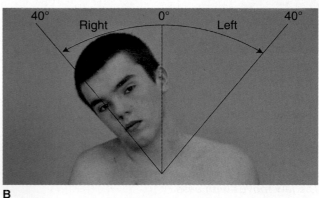

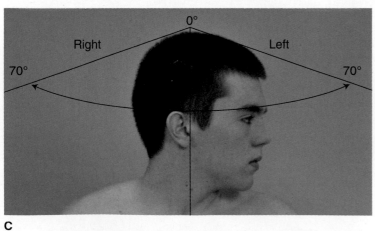

Figure 23.16 Assessing neck ROM.
A. Flexion. **B.** Testing lateral flexion or bending by moving the ear to shoulder left and right.
C. Assessing rotation by moving the chin to shoulder left and right.

Palpation. Stand behind the patient to palpate the cervical spine and neck. C7 and T1 spinous processes should be prominent. *The paravertebral, sternocleidomastoid, and trapezus muscles are fully developed, symmetrical, and nontender.*

ROM. Ask the patient to touch the chin to the chest (flexion), look up toward the ceiling (hyperextension), attempt to touch each ear to the shoulder without elevating the shoulder (lateral flexion or bending), and turn the chin to the shoulder as far as possible (rotation) (Fig. 23-16). *Neck ROM is normal: flexion 45 degrees, hyperextension 55 degrees, lateral flexion 40 degrees, and rotation 70 degrees to each side.*

Muscle Strength. Ask the patient to rotate the neck to the right and left, against the resistance of your hand. This tests cranial nerve XI. *Muscle strength is sufficient to overcome resistance.*

Clinical Significance 23-4

Following any trauma, do not move patients with neck pain until the neck is stabilized. Moving the patient could cause subluxation or dislocation of the cervical vertebrae and permanent injury to the spinal cord.

Osteoarthritis, neck injury, disc degeneration because of aging or occupational stress, and spondylosis can cause decreased ROM, pain, and tenderness on palpation. Pain on palpation may indicate inflammation of the muscles (**myositis**). Neck spasm may indicate nerve compression or psychological stress.

Pain or muscle spasms may impair ROM. Hyperextension and flexion may be limited because of cervical disc degeneration, spinal cord tumor, or osteoarthritic changes. Pain may radiate to the back, shoulder, or arms. Pain, numbness, or tingling may indicate compression of spinal root nerves.

Weakness or loss of sensation in arms may result from cervical cord compression.

Documentation of Normal Findings

Viewed from behind, the neck is straight and holds the head in alignment with the spine. Viewed from the side, the neck is slightly concave. Muscle size is symmetrical bilaterally. The neck has full ROM and moves smoothly and painlessly. Muscle strength is 5/5. The patient denies tenderness during palpation. C7, T1 spinous processes are prominent and palpable. The muscles are fully developed. No nodules, swelling, crepitus, or muscle spasms are noted. *C. Chin, RN*

Shoulder

Inspection. Compare both shoulders anteriorly and posteriorly for size and contour. Observe the anterior aspect of the joint capsule for abnormal swelling. *No redness, swelling, deformity, or muscular atrophy is present. Shoulders are smooth and bilaterally symmetric. Right and left shoulders are level. Each shoulder is at an equal distance from the vertebral column.*

Palpation. Stand in front of the patient and palpate both shoulders, noting any muscular spasm, atrophy, swelling, heat, or tenderness. Start at the clavicle and methodically explore the acromioclavicular joint, scapula, greater tubercle of the humerus, area of the subacromial bursa, biceps groove, and anterior aspect of the glenohumeral joint. *Muscles are fully developed and smooth.*

Shoulder joints may have some deformity because of arthritis, trauma, or scoliosis. Redness and swelling may indicate injury or inflammation. Unequal shoulder height may indicate scoliosis.

Tenderness may be because of inflammation of the muscles, overuse of unconditioned muscles, or sports injuries.

⚠ *SAFETY ALERT 23.5*
Suspect a cardiac origin for reports of shoulder pain without tenderness or inflammation. Assess for shortness of breath, nausea, and diaphoresis. If these symptoms are present, the patient needs to be sent to an emergency department for assessment of cardiac ischemia.

(text continues on page 656)

ROM. Ask the person to perform forward flexion, extension, hyperextension, abduction, adduction, and internal and external rotation (Fig. 23-17). Cup one hand over the patient's shoulder during ROM to detect any crepitus. *Movement is fluid. Normal ROM is forward flexion 180 degrees, hyperextension 50 degrees, abduction 180 degrees, adduction 50 degrees, internal rotation 90 degrees, and external rotation 90 degrees.*

Limited ROM, pain, crepitation, and asymmetry may be from *arthritis,* muscle or joint inflammation, trauma, or sports injury. Inability to externally rotate the shoulder suggests a rotator cuff injury.

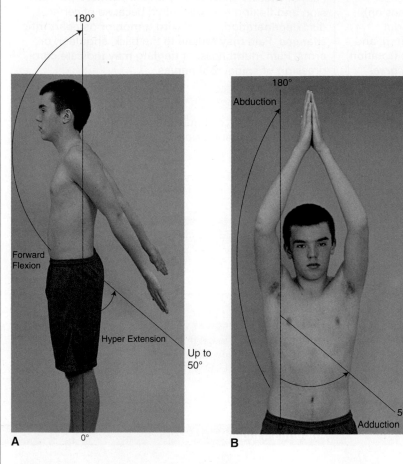

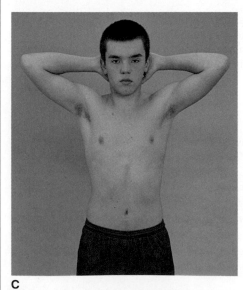

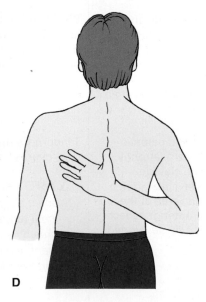

Figure 23.17 Assessing shoulder ROM. **A.** Extension. **B.** Abduction/adduction. **C.** External rotation. **D.** Internal rotation.

Technique and Normal Findings (continued)	Abnormal Findings (continued)
Muscle Strength. Ask the patient to shrug both shoulders, flex forward and upward, and abduct against resistance. Shrugging the shoulders tests cranial nerve XI (spinal accessory). *Patient can perform full ROM against resistance.*	Decreased ability to shrug the shoulders against resistance may indicate compressed spinal cord root nerve or spinal accessory cranial nerve (CN XI).

Documentation of Normal Findings

Shoulders are equal height and equidistant from the spinal column. Muscle size is symmetrical bilaterally. Both shoulders have full ROM and move smoothly and painlessly. Muscle strength is 5/5. The patient denies tenderness during palpation. No nodules, swelling, crepitus, or muscle spasms are noted. *C. Chin, RN*

Technique and Normal Findings	Abnormal Findings
Elbow	
Inspection. Inspect the size and contour of the elbow in both the extended and flexed positions. Check the olecranon bursa for swelling. *Elbows are symmetrical with no swelling.*	Subluxation of the elbow shows the forearm dislocated posteriorly. This may occur when an adult tugs on a small child's forearm or swings the child holding onto the child's forearms. Swelling and redness of the olecranon bursa are easily observed because of the proximity to the skin. Effusion or synovial thickening is observed as a bulge on either side of the olecranon process and indicates *gouty arthritis*.
Palpation. Support the patient's forearm and passively flex the elbow to 70 degrees. Palpate the olecranon process and medial and lateral epicondyles of the humerus (Fig. 23-18). The tissues and fat pads should feel solid. Check for any synovial thickening, swelling, nodules, or tenderness. *Elbows are smooth with no swelling or tenderness.*	Epicondyles and tendons are common sites for inflammation and tenderness. Soft, boggy swelling occurs with synovial thickening or effusion. Local heat or redness may indicate synovial inflammation. Subcutaneous nodules at pressure points on the olecranon process or ulnar surface may indicate rheumatoid arthritis.

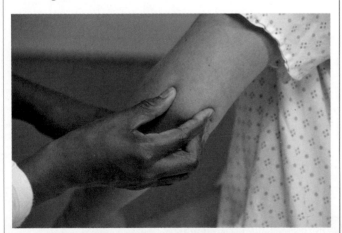

Figure 23.18 Palpation of the elbow.

ROM. Ask the patient to bend and straighten the elbow. Then have the person pronate and supinate the forearm by laying the forearm and ulnar surface of the hand on	Decreased ROM, pain, or crepitation may be from *arthritis*, muscle or joint inflammation, trauma, or sports injury. Redness, swelling, and tenderness of the olecranon

(text continues on page 658)

a table. Have the patient touch the palm and then the hand dorsum to the table (Fig. 23-19). *Normal ROM is flexion 150–160 degrees, extension 0 degrees; however, some people cannot extend the elbow fully (only to 5 to 10 degrees). Some people can hyperextend the elbow –5 to –10 degrees. Pronation and supination of 90 degrees is normal.*

process may be because of *bursitis. Lateral epicondylitis* (tennis elbow) is inflammation of the forearm extensor and supinator muscles and tendons, causing disabling pain at the lateral epicondyle of the humerus that radiates down the lateral side of the forearm. *Medial epicondylitis* (golf elbow) is the same as tennis elbow, except it affects the flexor and pronator muscles and tendons.

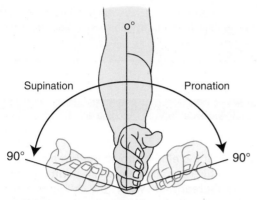

Figure 23.19 Supination and pronation of the elbow.

Muscle Strength. While supporting the patient's arm, apply resistance just proximal to the patient's wrist, and ask the patient to flex and then extend both elbows (Fig. 23-20). *Patient can perform full ROM against resistance.*

Decreased strength may be from pain, nerve root compression, or arthritic deformity. People may compensate for weakened biceps or triceps muscles by using the shoulder muscles.

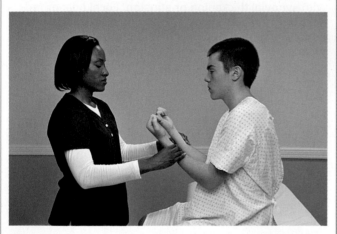

Figure 23.20 Assessing elbow muscle strength.

Documentation of Normal Findings

Elbows are equal in size and shape. Muscle size is symmetrical bilaterally. Both elbows have full ROM and move smoothly and painlessly. Muscle strength is 5/5. The patient denies tenderness during palpation. No nodules, swelling, crepitus, or muscle spasms are noted. *C. Chin, RN*

Wrist and Hand

Palpation. Hold the patient's hand in your hands. Use your thumbs to palpate each joint of the wrist and hand for tenderness (Fig. 23-21). *Joint surfaces are smooth without nodules, edema, or tenderness.*

Painful joints in the fingers are common in *osteoarthritis*. A firm mass over the dorsum of the wrist may be a *ganglion*. *Rheumatoid arthritis* may cause edema, redness, and tenderness of the finger and wrist joints.

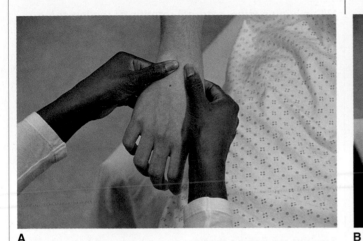

A

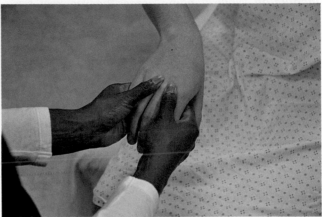

B

Figure 23.21 Palpating the joints of the **A.** wrists and **B.** hands.

ROM. Observe wrist and hand ROM (Fig. 23-22). *The wrist motions are flexion (90 degrees), extension (return to 0 degrees), hyperextension (70 degrees), and ulnar (55 degrees) and radial (20 degrees) deviation. The metacarpophylangeal joints motion are flexion (90 degrees), extension (0 degrees), and hyperextension (up to 30 degrees). Proximal and distal intraphalangeal joints perform flexion (making a fist), extension, and abduction. The thumb performs* **opposition** *with each fingertip and the base of the little finger.*

Joint or muscle inflammation may cause decreased or unequal ROM. Previous trauma may limit ROM.

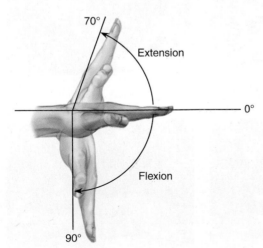

Figure 23.22 Wrist and hand flexion and extension.

(text continues on page 660)

Muscle Strength. Perform each motion above against resistance. Ask the patient to grasp your first two fingers tightly while you pull to remove your fingers. *Muscle strength is equal bilaterally and sufficient to overcome resistance.*

Weak muscle strength may be because of arthritic changes or fractures of the metatarsals or phalanges.

Hip

Inspection. While standing, assess the iliac crest, size and symmetry of the buttocks, and number of gluteal folds. Assist the patient to the supine position with legs straight. Look for any swelling, lacerations, lesions, deformity, size of the muscle, and symmetry. Look at the hips from the anterior and posterior views. *Hips are rounded, even, and symmetrical.*

When lying supine, external rotation of the lower leg and foot indicates a fractured femur. Unequal gluteal folds or unequal height of iliac crests may indicate uneven leg length or *scoliosis*.

Palpation. While the patient is supine, palpate the hip joints, iliac crests, and muscle tone. Feel for any bumps, nodules, and deformity. Ask if there is any tenderness with touch. Feel for crepitus when moving the joint. *Buttocks are symmetrical in size. Iliac crests are at the same height on both sides.*

Asymmetry, discomfort when touched, or crepitus during movement may occur with hip inflammation or *degenerative joint disease*.

ROM. Observe for full active ROM of each hip (Fig. 23-23): flexion (lift straight leg to 90 degrees or draw knee to chest to 120 degrees), extension (standing position or lying on the examination table with the leg straight), abduction (lift, if standing, or slide, if lying, foot and straight leg to the side, away from body to 45 degrees), adduction (swing foot and straight leg in front and past the other leg to 30 degrees), internal and external ROM (with the hip and knee flexed, move the leg medially 40 degrees and then laterally 45 degrees). Have the patient stand or positioned prone to test hyperextension. Ask the patient to move the straight leg backward, away from the body (15 degrees).

Straight leg flexion that produces back and leg pain radiating down the leg may indicate a *herniated disc*. When lying down, one leg longer than the other or limited internal rotation may indicate a hip fracture or dislocation.

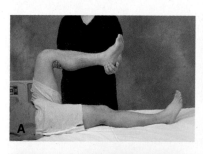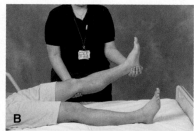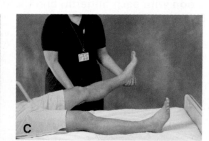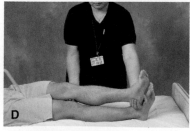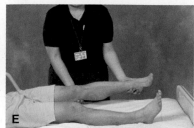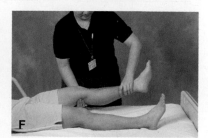

Figure 23.23 Hip ROM. **A.** Flexion. **B.** Extension. **C.** Abduction. **D.** Adduction. **E.** Internal rotation. **F.** External rotation.

Technique and Normal Findings (continued)	Abnormal Findings (continued)
Circumduction while standing or lying on one side moves the foot and leg in a circle beside the body is all movements, *Patient can perform full ROM without discomfort or crepitus.*	
Muscle Strength. With the patient lying down, apply pressure to the top of the leg while the patient flexes the hip. Apply pressure to the side while the patient abducts the hip. *Patient can perform full ROM against resistance.*	Asymmetry of strength may be from pain, or a muscle or nerve disease. ⚠ *SAFETY ALERT 23.6* *Do not test adduction or flexion greater than 90 degrees in anyone with a hip replacement. Doing so may cause dislocation.*

Documentation of Normal Findings

The muscles are well formed, firm to touch, and symmetrical. Hip joints have full active ROM through flexion, extension, hyperextension, abduction, adduction, circumduction, and internal and external rotation. Muscle strength is 5/5. Patient denies any discomfort while still or moving. *C. Chin, RN*

Technique and Normal Findings	Abnormal Findings
Knee	
Inspection. Inspect the knee both standing and sitting. Inspect contour and shape. Look for any swelling, lacerations, lesions, deformity, size of the muscle, and symmetry. Look for symmetry in the length of long bones: when the patient is standing, is one hip higher than the other? When seated, is one knee higher than the other? When seated, does one knee protrude further than the other? *Hollows are on each side of the patella. Knees are symmetrical and aligned with thighs and ankles.*	Swelling of the knee indicates inflammation, trauma, or *arthritis*. Muscle atrophy may accompany disuse or chronic disorders. A part of a limb twisted toward or out from the midline is labeled **varus** and **valgus,** respectively. For example, *Genu valgus* is knock-knee, while *genu varus* is bowlegged. Asymmetry in leg muscle size may be from disuse or nerve or muscle injury.
Palpation. With the knee flexed, palpate the quadriceps muscle for muscle tone. Palpate downward from approximately 10 cm above the patella; evaluate the patella and each side of the femur and tibia (Fig. 23-24).	Pain, swelling, thickening, or heat may indicate synovial inflammation, *arthritis*, or meniscus tear. Painless swelling may occur with *osteoarthritis. Bursitis* causes swelling, heat, and redness.

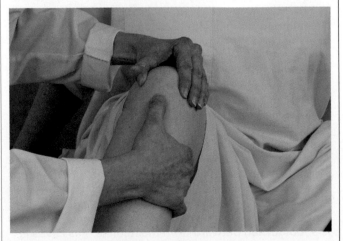

Figure 23.24 Palpating the knee.

(text continues on page 662)

Palpate the tibiofemoral joints with the leg flexed 90 degrees. Assess the tibial margins and the lateral collateral ligament. Feel for any bumps, nodules, or deformity. Ask if there is any tenderness during touch. Feel for crepitus when moving the joint. *The quadriceps muscle and surrounding tissue are firm and nontender. The suprapatellar bursa is not palpable. The joint is firm and nontender.*

An advanced practice nurse may perform the drawer test, bulge test, and **ballottement**. See Table 23-10.

ROM. Observe for full active ROM of each knee with the patient seated. Flex the knee to 130 degrees and return to extended position. *The knee can perform full ROM without discomfort or crepitus.*

Inability to perform full ROM may be from contractures, pain associated with trauma or inflammation, or neuromuscular disorders.

⚠ *SAFETY ALERT 23.7*
Do not encourage the patient to hyperextend or rotate the knee. Attempting to do so may cause injury.

Muscle Strength. With the patient seated, apply pressure to the anterior lower leg while the patient extends the leg. Also, with the leg bent, ask the patient to maintain that position while you pull the lower leg as if to straighten it.

Muscle strength is equal bilaterally and able to overcome resistance.

Injury or deconditioning may lead to asymmetry of strength.

Documentation of Normal Findings

The knees are aligned with the long axis of the leg. The muscles are well formed, firm to touch, and symmetrical. Joints have full active ROM through flexion and extension. No bulging or swelling is noted. Muscle strength is 5/5. Patient denies any discomfort while still or moving. *C. Chin, RN*

Ankle and Foot

Inspection. Inspect the feet with the patient both standing and sitting. Look for any swelling, lacerations, lesions, deformity, size of the muscle, and symmetry. Look for toe alignment. *Feet are the same color as the rest of the body. They are symmetrical, with toes aligned with the long axis of the leg. No swelling is present. When the patient stands, the weight falls on the middle of the foot.* Advance practice nurses may perform ankle anterior drawer test or talar tilt test to assess for ankle sprains, or the Thompson squeeze test to assess for a ruptured Achilles tendon. See Table 23-10.

An enlarged, swollen, hot, reddened metatarsophalangeal joint and bursa of the great toe indicates *gouty arthritis*. An ankle sprain or strain may cause pain on palpation and ROM. Crepitus may indicate a fracture. Often a sprain cannot be differentiated from a fracture without an x-ray. With *hallux valgus* (*bunion*), the great toe is angled away from the midline, crowding the other toes. Flexion of the proximal interphalangeal joint with hyperextension of the distal joint indicates *hammertoe*. A callus or corn forms on the flexed joint from external pressure. With *flatfoot* (*pes planus*), the arch of the foot is flattened and touches the floor. This may only be visible when the person is standing. *Pes varus* describes a foot that is turned inward toward the midline. *Pes valgus* is a foot turned outward from the midline. *Pes cavus* is an exaggerated arch height. A *corn* is a conical area of thickened skin from pressure. Corns may be painful and can occur between toes. *Callus* is thickened skin from pressure and usually occurs on the sole of the foot. Calluses are usually not painful.

Pain in the heel that occurs early in the morning or with prolonged sitting, standing, or walking may be *plantar fasciitis*, an inflammation of the plantar fascia where it attaches to the calcaneus.

An inward turning foot is *talipes equinovarus* (*club foot*).

Palpation. Palpate for muscle tone. Feel for any bumps, nodules, or deformity. Holding the heel, palpate the anterior and posterior aspects of the ankle, the Achilles tendon (calcaneal tendon), and the metatarsophalangeal joints in the ball of the foot (Fig. 23-25). Palpate each interphalangeal joint, noting temperature, tenderness, and contour. Ask if there is any tenderness during touch. Feel for crepitus when moving the joint. *Ankle and foot joints are firm, stable, and nontender.*

Pain or discomfort in the ankle or foot during palpation may indicate arthritis or inflammation. Pain and tenderness along the Achilles tendon may be from bursitis or tendonitis. Small nodules on the tendon may occur with rheumatoid arthritis.

Cooler temperature in the ankles and feet than in the rest of the body may be from vascular insufficiency, which will lead to musculoskeletal dysfunction (see Chapter 20).

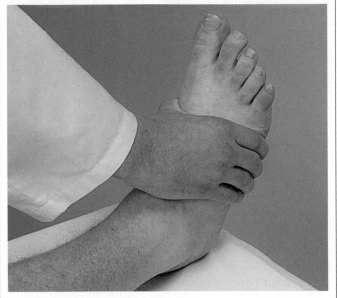

Figure 23.25 Palpating the ankle.

ROM. Observe for full active ROM of the ankle. Assess dorsiflexion by asking the patient to raise the toes toward the knee. Plantar flexion requires the patient to point toes downward toward the ground. Inversion occurs when the sole of the foot is turned toward the opposite leg. Eversion is when the sole of the foot is turned away from the other leg (Fig 23-26). Ask the patient to curl the toes and return them to straight position (flexion and extension). To assess hyperextension, ask the patient to keep the soles on the ground and raise the toes upward. For abduction, ask the patient to spread the toes wide open, as far apart

Limited ankle or foot ROM without swelling indicates arthritis. Inflammation and swelling with limited ROM indicates trauma.

(text continues on page 664)

from each other as possible. Adduction occurs when the toes return to their original position. *Normal ankle ROM is dorsiflexion 20 degrees, plantar flexion 45 degrees, inversion 30 degrees, and eversion 20 degrees. The toes can flex, extend, hyperextend, and abduct.*

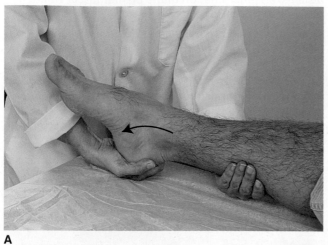

A

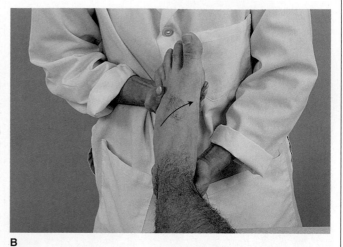

B

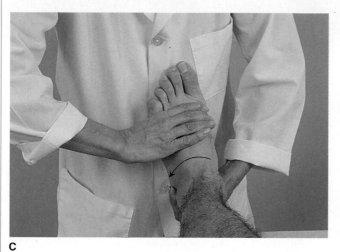

C

Figure 23.26 A. Plantar flexion. **B.** Foot inversion. **C.** Foot eversion.

Muscle Strength. Ask the patient to perform dorsiflexion and plantar flexion against the resistance of your hand. Then ask the patient to flex and extend the toes against your resistance.

Muscle strength is equal bilaterally and able to overcome resistance.

Asymmetry of strength may be from pain, inflammation, deconditioning, or chronic disease.

Documentation of Normal Findings

The ankles and feet are symmetrical and the same color as the rest of the body. The muscles are well formed, firm to touch, and symmetrical. The ankles have full active ROM through dorsiflexion, plantar flexion, inversion, and eversion. The toes abduct, flex, and extend. Muscle strength is 5/5. Patient denies any discomfort while sitting, standing, or walking. *C. Chin, RN*

Thoracic and Lumbar Spine

Inspection. With the patient standing, look at the patient from the side for the normal S pattern (convex thoracic spine and concave lumbar spine) (Fig. 23-27). Observe the patient from behind, noting whether the spine is straight (Fig. 23-28). Observe if the scapulae, iliac crests, and gluteal folds are level and symmetrical. Ask the patient to bend forward and reassess that the vertebrae are in a straight line and the scapulae are equal in height. *The spine is in alignment both standing and sitting.*

Kyphosis, a forward bending of the upper thoracic spine, may accompany *osteoporosis, ankylosing spondylosis*, and *Paget's disease*. Exaggerated curvature in the lumbar spine is lordosis, which is common in late pregnancy and obesity. A flattened lumbar curve may occur with lumbar muscle spasms. A list is a leaning of the spine to one side. This may occur with paravertebral muscle spasms or a herniated disc. Scoliosis is a lateral spinal curvature with a compensatory lumbar curve in the opposite direction.

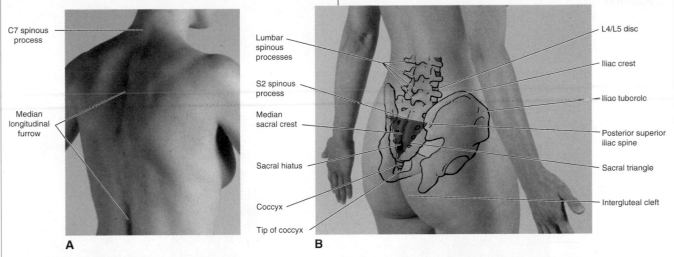

C7 spinous process

Median longitudinal furrow

Lumbar spinous processes

S2 spinous process

Median sacral crest

Sacral hiatus

Coccyx

Tip of coccyx

L4/L5 disc

Iliac crest

Iliac tuberole

Posterior superior iliac spine

Sacral triangle

Intergluteal cleft

A   **B**

Figure 23.27 Assessing the spine and upper back. **A.** Upper portion. **B.** Lower portion.

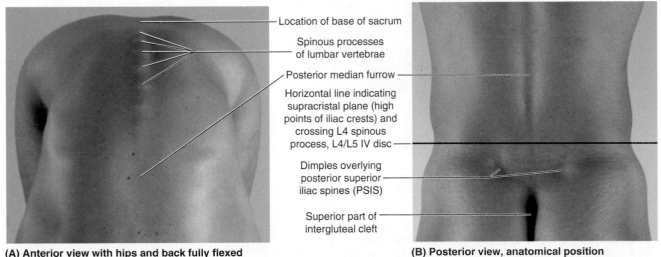

Location of base of sacrum

Spinous processes of lumbar vertebrae

Posterior median furrow

Horizontal line indicating supracristal plane (high points of iliac crests) and crossing L4 spinous process, L4/L5 IV disc

Dimples overlying posterior superior iliac spines (PSIS)

Superior part of intergluteal cleft

(A) Anterior view with hips and back fully flexed

(B) Posterior view, anatomical position

Figure 23.28 Lower back.

Palpation. Palpate the spinous processes. Feel for any bumps, nodules, or deformities. Ask if there is any tenderness during touch. Feel for crepitus when the spine bends. *The spinous processes are in a straight line. Patient denies tenderness. The paravertebral muscles are firm. There is no crepitus.*

Pain on palpation may indicate inflammation, disc disease, or *arthritis*. Unequal spinous processes may indicate subluxation.

(text continues on page 666)

ROM. Observe for full active ROM of the spine. Ask the patient to stand and bend forward to 75–90 degrees. Ask the patient to lean backward (hyperextend) to 30 degrees (Fig. 23-29). The spine assessment also includes lateral flexion (or abduction) to 35 degrees on either side. Ask the patient to slide a hand on one side down that thigh and bend away from the midline toward the side. Do this on both sides. To perform rotation of the spine, ask the patient to keep legs and hips forward facing while the shoulders move turn to the side (30 degrees). Repeat to the other side. *The patient can perform full ROM without crepitus or discomfort.*

Pain, back injury, *osteoarthritis*, and *ankylosing spondylitis* may result in limited ROM.

⚠ *SAFETY ALERT 23-8*

Stand beside the patient and be ready to provide support while the patient performs spine ROM. Patients may lose balance and fall.

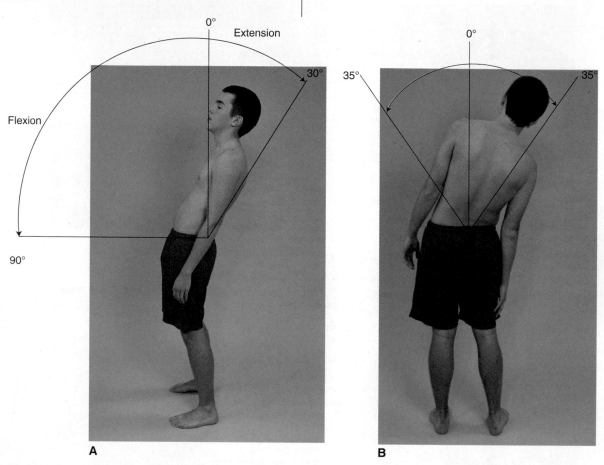

Figure 23.29 Spine ROM. **A.** Hyperextension. **B.** Lateral flexion.

Advanced practice nurses may perform the Straight Leg Test or the Milgram test to assess for a herniated disc. The Adams Forward Bend Test and a scoliometer are used to test for scoliosis. See Table 23-10.

Documentation of Normal Findings

The muscles are well formed, firm to touch, symmetrical. The spinous processes are straight and nontender. The thoracic and lumbar spines have full active ROM through flexion, extension, hyperextension, lateral flexion (or abduction), and rotation. Muscle strength is 5/5 Patient denies any discomfort while still or moving. *C. Chin, RN*

BOX 23.1 MORSE FALL SCALE

*N*ursing fall risk assessment, diagnoses and interventions are based on use of the Morse Fall Scale (MFS). The MFS is used widely in acute care settings, both in hospital and long term care inpatient settings. The MFS requires systematic, reliable assessment of a patient's fall risk factors upon admission, fall, change in status, and discharge or transfer to a new setting. MFS subscales include assessment of:

1. History of falling; immediate or within 3 months
   No = 0
   Yes = 25

2. Secondary diagnosis
   No = 0
   Yes = 15

3. Ambulatory aid
   None, bed rest, wheel chair, nurse = 0
   Crutches, cane, walker = 15
   Furniture = 30

4. IV/Heparin lock
   No = 0
   Yes = 20

5. Gait/transferring
   Normal, bed rest, immobile = 0
   Weak = 10
   Impaired = 20

6. Mental status
   Oriented to own ability = 0
   Forgets limitations = 15

Risk Level	MFS Score	Action
No Risk	0–24	None
Low Risk	25–50	See standard fall prevention interventions
High Risk	= 51	See high risk fall prevention interventions

Source: Morse, J. M. (2009). *Preventing patient falls*. (2nd ed.). New York: Springer.

Fall Risk

To assess if a patient is at risk for falling, nurses can use several tools. Most common are the Morse Fall Risk and Hendrich II Fall Risk model. A high score indicates a risk for falling and indicates a need for preventive interventions. Examples include frequent reminders, a bed alarm, or environmental cues. The Morse Fall Risk is more commonly used in hospitalized patients. See Box 23-1.

Lifespan Considerations

Pregnant Women

Lordosis shifts the weight back on the lower extremities and causes strain on the lower back muscles. Anterior flexion of the neck and slumping of the shoulder girdle compensate for lordosis. The upper back changes may put pressure on the ulnar and median nerves during the third trimester. Pressure on the nerves may cause aching, numbness, and upper extremity weakness in some pregnant women.

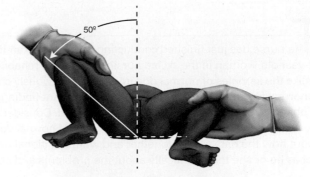

Figure 23.30 Testing for Allis' sign.

Newborns, Infants, and Children

At birth, newborns are assessed for congenital hip dislocation. The examiner performs either a Barlow-Ortolani maneuver or a test for Allis' sign.

In the Barlow-Ortolani maneuver, the infant is supine with flexed knees and hips so that the heels touch the buttocks. The examiner places his or her fingers on the baby's greater trochanter of the humerus and adducts the legs, moving the knees down and laterally. This maneuver is negative when the movement is smooth, with no clicking sound. If a clicking sound is audible, the maneuver is considered a positive indication of hip dislocation. See Chapter 28.

The examiner tests for Allis's sign by placing the infant supine with flexed hips and knees and both feet flat on the table. A negative Allis' sign is when the knees are at equal heights. A positive Allis' sign is when one knee is lower than the other, indicating hip dysplasia (Fig. 23-30).

The spinal column undergoes changes in contour as the child becomes more active. At birth the spine has a C shaped curve. The cervical curve develops by age 3 to 4 months as the child begins raising its head. The lumbar curve develops when the child stands, usually between 12 and 18 months (see Fig. 23-31).

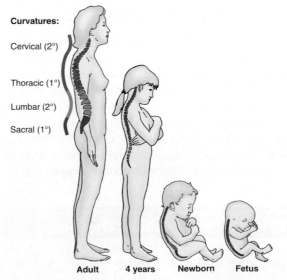

Curvatures:

Cervical (2°)

Thoracic (1°)

Lumbar (2°)

Sacral (1°)

Adult   4 years   Newborn   Fetus

Figure 23.31 Changes in spinal curvature from infancy through adulthood.

The nurse has just finished conducting a physical examination of Mrs. Runningbird, the 82-year-old woman in the skilled nursing facility for rehabilitation following a fall at home. Unlike the samples of normal documentation previously charted, Mrs. Runningbird has abnormal findings. Review the following important findings that were revealed in each step of objective data collection for Mrs. Runningbird. Consider how these results compare with the normal findings presented in the samples of normal documentation. Begin to think about how the data cluster together and what additional data the nurse might want to collect as he or she thinks critically about the problems and anticipates nursing interventions.

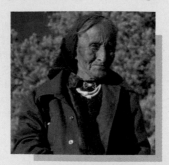

Inspection: Skin warm and pink. Mild kyphosis present. Heberen's nodes present at the distal interphalangeal joint; Bouchard's nodes present in the proximal interphalangeal joints in the hands. Diffuse swelling noted in all joints, most prominent in the hands. ROM approximately 50% of expected. Hip abduction and internal rotation are limited. Joints in knee and ankles are also swollen. Rheumatoid nodules are present. Gait slow but stable.

Palpation: Tenderness noted over joints in hands. Muscle strength 2/5 is decreased. Pulses ¾. Capillary refill 2 seconds. Identifies sharp and dull touch accurately. Muscle strength in feet and legs is 3/4.

V. Stark, RN

Examiners assess muscle tone in the newborn by observing flexion of the arms and legs and by holding the infant under the arms. With good muscle strength, the shoulders support the weight of the infant. Infants with poor muscle tone slide through the examiner's hands.

Older Adults

Examiners should allow extra time for older adults to complete each activity. They may divide the assessment into portions if an older patient appears fatigued.

Lifestyle affects the musculoskeletal system. Hardy et al. (2007) found that improved gait speed indicated better and longer survival and recommended assessment of gait speed as a vital sign for older adults.

Environmental Considerations

Some working conditions present potential risks to the musculoskeletal system. Workers required to lift heavy objects may strain and injure their backs. Jobs requiring substantial physical activity, such as construction work and fire fighting, increase the likelihood of sprains, strains, and fractures. Frequent repetitive movements may lead to misuse disorders such as carpal tunnel syndrome, pitcher's elbow, or vertebral degeneration. Musculoskeletal injuries may also occur when people sit for long periods at desks with poor ergonomic design.

Evidence-Based Critical Thinking

Organizing and Prioritizing

As with other systems, assessment of the musculoskeletal system usually proceeds from general to specific and from head to toe. Focused assessments may be more appropriate when the patient reports an injury to a specific area or joint.

Students need structure as they learn assessment skills. Medical students improved their skills in assessment of the musculoskeletal system when they were taught the GALS (Gait, Arms, Legs, Spine) locomotor screen (Doherty, et al., 1992; Fox, et al., 2000). The GALS is a method of quickly inspecting gait, arms, legs, and spine. The patient performs 11 tasks, and the examiner asks two questions: "Do you have any pain or stiffness anywhere?" and "Do you have any difficulty washing, dressing, or climbing stairs/steps?" Some educators and researchers have modified the first question to be more specific, that is, "Do you have any pain or stiffness in your muscles, joints, back, or neck?"

Laboratory and Diagnostic Testing

Laboratory tests can help identify specific musculoskeletal problems. Health care providers evaluate all test results within the context of other signs and symptoms. Common laboratory tests of muscle injury include evaluations of lactate dehydrogenase, creatinine kinase, alanine aminotransferase, and aspartate aminotransferaxe. Other tests can reveal responses to bone damage, such as alkaline phosphatase. Uric acid is elevated in gouty arthritis. Inflammatory markers such as erythrocyte sedimentation rate, C reactive protein, and rheumatoid factor are elevated with all inflammatory conditions, including rheumatoid arthritis and lupus.

Imaging tests are especially valuable in identifying musculoskeletal injuries and deformities. X-rays show bone fractures. Computerized tomography (CT) and magnetic resonance imaging (MRI) can reveal soft tissue damage, including ligament and tendon injuries. Bone density scans can help identify patients with osteoporosis and at risk for injury from falls.

Diagnostic Reasoning

When formulating a nursing diagnosis, it is important to use critical thinking to cluster data together and identify patterns that fit together. The nurse compares these clusters of data with the defining characteristics (abnormal findings) for the diagnosis to assure the most accurate labeling and appropriate interventions.

Nursing Diagnoses, Outcomes, and Interventions

A nursing diagnosis is a clinical judgment about responses to health problems or life processes. Table 23-11 compares nursing diagnoses, abnormal findings, and interventions commonly related to the musculoskeletal system assessment (Johnson, et al., 2005).

Nurses use assessment information to identify patient outcomes. Some outcomes that are related to system problems include the following (Moorhead, et al., 2004):

• Patient does not fall.

• Patient dresses, grooms, and eats independently.
• Patient ambulates in hall three times daily.

Once the outcomes area established, nursing care is implemented to improve the status of the patient. The nurse uses critical thinking and evidence-based practice to develop the interventions. Some examples of nursing interventions for the musculoskeletal system are as follows (Dochterman & Bulechek, 2004):

• Teach patient to call for help before ambulating to bathroom.
• Open packages and arrange tray prior to encouraging patient to eat independently.
• Communicate through documentation about the type of assistance needed.

The nurse then evaluates the care according to the patient outcomes that were developed, therefore reassessing the patient and continuing or modifying the interventions as appropriate. An accurate and complete nursing assessment is an essential foundation for holistic nursing care.

Table 23.11	Common Nursing Diagnoses Associated with the Musculoskeletal System		
Diagnosis and Related Factors	**Point of Differentiation**	**Assessment Characteristics**	**Nursing Interventions**
Impaired physical mobility (differentiate from impaired bed and wheelchair mobility)	Difficulty with being able to execute purposeful movements of the body or extremity without external supports	Limited ability to perform gross or fine motor skills, limited ROM, uncoordinated or jerky movements, difficulty with gait	Use footwear that facilitates waking and prevents injury. Use assistive devices. Screen for mobility skills (eg, transitions to sitting or standing).
Activity intolerance	Lack of energy to initiate, sustain, or perform daily routines and behaviors	Report of fatigue or weakness, abnormal pulse or blood pressure, shortness of breath, dizziness, chest pain	Determine cause of intolerance. Promote reconditioning when the result of immobility. Gradually increase activity according to symptoms.
Self care deficit: specify Bathing/ hygiene, Dressing/ grooming, Feeding, Toileting	Inability to perform activities of daily living for oneself	Grade ability to perform activity using a scale that includes being completely independent, requires use of equipment, requires help from another person, or completely dependent	Observe patient's ability to perform skill. Ask for input on habits and preferences. Encourage patient to do as much independently as possible. Use adaptive devices such as Velcro or elastic versus buttons or ties.
Impaired walking	Limitation of independent movement within the environment on foot	Cannot walk on even surfaces or uneven surfaces, climb stairs, or go required distances	Follow weight-bearing restrictions.* Use assistive devices such as a cane or walker. Obtain appropriate number of people to assist with walking the patient. Limit distractions during ambulation.

*Collaborative interventions.

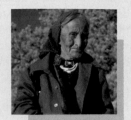

Remember Mrs. Runningbird, whose problems have been outlined throughout this chapter. The initial subjective and objective data collection is complete, and the nurse has spent time reviewing the findings and other results. The following nursing note illustrates how subjective and objective data are collected and analyzed and nursing interventions are developed.

Subjective: I feel stiff and cold. My legs and hands don't work the way that they used to.

Objective: Skin warm and pink. Diffuse swelling noted in all joints, most prominent in the hands. Rheumatoid nodules are present. ROM 50% in hands. Tenderness noted over joints in hands. Muscle strength 2/5 in hands and 3/5 in legs. CMS + all four extremities. Identifies sharp and dull touch accurately. Hip abduction and internal rotation are limited. Gait slow but stable. Needs one person assist and walker for ambulation to bathroom. Needs setup on fine motor skills for hygiene, dressing and eating.

Analysis: Impaired physical mobility related to reduced strength and ROM

Plan: Allow patient to perform as much independently as possible. Provide encouragement for participation in physical and occupational therapies and positive reinforcement for small increments in improvement. Remind her to use walker and call for help before ambulating to bathroom.

V. Stark, RN

Critical Thinking Challenge

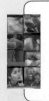

- What other assessments are important in addition to the musculoskeletal system?
- How will the nurse collect complete assessment information but avoid fatiguing Mrs. Runningbird?
- What functional patterns might the limited ROM and joint tenderness affect?
- Which is more of a concern for this patient—physiological or psychosocial assessment? Provide rationale.

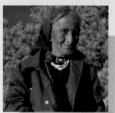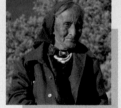

Both occupational and physical therapists work with patients to increase mobility and functional abilities for rehabilitation. Generally physical therapists focus on larger motor groups, while occupational therapists focus on fine motor skills and the upper body. Nurses may consult occupational therapists for patients with difficulties involving bathing, dressing, grooming, home and money management, assistive technology, or increasing ROM, tone, sensation, or coordination.

Mrs. Runningbird has been working with occupational therapy (OT) to increase function and to attain adaptive devices for her in the home. The following conversation illustrates how the nurse might communicate progress when OT comes.

Situation: Hi Cheryl. I'm taking care of Mrs. Runningbird today. She said that you were going to work with her in the kitchen today. (Cheryl confirms)

Background: She's a little discouraged because she doesn't feel like she's making progress.

Assessment: I had a discussion with her about how she's coping with her decline in function. She feels frustrated that she's not making faster progress because she really wants to go home.

Recommendations: I encouraged her and talked about how much improvement noted I've seen and she seemed encouraged by that. I think that if you also provided her with feedback on things that she is doing well, it will be motivating for her. We talked some about working with you today and seeing how she does in the kitchen because that's her biggest concern. She wants to be able to prepare her own meals but also is aware that a service that delivers meals might be an option. I told her how you would show her some tricks for cooking and also some ergonomic and lightweight cooking tools. Can you also work with her on opening jars? She's been having difficulty for awhile and thinks that you might be able to help her.

Critical Thinking Challenge

- Why didn't the nurse provide all of the physical assessment data to the OT?
- What is the role of the nurse in providing the psychosocial information to the OT?
- What types of assessments will need to be completed prior to discharging the patient to home?

The nurse uses assessment data to formulate a nursing care plan with patient outcomes and interventions for Mrs. Runningbird. Outcomes are specific to the patient, realistic to achieve, and measurable; they also have a time frame for completion. The interventions are actions that the nurse performs, based on evidence and practice guidelines. After implementation of these interventions, the nurse re-evaluates Mrs. Runningbird and documents the findings in the chart to show progress toward the patient outcome. The nurse uses critical thinking and judgment to continue or revise the diagnosis, outcomes or interventions. This is often in the form of a care plan or case note similar to the one below.

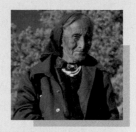

Nursing Diagnosis	Patient Outcomes	Nursing Interventions	Rationale	Evaluation
Impaired Physical Mobility related to joint swelling and tenderness as evidenced by limited ROM and reduced strength in hands	Demonstrates independent dressing, grooming, and toileting with assistive devices	Allow patient to do as much as possible. Provide positive feedback for progress each shift. Consult with OT on assistive devices. Collaborate on a plan for discharge and needed resources.	Independence provides increased control, functional ability, and a sense of accomplishment. OT can identify devices that might be helpful for discharge. A home care nurse may initially visit the patient to identify necessary resources.	Bathing and dressing with minimal assistance using elastic waist pants and Velcro shoes. Dressed the bottom half first and then the top. OT worked with patient today and identified assistive devices for the kitchen. Recommend home OT consult for at least one visit.

Using the previous steps of diagnostic reasoning, organizing, and prioritizing, consider all the case study findings woven throughout this chapter. When answering the following questions, begin drawing conclusions and see how the pieces of assessment must work together to create an environment for personalized, appropriate, and accurate care.

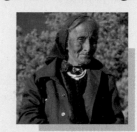

- How are physiological and psychological data connected?
- What nursing diagnoses might be activated on this patient's problem list? Provide rationale.
- What items will the nurse assess as part of a comprehensive musculoskeletal assessment? What additional assessments should the nurse add?
- What are expected findings for Mrs. Runningbird based on her age versus findings based on her osteoarthritis?

Key Points

- Functions of the musculoskeletal system include providing shape to the body and permitting movement.
- Identification of musculoskeletal risk factors is important for focused patient teaching aimed toward decreasing deformity or injury.
- Subjective data from the history and current condition guides performance of the physical assessment of the musculoskeletal system.
- The nurse should compare one side of the body to the other and determine if symmetry is present.
- The nurse assesses each joint for ROM and muscle strength.
- Gait, coordination, and balance involve both the musculoskeletal and neurological systems.

- Nurses use inspection and palpation to assess the musculoskeletal system. Advance practice nurses may use percussion to assess injured joints.
- During passive ROM, examiners do not force joints beyond the development of resistance or the development of discomfort.
- Patients with fragile bones require gentle handling to prevent fracture.
- Nurses consider abnormal findings in ROM and muscle strength when developing nursing diagnoses and planning interventions.
- Nurses individualize assessment of the musculoskeletal system according to the patient's condition, age, gender, and ethnicity.

Review Questions

1. Mr. Brown was playing soccer and hurt his right knee. It appears swollen. What is the first assessment the nurse should make?
   A. Palpate for crepitus in the knee
   B. Compare the swollen knee to the other knee
   C. Assess active ROM in the knee
   D. Feel the knee for warmth

2. Mrs. Johnson, a transcriptionist, reports pain and burning in her right hand. What assessment procedures should the nurse perform next?
   A. Trendelenburg's and drawer signs
   B. McMurray's and Thomas' tests
   C. Bulge test and ballottement
   D. Phalen's and Tinel's tests

3. Which of the following assessment tasks can you appropriately delegate to an unlicensed care provider?
   A. Height, weight, and vital signs
   B. Active and passive ROM
   C. History of current complaint
   D. Muscle strength

4. When doing an assessment of the spine of an older adult, the nurse can expect to see which variation?
   A. Lordosis
   B. Torticollis
   C. Kyphosis
   D. Scoliosis

5. When assessing the spine of a woman in her ninth month of pregnancy, the nurse would expect to see which variation?
   A. Lordosis
   B. Torticollis
   C. Kyphosis
   D. Scoliosis

6. To correctly document that ROM in the fingers is full and active, the nurse writes that the patient can
   A. perform rotation, lateral flexion, and hyperextension
   B. make a fist, spread and close fingers, and do finger-thumb opposition
   C. touch finger to own nose and to examiner's finger back and forth
   D. perform supination, pronation, and lateral deviation

7. When assessing a newborn, the nurse notes that one knee is lower than the other when the legs are flexed and the heels are together on the bed. The nurse should correctly document this finding as positive
   A. ballottement
   B. Thomas' test
   C. Allis' sign
   D. genu varus

8. A nurse is assessing a patient who has been diagnosed with a neuromuscular disorder. The nurse notes the patient cannot lift the right leg off of the bed when the nurse is applying resistance. The nurse would document the muscle strength in the right leg as
   A. fair
   B. 2/5
   C. 50%
   D. within normal limits

9. The nurse notes an adolescent has uneven shoulder height. To differentiate functional from structural scoliosis, the nurse will ask the patient to
   A. stand up straight while the nurse checks the height of the iliac crest
   B. flex the elbow and pull against the nurse's resistance
   C. shrug both shoulders while the nurse provides resistance
   D. bend forward at the waist while the nurse palpates the spine

10. A patient reports that a previous right hip replacement is suddenly painful. Which hip assessment technique should the nurse omit?
    A. Adduction
    B. Hyperextension
    C. Extension
    D. Circumduction

11. A female patient reports that her mother has osteoporosis and wants to know what she can do to prevent developing the disease. Which of the following responses is best for the nurse to provide?
    A. Engage in aerobic exercise at least three times per week
    B. Eat at least one serving of dark green leafy vegetables daily
    C. Consume three servings of dairy products per day
    D. Perform muscle strengthening exercises every other day

References

AHRQ. (2007). *Comparative effectiveness of treatment to prevent fractures in men and women with low bone density or osteoporosis.* Agency for Healthcare Research and Quality, Rockville, MD. Retrieved January 31, 2008, from http://effectivehealthcare.ahrq.gov/index.cfm/search-for-guides-reviews-and-reports/?pageaction=displayproduct&productid=73

Almstedt Shoepe, H., & Snow C. M. (2005). Oral contraceptive use in young women is associated with lower bone mineral density than that of controls. *Osteoporosis International, 16*(12), 1538–1544.

CACPF. (2008). *Child meal recommendations.* Retrieved March 25, 2008, from http://www.cacfp.com/child_meal_pattern.pdf

Dane, C., Dane, B., Cetin, A., & Erginbas, M. (2007). Comparison of the effects of raloxifene and low-dose hormone replacement therapy on bone mineral density and bone turnover in the treatment of postmenopausal osteoporosis. *Gynecological Endocrinology, 23*(7), 398–403.

Doherty, M., Dacre, J., Dieppe, P., & Snaith, M. (1992). The "GALS" locomotor screen. *Annals of the Rheumatic Diseases, 51*(10), 1165–1169.

Dochterman, J. M., & Bulechek, G. M. (2004). *Nursing interventions classification (NIC)* (4th ed.). St Louis, MO: Mosby.

Finkelstein, J. S., Brockwell, S. E., Mehta, V., Greendale, G. A., Sowers, M. R., Ettinger, B., et al. (2008). Bone mineral density changes during the menopause transition in a multiethnic cohort of women. *Journal of Clinical Endocrinology and Metababolism, 93*(3), 861–868.

Fox, R. A., Dacre, J. E., & Ingram Clark, C. L. (2000). Impact on medical students on incorporating GALS screen teaching into the medical school curriculum. *Annals of the Rheumatic Diseases, 59*(9), 668–671.

Gartner, L. M., & Greer, F. R. (2003). Prevention of rickets and vitamin D deficiency: New guidelines for vitamin D intake. *Pediatrics, 111*(4), 908–910.

Goebel, L. (2007). *Scurvy.* Retrieved March 25, 2008, from http://www.emedicine.com/med/topic2086.htm

Hampl, J. S., Taylor, C. A., & Johnston, C. S. (2004). Vitamin C deficiency and depletion in the United States: the Third National Health and Nutrition Examination Survey, 1988 to 1994. *American Journal of Public Health, 94* (5), 870–875.

Hardy, S. E., Perera, S., Roumani, Y. F., Chandler, J. M., & Studenski, S. A. (2007). Improvement in Usual Gait Speed Predicts Better Survival in Older Adults. *Journal of the American Geriatric Society, 55*(11), 1727–1734.

Healthy people 2010: What are its goals? (n.d.). Retrieved July 7, 2010, from http://www.healthypeople.gov/About/goals.htm

Hewett T. E., Ford, K. R., Gregory D., & Myer, G. D. (2006). Anterior cruciate ligament injuries in female athletes: part 2, a meta-analysis of neuromuscular interventions aimed at injury prevention *American Journal of Sports Medicine, 34*, 490.

Johnson, M., Bulechek, G. M., McCloskey Dochterman, J, & Maas, M. L. (2005). *NANDA, NOC, and NIC linkages: Nursing diagnoses, outcomes, and interventions.* St. Louis, MO: Mosby.

MacLean, C., Newberry, S., Maglione, M., McMahon, M., Ranganath, V., et al. (2008). Systematic review: Comparative effectiveness of treatments to prevent fractures in men and women with low bone density or osteoporosis. *Annals of Internal Medicine, 148*(3), 197–213.

Moorhead, S., Johnson, M., & Maas, M. (2004). *Nursing outcomes classification (NOC)* (3rd ed.). St. Louis: Mosby.

Morse, J. M. (2009). *Preventing patient falls* (2nd ed.). New York: Springer.

NIAMSD. (2006). *Strategic plan for reducing health disparities.* Retrieved March 25, 2008, from http://www.niams.nih.gov/About_Us/Mission_and_Purpose/strat_plan_hd.asp

National Osteoporosis Foundation. (2008). *Osteoporosis facts.* Retrieved March 25, 2008, from http://www.nof.org/osteoporosis/diseasefacts.htm

Pressler, J. L. (2008). Classification of major newborn birth injuries. *Journal of Perinatal & Neonatal Nursing, 22*(1), 60–67.

Swiontkowski, M. F., Engelberg, R., Martin, D. P., & Agel, J. (1999). Short musculoskeletal function assessment. *The Journal of Bone and Joint Surgery, 81-A*(9), 1245–1260.

Towheed, T. E., Maxwell, L., Anastassiades, T., et al. (2005). Glucosamine therapy for treating osteoarthritis. *Cochrane Database Systematic Review.* 2:CD002946.

Tylavsky, F. A., Ryder, K. A., Lyytikäinen, A., & Cheng, S. (2005). The influence of Vitamin D on bone health across the life cycle: Vitamin D, parathyroid hormone, and bone mass in adolescents *American Society for Journal of Nutrition, 135*, 2735S–2738S.

Valachovicova, T., Slivova, V., Bergman, H., Shuherk, J., & Sliva, D. (2004). Soy isoflavones suppress invasiveness of breast cancer cells by the inhibition of NF-kappaB/AP-1-dependent and -independent pathways. *International Journal of Oncology, 25*, 1389–1395.

van Schoor, N. M., Visser, M., Pluijm, S. M., Kuchuk, N., Smit, J. H., & Lips, P. (2008). Vitamin D deficiency as a risk factor for osteoporotic fractures. *Bone, 42*(2), 260–266.

Volpi, E., Nazemi, R., & Fujita, S. (2004). Muscle tissue changes with aging. *Current Opinion in Clinical Nutrition & Metabolic Care, 7*(4), 405–410.

Ward, K. D., & Klesges, R. C. (2001). A meta-analysis of cigarette smoking on bone mineral density. *Calcified Tissue International, 68*(5), 259–270.

Women's Health Care in the United States: Selected Findings From the 2004 National Healthcare Quality and Disparities Reports. Fact Sheet. AHRQ Publication No. 05-P021, May 2005. Agency for Healthcare Research and Quality, Rockville, MD. Retrieved January 31, 2008, from http://www.ahrq.gov/qual/nhqrwomen/nhqrwomen.htm

---

The Jensen suite offers these additional resources to enhance learning and facilitate understanding of this chapter:

- thePoint on line resource, http//thepoint.lww.com/Jensen1E
- Student CD-ROM included with the book
- *Laboratory Manual for Nursing Health Assessment: A Best Practice Approach*
- *Pocket Guide for Nursing Health Assessment: A Best Practice Approach*

Tables of Abnormal Findings

Table 23.12 Selected Musculoskeletal Problems: Onset, Gender, and Ethnicity

Problem	Age at Onset	Gender	Ethnicity
Amyotrophic Lateral Sclerosis (ALS)	Median age 55–66 years	More common in men	Most common in Caucasians
Ankylosing Spondylitis	Women 17–35 years; men 20–30 years	Three times more common in men	Most common in Native Americans
Bursitis	Older than 40 years	Occurs in men and women, related to chronic stress or acute injury	Occurs in all ethnicities
Carpal Tunnel Syndrome	25–50 years	Three times more common in women; especially prevalent in pregnant and menopausal women	Most common in Caucasians
Dupuytren's Contracture	After 40 years	More common in men	Most common in Caucasians of north European ancestry
Gout	Older than 70 years	Three times more common in men	Slightly more common in African Americans
Low Back Pain	30–50 years	More common in men	Affects all ethnicities
Multiple Sclerosis	Average age 18–35 years but can occur at any age	Twice as common in women	Most common in Caucasians, but the more aggressive form occurs more frequently in African Americans
Multiple Myeloma	Older than 50 years	More common in men	Two to four times more common in African Americans
Myasthenia Gravis	Women 18–25 years; men older than 60 years	Twice as common in women	Occurs in all ethnicities
Osteoarthritis	Older than 50 years in women; 40–50 years in men	More common in women, although hip osteoarthritis is similar	Most common in Caucasians
Osteoporosis Types I and II	Postmenopausal women; 50–70 years in men	Type I more common in women	Type I most common in Caucasians
Osteosarcoma	Younger than 20 years and also 50–60 years	Slightly more common in men	Slightly more common in African Americans
Paget's Disease	Older than 40 years	More common in men	Most common in Caucasians
Polymyalgia Rheumatica	Over 50 years	More common in women	Most common in Caucasians
Rheumatoid Arthritis	20–40 years	Two to three times more common in women	Most common in North American Indians
Scleroderma	30–50 years	Two to eight times more common in women	Most common in Choctaw Indians, followed by African, Hispanic, Caucasian, and then Japanese Americans
Scoliosis	10–15 years	Eight times more common in girls	Found in all ethnicities
SLE	20–30 years	Ten times more common in women	Most common in non-Caucasians

Sources: *Kelly's Textbook of Rheumatology*, 7th ed; *Campbell's Operative Orthopedics*, 10th ed.

Table 23.13 Abnormal Gait Patterns

Gait	Pathological Condition	Description
Antalgic	Degenerative knee or hip disease	Patient walks with a limp to avoid pain. The gait is characterized by a very short stance phase.
Ataxic	Cellebellar lesion	Patient shows unsteady, uncoordinated walking with a wide base, feet thrown out, and a tendency to fall to one side.
Short leg	Discrepancy in length of one leg, flexion contracture of hip or knee, congenital hip dislocation	Patient limps with walking unless he or she wears adaptive shoes.
Footdrop or steppage	Peroneal or anterior tibial nerve injury, paralysis of dorsiflexor muscles, lower motor neuron damage, damage to spinal nerve roots L5 and S1	Patient lifts the advancing leg high so that the toes may clear the ground. He or she places the sole of the foot on the floor at one time, instead of placing the heel first. This problem may be unilateral or bilateral.
Apraxic	Frontal lobe tumors, Alzheimer's disease	Patient has difficulty initiating walking. After starting to walk, the gait is slow and shuffling. Motor and sensory systems are intact.
Trendelenburg (compensated gluteus medius gait)	Developmental hip dysplasia, muscular dystrophy	The trunk lists toward the affected side when weight bearing is on that side. A waddling gait may develop if both hips are affected.

Other gait abnormalities are described in Chapter 24, Table 24-10.

Table 23.14 Comparison of Musculoskeletal Conditions Affecting Multiple Joints

Assessment	Rheumatoid Arthritis	Osteoarthritis	Gouty Arthritis	Fibromyalgia
Risk factors	Physical and emotional stress	Obesity, aging	Family history, diet high in purine-rich foods, alcohol, stress	Family history; Emotional stress
Pain	Upper extremities	Lower extremities	Base of big toe; may also affect feet, ankles, knees, elbows	Any joints, especially neck, back, shoulders, knees, hands
Onset	Young adulthood	50s–60s	Middle-age men	Adult women, 22–55 years
Stiffness	Significant in mornings and after inactivity	Worse later in the day and after inactivity	None in acute cases, develops with chronic cases	Some stiffness, especially in the morning
Generalized complaints	Weakness, fatigue, low fever	None	Painful, monoarticular, nocturnal joints, later more joints, great toe most often	Sleep disturbance and morning fatigue
Physical examination—joints	Tender, swollen, may be warm	May be tender	Swollen, warm, tender, shiny, red	No swelling, tender to touch
Diagnostic tests	Elevated serum proteins in blood and synovial fluid—rheumatoid factor	X-ray, CT, MRI	Elevated uric acid in blood and urine; Synovial fluid aspiration	Not definitive, rule out other diagnoses

Atrophy

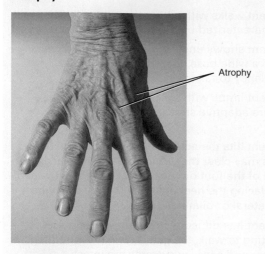

Atrophy

Hand of an 84-year-old woman

Decreased size can occur in any muscle. Causes include nerve damage, disuse, and nerve or muscle damage.

Joint Effusions

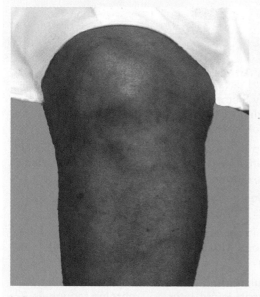

Inflammatory processes commonly resulting from trauma, joint overuse, and rheumatoid arthritis can cause synovial fluid to accumulate in a joint. When considerable fluid builds up, the joint appears swollen. The fluid is compressible, also called fluctuant. Treatment may involve rest, antiinflammatory agents, or surgical removal.

Joint Dislocation

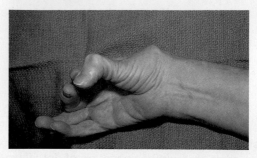

The ends of bones slip out of the usual position, usually from a sports-related injury, trauma, or a fall. Severe dislocation can cause tearing of the muscles, ligaments, and tendons that support the joint. Manifestations include swelling, pain, and immobility of the affected joint. Hand joints are most frequently dislocated, followed by shoulders. Hips, knees, and elbows are less commonly dislocated. Dislocations require medical intervention to prevent nerve damage.

Longstanding Rheumatoid Arthritis

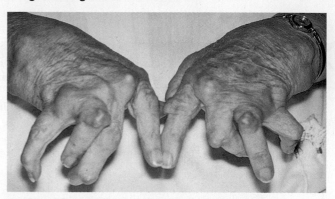

In this chronic, systemic, inflammatory disease of joints and connective tissue, inflammation causes thickening of synovial membrane. Fibrosis follows, with eventual bony ankylosis. The disorder is bilateral and symmetrical. Characteristics include heat, redness, swelling, and painful motion of affected joints. Associated symptoms include fatigue, weakness, anorexia, weight loss, low-grade fever, and lymphadenopathy.

Rotator Cuff Tear

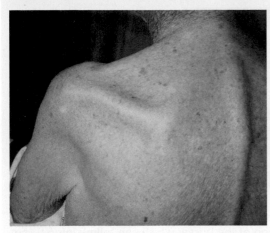

Manifestations include a hunched shoulder and limited arm abduction. A positive drop arm test (arm is passively abducted, person cannot maintain position, and arm falls to side) is diagnostic. This condition may result from trauma while arm is abducted, falling on shoulder, throwing, or heavy lifting.

Osteoporosis

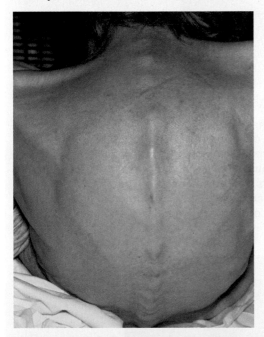

Osteoporosis occurs when bone resorption is faster than deposition. The weakened bone increases risk for fractures, especially in vertebrae, wrist, and hip. This occurs predominantly in postmenopausal Caucasian women. Risk factors include small bone frame, younger age at menopause, sedentary lifestyle, tobacco use, alcohol intake, and inadequate diet.

Osteoarthritis

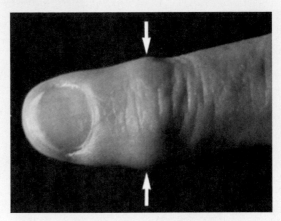

This localized, progressive, noninflammatory disease results in deterioration of articular cartilage and bone, and deposition of new bone at joint surfaces. Incidence increases with age. Commonly affected joints include hands, knees, hips, and lumbar and cervical vertebrae. Manifestations include stiffness, swelling, hard bony protuberances, pain with motion, and limited motion.

Genu Valgum ("Knock Knee")

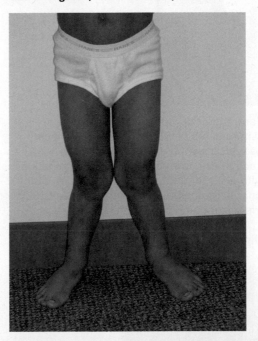

Many children have a temporary period of this condition, but persistent knock knee may be genetic or the result of metabolic bone disease. The patient may need to swing each leg outward while walking to prevent striking the planted limb with the moving limb. The strain on the knee frequently causes anterior and medial knee pain. Physical therapy and surgical intervention may be required.

(table continues on page 678)

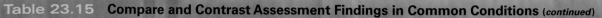

Ganglion Cyst

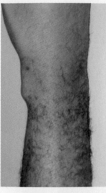

A soft, nontender, round nodule on the dorsum of the wrist that becomes more prominent during flexion. It is a benign tumor.

Epicondylitis

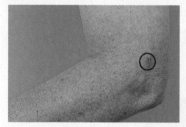

Epicondylitis

With this inflammation of the lateral epicondyle of the elbow, pain radiates down the extensor surface and increases with resisting extension of the hand. It results from activities combining excessive supination of forearm with an extended wrist. Inflammation of the medial epicondyle (golf elbow) is rarer and results from excessive wrist flexion and pronation.

Congenital Hip Dislocation

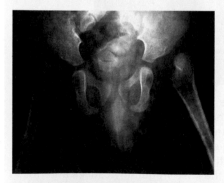

The head of the femur is displaced from the acetabulum. This condition is seven times more common in females. Signs include asymmetric gluteal creases, uneven limb length, and limited abduction when the thighs are flexed. Diagnosis for newborns is a positive Barlow-Ortolani's sign. Older children will have a positive Trendelenburg's sign.

Bursitis (Olecranon Bursitis)

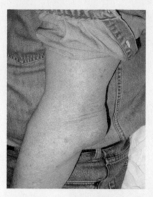

More than 150 bursae in the body cushion and lubricate joints, tendons, and ligaments. Bursitis is an inflammation of the bursa, which can follow injury, infection, or a rheumatic condition. Shoulders, elbows, and hip are common sites of bursitis; however, bursitis can occur in any joint, including knees, heels, and bases of big toes. Characteristics include swelling, tenderness, and pain that increases with movement.

Swan Neck and Boutonnière Deformity

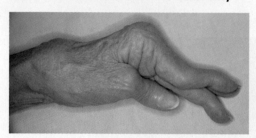

The fingers have a "swan-neck" appearance resulting from flexion contracture of the metacarpohyalangeal joint with hyperextension of the distal joint. Boutonnière deformity causes flexion of the proximal interphalangeal joint with hyperextension of the distal joint. Both conditions occur with chronic rheumatoid arthritis and are often accompanied by ulnar deviation of the fingers.

Polydactyly

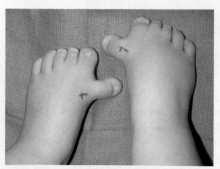

This congenital deformity results in extra fingers, usually at the thumb or fifth finger. Cosmetic removal is frequent, unless extra digit has full ROM and sensation.

Table 23.15   Compare and Contrast Assessment Findings in Common Conditions *(continued)*

Syndactyly

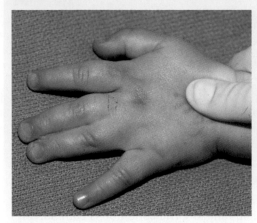

In this congenital deformity of webbed fingers, the metacarpals and phalanges of the webbed fingers are unequal in length and the joints do not align, which limits flexion and extension. Surgical separation is usual. Toes may also be webbed.

Dupuytren's Contracture

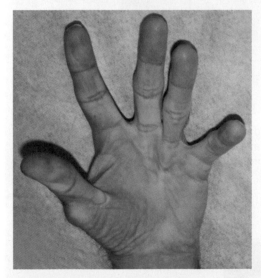

Hyperplasia of the palmar fascia causes painless flexion contracture of the digits, which impairs function. It usually starts in the fourth digit, then extends to the fifth and third. Dupuytren's commonly occurs in men older than 40 years and develops bilaterally. Incidence increases with diabetes, epilepsy, family history of Dupuytren's contracture, and alcoholic liver disease.

Herniated Nucleus Pulposus

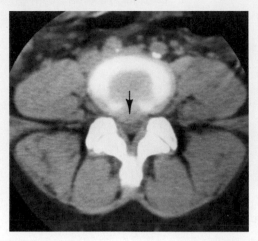

The intervertebral discs may slip out of position following trauma or strain. Rupture of the nucleus pulposus (soft inner portion) may put pressure on the spinal nerve root. Symptoms include sciatic pain radiating down the leg, numbness, parasthesia, listing from the affected side, decreased mobility, low back tenderness, and decreased motor and sensory function in the affected leg. Straight leg raises produce sciatic pain.

Talipes Equinovarus ("Club Foot")

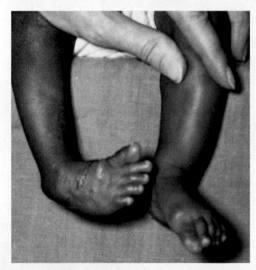

The foot is turned to the side, and the involved foot, calf, and leg are smaller and shorter than the normal side. One or both feet may be affected. This condition is not painful; however, if left untreated, significant discomfort and disability will develop. Treatment ranges from braces or casts to surgery.

(table continues on page 680)

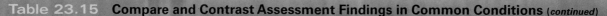

Ulnar Deviation

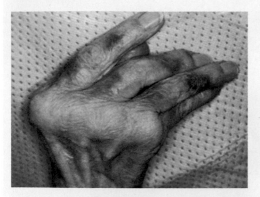

Stretching of the articular capsule and muscle imbalance in rheumatoid arthritis cause fingers to point in the ulnar direction.

Ankylosing Spondylitis

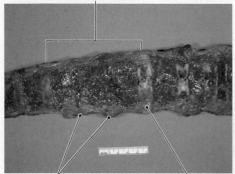

Three vertebrae fused into one

Approximate sites of destroyed intervertebral discs   Intervertebral disc

This chronic, progressive inflammation of the spine and sacroiliac and large joints in the extremities affects men 10 times more than women. It is characterized by bony growths. Muscle spasms pull the spine forward and eliminate the cervical and lumbar curves. Flexion deformities can also occur in knees and hips.

Acute Rheumatoid Arthritis

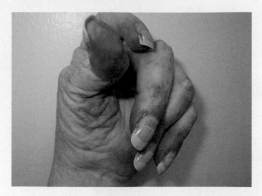

Inflammation results in painful, reddened, swollen joints and limited function. The condition is common in proximal intraphalangeal joints.

Heberden's and Bouchard's Nodes

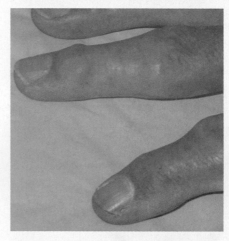

Hard, nontender bony growths on the distal (Heberden's) and proximal (Bouchard's) intraphalangeal joints. Frequently occurs with deviation of the fingers.

Carpal Tunnel Syndrome

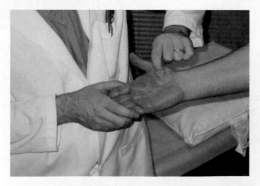

Carpal tunnel syndrome occurs from repetitive motion and develops in people 30–60 years. It occurs in women five times more frequently than men. Symptoms include burning, pain, and numbness from compression of the median nerve inside the carpal tunnel of the wrist. Atrophy of the thenar eminence at the base of the thumb is common. Diagnosis is made from a positive Phalen's test or Tinel's sign.

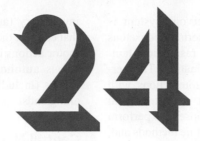

24

Neurological Assessment

Learning Objectives

1 Describe the structure and function of the central nervous system (CNS), including cellular components, brain, spinal cord, and supportive and protective elements.

2 Apply anatomic and physiologic concepts to nursing assessment of the neurological system.

3 Correlate the physiology of specific structures of the CNS with clinical presentation during the health history and physical assessment.

4 Identify teaching opportunities for health promotion and risk reduction related to the neurological system.

5 Summarize elements of a complete health history that contribute meaningful data to neurological assessment.

6 Discuss factors that influence the nurse's decision about which elements of the neurological examination to include for specific patients and situations.

7 Identify clinical situations that require urgent communication of neurological findings.

8 Demonstrate application of the Glasgow Coma Scale.

9 Describe assessment of at least one function of each of the 12 cranial nerves.

10 Outline testing of motor and sensory function for conscious and unconscious patients.

11 Use subjective and objective data to analyze neurological findings and plan interventions.

12 Document and communicate neurological findings using appropriate medical terminology.

13 Individualize neurological health assessment considering the condition, age, gender, and culture of the patient.

14 Use neurological findings to identify diagnoses and to initiate a plan of care.

*M*r. Gardner, a 56-year-old African American, has a history of hypertension, smoking, and mild baseline dementia. He was admitted to an acute care unit via the emergency department (ED) following a stroke. He lives alone, has poor hygiene, and is wearing multiple layers of mismatched clothing. He does not remember the last time he took his blood-pressure medication. Vital signs are T 36.8°C orally, P 88 beats/min, R 22 breaths/min, and BP 168/92 mm Hg. Mr. Gardner is alert, but appears somewhat fearful and agitated. He asks for cigarettes and is oriented to name only. Speech is comprehensible but slurred.

You will gain more information about Mr. Gardner throughout the chapter. As you study the content and features, consider the case and its relationship to what you are learning. Begin thinking about the following points:

- Is Mr. Gardner's condition stable, urgent, or an emergency?
- What immediate health-promotion and teaching needs are evident?
- How will the nurse focus, organize, and prioritize subjective data collection?
- How will the nurse focus, organize, and prioritize objective data collection?
- How will the nurse individualize assessment to Mr. Gardner's specific needs, considering his condition, age, and culture?

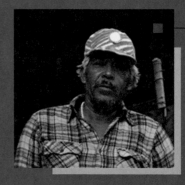

An intact, appropriately functioning nervous system is critical for all human endeavors. It exerts unconscious control over basic body functions, such as respiration, temperature regulation, and movement coordination. The nervous system also enables very complex interactions with people and the environment. Assessment of neurological functioning serves multiple purposes. All those who perform neurological assessments use some of the same methods and, at times, share the same goals (eg, detection of change in neurological status, particularly acute and life-threatening alterations). Generally, however, physicians assess neurological function primarily to localize pathology and to make a medical diagnosis. Nurses perform neurological assessment mainly to identify actual or potential health problems related to neurological dysfunction, and the patient's response to those problems.

Common to all settings and types of neurological assessment is use of an organized approach to maximize the value of information derived from collected data. This approach consists of general patient observation, data-gathering from the health history (often performed simultaneously), and a systematic neurological examination.

Structure and Function Overview

The nervous system is divided into the **central nervous system (CNS)**, consisting of the brain and spinal cord, and **peripheral nervous system**, which includes the cranial, spinal, and peripheral nerves. The nervous system also can be classified according to function as either voluntary or involuntary (autonomic). In the **voluntary** division, fibers that connect the CNS to muscles and skin facilitate deliberate motor actions in response to stimuli. In the primarily unconscious **autonomic** division, fibers connect the CNS with organs (including the heart and kidneys), smooth muscles, and glands.

Central Nervous System

Brain

The brain is a network of interconnecting **neurons** that control and integrate the body's activities. Each neuron contains a *cell body*, which serves as the control center; smaller receiving fibers called *dendrites*; and a connecting long fiber called an *axon*. Axons are white because they are covered with a *myelin sheath* that speeds impulse conduction. Cell bodies are on the outside of the brain (gray matter or cerebral cortex), while axons that connect to other parts of the nervous system (white matter or brain tissue) are directed toward the center of the brain. Neurons communicate with one another at *synapses*, small spaces between two neurons. Important parts of the brain include the cerebrum, brainstem, and cerebellum (Fig. 24-1).

Cerebrum. The cerebrum has two hemispheres, left and right, and contains 80% of the brain tissue. The left hemisphere is primarily analytical, while the right is more creative (Frishkoff, 2007). The *cerebral cortex*, which forms the outside of the cerebrum, contributes to motor and sensory function, intellect, and language.

Each hemisphere of the cerebral cortex has four lobes: frontal, temporal, parietal, and occipital (Fig. 24-2).

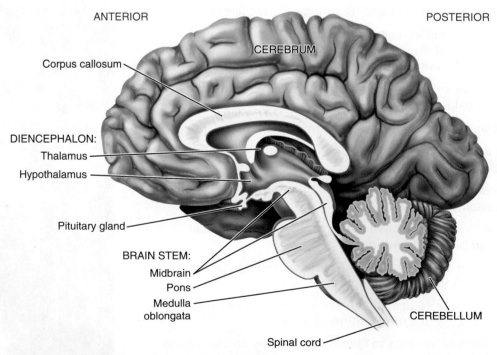

Figure 24.1 The brain and its important divisions.

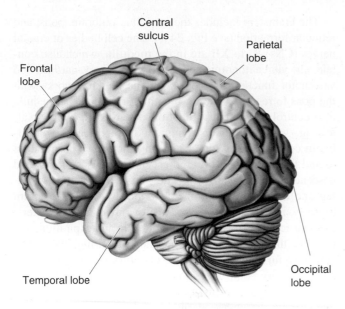

Figure 24.2 Lobes of the cerebral cortex.

The *precentral gyrus* in the frontal lobe controls *motor function* on the opposite side of the body; the left side of the brain controls the right side of the body, and the right side of the brain controls the left side of the body. The *postcentral gyrus* in the parietal lobe receives input on *sensory function* including temperature, touch, pressure, and pain, also from the opposite side of the body. Motor and sensory function is organized from head to toe on both the left and right sides, similar to a person hanging upside down (Fig. 24-3).

The cerebral cortex also is responsible for visual imaging, auditory processing, and language comprehension and expression. Each of the four lobes contributes to different functions. The **frontal lobe** is responsible for complex cognition (orientation, memory, insight, judgment, arithmetic, and abstraction); language (verbal and written); and voluntary motor function. It integrates this cognitive function with emotional responses, personality, impulse control, and social behavior. The motor function area, previously discussed, is located at the foot of the frontal lobe. The **parietal lobe** recognizes the size, shape, and texture of objects, and interprets touch, pressure, and pain. The sensory areas previously discussed are located at the front of the parietal lobe. Language is processed in Wernicke and Broca areas in the parietal lobe of the left hemisphere. **Wernicke area** integrates understanding of spoken and written words, while **Broca area** regulates verbal expression and writing ability. The primary visual area is the **occipital lobe** in the back of the brain, with visual associative areas that interpret and integrate stimuli. The **temporal lobe** registers auditory input and is responsible for hearing, speech, behavior, and memory. Additionally, some scientists identify a fifth lobe (Standring, 2004). The **limbic lobe** consists of the hippocampus and amygdaloid nucleus, a more primitive part of the brain. It is primarily concerned with

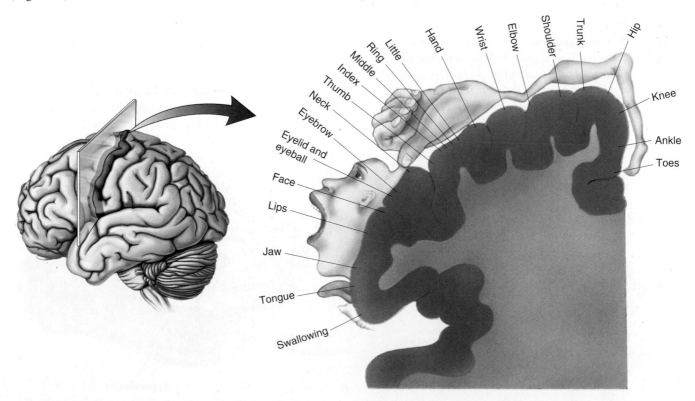

Figure 24.3 The homunculus, showing the organization of sensory function.

self-preservation, including recall of pleasurable, unpleasant, or potentially dangerous events. It also recalls mood and emotional responses in relation to events, including aggression, interpretation of smell, feeding and sexual behavior, and autonomic responses associated with emotion.

The cerebrum contains the basal ganglia, thalamus, hypothalamus, and limbic system (Standring, 2004). The **basal ganglia** are four paired tracts of gray matter on both sides of the thalamus deep within the brain tissue (Fig. 24-4A). They modulate automatic movements, receiving input from the cerebral cortex and sending output to the brainstem and thalamus to facilitate smooth motor function (eg, fluid swinging of the arms while walking). The **thalamus**, directly above the brainstem, is the major relay station and gatekeeper for both motor and sensory stimuli to the cerebral cortex. The **hypothalamus** controls vital functions of temperature, heart rate, blood pressure, sleep, the anterior and posterior pituitary, the autonomic nervous system, and emotions. It maintains overall autonomic control. The **limbic system** is more primitive and mediates survival behaviors such as fear, aggression, mating, and affection (Fig. 24-4B).

Brainstem. The **brainstem** is integral to intact neurological functioning. Both afferent and efferent fibers pass through it from the spinal cord to the cerebrum and cerebellum. **Afferent (sensory) stimuli** travel through the brainstem to the cerebral cortex; **efferent (motor) fibers** leave the cortex to pass through the brainstem and spinal cord.

The brainstem includes the medulla, midbrain, pons, and reticular formation (see Fig. 24-1). The cell bodies of cranial nerves (CNs) III to XII are in the **medulla**, which also contains the vital autonomic centers for respiratory, cardiac, and vasomotor function (Table 24-1). The medulla works with the pons to regulate smooth breathing rhythm. The medulla also controls involuntary functions such as sneezing, swallowing, vomiting, hiccoughing, and coughing. The **midbrain** contains many motor neurons and relays information to and from the brain through ascending sensory tracts and descending motor pathways. The **pons** contains the ascending and descending neuron tracts and assists the midbrain to relay information. It contains two respiratory centers: one that controls the length of inspiration and expiration, and the other that controls respiratory rate (Standring, 2004). The **reticular formation** relays sensory information, excitatory and inhibitory control of spinal motor neurons, and control of vasomotor and respiratory activity. It is responsible for increasing wakefulness, attention, and responsiveness of cortical neurons to sensory stimulation.

Cerebellum. The **cerebellum** is under the occipital lobe in the posterior part of the brain. It coordinates voluntary movement, posture, and muscle tone, and maintains special orientation and equilibrium. It ensures adjustments in movement to maintain overall balance and coordination through connections to the motor cortex, brainstem, and pathways. It integrates information from the cerebral cortex, inner ear, muscles, and joints. Alcohol intake can affect the cerebellum, causing the characteristic loss of balance and coordination. The cerebellum rests against the opening at the base of the skull known as the **foramen magnum**.

Protective Structures of the CNS

The *meninges* and *skull* cover and protect the brain. The *ventricles* of the brain are fluid-filled cavities that connect with the spinal cord. *Cerebrospinal fluid* (CSF) circulates within the space surrounding the brain, brainstem, and spinal cord. In addition to carrying nutrients, the CSF cushions and allows for shifts of fluid between the brain and spinal cord.

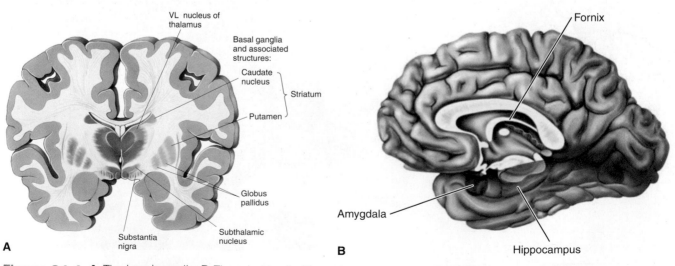

Figure 24.4 **A.** The basal ganglia. **B.** The primitive limbic system.

Table 24.1   Cranial Nerves

Cranial Nerve	Anatomy	Physiology
I. Olfactory (sensory)	Originates in the nasal mucosa; ends in the temporal lobe	Smell and smell interpretation, including peristalsis, salivation, and sexual stimulation
II. Optic (sensory)	Originates in the retinal cells in the optic disc; travels over the optic nerve to end in the occipital lobe	Vision, including visual acuity and peripheral vision
III. Oculomotor (motor)	Originates in the midbrain and supplies motor fibers to the eye, eyelid, ciliary muscles, and iris	EOMs: • Upward • Medial • Downward • Up and in Eyelid raising and pupil constriction
IV. Trochlear (motor)	Originates in the midbrain and supplies motor fibers to the superior oblique muscle of the eye	EOMs: Down and in
V. Trigeminal (sensory and motor)	Originates in the pons; has three branches: *ophthalmic* (sensory), *maxillary* (sensory), and *mandibular* (sensory and motor)	*Ophthalmic branch*: Sensation to the cornea, conjunctiva, nasal mucosa, forehead, and nose *Maxillary branch*: Sensation to the skin of the cheek and nose, lower eyelid, upper jaw, teeth, mouth mucosa *Mandibular branch*: Sensation to the lower jaw, and motor function to muscles of mastication
VI. Abducens (motor)	Originates in the pons and supplies motor fibers to the lateral rectus muscle	EOMs: lateral
VII. Facial (sensory and motor)	Originates in the pons and supplies sensory fibers to the anterior two-thirds of the tongue and soft palate and motor fibers to the muscles of the face	Taste and sensation for the anterior two-thirds of the tongue and soft palate; serves as the primary motor nerve for facial expression
VIII. Acoustic (sensory)	Cochlear sensory fibers originate in the cochlea and transmit auditory sensation to the ear, pons, and temporal lobe. Vestibular sensory fibers originate in the semicircular canals of the ear and vestibular ganglion and end in the pons	Hearing Equilibrium
IX. Glossopharyngeal (sensory and motor)	Sensory divisions from the external ear, tympanic membrane, upper pharynx, and posterior one-third of the tongue end in the medulla; motor divisions supply the pharyngeal muscle and parotid gland	Pharyngeal muscle elevation for swallowing and speech; parotid gland secretion; general sensory (pain, touch, temperature) function
X. Vagus (sensory and motor)	Major parasympathetic nerve of the body; originates in the medulla; sensory from larynx, esophagus, trachea, carotid bodies, thoracic and abdominal viscera, and stretch and chemoreceptors from the aorta; motor supplies the pharynx, larynx, thoracic, and abdominal viscera	Provides most parasympathetic innervation to a large region; effects include digestion, defecation, slowed heart rate, and reduced contraction strength
XI. Spinal accessory (motor)	Originates in medulla with two branches; cranial root innervates muscles of the larynx and pharynx; spinal root innervates trapezius and sternocleidomastoid muscles	Swallowing and speaking; innervates the muscles that turn the head and elevate the shoulders (shoulder shrug)
XII. Hypoglossal (motor)	Originates in the medulla and ends at the tongue	Tongue movement

Source: Standring, S. (2004). *Gray's anatomy: The anatomical basis for clinical practice* (39th ed.). London: Elseiver Churchill Livingstone; Kandel, et al., (2008). *Principles of neural science* (5th ed.). Philadelphia: Elsevier.

Spinal Cord

The spinal cord continues from the brainstem, exiting from the base of the skull and extending to the coccyx. The cells of the spinal cord are aligned so that there are specific ascending and descending pathways or tracts. The spinal pathways are named according to point of origin and destination (eg, spinothalamic, corticospinal). Similar to the brain, the cell bodies of the spinal cord are aligned so that there is gray (cell bodies) and white (axons) matter. The H-shaped gray matter is in the center, surrounded by white matter. The gray matter contains the cell bodies of voluntary motor neurons, autonomic motor neurons (parasymphathetic

neurons from S2 to S4 and sympathetic neurons from T1 to L2), and sensory neurons (Standring, 2004). The white matter contains the axons of the ascending and descending motor fibers. The axons are clustered into specific tracts for either ascending or descending fibers.

The **ascending tracts** generally carry specific sensory information from the periphery to higher levels of the CNS (Fig. 24-5). Input from sensory receptors in the skin, organs, and muscles travels through the peripheral nerves to the dorsal root of the spinal nerve and into the spinal cord. These **dorsal columns** (also called posterior columns) carry information about localized touch (stereognosis), deep pressure, vibration, position sense (proprioception), and movement (kinesthesia) (Standring, 2004). They travel up the same side of the spinal cord to the brainstem. At the medulla they synapse, cross to the opposite side of the body, and travel to the sensory cortex. Because of the crossing of the fibers in the medulla, right-sided sensations are perceived on the left side of the brain, and left-sided sensations are perceived on

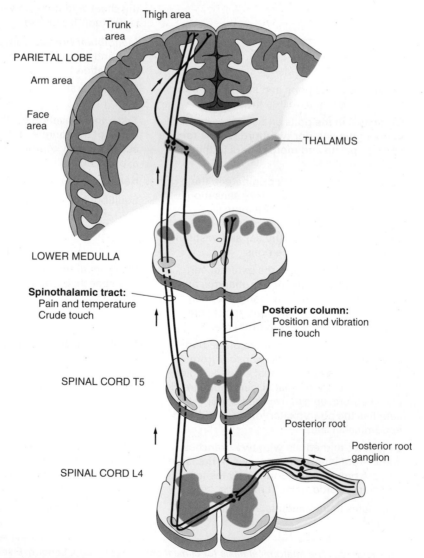

Figure 24.5 Ascending tracts of the brain carry sensory information from peripheral nerves to the central nervous system.

the right side of the brain. Additionally, specialized ascending tracts for pain and temperature (spinothalamic) and coordination of movement (spinocerebellar) enter the dorsal ganglia, synapse with another neuron, and cross the spinal column here (instead of in the medulla as with the dorsal columns). The information is carried to the sensory cortex on the opposite site of the brain. Thus, all sensory information is perceived on one side of the brain for the opposite side of the body.

Clinical Significance 24-4

When half of the spinal cord is severed (eg, with a gunshot wound), the patient may experience *Brown-Séquard's syndrome sensory loss.* Manifestations include loss of pain and temperature on the opposite side of the injury, because these fibers cross in the spinal cord. Localized touch, deep pressure, vibration, position sense, and movement remain on the same side of the body because these fibers cross in the medulla.

The **descending tracts** carry information related to motor function and muscle movement (Fig. 24-6). They control voluntary movement, carrying impulses from the cortex to the cranial (corticobulbar tract) and peripheral (corticospinal tract) nerves (Standring, 2004). The corticobulbar and corticospinal tracts are referred to as the **pyramidal tract**. Axons originate in the motor cortex, travel to the brainstem, and cross at the medulla. Similar to the sensory tracts, the motor tracts on the left side of the brain control the right side; those on the right side of the brain control the left. The neurons exit the spinal cord at the ventral root of the spinal nerve, and impulses are carried to the peripheral motor nerves.

Another group of fibers in the descending tract carries information involving all motor systems except those of the pyramidal tract. This **extrapyramidal tract** originates in the reticular formation and is modulated by the brainstem, basal ganglia, and cerebellum. It travels down and synapses in the ventral root of the spinal cord; however, it does not directly innervate the peripheral motor system. This tract

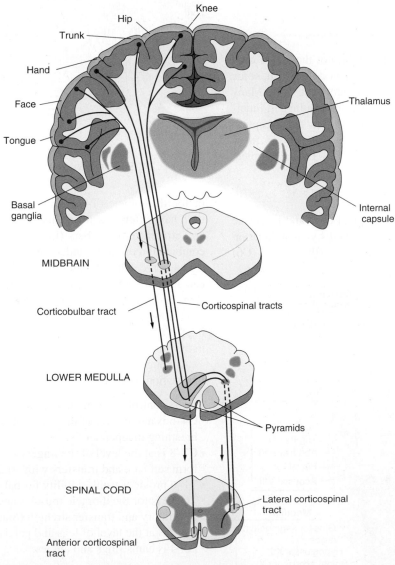

Figure 24.6 Descending tracts carry motor and muscle information from the cortex to the cranial and peripheral nerves.

controls gross automatic movements such as reflexes, walking, complex movements, and postural control.

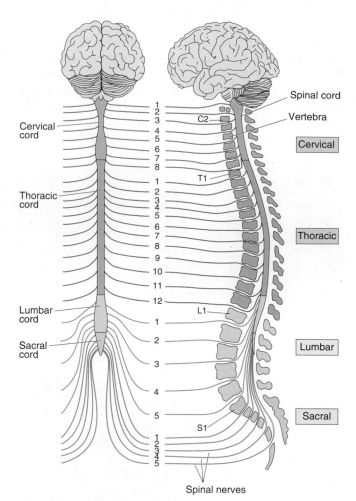

Figure 24.8 The spinal nerves.

Clinical Significance 24-5

Some medications prescribed to patients with psychiatric illnesses have extrapyramidal side effects. Such patients need ongoing assessment for involuntary and irregular muscle movements, restlessness, and spasms of the neck, tongue, or jaw. Patients with Parkinson's disease may have poor skeletal muscle tone, drooling, tremor, and shuffling gait related to loss of neurons in the extrapyramidal tract. Involuntary writhing movements related to damage to this tract also may accompany cerebral palsy.

Peripheral Nervous System

The peripheral motor system includes neurons outside the CNS. The CNs, spinal nerves, and autonomic nervous system all belong to the peripheral motor system.

Cranial Nerves

The 12 paired **CNs** exit from the brain, not the spinal cord (Fig. 24-7). Some CNs have only a sensory component, some have only a motor component, and others have both. Many CNs originate in the midbrains, pons, or medulla and innervate the eyes, ears, nose, mouth, and throat. An exception is the vagus nerve, which provides motor and sensory function to the heart and abdomen. See Table 24-1 for a complete description of the CNs.

Spinal Nerves

The **spinal nerves** arise from the spinal cord and innervate the rest of the body. They are described by their location in relation to the vertebrae, such as the sixth cervical (C6)

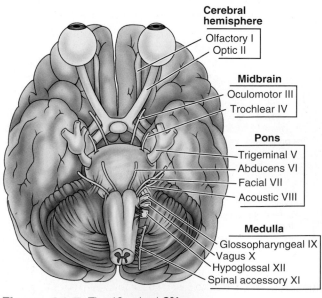

Figure 24.7 The 12 paired **CNs.**

or fourth thoracic (T4). Unlike the CNs, the spinal nerves each have afferent sensory fibers (located in the dorsal root) and efferent motor fibers (located in the ventral root). The combination of motor and sensory fibers is referred to as the spinal nerve. The 31 pairs of spinal nerves include 8 cervical, 12 thoracic, 5 lumbar, 5 sacral, and 1 coccygeal nerves (Fig. 24-8). Each level innervates a specific body part from head to toe on the right and left sides. This is seen by evaluating the area of skin innervated by the afferent sensory fibers in the dorsal root of a spinal nerve, called a **dermatome**.

Although the dermatomes provide a general idea of the innervation by each nerve, some overlap exists (Fig 24-9):

- C1–3 controls movement in and above the neck.
- C4–6 is at the level of the shoulder and diaphragm for breathing independently.
- C7–8 is at the level of the fingers and hand grasp to perform self care and transfers with arms.
- T1–6 provides trunk stability for balance when sitting.
- T6–12 is for the thoracic muscles and upper back for respiratory and transfer strength (Standring, 2004).
- L1–2 is at the level of legs and pelvis.
- L3–4 is hamstrings and ankles.

Level of injury to the spinal cord affects function at and below the site of trauma. Thus, a patient with an injury at T6 would

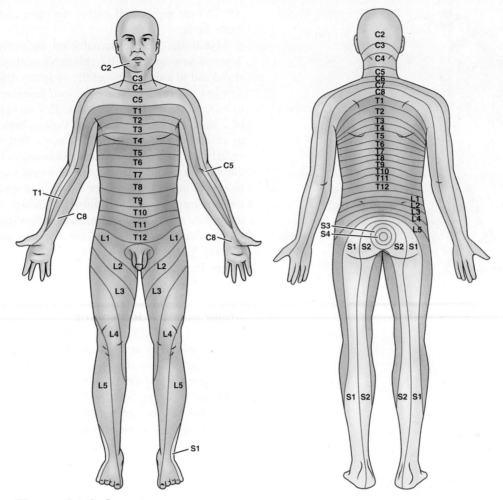

Figure 24.9 Dermatomes.

have arm movement and sensation but no leg movement or sensation. The patient with a lesion or spinal cord injury at L1–2 has varying control of the legs and pelvis. One with problems at L3–4 has weakened hamstrings and ankles, which may permit ambulation with braces and a cane.

Autonomic Nervous System

The autonomic nervous system maintains involuntary functions of cardiac and smooth muscle and glands. It has two components: sympathetic (fight or flight) and parasympathetic (rest and digest). These two systems balance the body and maintain homeostasis (Standring, 2004). The sympathetic ganglia are located in the spine from T1 to L2. The major neurotransmitter is epinephrine or adrenaline. The cell bodies of the parasympathetic nervous system are located in the brainstem and spinal segments S2–4. The ganglia are located near the structures that they innervate; the neurotransmitter is acetylcholine.

The autonomic system can both sense and make changes based on input. To regulate heart rate and blood pressure, it receives input from chemoreceptors and baroreceptors (see Chapter 19). Based on such input, the sympathetic system secretes epinephrine to increase blood pressure, heart rate, and contractility; the parasympathetic system secretes acetylcholine to reduce heart rate and force of contraction. Many times the two systems work in opposite ways to provide balance to the body's overall function.

Reflexes are involuntary responses to stimuli. They maintain balance and tone, such as the sucking reflex of a baby when the cheek is stroked. Reflexes also provide quick responses in potentially harmful situations, such as withdrawing of the foot when stepping on a sharp object. The simplest type of **reflex arc** involves a receptor-sensing organ, afferent sensory neuron, efferent motor neuron, and effector motor organ (Fig. 24-10). A commonly tested reflex is the "knee-jerk" reaction when the knee is tapped; this is a deep tendon reflex (DTR) as the patellar tendon is stimulated. The patellar tendon is the sensing organ, which travels through the sensory neuron to the dorsal root ganglion. It synapses in the spinal cord and travels out through the motor neuron to the quadriceps muscle, where this motor organ contracts and the knee jerks. The muscle also must be strong enough to cause the reflex. Other reflexes include the superficial (eg, corneal, abdominal), visceral (pupillary response to light), and neonatal (rooting, grasp, Babinski).

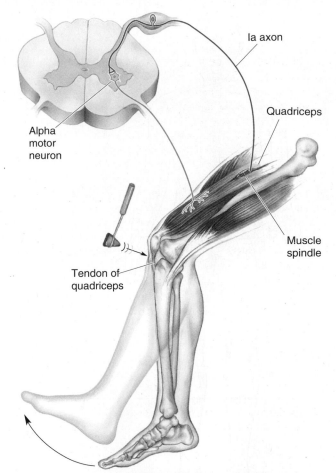

Figure 24.10 A commonly cited **reflex arc** is the "knee-jerk" reaction, which is a DTR that results with stimulation of the patellar tendon.

Labels: Ia axon, Alpha motor neuron, Quadriceps, Muscle spindle, Tendon of quadriceps

🔺 Lifespan Considerations

Pregnant Women

Little is known about neurological changes in pregnancy (Lowdermilk & Perry, 2007). Notably, changes in the hypothalamic-pituitary axis lead to elevated levels of estrogen, progesterone, prolactin, and oxytocin. Other changes are related to pressure on the peripheral nerves from the weight of the fetus and postural changes; these usually resolve after birth.

Newborns and Infants

The fetal nervous system grows rapidly. At birth the incompletely integrated nervous system is developed enough to sustain life, primarily through reflexes. The autonomic nervous system is critical during this period, because it stimulates the first respiration, assists in maintaining acid-base balance, and regulates temperature control (Hockenberry & Wilson, 2007).

Myelin is necessary for quick and efficient transmission of nerve impulses. Myelination is incomplete at birth; it develops from head to toe and centrally to peripherally. The earliest tracts are sensory (taste, smell, and hearing), cerebellar (balance and coordination), and extrapyramidal (pain).

All CNs are myelinated except the optic and olfactory (see Table 24-1).

Myelination of the spinal cord is nearly complete by 2 years, as manifested by children's ability to walk unassisted and to move purposefully in space. By the end of the first year, all brain cells are present; however, they continue to increase in size. Brain growth is 75% completed by the end of 2 years (Wong, et al., 2007). Various brain areas develop as children gain intellectual capacity. Milestones have an orderly and predictable sequence in healthy children. As toddlers begin talking, Broca area develops. Cortical areas for motor control of the legs, hand, feet, and sphincters grow as toddlers learn to walk and train the bladder and bowels. Initially their ability to attend to locomotion and elimination is limited; however, by 3 years, development and coordination of these functions allow toddlers to listen better and behave longer. Postural control continues to develop as the functions are integrated.

Children and Adolescents

School-age children are steadier on their feet than preschoolers. They are more coordinated with better posture that enables them to climb, ride bikes, and play games. Head circumference is decreased in relation to height. The skull and brain grow very slowly during this period; most of the growth has been completed (Wong, et al., 2007).

Although the number of neurons does not increase in adolescents, nourishing support cells for neurons continue to grow. Development of the myelin sheath "fine tunes" the neural system, coinciding with the adolescent's more advanced cognitive development.

Older Adult

Neurons of the CNS, brain size, and neurotransmitters decrease with aging. Results include slower thought processing, reduced response to stimuli, and delayed reflexes. Ability to respond to multiple stimuli and manage multiple tasks concurrently is reduced. Peripheral nerve function and impulse conduction decrease, with resultant decreased proprioception and potential for a Parkinson-like gait. Thus, older adults are at risk for poor balance, postural hypotension, falls, and injury. Light touch and pain sensation are reduced, with ischemic paresthesia common in the extremities. Overall cognitive function with aging varies greatly depending on overall lifestyle choices and heredity (ANA & John A. Hartford Foundation Institute, 2007).

🔹 Acute Assessment

Once baseline information has been gathered, it is often not practical or necessary to perform a complete neurological examination. Choice of elements to assess in a given setting depends on many variables. Recognition of situations requiring acute assessment and rapid communication of findings is critical to preventing or limiting negative outcomes for patients (Box 24-1).

BOX 24.1 SIGNIFICANT CHANGES IN NEUROLOGICAL STATUS

- Acute change in mental status: increasing restlessness, agitation, or confusion
- Changes in consciousness not explained by known causes (eg, sedatives). This ranges from patterns of increasing difficulty in arousing the patient to complete lack of responsiveness to any stimulus.
- Seizure activity
- Onset of flexor or extensor posturing, either spontaneously or in response to noxious stimuli
  - Flexor posturing = adduction of arm with flexion at elbow and wrist, extension and internal rotation of leg with plantar flexion of foot
  - Extensor posturing = adduction, internal rotation, and extension of arm; extension and internal rotation of leg with plantar flexion of foot
  - Change in size and decreased reactivity to light in one or both pupils
  - Onset of conjugate or dysconjugate eye deviation
  - Progressing weakness (paresis) or paralysis of an extremity or one side of the body; observe for facial weakness on the same side
- Changes in ability to identify sensation

- Significant changes in vital signs (beyond parameters established by physician)
- Changes in blood pressure may threaten tissue oxygenation or result in direct injury from hemorrhage. For example, a patient with cerebral vascular insufficiency who is usually hypertensive may suffer a cerebral infarction if blood pressure drops too low. In a patient with an untreated ruptured cerebral aneurysm or intracerebral hemorrhage, hypertension may trigger additional hemorrhage.
- Change in heart rate or rhythm may threaten adequate perfusion or indicate potential etiology (eg, atrial fibrillation with emboli, causing stroke).
- Fever may indicate infection or dysfunction of the autonomic nervous system and is associated with worsened outcome after traumatic brain injury and acute stroke.
- Significant or progressively rising blood pressure may lead to widening pulse pressure, decreasing pulse, and decreasing respirations, the classic signs of increased ICP (Cushing response); these are late signs of lower brainstem compression.
- Irregular breathing patterns may indicate progressing brainstem compression.

When situations such as those in Box 24-1 are identified, rapidly assessing key areas included in the neurological examination is the first step in determining the nature of the problem and possible acute interventions. This abbreviated acute assessment (details of each element are described more completely later) includes the following:

- Rapid assessment of **level of consciousness** (LOC) using the **Glasgow Coma Scale** (GCS), scoring verbal response, eye opening, and motor function. If the patient can respond verbally, basic orientation is assessed. This also allows a basic speech/language assessment (comprehension and production of spoken language and speech quality, such as garbled or slurred).
- **Pupillary reaction**: Assess size (before and after light stimulus) and speed of response to light.
- Gross assessment of **extremity strength**. If the patient can follow commands, ask him or her to lift each extremity off the bed, noting whether he or she can maintain limb elevation against gravity, and then against resistance from the examiner. Also note any facial asymmetry (either at rest or during facial movement).
- Gross assessment of **sensation** (only possible if the patient can communicate) by examining ability to identify presence and location of light touch on all extremities and both sides of the face.
- If consciousness is impaired, assessing selected other **CNs** may help differentiate neurological from metabolic causes, particularly **extraocular movements** (EOMs), **gag reflex**, and **corneal reflex**.

Vital signs are part of this acute assessment, because they may be either a cause or result of the acute change (see Box 24-1). As soon as is practical, obtaining health history information helps identify potential sources of the problem.

Subjective Data Collection

Areas for Health Promotion/ *Healthy People*

An important purpose of the health history is to gather information to promote health and provide health teaching. Health-promotion activities for the nervous system focus on preventing disease, identifying problems early, and reducing complications of existing or established diagnoses. See Table 24-2 for some areas related to health promotion for this body region.

Assessment of Risk Factors

Nurses obtain a history of past medical diagnoses, particularly head or spinal trauma, and known risk factors for common neurological conditions (eg, stroke). They note chronic or recent exposures to toxins; any recent viruses; vaccinations; and insect, spider, tick, snake, or scorpion bites or stings. While taking health history, nurses might elicit information that suggests a seizure disorder, stroke, or traumatic injury.

When questioning patients about risk factors, the goal is to identify how likely they are to develop or to already be experiencing consequences of neurological and neurovascular diseases. Such investigation creates an

Table 24.2 *Healthy People* Goals Related to Neurological Health

Goals	Patient Education Topics
Reduce stroke deaths. Increase the proportion of adults who are aware of the early warning symptoms and signs of a stroke.	Teach healthy behaviors; screen for risk factors. Teach patients to call 911 if they experience: • Sudden numbness or weakness of the face, arm, or leg, especially on one side of the body • Sudden confusion, trouble speaking or understanding • Sudden trouble seeing in one or both eyes • Sudden trouble walking, dizziness, loss of balance or coordination • Sudden, severe headache with no known cause (American Heart Association [AHA], 2007)
Increase the proportion of adults with high blood pressure who are taking action (eg, losing weight, increasing physical activity, and reducing sodium intake) to help control their blood pressure.	Encourage healthy weight, increased exercise, and reduced sodium intake. Approximately one-third of patients have difficulty maintaining adherence to their blood pressure medication (Nelson, et al., 2007); assess any reasons for not taking medications.
Increase the proportion of adults who are at a healthy weight and reduce the proportion of adults who are obese.	Patients with obesity, in particular abdominal obesity, are 1.6–1.8 times more likely to have an ischemic stroke (Hu, et al., 2007). Teach patients to reduce calorie intake.
Reduce the proportion of adults who engage in no leisure-time physical activity and increase the proportion of adults who engage regularly, preferably daily, in moderate physical activity for at least 30 minutes.	Patients with no leisure-time activity are 2.7 times more likely to have a stroke compared to those who exercise (Goldstein, et al., 2006). Encourage hesitant patients to start small and gradually increase activity.
Reduce tobacco use by adults.	Smokers are 1.8 times more likely to have a stroke than are nonsmokers (Goldstein, et al., 2006). Counsel patients at every visit about willingness to quit.

Source: *Healthy people 2010: What are its goals?* (n.d.). Retrieved July 7, 2010, from http://www.healthypeople.gov/About/goals.htm

environment in which health care providers can implement necessary interventions to control symptoms, direct education to prevent new problems or complications, and establish within the patient's record areas needing ongoing follow-up and emphasis. For example, overweight, physical inactivity, high blood pressure, high cholesterol, and diabetes mellitus are common causes of stroke (AHA, 2007). After assessment, nurses identify focused teaching areas and evaluate in ongoing visits the patient's progress toward change.

The following screening questions are important to establishing the patient's risk for neurological disease.

Questions on History and Risk	Rationales
From the chart obtain the following: • Age • Heredity • Gender • Date and result of last blood pressure reading • Date and result of last cholesterol level	Increased age and male gender increase risk for *stroke*. Another risk is stroke in a parent, grandparent, or sibling. African Americans have a higher risk of death from stroke than Caucasians, partly because blacks have higher risks of high blood pressure, diabetes, and obesity (AHA, 2007).
Have you ever been diagnosed with a neurological problem, such as seizure? • When did you have it? How often? • Seizure history: associated warning signs (aura), motor activity, loss of consciousness, incontinence, sleepiness after the seizure (postictal phase), precipitating factors • How was the seizure treated? • Was the treatment effective?	Various scales have been developed to identify *seizure* severity; criteria include seizure frequency, seizure type, seizure duration, postictal events, postictal duration, automatisms, seizure clusters, known patterns, warnings, tongue biting, incontinence, injuries, and functional impairment (Cramer & French, 2001).

Questions on History and Risk	Rationales
Have you ever had a head injury? • When? • How was it treated? • What were the outcomes?	A *head injury* is suspected if there is a: • Witnessed loss of consciousness of longer than 5 minutes • History of amnesia of longer than 5 minutes • Abnormal drowsiness • More than three episodes of vomiting • Suspicion of non-accidental injury • Seizure in a patient with no history of epilepsy (Thiessen, 2006)
Have you ever had a stroke? • When did you have it? • How was it treated? • What were the outcomes?	An exact time of onset, definite focal symptoms, neurological signs, and ability to lateralize the signs to the left or right side of the brain suggest a *stroke* (Hand, et al., 2006).
Have you ever had any infectious or degenerative diseases, such as meningitis or muscular sclerosis?	Symptoms of *meningitis* include high fever, stiff neck, drowsiness, and photosensitivity. Symptoms of *degenerative disease* include weakness, tingling or numbness, difficulty seeing, and elimination-control problems.
Have you had any changes in your emotional state or coping strategies related to your health? • Personality change • Alterations in level of independence • Loss of role function related to altered ability to carry out responsibilities, interact with others • Depression, apathy, or irritability • Change in ability to tolerate stress • Issues related to chronic conditions, progressive deterioration in function or hospitalization	Information regarding past and current emotional state and coping strategies is obtained through attention to functional health patterns. Family relationships and socio-economic background provide valuable clues to the patient's support system and capacity to manage the social and financial effects of disabilities frequently associated with neurological conditions.
Do you have a history of high blood pressure? • When was it diagnosed? • How is it being treated?	Systolic blood pressure >140, diastolic blood pressure ≥90, or both is a risk factor for *stroke* (Rothwell, et al., 2005).
Which of the following conditions place you at risk for neurovascular disease? • Diabetes mellitus • Carotid artery disease • Atrial fibrillation • Sickle cell disease	*Atrial fibrillation* increases risk for stroke, because quivering atria can lead blood to stagnate and form small clots. A clot that breaks off can circulate to the brain and block the artery, causing an *embolic stroke*. In *sickle cell disease*, blood cells tend to be stickier, causing clots to form more easily in narrowed arteries.
What lifestyle choices place you at risk for neurovascular disease? • Smoking • High-fat diet • Obesity • Physical inactivity	Many risk factors for stroke are the same as for cardiovascular disease (see Chapter 19).
What environmental or occupational hazards increase risks of neurological trauma? • Lack of seat belt use • No helmet when biking, snowboarding, engaging in high-risk sports • Incorrect use of car seats for children • Use of drugs or alcohol while driving • Falls (lack of window guards, pull bars, safety gates) • Ignorance of firearm safety	Males are almost twice as likely as females to sustain traumatic brain or spinal cord injuries, partly because they engage in riskier activities (National Center for Injury Prevention and Control, Spinal Cord, 2007).

Risk Assessment and Health-Related Patient Teaching

As mentioned, risk assessment helps to identify potential problems so that health care providers can give patients information that can influence behavioral choices. The most important focus areas for the neurological system involve prevention of stroke and unintentional injury.

Stroke Prevention

Risk factors for stroke are similar to those for cardiovascular disease; thus, prevention also involves modification of unhealthy lifestyle choices. Patients should control blood pressure through weight reduction, healthy diet, and use of antihypertensive medications as prescribed. At every visit, nurses should ask patients about smoking and, for those with a positive response, about the desire for cessation. Nurses should provide all patients with information about a diet low in saturated fat and high in fruits and vegetables. They should ask overweight and obese patients about their willingness to reduce calories. Additionally, nurses should advise all patients to exercise aerobically three to seven times a week for 20 to 60 minutes per session (Gordon, et al., 2004).

Injury Prevention

When investigating risk for traumatic injury, nurses also provide information about prevention. Nurses should recommend use of protective helmets and gear to patients who engage in sports involving physical contact. During assessment of driving habits, nurses advise patients about the importance of seat belts and discourage use of alcohol and drugs. They provide patient teaching materials to reinforce concepts, especially for adolescents and young adults who are at highest risk of brain and spinal cord injury.

Focused Health History Related to Common Symptoms

The history of the present illness or problem should elucidate a detailed account of each symptom, its nature (location, quality, and severity), date of onset, precipitating factors, and duration (constant, intermittent, or worse at any particular time of day). Nurses also should note what, if anything, makes the symptom worse or better, and what has been the general pattern of progression (rapid, static, progressively worse, remitting, exacerbating).

During assessment of the neurological system, nurses should inquire about common symptoms in all patients to screen for the early presence of disease. If a patient is concerned about specific neurological problems, nurses assess these focused areas with follow-up questions. A thorough history of symptoms assists with identifying the current problem or diagnosis. Nurses should direct questioning toward a history of problems with headaches, weakness or paralysis, loss of sensation, and involuntary movements or sensations.

Common Neurological Symptoms

- Headache or other pain (see Chapter 14)
- Weakness of single limb or one side of body
- Generalized weakness
- Involuntary movements or tremors
- Difficulty with balance, coordination, or gait
- Dizziness or vertigo
- Difficulty swallowing
- Change in intellectual abilities
- Difficulties with expression or comprehension of speech/language
- Alteration in touch, taste, or smell
- Loss or blurring of vision in one or both eyes, diplopia (double vision)
- Hearing loss or tinnitus (ringing in the ears)

Questions to Assess Symptoms	Rationales/Abnormal Findings
Headache or Other Pain Do you have a headache or other pain (see chapter 14).	
Limb or Unilateral Weakness Do you have any weakness on one side or in one limb? • How long does it last? • Is there any associated speech problem?	Unilateral weakness, disturbed speech, and symptoms longer than 10 minutes increase risk of *stroke* (Rothwell, et al., 2005). Report patients with positive findings to a physician for diagnosis and treatment.
Generalized Weakness Do you have generalized weakness? • Does it occur mostly in the hands and feet or core muscles? • Do any repetitive actions lead to such weakness? • Are there any associated symptoms such as rash or joint inflammation?	Causes may be infectious, neurological, endocrine, inflammatory, rheumatic, genetic, metabolic, electrolyte-induced, or drug-induced. *Neuropathy* primarily occurs in distal muscles. A rash is a sign of *lupus*. Repetitive actions exacerbate *myasthenia gravis*. Common neurological causes include *demyelinating disorders, amyotrophic lateral sclerosis, Guillain-Barré's syndrome, multiple sclerosis, myasthenia gravis*, and *degenerative disc disease* (Saguil, 2005).

Questions to Assess Symptoms	Rationales/Abnormal Findings
Involuntary Movements or Tremors Have you noted any shaking or tremors? • Do they occur at rest? With movement? While maintaining a fixed position?	Resting tremors worsen at rest and decrease with activity; they are usually a symptom of *Parkinson's disease*. Gradual onset of positional tremors suggests *essential tremor*; acute onset suggests a *toxic* or *metabolic disorder*. Intention tremors are worst with movement toward an object; they may result from *multiple sclerosis* (Bennet, et al., 2006).
Balance/Coordination Problems Do you have any difficulty with balance, coordination, or walking?	*Multiple sclerosis, Parkinson's disease, stroke*, and *cerebral palsy* are neurological causes of impaired gait. Refer to Chapter 23 for further information.
Dizziness or Vertigo Have you had any periods of dizziness? • Can you describe what it feels like without using the word dizziness? • Is it associated with nausea and vomiting? • Does changing positions make it better or worse?	Common causes include *multiple sclerosis, Parkinson's disease, cerebellar ischemia or infarction, benign or malignant neoplasms*, and *arterial-venous malformation of blood vessels in the brain*. Position changes usually worsen dizziness associated with the inner ear.
Difficulty Swallowing Have you had any difficulty swallowing? • Are any foods or liquids particularly difficult?	**Dysphagia**, associated with CN dysfunction, is a common symptom of *stroke* or *neuromuscular disease*. Generally soft foods are more easily tolerated than chewy foods or liquids.
Intellectual Changes Have you noticed intellectual changes or difficulty with concentration, memory, or attention? (Nurse also may ask family members or friends of patients about this.)	Common causes of memory loss include *Alzheimer's disease, dementia, depression, stroke, some medications*, and *metabolic imbalances*. Refer to Chapter 30 for more information.
Speech/Language Difficulties Do you notice any difficulties with expression or comprehension of speech/language? • Any difficulty understanding speech? • Any difficulty forming words? • Any difficulty finding words and putting sentences together?	**Aphasia** is a common symptom of *stroke*, especially when it affects the speech centers in the left hemisphere (Hand, et al., 2006). Neuromuscular disease also affects the speech center, such as with *Alzheimer's disease* or other forms of *dementia*.
Changes in Taste, Touch, or Smell Have you noticed alterations in touch, taste, or smell? • Any numbness, tingling, or hypersensitivity? • Where do you feel it?	**Paresthesia**, abnormal prickly or tingly sensations, is most common in the hands, arms, legs, and feet, but can occur over other body parts. Causes include *neurological disease* or traumatic nerve damage such as *carpal tunnel syndrome* or *cervical stenosis*.
Lost or Blurred Vision Have you had a loss or blurring of vision in one or both eyes, or double vision? • When do you notice it? • Are there associated symptoms such as weakness or impaired speech? • Does this create any safety issues? Can you drive?	Central causes of **diplopia** (double vision) include *stroke, vascular malformation, tumor, mass, trauma, meningitis, hemorrhage*, and *muscular sclerosis*.
Hearing Loss or Tinnitus Have you noticed any hearing loss or tinnitus (ringing in the ears)? • Do you have a history of hearing loss? • Was it a sudden or slow onset? • Is it in one or both ears?	Common causes of sensorineural hearing loss include noise, *autoimmune disorders, Meniere's disease, ototoxic medications*, and *head trauma* (Isaacson & Vora, 2003). Refer to Chapter 16 for more information.

▲ Lifespan Considerations

Additional Questions	Rationales/Abnormal Findings
Pregnant Women Do you have a history of seizures? • Have you noticed weight gain or edema? Have you had high blood pressure or tested positive for protein in your urine? • Are you taking any medications as prescribed?	Some pregnant women with epilepsy stop taking anticonvulsants because of their potentially harmful fetal effects, such as *neural tube deficits* (including *spina bifida*), *cleft lip or palate, congenital heart disease, developmental delay*, and *cognitive impairment* (Koren, et al., 2006). These patients must weigh the risk of having seizures while not taking anticonvulsants against the potentially teratogenic effects. Seizures from epilepsy must be differentiated from those of eclampsia.
Do you have a headache or any sensory, motor, or visual changes?	*Migraines* are more common during pregnancy, possibly from increased hormones.
Do you have a history of migraines, epilepsy, or multiple sclerosis?	Hormones influence the course of *multiple sclerosis*; relapse rate is lower during pregnancy, especially in the third trimester, with a marked increase in the first 3 months postpartum (Vukusic, et al., 2004).
Newborns and Infants • Is there any family history of genetic neurological disorders? • Were there any birth difficulties? • Was the baby premature? • Are there any congenital anomalies or developmental delays?	Neuroblastomas are associated with chromosomal abnormalities. Additionally, *Down's syndrome, muscular dystrophy, phenylketonuria,* and *Tay-Sachs' disease* are genetic neurological disorders. Also pay attention to the developmental history, including perinatal history (eg, difficult labor, prematurity). Risk of *cerebral palsy* increases with a history of maternal infection in pregnancy, preterm birth, and multiple pregnancies (Bax, et al., 2006).
Children and Adolescents Is there any history of head injury? • Does your child maintain eye contact and respond with appropriate facial expressions and gestures? • Is he or she meeting developmental milestones? • How well does your child interact and play with other children? • Would you describe your child as flexible or focused on routines?	The age groups at highest risk for *traumatic brain injury* are 0–4 year olds and 15–19 year olds (National Center for Injury Prevention and Control, Traumatic Brain, 2007). Falls, motor vehicle injuries, and bicycle injuries are common causes of brain injury in children (Dunning, et al., 2006). Children with *autism, ADD/ADHD*, and other psychiatric challenges are two to three times more likely to experience injuries needing medical attention (Lee, et al., 2008). Risk for autism increases with advanced maternal or paternal age, low birth weight, shortened gestation, and intrapartal hypoxia (Kolevzon, et al., 2007). Autism also is associated with breech presentation, low 5-minute Apgar's score, birth before 35 weeks' gestation, and parental psychiatric illness (Laarson, et al., 2005).
Does the child have fever, chills, headache, or vomiting? Has he or she received the meningococcal vaccine?	Children 11–18 years should receive this immunization, as should teens entering high school and college freshmen moving to dormitories (CDC, 2007). The new meningitis vaccine lasts approximately 8 years, compared to the 3- to 5-year protection that the older vaccine offered.

Additional Questions	Rationales/Abnormal Findings

Older Adults

Additional Questions	Rationales/Abnormal Findings
Do you have a history of Alzheimer's disease, dementia, stroke, Parkinson's disease, or epilepsy?	These conditions are increased in the elderly. *Hypertension; atrial fibrillation; diabetes; congestive, chronic renal disease;* female gender; *previous cerebrovascular disease;* and *ischemic stroke* increase risk of neurovascular disease (Arboix, et al., 2006).
Have you fallen or had a head injury? To the patient or caregiver: Have you noticed any cognitive impairment; language problems (slow, slurred, and difficult or impossible to understand speech); hearing, taste, smell, or vision losses; and balance or emotional problems?	Those 75 years or older have the highest rate of traumatic brain injury-related hospitalization and death (National Center for Injury Prevention and Control, Traumatic Brain, 2007). Falls are the most common cause, followed by car accidents.

Cultural Considerations

Additional Questions	Rationales/Abnormal Findings
From the chart, note ethnicity, gender, and area of residence.	These variables are relevant in some disorders (eg, incidence of *multiple sclerosis* is higher in temperate climates; *stroke* occurs more often in African Americans than in Caucasian Americans).
Is there any history of head injury?	Hospitalization rates for *traumatic brain injury* are highest among African Americans and American Indians/Alaska Natives (National Center for Injury Prevention and Control, Traumatic Brain, 2007). African Americans have the highest death rate from traumatic brain injury (National Center for Injury Prevention and Control, Traumatic Brain, 2007). Certain military duties (eg, paratrooper) increase risk for brain injury (National Center for Injury Prevention and Control, Traumatic Brain, 2007).
Are you exposed to pesticides at work or home?	Maternal exposure to pesticides is linked to increased incidence of *anencephaly* and *neural tube defects*. Living in areas of pesticide use also increases risks. Implications for farm workers, especially migrant workers, are particularly concerning (Rull, et al., 2006). Folic acid deficiency also is linked to neural tube defects. Incidence of spina bifida is highest among Hispanic women, partially as a result of exposure to pesticides (Williams, et al., 2005).
How old is your home? Do you know if the paint has lead in it?	The most common cause of lead exposure is dust and chips from deteriorating paint that included lead (before 1978). Exposure is higher in those living in old homes with poor repair (EPA, 2007). Exposure to lead paint also is of concern for children; lead has been found in toys (EPA, 2007). Severe lead exposure can lead to *encephalopathy*; mild exposure can lower IQ scores and contribute to attention problems (Committee on Environmental Health, 2005). Lead also can cause pregnancy difficulties and reproductive problems (in both men and women; EPA, 2007).

Therapeutic Dialogue: Collecting Subjective Data

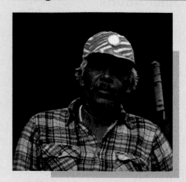

Remember Mr. Gardner, introduced at the beginning of this chapter, who was seen in the ED for acute stroke. He is confused, and healthcare providers are finding it challenging to communicate with him. The nurse needs to accurately assess the patient's neurological status; later, the nurse will interview Mr. Gardner to gather details about the lifestyle practices that have led to him having a stroke at a young age.

The following conversations give two examples of interview styles used by different nurses to obtain an assessment of orientation. One style is more effective than the other.

Less Effective

Nurse: Mr. Gardner, can you tell me where you are now?

Mr. Gardner: (Nods head yes)

Nurse: Can you tell me where you are?

Mr. Gardner: (Speaks slowly) Can I have a cigarette?

Nurse: Not now. Can you tell me where you are?

Mr. Gardner: (Nods head yes)

Nurse: Tell me where you are.

Mr. Gardner: I'm home. Who are you?

Nurse: I'm your nurse. Where are you?

Mr. Gardner: I'm home (smiles).

Nurse: Can you tell me what day it is?

Mr. Gardner: Is it Wednesday? (correct answer is Monday)

Nurse: No, can you tell me what your name is?

Mr. Gardner: Bill Gardner. Can I have a cigarette?

More Effective

Nurse: Mr. Gardner, I would like to ask you a few questions to find out more about your stroke. Is that alright?

Mr. Gardner: (Shakes head yes). (Speaks slowly) Can I have a cigarette?

Nurse: Your cigarettes are put away. I would like to ask you a few questions. Tell me where you are now.

Mr. Gardner: I'm at home. Who are you?

Nurse: I'm your nurse. My name is Boyd. You're in the hospital because you had a stroke. You're at Mountain View Hospital. Tell me what day it is today.

Mr. Gardner: Is it Wednesday? (correct answer is Monday)

Nurse: Today is Monday, July 10th, 2010. Tell me what your name is.

Mr. Gardner: Bill Gardner (smiles)

Critical Thinking Challenge

- Compare and contrast the data collected in the two dialogues. What approaches made the second dialogue more effective?
- Why did the more effective nurse provide information on the correct day, date, and place? Provide rationale.
- Considering this patient's speech deficits, should the nurse ask open- or closed-ended questions for orientation? Provide rationale.
- How would you respond to his request for a cigarette? Provide rationale.

Objective Data Collection

Equipment

- Penlight or flashlight
- Tongue blade
- Cotton swab
- Optional: Tuning fork, reflex hammer, supplies for CN testing

Preparation

Nurses anticipate that patients may attempt to minimize or to hide neurological deficits. For example, when a nurse asks, "What year were you born?" the patient might say, "Well, if I told you that, then you'd know how old I was (and laughs)." The nurse can return to this question later to evaluate long-term memory, or change the question slightly to get a different response.

Table 24.3 Common Versus Specialty/Advanced Neurologic Techniques

Comprehensive Assessment Technique	Purpose	Screening or Registered Nurse Assessment	Focused or Advanced Practice Examination
Assess LOC	Alertness	X	
Assess attention	Cognitive functions and processing	X	
Evaluate complex cognitive function	Orientation, cognition, memory		X
Assess communication/speech	Aphasia or dysarthria	X	
Inspect pupillary responses	CN II function and ICP	X	
Check for abnormal posturing	Severity of deficits	X	
Test function of CNs III–VII	Basic evaluation	X	
Check function of CNs I–XII	Comprehensive evaluation		X
Evaluate muscle tone and strength	Upper and lower motor function	X	
Check gait and balance	Basic cerebellar function	X	
Check coordination	Advanced cerebellar function		X
Assess deep tendon and superficial reflexes	Intact reflex arc		X

In healthy people, nurses can integrate the neurological examination with history taking. For example, they can evaluate function of the CNs during conversation and while observing the patient's facial expressions. Neurological screening is performed on patients at high risk for problems, such as following a motor vehicle collision, or for patients with a documented history of previous neurological illness. Nurses add techniques according to the specific injury or disease process as part of a focused neurological examination.

Common and Specialty/Advanced Techniques

The routine head-to-toe assessment includes the most important and common techniques of neurological assessment. Examiners add specialty or advanced steps if concerns exist over a specific finding, as the clinical situation demands, or as a regular part of advanced practice (see Table 24-3.)

Comprehensive Physical Examination

Physical examination of the nervous system provides information about its functional integrity. Because of how the nervous system is organized, a deficit or group of deficits often provides the information needed to localize the area of pathology. This information, combined with the history and diagnostic testing, allows determination of the nature (eg, traumatic, neoplastic, vascular, infectious, degenerative) of the pathological process.

Nurses mainly use inspection and palpation in neurological examination. Clinicians use percussion when testing DTRs; they limit auscultation of the nervous system to evaluation of vascular sufficiency.

Comprehensive neurological assessment begins with general observation of how the patient relates to the environment. Such observation may occur during initial contact, before the formal process of history taking begins. Often, however, observation occurs during the entire encounter with the patient. Observation of level of alertness and responsiveness necessitates focus on attention span, mood, and affect. Assessment of general appearance includes grooming, cleanliness and arrangement of clothing, use of prosthetics (eg, eyeglasses, hearing aids), and any visible evidence of trauma or other surface abnormalities (eg, birthmarks; skin tumors; asymmetry of face, gaze, or extremities). Often, this initial interaction also allows nurses to assess speech and language, general movement, and gait and balance. It often provides data that directs further focused assessment of individual functions during the physical examination.

Table 24.4 Assessment of Consciousness. Applying Stimulation

Order of Stimulation	Example
Spontaneous	Enter room and observe arousal.
Normal voice	State patient's name; ask him or her to open eyes.
Loud voice	Use loud voice if no response to normal voice.
Tactile (touch)	Touch patient's shoulder or arm lightly.
Noxious stimulation (pain)	Apply nailbed pressure to elicit pain response, telling patient that you will be applying pressure.

Technique and Normal Findings	Abnormal Findings

Level of Consciousness

Begin by assessing LOC. The initial outcome determines the extent and method of the rest of the examination. People visibly express LOC through degree of response to stimulus, with the highest level being spontaneous alertness. Be sure to apply stimulus in the correct order (Table 24-4), moving to a more intense stimulus only when the previous attempt is unsuccessful. First arouse the patient by speech, then by touch, and then by pressure to the nail beds (Fig. 24-11) or by pinching a large muscle mass on an extremity. (**Note: Do not pinch a small fold of skin, which may cause soft tissue trauma.**) Pressure to the nailbeds also can be useful in determining gross motor function when the patient's LOC makes formal strength testing impossible.

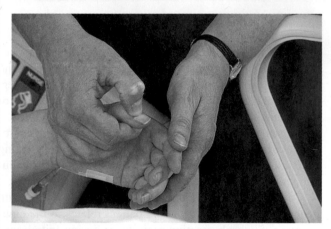

Figure 24.11 The nurse is applying pressure to the nailbeds to arouse a patient who has not responded to speech or touch.

The GCS (Box 24-2) has facilitated the assessment of patients with impaired consciousness. Primarily, the GCS determines the degree of conscious impairment by evaluating behavioral responses in three areas: motor responses, verbal responses, and eye opening. The examiner lists, for each category, the patient's best response. The GCS weights each response numerically to quantify overall response. The minimum score is 3; the maximum is 15.

- Motor response is scored according to the most functional response from either upper extremity (eg, if a patient follows commands with the right hand but not the left, the motor score indicates ability to follow commands).
- Verbal response includes orientation, conversation, speech, sounds, and no response as an indicator of cognitive function.
- Eye opening is in response to activity in the environment, verbal cues, non-noxious stimuli, or noxious stimuli pressure as an indicator of LOC.

BOX 24.2 GLASGOW COMA SCALE

The GCS is a tool for assessing a patient's response to stimuli. Scores range from 3 (deep coma) to 15 (normal).

Eye opening response	Spontaneous	4
	To voice	3
	To pain	2
	None	1
Best verbal response	Oriented	5
	Confused	4
	Inappropriate words	3
	Incomprehensible sounds	2
	None	1
Best motor response	Obeys command	6
	Localizes pain	5
	Withdraws	4
	Flexion	3
	Extension	2
	None	1
Total		3–15

Source: Teasdale, G. & Jennett, B. (1974). Assessment of coma and impaired consciousness. A practical scale. *Lancet, 304,* 81–84.

Table 24.5 Levels of Consciousness

Term	Definition
Alert wakefulness	Patient appreciates the environment and responds quickly to stimuli.
Confusion	Patient is disoriented to time, place, or person; has shortened attention span; shows poor memory; or has difficulty following commands.
Drowsiness	Patient responds to stimuli appropriately but with delay and slowness; may respond to some but not all (also described as **lethargy** or **obtunded** state).
Stupor	Patient is unresponsive and can be aroused only briefly by vigorous, repeated stimulation.
Coma	Patient is unresponsive and generally cannot be aroused.

Source: Hickey, J. V. (2002). The neurological physical examination and neurological assessment. In J. V. Hickey (Ed.), *The clinical practice of neurological and neurosurgical nursing* (5th ed., pp. 117–158 and 158–184). Philadelphia: Lippincott Williams and Wilkins.

Technique and Normal Findings (continued)

Objective description of the patient's response is critical to evaluating changes in LOC over time. A wide range of terms has been used to describe LOC (Table 24-5). Despite careful definition within a particular institution, these terms are by nature subjective and must be used carefully to allow accurate comparisons of serial assessments by different practitioners. Description of specific response to stimulus provides the best chance of identifying change that may initially be subtle. *Normal findings are "patient alert, opens eyes spontaneously."*

Cognitive Function

If results of LOC assessment show that the patient can interact, evaluate cognitive function (many components of which may have been done during history taking). Remember to conduct specific cognitive tests so that patients do not feel that their intelligence is being challenged.

Cognitive function includes basic orientation, concentration, and attention span, and more complex functions, such as memory, calculation ability, abstract thinking, reasoning, and judgment. Complex cognitive function can be tested informally whenever you interact with the patient, especially when teaching, establishing goals and priorities, and planning for home care. Doing so provides information about the patient's ability to learn, to reason, and to make judgments. See Chapter 10 for discussions of assessment of attention, concentration, memory, calculation, and abstract thinking.

Orientation. Assess orientation by directly questioning the patient about person, place, and time. Display sensitivity to the patient's environment and communication ability. Asking "What month (year, season) is it?" may be more reasonable than "What day is it?" if the patient has been hospitalized for several days with few cues about day of the week. Asking about place through yes or no questions rather than "Where are you?" may be

Abnormal Findings (continued)

Although accepted as a relatively objective assessment of consciousness, the GCS itself is also vulnerable to differences in scoring of the same patient situation, especially in the motor area (Heron et al., 2001; Gill, et al., 2004). Consistency in training staff to use the GCS, with periodic review, may be needed to produce reliable results. GCS is predictive of outcome from a traumatic brain injury when combined with the patient's age and pupillary response (McNett, 2007).

The Blessed Dementia Rating Scale and the Mini-Mental State Examination (MMSE) are tools used to assess dementia (see Chapter 10). Patients can also be asked about items related to functional ability: telling the time using a clock face and counting change. Inability to name the time within 60 seconds or count change within 90 seconds is correlated with dementia (Inouye, et al., 1998).

necessary for patients with *aphasia* (impaired ability to interpret or use the symbols of language). Regarding person, as well as identifying himself or herself, ask the patient to identify visitors or family pictures. Also ask the patient about his or her age (NIH, 2003). *The patient is "oriented."*

Communication (Speech/Language)

Communication is another function to assess continuously throughout the interaction. Observe clarity and fluency of speech through basic conversation. Ask the patient to repeat words or phrases with multiple combinations of consonants and vowels (eg, "aggravating conversation") to test speech articulation. Formal testing includes assessment of comprehension, repetition, naming, reading, and writing (see Chapter 10). *Speech is clear and articulate.*

Deficits in articulation are referred to as **dysarthria**. In some cases, distinguishing speech/language deficits from confusion is difficult. Typically those with speech/language deficits behave appropriately to situation and environment, especially to visual cues. These findings are less likely in confused patients, but consultation with a speech pathologist for formal assessment of communication and cognitive function will clarify the type of deficit. Patients with a language deficit might be unable to express needs, but usually can follow simple commands (eg, "Open and close your eyes," "Squeeze your hand"; NIH, 2003). Confused states can be described as acute (delirium) or chronic (dementia, with multiple etiologies).

Pupillary Response

Basic assessment of pupils includes size, shape, and reactivity to light (see Chapter 15). Darken the room and instruct the patient to gaze into the distance to dilate the pupils. Ask him or her to keep looking ahead. Hold a light on the side (avoid pointing it into the eye). Observe for nystagmus in one or both eyes. Bringing the light in quickly from the side, observe the reaction of the same and then the other pupil for the consensual light reflex. Use a preprinted guide or scale on a penlight to identify the size. Record both the initial size and response size as R 6→4, L6→4. *Pupils are round, equal, and constrict briskly (within 1 second) in response to light, both directly and consensually (when one pupil constricts to light, the other does, too).* This is also recorded as PERRL (pupils equal, round, reactive to light).

Test accommodation by having the person shift the gaze from a distant to near object. *Accommodation includes constriction of the pupils and convergence of the eyes bilaterally.* When documented with the pupils, it is charted as PERRLA (A is for accommodation).

Also assess the gaze for eye contact and drifting. If the eyes deviate, assess if it is conjugate (move together) or dysconjugate (move separately). *Gaze is purposeful and conjugate.*

Nystagmus is a jerking movement of the eye that can be quick and fluttering or slow and rolling, similar to a tremor. Causes include *medications* (eg, antiseizure medications), *cerebellar disease, weakness in the extraocular muscles*, and *damage to CN III*. See also Chapter 15 and Table 24-9 at the end of this chapter.

Abnormal Movements

Observation of abnormal movements is an additional element of inspection. They include abnormal reflex posturing (spontaneous or in response to painful stimuli) and involuntary movements caused by various neurological disorders affecting the extrapyramidal motor system. *Movements are smooth and symmetric.*

Abnormal posturing includes flexion abnormal, extension abnormal, hemiplegia, quadriplegia, and paralysis (see Table 24-10 at the end of this chapter). Abnormal movements include tic, myoclonus, fasciculation, dystonia, tremor, chorea, and athetosis (see Table 24-11 at the end of this chapter).

Cranial Nerve Testing

There are 12 pairs of CNs. Each member of the pair innervates structures on the same side from which it arises (the ipsilateral side). A lesion of the CN or its nucleus results in an ipsilateral peripheral nerve deficit. A lesion in the cerebral cortex in the area that supplies the CN nucleus, or the tracts traveling from the cerebral cortex to the CN nucleus, results in a contralateral CNS deficit. Example: Facial weakness caused by a lesion in the right frontal motor control center occurs on the left side of the face. A lesion affecting the right facial nerve itself produces weakness on the entire right side of the face.

Aside from a thorough screening assessment for a suspected problem, it is rarely necessary to assess complete CN function (Table 24-6). Examples of selected testing include the following:

- Observe functional near and far vision; assess pupil constriction and extraocular movements (EOMs); assess corneal reflexes (included above under acute assessment) if LOC is acutely impaired.
- Observe facial expression, test facial strength and sensation, observe uvula rise with "ah," test gag reflex and observe tongue movement when assessing potential for dysphagia (difficulty swallowing). Alertness and attention span are also relevant for this purpose.

Findings are PERRLA, EOMs intact. Positive gag and corneal reflexes. Facial strength 4+ with intact sensation bilaterally.

Use of the gag reflex as part of assessment varies widely (Mathers-Schmidt & Kurlinski, 2003). Many practitioners continue to use absence of gag reflex as an indicator for risk of aspiration; however, they may overestimate risk when absence of gag reflex is the only deficit found. Conversely, they may miss other risks if gag reflex is the only function tested and found intact (Leder, 1997). Refer to Table 24-6 for a description of abnormal findings.

Motor Function

Examination of the motor system focuses on assessment of symmetry of muscle bulk, tone, and strength.

Distinct patterns of abnormality are found with CNS motor pathway (**upper motor neuron [UMN]) lesions** compared to peripheral motor nerve pathway (**lower motor neuron [LMN]) lesions**. See Table 24-12 at the end of this chapter for a description of UMN and LMN deficits.

Muscle Bulk and Tone. Inspect muscle bulk by observing and palpating muscle groups to check for any wasting (atrophy). This inspection provides some information about muscle tone as well. The relaxed muscle shows some muscular tension. To further assess tone, determine degree of resistance of muscle groups to passive stretch. Instruct the patient to relax totally and to let the examiner move his or her limbs. Commonly tested groups include deltoids, biceps, triceps, hamstrings, and quadriceps. *Findings are good muscle bulk and tone.*

If there is absolutely no resistance to movement, the muscles are said to be **flaccid** or **atonic**. If the tone seems to be only decreased or "flabby," note the finding as **hypotonia**. Increased resistance of the muscles to passive stretch is called **hypertonia**. **Spasticity** also can occur with UMN disorders. It is characterized by increased resistance to rapid passive stretch, especially in flexor muscle groups in the upper extremities, resulting from hyper-excitability of the stretch reflex. In certain conditions, this resistance is strongest on initiation of the movement and "gives way" as the examiner slowly continues the movement. This characteristic has prompted the use of the term **clasp-knife spasticity**, and describes the type of hypertonicity noted in patients with Parkinson's disease.

(text continues on page 706)

Table 24.6   **Summary of Cranial Nerve Assessment**

Cranial Nerve	Technique	Abnormal Findings
I. Olfactory (sensory)	Usually deferred, CN I is tested when symptoms involve smell or abnormal findings warrant evaluation. First assess patency by closing off one nostril and asking the patient to inhale; perform the same technique on the opposite side. Occlude one naris. Tell the patient to close the eyes, place a familiar scent near the open naris, and ask the patient to inhale and identify the scent. Repeat on the opposite side. Commonly used fragrances include orange, peppermint, cinnamon, and coffee.	Only a few neurological conditions are linked with deficits. It is important to test for patency of the naris, which can influence ability to smell. Other influences include allergies, mucosal inflammation, increased age, and excessive tobacco smoking. An olfactory tract lesion may compromise ability to discriminate odors (anosmia).
II. Optic (sensory)	Monitor while working with the patient. Ask him or her to identify how many fingers you are holding up. Use the Snellen chart to evaluate far vision and near vision with small print. Test visual fields using confrontation. See Chapter 15 for tests of visual acuity and visual fields.	Visual acuity <20/20 is abnormal. Inability to read small print is common in older adults, as a result of age-related loss of accommodation.
III. Oculomotor (motor), IV. troclear (motor), and VI. abducens (motor)	Assess pupils for size, shape, and equality. Assess the six cardinal positions of gaze. Observe for nystagmus in one or both eyes (see Chapter 15).	**Nsytagmus** may manifest as quick and jerky movements or slow pendulous movements, where the eye moves back and forth in the socket. Note if the movement is fine or coarse and constant or intermittent. Check if the plane of movement is either up and down or back and forth. Nystagmus is associated with disease of the vestibular system, cerebellum, or brainstem.
V. Trigeminal (sensory and motor), includes corneal	Evaluate sensory function by touch and motor function with movement. To evaluate the sensory component, ask the patient to close the eyes. Using a cotton swab and broken tongue blade or swab, ask the patient to identify sharp or dull sensations when he or she feels them. Be sure to evaluate all three divisions of the nerve at the scalp (ophthalmic), cheek (maxillary), and chin (mandibular) areas on each side. Evaluate motor function by observing the face for atrophy, deviation, and fasciculations. Ask the patient to tightly clench the teeth; palpate over the jaw for masseter muscle symmetry. Ask the patient to open the jaw against resistance; normal movement is symmetric. The corneal reflex is not normally tested unless motor or sensory abnormalities are noted. Have the patient remove any contact lenses. Instruct him or her to look up. Inform the patient that you will touch the eye with a cotton swab wisp. Bring the swab in from the side and lightly touch the cornea, not the conjunctiva. Normally the patient blinks bilaterally as stimulation is applied.	Decreased or dulled sensation, weakness, or asymmetric movements are abnormal findings associated with CN V. A weak blink from facial weakness may result from paralysis of CN V or VII. A depressed or absent corneal response is common in contact lens wearers.

| Table 24.6 | **Summary of Cranial Nerve Assessment** (*continued*) |

Cranial Nerve	Technique	Abnormal Findings
VII. Facial (sensory and motor)	Assess by evaluating taste. Place sweet, sour, salty, and bitter solutions on the anterior 2/3 of the tongue on both sides; also test the posterior 1/3 of the tongue for CN IX. The patient should properly identify the taste. Evaluate motor function by observing facial movements during conversation. Additionally, the patient completes facial movements and symmetry is observed. Ask the patient to raise the eyebrows, squeeze the eyes shut, wrinkle the forehead, frown, smile, show the teeth, purse the lips, and puff out the cheeks. Normal movements are strong and symmetric.	Fasciculations or tremors are abnormal. Asymmetric movements may be noted with the lower eyelid sagging, loss of the nasolabial fold, or mouth drooping. These findings are common following a stroke or with Bell palsy.
VIII. Acoustic (sensory)	Evaluate hearing during normal conversation using a simple whisper test, or with an audiometer. Refer to Chapter 16 for more information.	Inability to hear conversation is abnormal; note the presence of a hearing aid.
IX. Glossopharyngeal (sensory and motor)	Evaluate sensory function with CN VII. Evaluate motor function with CN X upon swallowing.	Impaired taste or swallowing is common following a stroke.
X. Vagus (sensory and motor), includes gag reflex	Evaluate the motor component by asking the patient to open the mouth and stick out the tongue, which should be symmetric. Place a tongue blade on the middle of the tongue and have the patient say "ah"; observe the uvula and soft palate for symmetry. Evaluate the sensory component by stimulating the gag reflex, which is tested only when a problem is suspected. Inform the patient that you will be touching the posterior pharyngeal wall, and it may cause gagging. Observe for upward movement of the palate and contraction of the pharyngeal muscles with the gag reflex.	Injury to the vagus or glossopharyngeal nerve causes the uvula to deviate from midline. Asymmetry of the soft palate or tonsillar pillars is also abnormal. An impaired gag reflex, coughing during oral feeding, and changes in voice after swallowing are all associated with aspiration. Closely evaluate patients with any of these symptoms (Terré & Mearin, 2006).
XI. Spinal accessory (motor)	Evaluate the sternomastoid and trapezius muscles for bulk, tone, strength, and symmetry. Ask the patient to press against resistance on the opposite side of the chin. Also ask the patient to shrug the shoulders against resistance. The movements should be strong and symmetric.	Weakness or asymmetry in movement accompanies neurological and musculoskeletal problems.
XII. Hypoglossal (motor)	Evaluate this function with CN X. First inspect the tongue; then ask the patient to stick out the tongue and observe for symmetry. Ask the patient to say, "light, tight, dynamite" and note that the letter l, t, d, and n are clear and distinct.	Fasciculations, asymmetry, atrophy, or deviation from midline may occur with general neuromuscular conditions or lesions of the hypoglossal nerve.

Rigidity is characterized by a steady, persistent resistance to passive stretch in both flexor and extensor muscle groups. This phenomenon has led to the descriptive phrases **"lead-pipe" rigidity** or "plastic" rigidity. **Cogwheel rigidity** is seen in patients with Parkinson's disease and is manifested by a ratchet-like jerking noted in the extremity on passive movement.

Muscle Strength. Assess muscle strength (pyramidal motor system) by asking the patient to move extremities or selected muscle groups both independently and against the examiner's resistance. In addition to the muscle groups mentioned above, evaluate strength by hand grasp, pronator drift, dorsiflexion, and plantar flexion. Grade strength of movement on a scale of 0–5+:

0—No muscle contraction

1—Barely detectable, flicker

2—Active movement with gravity eliminated

3—Active movement against gravity

4—Active movement against some resistance

5—Active movement against full resistance

Strength is 4–5+.

Motor strength of 0–3+ indicates weakness.

During conversation, observe for ptosis or facial palsy (NIH, 2003). An early or mild upper extremity weakness can be detected by observing for pronator drift. Ask the patient to close the eyes and outstretch the arms straight ahead with palms upward (supinated) for 10 seconds (Fig. 24-12). *The patient extends the hands for 10 seconds without drifting.*

Pronation of the hands and downward drift of the arm indicate weakness.

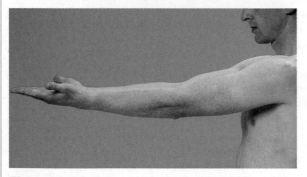

Figure 24.12 Assessing for pronator drift.

Also ask the patient to press the feet against resistance to assess strength or extend the leg at 30 degrees; drift is present if the leg falls before 5 seconds (NIH, 2003). Refer to Chapter 23 for a complete description of strength testing.

Gait and posture combine functions of the pyramidal and extrapyramidal motor systems, other cerebellar function, and sensory systems. If possible, ask the patient to walk down a corridor. Points to observe include smoothness of gait, position of feet (narrow versus wide base), height and length of step, and symmetry of arm and leg movement. Also ask the patient to walk on heels and toes, then tandem-walk (ie, heel-to-toe in a straight line) (Fig. 24-13). *The patient walks smoothly without swaying.*

Abnormal gaits include spastic hemiparesis, scissors, Parkinsonian, cerebellar ataxia, sensory ataxia, waddling, dystonia, and athetoid (see Table 24-13 at the end of this chapter).

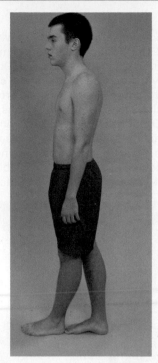

Figure 24.13 Assessing the tandem walk to evaluate gait and posture.

In the **Romberg test**, ask the patient to stand with feet together and arms at sides (Fig. 24-14). Note any swaying (stand close enough to prevent falling). Ask the patient to close the eyes during the Romberg for additional testing. Slight swaying may be normal, because visual cues help humans maintain balance. *The patient can maintain position without opening the eyes.*

Moderate swaying with eyes open and closed indicates *vestibulocerebellar dysfunction.* Pronounced increase in swaying (sometimes with falling) with the eyes closed usually indicates a *lesion in the posterior columns of the spinal cord.*

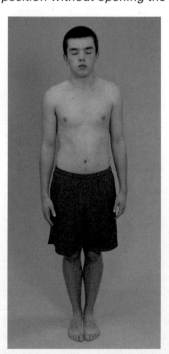

Figure 24.14 Positioning for the Romberg's test.

(text continues on page 708)

Cerebellar Function

Assessment of finger-to-nose coordination or rapid alternating movements tests upper extremity cerebellar function. Ask the patient to touch the tip of the examiner's finger with the tip of his or her forefinger (test each hand separately) and then to touch his or her own nose, and to repeat this maneuver several times while the examiner's finger is moved each time (Fig. 24-15). To assess rapid alternating movements, instruct the patient to slap his or her thigh with first the palm of the hand and then the back as fast as possible (Fig. 24-16). It is not uncommon for people to perform better with their dominant hand.

Ataxia is unsteady, wavering movement with inability to touch the target. During rapid alternating movements, lack of coordination is **adiadochokinesia**. Deficits in any of these maneuvers indicate an **ipsilateral cerebellar lesion**. Note any tremor. Other signs of cerebellar dysfunction can include hypotonia, nystagmus, and dysarthric speech. Dysarthric speech noted with cerebellar lesions may exhibit a peculiar quality called scanning speech, which is characterized by alternating patterns of slowness and explosiveness as each syllable is spoken. Refer to Table 24-13 at the end of the chapter.

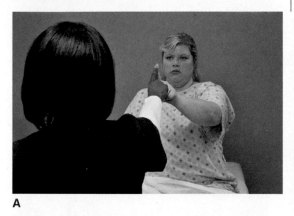 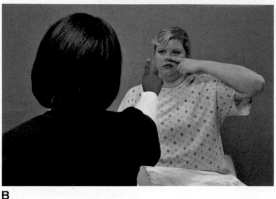

A B

Figure 24.15 Assessing cerebellar function. **A.** The patient touches the examiner's finger with her forefinger. **B.** The patient touches her own nose.

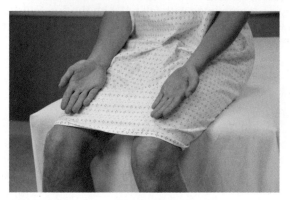

Figure 24.16 Assessing rapid alternating movements.

Assess lower extremities by the heel-to-shin test. With the patient seated or supine, ask him or her to take the heel of one foot and, without deviation, move it steadily down the shin of the other leg. *Normal responses are good coordination of movements.*

Sensory Function

When assessing sensation, it is important that the patient's eyes are closed to avoid visual cues from influencing responses. Have the patient identify where he or she feels the sensation, but avoid cueing the patient by asking, "Do you feel this?" Allow 2 seconds between each stimulus to avoid summation, in which the patient perceives frequent, small stimulations as one-long stimulation. Begin with light stimulation and proceed with increased pressure until the patient reports

Interpret sensory deficits considering that this testing includes the peripheral nerves, sensory tracts, and cortical perception. Consider the patient's clinical situation and whether the problem is generalized or specific, such as trauma to a nerve. *Spinal cord injury* generally follows the pattern of the dermatome, while sensory loss in *diabetic neuropathy* is distal. See also Table 24-14 at the end of this chapter.

a sensation. Stronger stimulation is needed over the central torso and back than on the more sensitive hands. Observe areas of sensory decrease or loss. Compare findings between sides. Screening may be performed by testing the most distal areas and proceeding centrally if deficits are noted. Testing involves the arms (not hands), legs, trunk, and face (NIH, 2003). Complete testing of all nerves is rare. Clinically, patterns of sensory loss are assessed depending on the problem or area of injury.

Light Touch. Pull the end of a cotton swab so that it is wispy. Ask the patient to close the eyes, and apply light touch to the skin with the swab (Fig. 24-17). Ask the patient to state where he or she feels the sensation. *Patient correctly identifies light touch.*

Hyperesthesia refers to increased touch sensation. **Anesthesia** refers to absent touch sensation. Reduced touch sensation is **hypesthesia**.

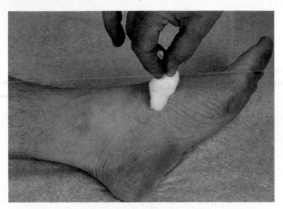

Figure 24.17 Applying a cotton swab to assess light touch sensation.

Superficial Pain Sensation. Break a tongue blade or cotton swab so that the end is sharp. Ask the patient to close the eyes; lightly touch the patient's skin with the sharp end. Ask the patient to state where he or she feels the sensation. *Pain sensation is intact.*

Hyperalgesia refers to increased pain sensation. **Analgesia** refers to absent pain sensation. Reduced pain sensation is **hypalgesia**.

⚠ *SAFETY ALERT 24.1*

Patients with neuropathy need to be taught to visually inspect their feet, because they may have injuries that go unnoticed.

Temperature Sensation. Test temperature sense only if pain or touch is abnormal. Use one prong of a tuning fork that has been warmed with the hands or test tubes containing warm and cold water. Ask the patient to close the eyes. Touch the skin with warm or cold objects. Have the patient identify when he or she feels warm or cold. *Temperature sensation is intact.*

Abnormal temperature sensation is common in *neuropathies.*

⚠ *SAFETY ALERT 24.2*

Patients with neuropathy need to learn to use a body part with good sensation to determine the temperature of hot surfaces. Getting into a too-hot bath can cause inadvertent burns to the feet. Similarly, a patient with neuropathy can be easily burned with too hot of a heating pad.

Point Localization. Ask the patient to close the eyes. Using a finger, gently touch the patient on the hands, lower arms, abdomen, lower legs, and feet. Have the patient identify where he or she feels the sensation, but avoid cueing the patient by asking, "Do you feel this?" Observe areas of sensory loss. Compare side to side. *Point localization is intact.*

Observe the pattern of sensory loss by mapping it out during testing. "Stocking-glove" distribution suggests peripheral nerves; dermatomal distribution suggests isolated nerves or nerve roots; reduced sensation below a certain level is associated with the spinal cord. A crossed face-body pattern suggests the brainstem, and hemisensory loss suggests a stroke (Hickey, 2002).

(text continues on page 710)

Vibration Sensation. Strike a low-pitched tuning fork on the side or heel of the hand to produce vibrations. Ask the patient to close the eyes. Holding the fork at the base, place it over body prominences, beginning at the most distal location. The toes, ankle, shin, finger joints, wrist, elbow, shoulder, and sternum can all be tested (Fig. 24-18). If the sensation is felt at the most distal point, no further testing is necessary. Ask the patient to state where the sensation is felt and when it disappears. To stop the sensation, dampen the tuning fork by pressing on the tongs. *Vibration sense is intact.*

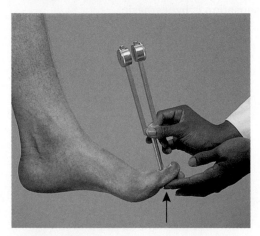

Figure 24.18 Testing vibration sensation.

Motion and Position Sense. Ask the patient to close the eyes. Move the distal joints of the patient's fingers and then the toes up or down. If the patient cannot identify these movements, test the next most proximal joints (eg, wrist if finger movement is not sensed). *Motion and position sense are intact.*

Stereognosis. This test evaluates cortical sensory function. Ask the patient to close the eyes and identify a familiar object (eg, coin and key) placed in the palm (*stereognosis*; Fig. 24-19). *The patient correctly identifies the object.*

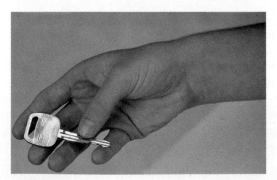

Figure 24.19 Testing stereognosis.

Graphesthesia. This test also evaluates cortical sensory function. Use a blunt object to trace a number (eg, "8") on the patient's palm. Ask the patient to identify which number has been traced (*graphesthesia*) (Fig. 24-20). *The patient correctly identifies the number.*

Peripheral neuropathy is more severe distally and improves centrally. It is a common consequence of *peripheral vascular disease* and *diabetic neuropathy.* Often vibration sense is the first lost.

With damage to a specific dermatome, the line of sensory loss is usually marked and specific.

Involuntary writhing, snakelike movements of a limb (athetosis) result from loss of position sense. The brain cannot sense where the limb is in space so the limb moves on its own; the patient must use vision to consciously control the limb's movements.

Inability to identify objects correctly (**asereognosis**) may result from damage to the sensory cortex caused by *stroke.*

Cortical sensory function may be compromised following a *stroke.*

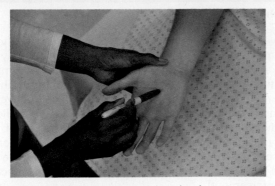

Figure 24.20 Assessing graphesthesia.

Two-point Discrimination. Ask the patient to close the eyes. Hold the blunt end of two cotton swabs approximately 2-in apart and move them together until the patient feels them as one point (the ends of an opened paperclip may also be used). The fingertips are most sensitive, with a minimal distance of 3–8 mm, while the upper arms and thighs are least sensitive, with a minimal distance of 75 mm. *Generally there is more discrimination distally than centrally.*

Cortical sensory function may be lost with a stroke.

Extinction. Ask the patient to close the eyes. At the same time, touch a body area on both sides. Ask the patient to state where he or she perceives the touch. *Sensations are felt on both sides.*

Cortical sensory function may be lost with a *stroke*. The stimulus on the opposite side of the damaged cortex may be lost or reduced.

Reflex Testing

Reflex testing includes muscle stretch reflexes (DTRs), superficial (cutaneous) reflexes, and other pathological reflexes that may or may not be tested along with the others.

DTRs. Advanced practice nurses and physicians generally test DTRs. Nevertheless, direct care nurses should understand how to test them to better incorporate the findings of other practitioners into identifying patterns of neurological deficit.

DTRs tested include biceps, triceps, brachioradialis, patellar, and Achilles (Table 24-7). These reflexes are observed for symmetry when tested bilaterally and for briskness of reflex movement. DTRs are graded on a scale of 0–4, with 0 representing absent reflexes and 4 corresponding to significantly hyperactive responses.

- 4+—Very brisk, hyperactive with clonus
- 3+—Brisker than average
- 2+—Average, normal
- 1+—Diminished, low normal
- 0—No response

The reflex response depends on the force of the stimulus, accurate location of the striking area over the tendon, and patient's relaxation level. Refer to Chapter 4 for use of the reflex hammer and technique. To ensure accurate location, have the patient flex the muscle to find the tendon and then relax it for testing. Pathologic reflexes are primitive responses and indicate loss of cortical inhibition (see Table 24-15 at the end of this chapter). *DTRs are 2+ bilaterally without clonus.*

Clonus is characterized by alternating flexion/extension movements (jerking) in response to a continuous muscle stretch. In unconscious patients, DTRs may be tested in the usual manner; however, depth of coma alters the response. Deep coma is associated with loss of all reflexes, as well as loss of muscle stretch and tone.

(text continues on page 713)

Table 24.7   **Deep Tendon Reflexes**

DTR: Level Tested	Technique

Biceps: C5 and C6

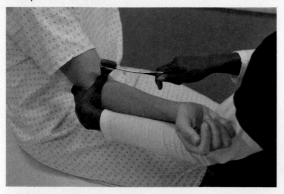

Have the patient partially flex the elbow and place the palm down. To assist with relaxation, the patient may rest the arm against the nurse's. Place one finger or thumb on the biceps tendon. Strike the finger or thumb with the reflex hammer briskly so that the impact is delivered through the digit to the biceps tendon. Observe for flexion at the elbow and contraction of the biceps muscle. If the patient's reflexes are symmetrically diminished or absent, ask the patient to clench the teeth or squeeze one hand tight with the opposite hand to aid in detection (reinforcement).

Triceps: C6–8

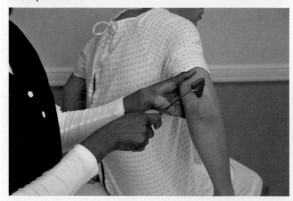

Have the patient flex the arm at the elbow and turn the palm toward the body if supine. If the patient is seated, it may be easiest for the nurse to hold the patient's arm in a relaxed dangling position. Palpate the triceps muscle and strike it directly just above the elbow. Observe for extension of the elbow and contraction of the triceps muscle.

Brachioradialis: C5 and C6

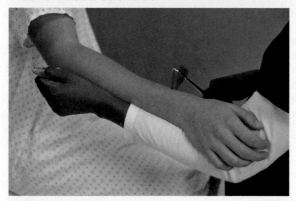

Have the patient flex the arm (up to 45 degrees) and rest the forearm on the nurse's arm with the hand slightly pronated. Palpate the brachioradial tendon approximately 1–2 in above the wrist and strike it directly with the reflex hammer. Observe for pronation of the forearm, flexion of the elbow, and contraction of the muscle.

Patellar: L2–4

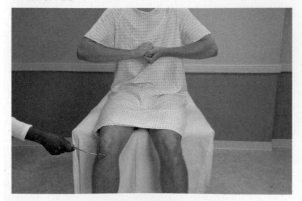

Have the patient flex the knee at 90 degrees, allowing the lower leg to dangle. Support the upper leg with the hand. Palpate the patellar tendon directly below the patella. Observe for extension of the lower leg and contraction of the quadriceps muscle. If the patient's reflexes are symmetrically diminished or absent, ask the patient to lock the fingers in front of the chest and pull one hand against the other (reinforcement).

Table 24.7 Deep Tendon Reflexes (continued)

DTR: Level Tested	Technique
Achilles: S1 and S2 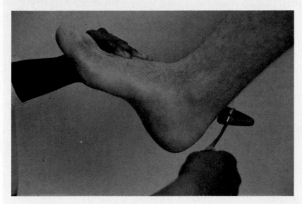	With the patient sitting and legs dangling, hold the patient's foot. (The patient may also kneel on a stool with the feet dangling.) Palpate the Achilles tendon; strike the tendon directly near the ankle maleolus. Observe for plantar flexion of the foot and contraction of the gastrocnemius muscle.

Technique and Normal Findings (continued)	Abnormal Findings (continued)

Superficial Reflexes. Superficial reflexes are elicited by stimulation of the skin. Record the response to stimulation as present, absent, or equivocal (ie, present or difficult to determine).

Plantar Response. Test by stroking the sole of the foot with a blunt instrument such as the edge of a tongue blade or the handle of a reflex hammer. Apply the stimulus firmly but gently to the lateral aspect, beginning at the heel and stopping short of the base of the toes. The toes flex (a flexor-plantar response).

Pathological reflexes include **abnormal plantar reflexes** and the **triple flexion response** (Fig. 24-21).

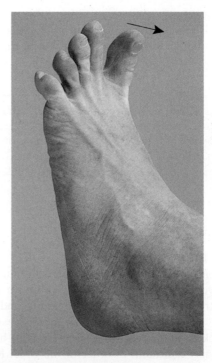

Figure 24.21 Babinski's sign.

With abnormal plantar reflexes, the great toe extends upward and the other toes fan out (an extensor-plantar response, or Babinski's sign). Triple flexion describes reflex withdrawal of the lower extremity to plantar stimulus through flexion of ankle, knee, and hip.

(text continues on page 714)

Technique and Normal Findings (continued)	Abnormal Findings (continued)
Upper Abdominal. This test is to identify the integrity of T8–10. Stroke the upper quadrants of the abdomen with a tongue blade or reflex hammer. *The umbilicus moves toward each area of stimulation symmetrically.*	Depression or absence of this reflex may result from a *central lesion, obesity,* or lax skeletal muscles (eg, postpartum). It also may be noted with *spinal cord injury.*
Lower Abdominal. This test is to identify the integrity ofT10–12. Stroke the upper quadrants of the abdomen with a tongue blade or reflex hammer. *The umbilicus moves toward each area of stimulation symmetrically.*	Abnormal findings are the same as for the upper abdominal region.
Cremasteric (Male). This test helps identify the integrity of L1–2 in male patients. Stroke the inner thigh of the male patient. *The testicle and scrotum rise on the stroked side.*	Response is diminished or absent.
Bulbocavernous (Male). This test helps identify the integrity of S3–4 in male patients. Apply direct pressure over the bulbocavernous muscle behind the scrotum. *The muscle should contract and elevate the scrotum.*	Response is diminished or absent.
Perianal. This test helps identify the integrity of S3–5. Scratch the tissue at the side of the anus with a blunt instrument. *The anus should pucker.* **Note: The anal reflex also can be tested when administering rectal medications.**	Response is diminished or absent.
Carotid Arteries	
Auscultation over the carotid artery may elicit a bruit that indicates stenosis and turbulent flow in the artery. Refer to Chapter 19 for technique. *No bruit is heard.*	A bruit is associated with an increased risk of *stroke* (Gillett, et al., 2003).

Documentation of Normal Findings

> Well-groomed and relaxed with good eye contact. Alert and oriented with good attention span and judgment. Speech clear and appropriate. Immediate and recent memory intact. CNs II–XII grossly intact. PERRLA with L5→3 and R5→3, EOMs intact without ptosis or nystagmus. Can correctly identify light touch on face, arms, and legs; strength 5+ bilaterally. Gait smooth and coordinated, no tremors.
> *B. Bolt-Hasen, RN*

 Lifespan Considerations

Newborns, Infants, and Children

The neurological system develops dramatically during the first 2 to 3 years as children lose their primitive reflexes and gain control of bowel, bladder, locomotion, and speech (Fig. 24-22). At birth, newborns have protective reflexes including sucking and swallowing. Depressed or hyperactive reflexes may indicate a disorder of the CNS. Refer to Chapter 28 for more information and a complete description of neonatal reflexes. Spontaneous motor activity is noticeable, especially during crying. Transient tremors are normal and should disappear by 1 month of age. Muscle tone and strength are usually related. Depressed LOC may result from maternal sedation; this should be differentiated from hypoglycemia or CNS disorders.

Variations in state of consciousness for infants are called *sleep-wake states.* They range from deep sleep to extreme irritability. Infants use purposeful behavior to maintain the optimal arousal state by withdrawing, fussing, and crying. A weak or high-pitched cry may indicate CNS abnormality. Refer to Chapter 28 for additional abnormal findings.

Persistent tremors, increased tonicity or spasticity, or twitching of the facial muscles may indicate seizures and should be evaluated. Tremors of hypoglycemia or CNS disorders should also be evaluated. Birth trauma may cause nerve damage that results in asymmetry or paralysis. CN testing is modified for newborns and infants; refer to Chapter 28.

Cognitive abilities and speech articulation develop during preschool and early childhood. Fine and coarse motor skills follow developmental milestones. Expected motor function by

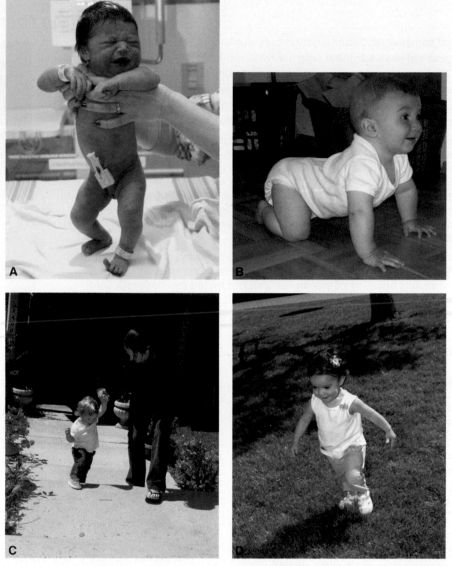

Figure 24.22 As children grow, their neurological system develops to enable more complex behaviors and movements. **A.** The newborn must be held by someone at all times. **B.** The 8-month-old child is capable of crawling. **C.** After the first birthday, the child begins to walk, at first with assistance and then independently. **D.** By 2 years of age, the child achieves independent ambulation.

2 to 3 years includes grasping, sitting, crawling, standing, and walking. Further investigation is warranted with reduced amount of rotation during crawling, delayed balance, and delayed onset and poor quality of early walking behavior (Fallang & Hadders-Algra, 2005). Refer to Chapter 28 for more information.

Adolescence is also a period of cognitive growth and completion of myelinization of the nerve fibers. From preschool through adolescence, learning disabilities, hyperactivity, and tic disorders may develop (see Chapters 28 and 29). Motor delay and disorders of gait may also occur.

Older Adults

As discussed earlier, normal changes in neurological function accompany aging. Examples include lost nerve cell mass, atrophy in the CNS, decreased brain weight, and fewer nerve cells and dendrites. Such changes lead to slower thought, memory, and thinking; however, plasticity enables the lengthening and production of dendrites to accommodate for this loss. Demyelinization of nerve fibers leads to delayed impulse transmission. An increased latency period (period before next stimulation) causes slowed reflexes, which may produce mobility and safety issues. Fewer cells are in the spinal cord, although this does not appear to reduce function. Peripheral nerve conduction slows. Therefore, assessment techniques, interpretation of findings, and linked interventions may require adjustments as appropriate. Refer to Chapter 30 for more information.

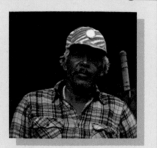

Unlike the normal samples of documentation previously charted, the samples for Mr. Gardner, the 56-year-old man admitted with a stroke, reflect abnormalities. Review the following important findings revealed during each step of objective data collection for this patient. Compare these results with the normal findings presented in the samples of normal documentation. Begin to think about how the data cluster together and what additional data might be needed to anticipate appropriate nursing interventions.

Inspection: A 56-year-old African American man with a history of hypertension, smoking, and mild baseline dementia. Lives alone, with poor hygiene and multiple layers of mismatched clothes. Does not remember the last time he took "high pressure pills." Is alert, appears somewhat fearful and agitated, asking for cigarettes, oriented to name only. Speech is comprehensible but slurred. Patient can follow 1-step commands only—is easily distractible. Impaired short-term memory—remembers zero of three objects after 1 minute. Pupils equal, round, briskly reactive. Appears to have left visual field loss, EOMs intact. Left lower facial weakness, left tongue deviation.

Palpation: Muscle bulk symmetrical, tone slightly increased on left arm/leg. Strength 5/5 right arm/leg, 2/5 left arm, 3/5 left leg, left Babinski. Right arm/leg coordination grossly intact, left arm/leg not tested because of weakness, gait not tested (on bedrest). Diminished attention to objects/people on left side of bed, difficult to assess sensation because of varying patient attention. Remains hypertensive—see flow sheet for vital signs (VS).

B. Bolt-Hasen, RN

Neurological Assessment in Selected Situations

Screening Examination of a Healthy Patient

Experienced nurses may complete a thorough screening assessment of a healthy patient in 10 to 15 minutes or less. Problems with perfusion and autonomic dysfunction are implicated in several neurological conditions. Following a history and general observations (as described earlier), the nurse notes vital signs, including right and left radial pulses; right and left brachial blood pressures; and lying and standing blood pressure (immediate, and after 3 minutes). See Box 24-3 for the components of a screening examination in a healthy patient.

Serial Neurological Assessment and Documentation

Although some neurological changes are evident instantaneously, most progress over time. Consistent, accurate serial assessment is critical for timely identification and intervention. When orders for "neuro checks" are written, these usually comprise signs that, if deterioration were to occur, would signify a critical or potentially life-threatening event. These signs typically include the patient's LOC (GCS score), pupillary size, equality and light responses, motor ability, and, when appropriate, additional elements linked to location of pathology or existing deficits (eg, other selected CNs or sensory function). When intracranial pathology is not present (eg, postoperative laminectomy), it is sufficient to observe for motor and sensory changes only and not use the GCS.

The patient's specific risk for acute neurological deterioration dictates the frequency of assessment. Even mild neurological decline should trigger increased frequency of assessment to observe for development of a pattern of deficits that may indicate urgent or emergent intervention.

Communication of findings is critical. Documentation of the neurological examination may be handwritten or entered electronically. Nurses typically use a flow sheet to track assessment changes over time, supported by a narrative note to detail assessments not addressed by the limitations of a flow sheet. A written note should be succinct but clearly describe relevant findings. Repetition of information recorded on a flow sheet is unnecessary.

Assessment of Meningeal Signs

A stiff neck (nuchal rigidity) is associated with *meningitis* and *intracranial hemorrhage* from irritation of the meninges. Ask the patient to relax and lie down. With the patient supine, slide your hand under and raise the patient's head gently, flexing the neck. Pain and resistance to movement are associated with nuchal rigidity. If neck stiffness is present, the Brudzinski's sign may be present. The sign is positive if there is resistance

---

BOX 24.3 NEUROLOGICAL SCREENING EXAMINATION IN A HEALTHY PATIE

- Vital signs (temperature, pulse, respiration, blood pressure, pulse oximetry)
- LOC
- Communication/speech
- Orientation
- Motor (strength, pronator drift, balance, and coordination)
- Sensory (gross assessment of limbs and face)
- Pupillary reaction

National Clearinghouse Guidelines (2007). Stroke assessment across the continuum of care (2007). Retrieved August 12, 2007, from http://www.guideline.gov/summary/summary.aspx?doc_id=7426

---

or pain in the neck and flexion in the hips or knees. Evaluate for Kernig's sign by flexing the leg at the hip. With the patient supine, raise the leg straight up (or flex the thigh on the abdomen) and extend the knee. The sign is present if there is resistance to straightening or pain radiating down the posterior leg.

Assessing the Unconscious Patient

Assessment of unconscious patients deserves special consideration for the following reasons:

- Patients who present with acute unconsciousness require urgent evaluation to determine the cause of the impairment and, when appropriate, to implement prompt intervention.
- Unconscious patients are at risk for life-threatening complications secondary to loss of protective reflexes; these deficits may be noted during examination.
- They require special assessment techniques, because they cannot participate in the examination.

The nurse should quickly review the patient's history for possible causes of impaired consciousness. Review of recent medications and laboratory values may reveal potential causes. The nurse rapidly evaluates the patient's general cardiovascular and respiratory status so that any existing compromise can be treated promptly. The patient requires thorough inspection for any visible clues, such as trauma, that might be the cause of the loss of consciousness. Physical examination includes the following:

- LOC assessment via the Glasgow Coma Score
- Pupillary assessment
- Brainstem assessment—gaze, facial symmetry, corneal reflex, gag reflex, cough, oculocephalic reflex (doll's eye maneuver, Fig. 24-23) if cervical spine injury has been ruled out
- Motor function in addition to motor component of GCS (although formal strength testing cannot be done with an unresponsive patient, observe for hemiparesis/hemiplegia by comparing right and left extremity response to pain or noting frequency and location of any spontaneous movement)
- Close observation for patterns of dysfunction associated with progressing herniation

If LOC assessment progresses to application of painful stimulus (under eye-opening), the nurse must employ a method to elicit the desired response without causing harm. Noxious stimulus can be categorized as peripheral or central. Peripheral stimulation is performed first using nailbed pressure. Central stimulus is more reliable in evaluating patients with impaired LOC, and may be applied by pinching the trapezius or pectoralis muscle. Applying pressure to the supraorbital notch can be effective but is contraindicated if a facial fracture is suspected. Application of a "sternal rub" (knuckles applied to the skin over the sternum) also works, but can easily bruise the skin if use is prolonged.

The oculocephalic reflex (doll's eyes) assesses brainstem function in comatose patients. Ensure that the spinal cord is clear and intact before performing this test. Hold the patient's eyes open and turn the head first to one side quickly and then to the other. In a patient with an intact brainstem, the eyes move toward the opposite side. If brainstem or midbrain

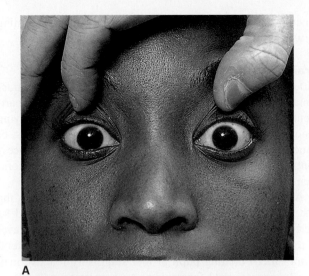

A

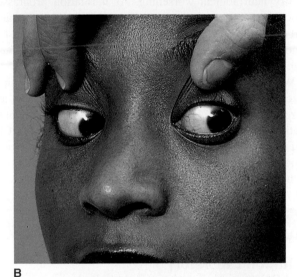

B

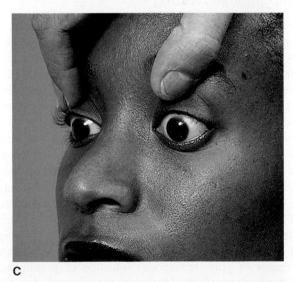

C

Figure 24.23 The oculocephalix reflex involves the doll's eye maneuver. **A.** The nurse holds the patient's upper eyelids open. The nurse then quickly turns the patient's head. **B.** If the eyes can move in the opposite direction of the head, this indicates that the brainstem in intact. **C.** In a comatose patient, the ability to move both eyes to one side is lost.

function is lost, the eyes move with the head, still pointing forward (similar to a doll with the eyes painted on).

Brain Herniation Syndromes

Patterns of neurological change occur when increasing intracranial pressure (ICP) causes tissue shifts between compartments within the brain. Mass effect from space-occupying lesions such as brain edema, hematoma, hydrocephalus, or tumor may occur bilaterally or unilaterally. If either process continues unchecked, the cerebellum down through the foramen magnum can herniate.

Altered mentation and decreasing LOC are usually the first signs of neurological deterioration. Nurses should be alert to even subtle changes in the patient's behavior and level of responsiveness. With *unilateral herniation*, an ipsilateral (same-sided) dilating pupil at first sluggishly reactive may signify neurological worsening. As herniation progresses, which it may do rapidly, response only to pain, contralateral (opposite-sided) posturing of extremities, and brainstem abnormalities may be noticeable. With *bilateral herniation*, pupil change and reflex posturing are on both sides.

With *cerebellar herniation*, the patient has fixed pupils (size depends on site of original lesion), flaccid muscles, and no response to pain. The patient may rapidly experience brain death, as well as respiratory and cardiovascular changes. Certain respiratory patterns may be seen with progressive neurological deterioration related to increased ICP or focal lesions of the brainstem (see Table 24-16 at the end of the chapter).

Evidence-Based Critical Thinking

Common Laboratory and Diagnostic Testing

Diagnostic tests serve to further define the precise location and often the nature and extent of a lesion. Many diagnostic tests also provide information regarding the integrity of surrounding areas. A wide variety of diagnostic tests can aid in the diagnosis of nervous system disease. Technological advances have made new equipment and techniques possible; such progress continues rapidly. Significant developments in genetic testing have allowed molecular diagnosis of infectious, congenital, and inherited neurological diseases, among multiple other applications. Although neurodiagnostic testing can be categorized in many ways, this review sorts tests as anatomic imaging, electrical conduction testing, and CSF/spinal procedures.

Computerized tomography (CT) continues to be the staple of neurodiagnostic imaging. It consists of passage of multiple x-ray beams through tissue in sequential planes, displayed in shades of gray. Intravenous injection of a radiopaque medium ("contrast") provides bright enhancement of vascular structures and areas of blood-brain barrier breakdown. CT detects potential causes of increased ICP and multiple other intracranial pathologies.

The MRI is a noninvasive, nonradiological test that delivers highly detailed images of neuroanatomy and associated pathology. Duration is usually significantly longer than CT. This, plus the effects of the strong magnetic field on most critical care monitors and equipment such as infusion pumps, makes MRI more problematic for critically ill patients. The procedure is noninvasive (barring intravenous infusion of contrast material for certain sequences), but patients may experience discomfort from the duration of the procedure, loud sounds, and possible feelings of claustrophobia. Patient movement disrupts the adequacy of images (as with CT), so sedation may also be indicated.

△ SAFETY ALERT 24.3

Pre-procedure considerations include removal of metallic objects from hair, wrists, fingers, and piercings. Providers also must screen the environment for metal that could possibly become a missile if exposed to the strong magnetic field in the immediate area of the MRI scanner. Objects such as oxygen tanks, scissors, forceps, and stethoscopes have been implicated in potential or actual patient injury.

Angiography, an invasive procedure, involves intra-arterial injection of contrast material to visualize the lumen of intracranial and extracranial vessels. It is the gold standard for identification of aneurysms, arteriovenous malformations, and vasospasm following subarachnoid hemorrhage (Perry, et al., 2006). Disadvantages of cerebral angiography are associated with risk for complications after arterial access of vessels that typically already contain pathology.

△ SAFETY ALERT 24.4

Pre-procedure nursing considerations include screening for allergy to shellfish or iodine or presence of renal disease (premedication to lower risk of anaphylaxis will be considered; an alternative contrast material can reduce risk of renal failure). The post-procedure focus is on observation and prevention of complications. Frequent serial assessment of the arterial puncture site, distal pulses, and limb color and temperature targets risk for bleeding, hematoma, or occlusion of the cannulated vessel.

The largely noninvasive EEG records spontaneous electrical impulses from scalp electrodes positioned over the brain surface area. EEG detects abnormal electrical activity such as seizures or alterations caused by neuronal damage from trauma, stroke, encephalopathies, or other cerebral pathology (Shiraishi et al., 2005). Electromyography records electrical activity in muscles at rest, during voluntary contraction, and with electrical stimulation via inserted small needle electrodes. Nerve conduction studies record speed of conduction in motor and sensory fibers of peripheral nerves using surface electrodes. They are used to evaluate for neuromuscular disorders such as myasthenia gravis, neuropathy, or other peripheral nerve dysfunction.

Lumbar puncture involves insertion of a hollow needle into the spinal subarachnoid space to examine and measure the pressure of CSF. Placement is between L4 and L5 or L3 and L4 vertebrae to avoid the spinal cord, which typically ends at L1. Lumbar puncture is usually performed at the bedside (or in a clinic if done as an outpatient procedure), under strict asepsis.

SAFETY ALERT 24.5

After lumbar puncture, patients typically must remain flat in bed for 6 to 8 hours. If headache develops or becomes severe when a patient first gets up, bed rest may continue for up to 24 hours. Headache typically results from loss of the cushioning effect of CSF or from leakage of CSF from the puncture site into surrounding tissue. If the ICP is significantly elevated, lumbar drainage of CSF could potentially precipitate downward herniation of the brain into the foramen magnum. Thus, patients need frequent assessment for headache and LOC following a lumbar puncture.

Diagnostic Reasoning

When formulating a nursing diagnosis, nurses use critical thinking to cluster data and identify related patterns. They compare clusters with defining characteristics (abnormal findings) for the diagnosis to ensure the most accurate labeling and appropriate interventions (see Table 24-8) (NANDA-I, 2009). Note how the potential interventions often include assessments. This illustrates how the nursing process is interwoven and assessment is a continuous part of nursing care.

Table 24.8 Common Nursing Diagnoses Associated with the Neurological System

Diagnosis and Related Factors	Point of Differentiation	Assessment Characteristics	Nursing Interventions
Impaired verbal communication related to aphasia	Compromised ability to use speech (whether receiving, transmitting, or both)	Difficulty forming words or sentences, difficulty expressing thoughts verbally, inappropriate verbalization	Observe behavioral cues for needs. Maintain eye contact. Ask yes and no questions. Anticipate patient's needs. Use touch as appropriate.
Acute confusion related to stroke	Abrupt onset of global, transient changes and disturbances in attention, cognition, and consciousness	Fluctuation in cognition, increased agitation or restlessness, lack of follow-through in behavior	Perform mental status examination. Provide environmental cues (eg, large clock and calendar). Orient to time, place, and person frequently.
Impaired memory related to dementia and stroke	Problems with recollecting or remembering information from levels ranging from short-term memory to basic behaviors	Inability to recall facts, remember recent or past events, or learn new information	Encourage patient to use a calendar, keep reminder lists, set alarm watches, and make signs for room number or bathroom.
Unilateral neglect related to left-sided muscle weakness	Lack of awareness and attention to one side of the body	Inattention to one side, inadequate positioning, leaves food on plate on affected side	Provide safe, well-lit, and clutter-free environment. Set up environment so that most activity is on unaffected side. Encourage patient to compensate for neglect.
Risk for aspiration related to muscle weakness and impaired swallowing	Risk for oropharyngeal secretions, food, or fluid entering into the tracheobronchial passages	Reduced LOC, facial droop, depressed cough and gag reflexes, drooling, choking, and coughing on food	Auscultate lungs before and after feeding. Request swallowing evaluation by speech therapy. Elevate head of bed when eating.
Risk for intracranial adaptive capacity related to potential increased ICP	Increased ICP in response to stimuli	Increases in ICP of more than 10 mm Hg for more than 5 minutes, resulting from brain injuries	Keep head and neck in midline. Avoid suctioning. Reduce environmental stimuli. Adjust sedation.*Provide adequate oxygen.
Ineffective brain tissue perfusion related to stroke	Decrease in oxygen or blood supply resulting in failure to nourish brain	Abnormal pupils, weakness or paralysis, changes in motor response, altered mental status	Monitor neurological status using neurological flow sheet. Notify physician for changes in condition. Prevent injury.

*Collaborative interventions.

Analyzing Findings

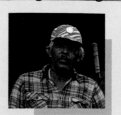

The problems of Mr. Gardner have been outlined throughout this chapter. Initial subjective and objective data collection is complete. The nurse is reviewing the findings and other results.

Mr. Gardner is reassessed on the acute care unit following his admission from the ED. The following nursing note illustrates the collection and analysis of subjective and objective data and the development of preliminary nursing interventions.

Subjective: A 56-year-old African American man with a history of hypertension, smoking, and mild baseline dementia. Lives alone, poor hygiene, wearing multiple layers of mismatched clothes. Does not remember last time he took "high pressure pills." Is alert, appears somewhat fearful and agitated, asking for cigarettes, oriented to name only. Speech is comprehensible but slurred.

Objective: Patient can follow 1 step commands only—is easily distractible. Impaired short-term memory—remembers zero of three objects after 1 minute. PERRLA. Appears to have left visual field loss, EOMs intact. Left lower facial weakness, left tongue deviation. Muscle bulk symmetrical, tone slightly increased on left arm/leg. Strength 5/5 right arm/leg, 2/5 left arm, 3/5 left leg, left Babinski. Right arm/leg coordination grossly intact, left arm/leg not tested because of weakness, gait not tested (on bed rest). Diminished attention to objects and people on left side of bed, difficult to assess sensation because of varying patient attention. Remains hypertensive—see flow sheet for VS.

Analysis: Findings consistent with right hemisphere stroke, complicated by baseline impaired cognitive function. Potential for further impaired cerebral perfusion. Probable left unilateral neglect, high fall risk, dysphagia, and aspiration risk.

Plan: Frequent neurological assessment to monitor for stroke progression. Monitor BP—currently not treated per stroke guidelines. Consult social work for support system and financial assessment—patient may be unable to return to independent living. Evaluate safe ADL performance with physical and occupational therapists. Implement fall prevention plan; discuss speech pathology consult for swallowing evaluation prior to starting diet.

B. Bolt-Hasen, RN

Collaboration with Other Health Care Providers

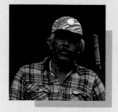

Mr. Gardner may be at risk for aspiration because of his facial droop and tongue deviation. The nurse contacts speech therapy to evaluate the patient's ability to swallow without choking or aspirating. Nurses consult speech therapy when patient needs are associated with:

• Swallowing evaluation/management and diet recommendations
• Cognitive communication and language evaluations
• Difficulty with communication
• Oral or facial trauma
• Aphasia

The nurse is contacting speech therapy at this time for the risk of aspiration, a safety issue. Speech therapy also may be involved during this patient's rehabilitation for issues related to communication. The following conversation illustrates how the nurse might organize data and make recommendations to speech therapy.

Situation: "Hello, I'm Boyd Bolt-Hasen, Mr. Gardner's nurse on 5 East."

Background: "Mr. Gardner was admitted yesterday with a right-sided stroke. He hasn't started a diet yet. He has some left lower facial weakness and left tongue deviation that might interfere with ability to chew and swallow. He wants to eat, but he still has an order for nothing by mouth."

Assessment: "I'm worried that he's at risk for aspiration. I would like you to evaluate his swallowing before we start feeding him."

Recommendations: "For now I'm going to keep him on nothing by mouth. After you see him, let me know what your evaluation is. We may have the physician change his diet order if he's safe to eat."

Critical Thinking Challenge

• Consider all the collected subjective data. Review the above report. Should the nurse communicate any other data to speech therapy?
• Critique the objective data. Is the organization logical? Would it be clearer to add to or take out any of the information?
• Critique the analysis and recommendations. What is the nurse's role in coordinating collaborative care with speech therapy?

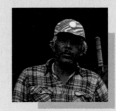

The nurse uses assessment data to formulate a nursing care plan with patient outcomes and interventions for Mr. Gardner. Outcomes are specific to the patient, realistic to achieve, measurable, and have a time frame. After interventions are completed, the nurse will re-evaluate Mr. Gardner and document the findings to show progress toward outcomes. The nurse uses critical thinking and judgment to continue or revise the diagnosis, outcomes, or interventions. This is often in the form of a care plan or case note similar to the one below.

Nursing Diagnosis	Patient Outcomes	Nursing Interventions	Rationales	Evaluation
Unilateral Neglect related to hemianopsia, left-sided weakness	Demonstrates measures to care for left side of body and keep it free from injury within 1 week	Assess neurological function every shift including muscle strength. Assist with dressing and grooming until strength returns. Place call bell on right side of bed.	The initial priority is patient safety and injury prevention. Assess function to determine improvements or decline. Assist patient with ADLs until he can care for himself.	Motor strength 2+ on left arm and leg; 4+ on right. Facial droop and tongue deviation persist. Needs assistance in two-handed tasks, such as bathing. Needs one-person assist with transfers. Continue to monitor; obtain PT consult to assess for readiness for rehabilitation.

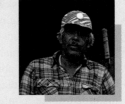

Using the previous steps of diagnostic reasoning, organizing, and prioritizing, consider all the case study findings woven throughout this chapter. When answering the following questions, begin drawing conclusions and see how the pieces of assessment must work together to create an environment for personalized, appropriate, and accurate care. Note how assessment forms the foundation for accurate, individualized, and holistic nursing care.

- Is Mr. Gardner's condition at the end stable, urgent, or an emergency?
- What ongoing health promotion and teaching needs are evident?
- How will the nurse focus, organize, and prioritize ongoing subjective data collection?
- How will the nurse focus, organize, and prioritize ongoing objective data collection?
- Compare and contrast nursing diagnoses to determine the highest priority.
- How will the nurse individualize assessment to Mr. Gardner's specific needs, considering the condition, age, and culture?

Nurses use assessment information to identify patient outcomes. Some outcomes related to neurological problems include the following (Moorhead, et al., 2007):

- Patient cares for both sides of the body and keeps affected side safe.
- Patient does not aspirate or fall and maintains a safe environment.
- Patient improves motor function and becomes independent with activities of daily living (ADLs).

Once outcomes are established, nursing care can be implemented. Nurse uses critical thinking and evidence-based practice to develop interventions. Some examples of nursing interventions for neurological care are as follows (Bulechek, 2007):

- Use cues and anchors to promote attention to the affected side.
- Assess neurological and mental status frequently; inform physician of changes.
- Orient patient to time, place, and person frequently.

Key Points

- Nurses use experience, knowledge of anatomy and physiology, and the patient's acuity, current deficits, and risk for deterioration to select elements of the neurological examination most appropriate for the situation.
- Although some neurological changes are evident instantaneously, most progress over time. Consistent, accurate, and clearly communicated serial assessments are critical for timely identification and intervention.

- Early recognition of events requiring urgent intervention maximizes the patient's chance of optimal outcome.
- Common areas of health promotion include reducing the risk of neurovascular disease and injury prevention.
- Common symptoms associated with the neurological system include headache, weakness, blurry vision, impaired motor function, and impaired speech.
- When collecting a headache history, characteristics such as pain worse in the morning on awakening and pain precipitated or made worse by straining or sneezing may indicate potentially elevated ICP.
- Clinical situations that require urgent communication of neurological assessment findings include a change in LOC, pupillary reaction, and verbal or motor response.
- Consciousness and cognition are assessed early in the neurological examination because these functions direct the method used to elicit further information.
- Use of the GCS helps to provide relatively objective information about LOC, but is most reliable with staff training.
- Assessment of the function of CNs is performed at the bedside through observation of vision, pupils, EOMs, facial expression and strength, and uvula and tongue movement.
- Spinal and peripheral nerve function may be assessed by testing for motor strength and sensation at different levels of the spinal cord according to the dermatomes.
- Abnormal reflexes include hyperactive or diminished DTR, decreased superficial reflexes, and abnormal reflexes such as a positive Babinski.
- Abnormal posturing occurs in late stages of injury, including abnormal flexion and abnormal extension responses.
- Abnormal motor function includes disorders of movement such as tremor and abnormal gait.
- Common nursing diagnoses are impaired verbal communication, acute confusion, impaired memory, unilateral neglect, risk for aspiration, risk for intracranial adaptive capacity, and ineffective brain tissue perfusion.
- While neurological assessment findings can highlight location and acuity of neuropathology, diagnostic testing provides the critical next step in assessing type and etiology of the condition. Knowledgeable pre and post procedure care aids in maximizing information obtained and reducing patient stress and complications.

Review Questions

1. Use of the GCS provides relatively objective assessment of LOC. The three functions assessed are
   A. pupil reaction, orientation, and sensation
   B. verbal response, eye opening, and motor response
   C. eye opening, motor response, and sensation
   D. verbal response, pupil reaction, and motor response

2. The patient with a head injury and increasing ICP is likely to have which assessment findings?
   A. Decreased LOC and sluggish pupil
   B. Left-sided weakness and facial droop
   C. Right ptosis and right-sided loss of vision
   D. Dilated left pupil and receptive aphasia

3. The chart states that a 62-year-old woman has a stroke in the right parietal area of the brain. The nurse expects to note which of the following?
   A. Tremors on the left side of the face
   B. Tremors on the right side of the face
   C. Weakness in the right arm
   D. Weakness in the left arm

4. The nurse performs blood pressure screening at the local community center. As part of the health promotion intervention, the nurse also discusses the following risk factors for stroke.
   A. Low blood pressure, lack of exercise, and diet high in fat
   B. High blood pressure and diet high in fat and smoking
   C. Diet high in fat, smoking, and walking five times weekly
   D. Obesity, swimming five times weekly, high blood pressure

5. If the great toe extends upward and the other toes fan out in response to stroking the lateral aspect of the sole of the foot, this is documented as which of the following?
   A. yporeflexia
   B. Normal plantar reflex
   C. Cushing response
   D. Babinski's sign

6. A 26-year-old man was in a motor vehicle accident and suffered a complete spinal cord injury to L3. The nurse assesses the patient for loss of motor function in the
   A. legs
   B. abdomen
   C. chest
   D. arms

7. A patient in a nursing home was admitted with a diagnosis of dementia. He started a fire because he was cooking at home and forgot that there was a pan on the stove. The nursing diagnosis that is highest priority is
   A. ineffective brain tissue perfusion
   B. risk for injury
   C. acute confusion
   D. impaired memory

8. While the nurse performs formal patient assessment, assistive personnel often observe changes when obtaining vital signs or assisting patients with ADLs. When discussing care for a patient with back pain, the nurse should particularly alert the assistant to watch for
   A. dizziness
   B. bowel/bladder incontinence
   C. difficulty swallowing
   D. arm weakness

9. When collecting a health history for the patient complaining of headache, the patient reports having as many as four episodes/day of severe right orbital pain lasting about 30 minutes with tearing and nasal congestion on the right. This is most consistent with
A. cluster headache
B. migraine with aura
C. tension headache
D. migraine without aura

10. Of the following changes, which is the earliest sign of progressing brain herniation that originates in the cerebral hemispheres?
A. An enlarging pupil that is sluggishly reactive to light
B. Altered mentation
C. Widening pulse pressure with bradycardia
D. Reflex posturing of extremities

References

American Heart Association. (2004). Physical activity and exercise recommendations for stroke survivors: An American Heart Association scientific statement from the Council on Clinical Cardiology, Subcommittee on Exercise, Cardiac Rehabilitation, and Prevention; the Council on Cardiovascular Nursing; the Council on Nutrition, Physical Activity, and Metabolism; and the Stroke Council. *Circulation, 109*(16), 2031–2041.

American Heart Association. Stroke risk factors. (2007). Retrieved August 1, 2007, from http://www.americanheart.org/presenter.jhtml?identifier=4716

American Nurses Association (ANA) and the John A. Hartford Foundation Institute. Normal changes in aging. (2007). Retrieved August 13, 2007, from http://www.geronurseonline.org/index.cfm?section_id=31&geriatric_topic_id=11&sub_section_id=77&page_id=166&tab=2#item_12

Arboix, A., Miguel, M., Císcar, E., et al. (2006). Cardiovascular risk factors in patients aged 85 or older with ischemic stroke. *Clinical Neurology and Neurosurgery, 108*(7), 638–643.

Bax, M., Tydeman, C., & Flodmark O. (2006). Clinical and MRI correlates of cerebral palsy: The European Cerebral Palsy Study. *Journal of the American Medical Association, 296*(13), 1602–1608.

Bennett, H. P., Piquet, O., Grayson, D. A., Creasey, H., Waite, L. M., Lye, T., et al. (2006). Cognitive, extrapyramidal, and magnetic resonance imaging predictors of functional impairment in nondemented older community dwellers: The Sydney Older Person Study. *Journal of the American Geriatrics Society, 54*(1), 3–10

Bulechek, G. B. & Butcher, H. K., McCloskey Dochterman, J. (2007). *Nursing Interventions Classification (NIC)* (4th ed.) St. Louis: Mosby.

Centers for Disease Control and Prevention. (2007). Revised recommendations of the Advisory Committee on Immunization Practices to vaccinate all persons aged 11–18 years with meningococcal conjugate vaccine. *MMRW Weekly, 56*(31), 794–795.

Committee on Environmental Health. (2005). Lead exposure in children: Prevention, detection, and management. *Pediatrics, 116*, 1036–1046.

Cramer, J. A., & French, J. (2001).Quantitative assessment of seizure severity for clinical trials: A review of approaches to seizure components. *Epilepsia, 42*(1). 119–129.

Dunning, J., Daly, J. P., Lomas, J. P., et al., for the Children's Head injury Algorithm for the prediction of Important Clinical Events study group. (2006). Derivation of the children's head injury algorithm for the prediction of important clinical events decision rule for head injury in children. *Archives of Diseases in Childhood, 91*, 885–891.

Environmental Protection Agency. (2007). *Lead in dust, paint and soil*. Retrieved August 15, 2007, from http://www.epa.gov/lead/pubs/leadinfo.htm#health

Fallang, B., & Hadders-Algra, M. (2005). Postural behavior in children born preterm. *Neural Plasticity, 12*(2–3), 175–182.

Frishkoff, G. A. (2007). Hemispheric differences in strong versus weak semantic priming: Evidence from event-related brain potentials. *Brain & Language, 100*(1), 23–43.

Gill, M. R., et al. (2004). Interrater reliability of Glasgow Coma Scale Scores in the emergency department. *Annals of Emergency Medicine, 43*(2), 215–223.

Gillett, M., Davis, W. A., Jackson, D., et al. (2003). Prospective evaluation of carotid bruit as a predictor of first stroke in type 2 diabetes: The Fremantle Diabetes Study. *Stroke, 34*, 2145–2151.

Goldstein, L. B., Adams, R., Alberts, M. J., et al. (2006). Primary prevention of ischemic stroke: A guideline from the American Heart Association/American Stroke Association Stroke Council: Cosponsored by the Atherosclerotic Peripheral Vascular Disease Interdisciplinary Working Group; Cardiovascular Nursing Council; Clinical Cardiology Council; Nutrition, Physical Activity, and Metabolism Council; and the Quality of Care and Outcomes Research Interdisciplinary Working Group. *Circulation, 113*(24), e873–e923.

Gordon, N. F., Gulanick, M., Costa, F., et al. (2004). Physical activity and exercise recommendations for stroke survivors: An American Heart Association scientific statement from the Council on Clinical Cardiology, Subcommittee on Exercise, Cardiac Rehabilitation, and Prevention; the Council on Cardiovascular Nursing; the Council on Nutrition, Physical Activity, and Metabolism; and the Stroke Council. *Circulation, 109*(16), 2031–2041.

Hand, P. J., Kwan, J., Lindley, R. I., Dennis, M. S., Wardlaw, J. M. (2006). Distinguishing between stroke and mimic at the bedside: The brain attack study. *Stroke,* 37, 769–775.

Healthy people 2010: What are its goals? (n.d.). Retrieved January 7, 2007, from http://www.healthypeople.gov/About/goals.htm

Heron, R., Heron, R., Davie, A., Gillies, R., & Courtney, M. (2001). Interrater reliability of the Glasgow Coma Scale score among nurses in sub-specialties of critical care. *Australian Critical Care, 14*(3), 100–105.

Hickey, J. V. (2002). The neurological physical examination and neurological assessment. In J. V. Hickey (Ed.), *The clinical practice of neurological and neurosurgical nursing* (5th ed., pp. 117–158 and 158–184). Philadelphia: Lippincott Williams and Wilkins.

Hockenberry, M. J. & Wilson, D. (2007). *Wong's nursing care of infants and children*. Philadelphia: Elsevier.

Hu, G., Tuomilehto, J., Silventoinen, K., Sarti, C., et al., (2007). Body mass index, waist circumference, and waist-hip ratio on the risk of total and type-specific stroke. *Archives of Internal Medicine, 167*(13), 1420–1427.

Inouye, S. K., Robison, J. T., Froehlich, T. E., & Richardson, E. D. (1998). The time and change test: A simple screening test for dementia. *Journal of Gerontology, 53*, M281–M286.

Isaacson, J. E., & Vora, N. M. (2003). Differential diagnosis and treatment of hearing loss. *American Family Physician, 68*(6), 1125–1132.

Kandel, E., Schwartz, J., & Jessell, T. (2008). *Principles of neural science* (5th ed.). Philadelphia: Elsevier.

Kolevzon, A., Gross, R., & Reichenberg, A. (2007). Prenatal and perinatal risk factors for autism: A review and integration of findings. *Archives of Pediatric Adolescent Medicine, 161*(4), 326–333.

Koren, G., Nava-Ocampo, A. A., Moretti, M. E., Sussman, R., & Nulman, I. (2006). Major malformations with valproic acid. *Canadian Family Physician, 52*, 441–442, 444, 447.

Laarson, H. J., Eaton, W. W., Madsen, K. M., Vestergaard, M., Olesen, A. V., Agerbo, E., et al. (2005). Risk factors for autism: Perinatal factors, parental psychiatric history, and socioeconomic status. *American Journal of Epidemiogy, 161*(10), 916–925.

Leder, S. B. (1997). Videofluoroscopic evaluation of aspiration with visual examination of the gag reflex and velar movement. *Dysphagia, 12*(1), 21–23.

Lee, L. C., Harrington, R. A., Chang, J. J., & Connors, S. L. (2008). Increased risk of injury in children with developmental disabilities. *Research in Developmental Disabilities, 29*(3), 247–255.

Lowdermilk, D. L., & Perry, S. E. (2007). *Maternity & women's health care* (9th ed.). St. Louis: Mosby.

Mathers-Schmidt, B. A., & Kurlinski, M. (2003). Dysphagia evaluation practices: Inconsistencies in clinical assessment and instrumental examination decision-making. *Dysphagia, 18*(2), 114–125.

McNett, M. (2007). A review of the predictive ability of Glasgow Coma Scale scores in head-injured patients. *Neuroscience Nursing, 39*(2), 68–75.

Moorhead, S., Johnson, M., Maas, M. (2007). *Nursing outcomes classification (NOC)* (4th ed.). St. Louis: Mosby.

National Center for Injury Prevention and Control. (2007). *Fact sheet: Spinal cord injury*. Retrieved August 1, 2007, from http://www.cdc.gov/ncipc/factsheets/scifacts.htm

National Center for Injury Prevention and Control. (2007). *Traumatic brain injury*. Retrieved August 1, 2007, from http://0-www.cdc.gov.mill1.sjlibrary.org/ncipc/factsheets/tbi.htm

National Clearinghouse Guidelines (2007). Stroke assessment across the continuum of care (2007). Retrieved August 12, 2007, from http://www.guideline.gov/summary/summary.aspx?doc_id=7426

National Institutes of Health. (2003). *NIH stroke scales and clinical assessment tools*. Retrieved August 14, 2007, from http://64.37.123.165/trials/scales/nihss.html

Nelson, M. R, Reid, C. M., Ryan, P., et al. (2007). Self-reported adherence with medication and cardiovascular disease outcomes in the Second Australian National Blood Pressure Study (ANBS2). *Medical Journal of Australia, 185*, 487–489.

Neural control of breathing (2007). Retrieved August 9, 2007, from http://www.meddean.luc.edu/lumen/meded/medicine/pulmonar/physio/pf11.htm

North American Nursing Diagnosis Association. (2009). *Nursing diagnoses, 2009–2011 Edition: Definitions and classifications (NANDA NURSING DIAGNOSIS)*. West Sussex UK: John Wiley & Sons.

Perry, J. J., Stiell, I. G., Wells, G. A., Mortensen, M., Sivilotti, M., Bullard, M., et al. (2006). Interobserver agreement in the assessment of headache patients with possible subarachnoid hemorrhage. *Academic Emergency Medicine, 13*, S138.

Pupillary abnormalities: Their recognition and diagnosis. (2007). Retrieved August 15, 2007, from http://www.opt.indiana.edu/riley/HomePage/Pupil_Abnormal/1_Saint_Pupil_Abnormal.html

Rothwell, P. M., Giles, M. F., Flossmann, E., et al. (2005). A simple score (ABCD) to identify individuals at high early risk of stroke after transient ischaemic attack. *Lancet, 366*, 29–36.

Rull, R. P., Ritz, B., & Shaw, G. M. (2006). Neural tube defects and maternal residential proximity to agricultural pesticide applications. *American Journal of Epidemiology, 163*(8), 743–753.

Saguil A. (2005). Evaluation of the patient with muscle weakness. *American Family Physician, 71*(7), 1327–1336.

Shiraishi, H. M., Ahlfors, S. P., Stufflebeam, S. M., et al. (2005). Application of magnetoencephalography in epilepsy patients with widespread spike or slow-wave activity. *Epilepsia, 46*(8), 1264–1272.

Standring, S. (2004). *Gray's anatomy: The anatomical basis for clinical practice* (39th ed.). London: Elseiver Churchill Livingstone.

Tang, Y.-W. (2003). Molecular diagnosis of herpes simplex virus infections in the central nervous system. *Abstract Interscientific Conference Antimicrobial Agents Chemotherapy*. 2003 Sep 14–17; 43rd conference.

Teasdale, G. & Jennett, B. (1974). Assessment of coma and impaired consciousness. A practical scale. *Lancet, 304*, 81–84.

Terré, R., & Mearin, F. (2006). Oropharyngeal dysphagia after the acute phase of stroke: Predictors of aspiration. *Neurogastroenterology Motility, 3*, 200–205.

Thiessen, M. (2006). Pediatric minor closed head injury. *Pediatric Clinics of North America, 53*(1), 1–26.

Vukusic, S., Hutchinson, M., Hours, M., Moreau, T., Cortinovis-Tourniaire, P., Adeleine, P., et al.; The Pregnancy in Multiple Sclerosis Group. (2004). Pregnancy and multiple sclerosis (the PRIMS study): Clinical predictors of post-*partum relapse*. *Brain, 127*(6), 1353–1360.

Williams, L. J., Rasmussen, S. A., Flores, A., Kirby, R. S., & Edmonds, L. D. (2005). Spina bifida and anencephaly by race/ethnicity: 1995–2002. *Pediatrics, 116*(3), 580–586.

The Jensen suite offers these additional resources to enhance learning and facilitate understanding of this chapter:

- thePoint on line resource, http//thepoint.lww.com/Jensen1E
- Student CD-ROM included with the book
- *Laboratory Manual for Nursing Health Assessment: A Best Practice Approach*
- *Pocket Guide for Nursing Health Assessment: A Best Practice Approach*

Tables of Abnormal Findings

Picture	Pathological Indication	Description
Unequal pupil size, physiological	Physiological anisocoria, not associated with any disease	May be congenital in 20% of the population
Unequal pupils size—abnormal	Anisocoria related to compression of the optic nerve	One pupil is 0.1 mm different from the other.
Constricted and fixed (pinpoint)	Miosis related to hemorrhage in the pons or opiate narcotics	Pinpoint pupils (<0.1 mm) or small pupils (1–2.5 mm) suggest damage to the sympathetic pathways or metabolic encephalopathy.
Dilated and fixed	Anoxia, sympathetic effects, atropine, tricyclics, amphetamines, or pilocarpine drops for glaucoma treatment; when associated with a head injury, prognosis is poor.	Pupils are >6 mm bilaterally.
Horner's syndrome	Preganglionic, central, or postganglionic lesion	Miosis (small pupil), ptosis (lid droop), anhydrosis (lack of sweat), and apparent enophthalmos (affected eye appears to be sunken)
Adie pupil	Denervation of the nerve supply from diabetic neuropathy or alcoholism	Both the pupillary response and accommodation are sluggish or impaired in one eye.
Argyll Robertson	Neurosyphilis, meningitis	Virtually no response to light, but brisk response to accommodation bilaterally. Pupils are small and frequently irregular in shape.
Third nerve palsy	Third nerve palsy	Sudden ptosis, diplopia, and pain are some of the symptoms. Pupil is fixed and dilated, and extraocular motility is restricted.

Source: Pupillary abnormalities: Their recognition and diagnosis. (2007). Retrieved June 17, 2010, from http://www.opt.indiana.edu/riley/HomePage/Pupil_Abnormal/1_Saint_Pupil_Abnormal.html; for more on abnormal pupils, see Chapter 15.

Picture	Pathological Indication	Description
Abnormal Extension Plantar flexed Flexed Pronated Extended Adducted	Damage to the midbrain or upper pons; more serious than abnormal flexion, because the patient is posturing toward rather than away from a noxious stimulus.	Very stiff, spastic movements may persist after noxious stimulation. Upper extremities are extended, adducted, and internally rotated; palms are pronated. Lower extremities are extended, back is hyperextended, and there is plantar flexion.
Abnormal Flexion Plantar flexed Internally rotated Flexed Adducted (Flexed)	Damage to the cerebral cortex	Very stiff, spastic movements may persist after noxious stimulation. Upper extremities are flexed and arms are adducted. Lower extremities are extended, internally rotated with plantar flexion.
Hemiplegia Externally rotated Flaccid	Stroke	Sensation and motor strength are lost unilaterally.
Flexion Withdrawal	CNS depression or injury	Gross movements of all body parts are away from the noxious stimulus. Rather than localizing pain to one side, the patient may withdraw both arms when nailbed pressure is applied.
Flaccid Quadriplegia	Nonfunctional brainstem	Sensation and muscle tone are completely lost.

	Common Associations	Description
Paralysis 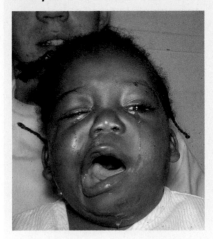	Stroke, spinal cord injury, chronic neuromuscular diseases, Bell palsy	Loss of motor function resulting in flaccidity over the area of damage; may be total, one-sided (hemiplegia), in all four extremities (quadriplegia), or in only the legs (paraplegia)
Resting Tremor 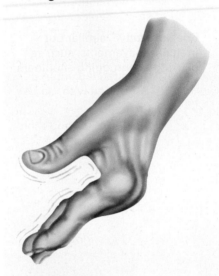	Parkinson's disease	Prominent at rest, may decrease or disappear with voluntary movement
Intention Tremor 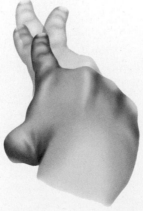	Multiple sclerosis with damage to the cerebellar pathways, or essential tremor	Absent at rest, increase with movement; may worsen as movement progresses

(table continues on page 728)

Table 24.11   Abnormalities of Movements (*continued*)

	Common Associations	Description
Fasciculation	Deterioration of the anterior horn cells	Fine, flickering, irregular movements in small muscle groups seen under the skin; may not cause movement at the joint. Because fasciculations occur under the skin, it is difficult to see them clearly.
Tic	Tourette's syndrome, use of psychiatric medications, and use of amphetamines (eg, methamphetamine)	Brief, repetitive, similar but irregular movements, such as blinking or shrugging shoulders
Clonus/Myoclonus	Seizures, hiccups, or just prior to falling asleep	Rapid, sudden clonic spasm of a muscle that may occur regularly or intermittently

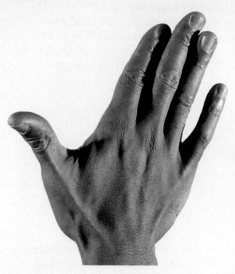

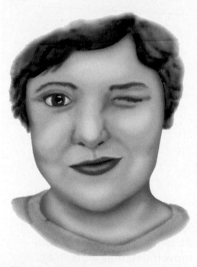

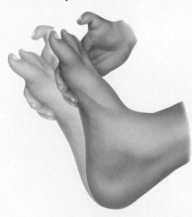

Table 24.11   **Abnormalities of Movements** (*continued*)

	Common Associations	Description
Dystonia 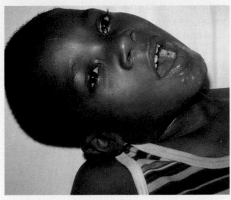	Use of psychiatric medications	Slow involuntary twisting movements that often involve the trunk and larger muscles; may be accompanied by twisted postures
Choreiform Movements 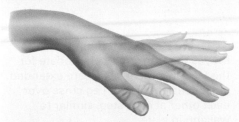	Huntington's disease	Brief, rapid, jerky movements that are irregular and unpredictable; commonly affect the face, head, lower arms, and hands
Athetoid Movements 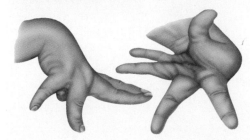	Cerebral palsy	Slow involuntary wormlike twisting movements that involve the extremities, neck, facial muscles, and tongue; may be associated with drooling and dysarthria

Signs	UMN Lesions (involve motor areas of cerebral cortex and white matter tracts connecting to motor nerve nuclei in brain or spinal cord)	LMN Lesions (involve brainstem or spinal cord motor nuclei, nerve roots or nerves)
Strength	Spastic paresis or paralysis (may be flaccid in acute phase)	Flaccid paresis or paralysis
Muscle tone	Increased (spasticity)	Decreased or absent (flaccidity)
Muscle stretch reflexes	Increased; presence of Babinski's sign	Decreased or absent
Muscle atrophy	Absent (although disuse atrophy may occur with prolonged deficit)	Present
Muscle fasciculation	Absent	Present

Table 24.13   Abnormal Gaits

Picture	Pathologic Indication	Description
Spastic Hemiparesis 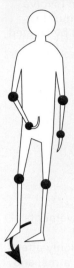	Stroke	One side is normal. The other side is flexed from spasticity. The elbow, wrist, and fingers are flexed; the arm is close to the side. The affected leg is extended with plantar flexion of the foot. When ambulating, the foot is dragged, scraping the toe, or it is circled stiffly outward and forward.
Scissors 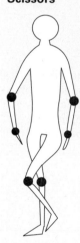	Spastic diplegia associated with bilateral spasticity of the legs	Moves the trunk to accommodate for the leg movements. Legs are extended and knees are flexed. Leg cross over each other at each step, similar to walking in water.
Parkinsonian 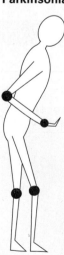	Parkinson's disease	Stooped posture, head and neck forward and hips and knees flexed. Arms are also flexed and held at waist. There is difficulty in initiating gait, often rocking to start. Once ambulating, steps are quick and shuffling. Has difficulty stopping once started.

Table 24.13   Abnormal Gaits (continued)

Picture	Pathologic Indication	Description
Cerebellar Ataxia 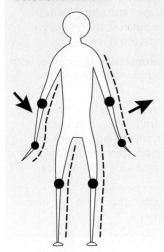	Cerebral palsy and alcohol intake	Wide-based gait. Staggers and lurches from side to side. Cannot perform Romberg because of swaying of the trunk.
Sensory Ataxia 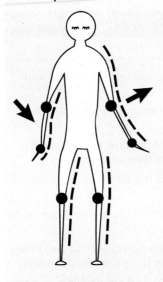	Cerebral palsy	Wide-based gait. Feet are loosely thrown forward, landing first on the heels and then on the toes. Patient watches the ground to help guide the feet. Positive Romberg from loss of position sense.
Dystrophic (Waddling)	Weak hip abductors	Wide gait. Weight is shifted from side to side with stiff trunk movement. Abdomen protrudes and lordosis is common.

Picture	Pathological Indication	Description
Peripheral neuropathy	Diabetes mellitus or peripheral vascular disease	Sensory loss is distributed peripherally in a characteristic "glove" or "stocking" pattern. More diffuse and less specific than injury associated with an individual nerve
Individual nerves	Trauma or injury	Follows the pattern expected in the nerve, with the cutaneous distribution that follows the dermatome.
Spinal cord hemisection	Brown-Séquard's syndrome from spinal cord injury, tumor, or mass	Because of how the nerves cross in the spinal cord, pain and temperature are lost below the level of the lesion on the opposite side. Position sense, vibration, and motor function are affected on the same side of the body.
Complete transection of the spinal cord	Spinal cord injury, tumor, or mass	All sensation and motor function is lost below the level of the lesion

! Table 24.15 Pathological (Primitive) Reflexes

Procedure	Abnormal Findings in Adults
Grasp reflex. Apply palmar stimulation.	A grasping response is associated with dementia and diffuse brain impairment.
Snout reflex. Elicit by tapping a tongue blade across the lips.	The snout reflex is present if tapping causes the lips to purse.
Sucking reflex. Touch or stroke the lips, tongue, or palate.	Observe sucking movement of the lips; this reflex also may be noted during oral care or oral suctioning.
Rooting reflex. Stroke the lateral upper lip.	The rooting reflex is present if the patient moves the mouth toward the stimulus.
Palmomental reflex. Stroke the palm of the hand.	It is present if stroking of the palm causes contraction of the same sided muscle of the lower lip.
Hoffman's sign. Tap the nail on the third or fourth finger.	A positive Hoffman's sign is if tapping elicits involuntary flexion of the distal joint of the thumb and index finger.
Glabellar's sign. Tap the forehead to cause the patient to blink.	Normally, the first five taps cause a single blink, and then the reflex diminishes.
	Blinking continues in patients with diffuse cerebral dysfunction.

Source: Hickey, J. V. (2002). The neurological physical examination and neurological assessment. In J. V. Hickey (Ed.), *The clinical practice of neurological and neurosurgical nursing* (5th ed., pp. 117–158 and 158–184). Philadelphia: Lippincott Williams and Wilkins.

Table 24.16 Abnormal Respiratory Patterns Associated with Intracranial Conditions

	Area of the Brain Affected
Cheyne-Stokes Respiration (Spindle Pattern)	
Breathing pattern with period of apnea (10–60 seconds) followed by gradually increasing depth and frequency of respiration, gradually decreasing in depth and frequency until period of apnea	Poor brain stem perfusion
Central Veurogenic Hyperventilation	
Rapid and deep respirations, sometimes >40/min	Medulla or pons malfunction
Apneustic Breathing	
Sustained inspiratory effort, usually <12/min	Medulla or pons damage
Gasping	
Rapid and quick, difficult breaths; irregular respirations with varying rate and tidal volume	Extensive pons damage, severe hypoxia
Biot Breathing (Cluster Pattern)	
Several short breaths followed by long irregular periods of apnea	Pons malfunction, increased ICP
Apnea	
Absence of breathing	High cervical cord or extensive medulla damage, brain death

Source: Neural control of breathing (2007). Retrieved August 9, 2007, from http://www.meddean.luc.edu/lumen/meded/medicine/pulmonar/physio/pf11.htm; for more on abnormal breathing patterns, see Chapter 18.

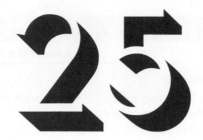

25

Male Genitalia and Rectal Assessment

Learning Objectives

1 Identify structures and functions of the male genitalia.

2 Identify the locations of male genital organs, the prostate, and the rectum.

3 Identify teaching opportunities for health promotion and risk reduction related to male genitalia.

4 Collect subjective and objective data on the male genitalia, rectum, and prostate, including present health status, past medical history, sexual history, and family history.

5 Identify normal and abnormal findings in the inspection and palpation of the male genitalia, prostate, and rectum.

6 Analyze subjective and objective findings to help plan interventions for men's health.

7 Document and communicate data from the male genitalia assessment using appropriate medical terminology.

8 Individualize health assessment considering the condition, age, gender, and culture of the patient.

9 Use assessment findings to identify diagnoses and to initiate a plan of care.

---

*M*r. Gardner, a 50-year-old Caucasian man, was diagnosed with benign prostatic hyperplasia (BPH) 3 years ago. He is visiting the clinic today because he is having increased difficulty with urination. Mr. Gardner has been married to his second wife for 3 months. He has two children from his first marriage and two stepchildren. Mr. Gardner's temperature is 37.0°C, pulse 84 beats/min, respirations 16 breaths/min, and blood pressure 122/68 mm Hg. Current medications include tamsulosin (Flomax) for the prostatic hyperplasia and lovastatin for his elevated lipid levels. Additional supplements include a multivitamin and fish-oil tablets that he takes to prevent cardiovascular disease.

You will gain more information about Mr. Gardner as you progress through this chapter. As you study the content and features, consider Mr. Gardner's case and its relationship to what you are learning. Begin thinking about the following points:

- Is Mr. Gardner's condition stable, urgent, or an emergency?
- How will the nurse work with Mr. Gardner to promote health and reduce risk for illness?
- Which nursing diagnosis is the highest priority? What is the rationale?

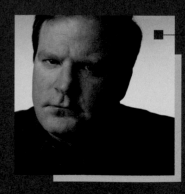

This chapter provides an overview of normal anatomy and focused physical assessment of the male genitalia, which includes the seminal vesicles, scrotum, penis, testicles, prostate gland, and epididymides (Fig. 25-1). While the rectum and anus are terminal structures of the gastrointestinal tract (see Chapter 22), nurses frequently integrate a holistic nursing assessment of these organs into the physical examination of the male genitalia. A basic understanding of pertinent anatomy assists nurses to perform assessments with confidence and knowledge.

During such very intimate assessment, it is important to provide patients with privacy. If desired, a patient has the right for a chaperone to be present during the examination. In language the patient will understand, remember to explain each step of the assessment. During assessment, education opportunities arise, and nurses can teach health promotion and risk reduction while collecting subjective and objective data. All findings should be documented as per protocol.

The design of this chapter is to provide the foundation for the nurse to conduct individualized health assessments, in which the nurse fully considers each patient's age, sexual orientation, and culture. Incorporated throughout are examples of evidence-based critical thinking, points of clinical significance, and key abnormal findings. A sensitive, tactful approach to examination of this area paves the way to providing excellent health care.

Structure and Function Overview

External Genitalia

The *penis* has two functions: (1) it is the final excretory organ of urination and (2) with sexual excitement, it becomes firm or erect to allow penetration for intercourse. It can be subdivided into the root, shaft (or body), and glan (Fig. 25-2).

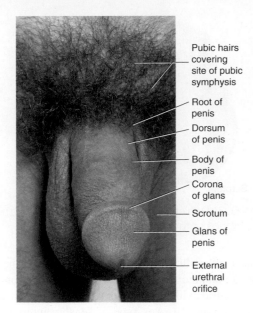

Figure 25.2 Surface anatomy of the penis.

Labels: Pubic hairs covering site of pubic symphysis; Root of penis; Dorsum of penis; Body of penis; Corona of glans; Scrotum; Glans of penis; External urethral orifice

The root of the penis lies deep within the perineum. The shaft has hairless, thin skin that adheres loosely, allowing for expansion of the erect penis. The glan (head of the penis) is lighter in pigmentation than the rest of the organ.

The penis contains three distensible structures: two *corpora cavernosa*, which form the dorsum and sides of the penis, and a single *corpus spongiosum*, which forms the bulb. The *urethra* is located in the middle of the corpus spongiosum, which ends in the cone-shaped glan with its expanded base, or *corona*. A small slit in the distal tip of the glan is the *urethra meatus*. The ridge of the corona separates the glan from the shaft.

When engorged with blood, the smooth, spongy tissue of the penis becomes erect. An erection is a complex neurovascular reflex that ensues when a decreased venous outflow and an increased arterial dilation cause the two corpora

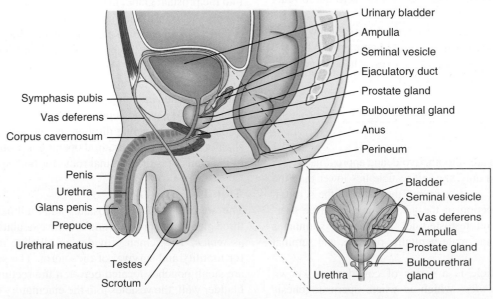

Figure 25.1 Overview of the male genitalia.

Labels (left): Symphasis pubis; Vas deferens; Corpus cavernosum; Penis; Urethra; Glans penis; Prepuce; Urethral meatus; Testes; Scrotum

Labels (right): Urinary bladder; Ampulla; Seminal vesicle; Ejaculatory duct; Prostate gland; Bulbourethral gland; Anus; Perineum

Inset labels: Bladder; Seminal vesicle; Vas deferens; Ampulla; Prostate gland; Bulbourethral gland; Urethra

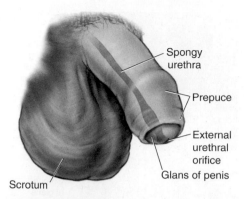

Figure 25.3 Depiction of an uncircumcised penis; note how the prepuce or foreskin covers the glan.

cavernosa to fill with blood. This reflex is under the control of the autonomic nervous system and depends on local synthesis of nitric oxide. Psychogenic and local mechanisms can induce an erection. Any type of sensory input, including auditory, tactile, visual, or imaginative can cause a psychogenic erection. Tactile stimuli initiate the local reflex mechanisms.

Ejaculation occurs with emission of semen from the epididymides, vas deferens, prostate, and seminal vesicles. Ejaculation follows constriction of the arterial vessels supplying blood to the corpora cavernosa. After ejaculation, the penis returns to its normal, flaccid condition.

In uncircumcised males, loose, hood-like skin called the *prepuce* or *foreskin* covers the glan (Fig. 25-3). Pulling back the foreskin or prepuce exposes the glan. Sloughed epithelial cells and mucus collect between glan and foreskin, forming a white, cheese-like substance called *smegma*. Circumcision is removal of the prepuce or foreskin.

The *scrotum* is a pouch covered with darkly pigmented, loose, rugous (wrinkled) skin. A septum divides the scrotum into two sacs, each of which contains a testis, epididymis, spermatic cord, and muscle layer known as the *cremasteric muscle*. The cremasteric muscle allows the scrotum to relax or contract.

Spermatogenesis requires a temperature below 37°C (approximately 2°C lower than core temperature). When the temperature rises, the scrotal sac relaxes; when temperature decreases, the scrotal sac rises closer to the body.

Internal Genitalia

Testes

The *testes* (*testicles*) are smooth, ovoid, and approximately 3.5 to 5 cm long. Commonly, the left testicle lies lower than the right. The spermatic cords suspend the testes in the scrotum (Fig. 25-4). The function of the testicles is to produce spermatozoa (sperm) and testosterone. Testosterone stimulates pubertal growth of the male genitalia, prostate, and seminal vesicles.

Inside each testicle is a series of coiled ducts known as *seminiferous tubules*, which is where spermatogenesis occurs. Mature sperm is generated approximately every

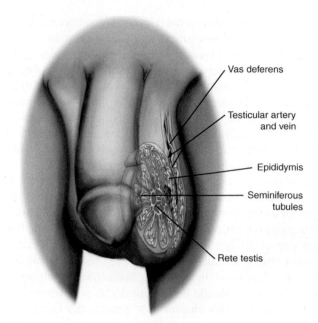

Figure 25.4 Anatomy of the testis.

90 days. As sperm are produced, they move toward the center of the testicle, traveling into the efferent tubules adjacent to the ductus epididymis.

Ducts

Ducts are responsible for moving sperm. The journey begins in the epididymides and continues to the *vas deferens*, ejaculatory duct, and urethra. The soft, comma-shaped *epididymis* is on the posterolateral and upper aspect of the testicles. This structure provides for storage, maturation, and transit of sperm. The *vas deferens* (*ductus deferens*) transports sperm from the epididymis to the ejaculatory duct. The vas deferens, arteries, veins, and nerves make up the *spermatic cord*, which ascends through the external inguinal ring and into the inguinal canal. Inside the canal and just before the entrance into the prostate gland, the vas deferens unites with the seminal vesicle to form the ejaculatory duct.

Once sperm enter the ejaculatory duct, they are transported downward through the prostate gland and into the posterior portion of the urethra. The urethra is approximately 7 to 8 in long, extending from urinary bladder to meatus. The urethra can be separated into three sections: (1) posterior, (2) membranous, and (3) cavernous or anterior. It extends from the base of the bladder, traveling through the prostate gland down the shaft of the penis. The urethral opening is a small slit at the tip of the penis; it is the terminal route for both sperm and urine.

Glands

The seminal vesicles, prostate, and bulbourethral are the three glands that produce and secrete ejaculation fluid known as *semen*. The semen provides an alkaline medium needed for motility and survival of the sperm. The seminal vesicles are small pouches located between the rectum and posterior bladder wall; the vesicles join the ejaculatory duct at the base of the prostate.

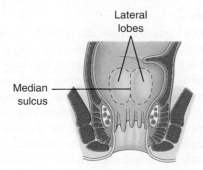

Lateral lobes

Median sulcus

Figure 25.5 The prostate gland.

The *prostate gland* contains muscular and glandular tissue (Fig. 25-5). It has five lobes and is approximately 3.5 × 3.0 cm. The prostate gland surrounds the urethra at the bladder neck; its shape resembles a large chestnut. The physiologic function of the prostate and its secretion is not fully understood; however, it produces the greatest volume of ejaculatory fluid. The right and left lobes of the prostate are divided by a slight groove known as the *median sulcus*. These two lobes are in close contact with the anterior rectal wall and palpable during digital rectal examination (DRE). The median lobe is anterior of the urethra and cannot be palpated on a rectal examination.

Clinical Significance 25-1

Usually, the middle and lateral lobes are above the ejaculatory ducts and typically involved in BPH. The exact cause of BPH is unknown, but the condition is believed to be associated with age-related hormonal changes. As men age, the fibromuscular structures of the prostate gland atrophy, and collagen gradually replaces the muscular element of the prostate.

The *bulbourethral glands* are located on either side of the urethra immediately below the prostate gland (Swartz, 2006).

Rectum and Anus

The rectum and anus constitute the terminal sections of the gastrointestinal tract and are included in the posterior portion of the male perineum examination.

Rectum

The rectum is approximately 12 cm long and is superior to the anus. The proximal end of the rectum is continuous with the sigmoid colon. The distal end, commonly referred to as the anorectal junction, is identifiable during a colonoscopy as having a saw-tooth–like edge. Located above the anorectal junction, the rectum dilates and turns posteriorly into the hollow area of the coccyx and sacrum; this forms the *rectal ampulla*, which stores flatus and feces. Three semilunar transverse folds, known as *rectal valves*, are located in the rectum. The valves extend across half the diameter of the rectum with the inferior valve palpable on digital examination. The exact functions of these valves are unknown; however, the valves may support feces while flatus is being expelled.

Anal Canal and Anus

The male's anal canal is approximately 2.5 to 4.0 cm long and extends from the anorectal junction to the anus. It is lined with mucous membrane arranged in longitudinal folds called *rectal columns*, which contain a complex system of veins and arteries commonly referred to as the *internal hemorrhoidal plexus*. Between each column is a recessed area identified as the anal crypt. The perineal glands empty into the anal crypt. Around the anal canal are two concentric rings of muscles, the internal and external sphincters. The internal sphincter contains smooth muscle and is under involuntary control. The sensation to defecate comes when the rectum fills with stool, which causes reflexive stimulation that relaxes the internal sphincter. The striated external sphincter consists of skeletal muscles and is under voluntary control; this allows for control of defecation.

The anal canal perceives pain differently; the autonomic nervous system controls the upper portion, which is relatively insensitive to stimuli. Conversely, the lower portion, which is controlled by somatic sensory nerves, is sensitive to stimulation.

The anus is the terminal portion of the rectum. The moist mucosal tissue is pink and surrounded by hyperpigmented perianal skin; hair may be present in the adult. Normally, the anus is closed except during defecation.

⚠ Lifespan Considerations

Infants and Children

Newborns usually pass the first meconium stool within 24 to 48 hours of birth. At this time, both the internal and external sphincters are under involuntary reflexive control because the myelination of the spinal cord is incomplete. It is common for infants to have a stool after each feeding because of the gastrocolic reflex. Commonly between 12 and 18 months of age, infants gradually achieve control of the external anal sphincter (Seidel, et al., 2003).

There is much debate over whether circumcision should be performed routinely. The American Academy of Pediatrics' (AAP) Circumcision Policy Statement (1999) states that several scientific studies show the benefits of circumcision. Recent evidence suggests fewer urinary tract infections (UTIs) in males who have been circumcised. A 2009 Cochrane review of observational studies presented strong evidence that male circumcision was associated with a reduced risk of acquiring HIV through vaginal intercourse (Siegfried, et al., 2009). Nonetheless, these benefits are not significant enough to recommend that all males be circumcised.

Because circumcision has potential benefits and risks, parents should determine what is in the best interest of the child. Often the decision is based on family tradition, culture, religious, and ethnic traditions. If parents decide to circumcise their son, the nurse needs to obtain informed consent before the procedure. The AAP states that analgesia should

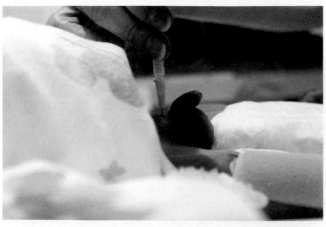

Figure 25.6 A health care provider is injecting a local anesthetic while preparing an infant boy for circumcision.

be provided for all circumcision procedures. More pain-relieving interventions are becoming part of routine practice: local anesthetics, dorsal penile nerve blocks, and subcutaneous ring blocks (Fig. 25-6).

Adolescents

With the onset of puberty, testicular growth begins and the scrotal skin thins and becomes pendulous. During puberty, the testes become active and begin to secrete testosterone, which promotes bone maturation and epiphyseal closure. Genital hair begins to appear at the base of the penis. As physical development continues, genital hair darkens and extends over the entire pubic area; it is at this time that the prostate gland enlarges. When maturation is complete, genital hair is curly, dense, and coarse, with a diamond shape from umbilicus to anus. Growth and development of the scrotum and testes are complete, and the length and width of the penis are increased.

> **Clinical Significance 25-2**
>
> Each adolescent has his own unique growth timetable and final growth results. The nurse must consider the patient's external environment and genetic predispositions. Nevertheless, chronological patterns are consistent for all. See Table 25-1 for the Tanner stages.

Table 25.1	Tanner Stages: Male Development	
Stage	**Male Development**	**Age Range (years)**
1	There is no pubic hair. Testes and penis are small (prepubertal).	<10
2	Sparse thin hair is at base of the penis. Testes enlarge. Scrotal skin becomes coarser and redder.	10–13
3	Scrotum and testes continue to grow. Penis lengthens, with diameter increasing slowly. Pubic hair increases, becoming darker, coarse, curly, and extending laterally.	12–14
4	Penis and testes continue to grow. Pubic hair extends across pubis but spares the medial thighs.	13–15
5	Penis is at its full size. Pubic hair is diamond shaped in appearance with adult color; texture extends to surface of medial thighs.	14–17

The Tanner stages present a scale of physical development for children, adolescents, and adults. The maturation process is based on external primary and secondary sex characteristics. Each person passes through each stage at different rates. See also Chapters 21 and 26.

Source: Tanner, J. (1962). *Growth at adolescence*. Oxford: Blackwell.

Older Adult

Older men may experience distention of the rectum from degeneration of afferent neurons in the rectal wall, which interferes with relaxation of the internal sphincter. The distention can cause an elevated pressure threshold for the feeling of rectal distention, causing retention of stool. At the same time the autonomically controlled internal sphincter loses tone, the external sphincter cannot, by itself, control the bowels; this may result in incontinence (Seidel, et al., 2003).

With aging pubic hair becomes finer, grey, and less plentiful. Pubic alopecia may also occur. Testosterone levels decline with aging, which may affect both libido and sexual function. Erection becomes more dependent on tactile stimulation and less responsive to erotic cues. The penis may decrease in size and testes drop lower in the scrotum. As the male ages, the fibromuscular structures of the prostate gland atrophy. Ironically benign hyperplasia of the glandular tissue often obscures the atrophy of aging.

🌐 Cultural Considerations

When a patient becomes ill, his recognition and reaction are rooted in cultural beliefs, values, social, and family structures. Illness is more than physical symptoms and pain. The concept of illness includes perceived problems with emotional, physical, and spiritual states (Leininger & McFarland, 2002). Appreciating the patient's perception of manhood, cultural beliefs, and sexual orientation helps the nurse understand how the patient perceives health, illness, and disease. Establishing an open and trusting relationship with a patient requires a nonjudgmental attitude. A dedicated nurse can develop an awareness of cultural beliefs and values through education, listening, and self-awareness.

In societies for thousands of years, piercings have occurred in various forms and fashions. In the last 10 years, genital piercing has increased in popularity (see Table 25-6). Nevertheless, it can be an unexpected finding for the nurse during assessment of the male genitalia. In a professional nonjudgmental manner, it is important to talk to the patient about the care of the piercing. Because this site is very prone to infection, discussion should involve how the patient cleans the piercing and ways to avoid infection. The nurse should inquire how the site feels to the patient—it is possible for him to lose sensation in the area of the piercing. It may also damage strategic nerves, thus leading to an inability to achieve an orgasm.

Investigate where the piercing was done; health risks such as hepatitis, tetanus, and tuberculosis among other diseases are possible when procedures are performed in an unsterile environment. U.S. laws concerning piercing vary in each state. The Associations of Professional Piercers Web site can provide further details (Anderson, et al., 2002).

Acute Assessment

⚠ SAFETY ALERT 25.1

Six conditions can result in an acute scrotum: ischemia, trauma, infectious conditions, inflammatory conditions, hernia, and acute situations accompanying a chronic condition (eg, testicular tumor with rupture). Although differential diagnosis is broad, an accurate physical assessment and history can often accurately define the condition. Imaging studies can correlate with the clinical assessment and expedite therapeutic decisions.

The signs and symptoms of the acutely ill genitourinary patient can range from subtle to obvious. An example of subtle signs is a patient complaining of fatigue or shortness of breath upon exertion (eg, anemia from rectal bleeding). More obvious behaviors are a patient who complains of sudden and severe testicle pain (eg, possible testicle torsion). Patients presenting with an acute problem are anxious and tense; staying calm will help the patient relax and promote clear thinking.

Anorectal problems can cause significant discomfort and concern. Because of the sensitive nature of this subject, patients often delay treatment. Colorectal cancer is common in adults and maybe present with a benign condition. All complaints need thorough investigation. Early detection has been clearly shown to lower the mortality rate for colorectal cancer.

All acute situations need immediate evaluation. It is important to compare two acute scrotal conditions: testicular torsion and epididymitis. Because torsion is a surgical emergency, it is imperative for health care providers to understand the difference (Cole & Vogler, 2004). Both diagnoses may present with the same chief concern of scrotal pain. See Table 25-5 at the end of the chapter for a discussion of the two disorders.

The patient with rectal bleeding needs rapid assessment. Bleeding associated with anorectal problems can resolve spontaneously or with local pressure. The patient undergoing anticoagulation therapy, however, may need hospitalization. Inquire about bleeding disorders.

Newborns with dark tarry stools or vomiting blood may have a vitamin K deficiency. Infants presenting with rectal bleeding could have necrotizing enterocolitis. This life-threatening disease needs immediate action.

Acute infection (eg, perirectal abscess) may require immediate hospitalization, especially for immune-compromised patients. Infection usually is associated with purulent discharge from the penis. Patients with HIV/AIDS or receiving chemotherapy are especially at risk (Dains, et al., 2003).

Subjective Data Collection

Subjective data collection includes health promotion, assessment of risk factors and health-related patient teaching, and a focused health history related to common symptoms.

Table 25.2 **Healthy People Goals Related to Male Health and Education**

Goals	Patient Education Topics
Reduce the prostate cancer death rate.	Recommend screening with DRE and prostate surface antigen for early detection.
Increase male involvement in pregnancy prevention and family planning efforts.	Provide information on family planning options (eg, condoms, oral birth control, vaginal ring).
Reduce the number of new AIDS cases among adolescent and adult men who have sex with men.	Teach safe sex practices including condom use.
Reduce the proportion of adolescents and young adults with *Chlamydia trachomatis* infections, gonorrhea, syphilis, and genital herpes.	Educate on modes of transmission and condom use.

Source: *Healthy people 2010: What are its goals?* (n.d.). Retrieved July 7, 2010, from http://www.healthypeople.gov/About/goals.htm

This includes assessments for prostate and testicular cancer. Additionally, it is important to assess risk for sexually transmitted infections (STIs).

Areas for Health Promotion/ *Healthy People*

Male health promotion is very important, because many problems such as STIs are preventable. Additionally, both testicular and prostate cancers have better outcomes if detected early. Table 25-2 includes pertinent goals and education topics for male patients. The goals relate to prostate cancer, family planning, and STIs.

Assessment of Risk Factors

Numerous factors affect the male genitalia, rectum, and anus. The nurse asks the patient about current problems, family history, personal history (including age, gender, and ethnicity), medications and supplements, and risk factors for infections or cancer. Knowledge of risk factors helps identify topics for health-promotion teaching.

Questions on History and Risk	Rationales
Family History Is there a family history of testicular cancer?	Risk for testicular cancer is greater in men whose brother or father had the disease (ACS, 2008). See Box 25-1.

BOX 25.1 RISK FACTORS FOR TESTICULAR, PROSTATE, AND PENILE CANCER

Testicular Cancer

- Age (highest incidence in young men ages 20–34)
- Ethnicity and culture (highest incidence among Caucasian men in United Kingdom and United States)
- Cryptorchidism (undescended testicle at birth)
- History of testicular cancer in other testicle
- Family history (increased risk if brother has had testicular cancer)

Prostate Cancer

- Second leading cause of cancer death in men
- Family history of prostate cancer
- Age: Highest incidence is in older men; 75% of new cases occur in men older than 65 years

- Ethnicity: African American men have highest incidence of prostate cancer—two times higher than white men. Worldwide, highest prevalence is in North America and northwestern Europe.

Penile Cancer

- Phimosis (the foreskin of the penis cannot be pulled back over the glans)*
- Age 60 years or older
- Poor personal hygiene*
- Sexual promiscuity*
- Using tobacco products*
- Possible link with HPV*

*This risk factor is modifiable.
Data from: American Cancer Society: What Are the Risk Factors for Testicular Cancer? Atlanta, 2008, American Cancer Society; www.nci.nih.gov and http:www.cancer.org
American Urology Association (www.urologyhealth.org); National Cancer Institute's Factsheets http://www.nci.nih.gov/cancertopics.

Questions on History and Risk	Rationales
Is there a family history of prostate cancer?	Prostate cancer in a first-degree relative increases the patient's risk. African American men have the highest incidence of prostate cancer—two to three times higher than Caucasian men. Prevalence is highest in North America and Europe (ACS, 2008). See Box 25-1.
Is there a history of penile cancer in your family?	Although rare in the United States, some studies suggest an association between penile cancer and human papillomavirus (HPV) (Palefsky, 2007). See Box 25-1.
Is there infertility in siblings?	Encourage the patient to review his family tree for signs of infertility, especially if he is having problems conceiving.
Is there a history of hernia in your family?	Congenital weakness may predispose the patient to develop a hernia.

Personal History

Do you have any current or chronic illnesses such as diabetes, hypertension, neurologic impairment, respiratory problems (asthma, chronic obstructive pulmonary disease (COPD), chronic bronchitis), or cardiovascular disease?

Men with these illnesses are at increased risk for erectile dysfunction (Lewis, et al., 2003).

Medical and Surgical History

- Was surgery ever performed on your penis, scrotum, or rectum?
- What type of procedure was performed (please include year and date)?
- How has this procedure affected you?

Surgery is used to treat enlarged prostate, testicular cancer, hydrocele, variocele, and undescended testicle. Some men choose permanent sterilization through vasectomy. Rectal or anal conditions requiring surgery include hemorrhoids, anorectal fissures, and carcinoma of the rectum and anus.

- Have you ever been treated for an STI?
- Where and when did you receive this treatment?
- What type of STI was diagnosed?
- How was it treated?
- Did you have a test of cure following the procedure?

There are more than 50 different STIs, which are sensitive but important subjects. Tactful direct questioning is an essential part of the assessment. See Box 25-2.

BOX 25.2 RISK FACTORS FOR SEXUALLY TRANSMITTED INFECTIONS

- Engaging in sexual relations with a new or multiple partners*
- Personal history of STIs or engaging in sexual activity with a partner with a history of STIs*
- Engaging in a relationship with a partner who has several partners*
- Failure to practice safe sex*

STIs can be transmitted through vaginal, rectal, or oral sex between homosexual or heterosexual partners.

*The risk factor is modifiable.

- Have you ever had an injury to or other problems with your scrotum, penis, or testes? If yes, please explain.

Examples include *testicular torsion*, *hydrocele*, *spermatocele*, and *varicocele*.

- Have you had a condition affecting the prostate gland such as BPH or prostatitis?

Identification of previous problems may help when documenting current health concerns.

- Do you have a history of cancer?
- When was the diagnosis?
- What treatment did you have?

See Box 25-1 for risk factors for testicular, prostate, and penile cancers (common cancers found in men). Even with removal of a cancerous testicle, cancer can recur in the other testicle.

(text continues on page 742)

Questions on History and Risk	Rationales

Sexual History

- How old were you the first time you had sexual intercourse?
- Was this by choice?
- Do you prefer sexual relationships with men, women, or both?
- In what type of sex do you engage (penile-vaginal, penile-rectal, recipient rectal, oral)?
- How frequently do you have intercourse?
- Do you have sex with multiple partners?
- How many partners have you had in the last 6 months?
- Do you or your partner frequently use drugs or alcohol before sexual intercourse?
- Are you satisfied with your sexual relationship?
- Do you use contraceptives? Do you use protective barriers every time you have intercourse?
- Have you ever gotten someone pregnant?
- What was the outcome of this situation?
- Have you ever been pushed, slapped, or had something thrown at you?
- Have you ever been kicked, bit, hit with a hand or object?

Often, nurses hesitate to initiate conversation about sexual history. Nevertheless, this information is important to help identify high-risk sexual practices, establish patient norms, and provide education. Sexual dysfunction can present as anxiety, anger, or depression. In addition, physical problems can lead to sexual problems (Swartz, 2006). The nurse must be careful not to impose personal standards on the patient.

⚠ SAFETY ALERT 25.2

Men and women can be victims of abuse, so it is important to ask these questions. Often it is difficult for men to admit that they are being victimized. See Chapter 12.

Medications

What medications do you currently take, including herbal supplements, recreational, and over-the-counter (OTC) drugs?

Many medications and supplements can affect the genitourinary tract and its function.

Additional Risk Factors

Do you wear protective gear during contact sports?

Lack of protection can lead to injury of sensitive genitalia. This question can provide a good teaching opportunity to encourage the use of protective equipment.

Have you received a hepatitis A or B vaccine?

⚠ SAFETY ALERT 25.3

The Centers for Disease Control and Prevention (CDC, 2006) recommend the hepatitis A vaccine for unimmunized men who have sex with other men. The CDC recommends the hepatitis B vaccine for all unimmunized people at risk for STIs.

Do you perform self-genital examination?

This question serves as an excellent teaching opportunity while stressing to the patient the importance of the self-examination.

Do you have regular clinical examinations by a health professional?

Primary prevention helps patients maintain health. Age-appropriate health screenings should be discussed during the appointment.

Risk Assessment and Health-Related Patient Teaching

It is important for men to screen themselves for testicular cancer by performing self-examination. Screening for prostate cancer is through laboratory blood testing and physical examination.

Testicular Self-Examination

The purpose of performing self-examination is not to find something currently wrong. By performing monthly self-examinations, men older than 14 years become familiar with what is normal for them. Once this "normal" is established, changes are easier to identify. Thus, testicular cancer can be detected at an early (and most often curable) stage.

Steps for testicular self-examination (TSE) are as follows:

1. TSE is best performed after a warm shower or bath. Heat relaxes the scrotum, which makes the TSE easier.
2. Examine each testicle one at a time with both hands. Place the index and middle fingers under the testicle with the thumbs placed on top. Roll the testicle gently from side to side. You should not feel pain. Remember that one testicle may be larger; this finding is normal (Fig. 25-7).
3. Cancerous lumps usually are on the sides of the testicle, but can show up on the front. Become familiar with the location of the epididymis; this soft, tubelike structure behind the testes collects and carries sperm. If you become familiar with this structure you won't mistake it for a lump.

4. Make an appointment with a physician, preferably a urologist, as soon as possible if you find a lump or any of the following warning signs: enlargement of the testes, pain or discomfort, heaviness in the scrotum, a dull ache in the groin, significant loss of size of one testicle, or a sudden collection of fluid in the scrotum (Testicular Cancer Resource Center, 2009).

Screening for Prostate Cancer

As per the U.S. Preventive Services Task Force and the National Cancer Institute, evidence is insufficient to conclude whether screening for prostate cancer with prostate-specific antigen (PSA) or DRE reduces mortality from prostate cancer (Harris & Lohr, 2002). The PSA screening test can detect cancer earlier, but it remains unclear if this leads to any change in the natural history and outcome of the disease.

Focused Health History Related to Common Symptoms

Common Symptoms of the Male Genitalia, Prostate, and Rectum

- Pain
- Problems with urination
- Erectile dysfunction
- Penile lesions, discharge
- Scrotal enlargement

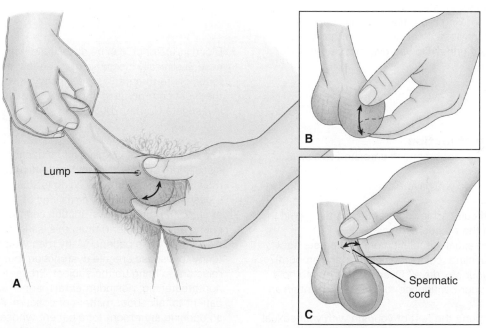

Figure 25.7 The TSE. **A.** The patient holds the penis in one hand away from the testicles while using the other hand to palpate one testicle at a time. The patient should roll the area side to side to feel for any lumps. **B.** He also should maneuver his fingers up and down. **C.** The patient should also run his fingers along the surface length of the spermatic cord to become familiar with how it feels, so that he does not mistake this for a lump.

Questions to Assess Symptoms	Rationales/Abnormal Findings

Pain

Please point to the painful area.

- Do you feel the pain anywhere else?
- When did it begin? How long have you had this pain? Have you ever experienced this pain before?
- Can you rate your pain on a scale of o to 10, with 10 being the worst pain you ever had?
- What does the pain feel like?
- Is the pain associated with nausea, vomiting, fever, abdominal distention, and burning on urination? Is your urine a different color?
- What makes the pain worse or what better? What have you done to help alleviate the pain, if anything? How well did this intervention help?
- What is your pain goal?

Have you ever had a prolonged painful erection?

Several problems can lead to pain in the lower abdominal, pelvic, or rectal areas. Sudden distention of the ureter, renal pelvis, or bladder may cause flank pain. Pain around the costovertebral angle may be from distention of the renal capsule. *Kidney-stone* pain may radiate down the spermatic cord and present as testicular pain. Pain in the groin or scrotum may result from a *hernia* or problems in the spermatic cord, testicles, or prostate. Testicular pain can occur secondary to any problem of the testes such as *epididymitis, orchitis, hydrocele, spermatic cord torsion,* and *tumor.* Understanding what interventions the patient does to relieve the pain assists with developing a treatment plan. Always ask about use of OTC medications, current prescriptions, and complementary substances.

A long and painful erection is called *priapism.* It can be seen in patients with *leukemia* or *hemoglobinopathies* (eg, sickle-cell anemia). This is not from sexual excitation—the prolonged erection results from vein thrombosis in the corpora carvernosa (Swartz, 2006).

Are you experiencing rectal or anal pain?

Perianal abscess, rectal fissure, and *hemorrhoids* are among the most painful problems of the anus and rectum.

Problems with Urination

- Do you have trouble starting a stream of urine?
- Is there a change in the flow of urine?
- Do you have sudden urges to urinate?
- Can you estimate how much urine is passed with each void or urination?
- Do you need to urinate at night?
- Are you straining to urinate?
- Have you been drinking more fluids than usual?
- Do you involuntarily lose small amounts of urine?
- What color is your urine? Do you ever notice red urine?

Urgency and frequency may be from *UTI, prostatitis, STI,* or low-grade *bladder cancer.* Prostate enlargement is common in older men. Because of the location of the gland, it can affect urine flow. The following are signs of partial prostate obstruction: recurrent acute UTIs, the sensation of residual urine, decreased caliber of the urine stream, hesitancy, straining, and terminal dribbling.

Blood in the urine can be associated with a benign disease, a clinically insignificant issue (eg, eating red-colored food), or life-threatening malignancy. It is therefore one of the most common and important signs for the nurse to investigate (Turner, 2008).

Male Sexual Dysfunction

- Do you have persistent erections unrelated to sexual stimulation?
- With an erection, do you have a curvature of the penis in any direction?
- Do you have difficulty achieving erection; is there pain associated with the erection?
- When you have sexual stimulation or intercourse, how often do you ejaculate (color, consistency, and amount)?
- How strong is your sex drive? Over the last month how would you rate your confidence to keep and maintain an erection?
- If you were to spend the rest of your life with your sexual function just the way it is now, how would you feel about that?

The main types of sexual dysfunction include premature ejaculation, erectile dysfunction (difficulty achieving or maintaining erection), low libido (sexual interest), delayed orgasm, and physical abnormalities of the penis (Albaugh, et al., 2002). Erectile dysfunction cannot be seen or felt during an assessment; thus, this issue is important to discuss with the patient. Many men welcome the opportunity to discuss erectile dysfunction, but often nurses are reluctant to bring up the subject. Presenting the topic in a nonthreatening, nonjudgmental manner encourages the patient to talk about matters of concern. An example of an opening statement for a patient whose hypertension is controlled with medication is, "High blood pressure medications often cause erectile dysfunction. Have you experienced any problems?" (Lewis, et al., 2003)

Questions to Assess Symptoms	Rationales/Abnormal Findings

Penile Lesions, Discharge, or Rash

- When did you first note the lesion? Is there more than one?
- Is pain, itching, burning, or stinging associated with the lesion?
- Is there discharge? When did discharge begin? Is there an odor or color associated with it?
- If you are sexually active, does your partner have the same symptoms? Has there been a change in sexual partners?

Direct, tactful questions about history of exposure to STIs are important. A lesion should alert the nurse to the possibility of STI. Ask if the patient has had *genital warts*, *syphilis*, *gonorrhea*, *trichomoniasis*, or other STIs. Assess if any discharge is continuous or intermittent. Bloody penile discharge is associated with *urethritis* and *neoplasm*. Tactfully explore if the patient has been with a new partner recently or if there has been a change in sexual habits.

Scrotal Enlargement

- When did you first notice the enlargement?
- Is there pain associated with it? Is pain intermittent or constant; associated with lifting or straining?
- Has there been any recent trauma to the groin?
- Have you ever had a hernia? Do you use a truss or any treatment?
- Have you had any problems with fertility?

Although rarely fatal, scrotal enlargement and pain carry a risk of morbidity from testicular atrophy, infarction, or necrosis. Any patient with scrotum pain should be presumed to have testicular torsion until this diagnosis can be proven otherwise. Accurate history and assessing skills contribute to an accurate diagnosis. Assess the patient for *varicoceles*, which are often linked with infertility.

Documentation of Normal Findings

Patient denies pain or discomfort. No difficulty problems with urination. States that he has no premature ejaculation, erectile dysfunction, low libido, delayed orgasm, or physical abnormalities of the penis. No lesions, discharge, or scrotal enlargement.
K. Kelly, RN

Lifespan Considerations

Additional Questions	Rationales/Abnormal Findings

Newborns, Infants, and Children

Has your infant ever had any genital defects, such as phimosis, hydrocele, failure of the testes to descend, hypospadias, epispadias, or ambiguous genitalia?

External genital defects are usually obvious at birth. Surgical correction may be necessary.

For toddlers: Is the child toilet trained? Is there any difficulty with wetting the bed at night?

Toilet training usually begins at around 2 years.

For adolescents: At around your age, boys often experience body changes, "wet dreams," and other issues related to sexuality. Do you have any concerns related to these issues?

Allow adolescents permission to discuss these sensitive issues. A boy may feel guilty about these things if he is not told that they are normal.

For adolescents: Have you ever had oral sex or sexual intercourse?

The AAP recommends asking adolescents about sexual activity at each annual clinic visit and offering STI screening to all sexually active teens. Adolescents are at higher risk for STIs than adults.

Older Adults

Are you noticing urinary dribbling, urgency, or frequency? Do you feel that your bladder does not completely empty?

Disorders of the prostate, including hyperplasia and cancer, are more common in older adults.

Often older adults may notice a change in their sexual function as they age. Have you noticed any such changes?

Older adults may notice that it may take longer to obtain an erection or ejaculate. Also consider coexisting illnesses and medications that may affect sexual function.

Additional Questions	Rationales/Abnormal Findings
Based on your age, ethnicity, and sexual preference, what do you perceive as your risk for developing HIV or STIs?	In young men who have sex with men, new HIV infections in blacks are 1.6 times the number in whites and 2.3 times the number in Hispanics (Quinn, et al., 2009). Men who have sex with men are also at higher risk for genital herpes. They should be offered STI screening at the annual visit.

Therapeutic Dialogue: Collecting Subjective Data

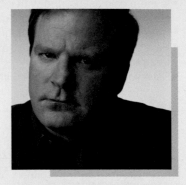

Remember Mr. Gardner, who was introduced at the beginning of this chapter. He is a 50-year-old man with a history of BPH and increasing symptoms. The nurse uses professional communication techniques to gather subjective data from Mr. Gardner. The following conversations give two examples of interview styles used by the nurse during the clinic visit. One style is more effective than the other.

Less Effective

Nurse: So what are you here for today?

Mr. Gardner: I'm having trouble urinating.

Nurse: What's it from?

Mr. Gardner: I think that it's related to my BPH.

Nurse: That's too bad. How did you get it?

Mr. Gardner: I think that it just happens when you get old like me.

Nurse: You're not old—I see here that you're married?

Mr. Gardner: Yes, I've been happily married for the past 3 months.

Nurse: Wasn't that at about the same time that you got the diagnosis?

Mr. Gardner: No, I've had BPH for 3 years.

Nurse: So are you a bit embarrassed about the trouble—I mean with your wife and all?

Mr. Gardner: You know, I'm having trouble urinating.

More Effective

Nurse: Hi, Mr. Gardner. It looks like you're here for difficulty with urinating. I see that you have BPH.

Mr. Gardner: Yes, I've had it for 3 years.

Nurse: Can you tell me more about your symptoms?

Mr. Gardner: Well, I am having more trouble with urination.

Nurse: So is that difficulty with starting your urine stream?

Mr. Gardner: Yes, and when I go, it seems like it starts and stops.

Nurse: And sometimes men also have some dribbling...

Mr. Gardner: Yes, I've had that too, and it's embarrassing. It also seems like my bladder never completely empties. I go and then I have to go back an hour or two later.

Nurse: That must be very uncomfortable.

Mr. Gardner: Yes, it is. I am newly married and I'm worried that this might affect my relationship if I have to have surgery.

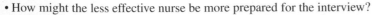

Critical Thinking Challenge

• How might the less effective nurse be more prepared for the interview?
• How will the more effective nurse discuss his concerns regarding these intimate issues?
• What concerns might Mr. Gardner have that could be further assessed?

Objective Data Collection

Equipment

- Latex gloves (check patient for allergies)
- Water-soluble lubricant
- Flashlight or penlight (for transillumination)
- Stethoscope (to listen for bowel sounds if hernia is suspected)
- Measurements of the nurse's index finger, which can be used as a ruler to measure the patient's penis, testes, and prostate gland

Preparation

As a nurse, it is important to maintain a confident, professional, matter-of-fact attitude throughout the examination. Upon entering the examination room, introduce yourself and include your title. Greet the patient by his full name and ask what he prefers to be called. Before beginning the genital examination, ask permission to perform it. This step is especially important if the nurse is female. Asking permission allows the patient to gracefully ask for a male nurse for this part of the examination.

If performing a complete history and physical assessment, conduct the genital examination last. Doing so allows the patient to become more comfortable with the overall interaction. A parent should always be present for a child's genital examination. An adolescent should have a choice whether he prefers a parent or guardian present. When accompanied by a companion, an adult man should be given the same option.

The patient should be examined in the spine position, on his side, and then standing. While the patient is standing, the nurse should be seated in front of him.

> ### Clinical Significance 25-3
>
> If the patient has an erection during the physical examination, reassure him that this is a normal physiologic response to touch that he could not have prevented. Do not stop the examination—doing so could cause further embarrassment.

Common and Specialty or Advanced Techniques

The routine head-to-toe assessment includes the most important and common assessment techniques. Table 25-3 summarizes those used in the comprehensive assessment, which are therefore essential to learn for use in clinical practice. Additional specialty techniques may be added if indicated by the clinical situation or in advanced practice for diagnosis. Note that the role of the registered nurse (RN) is primarily inspection. Advanced education is required for the more invasive genital examination.

Table 25.3	Checklist of Common Versus Specialty or Advanced Techniques			
Technique	**Purpose**	**Screening or RN Assessment**	**Focused or Advanced Practice Examination**
Inspect the genital hair, penis, and scrotum.		X	
Palpate the genital hair, penis, and scrotum.			X
Palpate the scrotum, testes, epididymides, and vas deferens.			X
Transilluminate the scrotum.			X
Palpate the inguinal canal.			X
Inspect the inguinal region and the femoral area.		X	
Palpate the anus.			X
Inspect the sacrococcygeal areas, perianal area, and anus.		X	
Palpate the sacrococcygeal areas, perianal area, and anus.			X
Palpate the anal canal and the prostate.			X
Examine stool.			X

Technique and Normal Findings	Abnormal Findings

Groin

With the patient supine, inspect the groin. Observe genital hair distribution. *Skin is clear, intact, and smooth. Hair is diamond shaped or in an escutcheon pattern. Hair appears coarser than at the scalp and has no parasites.*

Abnormal genital hair findings are no hair, patchy growth, or distribution in a female or triangular pattern with the base over the pubis. Observe for any infestations such as *pediculosis*, *scabies*, or any parasites. Look for inflammation, lesions, or dermatitis. *Candidiasis* infections cause crusty, multiple, red, round erosions and pustules; this infection is associated with immunological deficiencies (Albaugh & Kellogg-Spadt, 2003). *Tinea curis* (commonly referred to as "jock itch") is a fungal infection on the patient's groin and upper thighs. It appears with large red, scaly patches that are extremely itchy. Tinea cruris rarely involves the scrotum.

Penis

Observe the penis for surface characteristics, color, lesions, and discharge. Be sure to inspect the posterior side. *The dorsal vein is apparent on the dorsal surface of the penis. The penis has no edema, lesions, discharge, or nodules.*

Abnormal conditions include piercings, *phimosis* (foreskin cannot retract), *paraphimosis* (foreskin is retracted and fixed), and *blanitis* (related to diabetes). See Table 25-6 at the end of this chapter.

In the patient with an uncircumcised penis, the prepuce covers the glan. Ask him to retract the prepuce. *The prepuce retracts easily. Smegma (a thin, white, cheesy substance) may be normally present around the corona.*

In the patient with a circumcised penis, the glan and corona are visible, lighter in color than the shaft, and free of smegma. *Circumcised penises have varying lengths of foreskin: some have folds of skin, while others have no extra foreskin (see Fig. 25-1).*

Glan. Inspect the glan. *It is glistening pink, smooth in texture, and bulbous.*

Abnormalities of the glan include *hypospadias* (urethral meatus on underside) and *epispadias* (meatus on upper side). See Table 25-6.

Shaft. Inspect and palpate the shaft. *It feels smooth without lesions or pain. Normal variations include ectopic sebaceous glands on the shaft that appear as tiny, whitish-yellow papules.*

External Urethral Meatus. Inspect and palpate the external urethral meatus (Fig. 25-8). *It is located centrally on the glan. The orifice is slit-like and millimeters from the tip of the penis. The external urethral meatus has no discharge, stenosis, or warts.* The glan can be opened by pressing it between the thumb and forefinger. The patient can be instructed to do this. Next, strip or milk the penis from the base toward the glan or head. Note color, consistency, or odor of any discharge. *The glan is smooth and pink with no discharge.*

Discharge may be yellow, milky-white, or greenish and may have a foul odor. It needs immediate attention. See Table 25-7 at the end of the chapter.

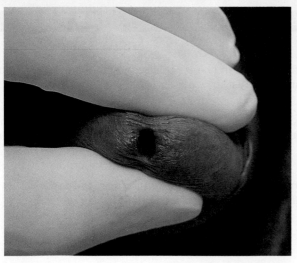

Figure 25.8 Inspecting and palpating the external urinary meatus.

Scrotum

Ask the patient to hold the penis out of the way, and inspect the scrotal septum. Inspect the anterior and posterior scrotum for any sores or rashes. *It is divided into two sacks. The scrotum could hang asymmetrically, with the left side lower than the right. Sebaceous cysts or sebaceous glands may be normally noted on the scrotal sac. The anterior and posterior scrotal skin appears darker in pigmentation with a rugous or wrinkled surface.*

Scrotal lesions, edema, and redness are abnormal. When examining the scrotum, certain diseases (eg, diabetic neuropathy, syphilis) may render the testes totally insensitive to pain. Renal, cardiac, and hepatic illness may result in scrotal edema. If there are inconsistencies in size or texture, be alert for possible infection, tumor, or cyst. Abnormal scrotal conditions include *testicular torsion, epididmytis, variocele, hydrocele,* and *spermatocele.* See Tables 25-6 and 25-8 at the end of the chapter.

Sacrococcygeal Areas

Inspect the sacrococcygeal areas for surface characteristics and tenderness. *Skin is clear and smooth with no palpable masses or dimpling.*

A dimple with an inflamed tuft of hair or a tender palpable cyst in the sacrococcygeal area suggests a *pilonidal cyst* or *sinus.* Generally, the patient is asymptomatic unless the area becomes infected. Once infected, redness, tenderness, and a cyst can be palpitated. When ruptured, the cyst drains purulent, mucoid secretions. Often the patient is febrile.

Perineal Area

With the patient on his side, spread the buttocks and inspect the perineal area. *Skin surrounding the anus is coarse with darker pigmentation. The anal sphincter is closed.*

A penlight assists in inspecting for *warts,* loose sphincter, lesions, *hemorrhoids,* fissures, fistulas, or polyps. Infestations from pinworms or fungal infections make this area appear irritated and erythemic. See Table 25-9 at the end of this chapter.

Inguinal Region and Femoral Areas

Instruct the patient to stand. Ask him to bear down. While he does so, inspect the inguinal canal area and femoral area for bulges or masses.

Bulges or masses suggest a **hernia**. If a bulge is noted, the inguinal canal needs to be palpated. See Table 25-10 at the end of the chapter.

Documentation of Normal Findings

Skin is clear, intact, and smooth. No masses or lesions noted. Foreskin intact. No phimosis or paraphimosis. Penis size is appropriate to age and smooth without lesions or pain. No discharge, edema, or redness. *K. Kelly, RN*

Special Circumstances or Advanced Techniques

Technique and Normal Findings	Abnormal Findings

Testicles

After inspection of the scrotal sac, palpate each testicle separately. *Note the smooth, rubbery consistency of each testicle; no nodules should be felt.*

The epididymis is located discretely on the posterolateral surface of each testicle. *It feels smooth and nontender.*

Vas Deferens

Next palpate the vas deferens, which is located in the spermatic cord and has accompanying arteries and veins (Fig. 25-9). It may be difficult to palpate; however, it should feel like a smooth, cord-like structure. *As the nurse palpates from the testicle to the inguinal ring, no nodules or lesions are palpable.*

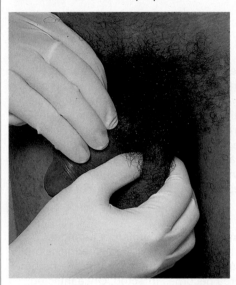

Figure 25.9 Palpating the vas deferens.

Transillumination of the Scrotum

Transillumination of the scrotum is done to assess for evidence of a mass or fluid.

The testes and epididymides do not transilluminate.

After palpating the scrotum for a mass or fluid, transilluminate each pouch. Use a bright penlight or transilluminator and press the light against the scrotal sac. *The sac does not contain additional fluids or contents.*

Hernias

Palpate the inguinal canal for hernia. With the patient relaxed, insert your finger into the scrotal sac and follow it upward along the vas deferens into the inguinal canal. Which finger the nurse uses depends on the age of the patient; for a child, the little finger is appropriate, but for an adult, the middle finger is used. Palpate the oval external ring. If a hernia is present, you should feel the sudden presence of a viscus against your finger (Fig. 25-10).

Irregularities in texture or size may indicate an infection, tumor, or cyst.

Note the place of any concerns with the epididymis and if the condition resolves itself when the patient is supine.

An unexpected finding is tenderness, tortuosity, thickening, or a mass-like structure. See Table 25-8.

Note any masses proximal or distal to the testes. Assess for any pain or tenderness. *Hydroceles* and *spermatoceles* contain fluid and transilluminate. Tumors, epididymitis, and hernias do not (Swartz, 2006) (see Table 25-8).

Hernia occurs when a loop of intestine prolapses through the inguinal wall or canal or abdominal musculature. The patient reports pain on exertion or lifting. On examination, pain increases when maneuvers or positioning increases intra-abdominal pressure. The only way to stop a hernia from worsening is to repair the defect surgically. Three of the more common hernias are direct/indirect inguinal and femoral. See Table 25-10.

Hernias are common, but not normal. There is no bulging or pain.

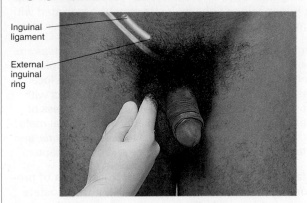

Inguinal ligament

External inguinal ring

Figure 25.10 Palpating for a hernia.

Perianal and Rectal Examination

A standing position is preferred for rectal examination, because it allows for visualization of the anus and palpation of the rectum. If the patient cannot stand, the rectal examination can be performed with the patient on his left side with the right leg flexed and the left leg semi-extended. This is also known as the Sims position.

Have the standing patient place both feet together, slightly flex both knees, and bend forward over the examination table (Fig. 25-11).

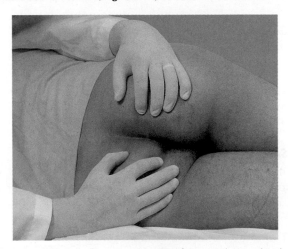

Figure 25.11 Sims positioning for rectal examination.

Anus. Spread the buttocks apart and inspect the anus. A penlight helps with visualization. Next, have the patient bear down. Observe the anus for lesions, warts, tags, hemorrhoids, fissures, and fistulas. It is helpful to use a clock for reference, 12 o'clock being ventral midline and 6 o'clock being dorsal midline.

Apply a lubricant to the index finger of the gloved hand. Explain to the patient the lubricant is used for his comfort and might feel cool. Further explain that initially he may feel like he is going to have a bowel movement; however, this will not happen. Have the patient take a deep breath while you insert the finger into the rectum. Rectal tone can be assessed at this time. *Full closure around the finger is palpable.* Rotate your index finger around the anal ring. *It feels smooth without nodules, masses, or irregularities.*

Look for thrombosed hemorrhoids, rectal fissures, or hard stool. Hemorrhoids can be classified as external or internal. Hemorrhoids are usually caused by constant or excessive straining upon defecation.

(text continues on page 752)

Continue to advance your index finger into the anal canal. *The lateral and posterior rectal walls feel smooth and uninterrupted. Internal hemorrhoids are usually not felt.*

Note any nodules, masses, irregularities, or polyps. Pay attention to any discomfort felt by the patient. Rotate your index finger to palpate the anterior rectal wall, repeating the above process. *There are no nodules, masses, irregularities, or polyps.*

Prostate. At this point of the examination, the posterior surface of the prostate gland can be felt (Fig. 25-12). Take time to explain to the patient that it may feel like he is going to urinate, but he will not. Note the prostate gland for its size, contour, consistency, and mobility. *The normal prostate gland has the consistency of a rubber ball. It is nontender, firm, smooth, and slightly movable. The diameter is approximately 4 cm; <1 cm protrudes into the rectum.* The lateral lobes should feel symmetric and divided by the median sulcus. The sulcus may be obliterated when the lobes are neoplastic or hypertrophied. The DRE of the prostate allows palpitation of the posterior surface, which is the area cancer often starts.

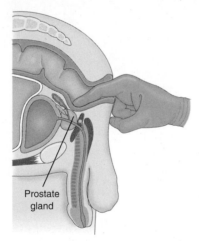

Prostate gland

Figure 25.12 Palpating the prostate.

Upon completion of the examination of the rectum, explain to the patient that you are going to remove your finger. Offer the patient a cleansing wipe and a private few minutes to redress.

Stool. Upon removing your finger from examining the rectum, inspect the gloved finger for consistency and color of the stool.

The stool is brown and soft.

*For 3 days prior to the examination, the patient should have refrained from eating red meat and ingesting vitamin C supplements. Use a guaiac test to evaluate for occult blood. See Box 25-3 instructions for testing.

A hypotonic or lax sphincter could be from rectal surgery, neurological deficit, or trauma (often associated with anal sex). Hypertonic or tight sphincter may be associated with inflammation, scarring, or anxiety about the examination.

Patients complain of pain when *anal fissures* or *fistulas* are present. Local anesthesia may be necessary to complete the examination. Extreme rectal pain is associated with local disease. Because the anterior rectal wall is in contact with peritoneum, you may be able to detect the tenderness of peritoneal inflammation and nodularity of peritoneal metastases. Abnormalities may be related to *BPH, prostatitis,* and *prostate cancer.* See Table 25-11 at the end of this chapter.

Prostate enlargement is classified by the amount of projection into the rectum (see Table 25-11). If the prostate feels hard, this may indicate *carcinoma, prostatic calcui,* or chronic fibrosis.

A rubbery or boggy glandular consistency may suggest BPH, a common finding in men older than 60 years. The gland may feel soft, tender, and boggy from infection. According to the National Institutes of Health, BPH is a condition of aging. 50% of men older than 60 years have BPH, as do 90% of men older than 70 years. Signs and symptoms of BPH are urine retention, hesitancy, urgency, dribbling, nocturia, and straining to void. If the problem becomes chronic, the patient can develop overflow incontinence from increased intra-abdominal pressure.

⚠ *SAFETY ALERT 25.4*

Acute urine retention needs immediate intervention (Dains, et al., 2003).

The seminal vesicles are not palpable unless they are inflamed (Uphold & Graham, 2003). Prostatitis is an inflammation or infection of the prostate gland.

⚠ *SAFETY ALERT 25.5*

Do not massage the prostate if acute prostatitis is suspected because of the possibility of releasing bacteria and producing septicemia.

Abnormal findings include stools with an unusual color, blood, purulent drainage, or mucus. Black tarry stool raises suspicion of upper GI bleeding. Very light tan or gray stool could indicate obstructive jaundice. A subtle loss of blood may not change the color of the stool; however, it may yield a positive guaiac test result, which is used to evaluate occult blood in the stool. A positive guaiac test may indicate occult blood in the stool.

BOX 25.3 INSTRUCTIONS FOR TESTING STOOL FOR BLOOD (GUAIAC)

The guaiac slide test is a qualitative test. Instructions are as follow:

- Obtain guaiac developer and slide.
- Open the flap of the cardboard guaiac slide.
- Dab the stool on the paper in the boxes of the slide (Fig. A).

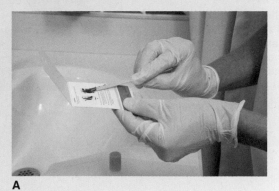

A

- Close the flap and remove your gloves.
- With clean gloves on, reverse the slide and open the flap.
- Apply two drops of developing solution to each box of guaiac paper (Fig. B).

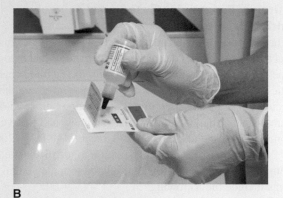

B

- Wait 30–60 seconds and note color of the paper (Fig. C). A bluish discoloration indicates a positive result, or that occult blood is present. This is a warning sign that a patient may have colorectal disease, including colon cancer. However, false positive guaiac results may occur from a diet of red or rare meats, dietary peroxidases, or both. Intake of vitamin C (ascorbic acid) may cause false negative results.

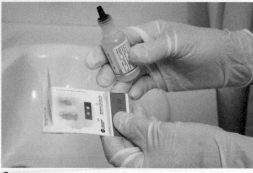

C

Lifespan Considerations

Infants and Children

Rectal examination is not performed routinely on infants or children. Symptoms that indicate a need for such examination include bowel abnormalities, abdominal distention, pelvic pain, a mass or tenderness, bleeding, bladder discomfort, pain, or distention.

If an examination is necessary, prepare the patient and guardian before it begins. The nurse must explain every step. Use your little finger when performing rectal examinations on infants or small children. Explain to the guardian that it is not unusual for the child or infant to have a small amount of bleeding directly following the examination. It is easier for the nurse to perform the rectal examination with the infant or child in a lithotomy position. Hold the feet together and flex the knees and hips on the abdomen. Routinely inspect the perineum, anal and surrounding areas for masses, redness, or ecchymosis. Inspect the anal area for abscess, perirectal tears, or fistulae.

When assessing an infant for rectal patency, assess whether the infant has passed meconium. If the infant has not passed any stool in the first 48 hours after birth, suspect rectal atresia.

If perirectal redness and/or excoriation are noted, remember to check for enterobiasis. Candida and other irritants can produce perineum excoriation. Rectal prolapse may be present from constipation, diarrhea, or sometimes from severe coughing. Hemorrhoids are rare in children; if they are present, it may suggest portal hypertension. Inspect the rectum for small flat flaps of skin that may be condylomas, which are syphilitic in origin. Finally, inspect the coccyx area for dimpling, sinuses, and tufts of hair in the pilonidal area, which would indicate lower spinal deformities. Lightly touching the anal area should produce an anal contraction. If no contraction is noted, assess for lower spinal cord lesion (Seidel, et, al. 2003).

Next, assess for rectal tone. It should feel tight but not loose. A lax sphincter could indicate lesions in the peripheral

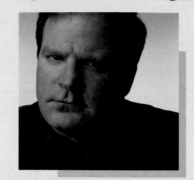

The APRN is assessing Mr. Gardner, the 50-year-old man with BPH. Unlike the samples of normal documentation charted previously, Mr. Gardner has abnormal findings. Consider how Mr. Gardner's symptoms are increasing. Consider what other data the nurse will collect while thinking critically and anticipating nursing interventions.

Inspection: Genital hair intact and appropriate to age. No odor. Glan and corona are visible, darker in color than the shaft of the penis, and free of smegma. Glan is slightly reddened around the meatus. The shaft of the penis is smooth without lesions or pain. Scrotum without swelling or inflammation. No masses or lesions in the inguinal or femoral area. Anal, sacrococcygeal area, perianal area, and anus are without redness, lesions, or masses. Skin is smooth and pink.

Palpation: The prostate is enlarged, symmetrical, firm, and smooth.

D. Hosseini, RN

spinal nerves or spinal cord. Bruises, scars, anal tears, and anal dilation could indicate sexual abuse and must be investigated. Lastly, feel for stool in the rectum; note if the stool is hard or soft. Following the examination, any stool on the nurse's examination glove should be tested for occult blood.

Older Adults

In older adults, pubic hair may be thin and gray. The testes may be smaller and feel softer. The scrotal sac has less ruggae and appears to droop more. Rectal tone is intact, but strength of the rectal reflex may be reduced slightly.

Cultural Considerations

Patients with darkly pigmented skin may have darker pigmentation in the scrotal and anal area. The pubic hair may also be darker and coarser.

Evidence-Based Critical Thinking

Nurses use assessment findings as the basis for ongoing care. An accurate and complete assessment provides a firm foundation for setting outcomes, providing individualized interventions, and evaluating progress.

Common Laboratory and Diagnostic Testing

The PSA test is a blood test that measures a protein produced by the prostate gland in men. Levels of PSA increase with infections, prostitis, hyperplasia, and cancer. The test is used in combination with the DRE. It can also be used as a marker for men with a previous history of cancer to see if the cancer recurs. Because prostate cancer is more common in older men, PSA is recommended for men older than 50 years. The test is controversial because it has many false positives

(positive but there is no disease) and false negatives (negative but prostate cancer is present).

Diagnostic Reasoning

Nursing Diagnosis, Outcomes, and Interventions

When formulating a nursing diagnosis, it is important to use critical thinking to cluster data and identify patterns that fit together. The nurse compares these clusters with the defining characteristics (abnormal findings) for the diagnosis to ensure the most accurate labeling and appropriate interventions. Table 25-4 compares nursing diagnoses, abnormal findings, and interventions commonly related to the male assessment (NANDA-I, 2009).

Nurses use assessment information to identify patient outcomes. Some outcomes that are related to male genital problems include the following:

• Patient will describe alternative safe sexual practices.
• Patient will remain free of infection.
• Patient will be continent of urine (Moorhead, et al., 2007).

Once the outcomes are established, nursing care is implemented to improve the status of the patient. The nurse uses critical thinking and evidence-based practice to develop the interventions. Some examples of nursing interventions for male genital system care are as follows:

• Assess the patient's knowledge and understanding of safe sexual practices.
• Teach care for the infection-prone site.
• Teach the patient exercises to strengthen the pelvic floor (Bulechek, et al., 2007).

The nurse then evaluates the care according to the patient outcomes that were developed, therefore reassessing the patient and continuing or modifying the interventions as appropriate. Even as a beginner, the nursing student can use the patient assessment to implement new interventions, evaluate the effectiveness of those interventions, and make a difference in the quality of patient care.

Table 25.4 Common Nursing Diagnoses Associated with the Male Genital System

Diagnosis and Related Factors	Point of Differentiation	Assessment Characteristics	Nursing Interventions
Ineffective sexuality pattern related to erectile dysfunction	Concern, dissatisfaction, or verbalized problems with sex life	Alteration in relationship with significant other, changes or limitations in sexual activities and behaviors	After establishing a relationship, give the patient permission to discuss issues by asking, "Are you concerned about sexual function because of changes in your health?"
Risk for infection	Potential for invasion by pathogens	Inadequate knowledge, urinary reflux, recent trauma, or urinary catheter placement	Teach safe sexual practices, warning signs of genital tract infections. Remove urinary catheters as soon as possible.
Urinary retention related to obstruction	Inability to completely empty the bladder	Increased urinary residual volume, slow stream, hesitant urination, dribbling	Obtain a postvoid bladder ultrasound. Teach double voiding and to avoid over the counter (OTC) cold medications with decongestant.
Risk for urge incontinence related to irritation of bladder	Involuntary passage of urine with a sudden desire to urinate	Voiding more than once every 2 hours, awakening at night	Assess the patient for functional barriers to continence; teach spacing of fluids in consistent quantities over the day. Avoid fluid late in the evening

*Collaborative interventions.

Analyzing Findings

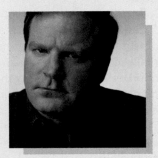

Remember Mr. Gardner, whose problems have been outlined throughout this chapter. Initial subjective and objective data collection is complete, and the nurse has spent time reviewing the findings and other results. Unfortunately, Mr. Gardner has urinary retention, so it is necessary to reassess him and document the findings. The following nursing note illustrates how subjective and objective data are collected and analyzed and nursing interventions are developed.

Subjective: I can't urinate and it feels like my bladder is full.

Objective: Urinary residual volume 250 mL, slow stream, hesitant urinary voiding, dribbling.

Analysis: Urinary retention related to partial obstruction

Plan: Inform urologist about residual volume. Teach the patient to avoid caffeine and alcohol because of the diuretic effects. Teach the patient to avoid pseudephrine and phenylephrine found in OTC cold medications. Teach double voiding. Teach to urinate every 2 to 3 hours and when first feeling the urge. Avoid rapid intake of fluids that may overdistend the bladder. Repeat bladder scan to ensure that residual volume is not increasing.

D. Hosseini, RN

Critical Thinking Challenge

- What can Mr. Gardner do to improve his health?
- How can Mr. Gardner talk with his wife about his symptoms?
- At what point will the nurse contact the urologist regarding an acute assessment?

Collaboration with Other Health Care Providers

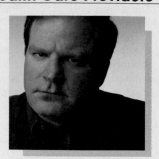

In this case, Mr. Gardner will need insertion of a urinary catheter if he cannot void. The nurse will need to talk with the urologist to obtain an order for a urinary catheter. Results that might trigger a consult with a urologist include urinary retention, incontinence, blood in the urine, prostate disease, kidney stones, infections of the urinary tract, infertility, and sexual dysfunction.

Mr. Gardner has been experiencing urinary retention; therefore, a urology consult will be indicated. The following conversation illustrates how the nurse might organize the data and make recommendations about the patient's situation.

Situation: Hi, I'm Denise, a nurse in the primary care clinic. Mr. Gardner is a 50-year-old man who has had BPH for the past 3 years.

Background: He came in today with symptoms of incomplete bladder emptying and he had a bladder scan that showed a residual volume of 250 mL. He is also having a slow stream, hesitant urinary voiding, and dribbling.

Assessment: I am concerned that Mr. Gardner is experiencing urinary retention and will be at risk for reflux and an infection.

Recommendations: He might be developing severe enough symptoms that he needs to have a urinary catheter inserted. When would you be able to evaluate him?

Critical Thinking Challenge

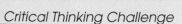

- When will the nurse intervene with health-promotion activities?
- At what point will the nurse talk with the wife about the patient's symptoms?
- What symptoms will prompt the nurse to call the urologist?

Pulling It All Together: Reflection and Critical Thinking

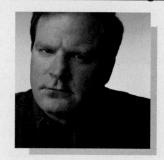

The nurse uses assessment data to formulate a nursing care plan with patient outcomes and interventions for Mr. Gardner. Outcomes are specific to the patient, realistic to achieve, measurable, and have a time frame for meeting the outcome. The interventions are actions that the nurse performs, based on evidence and practice guidelines. After these interventions are completed, the nurse reevaluates Mr. Gardner and documents the findings in the chart to show progress toward the patient outcome. The nurse uses critical thinking and judgment to continue or revise the diagnosis, outcomes, or interventions. This is often in the form of a care plan or case note similar to the one below.

Nursing Diagnosis	Patient Outcomes	Nursing Interventions	Rationales	Evaluation
Urinary retention related to obstruction	Patient will be free from urinary tract distress.	Teach the patient to double void by urinating, resting for 3–5 minutes, and then trying again to urinate.	Double voiding promotes more efficient bladder emptying by allowing the muscles to contract, rest, and then contract again.	Patient states that he has tried double voiding but he has discomfort and dribbling. Urologist contacted for evaluation of symptoms and possible surgery for retention.

Using the previous steps of diagnostic reasoning, organizing, and prioritizing, consider all the case study findings woven throughout this chapter. When answering the following questions, begin drawing conclusions and see how the pieces of assessment must work together to create an environment for personalized, appropriate, and accurate care.

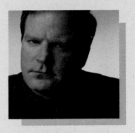

• Is Mr. Gardner's condition stable, urgent, or an emergency?
• How will the nurse work with Mr. Gardner to promote health and reduce risk for illness?
• Which nursing diagnosis is the highest priority? What is the rationale?

Key Points

• The anatomy of normal male genitalia includes external and internal structures.
• Tanner staging is used to determine the level of male sexual development for children and adolescents.
• Healthy People goals related to the male genital system include prevention of prostate cancer, appropriate family planning, and prevention of STIs.
• TSE and screening for prostate cancer are important health-promotion activities.
• Common symptoms of male genital problems include pain, problems with urination, erectile dysfunction, penile lesions or discharge, and scrotal enlargement.
• During the intimate male genital assessment, it is important to provide the patient with privacy.
• The role of the RN related to the male genital examination primarily involves inspection.
• The acute scrotum may be caused by ischemia, trauma, infections, inflammation, hernia, and chronic conditions with an acute exacerbation.
• Advanced practice nurses perform perianal, rectal, and prostate examinations.
• The stool is assessed for the appearance and presence of blood.
• Nursing diagnoses common following male genital assessment include ineffective sexuality patterns, risk for infection, urinary retention, and urge incontinence.

Review Questions

1. Where does spermatogenesis occur?
   A. Ductus epididymis
   B. Seminiferous tubules
   C. Ampulla of the spermatic cords
   D. Vas deferens

2. During a physical assessment, the nurse, using the handle of the reflex hammer, gently strokes the inner left thigh of the patient, which causes the ipsilateral testicle to rise. What superficial reflex is demonstrated?
   A. Abdominal reflex
   B. Babinski's reflex
   C. Brachioradialis réflex
   D. Cremasteric reflex

3. A 20-year-old Caucasian man complains of a mass in his left testicle. In addition to his age and race, what else is a risk factor for testicular cancer?
   A. Colon cancer in his mother
   B. Personal history of cryptorchidism
   C. Urinary tract infection last month
   D. Congenital hydrocele

4. Which of the following does the nurse recognize as an abnormal finding while performing the male genitalia examination?
   A. Smegma is present on the uncircumcised patient.
   B. Testes are palpable and firm within the scrotal sac.
   C. Impulse noted at the tip of nurse's finger during hernia examination.
   D. The urethral meatus has a slit-like opening central to the distal tip of the glan.

5. Which Tanner stage finds the base of the penis having sparse thin hair, testes beginning to enlarge, and the scrotal skin becoming coarser and redder?
   A. Stage 1
   B. Stage 2
   C. Stage 3
   D. Stage 4
   E. Stage 5

6. A 15-year-old boy presents with severe testicular pain. Which of the following is not consistent with testicular torsion?
   A. Elevation of affected testicle usually lessens pain.
   B. Testicular torsion pain is acute.
   C. There is no urethral discharge.
   D. The patient does not have a fever.

7. Upon ambulation, a patient complains of a soft, irregular mass on the left side of the scrotum. The nurse palpates a mass that feels distinctly like "a bag of worms." These findings are consistent with which condition?
   A. Hydrocele
   B. Varicocele
   C. Spermatocele
   D. Epididymitis

8. A 70-year-old man presents with the following symptoms: straining to void, nocturia, dribbling, and hesitancy when voiding. These signs are consistent with what condition?
A. BPH
B. Prostatitis
C. Testicular cancer
D. Phimosis

9. The nurse is inspecting the groin of an older adult man in a long-term care facility. Which of the following is a normal finding that the nurse documents?
A. Pediculosis in hair distribution
B. Hypospadias on glans
C. Yellow discharge from meatus
D. Smegma under foreskin

10. Which STI presents with painful red superficial vesicles along the penis or on the glans?
A. Gonorrhea
B. Chlamydia
C. Syphilis
D. Herpes II

References

Albaugh, J., Amargo, I., Capelson, R., Flaherty, E., Forest, C., Goldstein, I., et al. (2002). Health care clinicians in sexual health medicine: Focus on erectile dysfunction. *Urologic Nursing, 22*(4), 217–231.

Albaugh, J. A., & Kellogg-Spadt, S. (2003). Genital and dermatologic examination part II: The male patient. *Urologic Nursing, 23*(5), 366–367.

American Academy of Pediatrics. (1999). Circumcision policy statement. *Pediatrics, 103*(3), 686–693.

American Cancer Society. (2008). *Statistics for 2008*. Retrieved June 4, 2009, from http://www.cancer.org

American Cancer Society. (2008). *Cancer facts and figures 2008*. Retrieved June 4, 2009, from www.nci.nih.gov

American Gastroenterology Association. (2009). *Prostate specific antigen best practice statement: 2009 update*. Retrieved from http://www. auanet.org/content/guidelines-and-quality-care/ clinical-guidelines/main-reports/psa09.pdf

American Urological Association. (2009). *An AUA Best Practice Policy and ASRM Practice Committee Report*. Retrieved June 18, 2009, from http://www.auanet.org

Anderson, W. R., Summerton, D. J., Sharma, D. M., & Holmes, S. A. (2002). The urologist's guide to genital piercing. *BJU International, 91*, 245–251.

Bulechek, G. B., Butcher, H. K., & McCloskey Dochterman, J. (2007). *Nursing Interventions Classification* (*NIC*) (4th ed.) St Louis: Mosby.

CDC. (2006). *Sexually transmitted disease treatment guidelines, 2006*. Retrieved May 13, 2009, from http://www.cdc.gov/ STD?treatment/2006/clinical.htm database

Cole, F. L., & Vogler, R. (2004). The acute, nontraumatic scrotum: Assessment and management. *Journal of the American Academy of Nurse Practitioners, 16*(2), 50–56.

Dains, J. E., Baumann, L. C., & Scheibel, P. (2003). *Advanced health assessment & clinical diagnosis in primary care* (2nd ed.). Philadelphia: Elsevier.

Harris, R., & Lohr, K. N. (2002). Screening for prostate cancer: An update of the evidence for the U.S. Prevention Services Task Force. *Annals of Internal Medicine, 137*(11), 917–929.

Leininger, M., & McFarland, M. (2002). *Transcultural nursing: Concepts, theories, research, and practice* (3rd ed.). New York: McGraw Hill.

Lewis, J. H., Rosen, R., & Goldstein, I. (2003). Erectile dysfunction in primary care. *American Journal of Nursing, 10*(103), 48–57.

Moorhead, S., Johnson, M., & Mass, M. (2007). *Nursing Outcomes Classification* (*NOC*) (4th ed.). Philadelphia: Mosby.

North American Nursing Diagnosis Association. (2009). *Nursing diagnoses, 2009–2011 Edition: Definitions and classifications* (*NANDA NURSING DIAGNOSIS*). West Sussex UK: John Wiley & Sons.

Palefsky, J. (2007). HPV infection in men. *Disease Markers, 23*, 261–272.

Quinn, T. C., Bartlett, J. A., & McGovern, B. H. (2009). The global human immunodeficiency virus pandemic. Retrieved November 10, 2009, from Uptodate.

Seidel, H. M., Ball, J. W., Dains, J. E., & Benedict, G. W. (2003). *Mosby' guide to physical examination* (5th ed.). St. Louis: Elsevier.

Siegfried, N., Muller, M., Deeks, J. J., & Volmink, J. (2009). Male circumcision for prevention of heterosexual acquisition of HIV men. *Cochrane Database of Systemic Review 2009*, (2). Retrieved 06/03/2009, from database (Art.no.:CDoo3362. DOI:10,1002/14651858.CD003362.pub2.).

Swartz, M. H. (2006). *Textbook of physical diagnosis* (5th ed.). Philadelphia: Saunders, Elsevier.

Tanner, J. (1962). *Growth at adolescence*. Oxford: Blackwell.

The Testicular Cancer Resource Center. *How to do a testicular self examination*. Retrieved May 3, 2009, from http://tcrc.acor.org/ tcexam.html

Turner, B. (2008). Haematuria: Causes and management. *Nursing Standard, 23*(1), 50–56.

Uphold, C. R., & Graham, V. (2003). *Clinical guidelines in family practice* (4th ed.). Gainesvillem FL: Barmarrae Books, Inc.

The Jensen suite offers these additional resources to enhance learning and facilitate understanding of this chapter:

• thePoint on line resource, http//thepoint.lww.com/Jensen1E
• Student CD-ROM included with the book
• *Laboratory Manual for Nursing Health Assessment: A Best Practice Approach*
• *Pocket Guide for Nursing Health Assessment: A Best Practice Approach*

Tables of Abnormal Findings

Table 25.5   Testicular Torsion Versus Epididymitis

Testicular Torsion	Epididymitis
Pain is acute.	Pain is gradual.
Nausea and vomiting occur in 50% of patients.	Nausea and vomiting are rare.
Fever is rare.	Fever occurs in 50% of patients.
Voiding symptoms, urethral irritation, and urethral discharge are rare.	Voiding symptoms, urethral irritation, and urethral discharge occur in 50% of patients.
0%–30% of patients have abnormal urinalysis results.	Urinalysis will be diagnostic in 20%–95% of those with epididymitis.
Elevation of affected testicle does not lessen pain.	Elevation of affected testicle usually lessens pain.
Surgical intervention is immediately required.	Antibiotic therapy is indicated.

Table 25.6   Abnormal Conditions of the Penis

Genital Piercing

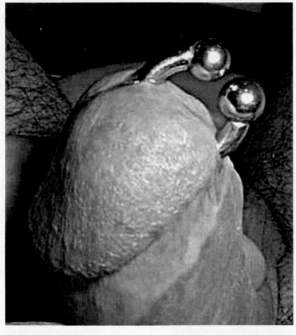

Phimosis

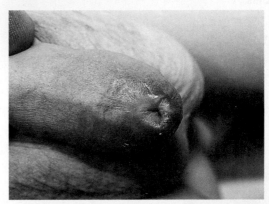

The prepuce cannot be retracted over the glan. It can occur during the first 6 years of life. It may be congenital or follow recurrent infections or *balanoposthitis* (inflammation of the prepuce and glan). Occasionally, the narrowed foreskin obstructs urinary flow, resulting in a dribbling stream or ballooning of the foreskin. Severe phimosis is treated by circumcision.

The Prince Albert is a common type of male genital piercing in which a ring is inserted through the urethra and out the bottom of the glans. The most common issue associated with piercing is infection. Other complications include bleeding and difficulty urinating.

(table continues on page 760)

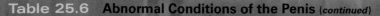

Table 25.6   Abnormal Conditions of the Penis (*continued*)

Paraphimosis

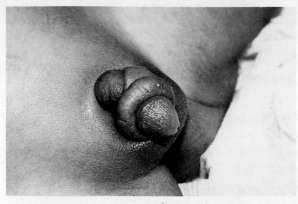

The retracted prepuce cannot be placed back over the glan. Paraphimosis may be severe enough to restrict circulation to the glan. An uncircumcised male would always have the foreskin pulled toward the urethral opening.

Balanitis or balanoposthitis

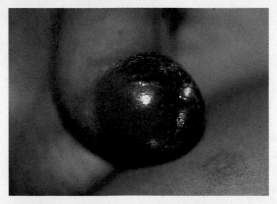

Inflammation of the glan and prepuce occurs in uncircumcised men. Many of these men have poorly controlled diabetes. Scars and narrowing of the urethral opening may cause inflammation, infections, and foul discharge. The scarring may make it difficult to clean under the foreskin.

Hypospadias

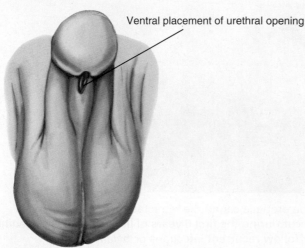

Ventral placement of urethral opening

The urethral meatus opens on the ventral side of the penis. The deviation of the meatus makes it difficult to urinate when standing. The physical appearance of the penis is altered, sometimes causing body image disturbances.

Epispadias

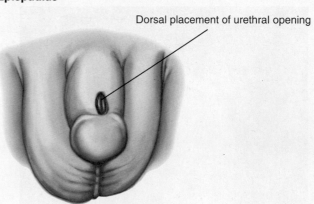

Dorsal placement of urethral opening

The urethral meatus opens on the dorsal surface of the penis. Epispadis may be associated with underlying congenital anomalies in genital urinary development. The lower urinary tract may be exposed in severe cases.

STI	Findings and Clinical Implications
Scabies infection 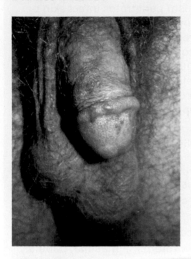	Scabies is a highly communicable skin condition caused by an arachnid, commonly known as the itch mite. It is transmitted by direct skin contact. The females live in burrows that appear as slightly darkened lines. There are associated papules, vesicles, pustules, and intense itching
Chlamydia 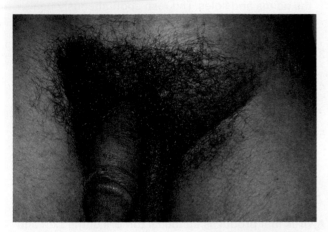	*C. trachomatis* is a bacterium with a variable incubation period, usually 1 week of exposure. The most frequently reported bacterial STI in the United States, **this disease is reportable in every state**. In men, the urethra has a mucopurulent discharge. There is burning on urination. Commonly chlamydia can present asymptomatically. A chlamydia infection can cause nongonococccal urethritis and acute epididymitis. If urethral discharge is present, obtain specimen for diagnostic testing.
Gonorrhea 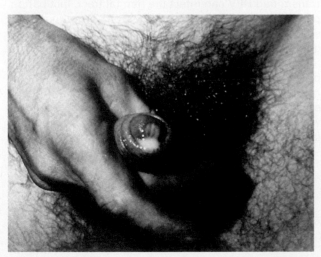	*Gonorrhoeae* organisms are Gram-negative diplococci present in exudates and secretions of infected mucous surfaces. Transmission results from intimate contact; incubation period is 2–7 days. **This disease is reportable in every state**. Men may present with dysuria, urethral discharge, rectal pain, or discharge. Common sites include the urethra, epididymis, prostate, rectum, and pharynx. If urethral discharge is present, obtain specimen for diagnostic testing.

(table continues on page 762)

Table 25.7 Sexually Transmitted Infections (*continued*)

STI	Findings and Clinical Implications

Syphilis

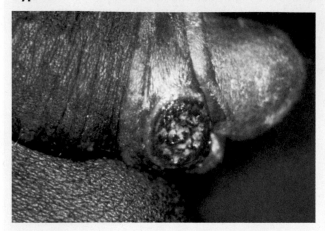

Syphilis is a thin, fragile organism with humans as the only host. The organism penetrates intact skin or mucous membrane during sexual contact, multiplies, and rapidly spreads to regional lymph nodes. Primary incubation period for acquired syphilis is about 3 weeks, but can occur 10–90 days after exposure. Secondary syphilis develops 6–8 weeks later. Latent and tertiary syphilis can occur years later. **Report all cases of syphilis to appropriate public health department**.

The five stages of syphilis are as follows:

1. With primary syphilis, genital lesions are usually indurated and painless. Reginal lymphadenopathy is usually present. Chancre persists for 1–5 weeks and heals spontaneously.
2. Secondary syphilis occurs 6–8 weeks later and is characterized by flu symptoms. A macular, papular, annular, or follicular rash is present, often involving the palms and soles. The rash spontaneously heals in 2–6 weeks. Secondary syphilis is the most contagious.
3. A latent stage occurs after the second stage. It can last from 2 to 20 years.
4. Tertiary syphilis has the most devastating effects on the cardiovascular, neurological, musculoskeletal, and ophthalmic systems of the body.
5. Congenital syphilis occurs from mother to child, usually when the mother has primary or secondary syphilis. Signs and symptoms in the infant include retinal inflammation, glaucoma, destructive bone and skin lesions, and central nervous system disorders.

HPV

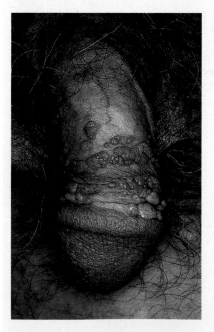

A virus that produces epithelial tumors of the skin and mucous membranes. More than 40 types of sexually transmitted HPV can infect the genital tract. Incubation period is unknown but can range from 3 months to several years. Most men with HPV never develop genital warts. Some strains of the virus can progress to genital warts. Although rare, a complication is penile or anal cancer. Visible genital warts usually result from HPV types 6 or 11. They can appear on the scrotum, perineum, perianal skin, and penis. Individual warts may become confluent and appear as a single, large fleshy lesion.

STI	Findings and Clinical Implications
Herpes Simplex Virus (HSV) Type 1 and 2 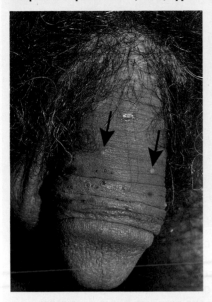	• HSV-1 and HSV-2 are epidermotropic viruses. Transmission is only by direct contact with active lesions or virus-containing fluid such as saliva. Incubation period is 2–14 days. HSV-1 is associated with infection of the lips, face, buccal mucosa, and throat. HSV-2 is associated with genitalia. There may be an overlap in site of infection; type 1 strains can be recovered from the genital tract, and type 2 strains could be recovered from the pharynx following oral-genital activity. The usual sequence is painful papules followed by vesicles, ulceration, crusting, and healing.

Note: There are more than 50 different STIs. Six common STIs are presented in the table.
Source: Information obtained from http://www3.niaid.nih.gov/topics/sti/ http://www.cdc.gov/std/stats07/toc.htm

⚠ **Table 25.8   Scrotum and Testes Abnormalities**

Abnormal Finding	Description
Testicular Torsion	**Epididymitis**
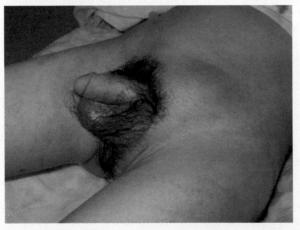	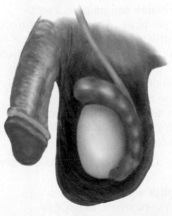
This sudden twisting of the spermatic cord typically occurs on the left side because the left cord is longer. Most common in late childhood or early adolescence, it is rare after 20 years and results from faulty anchoring of the testis on the scrotal wall, which enables rotation. The anterior part of the testis rotates medially toward the other testis. Blood supply is impaired, resulting in ischemia and venous engorgement. Because the testis can become gangrenous within a few hours, this *is considered a surgical emergency.*	This acute infection of the epididymis is commonly caused by chlamydia, gonorrhea, or other bacterial infection (eg, *E. coli*). In men younger than 35 years, the most common cause is an STI. Epididymitis is often linked to prostatitis, especially after surgical intervention/ urethral instrumentation. Uncommon causes include tuberculosis, trauma, systemic fungal infections, and use of the drug amiodarone. Pain in the scrotum is severe, accompanied by swelling and fever. The scrotum can become very enlarged, inflamed, and painful to touch. Treatment with antibiotics is often needed.

(table continues on page 764)

Abnormal Finding	Description

Varicocele

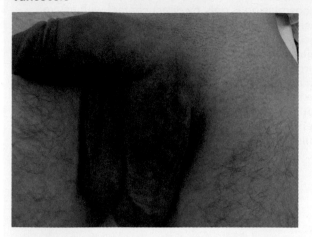

Hydrocele

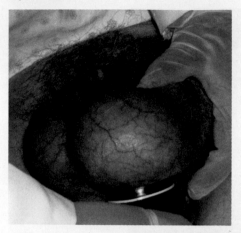

Dilated, tortuous varicose veins most often affect the left spermatic cord, which is longer and inserts at a right angle into the left renal vein. These are common in young males (5% of teens and 15% of adults) but rare before 10 years. In boys younger than 10 years, varicocele may correlate with malignancy. It is important for nurses to screen for varicocele in early adolescence, because this condition *is the most common cause of infertility*. Correction of testicular atrophy in early adolescence results in improved sperm count. Increased fertility has been noted in 80%–90% of those who undergo surgical correction. No visual abnormality may appear on the scrotum, but a bluish tinge may be seen in light-skinned patients. When the patient is upright, the nurse can palpate a soft, irregular mass that feels distinctly like a "bag of worms" posterior and superior to the testis. The varicocele collapses when the patient is supine but enlarges when the patient bears down or does the Valsalva maneuver. Testes on the affected side may be smaller because of impaired circulation, so the nurse needs to compare both testes (length, width, and depth). In advanced practice, orchidometers are often used to measure testicular volume in milliliters:

- Grade 3: "bag of worms" >2 cm in diameter and easily visualized
- Grade 2: 1–2 cm in diameter and easily palpable
- Grade 1: (most common) very small, difficult to palpate; Valsalva maneuver may help
- Asymptomatic:
- Grade 1 varicocele with normal testicular volumes usually do not require intervention in adolescents, but ultrasound is recommended every 6 months to evaluate size (American Urological Association, 2009).

This circumscribed collection of serous develops in the tunica vaginalis surrounding the testis. There are two types of hydroceles: noncommunicating and communicating. In *noncommunicating hydrocele*, fluid collects only in the scrotum but is persistent. A communicating hydrocele has a patent process vaginalis, so fluid can move from the abdomen to scrotum. Edema is intermittent, usually flat in morning, swollen during the day, or when the patient cries or performs the Valsalva maneuver. A communicating hydrocele is associated with a hernia. Incidence is 0.5%–2% of males, It primarily appears before 1 year of age; if it persists beyond 1 year, the nurse should assume it to be in conjunction with a hernia. In older children and adults, hydrocele may follow epididymitis, trauma, hernia, and tumor of testis. The patient will present with unilateral edema but no pain. He may complain of weight or bulk to the scrotum, which does not cause any apparent distress. On palpation of the scrotum, a large mass is noted, which can be transilluminated with a pink or red glow. If a hernia is involved, the hydrocele will not transilluminate. The nurse's fingers should be able to get around the mass; however, this is not possible if a hernia is present. If a noncommunicating hydrocele is present, no treatment is indicated unless the hydrocele is so large that it causes discomfort or persists for more than 1 year, because by then, there should be spontaneous absorption. A communicating hydrocele can resolve, but because of its association with hernia, this condition will need surgical repair. The nurse may order a scrotal ultrasound to help confirm the diagnoses (American Urological Association, 2009).

Abnormal Finding	Description
Spermatocele 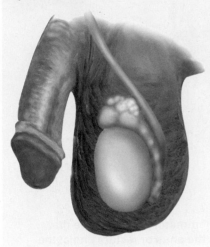	This benign scrotal mass or cyst develops on the head of the epididymis or testicular adnexa, which contains sperm. This uncommon finding occurs in <1% of all males from the neonatal period to a peak at 14 years. For the nurse, it is virtually impossible to differentiate from a simple epididymal cyst that does not contain sperm. Patients may complain of a lump in the scrotal sac or edema. Upon palpation, the nurse will find a mobile, cystic nodule usually <1 cm superior and posterior to the testis. The mass will transilluminate with a pink or red glow. The spermatocele will not change in size when the patient performs the Valsalva maneuver. The advanced practice nurse orders a scrotal ultrasound for diagnostic purposes.

! **Table 25.9   Conditions of the Anus, Rectum, and Prostate**

External Hemorrhoids	Internal Hemorrhoids
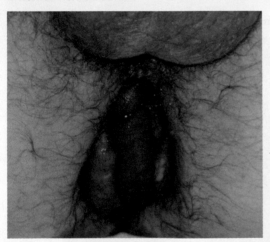	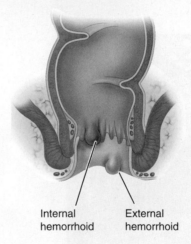 Internal hemorrhoid External hemorrhoid
External hemorrhoids are varicose veins that originate below the pectinate line and are covered by anal skin. Patients complain of rectal itching, pain, or burning. External hemorrhoids are usually not visible at rest but become visible upon standing or on defecation. If conventional hemorrhoid treatment proves ineffective or the hemorrhoids become edematous and thrombosed, surgery may be indicated. A thrombosed hemorrhoid presents as a blue, shiny, edematous mass on the anus. The patient is very uncomfortable and requires immediate attention.	Internal hemorrhoids can be painless unless they are thrombosed, infected, or prolapsed. They occur above the pectinate line and are covered by the mucosa of the anal canal. Internal hemorrhoids create soft swelling and are difficult to palpate on a digital examination unless they are prolapsed through the rectum. They can bleed daily with or without defecation. This can cause the patient to be anemic. This condition requires a referral for further treatment (American Gastroenterological Association, 2009)

(table continues on page 766)

Table 25.9   Conditions of the Anus, Rectum, and Prostate *(continued)*

Anorectal Fissure

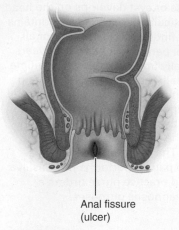

Anal fissure
(ulcer)

Anorectal fissure is a tear in the anal mucosa and can occur midline or posterior or anterior to it. Usually, a fissure is caused by the passage of large, hard stool. On observation, a sentinel skin tag may be seen at the lower end of the fissure. Ulcerations may appear at the site. The patient has bleeding, pain, and itching. As the internal sphincter is spastic, anesthesia of the site is necessary for examination.

Anal Fistula

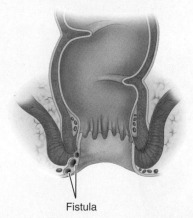

Fistula

Anal fistula is an inflammatory tract or tube that opens at one end in the anus or rectum and at the other end onto the skin surface. It originates in the anal crypts. The fissure can occur spontaneously or from perirectal abscess. On compression, serosanguinous or purulent drainage may appear. Externally, the area appears raised, red, and granular. This condition requires referral for further treatment (American Gastroenterological Association, 2009).

Rectal Polyp

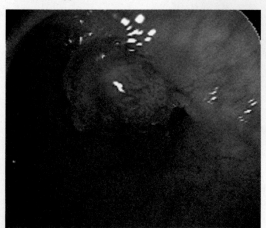

Polyps, common findings, can occur anywhere in the intestinal tract. They can be adenomas or inflammatory in origin, occurring singly or in clusters. They can cause rectal bleeding and be seen protruding through the rectum on examination. On DRE, polyps can felt as soft nodules and either be pedunculated or be sessile. Many times, the nurse cannot palpate polyps. Colonoscopy is needed to differentiate between a polyp and carcinoma. Older adults are more prone to rectal polyps and are at higher risk for carcinoma, making the rectal portion a significant part of the examination for them.

Carcinoma of the Rectum and Anus

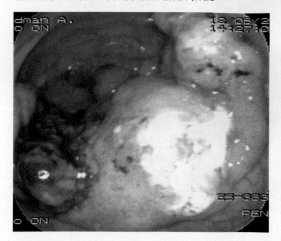

Although rare, cancers of the rectum and anus are becoming more common. The most common causes are anal intercourse, especially if associated with chronic irritation, such as with HPV. Symptoms of rectal or anal cancer include constant discharge, change in bowel habits, blood in the stool, and weight loss. On examination, a stony, irregular, sessile polypoid mass is felt. It is nodular with areas of ulceration. The cancer initially is asymptomatic, so routine clinical rectal examination and regular screening are key to early detection.

Table 25.9   Conditions of the Anus, Rectum, and Prostate *(continued)*

Rectal Prolapse

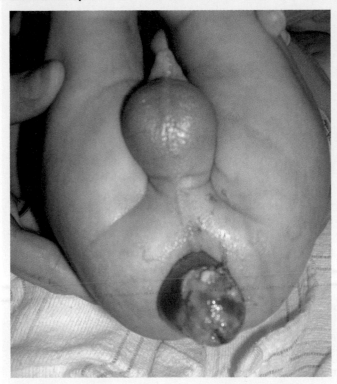

Rectal prolapse usually occurs with defecation; the rectal mucosa, with or without muscular wall, prolapses through the anal ring. On examination, a prolapse may present like a doughnut. A complete prolapse includes the muscular wall and is larger with circular folds. Cystic fibrosis is associated with children who present with rectal prolapse (Seidel, et al., 2003).

Prostatitis

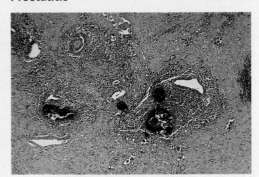

Inflammation or infection of the prostate gland can be acute or chronic. Acute **bacterial prostatitis** may result from ascending urethral infection, reflux of infected urine, extension of a rectal infection, or hematogenous spread. **Chronic prostatitis** results from autoimmune, allergic, neuromuscular, or psychological disorders of the bladder, detrusor hyperreflexia, or pelvic floor tension myalgia. Signs and symptoms for acute and chronic prostatitis are similar. Acute prostatitis usually presents with severe symptoms. Signs and symptoms include fever, chills, malaise, dysuria, frequency, inhibited urinary voiding, low back pain, suprapubic discomfort, and perineal pain. Many also complain of painful sexual intercourse, pain when defecating, and hematuria. On examination, the prostate is tender, warm, swollen, and boggy. Carefully and gently palpate because vigorous massage can disseminate bacteria in the bloodstream, resulting in bacteriemia. The patient with prostatitis is acutely ill and needs immediate intervention (Uphold & Graham, 2003).

Prostate Cancer

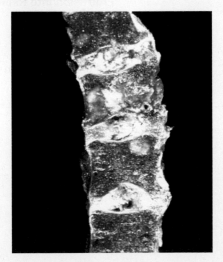

This second most common cancer among men (skin cancer is first) is also the second leading cause of death among men (exceeded by lung cancer). It is usually very slow growing and asymptomatic in the early stages. As the prostate enlarges, patients may develop hesitancy, dribbling, frequency, urgency, nocturia, retention, slow stream, or feeling of bladder fullness. Diagnosis is made with a PSA blood test and rectal examination.

Table 25.10 Types of Hernias

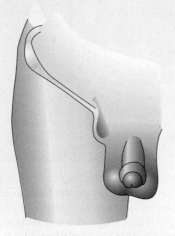
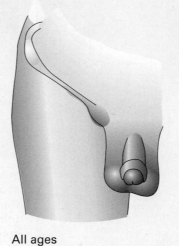
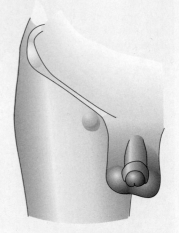

Feature	Direct Inguinal	Indirect Inguinal	Femoral
Affected population	Middle aged and elderly men	All ages	Least common, found more frequently in women
Bilaterality	55%	30%	Rare
Origin of swelling	Above inguinal ligament. Directly behind and through external ring.	Above inguinal ligament. Hernial sac enters inguinal canal at internal ring and exits at external ring	Below inguinal ligament
Scrotal involvement	Rare	Common	Never
Impulse location	At side of finger in inguinal canal	At tip of finger in inguinal canal	Not felt by finger in inguinal canal; mass; below canal

Table 25.11 Classifications of Prostate Enlargement

Grade	Protrusion into Rectum
I	1–2 cm or $^{3}/_{8}$–$^{3}/_{4}$ in
II	2–3 cm or $^{3}/_{4}$–1$^{1}/_{8}$ in
III	3–4 cm or 1$^{1}/_{8}$–1$^{3}/_{4}$ in
IV	>4 cm or 1$^{3}/_{4}$ in

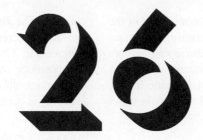

Female Genitalia and Rectal Assessment

Learning Objectives

1 Describe the normal physical characteristics of the female genitalia and rectum.

2 Describe the function of the female genitalia and rectum.

3 Differentiate developmental differences in the assessment of the female genitals and rectum.

4 Recognize age, ethnicity, and cultural differences in approaching the assessment of the female.

5 Collect subjective data with respect to, and consideration of, sensitive information.

6 Identify teaching opportunities for the female patient regarding current problems, risk reduction, and health promotion for the future.

7 Demonstrate knowledge of the pelvic examination and screening tests performed.

8 Identify normal and abnormal findings in the inspection and palpation of the internal and external genitalia.

9 Demonstrate the process of the physical examination of the rectum and the anus.

10 Effectively communicate and document techniques and findings using appropriate medical terminology.

11 Use assessment findings to identify diagnoses and to initiate a plan of care.

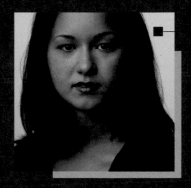

This chapter focuses on genital and rectal assessment of the female patient across the life span. By identifying key factors in the process of this assessment, the nurse can explore opportunities for positive communication and accurate information regarding women's health. Nurses can guide female patients in risk reduction and health promotion from the onset of puberty to the menopausal years and beyond.

Structure and Function Overview

The female genitalia can be subdivided as external and internal. External genitalia include the mons pubis, labia majora, labia minora, prepuce, and clitoris. The internal genitalia are the vagina, fornix, uterus, cervix, fundus, fallopian tubes, ovaries, and supporting tissues.

External Genitalia

The external genitalia are also called the *vulva* (Fig. 26-1). The **mons pubis** is the most anterior structure and is comprised of subcutaneous fatty tissue covered by pubic hair. The mons pubis lays directly over the pubic bone and creates a cushion that protects the bone during intercourse. The **labia majora** consist of two folds that extend from mons pubis downward to the perineum. The **clitoris**, an embryologic homologue of the penis, responds in an erectile fashion when stimulated. It consists of the glans that lies posterior to two crura. Nerve fibers in the clitoris respond to touch and produce pleasurable feelings for the female. The ventral surface of the **glans** is known as the **frenulum** and is where the **labia minora**, two small folds that extend from clitoral hood to the **posterior fourchette** of the vagina, fuse. The **vestibule** lies between the labia minora and is bound anteriorly by the clitoris and posteriorly by the perineum. Within the vestibule lie the urethra at the upper middle area, with bilateral **paraurethral Skene's glands** at the 7 and 5 o'clock positions respectively. The Skene's glands produce clear fluid that aids in lubrication during intercourse. The **vaginal introitus** lies posterior to the

urethra. The **Bartholin's glands**, located at the base of the vestibule, secrete clear mucus into the vaginal introitus during intercourse. They are positioned at 7 and 5 o'clock positions of the posterior vestibule. The **perineum** is the area between the vaginal introitus and rectum. This is the location where an episiotomy is occasionally done to facilitate difficult childbirth.

Internal Genitalia

Vagina

The **vagina** is a tube of muscular tissue that extends from vaginal introitus to uterus. The three-layer vaginal muscle wall is extremely expandable especially during childbirth. It is lined by glandular mucous membrane, within which are folds called **ruggae**. These ruggae become less prominent in advanced years. The vagina is approximately parallel to the lower portion of the sacrum. This position is the reason the anterior wall of the vagina measures 7 cm while the posterior wall is about 9 cm. The **vesicovaginal septum** separates the anterior wall of the vagina from the urethra and bladder. The **rectovaginal septum** separates the posterior wall of the vagina from the rectum.

Uterus

The hollow **uterus**, often referred to as the "womb," is the organ that holds the endometrial lining and is prepared to accept an implanted ovum (Fig. 26-2). It lies between the bladder and rectum and is approximately 7 to 8 cm long and 4 to 5 cm at its widest part. The uterine walls consist of an outer layer called the **peritoneum**, a muscle layer called the **myometrium**, and an inner layer called the **endometrium**.

The uterus has two parts separated by a narrow isthmus: the corpus (body) and the cervix. If implantation occurs, the uterus accommodates the growing fetus for the remaining 9 months. If no fertilization occurs, the endometrial lining sheds and the patient will have a menstrual period. The freely mobile uterus is supported bilaterally by the **round, cardinal, uterosacral, and broad ligaments**.

Cervix

The **cervix** is the posterior portion of the uterus that protrudes into the vagina. The cervix is smooth, rounded, and has a midline opening called the **os**. In a nonpregnant female, the os resembles a donut with a small hole in the middle. Once a pregnancy has occurred and thereafter, the opening resembles a horizontal slit.

Fallopian Tubes

The **fallopian tubes** transport ova from the ovary to the uterus. They are approximately 12 cm long and 1 mm in diameter. The tubes are composed of four layers of tissues: **peritoneal** (serous), **subserous** (adventitial), **muscular**, and **mucous**. These layers are responsible for the blood and nerve supply as well as providing the peristaltic condition necessary to move the ovum towards the uterus. The fallopian tubes are divided into three parts: **isthmus, ampulla, and the fimbriae**. Fertilization most often occurs in the ampulla portion of the fallopian tubes.

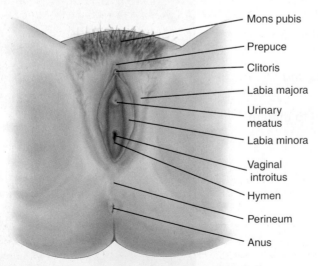

Figure 26.1 Anatomy of the external genitalia.

— Mons pubis
— Prepuce
— Clitoris
— Labia majora
— Urinary meatus
— Labia minora
— Vaginal introitus
— Hymen
— Perineum
— Anus

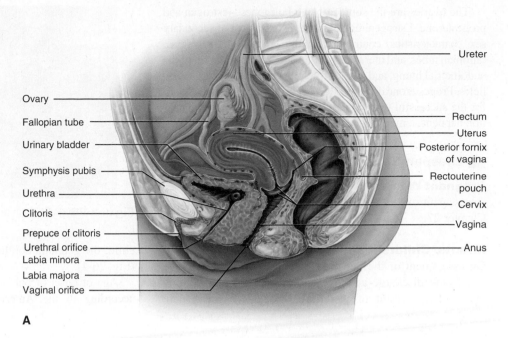

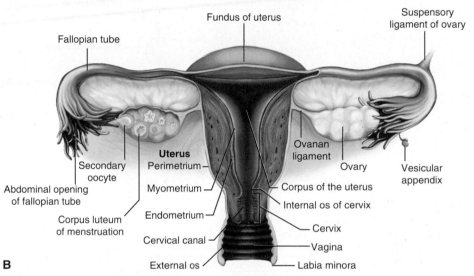

Figure 26.2 Internal female genitalia. **A.** Side view. **B.** Frontal view.

Ovaries

The **ovaries** are two almond-shaped structures measuring approximately 3 cm by 2 cm. They develop after puberty and reduce in size (atrophy) after menopause. The ovaries are held in place by ligaments called the **infundibulopelvic and ovarian ligaments**. The ovaries provide ova to be fertilized by sperm and secrete the hormones estrogen and progesterone (discussed later).

Rectum, Anal Canal, and Anus

Anatomy and physiology of the rectum, anal canal, and anus are covered in detail in Chapter 25.

Hormone Regulation

Many hormones regulate the female reproductive system. The main sources of these hormones are (1) the **anterior pituitary**, (2) the **hypothalmus**, and (3) the **ovaries**.

The anterior pituitary secretes **follicle-stimulating hormone (FSH)** and **lutenizing hormone (LH)**. The function of FSH is to stimulate the growth and maturation of the ovarian follicle and the production of testosterone, which maintains spermatogenesis in the male. LH functions to lutenize the follicle, which increases production of progesterone by the granulose cells (Speroff & Fritz, 2005). The lutenizing process ultimately produces the corpus luteum.

The hypothalamus is responsible for the release of FSH and LH by way of the **gonadatropin-releasing hormones (GnRH)** and lutenizing-releasing hormones (LnRH). The hypothalamus acts as an inhibitor of prolactin release. This is referred to as the **prolactin inhibiting factor** as well. These cyclic hormones drive the function of menstruation, reproduction, sexuality, and physical as well as emotional health (Speroff & Fritz, 2005). The pelvic organs are the recipients of the hormones.

The ovaries are the source of two hormones—estrogen and progesterone. Estrogen regulates the development of secondary sex characteristics, contributes to the growth of the vagina, fallopian tubes, and uterus, contributes to the proliferation of the endometrial lining, and plays a role in maturation of ovarian follicles. Progesterone develops the corpus luteum and is necessary for the successful implantation of the embryo. If no implantation happens, a menstrual cycle occurs. See also Figure 26-3.

 Lifespan Considerations

Pregnant Women
Assessment of the pregnant woman is discussed in detail in Chapter 27.

Infants, Children, and Adolescents
On assessment of the newborn, it is not uncommon to see some pink discharge at the opening of the vagina. This is most often a result of maternal estrogen. In the female

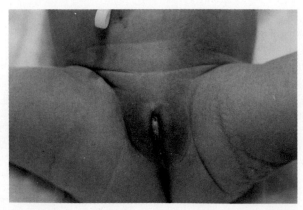

Figure 26.4 Surface anatomy of the female infant genitalia.

child, the genitalia continue growing, except for the clitoris (Fig. 26-4).

Age of onset of puberty in girls has continued to decline, according to the American College of Obstetricians and

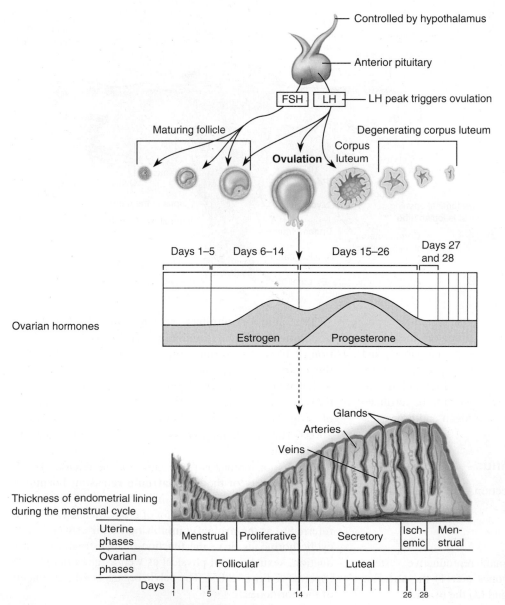

Figure 26.3 Diagram of the relationship between hormonal levels and (**top**) follicular development and (**bottom**) the menstrual cycle.

Gynecologist Committee on Adolescent Health Care. The U.S. median age at menarche is 12.4 years. African American girls may begin puberty before 8 years. Onset of menses correlates with estrogen release by the **hypothalamic-pituitary-ovarian** axis (Speroff & Fritz, 2005). Budding of the breast occurs first, followed by development of pubic hair (see Chapter 21). Onset of menses follows breast budding by approximately 2 to 3 years. Tanner's stages of maturation are used in the assessment of preadolescent and adolescent females (Marshall & Tanner, 1969). Female pubic hair stages are reviewed in Table 26-1.

Genital assessment of the adolescent is not required unless there has been initiation of sexual activity or there are genital tract problems. The opportunity for nurse education is greatest at this time, however. The adolescent is experiencing body changes, self-identity exploration, and relationship questions. The nurse should be direct and honest with the teen. Establishment of a trusting and confidential nurse-patient relationship is vital. Sexually active adolescent females should have an annual examination.

Table 26.1	Tanner Staging: Female Pubic Hair
Stage	**Description**
Stage 1: Preadolescent 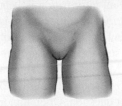	The vellus over the pubes is not further developed than that over the anterior abdominal wall (ie, no pubic hair).
Stage 2 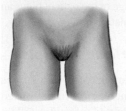	Long, slightly pigmented, downy hair that is straight or only slightly curled appears chiefly along the labia.
Stage 3 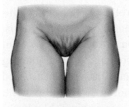	Hair is considerably darker, coarser, and more curled. It spreads sparsely over the junction of the mons pubis.
Stage 4 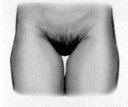	Hair is now adult in type, but the area covered by it is still considerably smaller than in most adults. There is no spread to the medial surface of the thighs.
Stage 5 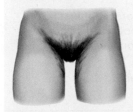	Hair is adult in quantity and type, distributed as an inverse triangle of the classically feminine pattern. Spread is to the medial surface of the thighs, but not up the linea alba or elsewhere above the base of the inverse triangle.

Older Adults

Women older than 50 years represent more than 81% of the female population (U.S. Census Bureau, 2007). As women age, they experience many changes in the genitourinary tract. Most of these are related to limited or absent estrogen in the system.

Menopause is defined as 12 consecutive months without menses (Speroff & Fritz, 2005). As estrogen levels decrease, the uterus becomes smaller, the ovaries shrink, the normal vaginal ruggae flatten, and the epithelium atrophies. These normal changes may lead to problems such as vaginal infections, urinary tract infections, **dyspareunia**, and lowered libido (Anderson & Must 2005). Older women are at increased risk for endometrial cancers and need education regarding abnormal signs and symptoms. The nurse has an opportunity to provide counseling and education regarding intimacy problems and physiologic changes, and to answer the patient's questions.

Acute Assessment

If the patient is experiencing severe pain or excessive bleeding, the assessment needs to be truncated to involve only questions pertinent to the immediate condition and necessary for current care. Severe pain may be related to an acute infection, urinary tract problem, gastrointestinal illness, or musculoskeletal trauma. It is important to perform a thorough symptom analysis to evaluate these problems. A ruptured ovarian cyst may be present and needs to be assessed quickly.

Subjective Data Collection

Subjective data collection begins with the health history, continues with questions about specific genital and rectal conditions, and ends with detailed collection of information about areas of concern. Each assessment of the female genitalia is unique to the individual patient. When beginning the history portion of the assessment, it is important to establish a trusting relationship with the patient. The assessment of the female is very invasive and can be uncomfortable to both patient and nurse. In initiation of the health history, you allow the patient to become comfortable with you; at the same time, the acquisition of important data instills confidence in the nurse. The establishment of a respectful, nonjudgmental demeanor is imperative.

When obtaining the history, the room should be private and comfortable, and the nurse should be seated at eye level or lower to the patient. Reassure the patient that all information is kept confidential. It is best to obtain the history while the patient is still dressed. This reduces embarrassment and vulnerability of the patient. If this is not possible, make sure the patient is completely covered, warm, and comfortable. Make eye contact but be careful of nonverbal communication. It is important to listen to the patient without thinking of your next question. Often minor cues give the greatest amount of information. Begin the interview with basic biographical data. The age of the patient plays an important role in the direction of examination and counseling.

Areas for Health Promotion/*Healthy People*—

Specific to the female population, an integral part of the assessment is the sexual behavior indicator. An estimated 15 million new cases of sexually transmitted infections (STIs) are reported each year. Of these, nearly 4 million occur in adolescents (Center for Disease Control [CDC], 2008). Complications of STIs include cervical cancer, pelvic infections, infertility, and pelvic pain. Education is the most powerful tool the nurse can offer regarding prevention. Maintaining confidentiality and offering the most current, evidence-based information ensure greater understanding from the patient. The indicators of *Healthy People* are covered in Table 26-2.

Table 26.2 *Healthy People* Goals: Female Genital Health and Education	
Goals	**Patient Education Topics**
Increase the proportion of adolescents who abstain from sexual intercourse or use condoms if currently sexually active.	Health education can occur in the schools by the school nurse or in health courses.
Increase the proportion of sexually active persons who use condoms.	Teach safe sex strategies if sexually active. Refer to resources if budget is an issue.
Reduce the proportion of adolescents and adults with chlamydia, gonorrhea, syphilis, genital herpes, PID, and HIV infections.	Teach that birth control does not protect against STIs. Provide adolescents information about oral sex and its risks. Advise on always using condoms especially if not in a monogamous relationship.
Increase by at least 97% those women age 18 and older who have ever had a Pap smear.	Include health promotion and screening during the annual visit.

Source: *Healthy people 2010: What are its goals?* (n.d.). Retrieved July 7, 2010, from http://www.healthypeople.gov/About/goals.htm

Assessment of Risk Factors

Questions on History and Risk	Rationales
Family History Tell me about your family history of the following, including two generations: • Diabetes • Heart disease • Cancer • Thyroid problems • Gynecologic conditions • Hypertension • Asthma • Allergies • Diethylstilbesterol (DES) use in mother • Multiple pregnancies • Congenital anomalies	Current studies show that the major factors in breast and ovarian cancer are the BRCA1 and BRCA2 genes. These genes may be transmitted from the father's side as well as the mother's side (Kolesar, 2004). DES was a hormone given to pregnant women to prevent miscarriages from 1940 to 1970. Maternal DES use is associated with higher risks of clear cell cancers as well as breast cancers in older women. Ongoing studies continue regarding DES exposure (CDC, 2008).
Personal History ***Menstrual History.*** Ask about menstrual history first. • How old were you when you got your first menstrual period? • What was the first day of the last menstrual period? • What is the character or consistency of your flow? • Do you use tampons? • How many days do you experience flow during your cycle? How many pads or tampons do you use per day? How many days is there heavy flow, moderate flow, or light spotting?	Menarche usually begins around 12 years of age. If a patient has not had menarche by 16 years, an endocrine evaluation is recommended. The menstrual cycle is calculated from the first day of the last menstrual period to the first day of the next menstrual period. Usual cycle is 28–32 days, but cycles can be as short as 20 days or as long as 40 days without intervention necessary. Flow is approximately 25–60 mL per menstrual period. Normal length is 2–8 days.
Obstetrical History • Have you ever been pregnant? • If so, how many times? • How many living children do you have? • Did you give birth vaginally or through cesarean section? • Were there any complications before, during, or after your pregnancy? • Have you ever had a miscarriage? • Have you ever had an abortion? If yes, was it an elective termination, spontaneous miscarriage, or incomplete miscarriage?	**Gravida:** The number of pregnancies a woman has had, including if she is presently pregnant. **Para:** The number of births a woman has had after 20 weeks even if the fetus died at birth. **Term:** Infant born after 37 weeks' gestation. **Preterm:** Infant born after 20 weeks but before 37 weeks. **Abortion:** Number of pregnancies that ended spontaneously or for therapeutic reasons. **Living:** Number of living children either delivered or adopted. A woman could be a **Gravida 1** (one pregnancy), and have two children. How? Twins!
Menopause • Have you stopped having menstrual periods? • Are your menstrual cycles irregular? • Do you experience any symptoms of irregularity or absence of menses?	**Menopause** is the cessation of menstrual periods for 12 months or more. **Perimenopause** is irregularity of menstrual cycles and accompanying symptoms (hot flashes, night sweating, mood swings, vaginal dryness, decreased sexual drive, or **libido**) between 40 and 55 years and before actual cessation of menses (Amin, et al., 2003).
Gynecologic History • Have you ever had a Pap smear? If so, when was it done? • Have your Pap smears always been normal? • If not, did you receive any treatment for it and when? • Have you had any previous procedures or surgeries?	**Papanicolaou smear** is a cytologic evaluation of the cells of the cervix to screen for precancerous cervical lesions. It does NOT screen for STIs or any cancers other than cervical cancer. In 2006, the American Cancer Society estimated 9,710 new cases of cervical cancer and approximately 3,700 deaths from it in the United States. The nurse needs to provide the most up-to-date evidence-based information. By educating the patient regarding the importance of follow-up and collaborating with health care providers to ensure compliance, the nurse plays a part in the reduction of cervical cancers (Martin, 2008).

(text continues on page 776)

Questions on History and Risk	Rationales
• Have you ever been treated for any vaginal infections? • Do you have frequent vaginal infections?	A patient with recurring yeast infections should be evaluated for diabetes and HIV (ADA, 2008).
• Do you use over-the-counter vaginal medication? • Have you ever had any pelvic infections?	Frequent use of over-the-counter (OTC) vaginal creams or suppositories can possibly mask other more serious infections.
• Do you use scented vaginal products such as sprays or scented tampons or pads?	Use of scented products may result in a **contact dermatitis** of the vulva or vagina.
• Do you douche? How often do you douche?	Nurses should educate the patient about problems that can arise from douching, such as vaginal infections, imbalance of normal vaginal flora (pH), and the possibility of transferring a vaginal infection into the uterus. The consequence can be pelvic inflammatory disease (PID).
Immunizations. Have you received the vaccine against the **human papillomavirus (HPV)**? • When did you receive it? • Did you receive all three doses?	Recommendations are to give quadrivalent HPV (types 6, 11, 16, 18) recombinant vaccine to females aged 9–26 years in three doses: the second dose 2 months after the first and the third dose 6 months after the first (CDC, 2008).
Sexual History • Have you ever had sex? • What type (vaginal, oral, anal)?	Frank discussion opens opportunities for inquiry otherwise not brought up by the patient. Current statistics show that adolescents may not engage in vaginal intercourse but may have anal or oral sex (CDC, 2008).
• Approximately how many sexual partners have you had? Male, female, or both? • Are you currently in a sexual relationship? Is it monogamous?	Ascertaining a patient's experience is important to determine risks. It is important to provide accurate and health-promoting information to homosexual, bisexual, and heterosexual females (Clark & Marrazzo, 2006).
• Have you ever experienced any type of sexual abuse?	Obtaining history of sexual abuse not only opens discussion about it and the patient's current feelings but also allows the nurse to proceed to the examination giving the emotional support necessary (Laumbach, 2004).
• Do you experience any pain or bleeding with or after intercourse?	Bleeding during intercourse may indicate an infection or possibly a cervical polyp.
• Do you experience urinary burning or infections related to intercourse?	**Dysuria** (burning with urination) or frequent UTIs may be related to bladder trauma from intercourse. Educate the patient to empty her bladder before and after intercourse to reduce trauma and introduction of bacteria into the urethra.
Contraception • Do you use condoms or other barrier methods during sexual intercourse? Sometimes or always? • Do you use any contraception? • If so, what is currently used? • Have you used anything different in the past? • Have you had any problems with any contraceptive forms?	Condoms provide some but not complete protection against STIs. They provide protection only if used consistently. It is just as important for homosexual females to use barrier methods to prevent transmission of certain infections. Contraceptive use is different than practicing "safe-sex." The only 100% safe sex practice is abstinence. Contraceptives ONLY protect against pregnancies, not STIs.

| Questions on History and Risk | Rationales |

Medications and Supplements
- Are you currently taking any prescribed medications?
- Are you taking any OTC medications?
- Have you recently been on any antibiotics?
- Do you use any herbal therapeutics?
- Do you currently take any vitamins?

Certain medications including oral contraceptives, antidepressants, and antihypertensive agents can cause changes in menstrual cycles, appetite, and libido. Certain antibiotics can strip the vagina of its normal flora and create an environment that promotes yeast infections. Antibiotics can interfere with the absorption of oral contraceptives. A backup method of contraception or abstinence is advised during the treatment period. Use of herbal therapy requires caution. Although there have been some reported positive effects with herbal preparations, there are also reported herb-drug interactions. Often herbal products affect other medications being taken. Patients taking anticoagulants, digoxin, oral contraceptives, statins, and HIV medications should exercise caution. All herbal products should be avoided during pregnancy (Low Dog, 2005).

Risk Factors
STIs
- Do you engage in unprotected sex?
- Do you have multiple sexual partners?
- Are you between 15 and 24 years?
- Are you experiencing any pain within or discharge from the pelvic region?

Screening, treating, and counseling of and about chlamydia and gonorrhea are currently recommended for all sexually active adolescents (Burns, et al., 2007). **Chlamydia trachomatis** is currently the most common and frequently reported bacterial **STI** in the United States. Approximately 2.8 million cases are reported annually. Of those, occurrence is highest in patients 15–24 years (CDC, 2008). Because of the asymptomatic nature of this infection, risk for infection is high. Long-term infection can cause **PID** and subsequent potential infertility.

Obesity. Obesity is considered an independent risk factor for coronary heart disease. **Central obesity** (apple shape) increases this risk. Women with pear shaped bodies are thought to be at less risk.

A **body mass index (BMI)** of 18.5–24.9 is considered normal, a BMI of 25–29 is overweight, and >30 is considered obese (see Chapter 8). The Women's Health Study (Mosca, et al., 2007) showed that just 1 hour of walking per week reduces the cardiovascular risk in women.

Osteoporosis. Osteoporosis is a bone disorder characterized by decreased bone mass, which leads to fragility and potential fracture especially in females. This condition contributes to approximately 1.5 million fractures annually and 500,000 related hospitalizations (USDHHS, n.d.)

Bone mineral density screening is a simple and cost-efficient test recommended for all women 65 years or older. Those at risk for osteoporosis (Caucasian or Asian women with a family history of osteoporosis, thin frame, tobacco use, glucocorticoid use, or any fracture after age 45 years) should be screened as well (National Osteoporosis Foundation, 2007).

Hormonal Contraceptive and Tobacco Use
- Do you smoke?
- Are you using hormonal contraceptives?
- How old are you?

Tobacco is contraindicated for any patient 40 years or older who uses hormonal contraceptives. The combination of tobacco and hormonal contraceptives increases risk for vascular problems (eg, deep vein thrombosis, pulmonary emboli) as well as risk for cardiovascular incident. More than 20 million U.S. women smoke. First-time myocardial infarction in women who smoke precedes that for non-smokers by 19–20 years. Even light or "social" smoking doubles a female patient's risk of cardiovascular mortality (Mosca, et al., 2007).

Risk Assessment and Health-Related Patient Teaching

Reducing risk factors can occur through the provision of accurate, evidence-based information. Giving women throughout the lifespan an opportunity to ask questions and allowing open and nonjudgmental discussion about sexuality are important.

Any woman with a history of multiple partners has the highest risk of developing HPV and cervical cancer. Discussing this factor and recommending monogamy, abstinence, or consistent use of condoms with each act of intercourse is important.

Women currently using oral contraceptives are less likely to use any barrier methods such as condoms or diaphragms. When counseling women on oral contraceptive use, it is important to stress that the pills do not protect against STIs.

Incidence of cervical cancer has decreased in the past decades because of widespread use of pap screening. The greatest risk factor for cervical cancer is infection with HPV. More than 100 types of HPV cause genital warts, some of which can lead to cancer of the cervix. Having unprotected sex increases the chance of contracting HPV. Not everyone infected with HPV develops cancer of the cervix. Other risk factors influence the likelihood of cervical cancer, such as tobacco use, infection with Chlamydia or HIV, poor diet, low income, and family history of cancer. HPV testing is a simple swabbing of the external and endocervical areas. This testing captures the types of HPV (16, 18, 31, 33, 35, 45, 51, 52, and 56) that cause high-grade cervical lesions that lead to cancer.

The HPV vaccine has been available since 2006 (CDC, 2008). As discussed previously, the vaccine consists of three separate doses and is recommended for females 9 through 26 years. Patients (and, in the case of minors, their parents) should be counseled regarding the availability. The FDA still recommends annual screening even if the patient has received a vaccine.

Focused Health History Related to Common Symptoms

When assessing the patient who presents with a specific complaint, the nurse performs a focused assessment. He or she asks questions relating to the reason for seeking care systematically. Begin with asking about the onset of the symptom. It is best to get specifics such as the number of hours, days, or weeks that the patient has been experiencing the symptom(s). If bleeding is the problem, inquire about the number of pads or tampons used per hour or day. Ask about the location. Many patients are not comfortable with anatomical descriptions and just say "down there." Use appropriate terminology in a matter-of-fact manner. Ask if pain involves the abdomen, bladder, vagina, urethra, uterus, or rectum. If possible, have the patient point to the area of concern. Inquire about the duration of the problem. Again, specifics help: How long does the symptom last? Is it ongoing? Ask about the character of the pain, bleeding, itching, discharge, or lesion.

The nurse can provide the patient with a laundry list of descriptions such as dull, sharp, burning, stinging, color and consistency of blood, presence of clots, thick or thin discharge, odor, or not. Find out if there are any associative factors such as nausea, vomiting, fever, malaise, fainting, or change in urinary or bowel habits. Inquire about things that might aggravate symptoms such as intercourse, menses, physical activity, hygiene products, or self-treatment. If the patient has experienced any relief, ask what has made it better. Has the symptom been experienced before and when? What was done for it? Finally ask about the severity of the symptom. How bad is the pain, itching, bleeding on a scale of 0 to 10 with 10 being the greatest?

Common Female Genital or Rectal Symptoms

- Pelvic pain
- Vaginal burning, discharge, or itching
- Menstrual disorders
- Structural problems
- Hemorrhoids

Questions on Common Symptoms	Rationale/Abnormal Findings

Pelvic Pain

Do you have any pain or discomfort?
- Location
- Intensity
- Duration
- Description
- Aggravating factors
- Alleviating factors
- Functional impairment
- Pain goal

Measurable pain identification allows the nurse to address symptoms individually. Ask the patient to rate the pain or discomfort from 0 to 10 with 10 being the worst pain ever. Differences between acute and chronic pain may alter the course of intervention and goals set. Always ask the patient to point to the area of pain or discomfort to gather more accurate and reliable data. Many gynecological problems differ in the pain characteristics. The description of burning versus dull and gnawing can help the nurse and practitioner identify the problem sooner. Conditions involving the pelvic region increase in pain and intensity with activities such as exercise, intercourse, or prolonged standing. Relief may be in the form of OTC medications or remedies such as warm baths or a heating pad. If the current problem is impairing functional ability, the nurse needs to address this as a priority as much as if he or she had the pain or discomfort. The goal is to assist in expediting the relief of the presenting symptom and to contribute to the return of functionality in the patient.

Vaginal Burning, Discharge, Itching

- Have you ever been treated for an STI?
- If you were treated, were your partner(s) treated?
- Did you have a follow-up examination to confirm treatment?
- Are you aware of the different types of STIs?
- Do you currently have any vaginal discharge? If so, is there a color, odor, or consistency to it?
- Do you have any itching or burning of your pubic hair, vulva, or vagina?

An STI survey allows the nurse to educate the patient on all the infections possible. Differentiate itching between external and internal location. Vaginal discharge is a common symptom of STIs; however, a patient with an STI may have few or no symptoms. External itching can be caused from any number of sources: **pediculosis pubis** (commonly called "crabs"), **contact dermatitis, herpes simplex virus, condyloma acuminatum (external genital warts)**, or **atrophic vulvitis**.

Menstrual Disorders

- Have you ever experienced irregular menstrual cycles or skipped a cycle?
- Do you experience cramps during your menses?
- Do you take any medication for menstrual cramps? If so how much and how often? Does it help?
- Do you experience preflow bloating, mood swings, headaches, or breast tenderness? Does it go away once your flow begins?
- Are there any times other than your menstrual period that you experience bleeding or spotting?
- Do you experience any bleeding or spotting following intercourse?
- Do any menstrual conditions cause you to miss work, school, or social functions?

Amenorrhea is the absence of menstrual periods. The most common causes of secondary amenorrhea are pregnancy and anovulation. **Dysmenorrhea** is pain with menses. *Premenstrual syndrome* is the emotional and physical symptoms that occur at the same time before menses each month (Bader, 2005). Nonsteroidal anti-inflammatory drugs have been shown effective for dysmenorrhea. Intermenstrual bleeding or spotting or bleeding could be normal or could indicate an ongoing infection. Postintercourse bleeding or spotting could indicate an STI or possibly a cervical polyp.

Structural Problems

- Have you ever been treated for any cancer of the reproductive organs?
- Have you ever been treated for any gynecological conditions such as endometriosis, uterine fibroids, ovarian cyst, or abnormal bleeding?
- Have you noticed any change in the amount of hair you have in the vulva, abdomen, or around the nipples?
- Have you gained weight especially in the midabdomen in the past 6 months?
- Have you noticed changes in your skin?

Patients with a history of **endometriosis** have increased risk of infertility (Curtis, et al., 2005). Frequent ovarian cysts along with menstrual irregularities warrant evaluation for **polycystic ovarian syndrome**. In this condition, the patient presents with obesity, acne, **hirsutism** (increased hair along the abdomen and around the nipples), and **acanthosis nigricans** (areas of hyperpigmentation around the back of the neck and under arms). Vaginal ultrasound reveals multicystic ovaries. The patient may have variations in hormone levels, including increased free testosterone (Barron & Falsetti, 2008).

Hemorrhoids

Do you have hemorrhoids?

They are very common especially following childbirth. Hemorrhoids may be either external or internal.

Lifespan Considerations

Additional Questions	Rationales/Abnormal Findings
Pregnant Women	
Have you had any bleeding or cramping since you became pregnant?	Any bleeding or spotting following confirmation of pregnancy must be investigated further by a specialist.
Have you had any abnormal Pap smears in the past?	Patients who have had abnormal results may have a recurrence during pregnancy. Those who have had surgery to remove abnormal cells may have scar tissue, which needs to be released during labor in order to permit a vaginal delivery.
Have you had any STIs in the past?	Verify that any STIs were treated per protocol. Assess risk of reexposure (many STIs can harm the fetus).
What type of contraception have you used? When was the last time you used it?	If the patient was using hormonal contraceptives within three cycles prior to conception, it is difficult to assess when ovulation occurred. A patient taking such contraceptives does not have true menses but rather has "withdrawal bleeds" when she is not taking progesterone for 7 days. Even if pregnant, if she continues her birth control pills, she may have withdrawal bleeds at the usual time. If her conception date is not clear, ultrasound dating in the first trimester can be offered.
Have you had any problems with infertility?	If the response is positive, fully document the patient's history, including any medication taken and type of assisted reproduction. In vitro pregnancies have a somewhat increased risk of multiple gestation and fetal loss.
Do you have any common symptoms of pregnancy? or (See also Chapter 27.)	Morning sickness, growing pains, increased vaginal discharge or urination, breast tenderness/discharge, periumbilical pain, fetal hiccups, or Braxton Hicks contractions may be uncomfortable.
Newborns, Infants, and Children	
Do you use bubble baths for your child?	Just as with older females, contact with perfumed bath products or lotions may cause a contact dermatitis. For young girls, it is best to avoid bubble bath and fragrance products.
Does your child have frequent pain with urination?	Problems with bladder control may require a specialist. Sudden regression in bladder or bowel control may signal sexual abuse.
Does your child (older than 2½) have control over the bladder?	
Do you notice your child scratching his or her genitals?	Itching or scratching in the genitals could be infection, pinworm, abuse, or hygiene related.
Have you noticed any vaginal discharge on the underwear? Do you notice any odor in the genital area?	Young children especially toddlers many times insert foreign objects in orifices including the vagina.
Older Adults	
Have you noticed any bleeding since your menses stopped?	Any bleeding that occurs after the patient has had 1 year without menses should be investigated.
Have you noticed any vaginal problems such as dryness, itching, or vaginal secretions?	Loss of estrogen in the vagina along with loss of normal ruggae can lead to irritation and possible spotting from the vagina.
Are you currently having sexual relations? Have you experienced any pain with intercourse? Do you have a satisfactory sexual relationship with your partner?	Regular sexual activity is normal in older women and encouraged unless it causes pain. Recommendation of vaginal lubricants will help provide relief from vaginal dryness. The practitioner may prescribe local estrogen to help with dryness.

Additional Questions	Rationales/Abnormal Findings
Have you noticed any vaginal pressure or loss of urine if you cough or sneeze? Have you noticed any rectal pressure or experienced difficulty with bowel movements or incontinence of feces?	Vaginal pressure may indicate *uterine prolapse*. With accompanying if bladder symptoms, there may be bladder support (*cystocele*) issues. Rectal pressure may indicate a *rectocele*, *prolapsed rectum*, or mass and should be evaluated.

🌐 Cultural Considerations

Have you ever had a pelvic examination? Would you prefer a female practitioner?	Some cultures and religions have rules about who can see women unclothed and when pelvic examinations are allowed (Hahm, et al., 2007).

Therapeutic Dialogue: Collecting Subjective Data

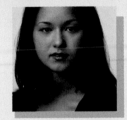

Teresa Nguyen, introduced at the beginning of this chapter, is a 28-year-old woman with vaginal discharge, pelvic pain, and fever. The following conversations give examples of interview styles used by different nurses. One is more effective than the other.

Less Effective

Nurse: Hi, Teresa. How are you today?

Teresa: Good, thank you.

Nurse: (Looks at chart). So it looks like you've been having some pain. Do you have any other symptoms?

Teresa: No, not really.

Nurse: Oh. It says that you also are having some vaginal discharge. Is that right?

Teresa: Yes.

Nurse: So what do you think that might be from?

Teresa: I don't know.

Nurse: Are you sexually active?

Teresa: No, I usually just lay there.

Nurse: I mean, are you having intercourse?

Teresa: Just with my boyfriend. I have been with him for a year and a half. My parents don't know because we're not married.

Nurse: Well, you don't have to be married to have sex. It's very common these days.

Teresa: My parents wouldn't approve.

Nurse: Don't worry—we won't tell anyone.

More Effective

Nurse: Good morning, how are you today?

Teresa: Good, thank you.

Nurse: What name would you like me to call you?

Teresa: You can call me Teresa.

Nurse: Good, and you can call me Shelly. Let me look over your chart (looks at chart). It looks like you've been having some pelvic pain and vaginal discharge.

Teresa: Yes.

Nurse: Tell me a little more about those symptoms.

Teresa: Well, I really notice that the pain is bad when my boyfriend has sex with me.

Nurse: (Listens)

Teresa: I'm really afraid that I have an STD. My friends really don't like my boyfriend and they said that he cheated on me.

Nurse: You sound very concerned.

Teresa: I just don't want my parents to know. They are very traditional.

Nurse: You are protected by privacy laws, but we may need to notify the health department if there is an illness that needs to be reported.

Critical Thinking Challenge

- How should the nurse proceed with questioning about privacy?
- What questions should the nurse ask regarding sexual activity and sexual practices? Give specific examples.
- What are your thoughts about Teresa's relationships with her parents? How might those affect the care?

Objective Data Collection

Equipment

- Examination gown
- Sheet or drape
- Nonsterile examination gloves (both latex and nonlatex)
- Water-soluble vaginal lubricant
- Light unit either goose neck or speculum attachment
- Wooden/plastic spatula
- Cervical brush (broom)
- Endocervical brush
- Glass slide
- Slide fixative
- Liquid pap base
- Culture tubes (DNA) for chlamydia and gonnorhea
- Sterile cotton swabs
- Large cotton swabs
- Small bottles with tops, one containing saline solution, one containing potassium hydroxide (KOH), and one containing acetic acid solution (white vinegar)
- Speculum (preferably warmed via heat source in examination drawer)
  - Pederson: narrow blades
  - Graves: wider blades
  - Pediatric: smaller Pederson with narrow blades and shorter length
  - Can be either metal or plastic

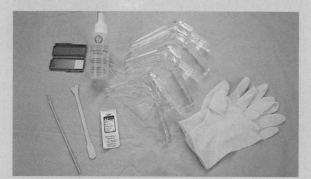

Materials used in the female examination.

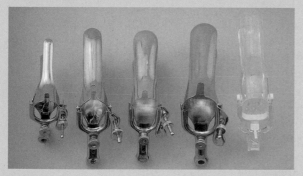

Specula.

Preparation

It is important to provide a comfortable environment. The nurse should display confidence while staying in tune with the patient's feelings of fear or embarrassment. A room containing information pamphlets and three dimensional models encourages inquiry and lessens anxiety. Ensure privacy throughout the examination. The table should be facing away from the door and instructions given not to disturb during the examination.

It is important to make sure the patient is not menstruating or has not had intercourse or douched before the Pap test. These conditions interfere with the cytology reading. Unless otherwise indicated, allow the patient to keep her socks on during the examination. Covers should be provided for table stirrups.

The patient should not have to sit too long in the examination room. If there is a cause for practitioner delay, offer the patient the opportunity to remain dressed until time for her examination.

Offer a step-by-step description of what will occur during the examination. Allow the patient to see all the instruments to be used and explain what they are for. The nurse should take time, especially if this is the first examination for the patient, to answer all the questions and concerns verbalized. Reassure the patient that if she is uncomfortable at any time to let you know, as the examination will stop or be altered. Empowering the patient and allowing patient control will enhance the examination experience and will ensure that the patient returns in the future. It is important to ask the patient to empty her bladder before the examination. Make sure all equipment is set up and within reach.

The nurse assists the patient into a semilithotomy position, helps her to move down just before the examination (Fig. 26-5), and assists the patient in placing her feet into

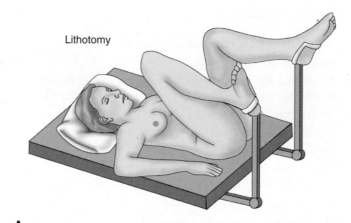

A

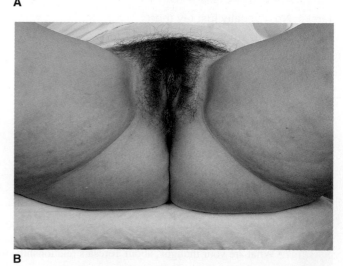

B

Figure 26.5 Lithotomy positioning for the examination of the female genitalia. **A.** Illustration showing the positioning of the lower extremities and buttocks. **B.** Frontal view of surface anatomy.

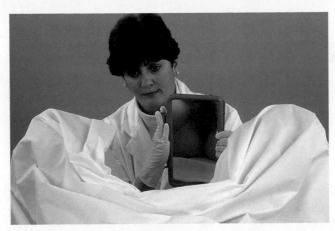

Figure 26.6 The nurse or health care practitioner may want to offer to the patient a mirror during the examination, so she can watch what is happening.

the stirrups. It is a good idea to make sure she is comfortable after the feet are placed. Elevating the patient's head and shoulders allows visualization of the examination by the patient. It is helpful to provide a mirror so that she might better see the examination (Fig. 26-6). Take time to encourage the patient to ask questions during the examination. When draping the patient, keep the genitals visualized without completely exposing the legs and knees. Also, keep in mind the importance of making sure she can see your face and you hers.

The nurse washes hands and puts gloves on both hands. At this point, the examination chair can be positioned in front of the examination table. Slowly have the patient move toward the end of the table. It is a good idea to reassure her that you will not let her fall. Holding the gloved hands out to the side of each knee, instruct the patient to allow her knees to drop into your hands, or allow her legs to go limp. It is important never to force the legs apart with your hands or arms. Also, the nurse should talk through each step and let the patient know what you are going to do next.

Common and Specialty or Advanced Techniques

The routine head-to-toe assessment includes the most important and common assessment techniques. Examiners may add specialty or advanced steps if concerns exist over a specific finding. Table 26-3 summarizes the most common techniques used in the comprehensive RN assessment, which are therefore essential to learn for use in clinical practice. In clinical practice, the RN assessment includes inspecting the external genitalia. This is important because yeast infections are common during antibiotic treatment or with incontinence where there may be skin irritation. Inspection of the internal vagina, obtaining a Pap smear, and a bimanual examination are within the scope of practice of the nurse practitioner. These examinations require additional training and skill (Table 26-3).

Table 26.3	Common Versus Specialty or Advanced Techniques		
Technique	**Purpose**	**Screening or Registered Nurse Assessment**	**Focused or Advanced Practice Examination**
Inspect external genitalia	To observe for deformities, drainage, rashes, or lesions	X	
Palpate internal genitalia	To palpate vaginal wall for weakness, masses, or tumors		X
Perform speculum examination	To increase visibility of vaginal walls and cervix		X
Inspect cervix and os	To observe for redness, lesions, or drainage		X
Perform Pap smear and cultures	To detect atypical cells and cancer (Pap smear) and infections (culture)		X
Inspect vaginal wall	To inspect for lesions, irritation, drainage		X
Perform bimanual examination	To palpate for masses, tumors, pain, organs		X
Perform rectovaginal examination	To palpate vaginal wall for rectocele		X
Perform rectal examination	To palpate for masses, tumors, pain		X

Technique and Normal Findings	Abnormal Findings

External Genitalia

Inspection begins with the mons pubis. Inspect the pubic hair for amount and distribution. The pubic hair of the older woman becomes thinner with age. Look at the hair and skin for lice or nits. *Hair is evenly distributed and growing in a downward direction. No lice or nits are seen.*

Inspect the skin for any redness, breakdown, papules, or vesicles. Bilaterally observe the inguinal area for erythema, fissures, or enlarged inguinal lymph nodes. Inspect the clitoris, noting size and shape. *The clitoris is 1–1.5 cm long.*

Inspect the labia majora for size and symmetry. Look for any swelling or redness. Because both labia majora and minora are composed of sebaceous and apocrine glands, they are prone to form small inclusion cysts. These are common and may come and go without notice.

Inspect the vaginal opening for swelling or redness (Fig. 26-7). *No protrusions are seen from the vagina.*

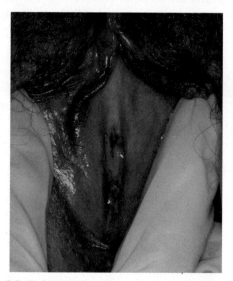

Figure 26.7 Inspecting the vaginal opening (introitus).

Inspect the vestibule for color, redness, swelling, odor, or discharge. Inspect the urethra for position and patency. *There is no discharge or redness.* Observe the Skene's glands at the 1 and 11 o'clock positions lateral to the urethra. *They are small, noninflamed, and occasionally not seen.*

Inspection is completed with the perineum. *The area between the introitus and anus is smooth with no lesions or tears. Scars from any episiotomies are healed. The anus is intact with no swelling, lacerations, or protrusions.*

Abnormal Findings:

Pediculosis pubis (crab lice) commonly presents with itching (see Table 26-6 at the end of the chapter).

Symptoms of herpes simplex virus 2 include vulvar or vaginal pain, flu-like symptoms such as chills or fever, sores on the vulva or genital region, scattered vesicles along the labia, matching vesicles on the labia reflecting "kissing" lesions, surface ulcerations or crusted healing lesions, and inguinal lymphadenopathy (see Table 26-5 at the end of the chapter).

Symptoms of condyloma acuminatum (warts) include vulvar or vaginal itching, vaginal secretions, and growths along the vagina or rectum. Examination may reveal fleshy pink or grey papilloma or wart-like projections at the vulva, vagina, or anus (see Table 26-5).

Cancer of the vulva is usually asymptomatic until the lesion becomes large enough that there may be itching, burning, pain, and bleeding or watery discharge from the lesion. Any discharge or mucus is considered abnormal and requires a culture (Kellog-Spadt, 2004).

Candidiasis is associated with vulvovaginal and possibly rectal puritus and dyspareunia. Examination may reveal vulvovaginal edema, erythemia, excoriation, and thick white secretions, sometimes only along the inner vaginal walls (see Table 26-5).

Look for abnormalities such as contact dermatitis and chancres of syphyllis (see Table 26-6).

Internal Genitalia

Using the thumb and middle finger of the gloved hand separate the inner portion of the labia minora, insert the index finger approximately 1 cm, and rotate the finger so that it is facing upward. Gently press the index finger forward to assess the urethra and Skene's glands (Fig. 26-8). Do not do this for a lengthy period because it will irritate the urethra and cause the patient discomfort.

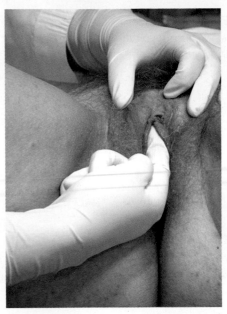

Figure 26.8 Palpating the Skene's glands and urethra.

With the index finger still inserted approximately 1 cm into the vagina, rotate the finger downward again and palpate with the index finger and the thumb finger the Bartholin's glands on each side (Fig. 26-9). The Bartholin's glands are located bilaterally in the lower labial areas at approximately 8 and 4 o'clock positions. *No swelling or tenderness is noted on either side.*

Abnormal findings include an abscess of Bartholin's gland or urethral caruncle (see Table 26-6).

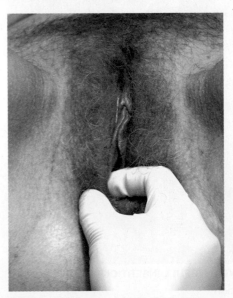

Figure 26.9 Palpating the Bartholin's glands.

(text continues on page 786)

While the finger is inserted, it is a good idea to advance it to locate the cervix. Explain to the patient what you are doing. This will help avoid inaccurate placement of the speculum around the cervix. While the index finger is still in place ask the patient to squeeze the vaginal muscles around your finger to check vaginal tone. Ask the patient to then bear down slightly to assess for pelvic organ prolapsed.

Speculum Examination

The speculum is chosen based on the patient's history, not weight or outward appearance. The speculum should be warmed in the examination table drawer if possible; if not, run the speculum under warm water. Hold the speculum between the index and middle finger of the dominant hand. Make sure the blades are pushed together and stay together during insertion to ensure comfort and to avoid pinching any part of the labia or vaginal walls between them. Place the thumb under the thumbscrew on the metal or the lever on the plastic type of speculum. The opposite hand will insert the index finger as done in the initial vaginal examination and place slight pressure downward.

The speculum is then inserted in an oblique position along the top of the finger (Fig. 26-10). A constant downward insertion prevents the anterior blade of the speculum from hitting the urethra or bladder and causing discomfort or pain. As the speculum moves in and downward, slowly remove the index finger. Have the patient exhale slowly as the speculum is inserted. This helps in relaxing the pubococcygeal muscles. Slowly rotate the speculum so that it is in a horizontal position with the bottom blade continuing to be pressed in a downward position at 45 degrees. Once the blade is completely inserted, slowly open the speculum blades while continually keeping a posterior pressure on the lower blade.

Assessment of vaginal tone is important, especially if the patient has complaints of pelvic relaxation or urinary incontinence. Pelvic organ prolapse is not limited to older women; many times, obesity and gravity are factors (Smith, 2007).

⚠ *SAFETY ALERT 26.3*
Do not use lubricants on the speculum because it can interfere with the cytology and culture readings.

⚠ *SAFETY ALERT 26.4*
Do not try to force the complete blade in if it causes the patient discomfort or pain.

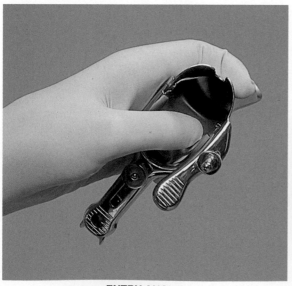
ENTRY ANGLE

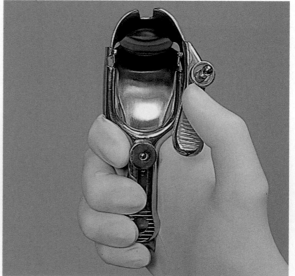
ANGLE AT FULL INSERTION

Figure 26.10 The speculum. **A.** Angle at entry. **B.** Angle at full insertion.

For most women the speculum most often used is the Pederson. The length of this speculum is approximately 6 cm, which is the usual length of the vagina. Once the speculum is inserted fully, the blades are opened slowly by pressing on the thumbpiece until the cervix comes into view at the end of the blades. As the cervix comes into view, the speculum is locked into place by tightening the screw on the thumb piece. Check with the patient at all steps to make sure she is comfortable (Fig. 26-11).

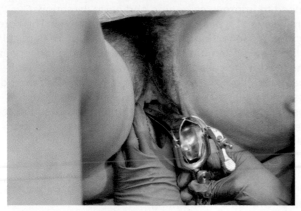

Figure 26.11 Inserting the speculum.

Cervix and Os. Inspect the cervix and vaginal walls (Fig. 26-12). *The cervix is smooth and pink and positioned midline in the vagina.* The position is based on the angle of the uterus and may tilt anteriorly or posteriorly as well. The cervix of a nulliporous woman has a small round os, while the parous woman has a horizontal or fish-mouth-looking slit. Inspect the cervix and surrounding area for increased discharge. Clear secretions are present normally and may be more or

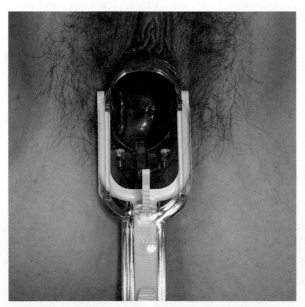

Figure 26.12 View of the normal cervix through the speculum.

If the cervix is not visualized, the speculum may be too high. Repositioning with the blades pressed posterior may be necessary.

If there have been any birth traumas, there may be a tear of the cervix resulting in an irregular slit. It is common in women who have had vaginal births to have one or several **nabothian cyst**. These small benign nodules resemble yellow pustules. These are not treated but documented as findings. There may be a small polyp at the opening or the os. It may be removed in the office and sent to pathology for testing (Fig. 26-13). Additional abnormal findings include *cervical polyps, DES syndrome, cervical dysplasia, carcinoma in situ*, and *cervical cancer* (see Table 26-8).

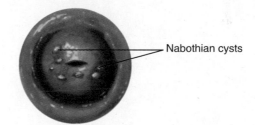

Nabothian cysts

Figure 26.13 Nabothian cysts.

(text continues on page 788)

less productive based on the woman's cycle or menstrua l history. It is best not to remove too much of this secretion because doing so may compromise cervical cells needed for the Pap smear. If the woman has an intrauterine device, this is the time to check for the strings (two strings clear in color).

Pap Smear and Cultures. The Papanicolaou (named after Dr. Nicholas Papanicolaou) or Pap smear is a screening tool for cervical neoplasia. An Ayers spatula (either wood or plastic) is used in conjunction with an endocervical brush for glass slide examinations. A plastic cytology broom is used to obtain both exocervical and endocervical cells for a liquid pap examination. The longer portion of the spatula is inserted into the cervical os and rotated 360 degrees as it is pressed against the cervix to gently scrape the cells from the **squamocolumnar junction** of the cervix (Fig. 26-14). This is also called the *transformation zone* and includes the outer and inner areas of the endocervix. It is the area of highest neoplastic involvement. Secretions obtained from the spatula are then spread on a clear glass slide and a fixative spray is applied. The endocervical brush is then inserted into the endocervix and rotated 720 degrees to ensure an adequate cell sample (Fig. 26-15). The endocervical brush is then gently rolled out on a clean glass slide, avoiding cell destruction. A spray fixative is applied and the slide labeled for cytology. If a liquid base pap is taken, the plastic broom is used. The tip of the broom inserted into the endocervix and rotated 720 degrees. The tip of the broom is removed and placed into the liquid solution (Fig. 26-16).

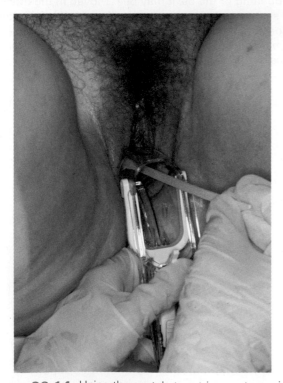

Figure 26.14 Using the spatula to retrieve ectocervical cells.

The Pap smear is used to evaluate cells from the cervix for precancerous or cancerous status. Newer technologies and techniques for obtaining the cervical cells have helped to improve screening and early detection. Currently several types of cytological testing exist. The conventional pap testing consists of acquisition of cervical cells by a wooden or plastic spatula and an endocervical brush, with the cells then "smeared" onto a slide with fixative applied. The conventional smear to slide method has a 20% false negative rate. (ACOG, 2008). Liquid-based cytology (Thin-Prep) uses similar technique except the practitioner uses a plastic spatula or broom and the cells removed are placed into a liquid solution.

Collection of cells from the endocervix or cervix may cause some spotting or bleeding; this can occur with a pap or with an STI screening.

⚠ *SAFETY ALERT 26.5*

It is important to do the Pap smear first so that bleeding is minimal on the cytology specimen. The cultures for chlamydia (CT) and gonorrhea (GC) are done after the Pap smear.

Most commonly, a DNA-based probe is used. This cultures both CT and GC at the same time. The Dacron probe is inserted into the endocervical canal and kept there for 30 seconds to 1 minute. Remove the probe, avoiding contact with vaginal secretions, and place the specimen into the culture tube.

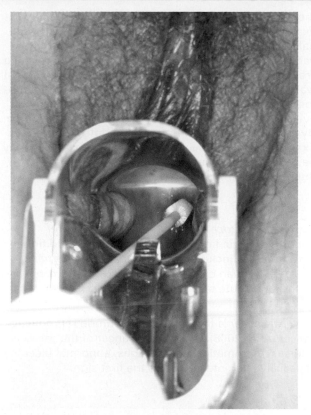

Figure 26.15 Using the endocervical brush.

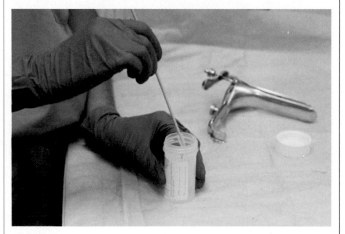

Figure 26.16 Collecting cells in the solution during liquid-based Pap testing.

Vaginal Wall. The vaginal wall is inspected during insertion and removal of the speculum. The lateral and anterioposterior walls are inspected for lesions, bleeding, erythema, or edema. In the older patient, it is not uncommon to see atrophic changes to the lining of the vagina from lack of estrogen. The examiner will notice a lack or thinning of the vaginal ruggae. This is very tender and uncomfortable and so should be examined gently. The speculum should be removed in

Any secretion abnormal in amount, color, or odor is sampled for infection (see Table 26-5). *Trichomoniasis* often presents with vaginal purities, thin or thick secretions, a foul vaginal odor, purulent yellow to green frothy discharge, pain on pelvic examination, cervical redness (strawberry looking), contact bleeding, pH > 4.5, and occasional dysuria. *Gonnorrhea* is indicated by yellow vaginal secretion, pain with urination (dysuria), and dyspareunia. In addition, there is purulent discharge from

(text continues on page 790)

the reverse order of insertion, with careful attention given to keeping the blades open until the cervix is slid away from the blades. The thumb stays on the lever and is slowly released. As the speculum is rotated to an oblique position, the blades are slowly closed avoiding pinching the vaginal walls or labia, or pulling the pubic hair.

Bimanual Examination

Inform the patient that this part of the examination is to assess the organs by manually palpating from the inside and outside the size, shape, and position of the uterus and ovaries as well as assessing general support of the organs.

At this time, the examiner removes the gloves and places a new glove on the hand doing the internal examination. The index and second fingers are inserted in a downward fashion and slowly turned upward once the fingers reach the cervix. The thumb is kept upward or tucked in during this time to keep it from pressing on the clitoris. The fingers rest internally at the posterior area of the cervix. The cervix is palpated for size, shape, and movement. The nonexamining hand is placed midway between the symphysis pubis and umbilicus (Fig. 26-17).

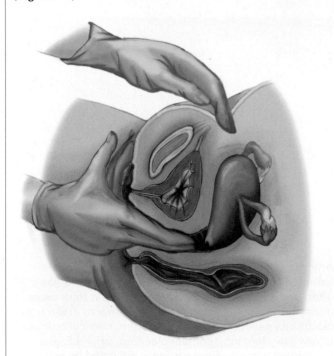

Figure 26.17 Positioning of the hands in bimanual palpation of the cervix.

the cervix and tenderness or pain with the pelvic examination. *Bacterial vaginosis* presents with vaginal secretions that have a strong "fishy" odor and vaginal itching or burning. Examination may reveal a creamy white to gray secretion that coats the vaginal walls (Elkins, et al., 2006). *Chlamydia* is often asymptomatic. Occasional clear or white secretion may be evident, and there may be bleeding after intercourse. Dyspareunia (pain with intercourse) may be present. Examination shows changes in the cervix, which may be reddened or bleed easily. There may be pain with the pelvic examination.

Cystocele, rectocele, and *uterine prolapse* are abnormal pelvic findings (see Table 26-7). Additional abnormalities include *endometriosis, leimyoma* (fibroid), *ovarian cyst,* solid ovarian mass, ectopic pregnancy, and acute salpingitis. These may or may not be related to pain.

Cervical cancer is the third most common reproductive cancer (ACS, 2008). Preinvasive cancer of the cervix is often asymptomatic. In later stages, abnormal bleeding, especially after intercourse, is the first sign.

The uterus is now palpated between the pads of the fingertips. The uterus is moved upward so that the examining fingers can palpate between the top and back of the uterus (Fig. 26-18). This position allows for evaluation of the size and shape of the uterus as well as its ability to move without tenderness or resistance. *Normal size is approximately 7 x 4 cm (size is occasionally larger in mulitgravid women). The uterus feels pear shaped and smooth and is freely mobile.*

Leiomyomas (fibroid tumors) can cause abnormal uterine bleeding and backage, abdominal pressure, constipation, incontinence, and dysmenorrhea if large.

Endometrial cancer is the most common malignancy of the reproductive system (ACS, 2008) and is associated with abnormal uterine bleeding, uterine enlargement, or mass.

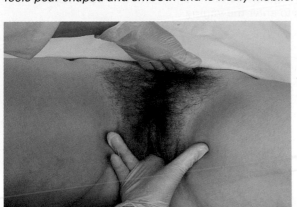

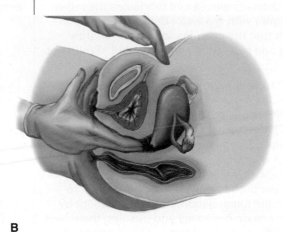

A   B

Figure 26.18 Bimanual palpation of the uterus. **A.** External view. **B.** Internal position of the hands.

Once the uterus has been assessed, let the patient know that you are now going to check her ovaries. With the two fingers still deep in the vagina and facing upward, move to the lateral side of the uterus. If the right hand is examining, the fingers move first to the patient's right and the hand on the abdomen is placed medial to the anterior superior iliac spine. The two hands are brought together as close as possible. With a slow sweeping motion, the fingers are moved down toward the introitus while allowing the adnexae to be palpated between them (Fig. 26-19). This is repeated on the patient's left side. The palpation is done quickly and gently. *The ovary is often not felt, especially in older*

With *ovarian cyst*, there may be pain, tenderness over the ovary, irregular menses, and intraperitoneal bleeding if it ruptures. A solid ovarian mass raises the possibility of ovarian cancer, which is the second most frequent reproductive cancer (ACS, 2008).

⚠ SAFETY ALERT 26.6

In an ectopic pregnancy, the most common symptoms are lower quadrant pain, nausea, and referred pain in the neck or shoulder from blood beneath the diaphragm. If severe hemorrhage occurs, the patient is at risk for shock.

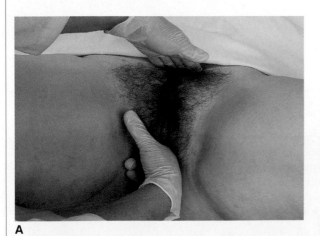

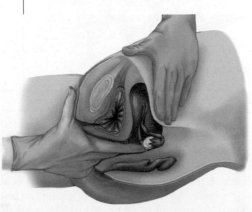

A   B

Figure 26.19 Bimanual palpation of the ovaries. **A.** External view. **B.** Internal position of the hands.

(text continues on page 792)

menopausal women. *If palpated, it feels like a small almond.* As stated above, this part of the examination should be brief because the ovaries are similar to gonads in their sensitivity.

Rectovaginal Examination

After completing the vaginal examination, circumstances may warrant a rectovaginal examination (see Chapter 25 for a complete rectal examination). The examiner changes gloves and lubricates the index and middle fingers with the water-based gel. He or she tells the patient that the examination will be slightly uncomfortable and may create pressure, but should not be painful.

Ask the patient to bear down slightly as the fingers are inserted. The index finger is inserted into the vagina and the middle finger is placed into the rectum (Fig. 26-20). *The septum is palpated with the two fingers and feels smooth and intact. The posterior portion of the uterus may be felt and is smooth.* Withdraw the gloved fingers and keep the hand lower while removing the glove and disposing it. Have tissues available for the patient to clean with after the examination. Assist the patient by placing your hands on her knees and pushing them back on the table. At the same time, extend your hand to help her sit up.

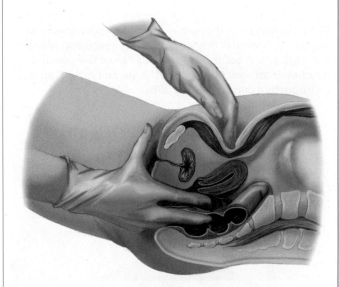

Figure 26.20 Rectovaginal examination.

Salpingitis is also referred to as *pelvic inflammatory disease.* Infection spreads throughout the uterus and up into the tubes. See Table 26-9.

This examination is used to evaluate any *rectocele* (bulging of rectum into the vagina) or *rectovaginal fistula* (opening between the vagina and the rectum allowing feces to enter the vagina).

Documentation of Normal Findings

External genitalia: Even hair distribution, no lesions present. Bartholin's glands, urethra, and Skene's glands (BUS): with no erythema, edema, or discharge. Vaginal introitus and walls: pink, moist with normal ruggae, good anterior and posterior wall support, no discharge present. Cervix: smooth round with no lesions and no tenderness upon movement. Uterus: normal size, shape, mid position, and freely mobile. Adnexa: No palpable masses, no tenderness to examination. Perineum: smooth. Anal area: pink, with no hemorrhoids, fissures, or bleeding. Rectal wall: smooth without masses or nodules, and good sphincter control.
F. Robbins, RN

The nurse has just finished a physical examination of Teresa Nguyen, the 28-year-old being seen with vaginal drainage and pelvic pain. Unlike the samples of normal documentation previously charted, Ms. Nguyen has abnormal findings. Review the following important findings revealed in each of the steps of objective data collection for her. Consider how these results compare with the normal findings presented in the samples of normal documentation. Begin to think about how the data cluster together and what additional data the nurse might want to collect as the nurse thinks critically about her problems and anticipates nursing interventions. This note is documented by the nurse practitioner who will work collaboratively with the RN.

Inspection: External genitalia has even hair distribution, no lesions present. BUS with no erythema, edema, or discharge. Vaginal introitus and walls pink, moist with normal ruggae, good anterior and posterior wall support, moderate clear discharge present.

Palpation: Cervix smooth round and red, some tenderness upon movement. Clear drainage present. Uterus normal size, shape, mid position, and freely mobile. Adnexa with no palpable masses, but positive tenderness to examination. Perineum smooth. Anal area pink, with no hemorrhoids, fissures, or bleeding present. Nonspecific tenderness present over lower half of abdomen during bimanual examination.

S. Captaris, APRN

Lifespan Considerations

Pregnant Woman

The physical examination of the pregnant female is discussed in Chapter 27. To review quickly, the first assessment the nurse makes is whether the membranes are ruptured or not. This can be done by inspection, in the case of gross rupture; using nitrazine (either paper or swab) to test the pH of the discharge; or through a sterile speculum examination if the nurse has received special training. Vaginal examinations by the nurse are deferred if the membranes are ruptured, especially if the patient does not appear to be in active labor.

Even with ruptured membranes, the nurse would perform a vaginal examination if requested to do so by the provider, or if he or she suspected that birth might be imminent. The nurse documents cervical dilation (in centimeters), effacement (in centimeters), station (degree of descent into the pelvis of the presenting part), consistency of the cervix (firm, medium, soft) and position (posterior, mid position, anterior). Together, these values can be used to calculate a Bishop's score. A Bishop's score above 9 suggests that vaginal birth is very likely, even if induction or augmentation is necessary.

Child

Allow the parent to hold the child and have the child place her feet together positioned like a frog. Allow the child to take part in the examination. Have the parent let the child know it is OK to allow this examination by a practitioner, especially if she has been taught not to allow anyone to touch her genitals.

Adolescent

Ask the patient if she would like her mother or a friend to be present during the examination. Provide a mirror so that she may observe the examination and have opportunities to ask questions. By placing the examining finger just at the posterior fourchettte and gently pressing downward, the pubococcygeal muscle will gradually relax allowing the insertion of the finger. The patient can identify the muscles to relax when the practitioner is inserting the speculum. Do a one-finger vaginal examination before inserting the speculum. This allows the practitioner the ability to estimate the vaginal capacity as well as the position of the cervix and ensures a more comfortable examination. Inform her that the speculum you will use will be no larger than your index finger, which she just felt. Avoid using words such as "pain"; instead use words such as "mild pressure" (Hewitt, 2006).

Older Adult

Menopause usually occurs between 48 and 51 years, although variability is wide. The ovaries stop producing estrogen and progesterone, causing the uterus to droop and the cervix to shrink. There is a thinning of the genital hair, thinning and loss of elasticity of vaginal mucosa, and diminished vaginal secretions as a result of lower estrogen levels. The fat pads atrophy and the labia and clitoris decrease in size.

Evidence-Based Critical Thinking

The RN and APRN work collaboratively to provide care for a patient with issues related to the female genital system. After collecting data, abnormal findings and health promotion areas will be identified. The data will be clustered to reveal significant patterns and make clinical judgments about outcomes and potential interventions.

Common Laboratory and Diagnostic Testing

Because the annual gynecological visit by the female patient is commonly the only physical examination she has, complete laboratory work will be done, including tests for anemia, cholesterol, thyroid, diabetes, and to rule out elevated WBC's in the case of infections. A urinalysis is commonly done at each visit. If the patient has signs or symptoms of urinary tract problems, a clean catch urinalysis and culture and sensitivity are done. If the patient is having any bleeding or lack of menses, a serum hCG is drawn to rule out pregnancy. The wet mount analysis of vaginal secretions is done to identify what, if any, vaginal infections are present. A slide is made with the vaginal secretions and either or both single drop of KOH and saline. The examination findings are then matched with the signs and symptoms and the wet mount findings. Blood tests, such as LH, FSH, and GnRH, are drawn if there are any endocrine irregularities. The vaginal and abdominal ultrasounds are the gold standard diagnostic tests for abnormalities of the fallopian tubes, ovaries, uterus, and the endometrial lining. More in-depth testing is done if the woman has infertility problems.

The American Cancer Society's current Pap smear screening recommendations are as follows. For initial screening, women should undergo a Pap test within 3 years of onset of sexual activity or at age 21 (whichever comes first). Women who have no sexual activity should still be screened. Women younger than 30 years should have a pap annually. Women older than 30 years who have three normal Pap tests in a row

have two options. They may receive a liquid-based pap every 2 to 3 years; but if the patient has any history of DES exposure, HIV, or any previous cervical cancer diagnosis, she should continue annual pap testing. The second option is to receive a screening with a liquid-based pap and a HPV DNA hybrid capture (HC2) testing. This hybrid capture is a culture specifically for the HPV virus. If both tests are normal, the patient can go 3 years without screening. The American Cancer Society recommends discontinuation of pap testing after 70 years. Women who have had total hysterectomy (for noncancerous reason) do not require pap testing (ACS, 2008).

Nursing Diagnosis, Outcomes, and Interventions

The formation of the nursing diagnosis is based on all the information given. Many times, it is considered a presumptive diagnosis, especially if the patient has multiple problems. Validation of the data is needed in order to analyze the findings and the subsequent management of the patient's symptoms. The nurse sees not only the condition of the patient but the possibilities for education and long-term benefits to the patient. Table 26-4 provides a comparison of nursing diagnoses, abnormal findings, and interventions commonly related to assessment of the female genitalia (NANDA-I, 2009).

Nurses use assessment information to identify patient outcomes. Some outcomes that are related to female genitalia problems include the following:

- Expresses ability to perform sexually despite physical imperfections
- States the risk factors for, causes of, and ways to prevent STIs

Table 26.4 Common Nursing Diagnoses Associated with the Female Genital System			
Diagnosis and Related Factors	**Point of Differentiation**	**Assessment Characteristics**	**Nursing Interventions**
Ineffective sexuality patterns related to illness and altered body function	Limitations from disease or therapy, alteration in sex role, change in interest of self or others	Altered body function, recent childbirth, reproductive surgery, medications, abuse	Gather sexual history. Determine patient and partner's knowledge. Observe for stress, loss, or depression. Explore physical causes with chronic disease.
Risk for infection	Potential for invasion by pathogens	Chronic illness, unsafe practices, rupture of amniotic membranes, recent surgery	Consider risk for MRSA. Observe and report signs of infection. Use appropriate hand hygiene and follow standard precautions. Avoid use of indwelling catheters when possible.
Ineffective health maintenance related to deficient knowledge	Lack of adaptation to changes, lack of knowledge, lack of interest in improving health behaviors	Inability to make appropriate judgments, ineffective family coping, unachieved developmental tasks	Assess the patient's feelings about not following safe practices. Assess family patterns. Assist the patient to community groups. Assess access to health services.

*Collaborative interventions.

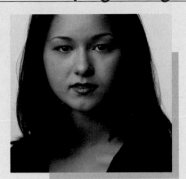

Remember Teresa Nguyen, whose problems have been outlined throughout this chapter. The initial subjective and objective data collection is complete, and the nurse practitioner has spent time reviewing the findings and other results. Unfortunately, Ms. Nguyen has a Chlamydia infection, so it is necessary for the nurse practitioner to treat her with antibiotics. The following nursing note illustrates how data are collected and treatment is prescribed by the nurse.

Subjective: States has pelvic pain and vaginal discharge. Increased during intercourse. Is present in the lower half of the abdomen, increases with palpation. States is 3/10 at rest, 8/10 with intercourse. Has had pain for 2 weeks, increasing in intensity. Pain has limited intercourse over the past 1½ weeks. Taking acetaminophen for pain with minimal effect. States that discharge is clear and increasing in amount.

Objective: Temperature 38.8°C orally, appears flushed. Culture is positive for *C. trachomatis*. White blood cell count and erythrocyte sedimentation rate elevated.

Analysis: Knowledge deficit related to *C. trachomatis* infection.

Plan: Obtain prescription for broad-spectrum antibiotic. Teach to take acetaminophen for pain and fever, drink 2 L of fluid and get additional rest. Teach to abstain from intercourse until treatment is complete. Assess knowledge level of safe sexual practices and provide accurate information. Report results to public health department and initiate partner notification process. Allow time for her to express her feelings and role play the words she will use when talking with partner.

L. Losey, RN

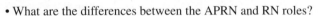

Critical Thinking Challenge

- What are the differences between the APRN and RN roles?
- What nursing diagnoses might be appropriate given the new medical diagnosis?
- How will the effects on Teresa, her family, and her partner be assessed? What specific questions would the nurse ask?

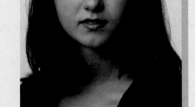

Teresa Nguyen will need to have further teaching based upon her new diagnosis. Unfortunately, the nurse assesses that Teresa does not have coverage to pay for the prescription. The following conversation illustrates how the nurse might communicate with pharmacy to get funding.

Situation: Hi, I'm Linda in the clinic and have a patient who does not have money to pay for her prescription.

Background: She hasn't been here before and was just diagnosed with PID and Chlamydia infection. The nurse practitioner has prescribed an antibiotic and Tylenol for symptoms.

Assessment: She needs to get started on antibiotics soon, and I would like her to have them before she leaves today.

Recommendations: Do you have any programs that she would be eligible for free or reduced price prescriptions?

Critical Thinking Challenge

- What additional issues should be assessed when considering her future care?
- What questions will the nurse use to assess Teresa's knowledge of PID and Chlamydia?
- What will be the top three priorities of assessment and teaching?

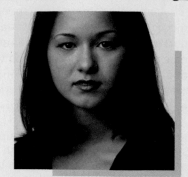

The nurse uses assessment data to formulate a nursing care plan with patient outcomes and interventions. Outcomes are specific to the patient, realistic to achieve, measurable, and have a time frame for completion. After interventions are completed, the nurse reevaluates and documents the findings in the chart to show progress toward the patient outcome. The nurse uses critical thinking and judgment to continue or revise the diagnosis, outcomes, or interventions. This is often in the form of a care plan or case note similar to the one below.

Nursing Diagnosis	Patient Outcomes	Nursing Interventions	Rationale	Evaluation
Anxiety related to effects on sexual relationships and family processes	Patient states that she feels prepared to discuss situation with partner. Patient identifies one person with whom she feels comfortable sharing her concerns.	Rehearse words to use when telling partner about infection. Discuss which family or friends she would feel comfortable talking with. Offer assistance and time for processing the issues.	Practicing in advance can reduce anxiety. Talking about her concerns is therapeutic. During the initial crisis, the nurse can provide therapeutic communication.	Expressing anger at boyfriend and feeling betrayed. Able to state she feels prepared to notify partner. Has a sister who is very supportive that she can talk with. Given phone number to clinic if she has questions or needs to talk more.

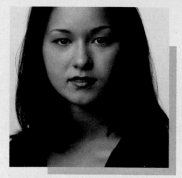

Using the previous steps of diagnostic reasoning, organizing, and prioritizing, consider all the case study findings woven throughout this chapter for Teresa Nguyen. When answering the following questions, begin drawing conclusions and see how the pieces of assessment must work together to create an environment for personalized, appropriate, and accurate care.

- What is the role of the nurse in assessing physiological symptoms versus psychosocial issues?
- What are some questions that the nurse should ask? What language or words might the nurse use?
- What cultural considerations should the nurse incorporate into the care provided?

- States disease process, treatment effects, and side effects (Moorhead, et al., 2007).

Once the outcomes area established, nursing care is implemented to improve the status of the patient. Some examples of nursing interventions for the female genitalia are as follows:

- Normalize the experience of problems related to sensitive sexual topics and allow time for patient to express concerns.
- Offer a variety of options for safe sex practices to provide choices and promote respect for differences.

- Teach about disease process, treatment effects, side effects, and expected outcomes (Bulechek, et al., 2007).

The nurse evaluates the care according to the patient outcomes that were developed, therefore reassessing the patient and continuing or modifying the interventions as appropriate. This is a sensitive and embarrassing topic for many patients and their nurses. It is important to include the psychosocial dimensions and become comfortable talking about the topic. The process can be modified to the individual so that outcomes can be positive for all those involved.

Key Points

- Examination of the female genitalia provides opportunity for open communication, exchange of information, and education between patient and nurse.
- Women have ongoing needs and concerns throughout the lifespan.
- Evidence-based research and protocols are the driving forces for health promotion and disease prevention.
- *Healthy People* has specific indicators by which the U.S. government hopes to shape the trends in communities towards healthy life choices.
- A genital examination does not need to cause anxiety or pain; through empathetic exchange and respect, the nurse can make it a positive experience.
- Adolescents struggle with issues of self-esteem to early experimentation with drugs, sex, and risk-taking behaviors. Nurses can attend to the physiologic and psychological needs of the adolescent female during this annual visit.
- The older female represents a great portion of the female population. As the average life span becomes greater, nurses must stay current with newer screening, therapeutics, and interventions that allow the greatest quality of life.

Review Questions

1. The nurse is taking a menstrual history. What would be an appropriate question to ask?
   A. Do you have any history of cancer in your family?
   B. Do you ever skip periods?
   C. Do you use condoms during intercourse?
   D. How many sexual partners have you had?

2. The nurse is inspecting the urethra and the Skene's glands. She knows these are a part of what area?
   A. Mons pubis
   B. Vulva
   C. Posterior fourchette
   D. Vestibule

3. An annual Pap smear is recommended to screen for what condition?
   A. Cervical cancer
   B. Ovarian cancer
   C. Endometrial cancer
   D. Vaginal cancer

4. After completing a history on a 45-year-old patient, the nurse suspects she may have uterine fibroids. What information might have led her to this?
   A. History of STIs
   B. History of multiple births
   C. Vaginal discharge
   D. Heavier than usual menstrual periods

5. The practitioner has decided to place the patient on Accutane for her acne problems. The nurse is going to counsel the patient. What is the most important information she needs to tell the patient?
   A. She needs to take the medication daily and avoid missing a dose.
   B. She should not take this medication with antibiotics.
   C. She needs to be on two forms of birth control or abstain 1 month before, during, and 1 month after taking this medication.
   D. She needs to take a weekly pregnancy test to make sure she hasn't gotten pregnant while on this medication.

6. What is the organism that contributes to salpingitis?
   A. Trichinosis
   B. *C. trachomatis*
   C. *Candida albicans*
   D. *Condyloma acuminata*

7. The nurse is preparing the patient for her examination. What position will the nurse assist the patient into for a comfortable genital examination?
   A. Semi-Fowler's
   B. Prone with her knees bent
   C. Supine with her knees bent
   D. Semi-lithotomy

8. The nurse is a part of a health-promotion fair. One of the guests asks her what the greatest killer of women is. The nurse knows by current evidence that it is
   A. cardiovascular disease
   B. lung cancer
   C. breast cancer
   D. osteoporosis

9. What other tests would the nurse know is important in a woman with frequent candidiasis?
   A. Cultures for chlamydia
   B. Blood test for glucose
   C. Blood test for syphilis
   D. Vaginal ultrasound

10. Upon inspection, the nurse sees flesh-colored lesions surrounding the anal area. What are these most likely indicative of?
    A. Hemorrhoids
    B. Herpes simplex II
    C. AIDS
    D. *C. acuminata*

References

American Cancer Society. (2008). *Cancer facts and figures 2008.* Atlanta, GA: Author.

American College of Obstetricians and Gynecologists (ACOG). (2008). *Revised cervical cancer screening guidelines require reeducation of women and physicians.* Retrieved March 9, 2008, from http://acog.org

American Diabetes Association (ADA). (2008). *Nutritional recommendations and interventions for diabetes.* Retrieved February 17, 2008, from http://care.diabetesjournals.org

Amin, S. H., Kuhle, C. L., & Fitzpatrick, L. A. (2003). Comprehensive evaluation of the older woman. *Mayo Clinic Proceedings, 78,* 1157–1185.

Anderson, S. E., & Must, A. (2005). Interpreting the continued decline in the average at menarche: Research from two nationally representative surveys of U.S. girls studied 10 years apart. *Journal of Pediatrics, 147*(12), 753–760.

Bader, T. (2005). *OB/GYN Secrets* (3rd ed.). Philadelphia: Elsevier Mosby.

Barron, A., & Falsetti, D. (2008). Polycystic ovary syndrome in adolescents: A hormonal barrage and metabolic upheaval. *Advance for Nurse Practitioners, 16*(3), 49–53.

Bulechek, G. B., Butcher, H. K., & McCloskey Dochterman, J. (2007). *Nursing Interventions Classification (NIC)* (4th ed.). St Louis: Mosby.

Burns, N., Briggs, P., & Gaudet, C. (2007). Chlamydia screening in teenage girls. *The Nurse Practitioner, 32*(6), 41–43.

CDC. (2008). *The History of DES.* Retrieved June 26, 2008, from http://www.cdc.gov/DES/hcp/nurse/history

Clark, B., & Marrazzo, J. (2006). Reproductive health and sexually transmitted infections in lesbian women. *The Female Patient, 31*(8), 38–40.

Curtis, M., Overholt, S., & Hopkins, M. (2005). *Glass' office gynecology* (6th ed.). Philadelphia: Lippincott Williams & Wilkins.

Elkins, B., Mayeaux, E. J., & Koduru, S. (2006). *Bacterial vaginosis*: Diagnosis and therapy. *The Female Patient, 31*(8), 41–46.

FDA. (2006). *iPLEDGE information.* Retrieved June 22, 2010, from http://www.fda.gov/Drugs/DrugSafety/Postmarket DrugSafetyInformationforPatientsandProviders/ucm094307.htm

Hahm, H. C., Lee, J., & Ozonoff, A. (2007). Predictors of STDs among Asian and Pacific Islander young adults. *Perspectives on Sexual and Reproductive Health, 39*(4), 231–239.

Hewitt, G. (2006). The young woman's initial gynecologic visit. *The Female Patient, 31*(9), 25–29.

Kellogg-Spadt, S. (2004). Performing a comprehensive external genital exam. *Women's Health Care: A Practical Journal for Nurse Practitioners, 3*(1), 18–19.

Kolesar, J. (2004). Clinical implications of BRCA1and BRCA2 genes in hereditary breast and ovarian cancer. *The Female Patient, 29*(6), 39–45.

Laumbach, S. (2004). Detecting domestic violence: To screen or not to screen? *The Female Patient, 29*(6), 30–34.

Low Dog, T., (2005). *Women's health in complementary and integrative medicine.* St. Louis, Mo: Elsevier.

Marshall, W. A., & Tanner, J. M. (1969). Variations in pattern of pubertal changes in girls. *Archives of Diseases in Childhood, 44*(235), 291–303.

Martin, J. (2008). Do women comply with recommendations for Papanicolaou smears following colposcopy? *Journal of Midwifery & Women's Health, 53*(2), 138–142.

Medscape. (2010). *HPV cervical vaccine and resource center.* Retrieved March 2, 2010, from http://www.medscape.com/resource/hpv-cervical-cancer

Moorhead, S., Johnson, M., & Mass, M. (2007). *Nursing Outcomes Classification (NOC)* (4th ed.). Philadelphia: Mosby.

Mosca, C, et al. (2007). Evidence-based guidelines for cardiovascular disease prevention in women. 2007 Update. *Circulation Journal of the American Heart Association, 115,* 1481–1501.

National Osteoporosis Foundation. (2008). *America's bone health: Physician's guide to prevention and treatment of osteoporosis.* Retrieved April 8, 2008, from www.nof.org

North American Nursing Diagnosis Association. (2009). *Nursing diagnoses, 2009–2011 Edition: Definitions and classifications (NANDA NURSING DIAGNOSIS).* West Sussex UK: John Wiley & Sons.

Smith, D. A. (2007). Pelvic organ prolapse. *Advance for Nurse Practitioners, 15*(8) 39–42.

Speroff, L. & Fritz, M. A. (2005). *The clinical gynecology and infertility* (7th ed.). Philadelphia: Lippincott.

U.S. Census Bureau. (2007). *National population estimates.* Retrieved March 22, 2008, from www.census.gov/popest/national/asrh

U.S. Department of Health and Human Services. (2008). *Bone health and osteoporosis: A report of the Surgeon General.* Retrieved April 8, 2008, from http://www.surgeongeneral.gov/library/bonehealth

U.S. Department of Health and Human Services, Center for Disease Control and Prevention, National Center for Health Statistics. (n.d.). *Healthy People 2010.* Retrieved March 22, 2008, from http://healthypeople.gov/document

---

The Jensen suite offers these additional resources to enhance learning and facilitate understanding of this chapter:

- thePoint on line resource, http//thepoint.lww.com/Jensen1E
- Student CD-ROM included with the book
- *Laboratory Manual for Nursing Health Assessment: A Best Practice Approach*
- *Pocket Guide for Nursing Health Assessment: A Best Practice Approach*

Table 26.5 Common Infections

Condition and Presentation	Physical Examination and Wet Mount Findings	Diagnostic Follow-up
Candidiasis 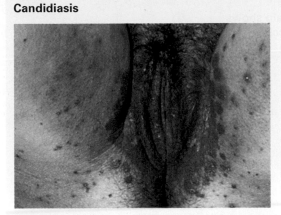 The patient reports vulvovaginal and possibly rectal puritus and dyspareunia. Vaginal secretions can be thick or thin.	*Examination:* Vulvovaginal edema, erythemia, and excoriation; thick white secretions, sometime only along inner vaginal walls *Wet Mount:* Pseudohyphae, occasional budding yeast	If chronic infection needs serum glucose to rule out diabetes and possibly HIV testing (seem often in immunocompromised patients)
Bacterial Vaginosis 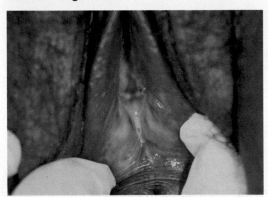 Signs and symptoms include vaginal secretions with a strong "fishy" odor and vaginal itching or burning.	*Examination:* Creamy white to gray secretions that coats the vaginal walls *Wet Mount:* Positive findings of clue cells on microscopy; possibly WBCs present as well	Positive amine (fishy odor) when secretion is mixed with KOH pH > 4.5 Gram stain
Chlamydia 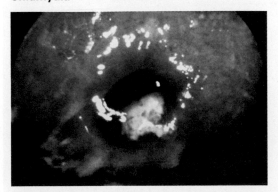 Many times, this is asymptomatic, although there are occasionally clear or white secretions. The patient reports dyspareunia, bleeding after intercourse, or both.	*Examination:* Changes in the cervical condition—reddened, mucopurulent from os, may bleed easily; possibly pain with pelvic examination *Wet Mount:* Increased WBCs and RBCs on slide	DNA probe for CT and GC Serology for syphilis HIV testing Hepatitis B and C testing

(table continues on page 800)

Table 26.5   Common Infections (continued)

Condition and Presentation	Physical Examination and Wet Mount Findings	Diagnostic Follow-up
Gonorrhea 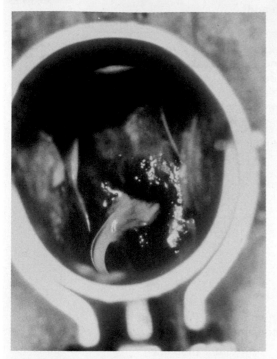 Vaginal secretions are yellow. The patient reports pain with urination (dysuria) and dyspareunia.	*Examination:* Purulent discharge from the cervix; tenderness or pain with the pelvic examination *Wet Mount:* Gram stain shows intracellular diplococci	Same testing as Chlamydia
Trichomoniasis 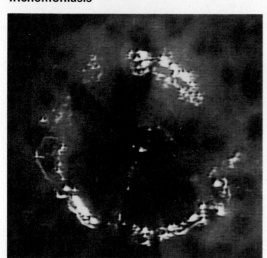 The patient has vaginal pruritis, thin or thick vaginal secretions, a foul vaginal odor, and occasionally dysuria.	*Examination:* Purulent yellow to green frothy discharge with foul odor; pain on pelvic examination; cervical redness (strawberry looking) and contact bleeding *Wet Mount:* Motile organisms >10 WBCs per high powered microscopy	Cultures for CT, GC Serology for syphilis. HIV testing UA

Table 26.5 Common Infections (*continued*)

Condition and Presentation	Physical Examination and Wet Mount Findings	Diagnostic Follow-up
Herpes Simplex Type 2 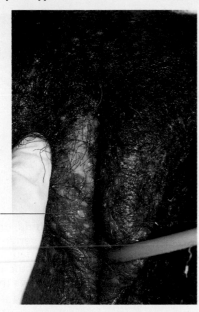 Shallow ulcers on red bases The patient reports vulvar or vaginal pain, flu-like symptoms (eg, chills, fever), and sores on the vulva or in the genital region.	*Examination:* Scattered vesicles along labia or matching vesicles on labia reflecting "kissing" lesions; surface ulcerations or crusted healing lesions; inguinal lymphadenopathy *Wet Mount:* >10 WBCs per high-powered microscopy	Viral culture from freshly incised vesicle Serology for syphilis HIV testing
Condyloma Acuminatum 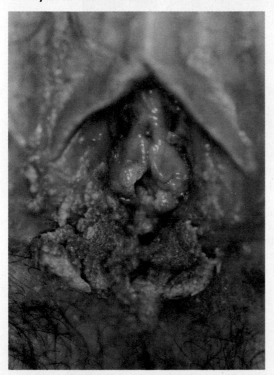 Common reports include vulvar or vaginal itching, vaginal secretions, and growths along the vagina or rectum.	*Examination:* Fleshy pink or grey papilloma or wart-like projections at vulva, vagina, or anus *Wet Mount:* Direct visualization	Application of 5% acetic acid (white vinegar) enhances visibility

Table 26-6 Abnormalities of the External Genitalia

Problems with the external genitalia can be isolated or part of another infectious process involving the internal genitalia as well. Listed are some examples of external findings.

Pediculosis Pubis (Crab Lice)

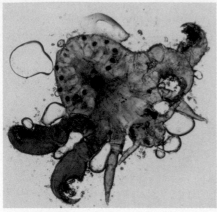

The patient presents with mild to severe itching, especially in the mons pubis and perineum. The external genitalia are excoriated based on the amount of itching. Tiny spots of blood may be seen on the underwear and possible lice not only on the underwear but around the pubis. Nits, which are the eggs, normally adhere to the pubic hair and can appear as small dark specks or may be translucent. The photo is an enlarged view of a single louse.

Chancre

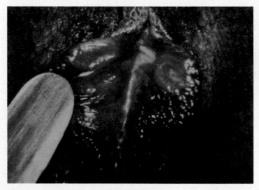

Seen in primary syphilis, this 1-cm button-like papule forms at the area of inoculation. This painless lesion with raised borders has a center of serous exudate. Present for 10–90 days.

Abscess of the Bartholin Gland

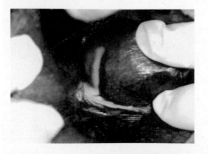

Urethral Caruncle

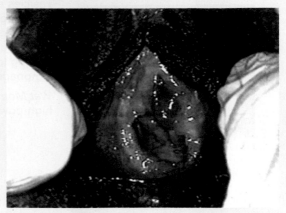

The patient usually has dysuria, **hematuria**, or frequently no response to antibiotics given for UTI. This condition is seen primarily in postmenopausal women. The caruncle develops from **ectropion** of the posterior urethral wall, which commonly develops as the vaginal tissue atrophies.

Contact Dermatitis

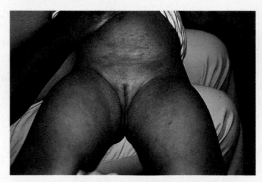

The patient has acute symptoms of external itching or burning, which may extend to the inner thigh. The perineum may be erythematous and possibly excoriated. Occasionally, the perineum has localized wheals or vesicles with possible drainage where the source of the inflammation came in contact with it. Scented sanitary pads can cause this type of inflammatory response, which will appear in the shape of the pad.

The patient has pain or tenderness in the Bartholin's area. Some abscesses develop gradually but usually very quickly within 2–3 days. They may rupture spontaneously or may need to be incised and drained.

Table 26.7 **Pelvic Organ Prolapse Conditions**

Cystocele

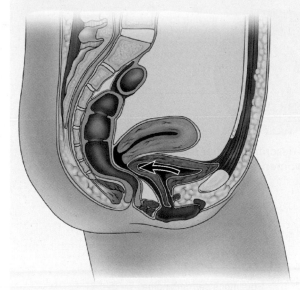

Protrusion of the bladder into the anterior vaginal canal and beyond is most common in women 40 years and older. It usually results from weakening of the supporting pelvic tissues (Smith, 2007). To evaluate this condition, the patient needs to be examined while standing as well as while lying down. The patient may have such symptoms as stress incontinence, urge incontinence, and discomfort with intercourse.

Rectocele

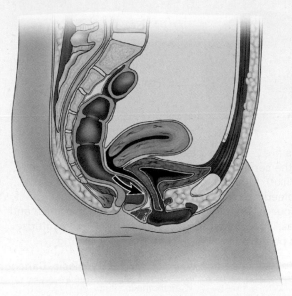

Prolapse of the rectum into the posterior vaginal wall can result from a lack of pelvic tissue support, which commonly follows lengthy vaginal labors and births. The patient has difficulty with bowel movements, pain with intercourse, and rectal pressure.

Uterine Prolapse

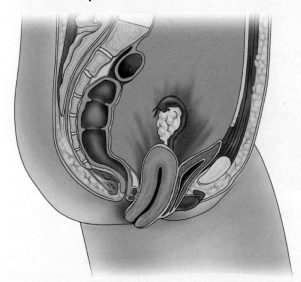

Descent of the uterus into the vagina and beyond results from pelvic relaxation and gradual weakening of uterine ligaments supporting the uterus. It may be a consequence of multiple vaginal births or an enlarging uterus. The patient presents with low pressure, fecal impaction, and vaginal and uterine irritation.

Cervical Polyps

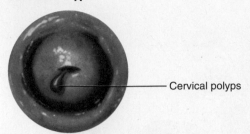

Cervical polyps

Polyps are 2–5 cm red lesions that sit at or protrude from the cervical os. Some polyps are pedunculated (stalk like). Most are benign. The patient may present with bleeding between menses or bleeding after intercourse. The polyp can be removed in the office and the base touched with silver nitrate AgNO$_3$ to cauterize it. The polyp is then set to pathology for testing.

DES Syndrome

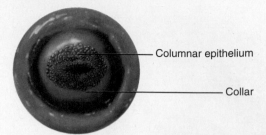

Columnar epithelium

Collar

DES as described earlier caused changes in the cervix in some women who were exposed to it.

Cervical Dysplasia, Caricnoma In Situ, and Cervical Cancer

Carcinoma in situ

Squamous cell carcinoma

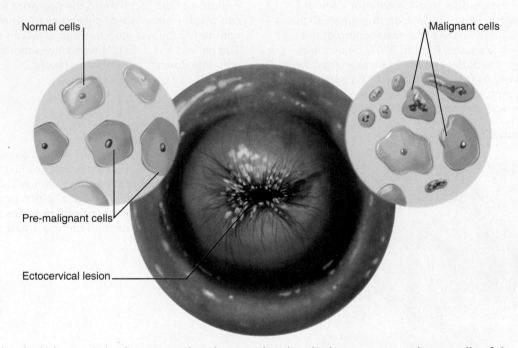

Normal cells

Malignant cells

Pre-malignant cells

Ectocervical lesion

- Cervical dysplasia is a neoplastic process that does not involve the basement membrane cells of the cervix. It may also be referred to as cervical intraepithelial neoplasia.
- Carcinoma in situ involves the full thickness of the epithelium.
- Cervical cancer is the diagnosis when carcinoma in situ invades the basement membrane.

Table 26.9   Abnormalities of the Internal Reproductive Organs

Endometriosis

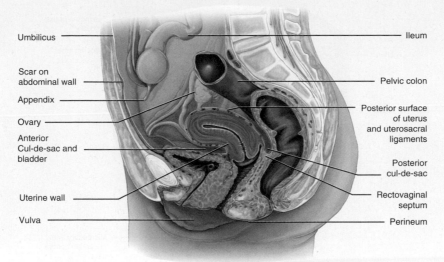

Umbilicus

Scar on
abdominal wall

Appendix

Ovary

Anterior
Cul-de-sac and
bladder

Uterine wall

Vulva

Ileum

Pelvic colon

Posterior surface
of uterus
and uterosacral
ligaments

Posterior
cul-de-sac

Rectovaginal
septum

Perineum

Endometrial tissue is found outside the uterus because of a retrograde flow of menstruation into the peritoneal cavity. This tissue adheres to other organs and causes pelvic pain, dyspareunia, dysmenorrhea, and many times infertility. Treatments range from drug therapy to surgical removal.

Leiomyoma: Uterine Fibroids

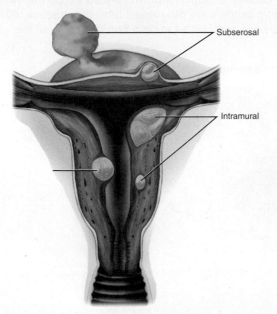

Subserosal

Intramural

This benign (99%) condition of the uterus and uterine walls appears as single or multiple tumors within the wall of the uterus, often extending from it on stalks (pedunculated). Fibroids are suspected when a patient presents with heavy flows, irregular bleeding, or pelvic pressure. Many women with fibroids are asymptomatic. Symptoms guide intervention, which usually involves surgery. If a woman is considering pregnancy and has fibroids >8 cm, surgical removal prepregnancy is often advised. Uterine fibroids are estrogen sensitive, which means they often enlarge with exposure to estrogen. Fibroids occur in 25% of Caucasian women and 50% of African American women (USDHHS, 2008).

Fluctuant Ovarian Cyst

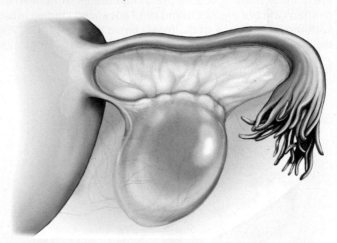

The ovarian follicle fails to rupture during the maturation phase. A fluid-filled cyst develops and either stays the same size or grows to be greater than the ovaries. The patient does not ovulate and has secondary amenorrhea (no menses). The cysts usually resolve spontaneously within two cycles. If the cyst enlarges, the patient presents with amenorrhea and low pelvic tenderness. Once pregnancy is ruled out and an ultrasound is done to confirm the presence and size of the cyst, treatment is implemented. Most commonly, the patient is put on two or more cycles of a low-dose hormone contraceptive to suppress the gonadotropin stimulation of the cyst.

(table continues on page 806)

Solid Ovarian Mass

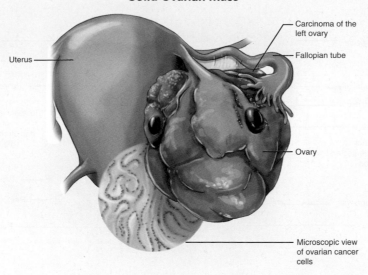

Uterus —

Carcinoma of the left ovary

Fallopian tube

Ovary

Microscopic view of ovarian cancer cells

There are many types of solid masses but the two most common will be discussed. The first is a **benign cystic teratoma**. This tumor forms in the ovaries and contains structures such as bone, cartilage, or teeth. Many of the tissues come from dermoid derivatives such as skin, hair follicles, and sebum. This is why it is also known as a **dermoid** cyst. The second mass is a malignant ovarian neoplasm. Approximately 21,000 cases of ovarian cancer are diagnosed each year in the United States (American Cancer Society, 2008). Symptoms are so vague that many ovarian cancers are not found until advanced stages. Most ovarian cancers are diagnosed after menopause (80%), with the median age of diagnosis being 62 years (ACS, 2008). The greatest risk factor is a family history of the disease. To date, there are no cost-effective screenings available.

Ectopic Pregnancy

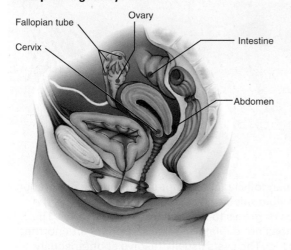

Fallopian tube

Ovary

Cervix

Intestine

Abdomen

A fertilized ovum implants in a site other than the uterine endometrium. Risk factors include previous ectopic pregnancy, past pelvic infection, endometriosis, or abnormalities of the tube. The patient presents with symptoms of a normal pregnancy initially. As the ectopic pregnancy grows larger, there are internal hemorrhage and subsequent lower quadrant pain. The most common symptoms are lower quadrant pain, nausea, and referred pain in the neck or shoulder from blood beneath the diaphragm. If hemorrhage is severe, the patient is at risk for shock.

Acute Salpingitis

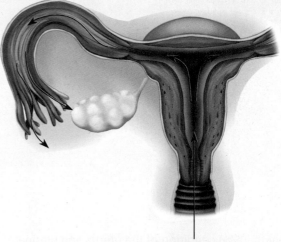

Spread of gonorrhea or chlamydia

The most common cause of fallopian tube disease, salpingitis is also referred to as PID. Infection spreads throughout the uterus and up into the tubes. The tubes become swollen and rupture. Scarring can occur even with treatment implemented; potential for infertility is high. *C. trachomatis* and *Neisseria gonorrhoeae* are the most common organisms that cause salpingitis. Chronic infections with either of these organisms can lead to tubal occlusion or obstruction. The patient presents with pain in the lower quadrant, chills, fever, dysuria, pyuria, and often vaginal discharge (CDC, 2008).

Special Populations and Foci

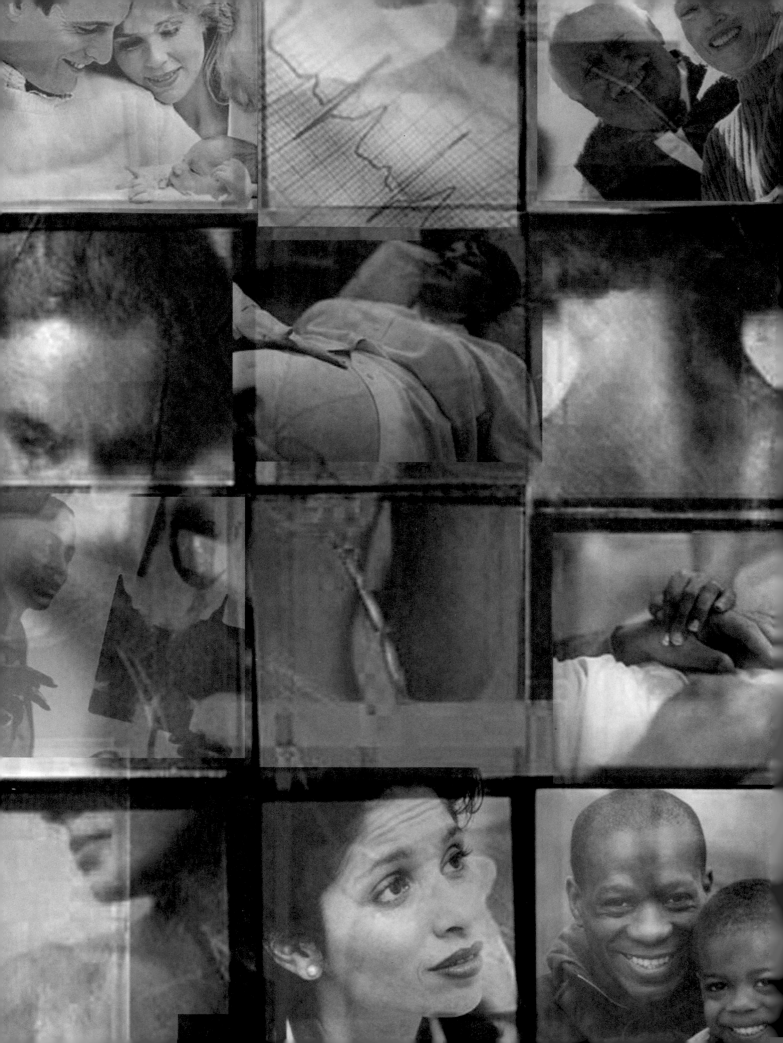

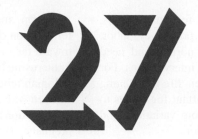

Pregnant Women

Learning Objectives

1 Describe how preexisting conditions are affected by and affect pregnancy.

2 Create strategies to minimize physical and psychosocial complications of pregnancy.

3 Describe changes in the pregnant abdomen over the course of the gestation.

4 Describe expected weight gain during each trimester of pregnancy.

5 List common laboratory and diagnostic tests for a normal pregnancy, and additional tests for common diagnoses found during pregnancy.

6 Identify risk-reduction opportunities and teaching strategies to address the risks.

7 List common complaints of pregnancy and methods to treat them.

8 Describe subjective data collected for urinary tract infection (UTI), pyelonephritis, round ligament pain, periumbilical pain, back pain, Braxton Hicks contractions, and labor.

9 Document subjective and objective findings using appropriate terminology.

10 Individualize the health assessment of the pregnant woman, considering her age, past and current medical history, and culture.

11 Use assessment findings to identify nursing diagnoses and initiate a nursing plan of care for a pregnant woman.

*M*ichelle Sherman is visiting the clinic following a positive home pregnancy test. She is a 21-year-old Native American, accompanied by her male partner and their 22-month-old son. Ms. Sherman, 5'4", is concerned because she has not yet lost all the weight she gained during her first pregnancy and is starting this pregnancy at 205 lb. She reports that she quit smoking during her last pregnancy but resumed smoking a half pack each day after the baby was born to manage the high stress while being a new mother. She thinks her last menstrual period (LMP) was 6 weeks ago and reports that it was lighter than usual.

- What additional history does the nurse need to gather from Michelle today?
- What physical assessment data are the nurse's responsibilities to gather and assess?
- What health-promotion needs does Michelle have today?
- What findings would indicate that Michelle's condition is stable, urgent, or emergent?
- What factors does the nurse need to consider to individualize Michelle's care?

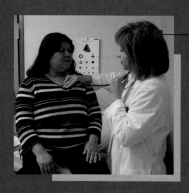

This chapter is based on the premise that, for most patients, pregnancy is not an illness. Usually, pregnancy, labor, childbirth, and postpartum recovery are normal and need only health-promotion and risk-reduction interventions. For some patients, however, serious and even life-threatening problems can occur. Therefore, it is important for nurses to be able to distinguish normal findings from variations and from conditions that require further attention.

This chapter describes normal anatomical and physiological changes of pregnancy, as well as expected variations based on age, risk factors, and environment. It considers how cultural variations can affect care during pregnancy. It also explores specific symptoms common to pregnancy and the nurse's role in their identification and management.

Structure and Function Overview

Preconception

The left and right ovaries typically ovulate in alternate cycles. Either ovary releases one egg into the fallopian tube approximately 14 days before the next menstrual period is expected (Fig. 27-1). After the release of the egg, the corpus luteum forms on the ovarian surface and produces progesterone, which supports the uterine lining until the placenta is formed. Without sufficient progesterone, the woman menstruates and there will not be a successful pregnancy.

Sperm meet the egg in the fallopian tube, where fertilization occurs. Cilia in the fallopian tube assist the egg toward the uterus. Factors that can delay progression of egg to uterus include cigarette smoking and inflammation of the fallopian tube, most commonly by chlamydia or gonorrhea. Women with histories of smoking or these sexually transmitted infections (STIs) are at increased risk for ectopic (tubal) pregnancy (see Chapter 26).

⚠ SAFETY ALERT 27.1

Ectopic pregnancy occurs when the egg never leaves the fallopian tube. Signs of this potentially life-threatening condition include lower abdominal pain on one side and spotting of blood. Confirmation of ectopic pregnancy is considered an obstetric emergency requiring hospitalization and termination of the pregnancy to save the mother's life.

First Trimester

The embryo travels from the fallopian tube and implants in the uterine lining, often with a resulting small bleed. Typically, the process from ovulation to implantation takes approximately 2 weeks, so implantation bleeding can occur at the same time the woman expects her period. Implantation bleeds are usually lighter and shorter than a normal period. Bleeding after implantation is a potential concern that requires investigation.

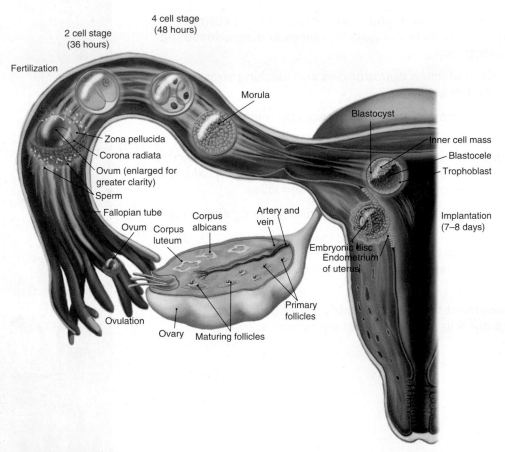

Figure 27.1 Follicular development and release.

The outer layer of the developing embryo produces human chorionic gonadotropin (hCG). Pregnancy tests (both urine and blood) measure levels of this hormone, whose presence validates the existence of a pregnancy and initiates a feedback loop that preserves the corpus luteum for longer than the normal 14 days.

At implantation, the embryo is far too small to be seen on ultrasound. One way to evaluate normal progression of early pregnancy is by checking levels of hCG and progesterone. Serum hCG levels should double every 48 hours, and progesterone levels slowly increase.

From weeks 2 to 8 after conception, all major fetal organs form. Therefore, it is very important for women to avoid teratogens during this period (which can be difficult because many are not even aware that they are pregnant this early). **Teratogens** are substances or infections that can cause malformations in the embryo. Examples of teratogens include tetracycline drugs, thalidomide, DES, alcohol, x-rays and other radiation, rubella vaccine, isotretinoin (Accutane), lithium, and some anticonvulsants. The Food and Drug Administration lists teratogenic drugs as Pregnancy Category X to indicate that they should not be used during pregnancy.

Between 25% and 50% of conceptions do not result in a viable pregnancy. Eighty percent of miscarriages (spontaneous abortions) occur during the first trimester, and more than half of these miscarriages are the result of chromosomal abnormalities. Another 40% have abnormal development of the egg just after fertilization, sometimes characterized as a "blighted ovum" or "chemical pregnancy." Nearly all first-trimester miscarriages cannot be prevented, either by mother or clinician. Nevertheless, women commonly wonder if they could have done something to prevent the tragedy and blame themselves. The ready availability of home pregnancy tests does not help. In the past, most women did not even know for sure that they were pregnant before they miscarried. Now, women bond before it is clear that the pregnancy is viable. Given these facts, reassurance from nurses that early miscarriages are not preventable can help women to grieve and heal from their losses.

Rate of miscarriage drops dramatically after the first trimester. At 10 weeks, the placenta weighs only on average 20 g, yet this may be sufficient for it to produce enough progesterone to maintain a pregnancy. By 12 weeks' gestation, the placenta has grown sufficiently to take over production of progesterone, and the corpus luteum is reabsorbed. Most women who have had morning sickness start feeling better once the placenta takes over progesterone production.

Second Trimester

During the second trimester, fetal growth is significant. The fetus begins this trimester 3 in long and weighing less than 1 oz (0.8 g). By the end of the second trimester, the fetus is about 15 in long and weighs more than 2 lb (1,000 g). Major organs develop to the point that the fetus may survive (with help) outside the womb.

At the beginning of the second trimester, the maternal uterus is large enough to extend beyond the pelvic bone into the abdomen. Many providers perform a fetal survey by ultrasound at 20 weeks' gestation, or halfway through the pregnancy. By this time, the fetus is large and developed enough that all major organs are visible on ultrasound, including the sex organs that indicate gender. In some cases, functionality of organs (eg, cardiac output) can also be assessed (Fig. 27-2). In addition, if ultrasound identifies certain abnormalities, such as gastroschisis (intestines formed outside the abdomen) or spina bifida (defect of the spinal canal), preparations can be made to improve fetal chances for survival at birth.

The fetal survey also indicates placement, functional grade, and size of the placenta. At week 20, it is not uncommon for the placenta to be close to the cervical os, or "low lying." Usually, as the uterus continues to expand, the placenta moves away from the os. When the placenta actually covers the os (**placenta previa**) at the end of the pregnancy,

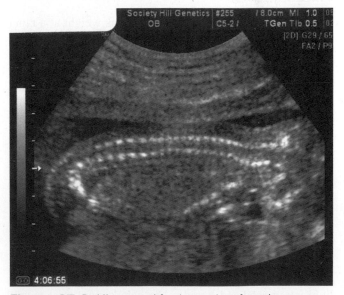

Figure 27.2 Ultrasound fetal scanning, focusing on spinal development, which in this case is progressing normally.

safe vaginal birth is not possible, and a cesarean is planned. Normally, the placenta is Grade 1 early in pregnancy and Grade 3 at birth. If the placenta is "old" or small early in pregnancy, the fetus may need to be delivered early, because the placenta may not be able to support normal third-trimester growth.

Two milestones for the healthy first-time mother (primipara) occur at about 20 weeks. Her uterus reaches the umbilicus, and she begins to "show." She also clearly feels fetal movements. In the 2 weeks leading up to the 20-week mark, she may feel "flutters" that she confuses with gas. By 20 weeks, however, most women feel definite kicks or "**quickening**."

Clinical Significance 27-3

Women who compare notes with friends or search the Internet may worry if they do not feel distinct kicks by 20 weeks. The most common reason a woman does not sense kicking by 20 weeks is that her dates are wrong. The second most common reason is that the placenta has randomly implanted on the anterior aspect (belly side) of the uterus.

Unless a cesarean is required, it makes no difference where the placenta implants as long as it does not cover the **cervical opening** (os). The anterior abdomen has many more sensory nerves than the posterior, so it is much easier to feel kicks in the front. The anterior placenta blunts the force of the fetal kicks on the anterior sensory nerves. The mother with an anterior placenta feels the kicks when the fetus grows big enough to kick the anterior abdomen around the edges of the placenta, usually at about 22 weeks. As the fetus continues to grow and gain strength, the mother can feel the kicks through the "padding" of the placenta.

Third Trimester

During the third trimester, the fetus gains weight at a rapid pace, but proportionally not as rapidly as during the second trimester. It begins the trimester weighing about 2 lb and at birth averages about 7½ lb in the United States (with a range for healthy term newborns of 6 to 9 lb). In the first two trimesters, most fetal growth is in the head and skeleton, but during the third trimester, fetal organs grow and mature, muscles increase in size and strength, and a protective fat layer forms to assist with temperature control after birth. Fetal skin thickens and forms a more protective barrier than during the second trimester. During the last 4 weeks of pregnancy, the mother transfers IgG antibodies to the fetus to assist in the formation of the fetal immune system. Integration of the nervous and muscular functions proceeds rapidly during the third trimester.

Near term, a normal fetus swallows nearly half the amniotic fluid volume each 24 hours, and insoluble debris in the fluid is removed and stored as the baby's stool (meconium) before the fluid is returned to the amniotic sac via fetal urine.

Clinical Significance 27-4

If the fetus does not swallow a normal amount of amniotic fluid (as can occur with maternal diabetes), then excess fluid collects in the amniotic sac (polyhydramnios). If the renal system is not normally formed and fetal urination is decreased, a deficiency of amniotic fluid results (oligohydramnios). Oligohydramnios is a risk factor for poor lung development.

A key task of the third trimester is maturation of the fetal lungs. Growth factors in amniotic fluid promote growth and differentiation of lung tissue. With normal amniotic fluid volume, functionality of the lungs depends on their ability to form surfactant, which prevents collapse of the alveoli upon expiration. If a fetus must be delivered between 28 and 34 weeks, a glucocorticosteroid injection is given to the mother to promote formation of surfactant.

Determining Weeks of Gestation

Human pregnancies last an *average* of 266 days after fertilization. By convention, pregnancies are dated from the first day of menstruation in a 28-day cycle, so 14 days are added (for a total of 280 days from the LMP) to calculate the "due date," or estimated date of birth (EDB). Thus, a woman who says that she is 6 weeks pregnant conceived 4 weeks ago.

Due date may be estimated by using **Naegele's rule**, which says to subtract 3 months from the first day of the LMP and add 7 days to the result. Thus, a woman whose LMP began April 17, 2010 would have an EDB of January 24, 2011. Another way to calculate EDB is with a pregnancy wheel (Fig. 27-3), which is turned to line up the LMP on the inner wheel with the corresponding EDB on the outer wheel. The marker on the inner wheel then aligns with the probable date of delivery, which corresponds to a 40-week pregnancy (38 weeks since conception).

If a woman is known to have a longer or shorter menstrual cycle than 28 days, adjustments should be made to her EDB. For instance, if her cycle averages 32 days, her EDB will be 4 days later than the date calculated using the LMP on the pregnancy wheel. Because women usually do not know exactly how long their cycles are or when they ovulated, and there are variations in how each woman carries her pregnancy, "due date" is only an approximation. The nurse plays an important role by asking detailed questions to ensure that all pertinent facts are considered to establish a probable due date. Accurate dating prevents early induction or post-term complications.

Clinical Significance 27-5

Inducing labor too soon can result in premature birth, difficult labor, and complications such as cesarean surgery. Failing to induce a post-term fetus can result in postmaturity syndrome or even stillbirth. The nurse can help prevent difficulties by explaining at the first visit that a baby is not premature after 37 weeks and is not "late" before 42 weeks. Babies born anytime during this 5-week window are considered "on time."

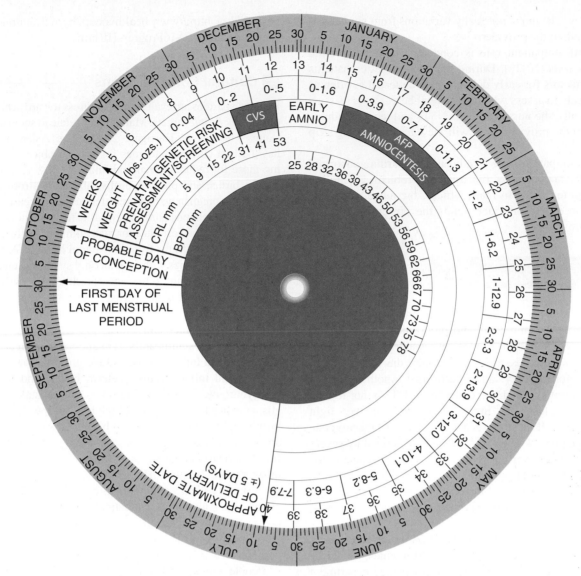

Figure 27.3 A pregnancy wheel can be used to find the EDB on the outer wheel by lining up the date of the LMP on the inner wheel.

Role of the Nurse in the Outpatient Setting

Health care for most pregnant women occurs in outpatient settings, in which registered nurses (RNs) may be responsible for conducting intake interviews. Associated tasks include dating the pregnancy, taking a very detailed history, obtaining consents for prenatal testing, arranging for referrals if needed, and educating the patient about the practice. An intake visit typically lasts 60 to 90 minutes and gives the patient an idea of how the practitioner will care for her. A caring, nonjudgmental, open attitude from the nurse can not only reassure the patient, but also increase the chances that she will reveal personal information that will improve her prenatal care. Development of a trusting relationship requires that the nurse use his or her best communication skills at a time when a patient usually has many questions, and sometimes fears.

Another outpatient role for nurses is triage. Pregnant patients are understandably worried about events they think might be abnormal. It is impossible for busy providers to see a patient each time she has a concern; therefore, the nurse handles many questions from pregnant women over the telephone or, increasingly, via secure email. The nurse must know which concerns can be handled by phone or computer; which require a visit to identify or confirm a diagnosis, and if so, the urgency; and which require that the patient proceed immediately to a hospital or birth center. Consequently, the nurse must be familiar with the symptoms of common diagnoses in pregnancy and be able to ask questions necessary to make safe recommendations to the patient.

A third outpatient role is to gather preliminary data before a provider sees the patient for her prenatal visit. Typically, the nurse weighs the patient, records her blood pressure, assesses her urine for protein and glucose, and identifies any problems or concerns. The nurse notes any variations from normal and reports them to the provider.

A fourth outpatient role is conducting and interpreting **nonstress tests** (NSTs). During the third trimester, patients with risk factors for early delivery may be tested as often as twice weekly to assess whether the fetal heart rate is reassuring. Typically, the nurse conducts NSTs and reports findings verbally to the provider, who will view the monitoring strip later.

A fifth outpatient role is education regarding abnormal test results and options for treating problems, including medication teaching. In many offices, the nurse, under the supervision of the provider, sends the prescription to the pharmacy.

Acute Assessment

Some conditions in pregnancy require immediate attention from a provider, immediate hospitalization, or both. For example, ectopic pregnancy is an obstetrical emergency, because if it ruptures, the woman may die from internal bleeding before surgery can be performed. Another example is pyelonephritis, which occurs when a UTI is not treated promptly. Because the immune system does not fight infections as well during pregnancy, a bladder infection can quickly become a kidney infection, characterized by severe flank pain and a fever above 100.4°F. While pyelonephritis is often treated on an outpatient basis for nonpregnant clients, during pregnancy pyelonephritis requires IV antibiotics immediately to prevent generalized sepsis, which is potentially fatal.

Any nonhospitalized patient with *hemorrhage*, defined as soaking a menstrual pad in less than 30 minutes, should be referred immediately to the nearest emergency department (ED) for evaluation and treatment. Also, any woman who has lost enough blood to be symptomatic (light-headed, dizzy, cold, confused, diaphoretic, anxious) should be referred immediately to the ED. If a woman is having regular, painful contractions before 37 weeks, she should be seen immediately for evaluation, preferably in an acute care setting with appropriate nursery facilities.

Subjective Data Collection

Areas for Health Promotion/*Healthy People*

All ten of the leading health indicators that were identified as priorities for action directly affect pregnant women (see Table 27-1). As is clear from *Healthy People*, much work is needed to improve the health of pregnant women, fetuses, and newborns in the United States. The nurse who is aware of these goals can do much to help achieve them by educating both pregnant and nonpregnant patients. In addition, related objectives from other focus areas for *Healthy People* are also important for pregnancy. Further information can

be found at http://www.healthypeople.gov/Data/midcourse/html/focusareas/FA16ProgressHP.htm.

Cultural Considerations

Racial disparities are evaluated in progress toward achievement of *Healthy People* targets. Many issues relate to socioeconomic status (Headley & Harrigan, 2009). The Asian population has the best current outcomes for several objectives, including those for reducing fetal and infant deaths, very low birth weight births, and preterm births; abstaining from cigarette smoking in pregnancy; and breastfeeding in the early postpartum and 6-month postpartum periods. The white non-Hispanic population has the best rates for many other objectives, including fewest infant deaths from congenital heart defects, maternal deaths, and babies with fetal alcohol syndrome and highest rates of prenatal care, attendance at childbirth classes, consumption of folic acid, and breastfeeding at 1 year.

Disparities in infant deaths among the Asian, Hispanic, white non-Hispanic, and black non-Hispanic populations have increased significantly (Headley & Harrigan, 2009). The American Indian/Alaska Native groups show high rates of fetal and infant deaths, preterm births, and fetal alcohol syndrome, as well as low rates of prenatal care. Non-Hispanic black women are at high risk for low and very low birth weight babies and preterm births. Of particular concern are the increased disparities in smoking during pregnancy for American Indian/Alaska Native, Native Hawaiian or other Pacific Islander, Hispanic, black non-Hispanic, and white non-Hispanic populations, compared with the Asian population. Although Asian patients met the target of 99% of pregnant women abstaining from smoking, other racial and ethnic populations are making little progress toward this target (Headley & Harrigan, 2009).

People with at least some college education have the best rate for all objectives except for cesarean births to low-risk patients. Women with less than a high school education demonstrate rates that are at least twice as high as those with at least some college education for postneonatal deaths and deaths from SIDS, but only half the rates of early entry into prenatal care, attendance at childbirth classes, abstinence from smoking during pregnancy, and breastfeeding during the early postpartum period. Patients with less than a high school education also have the lowest median RBC folate level (Healthy People, 2010). In many practices, RNs play key roles in providing the education essential to reducing such disparities.

Assessment of Risk Factors

As discussed earlier, the nurse gathers basic information during the intake interview, such as medical and obstetric history and personal history that might affect the pregnancy. The nurse asks about current problems, family history, age, gender, ethnicity, medications and supplements, and additional risk factors. Knowledge of risk factors helps identify topics for health-promotion teaching.

Table 27.1 *Healthy People* Goals Related to Pregnancy

Goals	Patient Education Topics
Encourage physical activity during pregnancy.	Patients may continue normal exercise so long as it does not involve a risk for falls (eg, skiing) or excessive fetal shaking (eg, horseback riding). Those who exercise at least 30 min/day during pregnancy are more likely to have better overall health, maintain good circulation to the placenta and fetus, gain appropriate weight, and thus have fewer complications.
Increase the proportion of mothers who achieve a recommended weight gain during their pregnancies.	Obesity increases risk for gestational diabetes, large gestational age (LGA) (>4,000 g for girls, >4,200 g for boys at 40 weeks' gestation) *and* small gestational age (SGA) (<2,500 g) babies, more difficult vaginal deliveries, and complications should a cesarean be necessary.
Reduce tobacco use during and after pregnancy.	Nicotine constricts blood vessels, and therefore reduces placental perfusion and oxygen transport to the fetus. Heavy smokers are at increased risk for placental infarcts (places where there is no blood supply) and placental abruptions.
Reduce the proportion of low birth weight (LBW ≤ 2,500 g) and very low birth weight (VLBW ≤ 1,500 g) babies	Obtain a detailed diet history and make culturally appropriate suggestions for improvement if necessary. Assist with smoking, alcohol, and illicit drug cessation. Emphasize the importance of regular prenatal care so that any issues can be identified and corrected early. Refer to social work if necessary for problem-solving to reduce stress.
Reduce cesarean births among low-risk (full-term, singleton, vertex presentation) patients – Patients giving birth for the first time – Patients with a prior cesarean birth	Encourage "getting in shape" prior to conception. Offer clients the 5-minute video: http://www.youtube.com/watch?v=EZy0JPtubiQ Avoid "convenience" inductions. Encourage pain relief options during labor that permit upright positioning. Consider referral to a certified doula for additional labor support. Patients with prior cesareans should wait 2 years for their next pregnancy.
Reduce the occurrence of spina bifida and other neural tube defects	Encourage patients to take prenatal vitamins for three months prior to conception. For healthy patients, consider offering prenatal vitamins throughout the childbearing years.
Increase the proportion of mothers who breastfeed their babies until 1 year of age	Educate mothers in the prenatal period about how to achieve a proper latch, the importance of colostrum, management of engorgement, and the effect of their child's "growth spurts" on milk supply. Demonstrate various positions for breastfeeding and how to assist the baby. Refer to a lactation consultant if necessary.

Source: *Healthy people 2010: What are its goals? (n.d.)*. Retrieved July 7, 2010, from http://www.healthypeople.gov/About/goals.htm

Questions on History and Risk	Rationales
Family History Do you have a family history of diabetes, hypertension, twins, or genetic illnesses?	Positive family history of these findings may increase the patient's risk for them.
Personal History *Age.* What is your date of birth? What is your age?	Pregnant teens have increased nutritional requirements because they, too, are still growing. In addition, their pelvises may not be fully developed. Pregnant teens are at increased risk for complications, especially preeclampsia, probably from inadequate nutrient intake. Mothers of advanced maternal age are those who will be 35 years or older at the EDB. They are at increased risk for miscarriage and genetic anomalies and may have increased preexistig health problems (eg, fibroids, advanced endometriosis, hypertension).

(text continues on page 816)

Questions on History and Risk	Rationales

Culture. With what ethnic group do you identify? Do you have a religious preference?

Some cultures or religions have important childbirth rituals, which may influence the role of the baby's father during labor, preferred anesthesia for surgery, handling of the newborn, or required or prohibited foods during the postpartum period. Some cultures may consider the violation of such norms as potentially harmful for mother or fetus. Some genetic diseases or pregnancy complications (eg, gestational diabetes, hypertension) are more prevalent in certain ethnic groups.

> **Clinical Significance 27-6**
>
> Examples of beliefs that can affect the care of pregnant women include that Jehovah's Witnesses accept no blood products, even to save the life of mother or baby; women from many parts of Africa are circumcised; and Russian patients often refuse cesarean for breech presentation.

Pregnancy History. What previous miscarriages, terminations, or pregnancies have you had?

Document each pregnancy (including miscarriages and terminations) by date, length of gestation, length of labor, type of delivery (vaginal, forceps/vacuum, or cesarean), type of anesthesia and any adverse reaction, sex and weight of the infant, and any complications. Past patterns can suggest possible current issues.

Pap Smears. Have you had any abnormal Pap smears in the past?

Patients with past abnormalities may have a recurrence with pregnancy. Those who have had surgery to remove abnormal cells may have scar tissue that needs to be released during labor to permit vaginal birth.

STIs. Have you had any past STIs?

Verify that prior STIs were treated according to protocol. Assess risk of reexposure, because many STIs are potentially harmful to the fetus.

Breast History. Have you had any breast reductions or implants? Any abnormal mammogram results?

Document augmentation or reduction surgeries, and whether an attempt was made to preserve ability to breastfeed. Document any other breast health issues (discharge, abscesses) and type of nipple (everted, flat, inverted). Document any past difficulties with nursing.

Infertility. Have you had any problems with infertility?

If it was difficult for the woman to conceive or maintain the pregnancy, fully document her history, including any medication that she took and what, if any, type of assisted reproduction was used. In vitro pregnancies have a somewhat higher risk than spontaneous pregnancies of multiple gestation and fetal loss.

Psychological Issues. Do you have depression, anxiety, or eating disorders?

Patients with a history of these psychiatric conditions are at risk for exacerbations during pregnancy and postpartum.

Headaches. Have you had headaches or migraines?

Only acetaminophen is recommended during pregnancy, so patients with frequent headaches may need to change their medication, especially in the third trimester. Those with frequent migraines are at somewhat increased risk for postpartum stroke. Severe headaches may be a sign of preeclampsia.

Allergies. Do you have any allergies? What is your reaction?

Note both the allergen and reaction to it. Although providers minimize medications prescribed during pregnancy and labor, some conditions common in pregnancy (ie, UTIs, positive Group B Strep status) are treated with antibiotics, to which a patient may be allergic.

Violence. Because violence is so common for so many people, I routinely ask all patients about violent experiences—in the past and currently? I wonder if you have experienced or are experiencing violence? (See Chapter 12.)

In the initial interview, it is common for patients to minimize their experience with violence and abuse. Nevertheless, pregnancy and labor can elicit painful memories or cause overprotective behavior. In severe cases, a patient may experience flashbacks or psychotic episodes during labor. Also, pregnancy is a time when domestic violence increases.

Questions on History and Risk	Rationales
Medications and Supplements ***Contraception.*** What type of contraception have you used? When did you last use it?	If the patient was using hormonal contraceptives within three cycles of conception, it is difficult to assess when she ovulated. Patients using hormonal contraceptives do not have true menses, but have "withdrawal bleeds" when they do not take progesterone for 7 days. Even if a woman is pregnant, she may have withdrawal bleeds at the usual time if she continues her birth control pills. If her conception date is unclear, ultrasound dating in the first trimester can be offered.
Additional Risk Factors ***Support System.*** What type of support system do you have?	Patients without a stable support system are at risk for poor nutrition, domestic violence, poor housing, and increased stress. Some patients achieve stability in marriage, others with a supportive family.
Personal Habits. Do you use tobacco, alcohol, or other drugs?	Pregnancy is a time when patients are more likely to discontinue habits known to be harmful for their child. The nurse provides support and cessation resources to patients who want them.
Recent Immigration. How long have you lived in this country?	Immigrants may have been exposed to infections that can harm them or the fetus. A refugee may have had inadequate nutrition when the bony pelvis was forming, resulting in a small or misshapen pelvis. With better nutrition in this country, she may be at increased risk for cephalopelvic disproportion, which would require cesarean surgery for a safe delivery. Immigrants from certain areas may have had female circumcision, which reduces the size of the introitus.
Access to Care. Do you have any financial concerns? Are you able to come to appointments?	Patients with no access to medical care before pregnancy are less likely to have had a preconception visit to address any issues that might affect the pregnancy. On average, they begin care later and receive less prenatal care in pregnancy (Stewart, et al, 2007). In some areas, assistance with transportation to medical appointments is available.

Focused Health History Related to Common Symptoms

The nurse responsible for triaging pregnancy-related calls can make an enormous difference in how a patient views her competence as a mother, in how much trust she has in her provider and the staff where she plans to give birth (home, hospital, or birth center), and in how well she will labor. Use of sound therapeutic communication is especially important during pregnancy, because a pregnant woman is understandably concerned not only about her own health, but also that of the fetus. What may seem like a "common complaint" of pregnancy to an experienced nurse may seem much more ominous to the pregnant patient. So-called "common complaints" of pregnancy are annoying, but not dangerous for

either mother or fetus. Supportive care is normally all that is required. Often, simple reassurance by the nurse is all the mother needs.

Focused Health History Related to Common Symptoms in Pregnancy

- Morning sickness
- Growing pains
- Increased vaginal discharge
- Increased urination
- Breast tenderness or discharge
- Periumbilical pain in the second trimester
- Fetal hiccups
- Braxton Hicks contractions

Questions to Assess Symptoms	Rationales/Abnormal Findings

Morning Sickness

Have you been experiencing any nausea, vomiting, or other physical symptoms with this pregnancy?

- Is there a particular time of day in which you have physical symptoms?
- Does anything help relieve symptoms?
- Does anything seem to make symptoms worse?

△ SAFETY ALERT 27.2

Some women have severe morning sickness (hyperemesis gravidarum). They cannot keep anything in their stomachs long enough to digest. As a result, they lose weight and their fluid and electrolyte balance is abnormal. These patients may require IV fluids or even hospitalization to restabilize. Utreated hyperemesis gravidarum can be fatal.

It is unknown why some women with normal pregnancies have morning sickness. This condition is thought to be associated with high estrogen levels, but it is also influenced by diet and emotions. Tense or anxious patients seem to be at risk, as are those who do not drink enough water or get enough B vitamins in early pregnancy. Usually, morning sickness can be managed on an outpatient basis if the woman increases B vitamins and fluid intake (sips only, not large glasses at a time) and uses methods of relaxation (eg, meditation, yoga, prayer). The nurse does the necessary teaching if the mother reports her problem in time. Once the woman can keep down sips of water, the nurse advises her to try the BRAT diet—bananas, rice, applesauce, or toast—starting with one bite and increasing intake by an additional bite every 15 minutes so long as there is no emesis. For most patients, nausea and vomiting is a self-limiting condition that does not require medical intervention.

Growing Pains

- Have you experienced pains or other sensations in your lower abdomen?
- If so, describe how they feel and how long they last.
- Does any movement or activity seem to trigger the pains?
- How often do they occur?

△ SAFETY ALERT 27.3

Appendicitis, pyelonephritis, ectopic pregnancy, and miscarriage can also present with abdominal pain. With these conditions, pain is more constant, increasing in severity, or less sharp.

In the first trimester, sharp pains in the lower abdomen are common. Stretching of the round and broad ligaments that support the growing uterus causes them, which are usually very short (<5 seconds) and have a stabbing quality. They are not repetitive, but often associated with position changes or, later, fetal movements. However, there are many other sources of abdominal pain during pregnancy, some of which are potentially fatal.

Increased Vaginal Discharge

- Have you noticed any increase in vaginal discharge with this pregnancy?
- If so, describe the quantity and quality.
- Does it have a particular odor or color?
- Do you have any itching, burning, or discomfort associated with it?

It is normal for pregnant women to have increased clear vaginal discharge from increased estrogen production. Patients describe this discharge as just like their normal vaginal discharge, except that there is more of it. If the discharge is like nasal mucus or cottage-cheese, is any color other than clear, or has a foul odor, it may be a sign of a vaginal infection or STI. Infections during pregnancy should be diagnosed and treated promptly, because some can affect the fetus. Patients who report such symptoms need evaluation.

Increased Urination

- Have you noticed a need to urinate more frequently with this pregnancy?
- How much water are you drinking every day?
- How often do you urinate?
- Is urination accompanied by any pain or pressure?
- Have you noticed any blood in your urine?

Increased urination in pregnancy is common, as a result of the relaxation of the urinary system by increased progesterone. This is one reason why it is important for the woman to drink 2 L/day of water. If urinary frequency is accompanied by suprapubic pressure, dysuria (painful urination), hematuria (blood in the urine), or flank pain, she may have a UTI, which requires prompt treatment.

Questions to Assess Symptoms	Rationales/Abnormal Findings

Clinical Significance 27-7

Patients already urinating more than usual are reluctant to increase fluid intake. Nevertheless, doing so helps prevent UTIs and constipation and reduces morning sickness. Fiber intake is also important, especially in later pregnancy when the growing fetus compresses the intestines, and therefore, transit time increases.

Breast Tenderness and Discharge

- Have you noticed any change in the size of your breasts?
- Have you experienced any breast pain or feelings of fullness?
- Have you noticed any nipple discharge? If so, please describe it.

Some patients can feel breast changes even before the pregnancy test is positive. Rapid growth of alveoli, addition of a fat layer, and construction of the duct system for breastfeeding can result in feelings of fullness or even pain. The nurse teaches the patient to use a supportive, properly fitted bra and to take acetaminophen if necessary for pain relief. Later in pregnancy, the patient may notice nipple discharge. This is almost always colostrum leaking in preparation for birth, but the nurse instructs the patient to mention the discharge when she sees the provider. The provider should evaluate to verify that discharge is not from infection or a tumor.

Periumbilical Pain

- Have you experienced any pain or pressure around your umbilicus?
- If so, does any movement or activity trigger the pain?

About halfway through pregnancy, women commonly feel a stretching pain all around the umbilicus. The pain is similar to "growing pains," which usually subside by the end of the first trimester. However, these second-trimester pains are similar in origin, resulting from additional ligaments stretching as the uterus accommodates the growing fetus.

Fetal Hiccups and Other Spasms

- Do you notice any regular fetal movements?
- Do you think that the fetus might be having hiccups or sucking his or her thumb?

By the third trimester, the patient may be aware of fetal hiccups, which result from spasms of the fetal diaphragm triggered by an immature neurological system (Popescu, et al., 2007). Hiccups can be thought of as "practice breathing," and they tend to resolve as the neurological system matures. Mothers sometimes report that it feels as if the fetus is having a seizure. Rarely, this is true. Usually, the rapid movement is again from the immature neurological system: the fetus has a hypersensitive startle reflex and "jumps" when stimulated. Such symptoms tend to resolve near term. Upon further questioning by the nurse, it may become obvious that what the mother feels is rhythmic thumb sucking by the fetus.

Braxton Hicks Contractions

- Have you experienced any irregular contractions with this pregnancy?
- If so, how often do they occur and how long do they last?
- How painful are these contractions?
- Is there anything you do that resolves the contractions?

Braxton Hicks contractions prepare the body for labor. They are usually irregular in frequency and duration, with fewer than five in 1 hour. They are also short (<30 seconds) but may be painful. These contractions may begin as early as the second trimester, especially for patients who have had babies before, but are more common in the third trimester. They often resolve with position changes, a hot shower, hydration, or relaxation. They are to be differentiated from preterm labor contractions, which are regular, do not resolve with comfort measures, occur more frequently than four in 1 hour, get longer and stronger over time, and result in cervical change. The triage nurse must be able to distinguish between Braxton Hicks and preterm labor contractions.

Therapeutic Dialogue: Collecting Subjective Data

Michelle calls the hospital on a Sunday when she is 30 weeks of gestation and says she is afraid she is in labor, but that she knows it is too early for the baby to come.

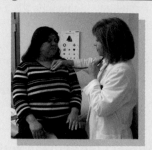

Less Effective

Nurse: You are only 30 weeks. It's unlikely anything serious is going on, but let me ask you a few questions to make sure.

Michelle: OK.

Nurse: You don't have any cramping?

Michelle: Actually, the pains have been coming all day.

Nurse: Oh (pause). How often?

Michelle: Every few minutes and they hurt.

Nurse: You're only 35 weeks, so they are pretty short?

Michelle: No, they last a long time.

Nurse: Oh, you've timed them?

Michelle: No, I don't have a watch.

Nurse: OK, then you'd better come in right away so that I can see what's going on.

Michelle: OK, whatever you think is best. Should I be worried?

Nurse: No, everything is probably ok. We'll take care of you. Sometimes it's something bad but not usually.

More Effective

Nurse: Tell me more about what has happened so far and how you are feeling.

Michelle: Well, I am cramping.

Nurse: How long have you been cramping?

Michelle: They have been coming all day.

Nurse: Have you been timing them?

Michelle: Not really, but it seems like every few minutes, and they hurt!

Nurse: I'm sorry. Could you tell me when one is starting?

Michelle: Well, one is starting now.

Nurse: Can you tell me where you are feeling it and what it feels like?

Michelle: All over my tummy, and it feels kind of like menstrual cramps.

Nurse: Can you tell me when it's over? It's over now? Ok, then that lasted about 20 seconds. Let me know if you feel another one.

Michelle: Should I be worried? It's too early to have the baby. Will my baby be OK?

Nurse: We'd like to see you as soon as you can get a ride, just to be sure, but you are not telling me anything that makes me sure that something is wrong. So far, everything you are saying could happen in a normal pregnancy. We will do some tests so that we know everything is OK. When could you get here?

Critical Thinking Challenge

- How does the more effective nurse show concern and avoid false reassurance?
- Why does the more effective nurse assess social issues?
- What knowledge base is important for a nurse to have to perform a complete assessment?

Objective Data Collection

Assessment During the Initial Visit

A maternity provider usually conducts the initial full physical assessment, with a pelvic examination (see Chapter 26), at the first or second visit. Ideally, this happens during the first trimester. For the healthy gravida (pregnant mother), examination includes the following:

- General survey and vital signs
- Nutrition
- Skin integrity, with any abnormalities (including large moles, piercings, or tattoos) noted or charted
- Head for abnormal bumps, lesions, or infestations

- Eyes to test pupils for PERRLA and the ocular fundus (see Chapter 15)
- Ears for a clear canal and pearly grey tympanic membrane
- Mouth for lesions, signs of infection, unusual anatomy, and oral/dental health
- Neck for size, smoothness, and placement of the thyroid
- Lung fields to make sure they are clear
- Heart sounds (mild systolic ejection murmurs are common in normal pregnancies)
- Extremities to note any vascularities
- Breasts and axilla for any abnormal lumps or lesions
- Abdomen for scars, adipose tissue, symmetry, striae, and fetal heart tones past 10 weeks
- Reflexes (see Chapter 24)
- External genitalia for signs of infection, and details of any female circumcision
- Vagina and cervix with a speculum. Samples for a wet mount or cultures may be collected if infection is suspected. Samples may also be taken for Papanicolaou, human papilloma virus, chlamydia, and gonorrhea tests if these have not been done in the last year (see Chapter 26).
- Uterus and adnexa (ovaries) with a bimanual examination (see Chaptrer 26).
- Pelvis, to assess the size and shape of the birth canal. See advanced techniques.
- Rectum for hemorrhoids (see Chapter 25).

If this is the patient's first assessment, the nurse explains the procedures, showing instruments that will be used, and answers any questions. If the provider is male, a female RN may be asked to stay in the room during examination to serve as a chaperone. The RN may hand instruments and specimen containers to the provider during the examination. The RN clearly labels specimens before they are removed from the examination room after verifying the patient's name and birth date. He or she also performs assessments and teaching related to nutrition and changes in the skin, breast, abdomen, urine, and vaginal secretions.

Technique and Normal Findings	Abnormal Findings
General Survey and Vital Signs Document weight, blood pressure, other vital signs, and pain level (Fig. 27-4). Although randomized trials have not shown a benefit for obtaining a urine sample from pregnant women with each visit, it is the standard of care in many communities. Test urine for glucose and protein, and chart the findings. 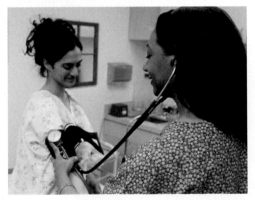 **Figure 27.4** Assessing the patient's blood pressure during the initial pregnancy visit. **Nutrition** Most women gain very little weight (if any) in the first trimester. Typical gains are <7 lb, partly because of morning sickness for those who have it. In addition, not much structural change is necessary for the woman to accommodate the fetus and uterus, which are still small enough to fit behind the pubic bone. A simple rule of thumb for a woman of normal prepregnant weight is that she will gain about 10 lb by 20 weeks and about 1 lb/week for the remaining 20 weeks, for a total of 25–30 lb (see Table 27-2).	Call excessive (or not enough) weight gain to the attention of the provider.

(text continues on page 822)

Table 27.2 Weight Distribution

This weight is distributed approximately as follows:

Tissues and Fluids	Average at Term (g)	Pounds/Ounces
Fetus	3,400	7 lb/8 oz
Placenta	650	1 lb/7 oz
Amniotic fluid	800	1 lb/12 oz
Uterus enlargement	970	2 lb/2 oz
Breasts	405	12 lb/5 oz
Blood (excess volume)	1,450	3 lb/3 oz
Extravascular fluid volume increase	1,480	3 lb/4 oz
Maternal stores (fat)	3,345	7 lb/6 oz
Total	12,500	27 lb/8 oz

Nutritional requirements to produce a healthy baby and associated weight gain include increasing intake by about 300 cal/day in the second and third trimesters, increasing complete protein intake to 60 g/day, increasing elemental iron intake by 27 mg/day, and increasing vitamin intake, especially for women with multiple fetuses, who smoke, or who use alcohol or drugs. A good resource for women to check dietary adequacy is www.mypyramid.gov. Women with healthy preconception diets provide an optimal start toward healthy child development.

Women who fail to meet these nutritional requirements risk *low–birth-weight* or *intrauterine growth–restricted babies* and increased difficulties with breastfeeding.

Skin

Increased melanization in the first trimester may lead to **linea nigra** (a hyperpigmented line between the symphysis pubis and the top of the fundus) and **chloasma** (mask of pregnancy—a blotchy hyperpigmented area on the cheeks, nose, and forehead.

Abdomen

Smooth muscles (ie, intestines and kidneys) relax and dilate as a result of increased circulating progesterone levels.

Stasis can result, causing *constipation* and *UTIs.*

By 10–12 weeks, it is common to be able to hear the fetal heartbeat with a Doppler (Fig. 27-5). Ultrasonic gel is placed on the Doppler's transducer, which is then placed with some pressure on the woman's abdomen. In the first trimester, the fetal heartbeat usually is audible just above the symphysis pubis. If the uterus is palpable superior to the pubic bone, the heartbeat may be heard higher in the abdomen as well.

For overweight women, it may take until 14 weeks to hear the baby's heartbeat with a Doppler. Morbidly obese women may need serial ultrasounds to monitor fetal well being.

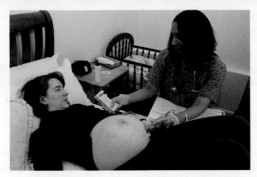

Figure 27.5 Assessing the fetal heart rate through use of Doppler ultrasound.

As pregnancy progresses, the experienced RN can palpate the fetal back, which feels firm and smooth. Usually, it is easiest to hear the fetal heart by placing the Doppler on the fetal back, because the bony skeleton transmits sound well. For Dopplers that do not give a digital read-out of fetal heart rate, the number of beats is usually counted for 15 seconds and then multiplied by 4 to obtain a rate per minute. Chart both the rate and place on the abdomen where the heartbeat was heard.

By the end of pregnancy, the uterus will have stretched and grown from its nonpregnant 40–70 g to 1,100 g, a more than 15-fold increase (Fig. 27-6).

Supporting ligaments also stretch, which can lead to sharp round ligament pain as soon as the first trimester. Extension of the pain to the inguinal area helps distinguish it.

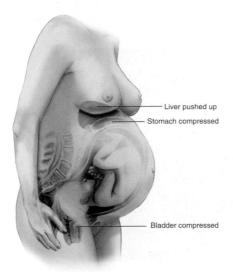

Liver pushed up
Stomach compressed
Bladder compressed

Figure 27.6 Growth of the uterus near term, with evident displacement of internal organs.

Breasts

First-trimester changes include increased breast size and more fullness and sensitivity. Areolae may darken, Montgomery glands may become more prominent, and nipples may be more erectile from increased progesterone and estrogen.

Breast changes may result in upper backache. As pregnancy progresses, some women notice the growth of accessory breast tissue, often near the axillae. While the appearance is unusual, such tissue poses no danger.

Genitalia

The woman may notice frequent urination and increased normal vaginal secretions.

Assessment During Routine Pregnancy Visits

Patients with normal pregnancies typically have visits once a month for the first two trimesters, then every other week until the last month, and then every week until delivery. Scientific evidence suggests that patients may have equally good outcomes with fewer visits, especially if they have had children before (ICSI, 2008).

Technique and Normal Findings	Abnormal Findings
General Survey and Vital Signs While collecting data, ask the patient how she is doing. Elicit a description of and chart any problems she may be having (ICSI, 2008).	Counsel patients who feel dizzy, especially when changing positions rapidly, to sit down in order to avoid possible syncope, falling, or both. Check for postural hypotension (see Chapter 6). Other possible causes of dizziness include dehydration, anemia, edema of the inner ear, and hypoglycemia.
Assist with diagnosis by checking the urine, including specific gravity to ensure that the patient is well-hydrated. Draw blood, if ordered, to check for low blood glucose level or anemia.	Proteinuria 1+ or greater may indicate *preeclampsia* and thus requires a provider's attention. Other signs of preeclampsia include significantly increased blood pressure as compared to baseline; sudden edema, especially of the face; persistent headache; and malaise.
Skin Changes over pregnancy are primarily attributable to the increasing fetus, uterus, and amniotic fluid volume (Fig. 27-7). As the abdomen continues to grow, the woman may get **striae gravidarum** ("stretch marks"). Striae may also appear on the enlarging thighs and breasts (Ghasemi, et al., 2007). Linea nigra may darken further, and terminal hairs may appear on the abdomen. Some women have **melasma** ("mask of pregnancy") as melanin production increases.	

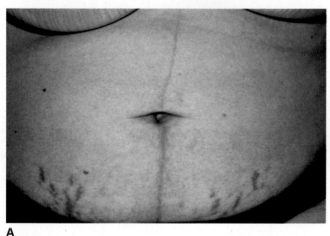 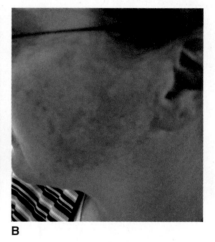

A   B

Figure 27.7 Skin changes in pregnancy. **A.** Evident linea nigra and striae. **B.** Melasma evident on the cheeks.

Nose, Mouth, and Throat Capillaries with lax walls proliferate from increased production of progesterone by the placenta.	Epistaxis (nosebleed) is a common result. Some women have nonpathological cervical spotting when a capillary breaks.
Thorax and Lungs Respirations increase, in response to both increased blood flow through the lungs and increased need for oxygen by the fetus and mother. The growing fetus limits the ability of the lungs to expand.	Toward the end of the second trimester, women may experience dyspnea with exertion.

Although respiratory rate changes very little during pregnancy, tidal volume and minute ventilation increase dramatically to meet the increased oxygen needs of both fetus and mother.

Heart

Maternal circulatory system changes significantly during the second trimester. Blood volume and cardiac output increase by about 40%; however, hematocrit falls. Increased work for the heart lead to a 10–15 beat increase in maternal heart rate.

Cardiac output decreases when the woman is supine, because the weight of the fetus impedes venous return, and increases when she is in lateral positions. Sitting and standing also decrease venous return from the extremities.

The mother may experience this change as shortness of breath.

The pregnant woman may subsequently experience palpitations.

Dependent edema may result. In the arms, it may lead to *carpal tunnel syndrome* when edematous tissues impinge on the nerve bodies. In the legs, standing for long periods can result in *varicosities*. Help prevent these problems by teaching ways to promote venous return. Examples include avoiding constrictive clothing (especially ankle hose/socks with tight tops); elevating the arms and legs whenever possible, ideally above the heart (lie on a sofa with feet elevated on the arm rest); and sleeping on the side. See Box 27-1.

BOX 27.1 PATIENT TEACHING—SLEEPING AND POSITIONING IN PREGNANCY

*P*regnant women are advised to sleep on their sides during the third trimester. Unfortunately, many women find this position uncomfortable, and feel like they wake up more tired than when they went to sleep. Help alleviate discomfort of it by teaching about strategic placement of pillows (as shown below). In addition to the pillow under her head, the woman can put a thick pillow between the legs, which raises the upper leg until it is parallel with the mattress and relieves strain on the abdominal muscles and ligaments. Wedging another pillow behind the woman's back allows her to lie at a 45-degree angle with her back supported, without impeding venous return. A pillow under the abdomen further supports the suspensory ligaments. When the nurse uses pillows to show the woman how this feels, most women can relax and are less anxious about getting a good night's sleep.

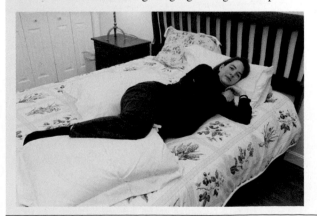

(text continues on page 826)

In the third trimester, rate of iron transfer from mother to fetus increases. The amount of iron required for a healthy pregnancy is not usually available from the woman's prepregnant iron stores and a healthy diet. FDA-approved prenatal vitamins provide the extra iron required to maintain health during pregnancy.

Clinical Significance 27-8

Mothers with a scheduled cesarean or at risk for postpartum hemorrhage (eg, multiple gestation) need teaching about eating iron-rich foods, taking prenatal vitamins daily, and using any prescribed iron supplements as directed. Iron is not as well absorbed with calcium (dairy) as with citrus (including vitamin C).

Peripheral Vascular

Decreased peripheral vascular resistance results in a somewhat lower blood pressure during the second trimester. Optimal circulation to the placenta (and fetus) is achieved in the left lateral position, but right lateral is also acceptable for sleeping once the woman is past 20 weeks.

Breasts

The Montgomery tubercles (sebaceous glands) on the areola may enlarge. Nipples may darken, enlarge, and begin to discharge colostrum (Fig. 27-8).

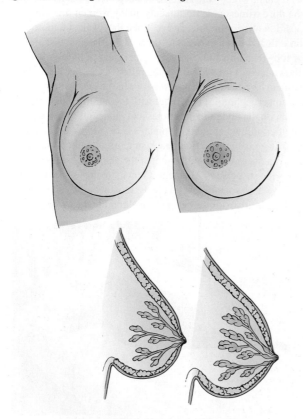

Nonpregnant　　　Pregnant

Figure 27.8 Comparison of the breasts in the nonpregnant versus pregnant states.

Women whose initial iron stores are low or who do not obtain sufficient iron during pregnancy become anemic. Women with anemia at the time of childbirth are at increased risk for transfusion, especially if they have a cesarean birth, because average blood loss for a cesarean is twice that for a vaginal delivery.

As blood volume increases and the growing fetus impedes venous return, pressure on valves in the lower extremities can result in their failure. *Varicose veins* form or worsen.

Spider veins may appear late in pregnancy, but disappear shortly after delivery.

Abdomen

By 20 weeks' gestation, the uterus is at about the umbilicus; by 36 weeks, it nears the bottom of the sternum (Fig. 27-9). Muscles of the abdominal wall may separate (**diastasis recti**) and not return to normal approximation until several weeks after childbirth.

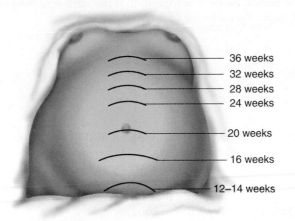

36 weeks
32 weeks
28 weeks
24 weeks
20 weeks
16 weeks
12–14 weeks

Figure 27.9 Growth in fundal height over the three trimesters of pregnancy.

The gallbladder does not contract as well as usual during pregnancy.

During the third trimester, the growing uterus mechanically displaces the intestines.

Musculoskeletal System

With fetal growth, the maternal center of gravity changes, and the woman's risk for falls increases. Pregnant women should not lift anything weighing more than 20 lb (including toddlers, groceries, and laundry). They should use good body mechanics when lifting anything.

Clinical Significance 27-9

One of the psychological tasks for a mother during a second pregnancy is to disengage sufficiently from her toddler so that the first child can become more independent. The best time to do so is by 20 weeks. This gives the toddler (and the mother!) an additional 20 weeks to adjust to new roles before the baby comes. Help by noticing if a mother is lifting the toddler, teaching the mother to protect her back, and helping her to think ahead about how she will cope once she has a newborn in her arms.

Gastric reflux (heartburn) is common during the third trimester, as sphincter tone decreases and gastric pressures increase from displacement of the stomach. Over-the-counter (OTC) antacids can usually relieve infrequent heartburn; however, frequent use of them during pregnancy causes a rebound effect, meaning that the woman needs more over time for less relief. Use of OTC H2 blockers (eg, ranitidine, Zantac) is both safe in pregnancy and more efficacious than antacids.

Retained bile salts can increase risk of gallstones. Stasis of bile salts can also occur in the liver, causing **pruritus gravidarum**, which produces a rash with intense itching often along the striae of the abdomen. The itching resolves soon after delivery, once normal circulation of bile salts is restored.

Pregnant women are at risk for constipation. Straining during bowel movements can also cause painful or itchy hemorrhoids. The primary way to prevent hemorrhoids is to prevent constipation by increasing exercise and intake of fiber and water.

Backaches are common during the second and third trimesters, partly from poor technique when lifting and also because of lack of back support when sleeping.

Not only is it physiologically prohibitive to maintain good back health while carrying both a rapidly growing fetus and a growing toddler, but carrying the toddler also sets up potential psychological difficulties for the toddler after the birth. Once the baby is born, the mother will not be able to carry both children, especially when nursing the newborn.

(text continues on page 828)

The musculoskeletal systems change noticeably at the end of pregnancy. The modest increase in the pelvic diameter that results from the relaxation of the cartilage allows the fetus to "drop," "lighten," or "engage" in the pelvis in preparation for childbirth.

Clinical Significance 27-10

Women often ask how soon the fetus will "drop." For many women, this process is gradual rather than sudden, so it is difficult to say exactly when engagement has happened. For a woman who has had children before, the fetus may not "drop" until labor has already progressed. Commonly, nulliparous mothers sense that their fetuses have dropped 2–3 weeks before birth.

Genitalia

As the woman's abdomen grows, couples may worry about the advisability of sexual relations. In the first trimester, before the woman was "showing," it was likely less of a psychological and practical concern. Couples with normal pregnancies benefit from being reassured that sexual relations do not hurt the fetus, which is well protected, and that receptors for any oxytocin produced with orgasm are inactive until pregnancy ends. Couples may find that certain positions for intercourse are more comfortable than others, and women can be encouraged to try new positions.

Increased weight from the fetus and breast tissue, with the accompanying change in the center of gravity, places increased strain on the abdominal muscles. The nurse teaches the pregnant woman exercises to strengthen her abdominal muscles ("cat stretch" and pelvic tilts against a wall), which may provide some relief. Also, hormonal changes near term, especially increased relaxin, loosen the cartilage between the pelvic bones. Women complain that they are waddling like a duck when they try to walk.

Research shows that women's interest in sexual relations during pregnancy varies. For many, there is no change; for others, libido increases, while for still others it decreases, possibly from fatigue, depression, or relationship problems that surface during pregnancy (DeJudicibus & McCabe, 2002).

Evidence-Based Critical Thinking

Common Laboratory and Diagnostic Testing

The nurse should be familiar with common laboratory tests administered during pregnancy and the significance of abnormal findings. The clinic will have protocols (either written or verbal) about how abnormal findings are treated. It is common for the nurse to explain findings to the mother and also the proposed treatment. Table 27-3 lists and describes common laboratory tests performed throughout pregnancy. Two advanced techniques are described below.

Nonstress Test

During the third trimester, the patient may be scheduled for a NST in conjunction with her prenatal visit. The purpose of the

Table 27.3	Laboratory Tests Performed During Pregnancy		
Test	**Rationale**		**Example of Plan/Treatment**
Blood type	If the mother needs an emergent blood transfusion during or after labor, the blood bank will need her blood type.		Mothers with Rh negative blood are offered RhoGam at approximately 28 weeks' gestation, or if they miscarry.
CBC	Checks for anemia, thalassemias, platelets, WBCs.		Anemia may be treated with iron supplementation or iron-rich foods. Thalassemias may require referral to specialists, because the condition poses some risks to the fetus. Patients with low platelet levels are at risk for disseminated intravascular coagulation and may not be candidates for epidurals. WBC counts are usually elevated in pregnancy; they may be as high as 12,000/mm^3 in the prenatal period, and during labor they may rise as high as 30,000/mm^3. WBCs in excess of these numbers suggest a potential infection.

Table 27.3 Laboratory Tests Performed During Pregnancy (*continued*)

Test	Rationale	Example of Plan/Treatment
Serology (VDRL, RPR)	Syphilis crosses the placental barrier to the fetus.	A positive result is usually verified by additional testing, and if those results also are positive, the mother is treated with antibiotics.
HBsAg (Hepatitis B surface antigen)	Hepatitis can be transmitted from the mother to the fetus.	Newborns of positive mothers are given an HBIG (IgG antibodies) injection and are immunized for hepatitis B shortly after birth.
HIV	HIV can be transmitted from the mother to the fetus.	Administration of retroviral medications to the HIV-positive mother during pregnancy significantly reduces the risk of transmission of the virus to the baby.
Rubella titre	Maternal infection with rubella during pregnancy (especially the first 2 months) can cause congenital heart malformations, intrauterine growth restriction, cataracts, and deafness in the fetus.	Patients without sufficient titres to protect them from infection cannot be vaccinated during pregnancy, because the vaccine is a live virus. However, they can be vaccinated promptly after delivery.
Triple- or quad-screen	Maternal blood drawn between 15 and 20 weeks screens for Down's syndrome and other trisomies, neural tube defects, gastroschisis, and other fetal abnormalities.	This test has a high false-positive rate; further testing is required for a definitive diagnosis. Test accuracy depends on accurately dating the pregnancy. Ultrasound can usually clarify dating issues and also help with identifying any abnormalities. Amniocentesis is offered if the ultrasound does not reveal any dating problems.
50-g glucose challenge	Maternal blood is drawn exactly 1 hour after the woman ingests a glucose drink. The test often is used to screen for (gestational) diabetes at 26–28 weeks, when maternal glucose metabolism changes. It may be done earlier for those at high risk for diabetes (obese or extensive family history). Patient does not need to fast prior to the test. Uncontrolled diabetes during pregnancy can result in macrosomia, difficult delivery, neonatal hypoglycemia, perinatal morbidity and mortality, and a host of other complications.	Patients with an elevated glucose level (135–140 mm/dL) are given a 3-hour glucose tolerance test, are referred to a dietician for diabetes counseling and education about blood glucose monitoring, or both. With strict diet control, many patients can control their blood glucose level; however, some will require oral medication or insulin injections to protect the fetus from glucose overload.
Group B Streptococcus (GBS)	Mothers with urine cultures positive for GBS are called "colonizers" and are at increased risk for fetal infection. Colonizers are treated with oral antibiotics immediately and offered IV antibiotics during labor for the current and all future pregnancies. For other mothers, a swab of the vagina and rectum is collected at 35–37 weeks (or sooner if prematurity is a risk). If the mother is GBS-positive, there is a small chance that the infant will be infected during prolonged rupture of membranes or a vaginal birth. If the infant is infected, there is a small chance it would not survive.	Protection for the infant results when antibiotics are administered 4 hours prior to delivery, so positive mothers are encouraged to notify their providers early in labor. (This is the current CDC guideline, but new evidence suggests that protection probably occurs much sooner.)

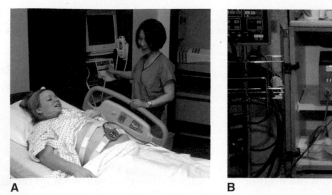

Figure 27.10 Nonstress testing. **A.** The nurse is observing external fetal monitoring of the patient. **B.** A reactive strip.

NST is to assess fetal well-being. If the patient is scheduled for an NST, the nurse will put the patient on the electronic fetal monitor (Fig. 27-10) after her usual data are gathered. The nurse puts the patient in a comfortable position, places the tocodyamometer on the fundus to measure uterine contractions, and places the ultrasound monitor where the fetal heart can be heard to measure its rate (FHR). The nurse checks periodically to make sure that the sensors are tracing accurately and that the mother is still comfortable. If the monitoring strip is not becoming **reactive**, the nurse may offer the mother a position change or a drink of juice in hopes of stimulating the fetus to react to these changes. The nurse reports any sign of fetal distress to the provider immediately.

Leopold's Maneuvers

Leopold's maneuvers are designed to estimate the position of the fetus. First, the nurse palpates the fundus of the uterus to determine whether it contains the head or the buttocks. The head moves independently of the torso, but the buttocks do not (Fig. 27-11A). Second, the fetal back

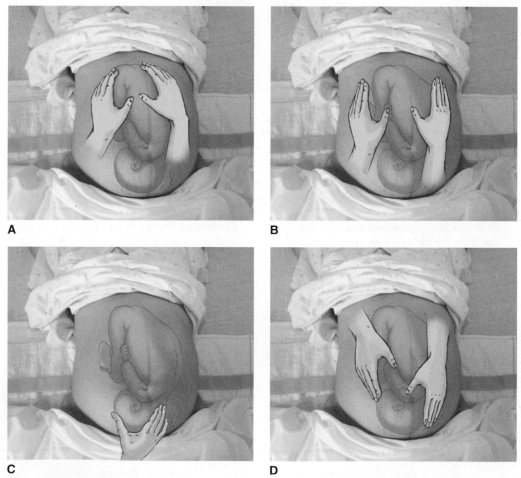

Figure 27.11 Leopold's maneuvers. **A.** First maneuver. **B.** Second maneuver. **C.** Third maneuver. **D.** Fourth maneuver.

is located by holding the fetus firmly on one side while the other is palpated, and then the procedure is reversed. The back feels firm and smooth; the opposite side contains "small parts" (arms and legs) that feel irregular (Fig. 27-11B). Third, palpating just above the symphysis pubis identifies the presenting part. It should be the part opposite that found in the fundus (Fig. 27-11C). Fourth and finally, the fetal head is palpated to determine whether it is flexed or deflexed. If it is properly flexed, a protrusion (the brow) will be palpated on the opposite side as the fetal back. If the head is deflexed, the protrusion (the occiput) will be palpated on the same side as the back (Fig. 27-11D). RNs usually only need to use the first and second maneuvers to locate the fetal heart rate and verify that the presenting part is the head.

Diagnostic Reasoning

Nursing Diagnosis, Outcomes, and Interventions

When formulating a nursing diagnosis, it is important to use critical thinking to cluster data together and identify patterns that fit together. Table 27-4 provides a comparison of nursing diagnoses, abnormal findings, and interventions commonly related to pregnancy (NANDA-I, 2009).

Nurses use assessment information to identify patient outcomes. Some outcomes related to pregnancy include the following:

• Family will affirm desire to improve parenting skills.
• Family will perform tasks needed for change.
• Family states positive effects of changes made (Moorhead, et al., 2007).

Once the outcomes area is established, nursing care is implemented to improve the status of the patient. The nurse uses critical thinking and evidence-based practice to develop the interventions. Some examples of nursing interventions for pregnancy are as follows:

• Assess the influence of cultural beliefs on the patient's perception of parenting.
• Teach family about the effects of pregnancy and adding a child to the family system.
• Identify resources for support and coping during this time of change (Bulechek, et al., 2007).

The nurse then evaluates the care according to the patient outcomes that were developed, therefore reassessing the patient and continuing or modifying the interventions as appropriate.

Table 27.4	Common Nursing Diagnoses Associated with Pregnancy		
Diagnosis and Related Factors	Point of Differentiation	Assessment Characteristics	Nursing Interventions
Health-seeking behaviors related to pregnancy	Actively seeking ways to move toward a higher level of health	Concern about environmental conditions on health status, desire for increased level of wellness, unfamiliarity with community resources	Educate on nutrition and overeating, develop exercise plan, teach stress management techniques. Instruct in smoking cessation, provide health screening.
Readiness for enhanced parenting	Providing an environment that encourages optimal growth and development of children	Emotional support of children, family attachment, physical needs of children are met	Use family centered care, encourage positive parenting, provide mother-to-infant skin contact, allow parent to assist in newborn's bath
Readiness for enhanced family coping due to new role	Effective task management with desire for enhanced growth and health	Moves toward enriching lifestyle, moves toward health promotion and optimal wellness	Assess the structure, resources, and coping abilities of families, encourage caregivers to become involved in support groups, acknowledge cultural influences.

Collaboration with Other Providers

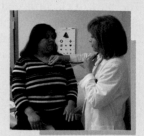

Michelle is tested for serum glucose because she is obese (body mass index [BMI] is 40.8). Further testing reveals that Michelle has gestational diabetes. The nurse also notes that recommended weight gain for Michelle is 15 lb or less for the pregnancy, but Michelle has already gained 26 lb (weight at last visit was 221 lb).

After the practitioner reviews laboratory values and determines the plan of care, the nurse calls Michelle to report the findings and conveys the recommendation that Michelle see a diabetes educator for nutritional counseling. The educator answers Michelle's questions about the potential effects of diabetes on her and the fetus. The educator also explains that Michelle should be retested when the baby is 6 weeks old to ensure that Michelle has not developed type 2 diabetes.

Below is the initial conversation between the nurse and the diabetes educator. The nurse uses SBAR to organize information for the educator.

Situation: Michelle is a 21-year-old Native American. She is 35 weeks pregnant by LMP dates and a 20-week ultrasound. Michelle did not pass either her 1-hour glucose test (150 mg/dL) or her 3-hour glucose tolerance test today.

Background: Michelle had a prepregnancy BMI of 35.2, so was given a 1-hour glucose test at her first visit, which was normal (132 mg/dL). Both her mother and her sister have type 2 diabetes. So far, Michelle has gained 26 lb since her initial visit.

Assessment: Michelle has gestational diabetes and is at risk for type 2 diabetes as evidenced by abnormal glucose test results.

Recommendation: Because she is pregnant, Michelle cannot wait the normal 1–2 months for placement in a regularly scheduled diabetes education class. Michelle needs immediate counseling regarding her diet, a diary to record everything she eats, a blood glucose monitor and instructions on its use, testing strips and lancets for the monitor, and a schedule for testing her blood glucose levels. If she cannot control her diabetes with her diet or does not keep her follow-up visits with the diabetes educator, please let us know.

Critical Thinking Challenge

- What additional assessments should the nurse perform related to the diabetes?
- Why did the nurse choose a food diary as the assessment tool?
- How might Michelle's cultural background and age affect her perceptions of her pregnancy?

Pulling It All Together: Reflection and Critical Thinking

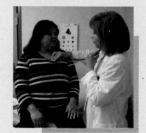

The nurse uses assessment data to formulate a nursing care plan with patient outcomes and interventions for Michelle. Outcomes are specific to the patient, realistic to achieve, measurable, and have a time frame for meeting them. The interventions are actions that the nurse performs, based on evidence and practice guidelines. After these interventions are completed, the nurse reevaluates Michelle and documents the findings in the chart to show progress toward the patient outcomes. The nurse uses critical thinking and judgment to continue or revise the diagnosis, outcomes, or interventions. This is often in the form of a care plan or case note similar to the one below.

Nursing Diagnosis	Patient Outcomes	Nursing Interventions	Rationale	Evaluation
Health-seeking behaviors related to pregnancy	Patient will limit weight gain to 16 lb	Assess the role that stress plays in overeating. Use nutritional guidelines to plan a diet high in protein, fiber, fruits, and vegetables.	People who eat under stress are more likely to gain weight and have elevated insulin and cortisol levels.	Goal has not been met. Patient has gained 26 lb. Discuss changes that patient is willing and able to make in her diet. Refer to diabetes educator.

Using the previous steps of diagnostic reasoning, organizing, and prioritizing, consider all the case study findings woven throughout this chapter. When answering the following questions, begin drawing conclusions and see how the pieces of assessment must work together to create an environment for personalized, appropriate, and accurate care.

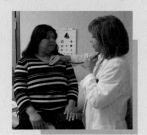

- What additional history does the nurse need to gather from Michelle today?
- What physical assessment data are the nurse's responsibilities to gather and assess?
- What health-promotion needs does Michelle have today?
- What findings would indicate that Michelle's condition is stable, urgent, or emergent?
- What factors does the nurse need to consider to individualize Michelle's care?

Key Points

- The due date is calculated using Naegele's rule. Subtract 3 months from the first day of the LMP and add 7 days, or about a 40-week pregnancy.
- The role of the RN includes conducting the intake interview, performing triage, gathering preliminary data, conducting NSTs, and educating patients and families.
- Acute conditions of pregnancy include ectopic pregnancy, pyelonephritis, hemorrhage, and contractions before 37 weeks.
- Health-promotion issues for pregnant women include physical activity, recommended weight gain, avoidance of tobacco, prenatal vitamins, and breastfeeding.
- Some cultures and religions have important rituals around birth.
- Common symptoms of pregnancy include morning sickness, growing pains, increased vaginal discharge, increased urination, breast tenderness, periumbilical pain, fetal hiccups, and Braxton Hicks contractions.
- A normal weight female will gain is 10 lb by 4½ months of pregnancy and about 1 lb a week for the remaining 20 weeks, for a total of 25 to 30 lb.
- Increased skin melanization occurs during pregnancy, resulting in linea nigra or choasma.
- By 10 to 12 weeks of gestation, the fetal heartbeat may be heard with a Doppler stethoscope.
- Breast changes include more fullness, sensitivity, darkened areola, more prominent Montgomery glands, and more erect nipples.
- Signs of preeclampsia include elevated blood pressure, sudden edema, headache, and malaise.
- As the abdomen enlarges, the pregnant woman may develop straie gravidarum, linea negra, and melasma.
- Women may experience dyspnea toward the end of pregnancy as the growing fetus limits the ability of the lungs to expand.
- Cardiovascular changes include lower hematocrit, weight gain, elevated pulse, edema, and varicosities.
- Gastric reflux is common in pregnancy from displacement of the stomach.
- Musculoskeletal changes include relaxed cartilage, lower back pressure, and a waddling gait.

- Nursing diagnoses commonly related to pregnancy include health-seeking behaviors, readiness for enhanced parenting, and readiness for enhanced family coping.

Review Questions

1. Michelle says that her last normal menstrual period was June 15. Using Naegele's rule, her EBD is
   A. September 8
   B. March 8
   C. March 22
   D. January 22

2. Michelle is half way through her pregnancy (20 weeks). The top of her uterus should be
   A. at the symphysis pubis
   B. half way between the symphysis and the umbilicus
   C. at the umbilicus
   D. at the xyphoid process

3. A normal electronic fetal monitoring strip shows
   A. a fetal heart rate of 90 beats/min
   B. variability of 0 to 5 beats/min
   C. two decelerations in 20 minutes
   D. three accelerations in 20 minutes

4. Which of the following conditions would be the highest priority to contact the health care provider about?
   A. Striae gravidarum
   B. Varicosities
   C. Contractions before 37 weeks
   D. More prominent Montgomery glands

5. A patient calls the provider's office to schedule an appointment because a home pregnancy test was positive. The nurse knows that the test identified the presence of which of the following in the urine?
   A. Estrogen
   B. Progesterone
   C. hCG
   D. Follicle-stimulating hormone

6. Important health promotion activities include recommending
   A. physical activity
   B. weight gain of 15 lb
   C. increase in intake of vitamin A
   D. shallow breathing

7. The patient comes for a NST, and the nurse notes that the fetal heart rate is 100 beats/min. Which of the following nursing actions would be appropriate to do first?
   A. Document the findings
   B. Notify the provider
   C. Inform the patient that everything is normal
   D. Instruct the patient to return to the clinic in 1 week for reevaluation of the fetal heart rate

8. The nurse is performing patient teaching about normal changes during late pregnancy. These include which of the following?
   A. Dark cloudy urine
   B. Waddling gait
   C. Vaginal bleeding
   D. Sudden edema

9. The nurse is caring for a patient who is admitted to the hospital with a possible ectopic pregnancy. Which of the following nursing actions is the priority?
   A. Monitoring daily weight
   B. Assessing for edema
   C. Monitoring the temperature
   D. Monitoring the blood pressure

10. The nurse assesses for common symptoms in pregnancy including
   A. headache
   B. high blood pressure
   C. gastric reflux
   D. hemorrhage

References

Bulechek, G. B., & Butcher, H. K., McCloskey Dochterman, J. (2007). *Nursing Interventions Classification (NIC)* (4th ed.) St Louis: Mosby.

DeJudicibus, M. A., & McCabe, M. P. (2002). Psychological factors and the sexuality of pregnant and postpartum patients. *Journal of Sexual Research, 39*(2), 94–103.

Ghasemi, A., Gorouhi, F., Rashighi-Firoozabadi, M., Jafarian, S., & Firooz, A. (2007). Striae gravidarum: Associated factors. *Journal of the European Academy of Dermatology and Venereology, 21*(6), 743–746.

Healthy People. (2010). *Progress towards elimination of health disparities.* Retrieved November 30, 2009 from http://www.healthypeople.gov/Data/midcourse/html/focusareas/FA16ProgressDisparities.htm

Headley, A. J., & Harrigan, J. (2009). Using the Pregnancy Perception of Risk Questionnaire to assess health care literacy gaps in maternal perception of prenatal risk. *National Medical Association, 101*(10), 1041–1045.

ICSI. (2008). *Routine prenatal care.* Retrieved November 29, 2009, from http://www.cochrane.org/reviews/en/ab000934.html

Moorhead, S., Johnson, M., Maas, M. (2007). *Nursing outcomes classification (NOC)* (4th ed.). St. Louis: Mosby.

North American Nursing Diagnosis Association. (2009). *Nursing diagnoses, 2009–2011 Edition: Definitions and classifications (NANDA NURSING DIAGNOSIS).* West Sussex UK: John Wiley & Sons.

Popescu, E. A., Popescu, M., Bennett, T. L., Lewine, J. D., Drake, W. B., & Gustafson, K. M. (2007). Magnetographic assessment of fetal hiccups and their effect on fetal heart rhythm. *Physiological Measurement, 28*(6), 665–676.

Stewart, A. L., Dean, M. L., Gregorich, S. E., Brawarsky, P., & Haas, J. S. (2007). Race/ethnicity, socioeconomic status and the health of pregnant women. *Journal of Health Psychology, 12*(2), 285–300.

The Jensen suite offers these additional resources to enhance learning and facilitate understanding of this chapter:

- thePoint on line resource, http//thepoint.lww.com/Jensen1E
- Student CD-ROM included with the book
- *Laboratory Manual for Nursing Health Assessment: A Best Practice Approach*
- *Pocket Guide for Nursing Health Assessment: A Best Practice Approach*

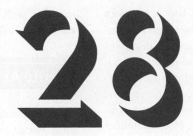

28

Newborns and Infants

Learning Objectives

1 Describe key features relevant to the infant's expected physical growth and motor and speech development.

2 List critical components of an acute assessment of the newborn and older infant.

3 Choose appropriate patient education topics for selected *Healthy People* objectives.

4 Collect pertinent subjective data for the most common symptoms encountered in infants.

5 Collect objective data using physical examination techniques adapted for the unique needs of infants.

6 Identify normal and abnormal findings in the inspection, palpation, percussion, and auscultation in the physical examination of the infant.

7 Use subjective and objective data about the infant to analyze findings and plan interventions.

8 Individualize health assessment considering the condition, age, gender, and culture of the patient.

9 Use assessment findings to identify diagnoses and to initiate a plan of care.

*K*eri Downs, 1-month-old, is visiting the clinic today for her well-child checkup and hepatitis B immunization. She was born at term and has had no health problems. Her mother is breastfeeding her; they have adjusted well.

Keri is the first child in a two-parent family. The mother is a nurse who plans on returning to work in 2 months; the father is an accountant. Paternal grandparents live in the area and provide child care 1 day a week.

As you consider this case study, begin thinking about the following points:

- What assessments will be the highest priorities?
- How should the nurse assess for growth?
- What reflexes should the nurse expect to see in this 1-month-old?

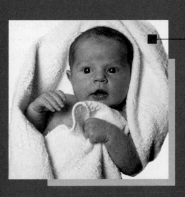

Infancy encompasses the first 12 months of life. A newborn is an infant 28 days old or younger. This chapter examines health assessment of newborns and infants. It discusses important past and present health history and pertinent findings of the physical examination. Because infants are preverbal and totally reliant on parents/guardians, the nurse must develop excellent observation skills and involve parents in the assessment and care planning. For ease of communication, the term "parents" is used throughout this chapter to indicate one or both parents or a guardian.

Structure and Function Overview

When assessing the individual child's physical, motor, and language development, it is important to determine whether these areas are progressing steadily. Using rigid timetables to measure the child's development is not helpful and does not provide an accurate assessment. Milestones serve only as guidelines so that developmental delays can be identified early and appropriate interventions instituted.

Chapter 9 explores physical growth, motor, and language development milestones in detail. A brief review is presented in the following paragraphs.

Physical Growth

Physical growth and development that began in utero continue rapidly after birth. In fact, during the first year of life, the growth rate is more accelerated than at any other time in childhood. Normal weight range for a full-term newborn is 5 lb 8 oz to 8 lb 13 oz (2,500 to 4,000 g). Average length is 19 to 21 in (48 to 53 cm). Most infants gain approximately 1 to 2 lb/month, double their birth rate by 6 months, and triple their birth rate by 1 year. By the end of the 12th month, most infants have increased their length by approximately 50% (Stantrock, 2006).

Motor Development

Motor development progresses in predictable patterns: cephalocaudally, central to distal, and gross to fine. For example, the infant develops head control before walking, can roll over before intentionally grabbing a toy, and can bat at a mobile before manipulating an object (Norberg, 2001). Nurses assess newborn and infant motor development using standardized developmental screening tools. An example is the Denver II, which is described in more detail in Chapter 29 (Stantrock, 2006).

Language, Psychosocial, and Cognitive Development

Speech development begins with vocalizations and babbling. The infant learns language through listening, watching, and interacting with the environment. The spectrum of normal language development is wide. More on language develop-

ment, as well as psychosocial and cognitive development of the infant, is discussed in Chapter 9 (Stantrock, 2006).

Acute Assessment

Acute assessment of the newborn is performed immediately after birth. Because the newborn must adapt rapidly to life outside the womb, the nurse must quickly make several key assessments. The American Academy of Pediatrics (AAP) in collaboration with the American Heart Association (AHA) outlines critical components of the initial assessment in the Neonatal Resuscitation Program. The ABCs of resuscitation, Airway, Breathing, and Circulation, are the same for infants as for adults; however, the assessments and interventions are modified to accommodate the infant's unique anatomical and physiological characteristics. The nurse must ask four key assessment questions about the newborn's health (AAP & AHA, 2006):

1. Is the newborn term gestation (37 weeks or greater)?
2. Is the amniotic fluid clear?
3. Is the newborn breathing or crying?
4. Does the newborn have good muscle tone?

If the answer to all four questions is "Yes," then the newborn is adapting well and may receive care at the bedside with his or her mother. If the answer to even one of the questions is "No," then the baby needs resuscitation. (See the *Neonatal Resuscitation Textbook*, AAP & AHA, 2006 for further information on neonatal resuscitation.)

Most emergent situations for the newborn involve respiratory decompensation. Signs of newborn respiratory distress include increased respiratory and heart rates, nasal flaring, and intercostal and substernal retractions. The first sign of respiratory distress in a newborn is often tachypnea (heart rate > 160 at rest). Moderate respiratory distress includes nasal flaring, retractions of the chest wall, grunting auscultated with a stethoscope, cyanosis on room air, and abnormal blood gas values. Severe distress is indicated by increasing work of breathing, deep retractions, audible grunting, and central cyanosis. Acute assessment of the infant is the same as for a small child (see Chapter 29).

⚠ SAFETY ALERT 28.1
Respiratory distress in the newborn and infant often progresses rapidly to severe distress requiring bag and mask or mechanical ventilation. Nurses must intervene early at the first sign of distress to avert an emergency resuscitation, if possible.

Subjective Data Collection

Areas for Health Promotion/*Healthy People*

Many *Healthy People* objectives apply to newborns and infants (Table 28-1). Health promotion for parents of newborns and infants focuses on prevention, early detection of illness and developmental delays, and early intervention to optimize

Table 28.1	*Healthy People* Objectives and Associated Education Topics for Parents of Infants
Goal	**Patient Education Topics**
Reduce the proportion of families that experience difficulties or delays in obtaining health care.	Discuss community resources for regular health care for children in the family, if the family is uninsured or underinsured or financially challenged. Medicaid and State Children's Health Insurance Program (SCHIP) are two such resources.
Reduce hospitalization rates for pediatric asthma, uncontrolled diabetes, and immunization-preventable pneumonia and influenza.	Discuss the importance of maintaining the home as a smoke-free zone. Provide influenza vaccine to all children older than 6 months.
Reduce vaccine-preventable diseases.	Educate about their dangers compared to the slight risks of the vaccine. Provide vaccines on schedule.
Reduce deaths caused by poisonings.	Teach parents how to childproof the home. Explain the importance of securing medications and other chemicals out of the reach of children. Encourage parents to keep the Poison Control number posted (1-800-222-1222).
Reduce deaths caused by suffocation and SIDS.	Educate parents on the importance of not sleeping with infants. Discuss safe sleep practices for infants. Always back to sleep, no pillows or excessively soft bedding or toys in cribs. Discuss choking prevention.
Increase the percentage of healthy full-term infants who are put down to sleep on their backs.	Alert parents to the increased risk of SIDS when infants are positioned prone for sleeping.
Increase use of child restraints.	Discuss with parents use of car seats, booster seats, and seat belts according to state laws.
Reduce residential fire deaths.	Explain the importance of maintaining functioning smoke alarms on every floor and in every sleeping area of the home. In homes with smoke alarms, residents are half as likely to experience a death from fire as are those without alarms.
Reduce drownings.	Instruct parents never to turn their backs on or leave an infant alone in any amount of water.
Reduce maltreatment and maltreatment fatalities of children.	Discuss shaken baby syndrome. Explore ways for parents to deal with frustration when the infant is fussy or inconsolable. Describe appropriate discipline techniques and community resources available for additional assistance.
Ensure appropriate newborn bloodspot screening, follow-up testing, and referral to services.	Collect specimens for newborn screening tests. Give parents instructions for and explain the importance of follow-up testing. When a developmental disorder is diagnosed, assist parents to enroll the infant in appropriate programs and services.
Increase the proportion of mothers who breastfeed.	Encourage mothers to breastfeed for as long as possible during the first 12 months. Discuss the advantages of breastfeeding. Assist mothers to find community resources supportive of breastfeeding, such as La Leche League.
Reduce growth retardation among low-income children under age 5 years.	Educate parents regarding the approximate amount of food that infants need as they grow. Explain how to determine if the newborn/infant is getting enough to eat and drink.
Reduce the proportion of children and adolescents who have dental caries in their primary or permanent teeth.	Discuss the prevention of baby bottle tooth decay. Describe good oral health: teeth are brushed at a minimum of twice per day and flossed once per day. A dental visit for the establishment of a dental home for children is recommended by age 1 year. Refer to a dentist who sees children.
Reduce the proportion of nonsmokers exposed to environmental tobacco smoke.	Emphasize that an infant exposed to second-hand smoke is more prone to upper respiratory infections and otitis media.

Source: *Healthy people 2010: What are its goals?* (n.d.). Retrieved July 7, 2010, from http://www.healthypeople.gov/About/goals.htm

Questions on History and Risk	Rationales
Current Problems	
• What brings you to the clinic today?	This question elicits the presenting issue in the parent's own words.
• When was the infant last known to be well? Alternatively, when was the infant last known to be his or her normal self?	These questions help identify how long any illness has been present and establish the infant's normal state of health.
• How and when did the problem begin? What was the infant's health immediately before symptom onset?	This line of questioning is designed to understand the course and progress of the present illness.
• How has the illness progressed?	
• What symptoms does the infant have? In what order did they appear?	
• Does anything seem to make the symptoms better or worse?	
• What treatments or medications (including over-the-counter [OTC]) have you given?	
• Has the child received medical attention for this illness (before the current visit)?	
Family History	
Tell me a little bit about your family and your home.	This broad question helps the examiner understand the socioeconomic situation, living conditions, other family members, and background and education of the parents. Follow up with questions to obtain desired information if the broader question fails to provide enough detail. Conversely, ask questions to gently refocus parents if they provide too much extra detail.
Personal History (Infant)	
• Were there any unusual circumstances or health problems during the pregnancy?	These questions help elicit the obstetric and birth history to identify risk factors.
• What was the duration of the pregnancy, type of labor and delivery, and type of anesthesia used for labor?	
• What was the Apgar score? Did the infant require any resuscitation?	
• What was the birth weight?	
• Did the infant go home with the mother? Did the infant spend any time in the neonatal intensive care unit (NICU)?	
• Has the infant had any infections, illnesses, hospitalizations, or surgeries since birth?	
• How often has the baby had well-child checkups?	
Medications and Supplements	
What medications is the infant taking (include OTC preparations and vitamins)? Is the infant current with immunizations?	This is to determine past medical history.
Risk Factors	
• Does your child sleep on his or her back?	This is to identify risk factors and promote health. Once risk factors are assessed, patient teaching can be performed.
• Does he or she fall asleep with a bottle?	
• Have you childproofed your home for choking hazards and secured poisons?	
• Do you have a car seat approved for infants? Is it in the back seat?	
• Have you learned CPR?	
• Has the infant had any accidents or injuries?	

outcomes. The nurse can help parents understand the importance of laying a foundation of healthy living and lifestyle choices that will help the infant achieve his or her potential.

Risk Assessment and Health-Related Patient Teaching

Infants should have regular examinations with a pediatrician or another health care professional with specialized pediatric training, such as a Pediatric Advanced Practice Registered Nurse. Ideally, parents schedule an initial visit before the baby is born. At this visit, the primary care provider obtains the family and prenatal history, gives anticipatory guidance, inquires about the chosen feeding method, and encourages breastfeeding.

After birth, the AAP recommends well-baby visits at 3 to 5 days of age, by 1 month, and then at 2, 4, 6, 9, and 12 months. This frequency gives the primary care provider an opportunity to identify potential developmental delays and other health problems, to continue anticipatory guidance, and to give immunizations on schedule.

The nurse performs a risk assessment to plan for care and teaching. Anticipatory guidance for parents of newborns and infants focuses on safety. Most unexpected deaths during infancy are related to injury, sudden infant death syndrome (SIDS), respiratory arrest, or near drowning. The leading cause of injury-related death for infants is choking and suffocation (AHA, n.d.). Parents require anticipatory guidance to avert preventable injury and illness. Major topics include safe sleep habits, choking prevention, immunization schedules, child safety car seats, CPR training for parents, syrup of ipecac/poison control, breastfeeding/iron rich foods, and preventing baby bottle tooth decay.

Safe Sleep Habits

Incorporating safe sleep habits for infants helps prevent SIDS. Infants should always be placed on their backs to sleep (Fig. 28-1). The mattress should be firm. Pillows, soft toys, excessive blankets, and bedding should not be in the crib when the infant is asleep. The infant should not sleep in the same bed in which an adult is sleeping. It is too easy for the tiny face to be covered inadvertently and for the infant to be smothered.

Choking

To prevent choking, parents should remain vigilant about the environment and remove choking hazards. The nurse should advise parents to get down on their hands and knees and survey the environment from the infant's perspective. Any small object within the infant's reach is a possible choking hazard. Anything that can fit in the infant's mouth and be inhaled should be removed from his or her reach. Examples include balloons, toys with small parts, safety pins, small balls, broken crayons, coins, and so on. Certain foods can increase the risk for choking. Firm or round foods, such as hot dogs, seeds, grapes, and raw carrots and apples, should be cooked or chopped into tiny pieces before serving to an infant or a very young child. See Chapter 29 for further discussion regarding safeguarding the home for small children.

Immunization Schedules

Newborns and infants need vaccines to protect them from diseases that can have serious consequences, such as seizures, brain damage, blindness, and even death. The Centers for Disease Control (CDC), the AAP, and the American Academy of Family Physicians collaborate to provide a schedule of immunizations recommended for infants and children. See Appendix A.

Because immunizations are normally administered in conjunction with routine checkups, determine if the parents are keeping regularly scheduled appointments. Next, check the immunization record. The initial record is typically provided to the parents before the newborn is discharged home when the first immunization is given. If the record is not up-to-date, ask if the parents are familiar with the immunization schedule. Provide a schedule, if needed, and help the parents determine where they can go to have the infant immunized.

Parents should be informed that it is important for their infant to receive vaccines at the ages and times recommended to ensure the highest level of protection against vaccine-preventable diseases. If the infant misses an immunization or gets behind schedule, there is a catch-up schedule available on the AAP Web site.

⚠ SAFETY ALERT 28.2

Many parents are concerned about the safety of vaccines; a few physicians do not subscribe to current scientific evidence in this regard. The evidence supports the safety of currently recommended vaccines. The diseases for which vaccines are protective can cause serious harm and even death. Encourage concerned parents to explore the evidence from the CDC and AAP.

Child Safety Car Seat

It is important to ask the parents how the infant is secured when riding in the car. Questions include: Is a car seat used? If so, is the restraint approved for use by infants? Is the restraint secured in the front or the back seat? Anytime

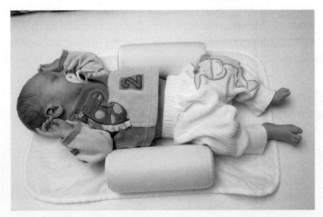

Figure 28.1 Placement of the infant on his back for sleep is a key SIDS prevention measure.

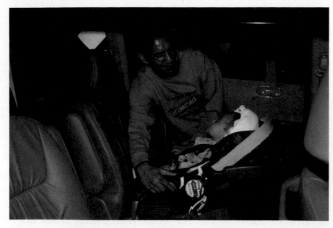
Figure 28.2 Infants should be in an appropriate sized car seat in the back seat of the vehicle.

an infant or a child younger than 4 years is in the car, the child should be restrained in a car seat for safety (Fig. 28-2). General guidelines can be found in Chapter 29; more detailed recommendations are listed on the AAP Web site. The article "Car Safety Seats: A Guide for Families 2009," available on the AAP Web site, can be printed and given to parents for reference.

CPR Training for Parents
Inquire if the parents know CPR. Traditionally, NICUs teach parents infant CPR before discharge because these infants are at higher risk than are healthy infants for respiratory and cardiac arrest. Nevertheless, it is important for all parents and babysitters to know CPR. Many communities offer CPR classes for nominal fees. A newer resource is *Infant CPR Anytime*. This self-directed learning kit, developed by the AAP in coordination with the AHA, contains a manikin for practicing CPR and a video demonstrating CPR that the learner can view and review, as needed.

Poison Control
The nurse asks the parents how they have secured medications, cleaning compounds, and other chemicals in the home. It is important to explain that safety locks should be placed on cabinets located close to the floor, and that it is wise to put medication and other toxic chemicals in high, locked cabinets. The nurse explains that ordering all prescription medications with childproof lids is another safety precaution. The nurse should ask if emergency numbers are posted near all phones in the home. The toll-free poison control number 1-800-222-1222 should be included in the list of emergency numbers.

Breastfeeding/Iron-Rich Foods
The nurse should ask the mother if she is breastfeeding. If she is, the nurse determines how long she plans to continue. If the mother has already returned to work, the nurse asks if she feels comfortable pumping her breasts at work and if there is a private place where she can do this. Many companies are becoming "breastfeeding friendly" work-

sites, providing private spaces for pumping, adequate time, and refrigeration for pumped breast milk. Alternately, some employers allow the baby to be brought to the workplace or the woman to go home for feeding.

Breast milk is the best food for the growing infant. For the first 4 to 6 months, it is the only food that the infant needs. Ideally, every baby should be breastfed for the first year of life. Iron-fortified infant formula is an acceptable alternative for mothers who cannot or choose not to breastfeed. The nurse cautions the parents that whole cow's milk is not an appropriate food for children younger than 1 year.

⚠ SAFETY ALERT 28.3
Honey should not be given to infants. It is a known reservoir for the bacterium that causes botulism. The spores the bacteria produce make a toxin that can cause infant botulism, a serious form of food poisoning. The toxin affects the infant's neurologic system and can lead to death.

As long as the woman has adequate iron stores, iron supplementation for exclusively breastfed infants is not necessary during the first 6 months. After 6 months, the parents may introduce meats or other iron-rich food sources to the infant's diet. This should ensure adequate iron intake without the need to supplement.

Baby Bottle Tooth Decay
The nurse should inquire regarding daily intake of sugar, especially the frequent consumption of sugary drinks (eg, soft drinks, punch, juice). He or should assess if the infant is ever allowed to go to sleep with a bottle of milk, formula, juice, or other sugary drink. This practice can lead to a condition known as **baby bottle tooth decay** (see Chapter 17). The problem is that the sugar sticks to the primary teeth and coats them. Bacteria in the mouth break down the sugars to use for food. As this breakdown occurs, the bacteria produce acids that attack the teeth and cause decay.

Some parents may not understand why the primary teeth are important. Unlike adult tooth decay, baby bottle tooth decay is most pronounced on the upper front teeth and is highly visible while the child's self image is forming. In addition, if the primary teeth experience significant decay, they may require extraction. Because the primary teeth serve as placeholders for the secondary teeth, if they are lost too early, the secondary teeth may come in excessively crooked.

Focused Health History Related to Common Symptoms

Common Newborn/Infant Symptoms
- Respiratory complaints and/or distress
- Fever
- Skin conditions
- Gastrointestinal distress
- Crying/irritability

Questions to Assess Symptoms	Rationales/Abnormal Findings

Respiratory Complaints/Distress

Has the infant had trouble breathing? Have there been any episodes in which the infant turned blue? Does the infant have frequent colds? Is there an associated cough or sneezing? Is there any sputum production or secretions? Has the infant had a stuffy or runny nose? Has the parent noticed any wheezing? What has been the infant's temperature pattern? Are the infant's immunizations up-to-date?

It is important to determine associated symptoms to identify severity and possible causation. This knowledge will guide the focused assessment.

Fever

In addition to the respiratory questions above, ask:

• Has the infant been exposed to anyone with a communicable illness?
• Has the infant traveled with the family recently? If so, where?
• Was the infant born prematurely or did the infant have a prolonged NICU stay?
• Has the child had previous infections or hospitalizations?
• Has the infant been pulling on one or both ears?
• Have the parents noticed any change in eating or behavior patterns, such as irritability or difficulty rousing?
• Has the child demonstrated any abnormal posturing?
• Has the infant had any periods when he or she stopped breathing momentarily (apnea)?
• Is there an unusual odor to the urine?
• Does there seem to be any pain associated with urination?
• What, if any treatments, have the family given?

Fever is associated frequently with infection, which can range in severity from mild to life-threatening. This line of questioning helps reveal the infant's risk factors for as well as possible causes of infection. The provider needs to determine if the fever likely has a respiratory origin (hence the respiratory questions). Could it be an *ear infection* (pulling on the ears) or *urinary tract infection*? Are there symptoms of *meningitis* (posturing), or is a blood infection likely? Although the nurse will not make a final medical diagnosis, these data will guide the nursing assessment and care planning (Wong, et al., 2008).

Skin Conditions

• When did the rash or hives begin? On what part of the body did it begin? Has it spread? If so, where?
• Has the parent noticed the infant scratching? Has there been any oozing, unusual odor, or puss-type material associated with lesions? Has there been crusting or erosion?
• Has there been a recent change in laundry detergents, soaps, or shampoos?
• Has there been a change in the texture or luster of the hair or nails?
• Is there an associated temperature elevation?
• Has the infant been exposed to anyone with a communicable disease?
• Are the immunizations up-to-date?

These questions help pinpoint possible causes. Many skin conditions have predictable patterns of spread, parts of the body affected, and associated symptoms, such as pruritis (itching). It is important to differentiate if the symptoms are localized versus systemic, or if there might be an infectious versus an allergic origin.

Gastrointestinal Distress

• Has there been vomiting? Is it projectile? What color and how much vomitus has there been?
• When was the last bowel movement? Describe the stool pattern and consistency. Has the stool been watery or unusually hard? What is the color and amount?
• Has the parent noticed a yellowish color to the skin?
• Does the child seem to be in pain? Has there been a fever?

Gastrointestinal symptoms can be associated with a wide range of conditions. In addition, infants can become dehydrated very quickly in the presence of vomiting or diarrhea.

Crying/Irritability

• What are the circumstances of crying? Has the parent found a way to calm the infant?
• Tell me about the infant's eating patterns.
• When was the last bowel movement? Has the pattern of bowel movements changed? How many wet diapers does the infant have in one day?
• What has been the infant's temperature?
• Has the infant been exposed to a communicable disease? Are any other friends or family members currently ill? If so, what is the illness?
• Are the immunizations current?
• What is the infant's activity level?

Crying and irritability are nonspecific symptoms implicated in conditions that range in severity from minor to life-threatening. It is important to identify associated symptoms, because this will guide the primary care provider's choice of diagnostic tests (Simon, 2009).

Additional Questions	Rationales/Abnormal Findings
Many families use home remedies to treat certain conditions. Are there any home remedies your family finds helpful?	If the parent describes a harmful practice (eg, giving the infant a bottle of water with honey), then respectfully educate about possible consequences. Follow up by negotiating with the parent for a healthier way to meet the particular need that fits the family's culture.

Therapeutic Dialogue: Collecting Subjective Data

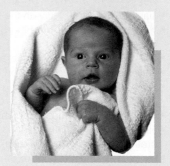

The nurse's role relative to subjective data collection is to gather information to improve the patient's health status and to help determine the cause of the patient's current symptoms. Remember Keri, who was introduced at the beginning of this chapter. This 1-month-old is visiting the clinic today for her well-child checkup and hepatitis B immunization.

The nurse uses professional communication techniques to gather subjective data from the mother, Diane Downs. The following conversations give two examples of interview styles used by different nurses. One style is more effective than the other.

Less Effective

Nurse: Boy, it's cold out today. I've been freezing to death since I've been here.

Mrs. Downs: Yeah, I'm cold too. They said that it was going to be this way the whole week. Did you hear that we might have some snow on Friday?

Nurse: I didn't hear that but those forecasters are always wrong. Remember the last time they said that it would snow and it didn't.

Mrs. Downs: Yeah, I don't know if things change or they just aren't good at predicting. (looks at chart)

Nurse: I see that you are a nurse and the baby is growing nicely, so it looks like you must be comfortable with breastfeeding. Right? Make sure to continue with breast milk only until Keri is 4–6 months old.

Mrs. Downs: Really?

Nurse: Yes. Now let's see. Keri is 1-month-old. She should be gaining weight and sleeping a lot. Is she sleeping through the night yet?

Mrs. Downs: No, she's waking up twice.

Nurse: I have a form I have to fill out that gives us information about your baby. Let's see. The first question is, "Were there any problems during the pregnancy or delivery?"

More Effective

Nurse: Good morning, Mrs. Downs. I am Keri's RN for today. I see you have Keri wrapped up snugly for the cold weather we're having!

Mrs. Downs: Yes, it's cold out.

Nurse: I will be asking you a few questions as part of the comprehensive assessment today, and I will be performing a physical examination of Keri. Before we get started, do you have any concerns or questions you would like to discuss today?

Mrs. Downs: No, but I'll ask if I have any.

Nurse: Great. Now during the first few weeks of life the parents and baby are getting to know one another and establishing routines. What is Keri's routine at home?

Mrs. Downs: She goes to bed around 8:30 pm and wakes up around 8 am, but is up twice during the night. During the day, she nurses every 2–3 hours. Do you think that she's getting enough milk?

Nurse: It looks like Keri is growing nicely. That usually means that she is getting plenty of milk. Please tell me about your breastfeeding experience. (Waits for Mrs. Downs to describe her experience.) How frequently is Keri nursing? Is Keri having any problems latching on?

Critical Thinking Challenge

- What strategies does the nurse with the more effective style use to gather and share information?
- What blocks to communication does the nurse with the less effective style use?
- What tips could you give him or her to improve communication with patients?

Objective Data Collection

After completing subjective data collection with the parent holding the infant, the nurse will collect equipment and prepare for the objective assessment. Well-child assessments include head-to-toe physical examinations, but the order is altered for infants, saving the least comfortable portions for last.

Equipment

Equipment that should be readily available includes a tape measure, stethoscope, thermometer, watch or clock with a second hand, infant scale, otoscope, and ophthalmoscope. A pacifier, if acceptable to the parent, may help keep the infant from crying during the examination.

Preparation

The examination should be performed in a well-lighted area. The environment should be comfortable, free of drafts, and quiet. There should be a place for both parent and nurse to sit while obtaining the history and performing parts of the examination that can be completed with the infant on the parent's lap.

After washing your hands, ensure that the parent and infant are comfortable. Introduce yourself and explain what the parent can expect. It may help to ease the parent if you comment on positive features of the infant. Engage the baby with friendly conversation while the parent continues to hold him or her. Sit at eye level and not tower above the family, a stance that can be viewed as threatening. It may be helpful to have a soft toy to offer the infant while you obtain the health history from the parent.

Warm your hands by placing them in warm water before touching the infant. This can be accomplished in conjunction with washing the hands just before the examination. Likewise warm the stethoscope with the hands before placing it on the infant's skin. For the older infant, let him or her hold the stethoscope and demonstrate listening to the heart on the parent to prepare the infant for what to expect. These measures can decrease the infant's stress during the examination.

Comprehensive Physical Examination

The physical examination typically is not completed in a head-to-toe fashion, as for adults. Order varies depending on the baby's developmental level, temperament, and individual needs. Nevertheless, the approach should be systematic to minimize the omission of parts of the examination. The most invasive techniques (ie, assessment of tonsils, uvula, ears) generally should be done at the end. If the infant is asleep or quietly alert, then count the respirations and listen to the heart, lungs, and abdomen before performing other parts of the examination that may disturb the infant, which can cause crying that disrupts your ability to hear clearly.

Two comprehensive assessments specific to newborns are also included below: the Apgar score assessment and the initial newborn assessment (including gestational age and reflexes). A complete head-to-toe assessment of the newborn occurs sometime in the first hour or two after birth and is similar to that for older infants.

Technique and Normal Findings	Abnormal Findings
Newborn: Apgar Score The Apgar score is one of the first newborn assessments the nurse makes. It is not used to guide resuscitation efforts but gives important clues about how well the newborn is adapting to life outside the womb. The newborn receives a score of 0–2 in each of 5 areas for a possible total score of 10. The score is calculated at 1 minute and again at 5 minutes of life. See Table 18-5. *A score of 7–10 indicates a vigorous newborn adapting well to the extrauterine environment.*	If the 5-minute score is <7, continue to score every 5 minutes until the score is above 7, the newborn is intubated, or the newborn is transferred to the nursery. If the 5-minute score is 4–6, the newborn is having some difficulty adapting and requires closer observation than a vigorous newborn. A score <4 signifies that the newborn is having severe difficulty adapting to life outside the womb and requires observation and care in a NICU.
Newborn: Gestational Age During pregnancy, gestational age is calculated from the date of the last menstrual period or by results of an early sonogram. After birth, physical characteristics and neuromuscular assessment are used to evaluate gestational age. The Ballard Gestational Age Assessment Tool (Fig. 28-3) is commonly used in newborn nurseries. *The New Ballard score ranges from −1 to 4 or 5 for each criterion. Possible totals range from −10 to 50, or a gestational range of 20–44 weeks. An increase in the score by 5 increases the age by 2 weeks.*	The New Ballard Scale includes extremely premature newborns and has been refined to improve accuracy in more mature newborns.

(text continues on page 844)

NEUROMUSCULAR MATURITY

NEUROMUSCULAR MATURITY SIGN	SCORE							RECORD SCORE HERE
	−1	0	1	2	3	4	5	
POSTURE								
SQUARE WINDOW (Wrist)	>90°	90°	60°	45°	30°	0°		
ARM RECOIL		180°	140°–180°	110°–140°	90°–110°	<90°		
POPLITEAL ANGLE	180°	160°	140°	120°	100°	90°	<90°	
SCARF SIGN								
HEEL TO EAR								
					TOTAL NEUROMUSCULAR MATURITY SCORE			

SCORE
Neuromuscular _____
Physical _____
Total _____

MATURITY RATING

Score	Weeks
−10	20
−5	22
0	24
5	26
10	28
15	30
20	32
25	34
30	36
35	38
40	40
45	42
50	44

PHYSICAL MATURITY

PHYSICAL MATURITY SIGN	SCORE							RECORD SCORE HERE
	−1	0	1	2	3	4	5	
SKIN	sticky, friable, transparent	gelatinous, red, translucent	smooth, pink, visible veins	superficial peeling and/or rash, few veins	cracking pale areas, rare veins	parchment, deep cracking, no vessels	leathery, cracked, wrinkled	
LANUGO	none	sparse	abundant	thinning	bald areas	mostly bald		
PLANTAR SURFACE	heel-toe 40–50 mm:−1 <40 mm:−2	>50 mm no crease	faint red marks	anterior transverse crease only	creases ant. 2/3	creases over entire sole		
BREAST	imperceptible	barely perceptible	flat areola no bud	stippled areola 1–2 mm bud	raised areola 3–4 mm bud	full areola 5–10 mm bud		
EYE-EAR	lids fused loosely: −1 tightly: −2	lids open pinna flat stays folded	sl. curved pinna; soft; slow recoil	well-curved pinna; soft but ready recoil	formed and firm instant recoil	thick cartilage, ear stiff		
GENITALS (Male)	scrotum flat, smooth	scrotum empty, faint rugae	testes in upper canal, rare rugae	testes descending, few rugae	testes down, good rugae	testes pendulous, deep rugae		
GENITALS (Female)	clitoris prominent and labia flat	prominent clitoris and small labia minora	prominent clitoris and enlarging minora	majora and minora equally prominent	majora large, minora small	majora cover clitoris and minora		
					TOTAL PHYSICAL MATURITY SCORE			

Figure 28.3 Ballard Gestational Age Assessment Tool for use in screening newborns.

Technique and Normal Findings (continued)	Abnormal Findings (continued)
Reflexes Evaluation of newborn reflexes gives information about neurologic status. Assess rooting, suck, Moro (startle), Galant's (trunk incurvation), stepping, palmar grasp, tonic neck, and Babinski reflexes (see Table 28-2).	Diminished reflexes indicate the possibility of neurological or developmental deficits.

Table 28.2 Newborn Reflexes

Rooting

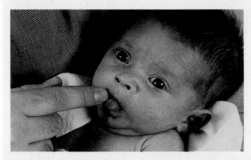

Gently stroke the cheek. The newborn turns toward the stimulus and opens the mouth. This reflex disappears at 3–4 months, although it may persist longer. Absence indicates a neurologic disorder.

Moro (Startle)

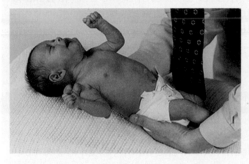

The Moro reflex occurs when the infant is startled or feels like he or she is falling. Sudden noise also can stimulate it, verifying that the infant can hear. Bring the infant to sit. Support the upper body and head with one hand; flex the chest. Suddenly let the head and shoulders drop a few inches while releasing the arms. The arms and legs extend symmetrically. The arms return toward midline with the hand open and the thumb and index finger forming a "C." Moro disappears by 4–6 months of age. Its absence or weakness points to an *upper motor neuron lesion*. An asymmetrical Moro occurs with *brachial plexus injury*.

Galant's (Trunk Incurvation)

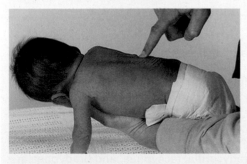

Place the newborn in ventral suspension. Stroke the skin on one side of the back. The trunk and hips should swing toward the side of the stimulus. Galant's reflex is normally present for the first 4–8 weeks of life. Its absence may indicate *spinal cord lesions*.

Suck

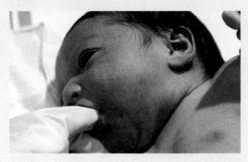

Place a gloved finger in the newborn's mouth. He or she should vigorously suck. The reflex may persist during infancy. A weak or absent reflex indicates a developmental or neurological disorder.

Tonic Neck

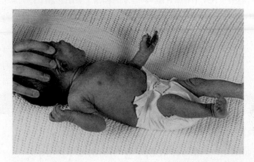

Turn the head of the supine infant to one side. The arm and leg extend on the side to which the face is pointed. The contralateral arm and leg flex, forming the classic fencer position. Repeat by turning the head to the other side—the position will reverse. This reflex is strongest at 2 months and disappears by 6 months. If still present at 9 months (an indicator of neurologic damage), the infant will not be able to support weight to crawl.

Palmar Grasp

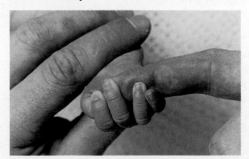

Place your finger in the newborn's palm; the infant's fingers will firmly grasp your finger. This reflex is strongest between 1 and 2 months. Persistence after 3 months indicates a *neurologic disorder*.

Table 28.2   Newborn Reflexes (continued)

Stepping

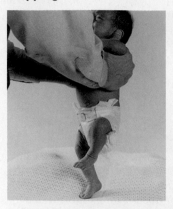

Hold the infant upright. Allow the soles to touch a flat surface. The legs flex and extend in a walking pattern. This reflex exists for the first 4–8 weeks of life and persists with neurological conditions (eg, *cerebral palsy*).

Babinski

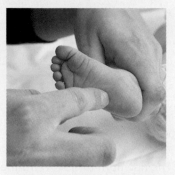

Stroke one side of the infant's foot upward from the heel and across the ball of the foot. The infant responds by hyperextending the toes: the great toe flexes toward the top of the foot and the other toes fan outward. This reflex lasts until the child is walking well. Persistence after age 2 years is associated with neurologic damage (eg, *cerebral palsy*).

Technique and Normal Findings (continued)	Abnormal Findings (continued)

General Survey

Begin the general survey, keeping in mind the age of the infant in months and the correlated expected development. Continue to collect data through observation during the entire visit. *The healthy infant has good muscle tone, a symmetrical appearance, and appears well. Respirations are unlabored with no signs of acute distress.*

Notice interactions between the infant and parent. If stranger anxiety is present, perform as much of the examination as possible with the infant on the parent's lap. *The parent picks up on cues from the infant. The infant appears alert and engaged in the environment, unless sleeping. A normal variant is stranger anxiety that begins around 9 months.*

The infant appears listless and uninterested in interaction. The parent pays little attention to the infant and does not pick up on cues, such as stress or readiness for interaction. Make note of any unusual odors. Certain diseases, such as *phenylketonuria, maple syrup urine disease*, and *diabetic acidosis,* have characteristic odors (see Table 28-5 at the end of this chapter). Poor hygiene or inappropriate dress for the weather should alert the nurse to watch for other signs of neglect.

Vital Signs

Axillary temperature measurement is appropriate for the newborn. After the first month of life, either axillary or tympanic temperatures are appropriate. Temperature is taken again after the first bath. *Range of normal is the same as for adults: 97.7°F–98.6°F (36.5°C–37°C).*

Both elevated and decreased temperatures can signal infection in the newborn because the regulatory mechanisms are not fully mature. The newborn may cool during bathing and cannot shiver to raise heat.

Apical pulse and respiratory rate should be measured for a full minute each with the infant at rest. *Normal pulse range for the newborn is 110–160 bpm, decreasing slightly to 80–140 for infants older than 1 month. Respiratory rate is 30–60 bpm for newborns and 22–35 for infants.*

Tachycardia, bradycardia, tachypnea, and bradypnea are abnormal findings at rest. These terms are defined as falling above or below the ranges listed.

Blood pressures are not measured routinely in the infant. If the blood pressures are taken, measure pressures in all four extremities. Make sure that the cuff fits appropriately. *Normal systolic pressures are 50–70 for newborns and 70–100 for infants older than 1 month.*

A difference between upper and lower extremity blood pressures may indicate *coarctation of the aorta.*

Pain

Assess for pain (see Chapter 7). *The infant without pain appears comfortable and not excessively irritable.*

Because the infant is preverbal, ask the parent to help interpret pain signals. Newborns cry indiscriminately when in pain. It may help to systematically eliminate other causes of crying, such us hunger or a soiled diaper.

Measurements

Weigh the infant using an infant scale that is calibrated regularly. Place a protective covering on it, zero the scale, and then position the infant with your hands just above, but not touching, to prevent a fall (Fig. 28-4). Use the tape measure and carefully measure from the crown of the head to the heel. Some nurses find it helpful to place the infant on the examination table, then using a pencil, place a mark at the crown and another mark at the infant's heel (with the hip and knee extended). Use the tape measure to measure the length between the two markings, which, if done properly, is an accurate

> #### Clinical Significance 28-1
>
> When plotting measurements for premature infants, use the corrected age for comparison instead of the chronological age for at least the first 24 months. For example, if the infant was born at 30 weeks' gestation, the birth was 10 weeks before term (40 minus 10). So at 12 weeks (3 months) chronological or postnatal age, the infant's corrected age would be 2 weeks (12 minus 10).

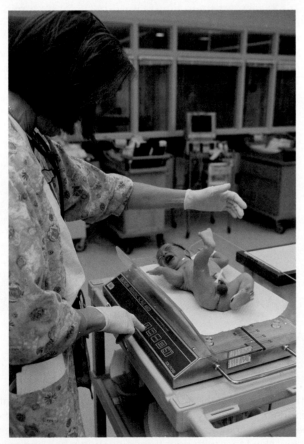

Figure 28.4 Weighing the newborn.

(text continues on page 848)

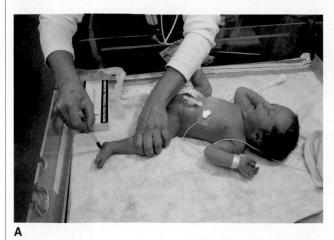

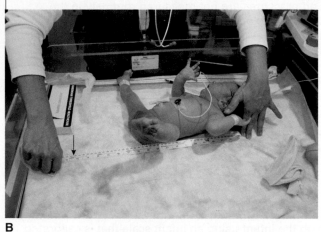

A   **B**

Figure 28.5 A. Marking the foot placement of the newborn with a pen. **B.** Using the tape measure to measure the length between the head and foot to arrive at an accurate length measurement.

measurement of length (Fig. 28-5). Measure head and chest circumferences (Fig. 28-6). Plot the measurements on a standardized growth chart. *In general, the measurements are above the 10th percentile and below the 90th percentile. Compare measurements with previous visits. The infant is gaining height and weight at a steady pace.*

Length varies depending upon heredity. A small head may indicate *microcephaly*, while a large head may be from *hydrocephalus* or *increased intracranial pressure.* A small chest circumference may be from prematurity.

Clinical Significance 28-2

One measurement in time is not a basis for determining appropriate growth. Only by comparing measurements over time are growth delays documented, because each infant grows as an individual guided by genetics and environment.

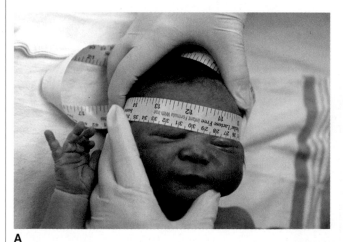

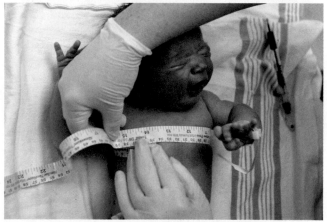

A   **B**

Figure 28.6 A. Measuring newborn head circumference. **B.** Measuring newborn chest circumference.

Nutrition

Inspect the general condition of the skin, hair, and nails. *A well-nourished infant has soft, supple skin and shiny hair.* Ask about urination and bowel movements. *On average, the infant getting enough to eat wets a diaper four to six times per day and has regular bowel movements that are soft and not watery.*

An indication that the infant is not eating enough is parental reports of fussing, crying, and not seeming satisfied after feeding. Other indications of inadequate nutrition include sallow skin tones with poor turgor, dry brittle hair and nails, losing weight or falling behind on growth charts compared to previous visits, and consuming <100 kcal/kg/day.

If the infant is bottle-feeding, ask the parent how many ounces per feeding and how many feedings per day. *The infant is consuming approximately 100 kcal/kg/day.* For example, if the infant weighs 10 lb (4.5 kg), then he or she should be eating approximately 450 kcal/day. Formulas for term infants contain 20 kcal/oz. So, the infant in this example should be consuming 22–23 oz/day (4.5 kg × 100 kcal/kg/day/20 kcal/oz = 22.5 oz). If the parent is having difficulty determining intake and there is a question as to adequacy, ask the parent to keep a diary of the infant's intake for the next 3 days and report back.

Failure to thrive is described as weight that falls below the fifth percentile for the child's age (El-Baba, et al., 2009). Causes to further evaluate include inadequate calorie intake, inadequate absorption, increased metabolism, or defective use of food sources. Be sure to differentiate inadequate intake from signs of acute dehydration, which include decreased skin turgor, sunken anterior fontanel, dry mucous membranes, no tears, and an acutely ill appearance. Ask the parent to describe how infant formula is prepared in the home. Improperly prepared formula is an important cause of inadequate nutrition. Safety issues related to infant formula preparation can be found on the U.S. Food and Drug Administration (FDA) Web site.

Mental Status

In infants, mental status is determined by observing sleep states and behavior throughout the examination. Observe for developmentally appropriate behavior. *For example, an alert 1-month-old engages with the eyes when face-to-face with the parent or nurse and responds to the voice by turning toward the sound or tracking with the eyes. An older infant reaches for an object the parent or examiner offers.*

During the first month or two, crying is a normal response to handling and undressing during a physical examination. Crying should stop with gentle rocking in the arms or while holding the infant against the shoulder. As the infant matures, the infant may smile and interact with the examiner, as long as movements are not sudden or threatening and the voice maintains a calm and reassuring quality.

Abnormal findings are when interaction between infant and parent does not seem synergistic and the older infant is excessively clingy or does not warm up to the examiner after a period of interaction. Excessive irritability and inconsolable crying may be early signs of a change in mental status. Later signs may be a high-pitched cry, or lethargy and listlessness.

⚠ SAFETY ALERT 28.4

If the infant cannot be aroused or does not move evasively when prodded during an examination, he or she is showing signs of a severe change in mental status. This infant needs immediate medical attention.

Violence

It is prudent to assess the parent for signs of domestic violence because children living in violent situations are much more likely to suffer abuse than children in households uncomplicated by violence. See Chapter 12. *Normal parental findings include a relaxed, confident demeanor with appropriate affect, good grooming, and appropriate interaction with and concern for the infant. Normal infant findings include appropriate grooming and dress, no injuries, and willingness to engage with the parent and the nurse.*

Signs that should raise the index of suspicion for child abuse and neglect are listed in Table 28-6 at the end of the chapter.

Clinical Significance 28-3

Of all age groups, infants are the most likely to be abused. Too often health care providers do not suspect or report suspected abuse. Long-term psychological and emotional sequelae from abuse are cumulative (Anda, et al., 2005). When the nurse reports suspected abuse and thereby prevents future episodes, he or she has made a significant difference in that child's lifelong health.

Skin, Hair, and Nails

Inspect skin, hair, and nails. *Healthy infant skin is soft, not excessively dry, and supple. It snaps quickly back to original shape after gentle pinching. It is free of rashes, lesions, bruising, and edema. Normal skin variants (eg,* **Mongolian spot**(s), *macular stains, spider nevi) are*

Investigate and describe any rashes, lesions, or bruising. Note if any rashes or lesions are macular, patchy, petechial, or vesicular. Is there excoriation from scratching? Does the skin seem sensitive to touch? Is there edema? Are any nails lifting off the nail bed? Are nails dry and

(text continues on page 850)

Table 28.3   Normal Skin Variants in Newborns and Infants

Mongolian Spots

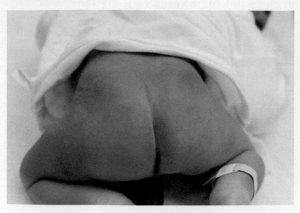

These bluish pigmented area(s) on the lower back or buttocks are common in infants of Asian, African, or Hispanic descent.

Macular Stains

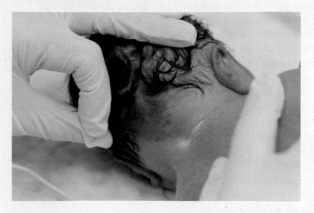

Also known as "stork bites," these capillary malformations appear on the eyelid(s), between the eyebrows, or on the nape of the neck. They tend to fade within 1–2 years.

Spider Nevus

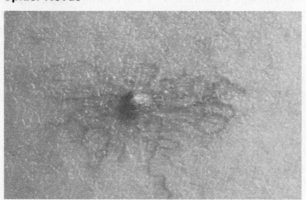

This benign lesion has a central arteriole from which thin-walled vessels radiate outward like spider legs. The lesion blanches when compressed.

Technique and Normal Findings (continued)	Abnormal Findings (continued)
illustrated in Table 28-3. Hair is soft and shiny. Some infants shed hair in the first 2 months of life. Nails are soft, of an appropriate length, and not growing inward. They are securely attached to the nail beds, which are pink, unless the child is dark-skinned.	brittle? Areas of inflammation around nails with nails poking into the skin suggest *ingrown nails*. Poor elasticity and tenting of the skin when lightly pinched over the calf muscles and on the abdomen are associated with *dehydration*. Pallor or pale mucous membranes may indicate *anemia*. Yellow, jaundiced skin tones require further investigation, because elevated bilirubin levels are toxic to the growing brain. Periorbital edema has various causes, such as crying, allergies, renal disease, or hypothyroidism. Dependent edema may occur with renal or cardiac disease. Multiple bruises in varied stages of healing, well-demarcated lesions, or bilateral burns may indicate physical abuse. See also Table 28-6 at the end of this chapter.

Head and Neck

Assess the head size and shape. Check for symmetry. Palpate the anterior and posterior fontanels and sutures (Fig. 28-7). Trace along each suture line with the tips of the fingers to ensure they have not fused prematurely. *The posterior fontanel usually is palpable until*

A head flattened from the back or one side may indicate positional *plagiocephaly* or *brachycephaly*, abnormal head shapes rom consistent positioning on the back or one side to sleep without enough "tummy time" while awake. It is important to differentiate positional plagiocephaly from

approximately 3 months of age, although it may be closed at birth. The anterior fontanel does not close until 9–18 months of age. The anterior fontanel is flat, not sunken or bulging, with the infant at rest and sitting. Sometimes, pulsations correlating with the infant's pulse can be felt while palpating the anterior fontanel. The fontanel may bulge slightly when the infant is crying. Suture lines are easily palpable. **Craniotabes**, soft areas on the skull felt along the suture line, are normal in infants, particularly those born prematurely.

plagiocephaly caused by *craniosynostosis*, premature closure of the cranial sutures. This condition can lead to impaired brain development if several sutures are involved and corrective surgery is not done in a timely fashion. See also Table 28-7 at the end of this chapter. Bulging fontanels with the infant at rest are a sign of increased cranial pressure or *hydrocephalus*, enlarged head from increased cerebrospinal fluid. Sunken fontanels are associated most commonly with acute dehydration.

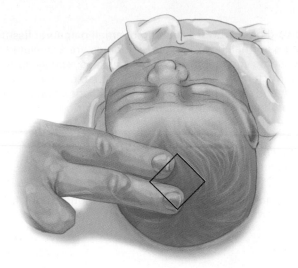

Figure 28.7 Assessing the fontanels and sutures.

Observe the infant's face. Look for symmetry of movement.

Asymmetrical facial movements may indicate *Bell's palsy* or a more serious heart condition. Bell's palsy sometimes results from traumatic birth or delivery assisted by instrumentation (eg, forceps). Bell's palsy typically fades over time, although occasionally it may persist.

Check range of motion by rotating the head toward the right shoulder and then the left, and then bending the neck so that the right ear moves toward the right shoulder and the left ear toward the left shoulder. *The neck has full range of motion. Head lag and head control correlate with expected development. For example, there is significant head lag in the newborn (Fig. 28-8A), whereas the 4-month-old can hold the head up without support (Fig. 28-8B).*

Persistence of head lag beyond the 4th month is a sign of developmental delay. Limited range of motion of the neck is associated with *meningeal irritation*. Webbing on the sides of the neck may indicate a congenital anomaly. An enlarged thyroid gland with a bruit is a sign of *thyrotoxicosis*.

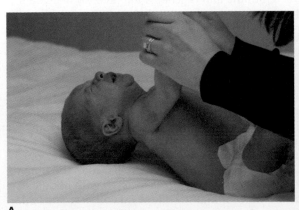

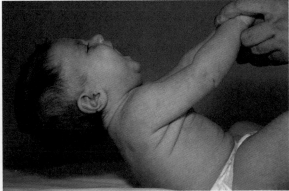

A   B

Figure 28.8 Head lag. **A.** The newborn has significant head lag. **B.** By 4 months of age, head lag has decreased noticeably.

(text continues on page 852)

Inspect and palpate the trachea. *The trachea is midline and no swelling or masses are palpable.* Auscultate for any bruits. *No bruits are present.* Palpate the clavicles in the newborn. *They are smooth with no pain or crepitus.* Palpate the following lymph node chains: preauricular (in front of the ear), suboccipital, parotid, submaxillary, submental, anterior and posterior cervical, epitrochlear (the area surrounding the elbow), and inguinal. *Any palpable lymph nodes are small, mobile, and nontender.*

A deviated trachea should be reported to the primary care provider. Crepitation over the clavicles in a newborn immediately after birth may indicate a *fracture*. By 3 weeks of age, a small lump may be felt on the bone following a clavicle fracture. Treatment usually is not indicated.

Eyes

Look for symmetry. Assess spacing of the eyes. Inspect the lids for proper placement and observe the general slant of the palpebral fissures. Inspect the inside lining of lids (palpebral conjunctiva), bulbar conjunctiva, sclera, and cornea. *Eyes are parallel and centered in the face. Ptosis is absent. Sclera are clear and white.*

Upward or downward slanting or small palpebral fissures can be normal; however, these findings are associated with some congenital conditions, such as *fetal alcohol syndrome (FAS)*. Eyes too close together, too far apart, or asymmetrical can occur with chromosomal abnormalities or illnesses. Exophthalmos is rare during infancy; its presence may indicate *thyrotoxicosis*. An eyelid that droops (ptosis) may indicate *oculomotor nerve (cranial nerve III) impairment*. It is important to correct any misalignment before 4–6 years to prevent visual loss.

Assess ocular alignment to detect strabismus using the corneal light reflex test or cover test. *Some strabismus is normal in the first few months of life.* Assess pupils for shape, size, and movement. *They are round, equal, and clear.* Test their reaction to light. Quickly shine a light source toward the eye and then remove it. *The pupils are equal and reactive to light.*

Abnormal pupils are asymmetrical, respond sluggishly, are "blown," or are pinpoint.

Use an ophthalmoscope to obtain the red reflex. Ensure that you have a +1 or =2 D lens. With the infant lying on the examination table or sitting in the parent's lap, approach from the side while looking into the ophthalmoscope. Shine the light into the eye from approximately 15–26 in away. If you do not visualize a red/orange reflection from the eye, make small adjustments with the instrument until you see the red reflex. Repeat in the opposite eye. *A red reflex is present.*

If the red reflex cannot be elicited in the newborn, the infant needs a complete eye examination by a specialist. Absence of the red reflex in newborns is associated with *congenital cataracts* and *neuroblastoma*.

Observe the infant for light perception and ability to fix on and follow a target. *Newborns are sensitive to light and often keep their eyes closed for long periods. They have a limited ability to focus, but by 3 months, they can follow objects.* An infant with any abnormal findings from the eye assessment should be referred to an advanced practitioner for further testing.

At birth, the visual system is the least mature of the sensory systems. Development progresses rapidly over the first 6 months and reaches adult level by 4–5 years. It is thought that visual acuity is sharpest at the distance from the infant to the mother's face.

Ears

Assess ear placement. *Ears are symmetrical. The top of the pinna lies just above an imaginary line from the inner canthus of the eye through the outer canthus and continuing past the ear.* Skin tags on the ears are a normal finding. Reassure the parent that these are easily removed, if desired for cosmetic reasons.

Ears that fall below the imaginary line are low-set and may indicate *chromosomal abnormalities*. It may be helpful to note if either parent has low-set ears. If so, then the low-set ears may be an inherited normal variant. One ear that is significantly smaller than the other or extra ridges and pits may be associated with middle ear abnormalities or congenital kidney disorders. See Table 28-8 for ear shapes associated with Down's or Turner's syndrome (Ranweiler, 2009).

At the end of the examination, use the pneumatic otoscope to visualize the tympanic membranes and to check the eardrums if otitis media is suspected. Test the pneumatic otoscope before each use to ensure there are no leaks. Squeeze the bulb, then place the tip against your fingertip and release the bulb. Suction on the fingertip confirms the integrity of the system.

Otitis media is common in infants. Early diagnosis and intervention result in the best outcomes (Waseem, et al., 2008). It is important to ensure that every ill infant has an otoscopic examination (Rennie, et al., 2009).

Position the infant. Ask the parent to hold him or her with the body facing the parent. Then the parent should wrap one arm around the infant to draw the body close and pin down the arms. The other arm should hold the infant's head against the parent's chest. Hold the bulb in one hand, and then use that hand to pull the pinna up and back. Gently insert the otoscope approximately ¼ in into the ear canal. Visualize the tympanic membrane and light reflex. *The tympanic membrane is convex, intact, and translucent and allows visualization of the short process of the malleus. The cone of light is visible in the anterior inferior quadrant.*

⚠ *SAFETY ALERT 28.5*
Always brace the hand holding the otoscope against the infant's face, so that if the infant moves, the otoscope moves with him or her to avoid injuring the tympanic membrane.

Then gently squeeze the bulb to blow a puff of air into the ear canal. *The tympanic membrane responds by moving.*

If there is no or diminished movement, suspect *otitis media.* Other conditions that can cause diminished movement include perforation (in one ear only) or tympanosclerosis. See also Chapter 16.

Screening for hearing acuity in infants and young children includes evaluation of developmental milestones, such as the Moro reflex in neonates.

Abnormal findings include lack of Moro reflex, inability to localize sound, or lack of understandable language by 24 months.

Nose, Mouth, and Throat

Inspect the nose. *It is in the midline of the face with symmetrical nares. The philtrum below the nose is fully formed (ie, not flat), and the nasolabial folds are symmetrical.* The best way to check patency is to hold a small mirror or specimen slide that has been chilled under the nose. Condensation on the glass is evidence of patency. *The nares are patent bilaterally.* Inspect the lips, mouth, and throat. Throat examination should be deferred to the end of the examination, unless the infant cries. The uvula can easily be visualized when the infant is crying. *The lips are symmetrical and fully formed. Young infants may have a white nodule on the upper lip. Sometimes referred to as a sucking blister, this is harmless. The tongue is of normal size and does not get in the way of feeding. The mucous membranes of the mouth, nose, and throat are moist and pink.*

Nasal flaring is a sign of respiratory distress. A flattened nasal bridge and macroglossia (enlarged tongue) are associated with *chromosomal abnormalities.* A flat philtrum and thin upper lip are associated with fetal alchol syndrome. A deviated uvula or a uvula with a cleft (rare), and red, inflamed tonsils should be noted.

Thorax and Lungs

Breathing movements are best observed in the abdomen from pronounced diaphragmatic excursion in the infant. *The thorax is symmetrical. Chest expansion is equal bilaterally.* Observe the infant's breathing

An asymmetrical chest wall, or an expanded anterior-posterior diameter (pigeon breast) or funnel shape (depressed sternum) should not be present. Retractions anywhere on the chest wall are a sign of respiratory

(text continues on page 854)

pattern. *There are no signs of distress or use of accessory muscles.* Auscultate all lobes of the lungs from the front, back, and under the arms on both sides. *Breath sounds are equal bilaterally and typically louder and more bronchial than in adults. Inspiration is slightly longer than expiration.*

Assess oxygenation. *Pink nail beds with crisp, <3 seconds, capillary refill time, and pink mucous membranes and tongue are all signs of adequate oxygenation. Blueness surrounding the mouth, circumoral cyanosis, can be normal, especially when the infant is crying, as long as the lips and tongue remain pink.*

distress. Wheezes, crackles, and/or grunting are always abnormal, as are absent or diminished breath sounds.

Central cyanosis, blueness in the center portions of the torso or of the lips, tongue, or oral mucous membranes, is a sign of poor oxygenation. Congenital heart disease is one possible cause.

Clinical Significance 28-4

If the infant is very pale and anemia is suspected, it is prudent to check the oxygen saturation. This is because it takes at least 5 g of reduced hemoglobin to produce the typical blueness of cyanosis. Anemic infants often do not have enough hemoglobin to exhibit cyanosis, even though they have very low oxygen saturation levels.

Heart and Neck Vessels

Palpate the point of maximum impulse (PMI). Auscultate the heart; inspect and auscultate the neck vessels. *The PMI may be difficult to palpate in the infant. The heart rhythm is regular with a single S1 and a split S2. Some murmurs are nonpathologic—typically they are soft and nonspecific in character (see Chapter 29 for discussion of innocent murmurs). The neck vessels are nondistended without bruits.*

Tachycardia at rest, persistent bradycardia, and clubbing should not be present. Abnormal findings suggestive of a cardiac defect include a single S2, ejection clicks, and some murmurs, particularly loud, harsh murmurs. If central cyanosis is present, evaluation of preductal and postductal oxygenation saturation is in order. Measure and compare readings in both upper extremities and one lower extremity. Oxygen saturation lower than 90% is abnormal, as are disparate readings between the upper and lower extremities. Infants with central cyanosis need a full cardiac evaluation by a cardiologist.

Peripheral Vascular

Note the character and quality of the brachial and femoral pulses. Compare left to right and upper with lower. *All pulses are equal; pulse rate matches apical heart rate.*

Weak, thready pulses indicate low cardiac output. Bounding pulses are associated with conditions characterized by right to left shunts (eg, *patent ductus arteriosus*). Palpable pulses in the upper extremities in correlation with diminished pulses in the lower extremities may indicate *coarctation of the aorta* or an *interrupted aortic arch*.

Breasts

Observe the nipples. *The areolae are full and the nipple bud well formed. It is normal for both male and female newborns to have swollen breasts that may even leak a watery fluid. The lingering effects of maternal hormones cause this.*

Check for any supernumerary (extra) nipples (see Fig. 13-4). These are usually found below the normal nipples and may not be recognized as nipples because they are usually small and not well formed. Although the condition is fairly common and usually benign, the number and location of the extra nipples should be documented. Reassure the parent that these nipples will not develop at puberty. See Table 28-8 at the end of the chapter for abnormalities related to Klinefelter's disease.

Abdomen

Inspect the abdomen. *It is cylindrical, protrudes slightly, and moves in synchrony with the diaphragm. Superficial veins may be visible in fair-skinned infants. The umbilical area is clean without discharge, bulging areas, or scarring.* Auscultate bowel sounds. *They are heard in all four quadrants and may be softer immediately after the infant has eaten.* Percuss the abdomen. *Dullness noted in the right upper quadrant helps outline the lower edges of the liver. Tympany is normal over an air-filled stomach and bowel.*

Palpate the abdomen. *It is soft, without rigidity, tenderness, or masses. The lower margins of the liver can be palpated from 1 to 2 cm below the right costal margin. The tip of the spleen may be palpable in the left upper quadrant.* Try to locate the kidneys using deep palpation in both upper quadrants. Be sure to palpate for hernias in the umbilical and inguinal regions. *Normally, the kidneys cannot be palpated and no hernias are present.*

Musculoskeletal

By this point in the examination, there have been many opportunities to observe for symmetry of movement and strength of the musculoskeletal system. Note shape and appearance of the hands, palms, fingers, feet, and toes. *The ankles have full range of motion, and feet return to a neutral position without assistance. Feet are flat before the infant begins walking*

Perform Ortolani's maneuver and elicit Barlow's sign to check for signs of hip dislocation. (Note that the maneuvers are performed in sequence, Barlow's directly after Ortolani's while maintaining the hand position.)

Ortolani's Maneuver. Position the infant supine on the examining table. With the baby's legs together, flex the knees and hips 90 degrees. Then, with your middle fingers over the greater trochanters and thumbs on the inner thighs, abduct the hips while applying upward pressure (Fig. 28-9). *No clicking or clunking sounds are heard.*

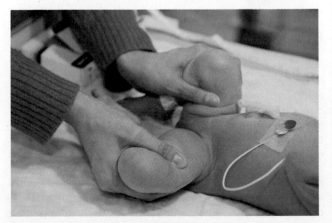

Figure 28.9 Performing Ortolani's maneuver.

A dull sound when percussing above the symphysis pubis may indicate a distended bladder. If abdominal distention is present, evaluate for a fluid wave. Note the size, shape, position, and mobility of any masses. Palpable kidneys indicate enlargement and should prompt further investigation by the primary care provider.

Loud, grumbling sounds may indicate hunger. Bowel sounds heard in the chest can indicate a diaphragmatic hernia.

The abdomen may be distended and firm with genitourinary masses or malformation. Gastrointestinal obstruction and imperforate anus are also the causes of a firm abdomen.

Throughout examination, note any asymmetrical movements. Crepitus with joint movement or any limitation of movement is abnormal. In *talipes varus (club foot)*, one or both feet are plantar-flexed and turn abnormally inward. In *talipes valgus*, seen less commonly, the foot or feet turn outward. See also Chapter 23.

Signs of congenital hip dislocation include positive Ortolani's and Barlow's maneuvers and asymmetrical thigh and gluteal folds. Infants with talipes varus, talipes valgus, or hip dislocation should be referred to an orthopedist for evaluation and treatment.

(text continues on page 856)

Barlow's Maneuver. Maintain your hold and the 90 degrees flexion; apply downward pressure while adducting the hips (Fig. 28-10). *The head of the femur remains in the acetabulum.*

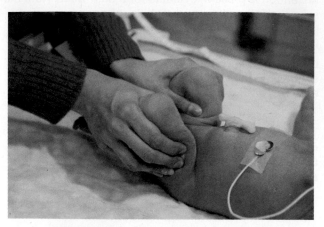

Figure 28.10 Performing Barlow's maneuver.

Neurological

Many assessments made throughout the examination give clues regarding intactness of the nervous system and cranial nerve function. These include motor function (muscle size, symmetry, strength, tone, and movement), developmental maturation, and reaction to touch. *The infant blinks when a bright light is shined in the eyes and when a loud noise, such as a clap, is produced close by.* Inspect, then palpate along the length of the spine. *There are no dimples or tufts of hair. Spine is midline.*

Clinical Significance 28-5

Infants can experience cerebral palsy despite having no risk factors. When the condition is identified early and therapy initiated promptly, long-term functioning is optimized. Watch for signs of neuromuscular dysfunction, such as hand preference before 1 year old, bilateral fist clenching after 3 months old, and involuntary or abnormal movements.

Genitalia

Female. Inspect the genitalia. *The labia majora cover the vestibule. The newborn girl may have an enlarged clitoris and labia, and the parent may have noticed a few drops of blood in the diaper.* These findings result from lingering effects of maternal hormones and should not be present after the first few weeks of life. Gently part the labia and observe the structures of the vestibule. Visualize the vaginal opening. *The genital area is clean and free of foul odors.*

Signs of neurological dysfunction include persistence of newborn reflexes (earlier discussion) past the time they normally disappear, involuntary movements, and abnormal posturing. Opisthotonos (Fig. 28-11) usually results from meningeal irritation that occurs with meningitis. Failure to blink when a bright light is shined in the eyes may be a sign of blindness, whereas absence of a blink upon production of a loud noise may denote deafness. Further evaluation is indicated in both instances. Dimpling or tufts of hair on the spine may indicate *spina bifida occulta.*

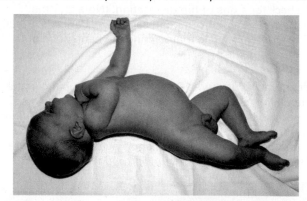

Figure 28.11 Opisthotonos, an indicator of meningitis.

Redness, swelling, bleeding (after 1 month of age), or torn tissue may indicate sexual abuse. The law mandates the reporting of signs of abuse to child protective services. When the hymen completely covers the vagina, the infant has an *imperforate hymen*, which requires minor surgery before puberty to allow exit of menstrual flow. Other abnormal findings include *labial adhesions/ fusion*, *lesions*, and foul-smelling discharge. If there is a foul smell, check for a foreign body in the vagina. This is done by placing a gloved finger in the rectum to palpate along the vaginal wall. If an object is located, use a gentle milking motion to gradually work the object out.

Technique and Normal Findings (continued)	Abnormal Findings (continued)
Male. Inspect the penis. Note cleanliness and placement of the urethral meatus. *It is at the top of the glans penis and midline.* For the uncircumcised penis, you will need to partially retract the foreskin to observe the meatus. Do not forcibly retract the foreskin. Evaluate the scrotum for size, color, and symmetry. *Testes are descended bilaterally; the area is free of edema, masses, and lesions.*	*Meatal stenosis,* an inadequate urethral opening, or a malpositioned meatus, *hypospadias,* or *epispadias,* should be referred to a pediatric urologist for evaluation. Note if the testes remain undescended. This condition requires evaluation if it persists into the toddler stage.
Anus and Rectum	
Inspect the anus. Use the little finger of a gloved hand to palpate it. *The anus is well formed with no redness or bleeding. The muscle contracts with light pressure to the area.* Rectal examination is not done routinely unless there is evidence of irritation, bleeding, or other symptoms.	Investigate redness, bleeding, or other signs of irritation for possible cause (eg, sexual abuse, fissures). Small white worms indicate a *pinworm infection.*

🌐 Cultural Considerations

The length and weight of the newborn and infant vary according to heritage, so ranges outside of usual may be normal for some patients. Mongolian spotting is more common in infants of African-American, Asian, and Native American origin.

Evidence-Based Critical Thinking

The nurse gleans a wealth of data throughout the examination. With the first observations of the infant and parent, the nurse begins to understand the child's emotional, musculoskeletal, neurological, and nutritional status as well as developmental level. As the examination progresses, additional detail adds to the nurse's understanding so that by the end, the nurse is ready to prepare the care plan. An approach that cultivates rapport with the infant and parent from the beginning and throughout the examination will facilitate the parent's willingness to collaborate with the nurse. Such involvement will help to ensure that the plan is culturally appropriate, which increases the likelihood that the family will follow the plan.

The nurse has enough data to communicate a concise, yet thorough description of the infant's health status. This information, when reported to the primary care provider, helps to guide diagnostic testing and subsequent medical diagnoses. In this way, the nurse helps to streamline the infant's care and increases the likelihood of timely and accurate diagnoses.

Nursing Diagnosis, Outcomes, and Interventions

When formulating a nursing diagnosis, it is important to use critical thinking to cluster data and identify patterns. The nurse compares these clusters of data with the defining characteristics (abnormal findings) for the diagnosis to ensure the most accurate labeling and appropriate interventions. Table 28-4 compares nursing diagnoses, abnormal findings, and interventions commonly related to newborn and infant assessment (NANDA-I, 2009).

Nurses use assessment information to identify patient outcomes. Some outcomes related to newborn or infant problems include the following:

- Bilirubin is normal for age when plotted on a nomogram.
- Infant is gaining weight with normal pattern of growth.
- Temperature is 36.5° to 37.2°C (Moorehead, et al., 2008).

Once outcomes are established, nurses implement care to improve the status of the patient. The nurse uses critical thinking and evidence-based practice to develop the interventions. Some examples of nursing interventions for newborn care are as follows:

- Protect the infant's eyes to prevent overexposure to phototherapy.
- Use valid and reliable tools to measure breastfeeding performance.
- Perform Apgar score after birth (Bulechek, et al., 2008).

Table 28.4   Common Nursing Diagnoses Associated with Newborns and Infants

Diagnosis and Related Factors	Point of Differentiation	Assessment Characteristics	Nursing Interventions
Neonatal jaundice related to destruction of fetal hemoglobin	Yellow orange tint of the skin resulting from accumulation of unconjugated bilirubin	Bilirubin high for age in hours or days (plotted on a nomogram), yellow-orange skin, yellow sclera	Prompt early feeding to stimulate stooling and removal of bilirubin. Administer phototherapy as ordered.*
Effective breastfeeding related to normal oral structure and gestational age	Mother and infant display proficient nursing behaviors	Appropriate weight for age, eagerness of infant to nurse, infant content after feeding	Facilitate skin-to-skin contact. Give positive feedback and encouragement. Refer to lactation consultant for assistance, if desired.
Ineffective thermoregulation related to immaturity of neurologic and endocrine systems	Difficulty maintaining normal temperature, easily becomes hypothermic in the newborn period; when ill during infancy, may become hypothermic or spike a very high temperature	Cool skin, cyanotic nail beds, pallor, piloerection, temperature below normal range; newborns do not shiver, which contributes to the hypothermia	Monitor temperature every 1–4 hours. Keep room temperature warm. Keep newborn's head covered. Use blankets.

*Collaborative interventions.

Analyzing Findings

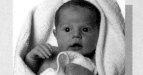

Remember Keri Downs, whose case has been outlined throughout this chapter. Two ½ months after the 1-month appointment, Keri's mother calls the office to state that Keri is losing weight. It is necessary for her to return to the clinic, so health care providers can reassess her and document findings. The following nursing note illustrates how subjective and objective data are collected and analyzed and nursing interventions are developed.

Subjective: Mother says that she is extremely frustrated with breastfeeding. At first, it went well, but now that she is back at work full time, she feels that she isn't making enough milk. Keri has been "fussy;" her weight has dropped by 1.2 lb.

Objective: Keri is irritable. Abdomen is soft and nondistended. T 37°C, P 138 beats/min, R 40 breaths/min. Mucous membranes are slightly dry, fontanels sunken. Mother states Keri is stooling twice per day but notes that diapers sometimes have dark urine. She changes five to six diapers per day. Weight is 12 lb, had been 13.2 lb at previous visit, so dropped by 5%.

Analysis: Ineffective breastfeeding related to changes in family schedule, new stressors, compromised milk production

Plan: Encourage mother to drink 2 L/day of fluid and get proper nutrition. Teach mother about pumping at work to keep milk supply. She does not want to supplement with formula. Provide pamphlet about how to manage breastfeeding while working. Provide Web address where patient can obtain more information and post questions for other working mothers to answer. Make referral to a lactation specialist.

J. Brown, RN

Critical Thinking Challenge

- How will the nurse assess the infant's other body systems that the weight loss might be affecting?
- What psychosocial issues might the nurse assess for this family?
- What other nursing diagnoses might be considered based on the data?

Collaboration with Other Health Care Providers

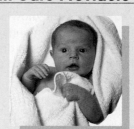

Results that might trigger a consult with a lactation specialist include pain while breastfeeding, a newborn who is wetting fewer than six diapers a day, a newborn having less than two bowel movements per day, a baby who is not gaining weight, or a baby who is not swallowing after milk is ejected.

Keri and her mother have been experiencing many of the problems outlined above; therefore, a consult is indicated. The following conversation illustrates how the nurse might organize the data and make recommendations about the patient's situation.

Situation: Hi, I'm Jan, a nurse in the outpatient clinic in primary care. We saw patients today, Keri Downs and her mother.

Background: Keri is 3⅓ months. Her mother, Diane, brought her to the office because she was concerned about her weight loss. She recently returned to work and is having difficulty with her milk production. She is also very frustrated. I think that it would be nice to give her some extra attention with this change. The baby is also somewhat irritable and not getting enough fluid or calories.

Assessment: Ineffective breastfeeding

Recommendations: I think that a 1-hour appointment would be helpful. She was successful before but needs some help with some strategies to improve her milk supply. I've already given her a pamphlet and access to a Web site.

J. Brown, RN

Critical Thinking Challenge

- How might the nurse assess the relationship between Diane and Keri?
- What are some other things that the nurse might want to assess?
- How does a team of nurses work together to coordinate care?

Pulling It All Together: Reflection and Critical Thinking

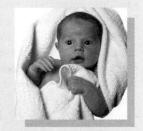

The nurse uses assessment data to formulate a nursing care plan with patient outcomes and interventions for Keri and her mother. Outcomes are specific to the patient, realistic to achieve, measurable, and have a time frame for completion. Interventions are actions that the nurse performs, based on evidence and practice guidelines. After completion of interventions, the nurse re-evaluates Keri and documents the findings in the chart to show progress toward the patient outcome. The nurse uses critical thinking and judgment to continue or revise the diagnosis, outcomes, or interventions. This is often in the form of a care plan or case note similar to the one below.

Nursing Diagnosis	Patient Outcomes	Nursing Interventions	Rationale	Evaluation
Ineffective breastfeeding related to return to work	Keri gains weight and wets six or more diapers per day.	Refer to lactation specialist. Encourage 2 L of water per day and appropriate nutrition.	Lactation specialist has the expertise and allotted time to provide personal support. Calories and fluids are necessary for milk production.	Patient seen by lactation specialist and stated that she was very helpful in getting her milk supply up. Will continue to pump at work and keep fluids at around 2 L/day.

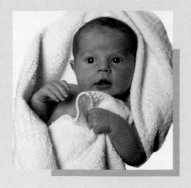

Using your knowledge of the nursing process and critical thinking, consider all the case study findings woven throughout this chapter. When answering the following questions, begin drawing conclusions and see how the pieces of assessment must work together to create an environment for personalized, appropriate, and accurate care.

- How will the nurse assess for growth?
- What reflexes will the nurse expect to see in a 1-month-old?
- What assessments will be the highest priority?

Key Points

- The infant's growth and development progresse in predictable ways: cephalocaudally, from central to distal, and from gross motor to fine motor control. It is important to evaluate patterns of growth and document steady progress.
- Emergent situations for the infant often have respiratory causes.
- Anticipatory guidance for parents of the infant includes education regarding immunization schedules, supporting breastfeeding, safe sleep practices, preventing baby bottle tooth decay, how to childproof the home, and other general safety topics.
- Infants commonly present with respiratory symptoms, fever, skin disorders, gastrointestinal distress, and crying. Interview questions for these symptoms should elicit information regarding severity and possible causation.
- Key assessments immediately after birth are vital signs including respiratory status, gestational age, and reflexes including muscle tone.
- Performing a physical examination on an infant requires the nurse to be flexible about the order and timing of specific assessments based on the developmental stage and the unique needs of the infant.
- Many assessment techniques are unique to the infant or newborn, such as Apgar scoring, evaluating reflexes, performing gestational age assessment, and maneuvers to identify congenital hip dislocation. Other techniques require adaptation to accommodate the infant's unique anatomical and developmental needs. Examples include use of the ophthalmoscope and otoscope, and examination of the throat.
- The nurse can glean a wealth of information about the infant's development and the mental, psychosocial, neurological, musculoskeletal, and nutritional status by carefully observing the infant's appearance, behavior, activity levels, and interaction with parents throughout the examination.
- Because infants are the age group most likely to be abused, screening for and identifying signs of child abuse and neglect are important ways the nurse can make a difference in long-term outcomes.

- A thorough skin assessment also reveals information about the infant's nutrition and hydration status, cardiac and respiratory function, and renal and lymphatic systems.
- Positional plagiocephaly and brachycephaly must be distinguished from craniosynostosis, which can lead to impaired brain development if not caught and treated early.
- Many abnormal findings in infants result from chromosomal defects or are acquired congenital conditions resulting from environmental conditions (eg, FAS).

Review Questions

1. A mother brings her 6-month-old to the clinic for a routine evaluation. At birth, the term infant weighed 7 lb 13 oz and was 20 in long. He now weighs 10 lb 2 oz. Which assessments are MOST important for the nurse to do next?
   A. Obtain a thorough obstetric and neonatal history and say, "I'm very worried that the baby hasn't gained more weight. What are you feeding him?"
   B. Measure head and chest circumference and length, then plot current weight, length, and head and chest circumferences on standardized growth charts.
   C. Review the immunization history, administer the Denver II assessment, and ask the mother if she has noticed any unusual patterns or behaviors.
   D. Screen for domestic violence and focus on the neurologic, cardiac, and abdominal portions of the physical examination.

2. The nurse is evaluating the growth pattern of a 5-month-old born at 27 weeks' gestation. Which of the following actions will yield the most accurate assessment of growth for this infant?
   A. Calculate how many kcal/day the infant is consuming, evaluate his bowel movement pattern, plot his measurements, and compare with the last 2 visits.
   B. Determine if he has gained at least 5 lb since birth, because infants should gain 1 to 2 lb/month in the first 6 months.

C. Plot the weight and length on a standardized growth chart for a 7-week-old and compare with birth measurements and measurements on previous visits.

D. Plot the weight and length on a standardized growth chart for a 12-week-old and compare with birth measurements and measurements on previous visits.

3. The nurse is assessing a 2-month-old whose mother brought her to the emergency department because the baby wasn't eating well and she "just looks sick." Which of the following assessment findings is most worrisome?
A. Stiff neck with an arched back
B. Circumoral cyanosis noted when crying
C. PMI not palpable, anterior fontanel bulges slightly when crying
D. T 97.5°F, heart rate (HR) 160 bpm, respiratory rate (RR) 38 breaths/min

4. The nurse is triaging infants who have presented to the emergency department on a Friday night. Which infant should the nurse take in for treatment FIRST?
A. A 2-week-old whose mother reports, "She just won't stop crying. I'm so worried." The cry is medium pitch. T 99°F, HR 160 bpm, RR 50 breaths/min. Abdomen moves with each breath.
B. A 6-week-old whose father reports, "He's vomited several times and he won't take his bottle." T 96.8°F, HR 70 bpm, RR 20 breaths/min. His lips are white. He is limp.
C. A 5-month-old with a stuffy nose who has been unusually fussy and has had 3 loose stools in the last 8 hours. T 99.8°F, HR 140 bpm, RR 45 breaths/min while crying.
D. An 8-month-old whose parents report he choked on a bean at dinner. The bean came out after five back pats. He turns blue around his mouth when he cries. T 98.6°F, HR 130 bpm, RR 30 breaths/min.

5. The nurse evaluates all the following children one morning in the clinic. Which should the nurse refer for further assessment?
A. A 6-week-old boy whose parents recently immigrated from Thailand; his head lags when pulled up by his arms; he has several dark spots that look like bruises on his lower back and buttocks
B. A 4-week-old African American girl whose liver margins are barely palpable along the right costal margin; her kidneys are easily palpable; her ears look "funny"
C. A 4-month-old Caucasian boy with loud breath sounds throughout the lung fields; auscultation of the heart reveals a split S2
D. A 9-month-old Latina who is fussy; her tympanic membrane is pearly gray and moves during pneumatic otoscopy

6. The nurse is teaching a parenting class, and the parents are sharing baby pictures. Which picture indicates that the parent may need additional education?
A. Baby is playing peek-a-boo in his car seat, which is installed in the middle part of the rear seat.
B. Daddy is brushing his son's two front teeth while baby is splashing in the bathtub.
C. Baby (10 months old) is in his high chair feeding himself banana cut in small pieces.
D. Baby is sleeping supine in her crib, no pillow, one blanket, bottle lying beside baby and a tiny dribble of milk at the corner of her mouth.

7. The infant has a new onset of rash, but otherwise seems well. Which interview question is BEST when trying to pinpoint a possible cause?
A. Was there a prolonged NICU stay?
B. What treatments have you given her for the rash?
C. Has anything changed lately, such as shampoos, soaps, or laundry detergent?
D. How many diapers is she wetting per day and what is the stool pattern?

8. Which of the following activities BEST facilitates anticipatory guidance?
A. Becoming very proficient in interviewing and performing the physical examination
B. Doing as much of the examination as possible with the infant in the parents' lap
C. Recognizing and reporting signs of physical abuse and neglect
D. Encouraging parents to make an appointment with the pediatrician before the baby is born

9. Which of the following infants has the most signs that point to possible abuse?
A. History of a long NICU stay for extreme prematurity, does not respond to loud clapping
B. Positive Ortolani's and Barlow's maneuvers; one leg looks shorter than the other
C. Small baby with large areas of denuded skin on his face and torso
D. When baby cries, mother says, "Shut up already." Baby has a foul odor and looks dirty

10. Which of the following 6-month-olds has the most markers for a possible genetic disorder?
A. Has large ears, is in the 95th percentile for weight and height, babbles
B. Has large scaly plaques on face and torso, redw reflex is absent in one eye, posterior fontanel has closed
C. Has significant head lag, one ear is small and malformed, nipples are unusually close together
D. Sits up alone, cranial sutures are palpable, back of the head is flat

References

American Heart Association. (n.d.). *Fact sheet: Infant CPR anytime*. Retrieved June 4, 2009, from http://www.americanheart.org/

Anda, R. F., Felitti, V. J., Bremner, J. D., Walker, J. D., Whitfield, C., Perry, B. D., et al. (2005). The enduring effects of abuse and related adverse experiences in childhood. A convergence of evidence from neurobiology and epidemiology. *European Archives of Psychiatry and Clinical Neuroscience, 256*(3), 174–186.

Anderson, M. L. (2005). Atopic dermatitis—More than a simple skin disorder. *Journal of the American Academy of Nurse Practitioners, 17*(7), 249–255.

El-Baba, M. F., Bassali, R. W., Benjamin, J., & Mehta, R. (2009). Failure to thrive. In M. R. Mascarenhas, M. L. Windle, J. Bhatia, M. P. M. Poth, & J. Bhatia (Eds.), *eMedicine*. Last updated May 04, 2009. Retrieved June 8, 2009, from http://emedicine.medscape.com/article/985007

Bulechek, G. B., Butcher, H. K., & McCloskey Dochterman, J. (2008). *Nursing interventions classification (NIC)* (5th ed.). St Louis: Mosby.

Giardino, A. P., & Giardino, E. R. (2008a). Child abuse and neglect: Physical abuse. In C. J. Johnson, M. L. Windle, C. Sylvester, & C. Pataki (Eds.), *eMedicine*. Last updated December 12, 2008. Retrieved May 30, 2009, from http://emedicine.medscape.com/article/915664

Giardino, A. P., & Giardino, E. R. (2008b). Child abuse and neglect: Sexual abuse. In C. J. Johnson, M. L. Windle, C. Sylvester, & C. Pataki (Eds.), *eMedicine*. Last updated December 11, 2008. Retrieved May 30, 2009, from http://emedicine.medscape.com/article/915841

Hornor, G. (2005). Physical abuse: Recognition and reporting. *Journal of Pediatric Health Care, 19*(1), 4–11.

Hurme, T., Alanko, S., Anttila, P., Juven, T., Svedstrom, E. (2008). Risk factors for physical child abuse in infants and toddlers. *European Journal of Pediatric Surgery, 18*(6), 287–291.

Kemp, A. M., Dunstan, F., Harrison, S., Morris, S., Mann, M., Rolfe, K. I., et al. (2009). Patterns of skeletal fractures in child abuse: Systematic review. *Child: Care, Health & Development, 35*(1), 141–142, 1365–2214.

Moorhead, S., Johnson, M., Mass, M. L., & Swanson, E. (2008). *Nursing outcomes classification (NOC)* (4th ed.). Philadelphia: Mosby.

NANDA International. (2009). *Nursing diagnoses: Definitions and classification*. West Sussex, UK: Wiley-Blackwell.

Nelson, K. E., & Williams, C. M. (2006). *Infectious disease epidemiology: Theory and practice* (2nd ed.). Sudbury, MA: Jones and Bartlett Publishers.

Norberg, S. (2001). Early signs of impaired motor development in infants and toddlers. *A Pediatric Perspective, 10*(5), 1–4.

Polonko, K. A. (2006). Exploring assumptions about child neglect in relation to the broader field of child maltreatment. *Journal of Health and Human Services Administration, 29*(3), 260–284.

Ranweiler, R. (2009). Assessment and care of the newborn with Down syndrome. *Advances in Neonatal Care, 9*(1), 17–24.

Rennie, C. E., van Wyk, F. C., Lee, M. S. W., & Toma, A. G. (2009). Pneumatic otoscope examination. In R. G. Bachur, M. L. Windle, & R. Kulkarni (Eds.), *eMedicine*. Last updated February 19, 2009. Retrieved June 1, 2009, from http://emedicine.medscape.com/article/1348950

Ricci, L., & Botash, A. S. (2008). Pediatrics, child abuse. In K. A. Bechtel, M. L. Windle, W. Wolfram, J. D. Halamka, & R. G. Bachur (Eds.), *eMedicine*. Last updated July 3, 2008. Retrieved May 30, 2009, from http://emedicine.medscape.com/article/800657

Santrock, J. (2006). *Life-span development* (10th ed.). New York: McGraw-Hill.

Shin, H. T. (2006). Diaper dermatitis that does not quit. *Dermatologic Therapy, 18*(2), 124–135.

Simon, H. K. (2009). Pediatrics, crying child. In K. A. Bechtel, M. L. Windle, W. Wolfram, J. D. Halamka, & R. G. Bachur (Eds.), *eMedicine*. Last updated May 1, 2009. Retrieved June 1, 2009, from http://emedicine.medscape.com/article/800964

Waseem, M., Aslam, M., & Wilson, L. A. (2008). Otitis media. In O. Brown, M. L. Windle, A. D. Murray, D. Rauch, Strafford, M. (Eds.), *eMedicine*. Last updated July 22, 2008. Retrieved June 1, 2009, from http://emedicine.medscape.com/article/994656

Wong, S. C., Scarfone, R. J., & Henretig, F. (2008). Fever in the neonate and young child. In K. A. Bechtel, M. L. Windle, W. Wolfram, J. D. Halamka, & R. G. Bachur (Eds.), *eMedicine*. Last updated October 2, 2008. Retrieved June 1, 2009, from http://emedicine.medscape.com/article/800286\

The Jensen suite offers these additional resources to enhance learning and facilitate understanding of this chapter:

- thePoint on line resource, http//thepoint.lww.com/Jensen1E
- Student CD-ROM included with the book
- *Laboratory Manual for Nursing Health Assessment: A Best Practice Approach*
- *Pocket Guide for Nursing Health Assessment: A Best Practice Approach*

Tables of Abnormal Findings

⚠ Table 28.5 Diseases with Characteristic Odors Evident in Infants

Odor	Disease or Condition
Rotten or offensive odor from the nose or vagina	Retained foreign body (eg, anything little hands can grasp and push into these body openings), poor hygiene
Mousy odor	Phenylketonuria (PKU)
Maple syrup odor to the urine	Maple syrup urine disease
Foul odor of umbilical area	Omphalitis
Noxious mouth odor	Ingestion of a chemical such as kerosene, bleach, glue, alcohol, etc.

⚠ Table 28.6 Red Flags for Child Abuse

Category	Details
Reported history of injury	The story keeps changing or is inconsistent between partners or over time.
	Details of the trauma do not correlate with the type or extent of injury.
	No history of trauma is given.
Delay in treatment	A significant delay elapses between the time of injury and when the parent seeks treatment.
"Doctor shopping"	Parent changes physicians, health care facilities, or both frequently.
Injuries consistent with abuse	Bruises appear on infants before they walk.
	Bruising or other injuries are in varied stages of healing.
	Multiple types of injuries appear.
	Injuries resemble an object, such as cigarette burns, burns in the shape of an iron, or loop marks.
	Grab or slap marks or human bite marks are visible.
	Evidence exists of immersion burns—these are usually well demarcated and bilateral (eg, both hands or feet) or occur on the buttocks and feet.
Fractured bone	Any fracture in an infant who is not walking should raise the index of suspicion for abuse, unless there is a verifiable cause (eg, motor vehicle collision, documented bone disorder predisposing to bone fragility).
Types of fractures associated with physical abuse	These include the following: • Multiple fractures • Fractured ribs ≃ 70% chance infant was abused • Fractured humerus (especially mid-shaft and spiral/oblique) ≃ 50% chance of abuse • Skull fracture ≃ 30% chance of abuse (Kemp, et al., 2009)
Pattern of injury consistent with shaken baby syndrome	Signs include subdural hematoma, retinal hemorrhages, rib fractures, and bilateral bruising in the rib cage.
Injuries consistent with sexual abuse	Any of the following in the genital area, anus, or both indicates sexual abuse: • Bleeding • Bruising • Redness
Signs of neglect	Examples include poor hygiene, clothes inappropriate for the weather, evidence of tissue wasting, signs of poor nutrition, failure to gain weight, and untreated illness.

Sources: Giardino & Giardino (2008a,b); Horner (2005); Hurme, et al. (2008); Polonko (2006); Ricci & Botash (2008).

Infections and Infestations

Pediculosis Capitis (Head Lice)

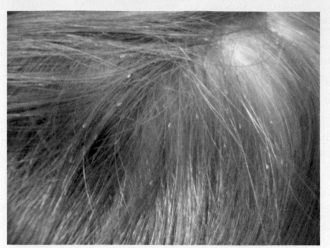

This highly contagious condition results from infestation with the human head louse, *pediculus humanus capitis*. Lice spread easily among children through close personal contact and sharing hairbrushes and other belongings.

Tinea Corporis (Ringworm)

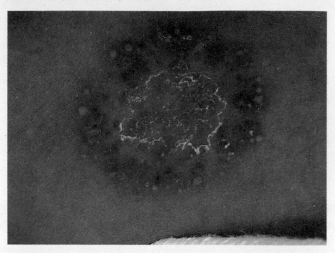

This fungal infection (dermatophytosis) is superficial. Because fungi prefer warm, moist environments, preventing ringworm involves keeping skin dry and avoiding contact with infectious material. Children are most likely to acquire the infection from an animal host, although human-to-human contact does occur as well.

Scabies

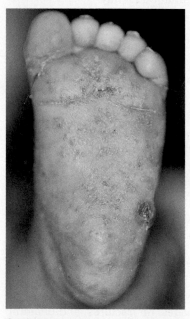

Scabies results from an allergic reaction to the *Sarcoptes scabiei* mite and her eggs. In infants, large blistering lesions and suppurative vesicles comprise the characteristic rash. The condition is highly contagious.

Staphylococcal Scalded Skin Syndrome

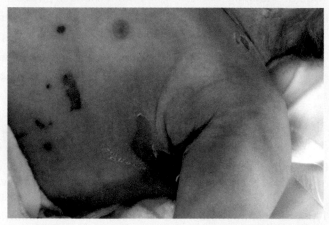

Acute exfoliation of the skin results from infection with a staphylococcal exotoxin. Pediatric populations are most susceptible to the condition, which usually heals within 2 weeks.

Table 28.7   Abnormal Skin Conditions in Newborns and Infants *(continued)*

Molluscum Contagiosum

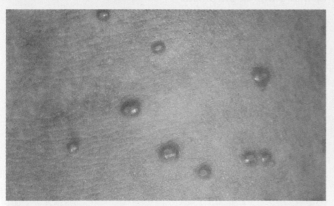

This virus spreads by direct contact; children with atopic dermatitis are especially vulnerable. The infection takes approximately 6–9 months to resolve.

Bullous Impetigo

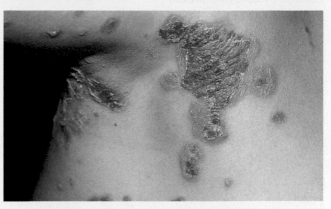

This common superficial staphylococcal infection is characterized by fluid-filled vesicles and blisters that easily rupture. It is a milder form of staphylococcal scalded skin syndrome (see next).

Contact Dermatitis and Inflammatory and Allergy-Related Conditions

Intertrigo

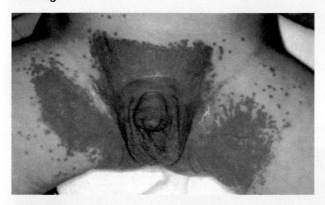

Inflammation of the skinfolds results from skin-on-skin friction. It can be a cause of diaper rash. Intertrigo frequently develops in obese people of older age groups as well.

Irritant Diaper Dermatitis

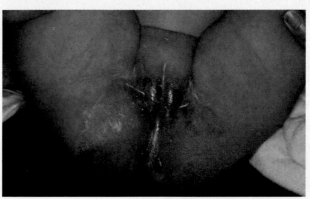

The typical "diaper rash" results from prolonged exposure of the affected areas to urine and stool. Aggravating factors include a diaper left on too long, a tight-fitting diaper, rubbing and chafing of the diaper, and diarrhea (Shin, 2006).

Candidal Diaper Dermatitis

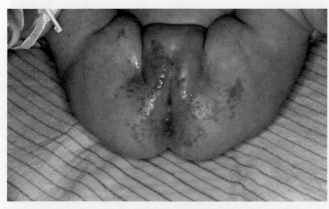

This type of diaper rash results from infection with *Candida albicans*, a fungus.

Allergic Contact Diaper Dermatitis

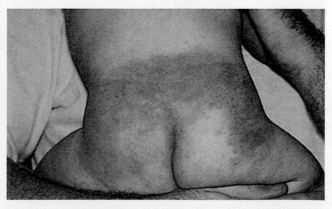

This type of diaper rash develops when the child's skin is in contact with an allergen.

(table continues on page 866)

Table 28.7   Abnormal Skin Conditions in Newborns and Infants (continued)

Eczema (Atopic Dermatitis)

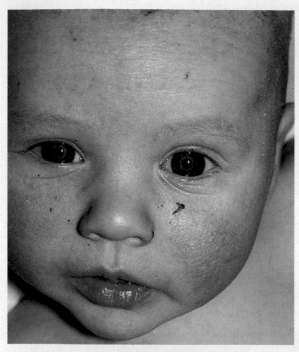

This skin condition usually appears in the first 6 months of life and typically resolves by age 5 years. It is characterized by dry, itchy, irritated skin. The exact cause is unknown, but a familial link and allergic component exist. Treatment, generally with topical corticosteroids, aims at controlling symptoms (Anderson, 2005).

Lichen Simplex Chronicus

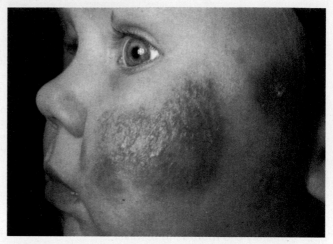

These discrete patches of eczema (thickened skin with scaling) result from irritation that follows repetitive rubbing or scratching. Secondary infections occasionally occur from breaks in the skin caused by excessive scratching.

Psoriasis

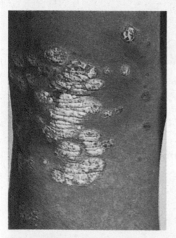

This proliferative, inflammatory, autoimmune disease is characterized by well-defined plaques covered by silvery scales.

Hives (Urticaria)

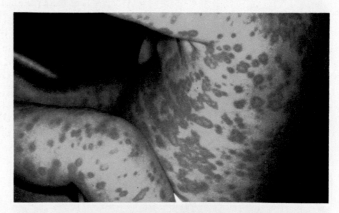

Hives are an allergic skin reaction characterized by pruritic plaques with pale centralized edematous wheals surrounded by erythematous areas, called flares. Hives are considered chronic if they last longer than 6 weeks.

Table 28.7 Abnormal Skin Conditions in Newborns and Infants (continued)

Skin Tumors/Hyperpigmented Lesions

Café Au Lait Spots

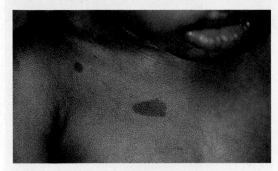

Spots start out as light brown pigmented lesions during infancy. They grow and darken as the child grows. If these spots are noted during an examination, the infant needs medical evaluation to rule out neurofibromatosis. Café-au-lait spots may be the only sign of this inherited disorder; however, the child needs close medical observation throughout childhood because of the devastating sequelae of neurofibromatosis.

Port Wine Stains

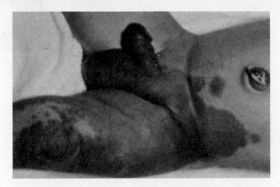

Also called *nevus flammeus*, these congenital capillary lesions are characterized by pink-to-purple or red patches anywhere on the body. The lesions can be disfiguring, particularly if they are large or on the face. Port wine stains grow proportionately with the child and often darken over time. Laser treatment is often effective.

Source: Nelson & Williams (2006).

Table 28.8 Genetic Disorders

Disorder	Description
Cystic fibrosis	This autosomal-recessive disorder is most common in Caucasians. It is characterized by abnormal transport of chloride and sodium in exocrine tissues. The result is thick viscous secretions in the lungs, pancreas, liver, intestine, and reproductive tract. Pulmonary complications generally lead to early death. Average life expectancy is 30 years.
Down's syndrome (Trisomy 21)	An extra chromosome 21 leads to moderate-to-severe mental retardation and affects almost every organ system. Common dysmorphic features include microcephaly, brachycephaly, up-slanting palpebral fissures, bilateral epicanthal folds, Brushfield's spots, flat nasal bridge, pronounced curve on the ear helix, protruding tongue, and abnormally placed nipples. Low-set thumbs, inward curvature of the little fingers, a simian (single palmar) crease, and a wide space between the great and second toes are other characteristics. Generalized hypotonia is noted in infants.
Fragile X syndrome	This most common cause of inherited mental retardation results from extra genetic material on the X chromosome. Dysmorphic features in infants include a prominent forehead, long narrow face with a high arched palate, and large ears, jaw, and testes. Young children demonstrate delayed development, hyperactivity, and autistic behavior.
Klinefelter's syndrome	A male inherits an extra X chromosome, with genotype XXY. The earlier the syndrome is diagnosed, the better the outcome; however, many patients are not diagnosed until adulthood when infertility becomes apparent. Characteristics include enlarged breasts, sparse hair, small testes, and no sperm production.
Triple X syndrome	A female inherits an extra X chromosome, with genotype XXX. This condition does not normally result in infertility. Some females experience learning disabilities and social difficulties; others are affected so mildly that they are never diagnosed.
Trisomy 13	The effects of an extra chromosome 13 are so devastating that only approximately 18% of infants with it live more than 1 year. Survivors are severely retarded. Physical characteristics include microcephaly, microphthalmia (small eyes), cleft lippalate, spina bifida, polydactyly, deafness, and heart defects.
Trisomy 18	An extra chromosome 18 severely affects all organ systems. Characteristics include profound retardation, microcephaly, prominent occiput, microphthalmia, epicanthal folds, short palpebral fissures, micrognathia (small jaw), ear malformations, and severe cardiac defects. Only approximately 10% of infants survive beyond 1 year of age.
Turner's syndrome	Caused by a missing X chromosome, this condition affects females only. Physical characteristics vary greatly, partly depending on how much X chromosome is missing. Characteristics include micrognathia, prominent ears, short neck with webbing, short fourth and fifth fingers, and heart and kidney defects. Incomplete sexual development and infertility are characteristics in adult women.

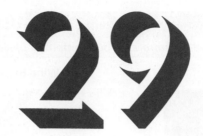

Children and Adolescents

Learning Objectives

1. Identify structures and functions of each body system that may be different in the child or adolescent than in the adult.

2. Identify teaching opportunities for health promotion and risk reduction in children and adolescents.

3. Collect pertinent subjective data including the health history and review of systems from the child's and caregiver's perspectives.

4. Identify normal and abnormal findings in the inspection, palpation, percussion, and auscultation of children and adolescents.

5. Individualize health assessment considering the condition, age, gender, and culture of the patient.

6. Use subjective and objective data about children and adolescents to analyze findings, identify diagnoses, and plan interventions.

7. Document and communicate data about children and adolescents using appropriate medical terminology.

Simon Chavez, a 4-year-old Hispanic boy, presents to the school-based health center for a preschool physical examination. Simon lives with his 20-year-old mother who stays home all day with him and his newborn sister. Simon's 21-year-old father is a delivery truck driver for a local grocery distributor; he leaves for work at 7 AM and returns most evenings by 5:30 PM, when he assists with care of the children.

Simon has not been in a structured preschool or day care environment. This fall will be his first exposure to care and formalized instruction outside the home. He seems excited about his new opportunity and is willing to discuss the new school with the nurse. Simon has never been hospitalized, but he has been treated in the emergency department twice for coughing and wheezing. He also has had frequent ear infections; the last one was 3 weeks ago. He has never had surgery. He has no known allergies; his only medication is a daily multivitamin with iron.

You will acquire more information about Simon's present health status and past health history as you progress through this chapter. As you study this content and features, consider Simon's case. Begin thinking about the following points:

- What health information and assessments are important for the toddler, preschooler, school-aged child, and adolescent?
- How do assessment findings differ between the child and adult?
- What adaptations will the nurse make when assessing a child?

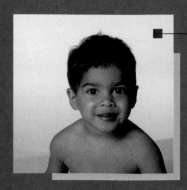

This chapter explores health assessment for children and adolescents. It highlights significant past and present health history along with related physical examination findings most pertinent for children and adolescents. These patients live with caregivers who have legal health care decision-making capacity for them. Therefore, caring for children and adolescents requires the nurse to involve both the parent/guardian and child/adolescent in assessment, diagnosis, planning, intervention, and evaluation.

Bright Futures (AAP, 2008) is a national health-promotion and disease-prevention initiative that addresses children's health needs within the context of family and community. It acknowledges that a multitude of support people and agencies is necessary to raise healthy children and to build the necessary foundation for them to develop into productive adult citizens. Therefore, health assessment of the child or adolescent also includes assessing community support, environmental exposures, and potential opportunities for health promotion (Table 29-1).

Structure and Function Overview

Physical Growth

Although children grow and develop at varying rates, they do both at predictable times according to previously established normal ranges. Health care providers must evaluate a child's physical growth with the use of **standardized growth charts**. These can be downloaded from the Centers for Disease Control and Prevention (CDC, 2008) or "thePoint" Web sites.

Growth charts are separate for boys and girls. Charts for children 0 to 3 years are for heights measured while recumbent; charts for children 2 to 18 years are for children measured upright with a stadiometer. Children are weighed on a calibrated scale. For children older than 2 years, health care providers calculate and plot body mass index (BMI) on the appropriate BMI chart. **Head circumference** is measured on children 0 to 3 years and plotted on similar growth charts (see Chapters 9 and 28).

Motor Development

Motor development of children is described as cephalocaudal (from head to toe) and proximal distal (from the center outward). For example, the infant gains head control before the ability to lift the chest off the bed. In addition, children master gross motor movements before attaining fine motor control.

Refinement of motor activity and skills continues throughout childhood and adolescence. Refer to Chapter 9 for more information. The Denver II is discussed later in the "Objective Data Collection" section as a tool for evaluating motor development.

⚠ SAFETY ALERT 29.1

Safety precautions in children change according to age group because of the variation in their developing motor abilities. For instance, covering electrical outlets is important once a child begins to sit well, while protecting the child from falls down stairs begins to matter more once the child can roll, crawl, or walk.

Language

A child develops speech and speech sounds in a predictable manner. Evaluation of the child's initiation and continuance of sounds, as well as articulation, is critical throughout the early years.

At birth the child cries. He or she then learns to coo and babble, as well as how to gesture. By 10 to 15 months old, the child says the first word; by 18 months, he or she has a vocabulary of approximately 50 words. Most children use two-word sentences by 2 years of age. By 3 years of age, their sentences are more complicated, and their speech is completely understandable to most people. Refer to Chapter 9 for more information.

A delay in **speech development** may signal a hearing loss or mental health concerns (eg, autism). Bright Futures recommends screening for autism at 18 months and 2 years of age with a tool such as the Modified Checklist for Autism in Toddlers (M-CHAT; Robins, et al., 1999) and with a structured developmental tool when the child is 2½ years old.

Clinical Significance 29-1

Children who babble at 4 to 6 months old and then stop babbling have an acquired hearing loss. Those who never babble may have a congenital hearing loss or a hearing loss since birth.

Psychosocial and Cognitive Development

Psychosocial and cognitive development related to and influential on the health of children and adolescents is discussed in detail in Chapter 9.

Acute Assessment

Children who present in physiological distress compensate with increased respiratory and heart rates. Physiological distress usually results from a respiratory disorder or significant blood loss (even children with a known congenital heart problem rarely present in acute distress from ischemic heart disease). Therefore, administration of oxygen and support of the child's ability to breathe are the first interventions. The child should remain sitting upright with the parent or in the parents' lap to promote optimal ventilation and to prevent the child from becoming upset, because crying requires additional oxygen and respiratory effort. Supplemental oxygen can be delivered by the parent via a mask held in place or close to the child's nose and mouth. The additional work of breathing is evidenced in a distressed child by nasal flaring accompanied by supracostal, intercostal, and subcostal chest retractions (Fig. 29-1) or abdominal breathing.

Transfer to a tertiary care center is indicated for children in distress; once they cannot compensate for oxygen requirements, they may soon require mechanical ventilation. Other acute situations include trauma, head injury, meningitis, and acute abdomen (eg, ruptured appendix).

American Academy of Pediatrics
DEDICATED TO THE HEALTH OF ALL CHILDREN™

Recommendations for Preventive Pediatric Health Care

Bright Futures/American Academy of Pediatrics

Bright Futures
Prevention and health promotion for infants, children, adolescents, and their families™

Each child and family is unique; therefore, these **Recommendations for Preventive Pediatric Health Care** are designed for the care of children who are receiving competent parenting, have no manifestations of any important health problems, and are growing and developing in satisfactory fashion. **Additional visits may become necessary** if circumstances suggest variations from normal.

Developmental, psychosocial, and chronic disease issues for children and adolescents may require frequent counseling and treatment visits separate from preventive care visits.

These guidelines represent a consensus by the American Academy of Pediatrics (AAP) and Bright Futures. The AAP continues to emphasize the great importance of continuity of care in comprehensive health supervision and the need to avoid **fragmentation of care.**

The recommendations in this statement do not indicate an exclusive course of treatment or standard of medical care. Variations, taking into account individual circumstances, may be appropriate.

Copyright © 2008 by the American Academy of Pediatrics.

No part of this statement may be reproduced in any form or by any means without prior written permission from the American Academy of Pediatrics except for one copy for personal use.

	INFANCY										EARLY CHILDHOOD						MIDDLE CHILDHOOD						ADOLESCENCE										
AGE[1]	PRENATAL[2]	NEWBORN[3]	3–5 d[4]	By 1 mo	2 mo	4 mo	6 mo	9 mo	12 mo	15 mo	18 mo	24 mo	30 mo	3 y	4 y	5 y	6 y	7 y	8 y	9 y	10 y	11 y	12 y	13 y	14 y	15 y	16 y	17 y	18 y	19 y	20 y	21 y
HISTORY Initial/Interval	●	●	●	●	●	●	●	●	●	●	●	●	●	●	●	●	●	●	●	●	●	●	●	●	●	●	●	●	●	●	●	●
MEASUREMENTS																																
Length/Height and Weight		●	●	●	●	●	●	●	●	●	●	●	●	●	●	●	●	●	●	●	●	●	●	●	●	●	●	●	●	●	●	●
Head Circumference		●	●	●	●	●	●	●	●	●	●	●																				
Weight for Length		●	●	●	●	●	●	●	●	●	●																					
Body Mass Index												●	●	●	●	●	●	●	●	●	●	●	●	●	●	●	●	●	●	●	●	●
Blood Pressure[5]		★	★	★	★	★	★	★	★	★	★	★	★	●	●	●	●	●	●	●	●	●	●	●	●	●	●	●	●	●	●	●
SENSORY SCREENING																																
Vision[6]		★	★	★	★	★	★	★	★	★	★	★	★	●	●	●	●	★	●	★	●	★	●	★	★	●	★	★	●	★	★	★
Hearing[7]		●	★	★	★	★	★	★	★	★	★	★	★	★	●	●	●	★	●	★	●	★	★	★	★	★	★	★	★	★	★	★
DEVELOPMENTAL/BEHAVIORAL ASSESSMENT																																
Developmental Screening[8]								●			●		●																			
Autism Screening[9]											●	●																				
Developmental Surveillance[8]		●	●	●	●	●	●		●	●		●		●	●	●	●	●	●	●	●	●	●	●	●	●	●	●	●	●	●	●
Psychosocial/Behavioral Assessment		●	●	●	●	●	●	●	●	●	●	●	●	●	●	●	●	●	●	●	●	●	●	●	●	●	●	●	●	●	●	●
Alcohol and Drug Use Assessment																						★	★	★	★	★	★	★	★	★	★	★
PHYSICAL EXAMINATION[10]		●	●	●	●	●	●	●	●	●	●	●	●	●	●	●	●	●	●	●	●	●	●	●	●	●	●	●	●	●	●	●
PROCEDURES[11]																																
Newborn Metabolic/Hemoglobin Screening[12]		●—————●																														
Immunization[13]		●	●	●	●	●	●	●	●	●	●	●	●	●	●	●	●	●	●	●	●	●	●	●	●	●	●	●	●	●	●	●
Hematocrit or Hemoglobin[14]						★			●or★			★		★	★	★	★	★	★	★	★	★	★	★	★	★	★	★	★	★	★	★
Lead Screening[15]							★	★	●or★		★	●or★		★	★	★	★															
Tuberculin Test[16]			★						★			★		★	★	★	★	★	★	★	★	★	★	★	★	★	★	★	★	★	★	★
Dyslipidemia Screening[18]												★	★	★	★	★	★	★	★	★	★	★	★	★	★	★	★	★	←—→			★
STI Screening[19]																						★	★	★	★	★	★	★	★	★	★	★
Cervical Dysplasia Screening[20]																													←—→			●
ORAL HEALTH[21]							★	★	●		●		●or★[22]	●or★[22]			●[23]															
ANTICIPATORY GUIDANCE[23]	●	●	●	●	●	●	●	●	●	●	●	●	●	●	●	●	●	●	●	●	●	●	●	●	●	●	●	●	●	●	●	●

1. If a child comes under care for the first time at any point on the schedule, or if any items are not accomplished at the suggested age, the schedule should be brought up to date at the earliest possible time.
2. A prenatal visit is recommended for parents who are at high risk, for first-time parents, and for those who request a conference. The prenatal visit should include anticipatory guidance, pertinent medical history, and a discussion of benefits of breastfeeding and planned method of feeding per AAP statement "The Prenatal Visit" (2001) [URL: http://aappolicy.aappublications.org/cgi/content/full/pediatrics;107/6/1456].
3. Every infant should have a newborn evaluation after birth, breastfeeding encouraged, and instruction and support offered.
4. Every infant should have an evaluation within 3 to 5 days of birth and within 48 to 72 hours after discharge from the hospital to include evaluation for feeding and jaundice. Breastfeeding infants should receive formal breastfeeding evaluation, encouragement, and instruction as recommended in AAP statement "Breastfeeding and the Use of Human Milk" (2005) [URL: http://aappolicy.aappublications.org/cgi/content/full/pediatrics;115/2/496]. For newborns discharged in less than 48 hours after delivery, the infant must be examined within 48 hours of discharge per AAP statement "Hospital Stay for Healthy Term Newborns" (2004) [URL: http://aappolicy.aappublications.org/cgi/content/full/pediatrics;113/5/1434].
5. Blood pressure measurement in infants and children with specific risk conditions should be performed at visits before age 3 years.
6. If the patient is uncooperative, rescreen within 6 months per AAP statement "Eye Examination in Infants, Children, and Young Adults by Pediatricians" (2007) [URL: http://aappolicy.aappublications.org/cgi/content/full/pediatrics;111/4/902].
7. All newborns should be screened per AAP statement "Year 2000 Position Statement: Principles and Guidelines for Early Hearing Detection and Intervention Programs" (2000) [URL: http://aappolicy.aappublications.org/cgi/content/full/pediatrics;106/4/798], Joint Committee on Infant Hearing. Year 2007 position statement: principles and guidelines for early hearing detection and intervention programs. Pediatrics. 2007;120:898-821.
8. AAP Council on Children With Disabilities, AAP Section on Developmental Behavioral Pediatrics, AAP Bright Futures Steering Committee, AAP Medical Home Initiatives for Children With Special Needs Project Advisory Committee. Identifying infants and young children with developmental disorders in the medical home: an algorithm for developmental surveillance and screening. Pediatrics. 2006;118(1):405-420 [URL: http://aappolicy.aappublications.org/cgi/content/full/pediatrics;118/1/405].
9. Gupta VB, Hyman SL, Johnson CP, et al. Identifying children with autism early? Pediatrics. 2007;119:152-153 [URL: http://pediatrics.aappublications.org/cgi/content/full/119/1/152].
10. At each visit, age-appropriate physical examination is essential, with infant totally unclothed, older child undressed and suitably draped.
11. These may be modified, depending on entry point into schedule and individual need.
12. Newborn metabolic and hemoglobinopathy screening should be done according to state law. Results should be reviewed at visits and appropriate retesting or referral done as needed.
13. Schedules per the Committee on Infectious Diseases, published annually in the January issue of Pediatrics. Every visit should be an opportunity to update and complete a child's immunizations.
14. See AAP Pediatric Nutrition Handbook, 5th Edition (2003) for a discussion of universal and selective screening options. See also Recommendations to prevent and control iron deficiency in the United States. MMWR. 1998;47(RR-3):1-36.
15. For children at risk of lead exposure consult the AAP statement "Lead Exposure in Children: Prevention, Detection, and Management" (2005) [URL: http://aappolicy.aappublications.org/cgi/content/full/pediatrics;116/4/1036]. Additionally, screening should be done in accordance with state law where applicable.
16. Perform risk assessments or screens as appropriate, based on universal screening requirements for patients with Medicaid or high prevalence areas.
17. Tuberculosis testing per recommendations of the Committee on Infectious Diseases. Testing should be done on recognition of high-risk factors.
18. "Third Report of the National Cholesterol Education Program (NCEP) Expert Panel on Detection, Evaluation, and Treatment of High Blood Cholesterol in Adults (Adult Treatment Panel III) Final Report" (2002) [URL: http://circ.ahajournals.org/cgi/content/full/106/25/3143] and "The Expert Committee Recommendations on the Assessment, Prevention, and Treatment of Child and Adolescent Overweight and Obesity: Supplement to Pediatrics. In press.
19. All sexually active patients should be screened for sexually transmitted infections (STIs).
20. All sexually active girls should have screening for cervical dysplasia as part of a pelvic examination beginning within 3 years of onset of sexual activity or age 21 (whichever comes first).
21. Referral to dental home, if available. Otherwise, administer oral health risk assessment. If the primary water source is deficient in fluoride, consider oral fluoride supplementation.
22. At the visits for 3 years and 6 years of age, it should be determined whether the patient has a dental home. If the patient does not have a dental home, a referral should be made to one. If the primary water source is deficient in fluoride, consider oral fluoride supplementation.
23. Refer to the specific guidance by age as listed in Bright Futures Guidelines. (Hagan JF, Shaw JS, Duncan PM, eds. Bright Futures: Guidelines for Health Supervision of Infants, Children, and Adolescents. 3rd ed. Elk Grove Village, IL: American Academy of Pediatrics; 2008.)

KEY
● = to be performed
★ = risk assessment to be performed, with appropriate action to follow, if positive
●———● = range during which a service may be provided, with the symbol indicating the preferred age

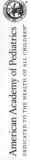

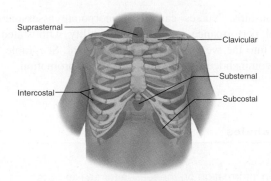

Figure 29.1 Sites of retractions.

Subjective Data Collection

Frequently several caregivers are involved with one child. The nurse should involve all interested adults who have a legal relationship with the child. If parents and child have agreed upon and given consent to include other family members or friends in care, the nurse also should share information with those designated people. This is especially true if the child is very young or has a chronic condition requiring adaptations to everyday life. This is less true as the child becomes an adolescent and begins to seek care for himself or herself alone.

Legal consent for health care treatment is 18 years of age. Most states, however, permit contraception and treatment for sexually transmitted infections (STIs) at 13 years.

Health assessment of a child or adolescent begins the moment that he or she enters the facility. Providers can ascertain much information by observing the patient's interactions with caregivers and providers. The nurse can evaluate the pediatric patient's ability to communicate along with movement capabilities when transferring from one room to the next. Children and teens demonstrate many developmental skills during the screening process. Focused observation of, and purposeful interactions with, children provide opportunities for nurses in the health care setting to assess children in a nonthreatening manner.

The nurse's assessment requires patience and skill to acquire the health information from both cooperative and noncooperative children. The health assessment should not be traumatic for patient or nurse. It is a time to learn about staying healthy and a chance for the nurse to reinforce positive lifelong health habits.

Areas for Health Promotion/*Healthy People*—

For children and adolescents, health-related patient teaching focuses on healthy lifestyle choices such as nutrition

Table 29.2	*Healthy People* Goals for Children and Adolescents with Associated Education Topics
Goals	**Patient Education Topics**
Increase the proportion of young children and adolescents who receive all vaccines that have been recommended for universal administration for at least 5 years.	Answer questions about vaccines recommended at each age; provide vaccines according to recommended schedule.
Reduce deaths of children, adolescents, and young adults.	Discuss health behaviors that affect morbidity and mortality for children and adolescents related to motor vehicles, drownings, weapons, assaults, suicides, mental health, HIV prevention, maltreatment, homicides, substance abuse, and infectious diseases.
Reduce the proportion of children and adolescents who are overweight or obese.	Discuss the BMI according to the child's sex and age. Intervene with nutritional and activity information early if the BMI is ≥85th percentile.
Reduce the proportion of children and adolescents who have dental caries in their primary or permanent teeth.	Describe good oral health: encourage tooth brushing at a minimum of twice per day and flossing once per day. A dental visit for the establishment of a dental home for children is recommended by 1 year of age. Refer to a dentist who will see children. Encourage dental sealants and topical fluoride treatments.
Increase the proportion of children with mental health problems who receive treatment.	Describe the many pressures and concerns of children and adolescents of today. Ask directly how the child feels today and in general. Consider a standardized mental health inventory. Once identified refer the child for treatment of the mental health issue; stress the importance of early intervention for the concern.
Increase the proportion of adolescents who abstain from sexual intercourse or use condoms if currently sexually active.	Answer questions regarding sexuality and sexual health. Encourage group activities and the normalcy of not engaging in sexual activity as a choice.

Source: *Healthy people 2010: What are its goals?* (n.d.). Retrieved July 7, 2010, from http://www.healthypeople.gov/About/goals.htm

and exercise. Teaching also includes information about the avoidance of unhealthy habits frequently acquired at early ages (eg, tobacco use). Additional information includes safety and the importance of emotional health and positive interpersonal relationships. Nurses can also incorporate assessment of school performance and its compatibility with stated life goals into the well-child health assessment. See Table 29-2 for recommended specific areas for health promotion.

Assessment of Risk Factors

Questions on History and Risk	Rationales
Reason for Seeking Care Tell me why you came to the clinic today. Or why did you have to come to the hospital?	Obtain information on the reason for seeking care. Ask follow-up questions if the child has pain or discomfort.
Family History Does anyone in your family have diabetes; hypertension; heart disease; elevated cholesterol level; asthma; allergies; cancer; liver, kidney, or gastrointestinal problems; arthritis; or learning problems?	A positive response to any of these increases the child's risk as well and may signal a need for additional testing (eg, serum cholesterol screening).
Has anyone in the family died before age 50 years?	Family history provides information about the seriousness of diseases reported above. Additionally, cardiac arrest of unknown origin may be associated with abnormal cardiac rhythms (eg, prolonged Q-T interval); an electrocardiogram may be indicated.
How is the health of the mother? Father? Siblings?	Illness in an immediate family member can affect the child/adolescent, causing changes in family functioning and dynamics and in the availability or accessibility of health care resources.
Prenatal History The nurse asks questions related to • Maternal health • Medications • Exposure to toxic substances, alcohol, or illicit drugs • Birth history • Birth weight • Birth date/due date • Labor and birth experience • Apgar scores at 1 and 5 minutes	Perinatal environment and exposures may affect the child's present health. Premature and small-for-gestational-age babies may have long-term sequelae if their transition to extra-uterine life was difficult (see Chapter 28). If they experienced anoxia, long-term sequelae are possible.
Postnatal History • Did the baby go home with the mother from the hospital? • Were there any difficulties once home? • Did the baby have jaundice? If so, did he or she require treatment?	The postnatal period is the time just after birth; the nurse can assume that the child's problems were limited if he or she went home with the mother 24–72 hours after birth. Extremely elevated postnatal bilirubin levels (≥25 mcg/dl) may be associated with neurological problems.
Developmental History • Did the child develop like other children? • At what age did he or she sit? Stand? Walk? • When was his or her first word? What was it? • When was the child toilet trained? Day? Night?	An accurate developmental history alerts the nurse to possible delays requiring further intervention. See Chapter 9.
Personal History Has the child been hospitalized? Has the child had surgery? What were the problems? What were the outcomes?	Significant past health problems may be related to a present problem.

Medications and Supplements

- Is the child taking any medications now?
- Is the child taking any prescription medications? How?
- Is the child taking any over-the-counter medications? How and how often?

All medications may affect the child's illness and also behavior. Medications taken together may interact. Children can be given too much or too little of an over-the-counter drug (eg, Tylenol).

Risk Factors

Lead-risk Screening

- Does your child live in or regularly visit a house or child-care facility built before 1950?
- Does your child live in or regularly visit a house or child-care facility built before 1978 that is being or has recently (within the last 6 months) been renovated or remodeled? (CDC, 2009)
- Does your child have a brother, sister, or playmate who has or had lead poisoning (AAP, 2008, p. 1074)?

"Yes" to any of these three questions requires health care providers to take a blood level on children 0–72 months old (and possibly beyond if at risk). Some toys may also contain lead (CDC, 2007).

Tuberculosis (TB) Screening

- Is the child infected with the human immunodeficiency virus (HIV)?
- Is the child in close contact with people known or suspected to have TB?
- Is the child in close contact with people known to be alcohol dependent or intravenous drug users or to reside in a long-term care facility, correctional or mental institution, nursing home/facility, or other long-term residential facility?
- Is the child foreign-born and from a country with high TB prevalence?
- Is the child from a medically underserved low-income population, including a high-risk racial or ethnic minority population (eg, African American, Hispanic, Native American)?
- Is the child/adolescent alcoholic dependent, an intravenous drug user, or a resident of a long-term-care facility, correctional or mental institution, nursing home/facility, or other long-term residential facility (Selekman, 2007)?

"Yes" to any of these questions requires the administration of a purified protein derivative tuberculin test to the patient.

Immunizations. Is the child current with immunizations?

Immunization schedules for children and adolescents can be found at the CDC Web site.

Car Safety. Does the child sit in an approved car seat? In the back seat? Does the adolescent always wear a seat belt (Fig. 29-2)?

A car seat is recommended for the newborn leaving the hospital and the next 4 years of life.

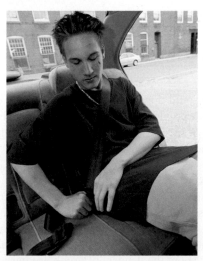

Figure 29.2 Adolescents need to understand the importance of the use of seat belts to optimize their protection while driving and as passengers.

(text continues on page 874)

Questions on History and Risk	Rationales
Poison Control. Are hazardous substances stored safely away from the child?	The house and other environments where the child spends significant time should be childproofed by locking up cleaning supplies and keeping all medicines out of the child's reach. For a child suspected of ingesting a nonfood substance, the national Poison Control Center (PCC, 2008) number is 1-800-222-1222.
Safety in the Home. Is the child protected from falls down stairs? From windows? Are guns in the home? Are they secured?	Children need to be protected from falls at windows and down stairs. Guns should not be loaded; they should be locked.
Fire Safety. Does your family have a fire escape plan?	Children need protection from burns related to open fire pits, campfires, grills, gas stoves, stovetop cooking of food, and matches.
Water Safety. Is the pool secured by fencing? Ask the child if he or she can swim. Can he or she swim to the side of the pool if he or she falls in the deep end?	Pools should have 6-ft fences and entrance gates with high locks.
Outdoor Safety. Has your child been taught to safely cross streets?	Child pedestrians are at risk for injury and need instruction about where and when to cross frequently traveled streets, as well as where and how to walk on the street.
Does the child wear a helmet for high-risk activities?	Bike helmets are encouraged when a child begins to ride a tricycle or a bicycle. Some states require bicycle helmets to be worn on state roads.
Does the child use sunscreen when outside?	Unprotected sun exposure increases risks for melanoma, basal cell carcinoma, and squamous cell carcinoma.
Drug and Alcohol Use. For the older child or adolescent, have you or your friends used drugs, alcohol, or tobacco?	People 12–20 years old drink 11% of all alcohol consumed in the United States. More than 90% of this alcohol is consumed as binge drinking (CDC, 2010).
Nutrition and Obesity. Describe what you would eat in a typical day.	Overweight and obesity have serious health consequences among children and adolescents including a greater risk of high cholesterol, hypertension, and diabetes.
Violence and Suicide. Ask children and teens if they feel threatened at school (see Chapter 12). Ask directly if the patient has thought about hurting self or others.	Youth violence includes bullying, slapping, or hitting. Other physical behaviors include robbery, assault, or rape.
Contraception and STIs. Ask adolescents, do you engage in oral sex or are you sexually active?	Adolescents are more likely than adults to have multiple sexual partners and short-term relationships, to engage in unprotected intercourse, and to have partners at high risk for STIs.

Risk Assessment and Health-Related Patient Teaching

In addition to taking family and individual history, the nurse performs health-related teaching to prevent disease or injury. Important education areas include immunizations, car safety, poison control, home safety, fire safety, water safety, outdoor safety, prevention of substance use, nutrition and prevention of obesity, and promotion of contraception and prevention of STIs.

Immunization Schedules

For children who have not received the full roster of recommended vaccines, the nurse should encourage catch-up doses.

He or she should document administration and dates of the vaccines and provide this information to caregivers/parents for their own records in addition to maintaining the health record at the place of regular health care.

Car Safety

The nurse should discuss with parents and children as appropriate the use of car seats, booster seats, and seat belts according to state laws. Car safety includes promoting car seats and booster seats for children from birth to 8 years and teaching adolescents about the dangers of drunk driving.

Promoting Use of Car Seats and Belts. The infant seat should be in the back facing backward for the first year

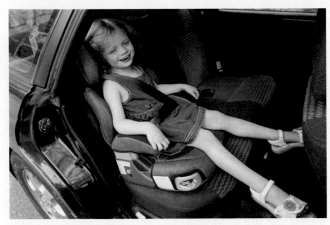

Figure 29.3 The booster seat requires the child to be restrained with a seat belt and for the seat to be in the back of the vehicle.

minimally. Depending upon the car seat, it may be in the back seat facing backward until the child is 30 to 35 lb. A child may be turned facing forward after 1 year of age if in the correct car seat. At 4 years of age or 40 lb, the child may graduate from a car seat to booster seat. He or she should be seated and restrained with a seat belt in such a seat, which is designed for use until children are at least 4'9" (Fig. 29-3).

Once out of the booster seat, children should ride in the back with a seat belt fastened securely. A child may move to the front seat after 12 years old if he or she is of adult size. Front air bags have been known to hurt younger and smaller children as a result of the force with which they are deployed. Although car seat and booster seat laws vary among states, the National Highway Traffic Safety Administration (2008) is a good resource for other information about child restraint in cars.

Preventing Drunk Driving. The nurse should discuss this topic by providing scenarios in which the adolescent has alternatives to riding with an impaired driver. He or she should encourage the use of a designated driver if the teen is in a situation in which he or she anticipates drinking or drug use.

Poison Control

The PCC provides information needed for the home or hospital treatment of a child who has ingested toxic substances. Recommendations might include use of ipecac syrup, activated charcoal, or both. Parents can buy these medications without a prescription; however, these should be used only if the PCC instructs them to do so. Presently, these medications are not recommended for home use because they have been used inappropriately in the past. The PCC can provide telephone stickers or magnets with its emergency phone number on it to be posted on or near telephones.

Safety in the Home

Signs of a home that has been modified to optimize child safety include the following:

- Open windows have well-maintained screens.
- Additional bars or barriers protect open low windows from which a toddler can reach and fall.
- Doors or gates block stairwells.
- Any guns in the home are locked and unavailable to children and adolescents.

Fire Safety

Children have a larger skin surface area than body weight. Burns on them make up a larger percentage of their surface area than for adults; therefore, burns are much more serious for children in terms of fluid replacement and potential for infection. Children and adolescents require protection against fire and must be taught the dangers of and significant respect for fire. The family should establish and discuss a family fire plan and escape routes from the house.

Water Safety

Once near a pool the young child unable to swim should always wear a life jacket. Around lake and murky water the necessity of a life jacket may continue until the adolescent can demonstrate strong swimming skills. Children should be encouraged to learn to swim and take swimming lessons to develop the ability to at least save themselves in water over their head.

Outdoor Safety

Outdoor safety includes safety while crossing streets, using helmets while riding tricycles, bicycles, or all-terrain vehicles, and using sunscreen.

Safe Street Crossing. Assess if the child walks to school or other places such as parks or playgrounds. The safest route and safe street rules should be discussed with the child. Discuss walking facing traffic and crossing the street.

Helmet Use. Most states require helmets for riders of motorized vehicles on state roads. A child on an all terrain-motorized vehicle is encouraged to always wear a helmet. Helmets should also be worn during high-risk sports, such as football, hockey, baseball, skiing, and snowboarding. Head trauma secondary to accidents is a common childhood injury with long-term sequelae. Wearing a bicycle helmets reduces the incidence of brain injury in children (Thomas, et al., 1994).

Use of Sun Screen. All children, no matter what their skin type or color, should apply sunscreen with SPF of at least 15 when exposing skin to the sun or be completely covered with clothing and a large brimmed hat to prevent skin damage and skin cancer. Sunglasses that block both UVA and UVB light are also recommended to prevent the development of cataracts.

Prevention of Drug and Alcohol Use

Nurses should continue to answer questions and counsel pediatric patients about the dangers of alcohol and drugs, emphasizing immediate over long-term risks. He or she also should assess for mental health issues, because drug-seeking behaviors are often ways in which people self-medicate for other problems (see Chapter 10). A potentially effective way to prevent young people from using substances is to explain how they interfere with the accomplishment of developmental tasks, which are difficult if the child or teen is impaired.

Nutrition and Prevention of Obesity

The nurse should discuss the child's BMI according to sex and age. Nutritional and activity information early is important if the BMI is at or above the 85th percentile. The family should receive nutritional information from the USDA (2005) **My Pyramid** guidelines (see Chapter 8). Children 2 years and older should consume daily at least two servings of fruit; three servings of vegetables, with at least one-third being dark green or orange; and six servings of grain products, with at least three being whole grains. Children 2 years and older should consume daily less than 10% of calories from saturated fat, no more than 30% of calories from total fat, and 2,400 mg or less of sodium; they also need to meet dietary recommendations for calcium.

Nurses can ask and educate families about multivitamins with iron for high-risk individuals, as well as about food choices at school and how they can correlate with the guidance offered by MyPyramid. Children and caregivers also need explanations about vigorous physical activity and assessment of their engagement in such activity. Young people need to exercise for at least 3 days/week for at least 20 minutes, with examples of appropriate activities.

Mental Health Issues

The nurse should discuss actions to deal with threats at school, conflict resolution, and school resources available. He or she needs to intervene immediately if a parent or child admits to concerns about hurting self or others. A patient or family member who describes a plan to complete suicide requires hospital admission for mental health concerns.

Promotion of Contraception and STI Prevention

The nurse should discuss abstinence, safe-sex practices, and avoidance of high-risk behaviors with sexually active adolescents and answer questions of all patients regarding sexuality and sexual health. The nurse can encourage group activities and normalize the decision not to engage in sexual activity. For those adolescents who choose to continue sexual activity, the nurse should encourage use of condoms.

The nurse also should educate adolescents on the signs, symptoms, and consequences of untreated STIs. He or she should urge immediate screening and treatment for symptoms and yearly examinations for sexually active adolescents even if they are asymptomatic.

Focused Health History Related to Common Symptoms

The following symptoms have been implicated as valid; however, they are also common in children attempting to avoid school. The pain goal is pain free (zero on FACES; see Chapter 7) and elimination of the contributing symptom. Also, the nurse should consider if the situation represents acute illness and requires immediate attention.

Common Symptoms in Children and Adolescents

- Abdominal pain
- Headache
- Leg pain

Questions on Common Symptoms	Rationale/Abnormal Findings
Abdominal Pain • Can you point to where it hurts? • How bad is the pain? • How long have you had this pain? • What does the pain feel like? Cues may need to be added (eg, sharp or dull). • Does anything make your pain worse? • Does anything make your pain better? • Has your pain stopped you from going to school, playing sports, or other things?	Children usually cannot isolate abdominal pain to one specific area. If the child points to the right lower quadrant or only tiptoes, *appendicitis* should be ruled out with abdominal scans. ⚠ *SAFETY ALERT 29.3* *Acute intense pain with vomiting may indicate appendicitis. A child who stops activity or play because of pain requires additional evaluation. If rest relieves the pain, life-threatening concerns are usually the problem.*
Headache • Can you point to where it hurts? • How bad is the pain? • How long have you had this pain? • What does the pain feel like? Cues may need to be added (eg, sharp or dull). • Does anything make your pain worse? • Does anything make your pain better? • Has your pain stopped you from going to school, playing sports, or other things?	For headaches children usually cannot isolate to one specific area. ⚠ *SAFETY ALERT 29.4* *Acute intense pain with vomiting may indicate a migraine or brain tumor. A child who cannot walk or stops activity or play because of pain requires additional evaluation.*

Leg Pain
- Can you point to where it hurts?
- How bad is the pain?
- How long have you had this pain?
- What does the pain feel like? Cues may need to be added (eg, sharp or dull).
- Does anything make the pain worse?
- Does anything make the pain better?
- Has your pain stopped you from going to school, playing sports, or other things?

For leg pain children usually cannot isolate to one specific area.

> ⚠ **SAFETY ALERT 29.5**
> *If the child consistently limps, then fractures, dislocations, and bone tumors should be ruled out.*

Therapeutic Dialogue: Collecting Subjective Data

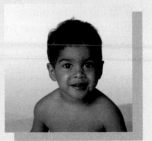

Simon, introduced at the beginning of this chapter, is 4 years old and undergoing a preschool assessment. The nurse uses professional communication techniques to gather subjective data from Simon. The following conversations give two examples of interview styles used by different nurses. One style is more effective than the other.

Less Effective

Nurse: Hello, Mrs. Chavez and Simon. How are you today?

Mrs. Chavez: We are very well, thank you.

Nurse: I see that you are here for Simon's physical for school, right?

Mrs. Chavez: Yes, that's right. Simon is excited about going to school.

Nurse: That's great! Simon, it looks like you have been very healthy from the chart. Weighed 7 lb 3 oz at birth, was breast-fed for about a year and developed like other children. He was walking at 1 year and toilet drained during the day 6 months ago. It says that he is still having difficulty at night about twice a week, so he wears a pull-up diaper to bed. Is this still the case?

Mrs. Chavez: Yes, that's correct.

More Effective

Nurse: It's nice to see you again, Simon and Mrs. Chavez. How are you today?

Mrs. Chavez: We are very well, thank you.

Nurse: Simon, how are you?

Simon: Chood.

Nurse: (Leans in closer to hear speech clearly) So, Simon, why are you visiting the clinic?

Simon: I am choing to go to shool! (speech is somewhat garbled)

Nurse: Mrs. Chavez, is it difficult for you to understand Simon sometimes?

Mrs. Chavez: Yes, but I thought that it might be because he speaks both Spanish and English. His father's parents visit from Chile once a year. They bring him toys and candy that I don't like. I try to keep him healthy. He only watches TV 1 hour a day. He eats meat only once a day. He brushes his teeth every night and saw a dentist last year.

Critical Thinking Challenge

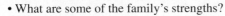

- What are some of the family's strengths?
- How will the nurse continue to assess Simon?
- What risk factors might be identified?

Cultural Considerations

Every child grows and develops in a family or care setting unique to that child regardless of racial background. Health habits are not race-related but defined culturally within the local community and family. Nevertheless, certain racial or ethnic groups are more prone than others to specific disorders or diseases. For instance, rates of obesity and type 2 diabetes are higher among Hispanics and African Americans than among Caucasians.

The norms of each family setting deserve assessment in regards to patterns of rest, activity, nutrition, illness intervention, health habits, and member roles. This includes who eats together, what is eaten, where food is obtained, who prepares food, and how food is prepared. These norms contribute to the health of the child and are important components of a nutritional assessment. Each area of assessment listed also contributes to or discourages the development of obesity. Some families do not prepare food at home and eat out most of the time, some families do not eat together, some eat in the front of the TV, some children eat only in their rooms, and some eat with grandparents. These norms are not known unless the provider asks about them. They are different for each family based not on race, but on familial cultural norms.

Another example of cultural differences in families concerns activity levels. One family would never consider walking to the grocery even if it is just one block away. Another family would consider themselves lazy if they did not hike at least 3 miles every Saturday in the park close to their house.

Assessment of language development is difficult if the provider is not bilingual and the child speaks another language. If a language other than English is spoken in the home, language development may be delayed if the child is attempting to develop two languages at the same time. These children will be bilingual and language delay is not of concern if hearing is normal.

Objective Data Collection

Equipment

In addition to the equipment needed for a head-to-toe assessment (see Chapter 4), the nurse needs to include selected developmental screening test equipment and a tape measure.

Preparation

Ensure that the room is a comfortable temperature and that chairs are available for the health care provider, parent, and child. During the health interview the child can be in the parent's lap or in his or her own chair. The toddler or very anxious small child can remain in the parent's lap for most of the physical examination. By age 3 years, most children enjoy the independence of climbing on the examination table. Most 4 year olds are able to climb on the examination table without

difficulty if the initial screening process is without trauma. While the child is climbing watch carefully and maintain a close hand to prevent a fall. Wash your hands prior to beginning the examination. The child is undressed at the beginning of the examination or after the assessment of the head and neck.

The examination of the child will start at the head and end at the toes. If, however, the child is predicted to become upset, listen to heart sounds first and then breath sounds. This is best done while the child is sitting on the parent's lap. Wipe the stethoscope with alcohol and warm the stethoscope first with your hand.

Children, and most specifically young adolescents, want to be reassured that everything evaluated is normal. They may frequently mention what seems to be a minor concern to the health professionals. To gain trust, it is important to evaluate or intervene for all stated concerns.

Denver Developmental Assessment

The **Denver Developmental Screening Test II** (DDST-II; Frankenburg, et al., 1992) is one of several standardized developmental screening tests used in the examination of the child and required for Early and Periodic Screening and Developmental Testing. The DDST-II is considered a gold standard for the developmental evaluation of children ages 1 month to 6 years. It evaluates four developmental areas of interest: personal-social, language, fine motor/adaptive, and gross motor.

During screening with the DDST-II, the examiner asks questions of the parent but the child also performs certain tasks. Toys and blocks provided with the screening tool assist in standardizing the assessment (Fig. 29-4). The DDST-II and accompanying required materials to perform it can be purchased at www.denverii.com/DenverII.html. A standardized evaluation such as the DDST-II is recommended, because behaviors or skills in a checklist are not standardized assessments. They are without validity or reliability, which makes results of the checklist difficult to interrupt and intervene.

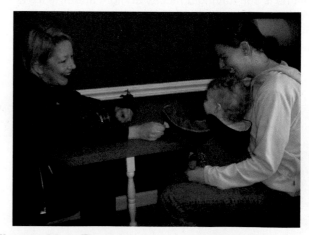

Figure 29.4 The nurse will use special toys and blocks to conduct the DDST-II.

Comprehensive Physical Examination

Technique and Normal Findings	Abnormal Findings

Vital Signs

Take the patient's height, weight, heart rate, respiratory rate, temperature, and blood pressure (Fig. 29-5). Plot height and weight on the appropriate growth charts; calculate BMI. Routine blood pressures with a cuff and sphygmomanometecter begin at 3 years of age if the newborn's blood pressure is recorded in the nursery as within normal limits in all extremities. Assessment of blood pressure includes the percentile according to height and sex. The blood pressure cuff covers 80% of the child's upper arm. *Charts for blood pressure norms are found on the National Heart, Lung and Blood Institute's (2004) and thePoint websites.*

Any blood pressure over the 90th percentile is considered borderline hypertensive and deserves follow-up. The 90th percentile is 1.28 SD, 95th percentile is 1.645 SD, and the 99th percentile is 2.326 SD over the mean.

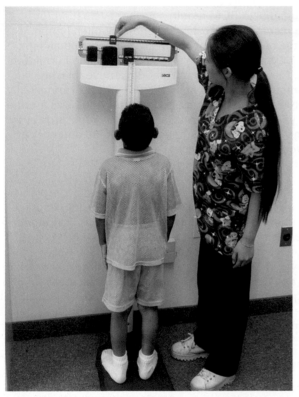

Figure 29.5 The child will typically enjoy standing on the scale and learning his progress from the last appointment.

General Survey

Observe the child's demeanor. Look for signs of distress, discomfort, or anxie ty. Note attentiveness and affect. *A 4 year old is generally talkative and engaged in the visit, and can answer simple questions about self and concerns.* Listen for speech difficulties. *By 2 years, the child uses two-word sentences; by 3 years, a child should speak in more complicated sentences with speech that is understandable 75% or more of the time (Drumwright, et al., 1973).*

There are assessments of the child's ability to understand and cognitive processing during the interview. Flat affect, no eye contact, and clinging to the caregiver may need further evaluation to assess for *autism* and other psychiatric concerns.

(text continues on page 880)

Observe for range of motion and musculoskeletal symmetry and coordination. *Range of motion is normally full with 4–5+/5 strength symmetrically.*

Asymmetry of movement and lack of coordination should be further evaluated.

Skin, Hair, and Nails

Inspect and palpate the skin, hair, and nails. *Skin is smooth and dry. Hair is smooth and evenly distributed. Nails are smooth and without clubbing.* Eccrine (sweat) glands begin to function by 2–18 days of life but become fully functional at adolescence. Apocrine (sex) glands do not become active until puberty.

Note any absence or overgrowth of nails. Dimpling, ripples, or discoloration in nails can be signs of *trauma* or *fungus.* There should be no unusual moles or hyperpigmented areas.

Note *acne* during adolescence; sebaceous glands work in utero and continue until the infant is 6–12 months. At this point they stop working and then begin activity again at puberty. With a gloved hand, feel any rash or skin complaints for elevation and size of papules, nodules, or cysts.

Head and Neck

Inspect the head and neck; observe range of motion of the neck. *The head and neck are normally symmetrical with full range of motion in neck.*

Palpate the head and neck. *Anterior and posterior cervical nodes may be palpable but not enlarged and also are nontender.* Palpate the head for nodules or pain due to infectious processes or trauma. *No nodule or tenderness is noted on the head.* Palpate fontanels of head on children up to 2 years old. *The anterior fontanel closes by 18 months, posterior fontanel by 6 months.*

Limited neck ROM requires further evaluation for possible meningitis or *torticolis.* Tender swollen lymph nodes of the neck and posterior head may indicate an infection. Lymph nodes are frequently palpable in children but they should be small, shoddy, moveable, and nontender. The lymphatic system grows exponentially between 6 and 12 years and reaches adult size around 12 years. Therefore, tonsils frequently look large at this time but will appear smaller as the head and neck grow throughout adolescence.

Eyes and Vision

Inspect the eyes. *The eyes are PERRL (A). Extraocular movements (EOMs) are at 180 degrees. Corneal light reflexes (CLR) are equal. There is no deviation during the cover and alternate cover tests. Fundoscopic examination reveals a distinct disk with no vessel nicking.*

Assessment of accommodation is difficult in young children. Unequal and nonreactive pupils may signify *increased intracranial pressure.* Unequal EOMs or CLR may indicate *esotrophia* or *exotropia* (see Chapter 15). Deviation with the cover test demonstrates an *esophoria* or *exophoria*, depending on direction. All these findings require further evaluation. By 3 years old, most children are cooperative enough for the nurse to obtain a quick glimpse of the retina.

Assess distance vision using a screening test based on developmental stage (Table 29-3). *Normal findings in toddlers are 20/200 bilaterally. Normal visual acuity in preschoolers is 20/40, improving to 20/30 or better by 4 years old. By 5–6 years old, normal visual acuity should approximate that of adults (20/20 in both eyes).*

Screen for color blindness in patients 4–8 years old.

Ears and Hearing

Inspect the ears. *They have a formed pinna, the top of which touches an imaginary straight line through both pupils* (Fig. 29-6).

Ear deformities are connected to kidney problems, because organogenesis for both ears and kidneys occurs about the same time in utero. Evaluate renal function if the ears appear malformed. Low-set ears are correlated with cognitive deficits and learning problems (Fig. 29-6B).

As head shape changes, visualization of the tympanic membrane requires alterations in technique. Before the child is 1 year old, pull the pinna down and toward

Infection is suspected if the tympanic membrane is erythematous or yellow, there is drainage in the canal, or there is limited mobility (see Chapter 16).

Table 29.3 Eye Screening Guidelines[a]

From Birth to 3 years of Age perform the following:

1. Ocular history
2. Vision assessment
3. External inspection of the eyes and lids
4. Ocular motility assessment
5. Pupil examination
6. Red reflex examination

For Children 3 years of Age and Older perform the following:

Numbers 1 through 6 above, plus:

7. Age-appropriate visual acuity measurement
8. Attempt at ophthalmoscopy

Children Ages 3–5 Years			
Function	**Recommended Tests**	**Referral Criteria**	**Comments**
Distance visual acuity	Snellen letters Snellen numbers Tumbling E HOTV Picture tests – Allen figures – LEA symbols	1. Fewer than 4 of 6 correct on 20-ft line with either eye tested at 10 ft monocularly (ie, <10/20 or 20/40)or 2. Two-line difference between eyes, even within the passing range (ie, 10/12.5 and 10/20 or 20/25 and 20/40)	1. Tests are listed in decreasing order of cognitive difficulty; the highest test that the child is capable of performing should be used; in general, the tumbling E or the HOTV test should be used for children 3–5 years of age and Snellen letters or numbers for children 6 years and older. 2. Testing distance of 10 ft is recommended for all visual acuity tests. 3. A line of figures is preferred over single figures.
Ocular alignment	Cross cover test at 10 ft (3 m) Random dot E stereo test at 40 cm		4. The nontested eye should be covered by an occluder held by the examiner or by an adhesive occluder patch applied to eye; the examiner must ensure that it is not possible to peek with the nontested eye.
	Simultaneous red reflex test (Bruckner test)	Any asymmetry of pupil color, size, brightness	Direct ophthalmoscope used to view both red reflexes simultaneously in a darkened room from 2 to 3 ft away; detects asymmetric refractive errors as well.
Ocular media clarity (cataracts, tumors, etc.)	Red reflex	White pupil, dark spots, absent reflex	Direct ophthalmoscope, darkened room. View eyes separately at 12–18 in; white reflex indicates possible retinoblastoma.

Table 29.3   Eye Screening Guidelines[a]   (continued)

Children 6 years of Age and Older			
Function	**Recommended Tests**	**Referral Criteria**	**Comments**
Distance visual acuity	Snellen letters Snellen numbers Tumbling E HOTV Picture tests – Allen figures – LEA symbols	1. Fewer than 4 of 6 correct on 15-ft line with either eye tested at 10 ft monocularly (ie, <10/15 or 20/30) or 2. Two-line difference between eyes, even within the passing range (ie, 10/10 and 10/15 or 20/20 and 20/30)	1. Tests are listed in decreasing order of cognitive difficulty; the highest test that the child is capable of performing should be used; in general, the tumbling E or the HOTV test should be used for children 3–5 years of age and Snellen letters or numbers for children 6 years and older. 2. Testing distance of 10 ft is recommended for all visual acuity tests. 3. A line of figures is preferred over single figures. 4. The nontested eye should be covered by an occluder held by the examiner or by an adhesive occluder patch applied to eye; the examiner must ensure that it is not possible to peek with the nontested eye.
Ocular alignment	Cross cover test at 10 ft (3 m) Random dot E stereo test at 40 cm Simultaneous red reflex test (Bruckner test)	Any asymmetry of pupil color, size, brightness	Direct ophthalmoscope used to view both red reflexes simultaneously in a darkened room from 2–3 ft away; detects asymmetric refractive errors as well.
Ocular media clarity (cataracts, tumors, etc.)	Red reflex	White pupil, dark spots, absent reflex	Direct ophthalmoscope, darkened room. View eyes separately at 12–18 in; white reflex indicates possible retinoblastoma.

[a]Assessing visual acuity (vision screening) represents one of the most sensitive techniques for the detection of eye abnormalities in children. The American Academy of Pediatrics Section on Ophthalmology, in cooperation with the American Association for Pediatric Ophthalmology and Strabismus and the American Academy of Ophthalmology, has developed these guidelines to be used by physicians, nurses, educational institutions, public health departments, and other professionals who perform vision evaluation services.

Source: Committee on Practice and Ambulatory Medicine, Section on Ophthalmology, American Association of Certified Orthoptists, American Association for Pediatric Ophthalmology and Strabismus and American Academy of Ophthalmology (2003 and reaffirmed in 2007). Policy statement: Eye examination in infants, children, and young adults by pediatricians. *Pediatrics, 111*(4), 902–907. Retrieved July 23, 2008 from http://aappolicy.aappublications.org/cgi/content/full/pediatrics%3b111/4/902

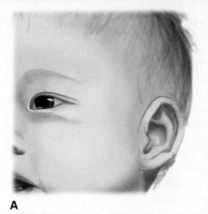
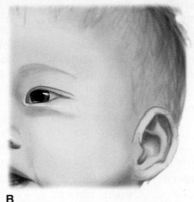

A   B

Figure 29.6 A. Normal positioning of the eyes in relation to the upper portion of the ears. **B.** Ear position that is much lower set than the outer canthus of the eye may be an indicator of genetic abnormalities or other health problems.

the face to straighten out the ear canal and promote visualization of the tympanic membrane. From 1 to 2 years, pull straight back on the pinna to straighten the ear canal for visualization of the tympanic membrane. After 2–3 years of age pull up and back on the top of the pinna to visualize the tympanic membrane. Once visualized, use the pneumatic bulb to test for movement of the tympanic membrane. *The tympanic membrane is gray, nonerythematous with the light reflex and landmarks visualized.*

Mobility is demonstrated with pneumoscopy. Palpate the pinna for tenderness and nodules. *The tympanic membrane is mobile; no tenderness or nodules are on the pinna* (Cunningham & Cox, 2003).

Screening for hearing acuity in infants and young children includes evaluation of developmental milestones, such as the Moro reflex in neonates (see Chapter 28). If there is a developmental lag or caregivers are concerned, a pediatric audiologist should perform a formal pediatric evaluation (Table 29-4).

Nose, Mouth, and Throat

Inspect the nose, mouth, and throat. *The nose is midline, nares are patent, and turbinates are pink with unrestricted air passage.* Note the number of deciduous and permanent teeth. *No caries are present.* In the mouth, tonsils are present and between +1 and +4 (see Chapter 17). *There is no erythema or exudate.*

Thorax and Lungs

Inspect the thorax and lungs. *There are no increased work of breathing and retractions.* Palpate the thorax. *There is no tenderness along intercostal spaces (ICSs).* Percuss the thorax and lungs. *The lungs are resonant.* Auscultate the thorax and lungs. *Breath sounds are clear in all lobes. No crackles, gurgles, or wheezes are noted.*

> **Clinical Significance 29-2**
>
> Children are prone to frequent cases of otitis media because the Eustachian tube is more horizontal than in adults (see Chapter 16). This is one reason why a child should never be put to bed with a bottle. Formula can pool in the back of the throat and ascend the Eustachian tubes, contributing to *otitis media.* As the head grows and shape changes, the Eustachian tubes become more vertical and the child is less prone to otitis media.

Tenderness with manipulation of the pinna may indicate *otitis externa.* Swollen, erythematous turbinates may indicate infection. Pale swollen turbinates may indicate *allergic rhinitis* and seasonal allergies.

Abnormal findings include lack of Moro reflex, inability to localize sound, or lack of understandable language by 24 months.

Dental caries are the most common infectious disease in childhood. Poor dental health is associated with poor physical health. Note any missing teeth. Erythema and exudate may be an infectious process.

Pain along ribs may be indicative of injury or viral infection such as costochondritis.

⚠ *SAFETY ALERT 29.6*
Respiratory distress requires immediate intervention and oxygen.

(text continues on page 884)

Table 29.4	Audiologic Tests for Infants and Children				
Developmental Age of Child	Auditory Test/ Average Time	Type of Measurement	Test Procedures	Advantages	Limitations
All ages	Evoked otoacoustic emissions test (OAEs), 10-minute test	Physiologic test specifically measuring cochlear (outer hair cell) response to presentation of a stimulus	Small probe containing a sensitive microphone is placed in the ear canal for stimulus delivery and response detection	Ear-specific results; not dependent on whether patient is asleep or awake; quick test time	Infant or child must be relatively inactive during the test; not a true test of hearing, because it does not assess cortical processing of sound
Birth to 9 mo	Automated brainstem response (ABR), 15-minute test	Electrophysiologic measurement of activity in auditory nerve and brainstem pathways	Placement of electrodes on child's head detects auditory stimuli presented through earphones one ear at a time	Ear-specific results; responses not dependent on patient cooperation	Infant or child must remain quiet during the test; not a true test of hearing, because it does not assess cortical processing of sound
9 months–2.5 years	Conditioned orienting response (COR) or visual reinforcement audiometry (VRA), 30-minute test	Behavioral tests measuring responses of the child to speech and frequency-specific stimuli presented through speakers	Both techniques condition the child to associate speech or frequency-specific sound with a reinforcement stimulus (eg, lighted toy); VRA requires a sound-treated room	Assesses auditory perception of child	Only assesses hearing of the better ear; not ear-specific; cannot rule out a unilateral hearing loss
2.5–4 years	Play audiometry, 30-minute test	Behavioral test measuring auditory thresholds in response to speech and frequency-specific stimuli presented through earphones, bone vibrator, or both	Child is conditioned to put a peg in a pegboard or drop a block in a box when stimulus tone is heard	Ear-specific results; assesses auditory perception of child	Attention span of child may limit the amount of information obtained
4 years to adolescence	Conventional audiometry, 30-minute test	Behavioral test measuring auditory thresholds in response to speech and frequency-specific stimuli presented through earphones, bone vibrator, or both	Patient is instructed to raise his or her hand when stimulus is heard	Ear-specific results; assesses auditory perception of patient	Depends on the level of understanding and cooperation of the child

Source: Adapted from Bachmann, K. R., & Arvedson, J. C. (1998). Early identification and intervention for children who are hearing impaired. *Pediatric Review*, 19, 155–165, with permission and Cunningham, M. D., & Cox, E. O. (2003). Clinical report: Hearing assessment in infants and children: Recommendations beyond neonatal screening by the Committee on Practice and Ambulatory Medicine and Section on Otolaryngology and Bronchoesophagology. *Pediatrics, 111*(2), 436–440.

Percuss the lungs if pneumonia is suspected. To encourage children to take deep breaths for an adequate assessment one may have a spinning pinwheel on which the child must blow so that the wheel spins.

Heart and Neck Vessels

Inspect for visible pulses on the thorax. Palpate and auscultate the point of maximal intensity (PMI). *The PMI is at the midclavicular line (MCL) in infancy and moves slightly laterally with age to the 4th ICS just to the left of the MCL in children younger than 7 years and then to the fifth ICS in children older than 7 years. There is no bounding PMI.*

If heart enlargement is suspected percussion can assist in determining size.

Auscultate the heart in all six designated areas on the chest and in the back. Assess with the child in two positions: lying and/or sitting and/or standing. *Closure of the tricuspid and mitral valves (S1) and the pulmonic and aortic (S2) valves is clear, crisp, and single. There are no murmurs, rubs, or gallops.* Observe the jugular venous pulsations. *The neck vessels are not distended or flat.*

The young child has a pliable skeletal system and the lung's functional reserve can be exhaled with a gentle chest squeeze. The next breath then is deep and longer than previous and assists with a complete assessment. Lower airway diameters in children are approximately half that of adults, which contributes to increased wheezing and *pneumonia*. The left main stem bronchus comes off at a more acute angle than the right in children. Therefore if a child aspirates, generally the foreign object is found in the right bronchus.

A visible PMI may signify increased cardiac load and increased oxygen requirements.

If a murmur is detected description of the murmur should include the intensity (Grades 1 through 6), timing, duration, quality, pitch, PMI, and if and to where it radiates (see Chapter 19). Characteristics of **innocent heart murmurs** and abnormal murmurs are noted in Box 29-1.

BOX 29.1 CHARACTERISTICS OF INNOCENT AND ABNORMAL HEART MURMURS

Innocent Murmurs

Innocent murmurs are associated with normal first and second heart sounds (S1 and S2). They occur in systole (except for the venous hum). They are usually very brief, well localized, and heard near the left sternal border. On a scale from 1 to 6, these usually are graded 1 or 2 without a thrill. The intensity changes with position, usually decreasing when standing. Innocent murmurs that may be auscultated in children are as follows:

• *Still's murmur*: a vibratory functional murmur, louder in the supine position
• *Pulmonary flow murmur*: increased flow, louder in the supine position, accentuated by exercise, fever, excitement
• *Venous hum*: continuous, loudest when sitting

Abnormal Murmurs

A murmur that sounds like a breath sound or is harsh or blowing (of any degree of intensity) signifies regurgitation of blood and pathology. Factors that increase the likelihood of an abnormal murmur include the following:

Symptoms such as chest pain, squatting, fainting, tiring quickly, shortness of breath, or failure-to-thrive

• Family history of Marfan's syndrome or sudden death in young (<50 years) family members
• Other congenital anomaly or syndrome (eg, Down's syndrome)
• Increased precordial activity
• Decreased femoral pulses
• Abnormal S2
• Clicks
• Loud or harsh murmur (>Grade 2)
• Increased intensity of murmur when the patient stands (McConnell, et al., 1999)

(text continues on page 886)

Peripheral Vascular

Inspect the peripheral vascular system. *The color is pink in all extremities and mucous membranes.* Palpate peripheral pulses (Fig. 29-7). *Pulses are equal in all extremities; there are no differences between upper-extremity and lower-extremity pulses.* Assess blood pressure in each extremity. *If there are slight differences, they are <10 mm Hg.*

Outside of the immediate newborn period, cyanosis requires immediate intervention. **Coarctation of the aorta** can present with unequal pulses between the upper and lower extremities (see Chapter 19). After the aorta leaves the heart, if there is a narrowing of the vessel then the lower extremities are not well oxygenated and pressure increases on the left side of the heart.

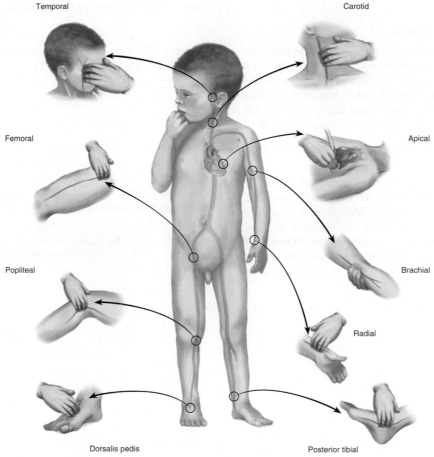

Figure 29.7 Location of peripheral pulses.

Breasts

Inspect the breasts. Refer to Chapter 26 for sexual maturity and Tanner staging for females. *Breast development begins with a "breast bud" or enlargement of the areola followed by enlargement of breast tissue.*

Onset of pubertal changes before 8 years in girls and 9 years in boys may be too early and needs further evaluation.

Abdomen

Inspect the abdomen. *No distension is noted.* A protuberate abdomen is a common finding in toddlers (Fig. 29-8). Palpate the abdomen. *There are no masses or tenderness.* Percuss the abdomen. *There is no tenderness with percussion and tympany throughout. The abdomen has a normal hollow or tympanic sound.* Percussion can assist in determining the size of the liver. *The liver is at the lower right costal margin.*

If distension is present assess for tenderness and ascities; if these are present, further intervention is required. Palpation of the abdomen to assess for abdominal masses is important, because *Wilms' tumors* of the kidney occur in toddlers and early school-age children. The normally protuberate abdomen, however, may interfere with detection of these tumors until they are of significant size. Significant abdominal tenderness requires further evaluation for *appendicitis*, *Crohn's disease*, *ulcerative colitis*, *gastroenteritis*, or other illnesses. Percussion can assist in determining the size of a palpable mass.

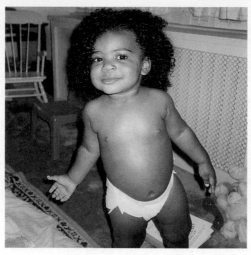

Figure 29.8 Note the protuberate abdomen, common in toddlers.

Musculoskeletal

Inspect the muscles and joints. Evaluation of scoliosis begins when the child can stand, but it is a focused part of the examination just prior to, and during, puberty (see Chapter 23). Observe range of motion (ROM) in all joints. Palpate the muscles and joints. *Normally the spine is straight. No joint tenderness is noted. ROM is full and symmetrical.*

Limited ROM in any joint requires further evaluation. Joint tenderness with palpation should be further evaluated for trauma and infection. Screening for scoliosis usually occurs during the school screening.

Neurological

Assess orientation. Observe for symmetry. Test deep tendon reflexes (DTRs) and evaluate for equality (Fig. 29-9). Ensure active movement and full strength in all extremities. *Older children are oriented to time and place. Movements are symmetrical; DTRs are 2+. Strength is 4–5+.*

Any noted asymmetry of gait, facial features, or movement needs further evaluation.

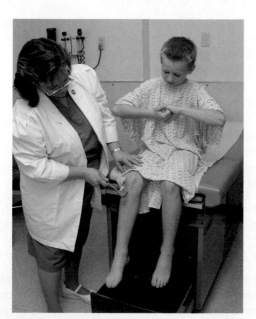

Figure 29.9 Testing DTRs in children.

(text continues on page 888)

| --- | --- |
Assess developmental progress for age. The Denver Developmental Screening Test is used for children 1 month to 6 years. For children older than 6 years, academic performance is noted. *Scores are within norms for the age.*	Confusion, unusual behaviors, delayed development progress, and poor academic performance need further assessment.
Male and Female Genitalia	
Inspect the genitalia. Refer to Chapter 25 and 26 for sexual maturity and **Tanner staging** for males and females. *In females, the genitalia show no signs of erythema, discharge, or irritation.*	Onset of pubertal changes before 8 years in girls and 9 years in boys may be too early and needs further evaluation. Visualization of the genitalia is recommended in a complete examination to detect early infections, trauma, or developmental concerns (eg, labial adhesions for girls, undescended testicles [*cryptochoidism*] for boys) that require intervention.
Note if the male is circumcised or uncircumcised with the urethra midline at the end of the glans. Palpate the male scrotum. *The testes are in the scrotal sac and are smooth with no nodules noted.*	The testes descend into the scrotal sac by age 6 months. If surgical repair is required, it should ideally happen before 2 years of age to prevent decreased fertility. *Hypospadias* requires intervention; it is usually diagnosed and treated in infancy (see Chapter 25). Adolescent boys should be assessed for testicular nodules; if found, they must be evaluated to rule out testicular cancer. Other testicular abnormalities (eg, hydrocele, varicocele, spermatocele) can be detected with testicular palpation.
Inspect the anus and rectum. *Skin on the anus and rectum is without irritation, erythema, or fissures.*	Rectal irritation or fissures require further evaluation for constipation, worms, or sexual abuse.

Evidence-Based Critical Thinking

Common Laboratory and Diagnostic Testing

No laboratory or diagnostic tests are recommended specifically for children and adolescents. Blood chemistry screening, hemoglobin (for anemia screening in patients 5 years or older), tuberculin skin screening (for children at average risk), and urinalysis are recommended when clinically indicated. The U.S. Preventive Services Task Force (USPSTF) states that screening for elevated blood lead levels is recommended only for symptomatic at-risk children 1 to 5 years.

Clinical Significance 29-3

A general hearing evaluation is required for children with speech difficulties prior to their being evaluated by a speech pathologist or undergoing speech therapy.

In the primary care setting, vision screening is recommended for children younger than 4 years old. By age 5 years, vision screening is part of the preschool assessment. Car seat and seat belt use is assessed. The BMI is calculated as a screen for overweight and obesity. Sexually active women younger than 25 years are screened for chlamydia (ICSI, 2009).

Diagnostic Reasoning

When formulating a nursing diagnosis, it is important to use critical thinking to cluster data and identify patterns that fit together. The nurse compares these clusters with the defining characteristics (abnormal findings) for the diagnosis to ensure the most accurate labeling and appropriate interventions. Table 29-5 provides a comparison of nursing diagnoses, abnormal findings, and interventions commonly related to assessment of the child.

Nurses use assessment information to identify patient outcomes. Some outcomes related to the child include the following:

- The family identifies health-promotion systems.
- The child achieves developmental tasks on schedule for age.
- The family seeks information regarding health promotion.

Once outcomes are established, nursing care is implemented to improve the status of the child. The nurse uses critical thinking and evidence-based practice to develop the interventions.

Table 29.5 Common Nursing Diagnoses Associated with the Child or Adolescent

Diagnosis and Related Factors	Point of Differentiation	Assessment Characteristics	Nursing Interventions
Readiness for enhanced family processes	Pattern of family functioning that supports the well-being of family members	Activities support individual and family growth	Assess the family's coping abilities and stressors. Encourage attendance at community groups and classes. Assess cultural beliefs and norms.
Delayed growth and development related to regression or lack of progression	Child or teen shows significant deviations from norms of peers	Delays exist in the skills typically found with children of the same age	Assess the influence of cultural norms, values, and beliefs on the parent's perceptions of development.
Health-seeking behaviors	Actively seeking ways to change health habits to improve health level	Concern about current conditions, unfamiliarity with wellness community resources	Discuss benefits and barriers to staying healthy, environmental factors to health, stress placed on the family.

Some examples of nursing interventions for the child are as follows:

• Provide information about community support systems available to the family during times of stress.

• Identify conditions that contribute to altered growth and development.

• Provide information that contributes to an improved state of health.

Analyzing Findings

Subjective: Simon's mother reports that he has been very healthy. The family speaks Spanish at home but English at church and with his maternal grandparents. His paternal grandparents live in Chile and visits once a year. The family lives in a large Victorian home built in the 1920s; they are renovating the house on the weekends.

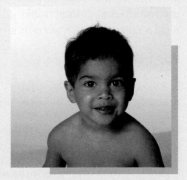

Objective: Cooperative 4-year-old child responds appropriately to questions and requests, generally pleasant. No complaints of pain, present discomfort, or health concerns. T 37°C, P 86 beats/min, R 20 breaths/min, BP 94/50 mm Hg left arm. Height 41 in. Weight 17.5 kg. BMI 16.3. Alert and cooperative; answers questions appropriately although difficult to understand at times. Knows what day it is and why he has come to the clinic for evaluation. Hearing = passed at 20 dB at 500, 1,000, 2,000, 4,000 Hz. However failed at 30 dB for 1,000, 2,000, 4,000 Hz. Passed DDST in personal-social, fine motor, and gross motor areas. Failed language area.

Assessment: Disturbed sensory perception, auditory. Hearing impairment detected. Immunizations recommended for children 4–6 years of age needed. At risk for elevated blood lead level. Speech difficulties.

Plan: Order blood lead level and refer for speech evaluation. Update immunizations. Provide information and handouts on nutrition, activity, limiting TV, reading, school readiness, immunizations, discipline, and safety. Refer to audiologist for further testing and treatment.

P. Singala, ARNP

Critical Thinking Challenge

• How do the subjective and objective data fit together?
• What findings of Simon's are abnormal?
• What is the nurse's role in his care?

Collaboration with Other Health Care Providers

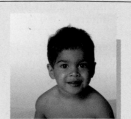

Hearing screening is becoming increasingly common in the newborn period. Without such testing, the average age of detection of hearing impairment is 14 months (ASLHA, 2010). If impairment is not detected until late in the preschool period, speech can be affected.

Simon's hearing loss was detected when he was 4 years old, which is likely contributing to his speech problems. The nurse needs to refer Simon to an audiologist in addition to speech therapy. The information below illustrates the nurse's communication with the audiologist.

Situation: Hello, I am Paula Singala, an advanced practitioner RN. I saw Simon Chavez earlier this morning.

Background: He is 4 years old and has some speech difficulties and hearing loss.

Assessment: Simon passed his hearing test at 20 dB at 500; however, he failed at 30 dB for 1,000, 2,000, and 4,000 Hz.

Recommendations: I would like you to evaluate him further.

Critical Thinking Challenge

- Why might Simon be having hearing loss?
- What other things would you assess as the nurse?
- How might his ability to speak two languages affect his speech?

Pulling It All Together: Reflection and Critical Thinking

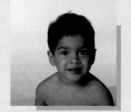

The nurse uses assessment data to formulate a nursing care plan with patient outcomes and interventions for Simon. This includes a diagnosis, outcomes, and interventions, which the nurse uses critical thinking and judgment to continue or revise. This is often in the form of a care plan or case note similar to the one below.

Nursing Diagnosis	Patient Outcomes	Nursing Interventions	Rationales	Evaluation
Disturbed sensory perception related to altered hearing	Patient uses assistive devices correctly. Speech becomes easier to understand.	Turn off TV and radio when communicating. Speak in lower tones if possible. Stand directly in front of the patient when talking.	Background noise interferes with hearing voices. The patient can use nonverbal cues, such as lip reading.	Patient obtained and is using hearing devices. Evaluate speech improvement at next visit.

Applying Your Knowledge

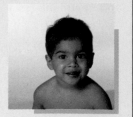

Using the previous steps of assessment and nursing process, consider all the case study findings presented in this chapter about Simon, who is undergoing a preschool physical examination. When answering the following questions, begin drawing conclusions and see how the pieces of assessment must work together to create an environment for personalized, appropriate, and accurate care. Consider Simon's case and answer the following questions.

- What health information and assessments are important for the toddler, preschooler, school-aged child, and adolescent?
- How do assessment findings differ between the child and adult?
- What adaptations will the nurse make when assessing a child?

Key Points

- Evaluation of a child's physical growth is performed with standardized growth charts.
- Head circumference is measured on children from birth to 3 years old.
- Motor development progresses cephalocaudally and from proximal to distal.
- Health-related teaching for families with children and adolescents includes obtaining immunizations; using child safety car seats, window/stair guards, pool fences, life jackets, and bike helmets; keeping a safe distance from firepits; crossing streets safely; following poison control measures; avoiding underage drinking and driving; contraception; and taking measures for adequate nutrition and sun screen.
- Most of the physical assessment of a toddler can be performed with the child sitting in the parent's lap.
- The DDST-II is the gold standard for developmental evaluation of children ages 1 month to 6 years.
- Innocent murmurs occur in systole, are brief and well localized, and are usually heard near the left sternal border.

Review Questions

1. What is the best time to assess the respiratory rate of a young child?
   A. While the child is crying
   B. While the child is playing in the playroom
   C. Immediately after taking the child's blood pressure
   D. While the child is quietly sitting on the parent's lap

2. Which factor places an infant at greater risk than an adult for developing otitis media?
   A. Introduction of solid foods
   B. Eustachian tubes that are more horizontal (flat) than vertical and wide
   C. Immature cardiac sphincter
   D. Feeding in a semi-Fowler's position

3. During assessment of a child's visual acuity, which finding may indicate myopia or nearsightedness?
   A. Holding a book close to the face
   B. Squinting
   C. Rapid eye movements
   D. Closing one eye

4. What is an easy way to determine whether a child has strabismus?
   A. Observe the red reflex.
   B. Check eyes for unequal pupil size.
   C. Shine the light in his or her eyes.
   D. Do a fundoscopic examination.

5. All the following may be symptoms of a child experiencing lead poisoning except
   A. Irritability
   B. Cardiomegaly
   C. Headaches
   D. Abdominal pain

6. As soon as the child can stand, begin to measure the height in the upright position.
   A. True, using the scale as soon as the child can stand on it is fine.
   B. False, measure the child standing starting between 2 and 3 years of age.
   C. It depends on when the child can stand independently.
   D. False, a child should always be measured in the recumbent position.

7. A child's head circumference is a measurement that should be obtained at every well-child visit until the child is 5 years old.
   A. True, this measure is indicative of brain growth.
   B. False, one or two measurements are the standard of care.
   C. True, it will provide information on the child's readiness for kindergarten.
   D. False, the charts for head circumference norms end at 36 months.

8. A blood pressure of 110/70 (left arm) was obtained in a 5-year-old boy. What would the nurse do about this blood pressure?
   A. Call the physician immediately.
   B. Bring the child back to the clinic two more times to ensure accuracy of the assessment.
   C. Determine the blood pressure percentile based on age, sex, and height percentile.
   D. It is normal, nothing needs to be done.

9. Health-promotion concepts for children that would affect their lifelong cardiovascular health include which of the following?
   A. Information on good nutrition
   B. Information on the prevention of illnesses
   C. Information on exercise
   D. All of the above

10. Children are usually brought for health care by a parent. At about what age should the interviewer begin to question the child regarding presenting symptoms?
    A. 5 years
    B. 7 years
    C. 9 years
    D. 11 years

References

American Academy of Pediatrics. (2008). *Bright futures: Guidelines for health supervision of infants, children and adolescents.* Retrieved July 13, 2008, from http://brightfutures.aap.org/3rd_Edition_Guidelines_and_Pocket_Guide.html

American Speech Language Hearing Association (ASLHA) (2010). *Hearing screening.* Retrieved March 4, 2010, from http://www.asha.org/public/hearing/testing/on

Centers for Disease Control and Prevention. (2009). *Lead prevention.* Retrieved June 23, 2010, from http://www.cdc.gov/nceh/lead/tips.htm

Centers for Disease Control and Prevention. (2010). *Quick stats: Underage drinking.* Retrieved February 14, 2010, from http://www.cdc.gov/alcohol/quickstats/underage_drinking.htm

Centers for Disease Control: Department of Health and Human Services. (2008). *Growth charts.* Retrieved July 13, 2008 from http://www.cdc.gov/growthcharts/

Centers for Disease Control: Environmental Health. (2007). *Toys and childhood lead exposure.* Retrieved July 23, 2008, from http://www.cdc.gov/nceh/lead/faq/toys.htm

Committee on Practice and Ambulatory Medicine, Section on Ophthalmology, American Association of Certified Orthoptists, American Association for Pediatric Ophthalmology and Strabismus and American Academy of Ophthalmology (2003 and reaffirmed in 2007). Policy statement: Eye examination in infants, children, and young adults by pediatricians. *Pediatrics, 111*(4), 902–907.

Cunningham, M. D., & Cox, E. O. (2003). Clinical report: Hearing assessment in infants and children: Recommendations beyond neonatal screening by the Committee on Practice and Ambulatory Medicine and Section on Otolaryngology and Bronchoesophagology. *Pediatrics, 111*(2), 436–440.

Drumwright, M. A., Drexler, H., VanNatta, P., Camp, B., & Frankenburg, W. K. (1973). Denver articulation screening exam. *JSHD, 38, 3.* Materials available and retrieved July 23, 2008, from http://www.denverii.com/DASE.html

Frankenburg, W. K., Dodds, J., Archer, P., Shapiro, H., & Bresnick, B. (1992). The Denver II: A major revision and restandardization of the Denver developmental screening test. *Pediatrics, 89,* 91–97. Materials available and retrieved July 15, 2008 from http://www.denverii.com/DenverII.html

Healthy people 2010: What are its goals? (n.d.). Retrieved July 7, 2010, from http://www.healthypeople.gov/About/goals.htm

Institute for Clinical Systems Improvement (ICSI) (2009). *Preventative services for children and adolescents (Guidelines).* Retrieved June 23, 2010, from http://www.icsi.org/guidelines_and_more/gl_os_prot/preventive_health_maintenance/preventive_services_for_children__guideline_/preventive_services_for_children_and_adolescents_762.html

McConnell, M. E., Adkins, S. B., & Hannon D. W. (1999). Heart murmurs in pediatric patients: When do you refer? *American Family Physician, 60*(2), 558–565.

National Heart, Lung and Blood Institute. (2004). *Blood pressure tables for children and adolescents from the Fourth Report on the Diagnosis, Evaluation, and Treatment of High Blood Pressure in Children and Adolescents.* Retrieved July 15, 2008, from http://www.nhlbi.nih.gov/guidelines/hypertension/child_tbl.htm

National Highway Traffic Safety Administration. (2008). Retrieved July 15, 2008, from http://www.nhtsa.dot.gov/

Robins, Fein, & Barton (1999). *M-CHAT Tool and scoring.* Retrieved July 13, 2008, from http://www.firstsigns.org/downloads/m-chat.PDF

Selekman, J. (2007). Changes in the screening for tuberculosis in children: Screening for TB. *Pediatric Nursing, 32*(1), 73–75.

Thomas, S., Acton, C., Nixon, J., Battistutta, D., Pitt, W. R., & Clark, R. (1994). Effectiveness of bicycle helmets in preventing head injury in children: Case-control study. *British Medical Journal, 308,* 173–176.

U.S. Department of Agriculture. (2005). *My Pyramid.* Retrieved July 13, 2008, from http://teamnutrition.usda.gov/Resources/mpk_poster2.pdf

---

The Jensen suite offers these additional resources to enhance learning and facilitate understanding of this chapter:

• thePoint on line resource, http//thepoint.lww.com/Jensen1E
• Student CD-ROM included with the book
• *Laboratory Manual for Nursing Health Assessment: A Best Practice Approach*
• *Pocket Guide for Nursing Health Assessment: A Best Practice Approach*

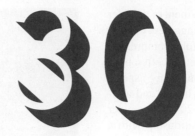

Older Adults

Learning Objectives

1 Identify normal changes that occur with aging.

2 Identify risk factors in older adults for malnutrition, mobility limitations, falling, polypharmacy complications, and skin breakdown.

3 Describe common symptoms in older adults, such as incontinence, sleep disturbances, pain, cognitive changes, depression, and elder abuse.

4 Identify teaching opportunities for health promotion and risk reduction in this population.

5 Collect subjective data, using interviewing techniques that include variations based upon age.

6 Collect objective data on the body systems including normal variations based on age.

7 Individualize health assessment considering the condition, age, gender, and culture of the patient.

8 Identify normal and abnormal findings from inspection, palpation, percussion, and auscultation of all body systems.

9 Use subjective and objective data to analyze findings, identify diagnoses, and plan interventions.

10 Use assessment findings to develop a plan of care for an older adult.

11 Document and communicate data using appropriate medical terminology.

*M*r. Ralph Monroe is a 76-year-old man with a history of Parkinson's disease. He has lived in a nursing home for the past 3 months because of functional limitations. He complains of "terrible constipation" and asks "What causes this?" His daily medications include Sinemet 25/250 four times before meals for Parkinson's, vitamin E 400 IU for prevention of heart disease, calcium 600 mg with vitamin D 800 IU for bone health, and Zestril 5 mg for his blood pressure.

Begin thinking about the following points:

- What are some causes of constipation that would immediately be apparent in this case?
- What health-promotion activities is Mr. Monroe already doing to stay healthy?
- What assessments might the nurse perform in addition to the screening examination?

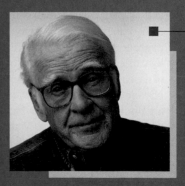

Conducting an accurate and complete assessment of an older adult is essential for the planning and management of care. **Geriatric** nursing experts identify the need for a comprehensive assessment of this population, because elders often have a unique presentation of illness. In addition, many aspects of the lives of older adults can affect their health and ability to cope with chronic changes (Amella, 2004). An older adult's social situation, living situation, relationship with a caregiver, access to transportation, mobility, financial or economic situation, understanding, expectation, and cultural or religious views on disease can influence health as much as his or her health history, past medical diagnoses, understanding of medications, physical examination findings, and functional ability (Lach & Smith, 2007).

In recent years, U.S. life expectancy has increased to 78 years (Kung, et al., 2008). This increase, careful management of chronic diseases, and prolonged periods of living with multiple chronic diseases have changed the U.S. population of older adults. As Baby Boomers age into their 70s and 80s, nurses can expect to see increasing numbers of older adults in community and all health care settings. By 2030, the United States will have 71 million people older than 65 years, accounting for 20% of the total population (Centers for Disease Control and Prevention and Merck Foundation, 2007).

This chapter begins with a review of physiologic changes associated with aging and then moves to a discussion of best practices for conducting an interview with an older adult. It includes some common assessment tools used to identify risk for specific geriatric symptoms. The chapter then discusses such tools in the context of physical examination findings. In that section, the normal aging process is separated from findings that represent abnormal changes commonly found in older adults. Previous chapters covered specific assessment considerations for older adults related to general survey, pain, nutrition/supplements/medications, developmental stages, mental status, social/spiritual/cultural concerns, and violence. Refer to Chapters 6 to 12 for more specific information on those areas.

Structure and Function Overview

Skin, Hair, and Nails

The epidermis thins with aging, and the epithelium renews itself every 30 days instead of every 20 days as in children and adults. This decreased mitotic activity of cells leads to a 50% reduction in rate of wound healing. In addition, there are degeneration of the elastic fibers providing dermal support, a loss of collagen, and a loss of subcutaneous fat. The number of sweat and sebaceous glands decreases as a result of atrophy, and vascularity and capillary fragility of the skin layer are diminished. Nail beds become more rigid, thick, and brittle, with slowed growth (Makrantonaki & Zouboulis, 2007).

It is important to note the difference between normal aging processes and the lifelong cumulative exposure to sun, called **photoaging** (Fisher, et al., 2002). For example, fine wrinkling

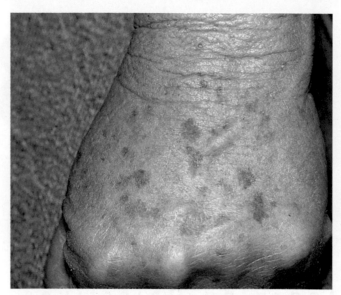

Figure 30.1 Solar lentigines, or "liver spots," are a common and normal skin finding in older adults.

of the skin is a normal part of aging, but coarse wrinkling is evidence of photoaging. Sun exposure also increases **solar lentigines** (age or liver spots, Fig. 30-1), mottled **dyspigmentation** areas, and **actinic keratoses**. Long-term smoking also alters skin by reducing dermal elastic fibers, reducing blood flow to the dermal layers, and slowing healing times for wounds.

Head and Neck

With aging, facial subcutaneous fat decreases, making the skeleton more pronounced. Skin may sag and wrinkle across the forehead, surrounding the eyes, at the tip of the nose, and on the cheeks, which alters facial appearance. Skin lesions are more likely, and careful assessment for possible cancers, especially in commonly sun-exposed areas, is important (CDC, 2010; see Chapter 13).

Thyroid function and thyroid hormones do not change with aging. Poor thyroid function in an older adult is related to thyroid dysfunction, not normal aging.

Eyes and Vision

Older adults have less fat in the orbital area, laxity of the orbital muscles, and decreased lid elasticity. They have fewer goblet cells that provide mucin, resulting in less lubrication for the eyes. Tear production decreases, which leads to dry eyes. Corneal sensitivity may diminish. Increased lipid deposits may be found at the periphery of the cornea around the iris. The ciliary body secretes less aqueous humor, and the ciliary muscle may atrophy, compromising the ability to focus the lens. The lens becomes less elastic, larger, and denser with age and can become progressively yellowed and opaque. The iris loses some pigment, and the pupil becomes progressively smaller. Slowed pupillary responses lead to a difficulty in accommodating to changes in light, difficulty with night driving, and problems with glare (Brodie, 2003).

Ears and Hearing

Physiological changes to ears and hearing include a widening and lengthening of the auricle, coarse wiry hair growth in the external ears (especially in men), narrowing of the auditory canal, and dry cerumen in the ear canal. The tympanic membrane in the middle ear becomes dull, less flexible, retracted, and gray. The organ of Corti atrophies, causing sensory hearing loss, and cochlear neurons are lost, causing neural hearing loss (Linton & Lach, 2007). Changes to the inner ear can reduce the older adult's ability to discriminate sounds, especially in noisy conditions (Bance, 2007).

Nose, Mouth, and Throat

Because of an age-related loss of olfactory receptor neurons, older adults have a decreased sense of smell, which can start as early as the fourth decade of life. The threshold for odors in older adults is 2 to 15 times greater than that for a younger person (indicating a need for a much stronger smell for recognition; Boyce & Shone, 2006). In addition, chronic medical conditions can alter the sense of smell. For example older adults with Alzheimer's or Parkinson's disease may have difficulty with odor recognition. Olfactory dysfunction can significantly reduce food intake, because smell and taste are important in the enjoyment of foods.

Teeth surfaces become worn with aging, which increases the risk of dental caries. Collagen and elasticity changes affect oral tissues, with mucosal thinning and smoothing of the tongue. Oral hygiene practices throughout the lifespan, however, greatly influence gum recession and tooth loss. Taste buds are replaced every 10 to 100 days. Many older adults experience changes in taste starting around 60 years old. Changes in taste detection and sensation were originally thought linked to a loss of taste buds; however, recent studies have shown that healthy older adults do not lose taste buds. Researchers now believe loss of taste sensation is more likely caused by medications, diseases, long-term smoking damage, or malnutrition. Older adults who regularly take medications or have diseases that create less saliva or xerostomia are more likely to have problems with taste (Boyce & Shone, 2006).

Thorax and Lungs

Changes to connective tissue related to aging are evident throughout the respiratory system. The chest wall is less elastic, and rigidity or lack of compliance limits chest expansion. Decreased respiratory muscle strength creates a less effective cough for older adults. Alveoli are thicker and fewer in older adult smokers, but the number of alveoli remains relatively constant in healthy older adults.

Loss of alveolar elastic recoil produces approximately a 20% decrease in lung vital capacity. Loss of alveolar surface area creates less area available for oxygen exchange and difficulties responding to hypoxic or hypercapneic episodes. Fewer cilia lining the airways create less efficiency in clearing the lungs. Residual volume (the volume of air remaining in the lung after a maximal expiration) increases with age. The forced expiratory volume in 1 second (FEV)/forced vital capacity ratio declines about 0.2% per year after 40 years (Sharma & Goodwin, 2006). Major changes in respiratory function are usually related to deconditioning and disease or damage from long-term smoking rather than the aging process itself.

Heart and Neck Vessels

Changes in connective and smooth muscle tissue affect the peripheral vessels and heart. Arterial walls are less elastic and stiffen. Subsequent decreased compliance affects blood pressure by increasing the afterload on the left ventricle. Systolic blood pressure increases, the left ventricle wall hypertrophies or thickens, and there is an increased dependence on atrial contraction. Coronary artery blood flow decreases by about one-third. The loss of atrial pacemaker cells and Bundle of HIS fibers may result in decreased heart rate. Intrinsic cardiac contractile function diminishes, reducing cardiac output, stroke volume, and cardiac reserves (Bernhard & Laufer, 2008). Responsiveness to beta-adrenergic receptor stimulation and reactivity of baroreceptors and chemoreceptors decrease, while circulating catecholamines increase. Jugular venous pulsations increase with fluid volume excess and decrease with fluid volume deficit.

Peripheral Vascular and Lymphatics

Calcification of the arteries, or *arteriosclerosis*, causes them to become more rigid (Fig. 30-2). Less arterial compliance results in increased systolic blood pressure (Porth, 2007). This is often compounded by the coexistence of atherosclerotic disease in the arteries supplying the brain, heart, and other vital organs. Incidence of peripheral arterial disease

Figure 30.2 Arteriosclerosis (hardening of the arteries) develops as people age. It can eventually progress to atherosclerosis, which can cause life-threatening complications.

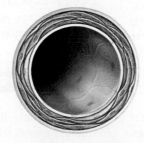
Normal vessel

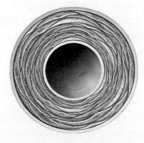
Arteriosclerosis

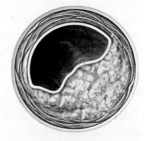
Atherosclerosis

(PAD) increases dramatically in the seventh and eighth decades of life (Porth, 2007). Prevalence of PAD in men and women is equal at this stage (Ostchega, et al., 2007). Patients with venous congestion may also develop edema from poor lymphatic drainage (see Chapter 20.)

Breasts and Lymphatics

Glandular breast tissue atrophies, becomes less dense, and is replaced by fat. As women age, glandular, alveolar, and lobular breast tissues decrease. After menopause, fat deposits replace glandular tissue that continues to atrophy as a result of decreased secretion of ovarian hormones, estrogen, and progesterone. The inframammary ridge thickens, making this area easier to palpate. Suspensory ligaments relax, causing the breasts to sag and droop. Additionally, breasts decrease in size and lose elasticity. Nipples become smaller, flatter, and less erectile. Axillary hair also may stop growing. These changes are more apparent in the eighth and ninth decades of life. Women who have had mastectomies may develop lymphedema in the affected arm.

Abdomen, Metabolism, and Elimination

Although it was previously thought that parietal and chief cells in the stomach decrease with aging, reducing hydrocholoric acid and pepsin, some studies now show that older adults actually have increased gastric acid secretion. Slowed peristalsis creates a delayed emptying of the stomach and delayed movement of food through the gastrointestinal system. Absorption of vitamin D, calcium, and zinc in the small intestine may be reduced (Elmadfa & Meyer, 2008). The number and size of hepatocytes decrease, and hepatic blood flow is reduced. Metabolism of medications on the first pass through the liver decreases, leaving older adults at risk for higher circulating medication levels. Secretion of bicarbonate and enzymes in the pancreas decreases, and the pancreatic duct becomes more dilated. The colonic transit rate is slower.

The size and function of the kidney decrease with age. Nephrons in the cortex of the kidneys are fewer, while abnormal glomeruli increase. The body responds to the sclerotic changes in the glomeruli by increasing the size of the remaining healthy glomeruli.

Older adults develop diverticular changes in the distal renal tubules. For older patients with vascular problems, the decrease in blood flow to glomerular units leads to a decrease in glomerular filtration rate (Lamb, et al., 2003). These changes are reflected in a decrease in creatinine clearance and a loss of ability to conserve sodium. Older adults also experience a general reduction in peak bladder capacity and a weakening of the bladder muscles, which can lead to incomplete emptying of the bladder.

Musculoskeletal

Older adults often lose height. Gradual compression of the spinal column is related to narrowing of intervertebral discs. Beginning at around age 30 years, bone absorption starts to exceed bone formation. In women, this bone loss accelerates in the decade immediately following menopause. Decreased lean body mass also occurs with aging. There is a loss of type II muscle (fast-twitch) fibers as compared with type I muscle (slow-twitch, fatigue-resistant) fibers, which leads to muscle wasting. Regeneration of muscle tissues slows with age, but studies show that exercise can increase lean muscle mass even in frail older adults (Peterson, et al., 2010).

Neurological

With aging, the number of neurons and glial cells gradually decline, and these cells show structural changes. Nevertheless, current studies do not support the notion of extensive brain atrophy in normal aging. Atrophy is common in people with degenerative neurological diseases. The overall number of neuronal synapses decreases, while lipofuscin granules in the nerve cells accumulate. There is increased production and accumulation of oxyradicals in all body systems (Foster, 2006).

Neurological changes are worsened in people who have changes to the vessels that supply the nervous system (eg, people with diabetes mellitus, smokers). Efficiency of the autonomic functions of the central nervous system decreases, so that recovery from stress becomes more difficult. Healthy older adults maintain cognitive function, but retrieval speed for information slows. Speed of brain processing on tests of psychomotor performance shows slowing with age. Reaction times are slower, but may be affected by other changes including vision and musculoskeletal changes. Postural control, decreased vibratory sense, and decreased righting reflex ability may affect the balance of older adults (Linton & Lach, 2007).

Male and Female Genitourinary

Age-related enlargement of the prostate can contribute to urinary retention or outlet obstruction. Genital hair thins. The vaginal mucosa thins and loses elasticity. Vaginal secretions diminish from lower estrogen levels with age (see Chapters 25 and 26).

Endocrine

The pituitary gland decreases in size, weight, and vascularity. Secretion of growth hormone and circulating levels of insulin-like growth factor decreases. Plasma levels of the adrenal steroids (DHEA and DHEA-S) show a significant decline with aging. Prevalence of glucose intolerance and type 2 diabetes increases. Older adults are more likely to have a decreased responsiveness to immunizations. Because of changes in the immune system, older adults may have more auto-antibodies and risks for autoimmune diseases (Chahal & Drake, 2007).

Acute Assessment

Falls, especially if accompanied by fracture, are the most common reason for admission of older adults to emergency departments (Hastings, et al., 2009). Chronic conditions also may be exacerbated; for example, worsening of COPD or congestive heart failure can be an acute condition. Infection, chest pain, abdominal pain, and delirium should be assessed and treated rapidly. Because older adults may not mount an immune response, infection may be present even in the absence of fever.

Subjective Data Collection

Areas for Health Promotion/*Healthy People*

Table 30-1 includes pertinent goals and education topics for the older adult based upon the *Healthy People* goals.

Interviewing the Older Adult

Before interviewing the older adult, the nurse should set up the room and create an environment that facilitates hearing and understanding of communication. Although some acute situations do not allow for finding a quiet space, an environment that is calm and quiet is essential for conducting an interview with an older person. It is essential to reduce or eliminate background noise as much as possible when carrying on conversations. This includes turning off the television or radio in the patient's room and closing the door to reduce sounds of telephones, beepers, alarms, or pagers. Cold or drafty environments are uncomfortable and can distract the older adult from tasks at hand. The older adult needs to be warm and comfortable during the interview (Ham, et al., 2007).

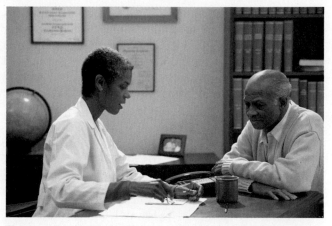

Figure 30.3 History taking with older adults needs to be at a slow and deliberate pace; it may need to be conducted over several visits for a comprehensive picture of the patient's health.

The interview of an older adult can take much longer than that for a younger, healthier person. It might not be completed in one encounter. Nurses need to allow additional time for an interview or health history (Lach & Smith, 2007; Fig. 30-3). Frail older adults may hesitate before answering questions. The nurse should not rush in to fill the silence. For an older adult with intact cognition, it is disrespectful to ignore him or her and address all questions to a patient's family member. The nurse should respectfully address questions directly to the patient and allow time for his or her responses. If the patient cannot provide information, the nurse may then address the family member with questions.

Table 30.1 *Healthy People* Goals Related to Older Adult Health	
Goals	**Patient Education Topics**
Reduce the proportion of adults with osteoporosis.	Encourage vitamin D and calcium supplementation as appropriate
Reduce the rate of new cases of end-stage renal disease.	Monitor and maintain blood pressure within American Heart Association guidelines.
Prevent diabetes.	Encourage diet that supports a normal BMI.
Increase the proportion of older adults who have participated during the preceding year in at least one organized health promotion activity.	Provide resources for classes on nutrition, exercise and health screening.
Increase the proportion of adults who are vaccinated annually against influenza and ever vaccinated against pneumococcal disease.	Provide opportunities for annual influenza and pneumococcal vaccines. Question about vaccine currency each fall.
Increase the proportion of adults who perform physical activities that enhance and maintain flexibility.	Assess availability of a gym or classes. Many facilities offer free or reduced price programs for seniors.
Increase the proportion of physician office visits for counseling or education related to diet and nutrition.	Assess desire for information on diet and nutrition and make appropriate referrals.

Source: *Healthy people 2010: What are its goals?* (n.d.). Retrieved July 7, 2010, from http://www.healthypeople.gov/About/goals.htm

Consideration of the patient's educational level is critical, and interview questions should match the older adult's knowledge level. It is not appropriate to ask an elderly patient with limited education "Have you noticed any signs of cerebrovascular or neurological changes?" Instead, questions need to be phrased in a way that might be better understood and specific to what is being asked. For example, "Have you ever noticed more clumsiness in one hand compared with the other?' or "Has your speech been slurred or jumbled?"

When older adults are hospitalized or more seriously ill, the nurse should gather as much information as pos-

---

BOX 30.1 CONDUCTING THE HEALTH INTERVIEW IN OLDER ADULTS WITH SPECIAL NEEDS

Hearing Impaired Older Adults

Before starting the interview, check that a hearing aid is in place and turned on and has a working battery. It is helpful to have a pocket amplifier and earphones available if you cannot locate the patient's hearing aid. Seat yourself directly in front of the person at eye level so that he or she can observe your face for visual cues (Lach & Smith, 2007). Do not stand and talk down to a seated patient. If necessary seat yourself on the bedside so that the patient can see you. Make certain that you have the patient's attention and are close enough to the person before you begin speaking. Hearing-impaired patients benefit from seeing your lips move, so keep your hands away from your face while talking. Speak normally or in a slightly louder fashion (ie, a soft-spoken person may need to speak a bit more boldly). Use a low-pitched, calm voice without shouting. If the person has difficulty understanding something, find a different way of saying the same thing, rather than continually repeating the original words. If the person has more profound hearing impairment, be prepared to write questions or messages if necessary. Use pictures, illustrations, body language, or gestures to facilitate communication. Do not assume that the hearing-impaired older adult is unreliable or has dementia. Try to gain as much information as possible within the limitations of his or her hearing impairment.

Visually Impaired Older Adults

If you are entering a room with someone who is visually impaired, identify yourself and your intentions. Avoid shouting or speaking too loudly (not all visually impaired older patients are also hearing impaired). If the patient wears corrective lenses, make sure these are clean. Repeat or reflect the patient's responses to your questions a little more frequently during the interview if he or she cannot see your face for the usual visual cues that indicate understanding. When you speak, let the person know whom you are addressing, especially if you are directing that question to an adult child or colleague and not to the patient. Ask what you can do to facilitate the interview, increasing the light, placing yourself in a different spot, and describing where things are. Be sure to say the person's name and tell him or her what you are going to touch or do during the physical examination. Keep in mind that people categorized as legally blind may have some vision. When you complete your interview and examination be sure to return items to their original location unless the person asks you to move them.

Older Adults with Aphasia

Patients who have experienced a stroke or another type of neurological injury or illness may have total or partial aphasia. Those with *expressive aphasia* may be able to partially or fully understand what you say but unable to respond to your questions. Use patience and allow plenty of time to communicate with a person with aphasia. You may want to seek out a picture board or communication device provided by a speech therapist to better facilitate the discussion. Let the patient know if you cannot understand what he or she is telling you. Allow the patient to try to complete thoughts, to struggle with words. Although it is recommended that you provide some words, avoid being too quick to guess what the person is trying to express. If possible, encourage the person to write the word he or she is trying to express and read it aloud. Use gestures or pointing to objects if helpful in supplying words or adding meaning.

Patients with Alzheimer's Disease or Related Disorders

As you conduct an interview with an older adult, you may find the patient has repeated the same story about three times within 20 minutes. This repetitive story telling is often an indicator of cognitive impairment. Patients who repeat the same story as if you have not heard it before should be screened with the MMSE. If you conduct an MMSE early in the interview, you can better determine whether it is wise to continue to seek information from the patient. People in early stages of Alzheimer's may be fairly accurate in their responses, especially about issues from early adulthood or childhood (remote memory). They are more likely to omit information about more recent issues (short-term memory). People with MMSE scores of 11 of less are unlikely to be reliable reporters for your interview.

When interviewing an older adult with known dementia, make sure that you approach from the front within the patient's line of vision. Provide the same respect that you would to any older patient, introduce yourself, and greet the patient by formal name. Be sure to face the person as you interview. A quiet calm environment is essential. Avoid a heavy traffic area, an area with multiple conversations, or a very noisy place. A low-pitched, calm tone of voice tends to be heard well and sets the tone. Ask only one question at a time. Repeat key words if the person does not understand the first time. As much as possible maintain eye contact and provide respect of personal space (Miller, 2008).

People with mild to moderate dementia who maintain language skills can still be accurate reporters of current symptoms and concerns. As dementia progresses, the patient may overestimate abilities to carry out self-care activities, IADLs, or safe and independent medication management. Be sure to clarify the accuracy of the patient's responses with a caregiver or family member. If the patient with dementia is more anxious and tends to wander or pace, you may need to walk with him or her while asking simple questions. Try to limit questions to yes or no for those with moderate to severe dementia; avoid open-ended questions or those that require abstract thinking or reasoning (Miller, 2008).

sible from previous records so that he or she can review and clarify findings with the older adult, rather than trying to gain all the information from the patient's memory (Lach & Smith, 2007). This helps the older person to conserve energy. If the older adult is acutely ill and fatigues easily, the nurse may need to return and complete the interview later.

Some older adults are reluctant to report symptoms that past health care professionals have dismissed or that they believe might be part of normal aging. For example, an older adult may avoid reporting knee pain because she has had the same pain for several years or believes that arthritis pain is normal for older people. It is best to use specific health screening questions to detect common complaints. Cues during the physical examination can help the nurse complete some of the health history. For example, when the nurse identifies three scars during examination of the abdomen, he or she might say "During our interview you told me that you had your appendix removed when you were 7, but could you tell me about these other two scars?"

When interviewing older adults with limited physical or mental abilities, the interview may need to be conducted somewhat differently to gain desired information. Box 30-1 presents suggestions for conducting interviews with hearing impaired or deaf older adults, visually impaired older adults, patients with aphasia, and patients with cognitive impairments (eg, Alzheimer's disease and other dementias).

🌐 Cultural Considerations

In many cultures, an older person would never be called by his or her first name at a first meeting and especially would not be addressed as "Sam" or "Nancy" by a young stranger. The nurse should set a tone of respect for the older person at the beginning of the interview by introducing himself or herself and then calling the patient by his or her formal name (Fig. 30-4). The nurse can then clarify how the patient would like to be addressed in the interview.

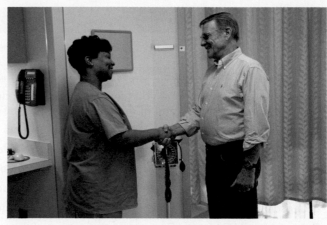

Figure 30.4 A respectful and pleasant introduction with an older patient can set the tone not just for the immediate health visit, but also for the overall nurse—patient relationship.

Assessment of Risk Factors

Nurses working with older adults should be familiar with instruments that have been developed to detect older adults' risk for the most common conditions or problems that accompany aging. These conditions or problems are often referred to as *geriatric syndromes* because of the interaction of multiple chronic diseases that contribute (Linton & Lach, 2007). Because these syndromes are common, nurses can provide a key role in early detection or an assessment of the problem so that interventions can be implemented (Linton & Lach, 2007). It is important to ask questions regarding family history, personal history, medications, and risk factors to detect the possibility of one or more of the following common syndromes seen in older adults:

• Nutritional changes
• Mobility impairments (activities of daily living [ADL] and instrumental activities of daily living [IADL] changes)
• Fall risk
• Polypharmacy
• Skin breakdown

Questions on History and Risk	Rationales
Current Problem The reason for seeking care is a brief statement, usually in the patient's own words, about why he or she is making the visit. Ask, "Tell me why you came to the clinic today" or "What happened that brought you to the hospital?" Records this information in the subjective part of documentation or put the statement in quotes.	If a patient replies by giving a medical diagnosis such as "heart attack," encourage the patient to describe symptoms such as "shortness of breath and chest pain."
Family History Ask the patient about the health of close family members (ie, parents, grandparents, siblings) to help identify those diseases for which patients may be at risk and to provide counseling and health teaching.	The following familial conditions are important to note: *high blood pressure, coronary artery disease, high cholesterol, stroke, cancer, diabetes mellitus, obesity, alcohol or drug addiction,* and *mental illness.*

(text continues on page 900)

Table 30.2   DETERMINE Nutrition Checklist

Possible Problem	Question to Answer	Score for "Yes" Answer (Circle if "yes")
Disease	Do you have an illness or condition that makes you change the kind and/or amount of food you eat?	2
Eating Poorly	Do you eat fewer than 2 meals per day?	3
	Do you eat few fruits, vegetables or milk products?	2
	Do you have 3 or more drinks of beer, liquor or wine almost every day?	2
Tooth Loss/Mouth Pain	Do you have tooth or mouth problems that make it hard for you to eat?	2
Economic Hardship	Do you sometimes have trouble affording the food you need?	4
Reduced Social Contact	Do you eat alone most of the time?	1
Multiple Medications	Do you take 3 or more prescribed or over-the-counter drugs a day?	1
Involuntary Weight Loss/Gain	Have you lost or gained 10 lb in the last 6 months without trying?	2
Needs Assistance In Self Care	Are you sometimes physically not able to shop, cook or feed yourself?	1
Elder Years > Age 80	Are you over 80 years old?	1
	TOTAL	_____

0 to 2—Good! Recheck your nutritional score in 6 months.
3 to 5—You are at moderate nutritional risk. See what can be done to improve your eating habits and lifestyle. Your office on aging, senior nutrition program (eg, Meals On Wheels), senior center or health department can help. Recheck your nutritional score in 3 months.
6 or more—You are at high nutritional risk. Bring this checklist the next time you see your doctor, dietitian or other qualified health or social service professional. Talk with them about any problems you may have. Ask for help to improve your nutritional health.
Source: From The Nutrition Screening Initiative, a project of the AAFP, ADA & NCOA, Washington, DC, 1992.

Questions on History and Risk	Rationales

Personal History

Nutritional Changes. The most commonly used instrument to identify elders at nutritional risk is the DETER-MINE instrument (Table 30-2; Posner, et. al., 1993). This simple 10-item checklist can be used to identify older adults who would benefit from health education about nutrition, or who have other issues that may affect their nutritional health. The screening tool also identifies older adults at high nutritional risk who may require interventions to improve nutritional status. If the DETERMINE shows risk, other tools may be used to follow up (See Chapter 8).

Nutritional screening is an abbreviated assessment of risk factors that identify older adults who may require a more comprehensive nutritional assessment. The combination of physiological changes with aging, physical or mental health issues, medications, or functional losses can significantly increase risk for weight loss in older adults. Almost one third of older adults suffer from nutritional deficiencies (Huffman, 2002). Chapter 8 reviews components included in a comprehensive dietary and nutritional history. Poor nutritional status indicators are linked to longer hospital stays, poor wound healing, and poor health outcomes (Stratton, et al., 2006; Thomas, et al., 2007).

Items in DETERMINE include such issues as "I eat fewer than 2 meals per day," "I eat alone most of the time," "I don't always have enough money to buy the food that I need." Higher scores correlate with increased risk.

Financial and transportation issues can limit an older adult's access to nutritional foods. Functional abilities or sensory losses can affect ability to physically prepare nutritious foods. Early cognitive losses that impair judgment, planning, foresight, or sequencing of complex tasks may reduce an older adult's ability to follow recipes or prepare complete meals. Recent weight loss can cause dentures to fit poorly and interfere with chewing. Medications can change tastes and interfere with appetite.

Mobility Level and Functional Abilities. The Katz Index of ADL (Katz, et al., 1963) was developed to quantify the degree of disability in a chronically ill population. Other measures of functional status include the Functional Independence Measure (FIM; Wright, 2000), the Jette

Nursing assessment of functional abilities is an essential component of a comprehensive assessment of an older adult and is included universally in every hospital, nursing home, or community-based comprehensive assessment form. Researchers who examine interventions for chronic

BOX 30.2 LAWTON INSTRUMENTAL ACTIVITIES OF DAILY LIVING

INSTRUCTIONS: Ask the patient to describe her/his functioning in each category; then complement the description with specific questions as needed.

Ability to Telephone

1. Operates telephone on own initiative: looks up and dials number, etc.
2. Answers telephone and dials a few well-known numbers.
3. Answers telephone but does not dial.
4. Does not use telephone at all.

Shopping

1. Takes care of all shopping needs independently.
2. Shops independently for small purchases.
3. Needs to be accompanied on any shopping trip.
4. Completely unable to shop.

Food Preparation

1. Plans, prepares, and serves adequate meals independently.
2. Prepares adequate meals if supplied with ingredients.
3. Heats and serves prepared meals, or prepares meals but does not maintain adequate diet.
4. Needs to have meals prepared and served.

Housekeeping

1. Maintains house alone or with occasional assistance (eg, heavy work done by domestic help).
2. Performs light daily tasks such as dishwashing and bed making.

3. Performs light daily tasks but cannot maintain acceptable level of cleanliness.
4. Needs help with all home maintenance tasks.
5. Does not participate in any housekeeping tasks.

Laundry

1. Does personal laundry completely
2. Launders small items; rinses socks, stockings, and so on.
3. All laundry must be done by others.

Mode of Transportation

1. Travels independently on public transportation, or drives own car.
2. Arranges own travel via taxi, but does not otherwise use public transportation.
3. Travels on public transportation when assisted or accompanied by another
4. Travel limited to taxi, automobile, or ambulette, with assistance.
5. Does not travel at all.

Ability to Handle Finances

1. Manages financial matters independently (budgets, writes checks, pays rent and bills, goes to bank); collects and keeps track of income.
2. Manages day-to-day purchases but need help with banking, major purchases, controlled spending, and so on.
3. Incapable of handling money.

Scoring: Circle one number for each domain. Total the numbers circled. The lower the score, the more independent the older adult is. Scores are only good for individual patients. It is useful to see the score comparison over time.

Questions on History and Risk

Functional Status Index (Jette, 1987), and the Barthel Index (Mahoney & Barthel, 1965). The FIM is a more sensitive measure and has been most frequently used in research settings. It has several well-tested and validated versions for use, including the original in-person version, short-form version, telephone version, and proxy report version (Wright, 2000).

When assessing an older adult returning to or living in the community, it is essential to identify his or her ability to manage IADL (Lawton & Brody, 1969; Box 30.2). Abilities measured by the Lawton IADL scale include use of the telephone, finance management, shopping, laundry, housekeeping and food preparation, and use of transportation. Older adults who can manage these tasks are more likely to be able to live independently in the community. The Lawton IADL instrument has been designed for older adults to self-report their abilities in these important tasks.

Rationales

diseases in older adults often use a measure of functional ability to measure efficacy of intervention outcomes (Kane, et al., 2004).

Many older adults define their health by their ability to perform self care, which health care providers identify as functional abilities. Functional ability in an older adult can vary widely during his or her later years. Some older adults require complete assistance with care, while others are completely functionally independent. Ability to carry out daily activities can be affected by depression, motivation, cognitive status, medical conditions, or sensory losses (Kresevic & Mezey, 2003).

Hospital discharge planners or community health nurses use the Lawton IADL instrument to identify appropriate matches of supportive services and family assistance that might allow an older adult to maintain independence in the community. Because the tool relies on accurate self-report by the elder, information can be misleading with cognitively impaired elders who lack insight into their functional losses. For example, an older woman with Alzheimer's disease may believe she can manage the telephone but in fact cannot demonstrate how she would call for help or assistance if needed.

(text continues on page 902)

CHAPTER **30** Older Adults **901**

Another option is to use the Direct Assessment of Functional Abilities (DAFA), a 10-item observational instrument designed for use with people with dementia (Karagiozis, et al., 1998). Occupational therapists sometimes use this performance-based instrument to measure IADL abilities. The DAFA requires the older patient to physically demonstrate tasks of meal preparation, money management, shopping, transportation use, reading, hobbies, and safety awareness.

For the patient with *dementia*, compare his or her perceived abilities with the report of a close family member when assessing IADLs.

Risk for Falls. Ask the patient, "Have you ever fallen before? Do you have any dizziness?" Several fall risk assessment instruments assist health care providers in identifying those older adults most at risk. The Morse Fall Scale developed for hospitalized elders (Morse, et al., 1987) is widely used in hospital settings and does not require major training of staff. Even modified, however, it does not include the risks posed by medications the elder is taking or potential environmental contributors (Morse, 2006). Another assessment instrument designed for hospitals is the Hendrich II Fall Risk Model (Hendrich, et al., 2003). This assessment tool measures intrinsic risk factors and does not include environmental factors. It does include higher risks for patients taking medications that might contribute to falling, although it limits this to two drug classes: seizure medications and benzodiazepines. The scale includes points for confusion or disorientation, depression, altered elimination, dizziness or vertigo, male sex, medications, and a partial use of the Get up and Go test.

More than one third of U.S. adults older than 65 years sustain a fall each year; of these, 20% have moderate to severe injuries, indicating that about 6% of all people who fall have moderate to severe injuries (Soriano, et al., 2007). Serious injuries related to falls increase with age and are four to five times greater in people 85 years or older compared to those 65–74 years (Stevens, 2006).

The Get Up and Go section of the Hendrich II is a portion of the Timed Get Up and Go test (Mathias, et al., 1986). However, the Hendrich II version does not time the subject in this section. The patient is simply asked to rise from sitting in a chair. If the patient can stand in a single movement without using her or his hands, the test score is 0. If the patient uses the hands to push up from the chair in one attempt, the score is 1. If the patient must make several attempts to push up but succeeds in standing, he or she receives three points. If the patient requires assistance to stand up, he or she receives a score of four points. See www.nursingcenter.com/AJNolderadults for a demonstration of how to use this instrument.

A patient receives four points under the "confusion, disorientation, impulsivity" section if he or she demonstrates any of the following: impulsive or unpredictable behavior; hallucinations; agitation; fluctuations in attention, cognition, psychomotor activity, or level of consciousness (delirium symptoms); unrealistic, inappropriate, or unusual behavior; disorientation to time person or place; inability to follow directions or retain instructions about self care or ADL care. Patients receive two points under "depression" if they demonstrate any of the following: prolonged feelings of helplessness, hopelessness, or being overwhelmed; tearfulness; flat affect or lack of interest; loss of interest in life events; melancholic mood; withdrawal; or statements about being depressed. The patient receives a point for altered elimination if he or she has any of the following: urgency or fecal incontinence, urgency or stress incontinence, diarrhea, frequent urination, or nocturia. Having an indwelling Foley catheter is not considered a risk unless the patient also has one of the symptoms listed above. When the patient receives a score of 5 or more, he or she is considered at risk for falling.

Medications/Polypharmacy. Ask the patient:

• "What medications are you taking?
• What is the dose of medication that you take?
• What is your schedule for taking your medications?
• Do you understand why you are taking each of your medications?"

Although older adults comprise only 13% of the population, they take more than 30% of prescription medications in the United States. For people older than 60 years, 28% of hospital admissions are linked to adverse drug events (Guay, et al., 2003).

Questions on History and Risk	Rationales
Ask the patient to bring in a bag of all medications that he or she has at home and to identify those currently being taken (Ham, et al., 2007). If this is not possible, phrase questions about medications based on body system. For example, "Do you take any medications for your heart or blood pressure? Do you take any medications for pain?" This approach is also useful when asking about over-the-counter (OTC) medications. "Do you take any medicine from the drugstore to help you sleep? Do you take anything from the drugstore to help your stomach or bowels? Are you taking any vitamins or minerals?" Be sure to specifically ask how frequently the patient takes each OTC medication or supplement.	While examining the label of each medication, determine whether the patient is taking the drug as prescribed and if he or she has medications that should not be used together because of interactions. Older adults with cognitive impairment may not take medications as scheduled, even though they report that they do. Nurses can identify accuracy by calculating how many days are between today's date and the refill date, noting how many pills the pharmacist included and counting out the number of tablets left in the container to obtain an estimate of pills taken.
In addition to asking about herbal or nutritional supplements, ask if any alternative health care providers have recommended other kinds of treatments.	Older patients may believe that drinking Chinese herbs boiled into tea is not considered a medication or supplement.
Finally, it is wise to ask, "Do you take any medications belonging to other people, including medications prescribed to a spouse, caregiver, friend, or neighbor?"	It is not unusual for elders living in retirement communities to share medications.
In addition to finding out what particular medications the patient takes, identify how often and when he or she takes each drug: • "Does your pattern of taking the medication follow the prescription on the bottle? If not, why not?" • "Are you experiencing side effects of the medication? If so, what kinds?" • "Do you take medications with food, water, or alcohol?" • Older adults with limited education may not understand a question about a "history of substance abuse" but would understand direct questions such as • "Do you take street drugs or drink alcohol?" • "Have you been treated in rehabilitation facility?" • "Do you need refills of prescription drugs because of withdrawal symptoms?"	This important information allows the nurse to identify how frequently the patient is missing doses or overdosing.
Skin Breakdown. Identify risk for skin breakdown, which is especially important in hospitalized and inactive patients. Many health care facilities use the Braden scale, with interventions based on the total score (Bergstrom, et al., 1987). See Table 13-16. Alternatively, the Norton scale includes incontinence and other variables (Defloor & Grypdonck, 2005).	The Braden scale scores patients from 1 to 4 in six subscales: sensory perception, moisture, activity, mobility, nutrition, and friction (Braden & Bergstrom, 1989). The Norton scale uses a 1–4 scoring system in each of five subscales: physical condition, mental condition, activity, mobility, and incontinence. A score <14 on Norton and 14–18 on Braden indicates a high risk for pressure ulcers.

Risk Assessment and Health-Related Patient Teaching

Teaching for older adults includes the use of sunscreen, adequate nutrition, management of polypharmacy, prevention of elder abuse, and falling prevention.

Skin cancers increase with age and lifelong exposure to the sun, with estimates that approximately 90% of cases result from ultraviolet light exposure (Schober-Flores, 2001). Nurses should especially observe for skin cancer changes in older adults with the following risk factors: fair, freckling skin;

light-colored eyes, red or blond hair, tendency to burn easily with sun exposure, male gender, and history of cigarette smoking. Patients should be taught to wear sunscreen at all times. Hats and clothing that covers the skin is also recommended. Teach patients to do a skin assessment and observe for cancers. Basal cell carcinoma is a common form of skin cancer in older Caucasians. Basal cell lesions in their early stage form a small smooth, hemispherical translucent papule covered by a thinned epidermis most often located on the face, the bridge of the check or below the eye. The papule gradually enlarges into a pearly nodule and has a central ulcerated lesion. Basal cells can be locally invasive if not treated (Stitt & Gilchrest, 2003). Squamous cell carcinoma usually starts as a hard red wart-like lesion with a raised or rolled gray yellow edge located on a highly sun exposed area. Look for these types of lesions on the auricle of the ear or face and neck areas with the most sun exposure. Malignant melanoma is a pigmented macule, papule, nodule, patches or tumor with the ABCD warning signs: Assymetry, Border irregularity, Color variegation, Diameter greater than 6 mm. This is a highly malignant form of cancer. Any suspicious lesions should be documented and the patient referred for follow-up (Byrd, 2008). Refer to Chapter 13 for more information.

Older adults need added vitamin D, because aging and smoking tend to impair vitamin D synthesis. Groups at risk for folate deficiency include patients with alcoholism, older adults, those who follow "fad" diets, and people of low socioeconomic status. Older adults also require special consideration during assessments of dietary requirements. They may compensate for diminished taste of sweet and salty foods by adding sugar and salt to their diet at a time when they are at increased risk for diabetes, hypertension, and heart disease. Their basal metabolic rate is declining concurrently with reductions in physical activity. When this occurs, caloric needs are significantly reduced. Older adults are also at increased risk for malnutrition as a result of social isolation. Eating alone is particularly problematic for people with reduced mobility, receiving social assistance, or both. They

may lack the resources required to maintain a nutritious and appealing diet. Poor dentition may also be an issue. Missing teeth, gum disease, or poor-fitting dentures can all detract from enjoying meals. Community programs such as Meals on Wheels offer food services to people with disabilities or chronic illnesses who live in social isolation.

Older adults often have multiple chronic conditions and are prescribed multiple medications, which makes medication management and assessment of patient knowledge and adherence to medication schedules especially complex. Safety also becomes important, ranging from assessment for elder abuse to assessment of safety in the home. The older adult may have stairs that are a risk for falling, cooking surfaces that can be a fire hazard, or cords that can easily be tripped over. Teaching should focus on keeping cooking surfaces clean and having cords out of the normal path of walking. Rooms should also be well lit. For hospitalized patients, a bed alarm may be a good reminder to call for help.

Focused Health History Related to Common Symptoms

- Incontinence
- Sleep deprivation
- Pain
- Cognitive changes
- Depression
- Elder abuse

Questions to Assess Symptoms	Rationales/Abnormal Findings
Incontinence • Have you ever leaked urine? • Have you ever lost control of your bladder?	There are three basic types of incontinence to assess: stress, urge, and functional. Incontinence is very common among hospitalized patients and those in long term care. Risks include increasing age, caffeine intake, limited mobility, impaired cognition, diabetes, and use of medications such as diuretics, obesity, Parkinson's disease, stroke, and prostate problems.
Sleep Deprivation • What time do you turn off the lights? • How many awakenings do you have in a night? • Do you feel rested upon arising?	Insomnia may be either acute or chronic. It may affect falling asleep, staying asleep, or early morning wakening. Risk factors include female gender, increased age, medical or psychiatric illness, and shift work.
Pain • Do you have pain or discomfort? If so, describe its location, duration, intensity, quality, and alleviating or aggravating factors. Also, describe your pain goal. • Has pain affected your ability to function normally? For example, has it affected diet, sleep, or mood?	Chronic illness such as osteoarthritis or diabetic neuropathy may increase pain in the older adult. The patient may be hesitant to report pain because of fear of dependence or wanting to be a "good patient." Pain may affect normal functions.
Cognitive Status Assessment of cognitive status helps guide nursing care in various settings and can give important information for discharge planning, patient and family education, interventions needed for safety, and general support. Some specific tips for using this examination in older adults are found in Box 30-3.	The Mini-Cog is a shorter and less stressful version while the Mini Mental Status Examination (MMSE) takes 10-15 minutes and is more thorough.

BOX 30.3 ASSESSMENT OF COGNITIVE STATUS

- Introduce the test. State "I am going to conduct a test of your thinking skills. This is a screening test and I want you to do your best."
- If a family member is present, it is wise to let him or her know that he or she is not allowed to answer for the older adult. Patients with mild dementia may look to a spouse or child to assist them with questions.
- If you detect that the patient is somewhat suspicious of your questions based on previous interactions, start with questions under the language section of the examination (ie, "What is this?" point to your watch, and have him or her identify watch). Usually these questions offer the patient some success in responses and allow you to complete more of the screening.

- Do not provide clues to answers. For example, when asking the orientation questions, simply say, "Can you tell me what month this is?" Do not say, "Well, we recently had our Thanksgiving break." If the patient is uncertain, simply restate the question. "Can you tell me the month?"
- Allow enough time for the patient to respond to the question that you have asked.
- Reassure the patient if he or she worries that the response might be incorrect. "It's OK if some of these are difficult for you." However, don't falsely tell patients that they are doing fine. Identify that this is simply a screening test and will help you better understand how to provide care for this patient.

Questions to Assess Symptoms	Rationales/Abnormal Findings

The Mini-Mental State Examination (MMSE) is the most widely used screening tool to detect cognitive impairment in older adults. It measures several areas of cognition: orientation (time and place), registration (ability to immediately register information), attention and calculation (ability to subtract sequential sevens), recall (short-term memory of three objects), language, ability to follow a three-step command, and visual-perceptual abilities (Folstein, et al., 1975). See Chapter 10.

Normal findings are a score of 24–30.

Depression

Although older adults are at risk for depression, the illness is not a normal or inevitable part of aging. To assess for depression, ask:
- "Do you struggle with depression?
- Have you ever suffered from depression?"

The Geriatric Depression Scale (GDS) provides a brief screening for depressive symptoms. The longer 30-item version of the GDS asks about symptoms, self-image issues, and losses in a yes/no format. The short-form 15-item GDS, also in a yes/no format, is used for patients with mild to moderate dementia (Yesavage, et al., 1982; Sheikh & Yesavage, 1986). Either version can be asked aloud (for visually impaired patients) or offered to the patient to read and complete privately. See Chapter 10.

If the screening examination reveals risk for or actual depression, assess for potential suicide risk. Mentally healthy older adults report that thoughts about death and suicide ideation are relatively rare. Chapter 10 discusses depression and suicide screening in more depth.

Elder Abuse

Many older adults are vulnerable to abuse by family members. Continued abuse may be compounded because of nondetection by professionals, in part because elderly patients often do not report violence. If indicated, ask "Injuries like yours could have been caused by someone hurting you. Did someone hurt you?"

Clinical Significance 30-1

Suspicious patients with mild to moderate dementia have difficulty with time orientation questions, so asking these questions first will highlight their deficits and may make them more likely to refuse to answer the rest of the examination.

Patients with *Parkinson's disease* may have a slow retrieval time and very delayed responses (Miller, 2007).

Depression may occur in older adults for various reasons. It is more common in people with multiple chronic health problems (Hybels & Blazer, 2003) or who have recently suffered the loss of a spouse, friend, family member, or pet. Decisions about moving out of a family home because of increasing care needs may also lead to depressive symptoms.

On the short-form GDS, a score above 6 suggests depression and a score above 9 indicates depression.

Factors that contribute to suicide in older adults include mental disorders (especially depression), physical illness, personality traits such as hostility, hopelessness, inability to verbally express psychological pain and dependency on others, and recent life events and losses (DeoLeo & Spathonis, 2003).

Many victims are isolated; some are ashamed and embarrassed or feel guilt and self-blame. In addition, some elders experience fear of reprisal, retribution from caregivers, or losing their home or independence. Others are pressured by relatives not to report.

Additional Questions	Rationales/Abnormal Findings
• Do you have any food preferences? • What is your primary language? • Do you have any favorite activities? • Do you feel part of your community?	Many older adults prefer to experience environments similar to those they had in younger years. Based on assessment findings, the nurse may provide interventions such as facilitating a Korean diet for a patient who prefers Korean food.

Therapeutic Dialogue: Collecting Subjective Data

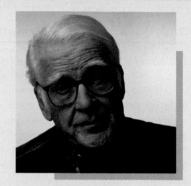

Remember Mr. Monroe, introduced at the beginning of this chapter. This 76-year-old man with a history of Parkinson's disease is complaining of constipation. The nurse uses professional communication techniques to gather subjective data from Mr. Monroe. The following conversations give two examples of interview styles used by the nurse during the visit. One style is more effective than the other.

Less Effective

Nurse: Hi, Ralph. How are you doing?

Mr. Monroe: Fine, I guess.

Nurse: What do you mean by I guess?

Mr. Monroe: I guess I'm fine.

Nurse: Good, well do you like living here? It's a great place.

Mr. Monroe: Who says it's a great place?

Nurse: What do you mean by that?

Mr. Monroe: Hmm … I don't like the people around here. I would rather just go home.

Nurse: Well, you can't go home because you can't take care of yourself there.

Mr. Monroe: Who said that? I can take care of myself just fine.

Nurse: That's not what your daughter said. She said that you were having trouble with cooking and cleaning.

Mr. Monroe: I just want to be able to do things my own way. People around here are too bossy.

More Effective

Nurse: Hello, Mr. Monroe. How are you?

Mr. Monroe: Not so well. How about you?

Nurse: I'm OK. How do you feel about your new living situation?

Mr. Monroe: I don't like my roommate. He snores all night. I don't like the people here.

Nurse: I noticed that you have been taking the wheelchair to your meals. Why is that?

Mr. Monroe: The aides say that it's faster. I would rather take my walker on my own.

Nurse: We can talk with them. How about your eating?

Mr. Monroe: I drink 1–2 glasses of milk or juice at each meal. But I have trouble eating their food because my dentures don't fit (pause).

Nurse: (nods head, waits)

Mr. Monroe: I also would like to move my bowels before breakfast but I can't because I need help with zipping and buttoning my pants and the aides don't have time.

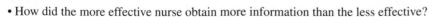

Critical Thinking Challenge

• How did the more effective nurse obtain more information than the less effective?
• What follow-up questions would you recommend for the less effective nurse?
• What additional assessments might the more effective nurse make?

Objective Data Collection

After completing subjective data collection, the nurse will collect equipment and prepare for the objective assessment. For a well assessment, a head-to-toe examination will be done. If the patient is being seen because of a problem, the highest priority assessment related to the patient's problem is performed first. The assessment may need to be broken into several sessions, because older adults tend to fatigue easily.

Equipment Needed

- Stethoscope
- Thermometer and BP cuff or electronic vital signs monitor
- Watch or clock with a second hand
- Otoscope
- Ophthalmoscope

Preparation

When assessing an older adult, nurses need to allow extra time. It is important to rely on general observations and focus on the patient's functional abilities. Some older adults with major health conditions and numerous abnormal physical findings describe their health as "very good" because they can still carry out daily activities.

Documentation of abnormal findings is very important for this population because of their frequent transitions across health care settings. Excellent documentation can assist health care providers in a new setting to evaluate and compare the patient's current examination findings.

Comprehensive Physical Examination

Technique and Normal Findings	Abnormal Findings
General Survey Observe normal changes that occur with aging. Assess for any decreasing abilities to function and care for self. Note any changes in mental status. *By the eighth or ninth decade, physical appearance changes, with sharper body contours and more angular facial features. Posture tends to have a general flexion, and the patient's gait tends to have a wider base of support to compensate for diminished balance. Steps tend to be shorter and uneven. The patient may need to use the arms to help aid in balance.*	Poor hygiene and inappropriate dress may indicate decreased functional ability or may result from medications, infection, dehydration, or nutritional status. Inappropriate affect, inattentiveness, impaired memory, and inability to perform ADLs may indicate *dementia* from Alzheimer's disease or another cause. Changes in mental status may be from medications, dehydration, poor nutrition, underlying infection, or hypoxia.
Height and Weight An essential component of assessing nutritional status is an accurate measure of height and weight. If possible, measure height with the person standing erect against a wall without shoes.	⚠ SAFETY ALERT 30.1 *Avoid having an older adult stand and balance on a weight scale when measuring height. Do not attempt to determine height when a frail older adult is standing on the weight scale. This creates a risk of falling because of the unsteadiness of the weight scale base.*
Height and weight are important components of the calculation for Body Mass Index. *BMI for older adults of 25 to 29 is linked to better health status and lower risks. This BMI is slightly higher than the recommended BMI for younger adults (Arterburn, et al., 2004).*	BMI above 29 increases health risks for older adults. BMI of 24 or less also is associated with increased mortality.
Vital Signs *Temperature.* Assess temperature. The *temperature of older adults is at the lower end of the normal range. Mean body temperature for older adults is 36°C–36.8°C (96.9°C–98.3°C).*	Because of changes in the body's temperature regulatory mechanism and decreased subcutaneous fat, the aging adult is less likely to develop a fever, but more likely to succumb to hypothermia. Temperatures within normal range for a younger adult may constitute fever in an older adult.

(text continues on page 908)

Pulse. Assess apical pulse for 1 minute. *The aging adult continues to have a normal range of 60 to 100 bpm.*

The pulse rate of older adults takes longer to rise to meet sudden increases in demand and longer to return to its resting state. Resting heart rate of older adults tends to be lower than for younger adults.

Respirations. Assess respirations. *Decreased vital capacity and inspiratory volume can cause respirations to be shallower and more rapid than in younger adults, with a normal respiratory rate of 16 to 24 breaths/min.*

Variation in rhythm may develop in some older adults. The radial artery may stiffen from peripheral vascular disease. A rigid artery does not indicate vascular disease elsewhere.

Heart sounds may be more difficult to assess and PMI more difficult to palpate because of increased air space in the lungs, which increases the anterior-posterior diameter of the chest.

Aging causes the costal cartilage to become more rigid, decreasing chest expansion and vital capacity. Decreased efficiency of respiratory muscles results in breathlessness at lower activity levels. Respiratory rates >24 are not normal and should be followed with further examination for cyanosis of the nail beds or the perioral area.

⚠ *SAFETY ALERT 30.2*

In older adults with chronic lung disease or congestive heart failure, observe for generalized distress, confusion, or an impression that the patient is working hard to breath. These symptoms may indicate decompensation.

Pulse Oximetry. Assess pulse oximetry. Placement of the pulse-oximetry probe can present a challenge in older adults. Sensors designed for the forehead or bridge of nose may be indicated. *Oxygen saturation is >92%.*

Peripheral vascular disease, decreased carbon dioxide levels, cold-induced vasoconstriction, and anemia may complicate assessment of oxygen saturation on the fingers.

Skin, Hair, and Nails

Inspect the skin, hair, and nails. The older adult's skin bruises and tears easily, exposing the patient to increased risk of infections of wounds. Nurses need to examine skin carefully for breakdown, especially in the perineal area of older adults who are incontinent, and in any area that is at risk for pressure ulcers (see Chapter 13).

Seborrheic keratoses are extremely common in older individuals. These dark brown, pigmented lesions are waxy appearing areas seen on the trunk of the body. They may appear on sun-exposed areas of the body.

Photoaging findings of the skin include coarse wrinkles over sun-exposed areas, solar lentigines (age or liver spots) on the face, hands, forearms, upper chest, or back and actinic keratosis (Fisher, et al., 2002). *There is increased wrinkling and skin is coarse in sun exposed areas. Scalp hair is thinned. The skin will be less elastic and may be dry (although dryness of skin is more often linked to poor hydration status). It is common to note thinning of the epidermal layer, more pronounced in the 8th and 9th decades. Nail beds may have ridges. Toenails may become thickened.*

Nurses should be alert for **bruising** in various stages of healing that might indicate abuse.

Pressure ulcers in any of the following areas should be staged and interventions begun immediately: sacral and ischial areas, greater trochanteric area, heels.

Patchy white scaly areas on the scalp are indicative of seborhhea, common in persons with Parkinson's disease and usually treated with corticosteroids. Very thick yellow overgrown toenails are usually a sign of onychomycosis (tinea unguium), a **fungal infection** of the nail beds. These infected nails are difficult to treat and may eventually fall off leaving a dry nail bed base.

Stasis dermatitis is another common finding in older adults with a history of varicosities, phlebitis, and trauma. Lower extremities have a reddish-brown ruddy appearance and are usually edematous, but are not inflamed or infected. Nurses often mistake stasis dermatitis with **cellulitis**, but the stasis changes do not respond to antibiotics. Stasis dermatitis may lead to leg ulcers on the lower shin area. These ulcers can become infected. Good assessment of the area includes the location, color and size of the area, size and depth of the ulcer (if present), presence of inflammation or warmth and presence and severity of edema.

Herpes zoster (shingles) is a red painful vesicular or pustular rash that follows the distribution of a dermatome along the trunk or even into the legs. Older adults have a less vigorous immune response and are at risk for developing this rash especially during times of illness or hospitalization. Prompt treatment is important to reduce post–herpetic neuralgia pain.

Head and Neck

Inspect the head and neck. *The appearance is symmetrical. Facial expression is appropriate to the situation.* Palpate the skull and hair. *The skull is smooth and there is no pain or mass. The hair is normally thin and gray in an older adult.* Palpate the sternocleidomastoid and trapezius muscles. *There is no pain or masses.* Palpate the thyroid. *The thyroid is not enlarged.*

A downward gaze with little eye contact may be a sign of depression. Any swelling, masses, or tumors are abnormal. Flat affect or facial tension may signify depression or anxiety. A patient who is extremely thin may have sunken hollows in their face. A patient with extremely thick structures may have thyroid problems. A goiter in the thyroid gland is also abnormal. Clicking or crepitus in the temporal mandibular joint may be associated with jaw or neck pain. Note limitations in movement in the neck.

Eyes and Vision

Inspect the eyes. *Senile ptosis or a sagging of the upper lid down across the eye, dry eyes that appear irritated and red, and a decrease in the corneal reflex may be present.*

Test vision, pupillary reflex, and extraocular movements. *Older adults may have difficulty focusing properly or presbyopia, and may have difficulty with glare and accommodating to changes in light. A smaller pupil size and a slower or sluggish pupillary accommodation to light are normal. Upward gaze is reduced because of muscle changes and laxity. Also commonly seen is a grayish yellow ring surrounding the iris, called arcus senilus. This was thought to be a normal change of aging, but more recently has been linked to elevated lipid deposits. Visual fields may be slightly diminished with confrontation but should not show unilateral differences.* Perform the ophthalmoscopic examination. See Chapter 15. *Retinal margins may be less distinct; drusen, yellow spots, may be on the macula (Brodie, 2003).*

Ectropian, a turning of the lid outward, or entropian, a turning of the lid inward may also be observed. **Entropian** can cause the eyelashes on the lower lid to scratch the corneal surface (Brodie, 2003; Fig. 30-5). Reduced visual fields, especially unilaterally, can be a sign of a stroke or central neurological lesion. Refer to Chapter 15 for more information. Loss of vision can significantly affect daily functioning including dressing, grooming, and ambulating safely.

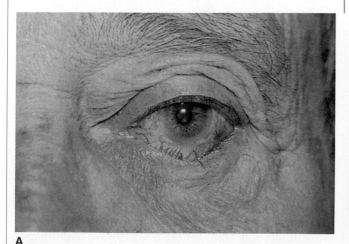
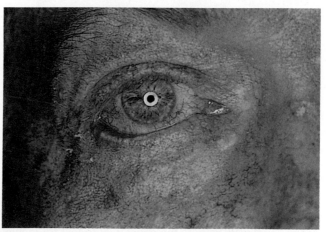

A   **B**

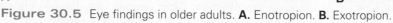

Figure 30.5 Eye findings in older adults. **A.** Enotropion. **B.** Exotropion.

Ears and Hearing

Inspect the ear for any lesions or changes to the auricle. *No pain, masses, or lesions are present.*

Ulcerated lesions on the auricle in older men with a history of sun exposure (eg, golfers, outdoor workers, farmers) may represent *squamous cell carcinoma* and should be evaluated. Refer to Chapter 16.

(text continues on page 910)

Perform the otoscopic examination (see Chapter 16). *There may be a gray tympanic membrane or an ear canal that is narrowed or occluded with wax. The patient may have conductive hearing loss and will lateralize hearing to the ear occluded with wax on the Weber test, or will hear bone conduction longer than air conduction in the ear occluded with wax on the Rinne' test.*

Loss of hearing is found in 30% of people older than 65 years, and in 47% of those older than 75 years (National Institute of Deafness and Communication Disorders, 2010). High-frequency sounds are lost most commonly for older adults, so they may have difficulty hearing a female examiner with a high-pitched voice. Hearing loss can affect emotional health and functional abilities. Early treatment of the causes of conductive hearing loss or information on assistive devices is important.

Nose, Mouth, and Throat

Inspect the nose, mouth, and throat. Test nasal patency (Fig. 30-6). *Deviation of the nasal septum is common in older adults.* Make note of the color and moisture of the mucosal membranes of the nose and oral cavity. *These are pink to pinkish red and moist. The tongue is pinkish red, moist, and has no fissures. A slightly dry oral mucosa is more common in older adults, but a fissured tongue is a sign of dehydration. Varicosities under the tongue are more common in older adults. The gag reflex is intact, although it may mildly diminish in frail older adults.*

Vasomotor rhinitis is common. Pale mucosal membranes can indicate *anemia* or *malnutrition*. Malodorous breath may indicate dental disease, poor dental hygiene, or underlying diseases. Poor dental condition, fractured teeth, or untreated dental caries should be referred to a dentist, because these can markedly influence nutritional intake. A bright red tongue can indicate *vitamin C or B1 deficiency*. An overgrowth of white patchy plaque on the tongue may be related to poor dental hygiene or may be a **fungal or yeast infection** (*oral candidiasis*). Any signs of poor oral care may be indicative of forgetting to manage ADLs, a symptom of cognitive impairment. An absent or markedly diminished gag reflex can be found in patients who have had a *stroke*, longstanding *alcoholism*, or *neurological disorders*. Patients with diminished or absent gag reflexes are at risk for aspiration pneumonia (see Chapter 17).

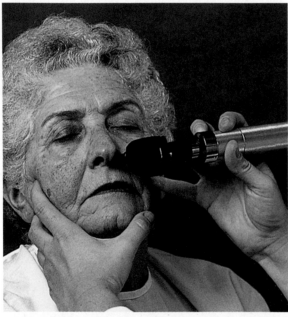

Figure 30.6 Assessing for nasal patency in the older adult.

Thorax and Lungs

Inspect the chest. *The older adult may have an increased anterior-posterior diameter related to rigidity of the chest wall.* Palpate the chest wall to test for tactile fremitus. Percuss the lungs. *Chest wall is free of pain, swelling, or masses. Tactile fremitus is not increased; percussion is resonant.* Auscultate breath sounds. *Older adults who can take good breaths should have normal breath sounds. Harsh rhonchi are sometimes found because of the difficulty of clearing materials from the lungs. Have the patient cough and then listen for breath sounds again. It is common for older adults to have some scattered fine crackles at the bases of their lungs.*

Increased fremitus or dullness with percussion, especially at the lung bases, can indicate fluid accumulation. Older adults with chronic lung disease have hyperresonance on examination. Older women may have kyphosis (curvature of the cervical or thoracic spine related to osteoporosis) that can affect the nurse's ability to hear lung sounds at the bases. The nurse may need to listen for breath sounds at the lateral sides of the posterior wall to hear the breath sounds. Lung sounds may be difficult to hear with advanced lung disease or may sound diminished and tight. Listening after a nebulizer treatment may give a clearer picture. See Chapter 18.

Technique and Normal Findings (continued)	Abnormal Findings (continued)

Heart and Neck Vessels

Auscultate heart sounds. *Pulse rates in the 50 to 60 range are common and often related to use of beta-blocker or other cardiac medications. Heart rate and rhythm are regular with no murmurs, rubs, or gallops. As older adults reach their 80s and 90s, murmurs are common, especially grade 2 systolic murmurs.* Observe neck vessels. *No jugular venous distention is present.*

⚠ SAFETY ALERT 30.3

Pulses >100 are abnormal and should be taken seriously. Because of their poor cardiac reserves, older adults do not tolerate these pulse rates well for long periods.

Loud (grade 3 or greater) or harsh holosystolic murmurs suggest valvular (usually aortic) stenosis and can sometimes be heard radiating up to the neck. Loud murmurs that can be heard radiating from the apex to around the side of the chest wall are usually mitral valve in origin. Findings from the whole examination should be considered when a patient has a loud murmur, specifically looking for lower extremity edema, abdominal distension, or other signs of fluid retention as well as a thorough respiratory examination to identify signs of *congestive heart failure.* Jugular venous distention is a sign of congestive heart failure. Arrythmias, especially **atrial fibrillation**, are common in older adults, but should be considered abnormal. Nurses need to note whether this is an irregularly irregular rhythm and specifically be concerned if the rate is >100. Abdominal aortic pulsations that extend over a wide area indicate an **aortic aneurysm.**

Peripheral Vascular

Palpate peripheral pulses. *Pulses are 2–3 on a 4-point scale and symmetrical.*

Absent peripheral pulses are of great concern and should be noted in the record. The primary provider should be contacted if this finding is new. It is more common in a person with a long history of smoking or who has diabetes; it can seriously interfere with wound healing. Vascular disease may be venous or arterial (see Chapter 20).

Breasts

Palpate breasts. Because breast tissue loses density with age, masses or nodules are easier to feel. *No masses or nodules are present.*

Mastectomy scars should be noted and palpated.

Abdomen and Elimination

Inspect, auscultate, palpate, and percuss the abdomen. Perform the rectal examination. *Take extra time to listen for bowel sounds in older adults with a history of constipation. Finding a mass of stool in the lower left quadrant is common. A flaccid or soft, distended abdomen is common, but can be related to deconditioning and loss of muscle control. Bowel sounds may be slow, but easy to hear. The rectal examination may show external hemorrhoids.*

A distended abdomen can signify excessive gas, stool, or fluid. Asymmetry or masses are important findings and may be signs of *severe constipation* or *cancer.* A rectal check should be performed for anyone with a lower abdominal mass. Patients with large amounts of abdominal ascites usually have *liver disease* or *cancerous involvement of the liver.* Hemorrhoids, internal or external are common, but should not be painful, fiery red, or inflamed. Fecal **incontinence** or involuntary passage of stool is abnormal in older adults. See Chapter 22.

Musculoskeletal System

Obtain height. *Loss of height of up to 6 inches can occur by 70–80 years of age.* Perform focused assessments of the bones, muscles, and joints as indicated. *Flexion and hyperextension of the neck are somewhat reduced. Likelihood of kyphosis of the spine is increased (more common in women than men). There may be a generalized decrease in strength and mildly decreased ROM. Older adults with arthritis may have enlarged*

Examination of range of motion of the upper extremities is important, especially for hospitalized older adults. Limited abduction of the shoulder can be addressed immediately to prevent "frozen shoulder," a condition that commonly occurs during or after a hospital stay. Pain on palpation of the spine after a fall should raise concerns about possible *compression fracture* of the spine. Large nodules in the distal interphalangeal joints are *Heberden nodes,*

(text continues on page 912)

joints, especially at the knees and in the hands. When possible, nurses should test the patient's ability to stand from a seated position, walk a short distance, and turn around. *Patients should be able to do this smoothly, without balance problems, stumbling, or assistance.*

Neurological

Cranial Nerves. Test cranial nerves. *Common normal findings in older adults include decreased upward gaze.*

Balance and Coordination. Test balance and coordination. *There may be slowing of psychomotor finger-nose testing, or finger-to-finger testing. Heal-to-toe walking may be impaired related to musculoskeletal conditions. Observation of gait with or without an assistive device shows smooth steps that may be wide based.*

> △ *SAFETY ALERT 30-4*
>
> *The Romberg test should only be done with an older adult when a chair is directly behind the patient and the examiner is at the patient's side to assist if the patient begins to fall.*

Test sensation. *Peripheral sensation and proprioceptive (position) sense may diminish slightly with aging.*

Reflexes and Muscle Strength. Test reflexes and muscle strength. *Reflexes normally diminish with aging, and muscle strength against resistance may be slightly diminished in those with musculoskeletal conditions.*

Male and Female Genitourinary

Inspect genitals. *Thinning of genital hair and testicular or penile atrophy is common. Skin in the vaginal area may be thinned.*

Endocrine, Immunologic, and Hematologic Systems

Evaluate laboratory data. *Older adults are likely to demonstrate decreased lean muscle and bone mass, increased fat mass and vasomotor symptoms, fatigue, depression, anemia, erectile dysfunction, decreased libido, and decline in immune function (Chahal & Drake, 2007).*

while enlargements of the proximal interphalangeal joints are *Bouchard nodes*, common with *arthritis* (Felson, 2004). Contractures of the hips and knees are abnormal but common in patients who spend much of their day in a wheelchair. These contractures change the structure of gait and balance and place the patient at risk for further immobility. See Chapter 23.

Older adults who appear to have a blank or blunted affect may have *depression, dementia,* or *Parkinson's disease.*

Abnormal gait changes include difficulty initiating gait; a small, short, stepped gait that gradually becomes normal is a sign of **Parkinson's disease**. A wide-based gait with a heel-to-toe foot slap to the floor is a sign of a cerebellar disorder; a gait in which the leg does not swing through smoothly, catches on the floor, drags, or stops next to the other foot is a sign of *cerebrovascular disease* (Miller, 2007). See Chapter 24.

> ### Clinical Significance 30-2
>
> Unilateral findings on neurological examination are always important and may be evidence of a previous cerebrovascular accident.

Tremors are abnormal. Determine if the tremor occurs only at rest and if it involves only one limb, one side, or all extremities. *Parkinson's disease* has a resting tremor that usually starts unilaterally and does not include the head and neck. Tremor of the hand or neck, that is heard in changes in the voice, or occurs in the hand only when the person is initiating an action is intentional or "essential" and has a very different treatment (Miller, 2007). Diminished grip strength or unilateral loss of strength against resistance is abnormal. Severely diminished or absent sensation or proprioception indicates *peripheral neuropathy.*

Observe for a distended lower abdomen with resonant-to-dull percussion of fluid. A full bladder after recently voiding is a sign of **urinary retention**. Underwear smelling of urine, staining of urine, or leaking urine indicates incontinence, which is common but not normal in older adults and should be treated. See Chapters 25 and 26.

Nurses may find that older adults do not mount a very high **febrile response** in the presence of *infection*. Total white lymphocyte count may remain low despite infection.

Cultural Considerations

Common integumentary findings in African Americans include curly hair that tends to be coarser than in Caucasians because of an impaired ability of secreted sebum to travel along the hair shaft to the skin. Skin is commonly excessively dry, resulting in ashy dermatitis. Pityriasis rosea, a macular hyperpigmented viral dermatitis in Caucasians, commonly presents as papular, maroon to purplish lesions in African Americans. Skin cancers are more common on the palms, soles, and nail beds in African Americans (Hemenway, 2006).

Southeast Asian men have less body and facial hair than patients of other genetic heritage. Tattoos, body piercings, and other skin adornments are common in various Asian cultures. Skin discolorations from cupping or coining are commonly found. Henna tattoos are common in Arabic and Indian females.

Evidence-Based Critical Thinking

Common Laboratory and Diagnostic Testing

The U.S. Preventative Services Task Force (2010) recommends the following screening as part of the well visit:

- Blood cholesterol
- Fecal occult blood test and/or sigmoidoscopy
- Mammogram for women 50 to 74 years every 2 years
- Papanicolaou (Pap) test (women) for those who have been sexually active and have a cervix

Routine testing of prostate-specific antigen (PSA) to screen for prostate cancer in men is debated, because false positives are common.

Diagnostic Reasoning

Nursing Diagnosis, Outcomes, and Interventions

When formulating a nursing diagnosis, it is important to use critical thinking to cluster data and identify patterns that fit together. The nurse compares these clusters with defining characteristics (abnormal findings) for the diagnosis to ensure the most accurate labeling and appropriate interventions. Table 30-3 provides a comparison of nursing diagnoses, abnormal findings, and interventions commonly related to the older adult assessment.

Nurses use assessment information to identify patient outcomes (Moorehead, et al., 2007). Some outcomes related to the older adult include the following:

- Patient maintains current weight.
- Patient has appropriate conversation that flows smoothly.
- Patient eats at least 75% of ordered meals.

Once outcomes are established, nursing care is implemented to improve the status of the older adult. The nurse uses critical thinking and evidence-based practice to develop interventions (Bulechek, et al., 2008). Some examples for older adult care are as follows:

- Provide between-meal snacks for smaller more frequent meals.
- Locate and clean eyeglasses.
- Place hearing aid in patient's ear.
- Assess food preferences and obtain favorite foods.

Common nursing diagnoses are in Table 30-3 (NANDA, 2009).

Table 30.3	Common Nursing Diagnoses Associated with the Older Adult		
Diagnosis and Related Factors	**Point of Differentiation**	**Assessment Characteristics**	**Nursing Interventions**
Adult failure to thrive related to depression	Progressive deterioration of functional abilities, physical skills, and cognition	Change in mood, decreased food intake at meals, neglect of home, finances, or other responsibilities	Assess for depression, complete minimental exam, Provide cues in the environment for food intake. Provide reality orientation. Encourage patients to reminisce and share life histories.
Disturbed sensory perception: visual or auditory, related to aging process	Change in stimuli	Reduced vision or hearing	Provide adequate lighting. Keep background noise now, such as turning off the TV when talking. Make sure that patient has devices such as glasses or hearing aid
Imbalanced nutrition, less than body requirements relating to isolation	Insufficient nutrient intake for metabolic needs	Nausea, vomiting, diarrhea. Anorexia. Lack of food. Eating alone. Shopping, cooking, and cleaning functional abilities are reduced	Note laboratory tests such as total protein, albumin and prealbumin. Weigh patient daily. Monitor food intake and record the percentage of meal eaten.

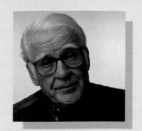

Mr. Monroe's problems have been outlined throughout this chapter. Initial subjective and objective data collection is complete, and the nurse has spent time reviewing the findings and other results. The following nursing note illustrates how the nurse collects and analyzes subjective and objective data and develops nursing interventions.

Subjective: A 76-year-old man, 10-yr history of Parkinson's disease, mild dementia, seen for new constipation. Has large, hard, dry, brown stool every fourth day. New admission to skilled care facility 3 months ago; "still adjusting"; does not like roommate. Can ambulate with walker. Takes wheelchair to meals "because it's faster." Ambulates in room. Fluids at meals 3 to 5 glasses milk or juice total, no additional water. Denies swallowing problems. Weight loss 16 lbs over past year, dentures uncomfortable, prefers soft foods, no fresh fruit. Previous BM after breakfast, states toilet not available before breakfast, needs help with pants zipping and buttoning. Medications: Sinemet 25/250 four times daily before meals, Vitamin E, 400 IU daily, Calcium 600 mg with Vitamin D 800 IU daily, Zestril 5mg daily.

Objective:

- Vitals: weight 156 lbs (decreased 4 lbs since admission), BP 104/60 mm Hg, P 76 beats/min, R 12 breaths/min, afebrile.
- General survey: Alert, conversant, thin man with resting tremor of hands bilaterally.
- Skin: dry, flaky, red raised areas on posterior scalp 3 × 5 cm.
- HEENT: dry oral mucosa, ill-fitting dentures, no oral sores or open areas, thyroid not enlarged, diminished gag reflex.
- Respiratory: no cough, clear to auscultation.
- Cardiac: S1, S2, RRR, no murmurs rubs or gallops.
- Abdomen: soft, nondistended, tender LLQ, with mass palpable. Approx 4 cm diameter, BS + all 4 quads.
- Rectal: 2 to 3 cm external hemorrhoid, no fissures, sphincter tone within normal limits, large amount hard stool high in rectal vault.
- Neurological: Decreased blink, blunted affect, increased tone, rigidity in all extremities, short stepped gait with walker, steady, slow, difficulty rising and sitting.

Analysis: Constipation related to immobility, medications, dehydration related to disease processes, and medications as evidenced by frequent use of wheelchair, limited walking, poor fiber intake, poor liquid intake, use of Sinemet, calcium, vitamin E, and Zestril (all potentially constipating medications).

Plan: *Goal*: Resident will have one bowel movement within 2 to 3 days without straining. *Interventions:* Ambulate to meals with walker three times daily. Increase fluids to more than 1.5 L every day. Offer 4 to 6 oz water at 10:00 AM, 2:00 PM, and 4:00 PM. Start fiber pudding 2 oz every day. Routinely schedule time for BM, find private bathroom near dining room.

Evaluate need for Zestril with primary provider. Evaluate need for multivitamin with iron and Vitamin E. Refer to dietician to increase dietary fiber. Refer to dentist for denture repair and refitting.

P. Jackson, APRN

Critical Thinking Challenge

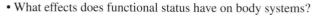

- What effects does functional status have on body systems?
- Provide rationales for the abnormal abdominal and rectal assessment findings.
- Interpret the neurological findings in the context of the patient's Parkinson's disease.

Collaboration with Other Health Care Providers

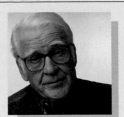

In many facilities, nurses initiate referrals based on assessment findings. Results that might trigger a dental consult include chipped or loose teeth, dental caries, tooth pain, denture care, bad breath, snoring or sleep apnea, and dry mouth.

Mr. Monroe has been experiencing loose dentures stemming from weight loss; therefore, a dental consult is indicated. The following conversation illustrates how the nurse might organize data and make recommendations about the patient's situation.

Situation: Hello, I am Pat Jackson, the nurse practitioner who is caring for Mr. Ralph Monroe, date of birth 2-10-1934.

Background: He was admitted 3 months ago with a loss of functional status related to Parkinson's. He has been complaining of difficulty in chewing, and he has lost 4 lb.

Assessment: I noticed that his oral mucosa is very dry. His dentures are loose and malfitting, although he has no oral sores or open areas.

Recommendations: Would you have an opening to see him for denture fitting in the next week?

Critical Thinking Challenge

- How did the nurse prioritize which information to include and delete in her report?
- What related assessments might be considered related to Mr. Monroe's nutrition?
- What nursing diagnoses are appropriate related to his mouth and dentures?

Pulling It All Together: Reflection and Critical Thinking

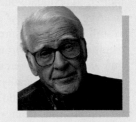

The nurse uses assessment data to formulate a nursing care plan with patient outcomes and interventions for Ralph Monroe. Outcomes are specific to the patient, realistic to achieve, measurable, and have a time frame for completion. Interventions are based on evidence and practice guidelines, and after their implementation, the nurse re-evaluates Mr. Monroe and documents findings in the chart to show progress. The nurse uses critical thinking and judgment to continue or revise the diagnosis, outcomes, or interventions. This is often in the form of a care plan or case note similar to the one below.

Nursing Diagnosis	Patient Outcomes	Nursing Interventions	Rationale	Evaluation
Constipation related to multiple medications, inactivity, and low fluid/bulk intake	Patient will have one BM in next 2–3 days without straining. Patient eliminates moderate amount of soft brown stool every 2 days.	Ambulate with walker tid, offer fluids every 2 hours, order fiber pudding with lunch, schedule time for BM, initiate diet consult.	Activity stimulated peristalsis, ensure that patient is well hydrated, increase bulk in the diet.	Patient had bowel movement of moderate hard brown stool. Will continue to monitor for improvement and re-establishment of regular patterns.

Applying Your Knowledge

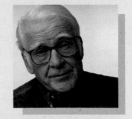

Using the previous steps of diagnostic reasoning, organizing, and prioritizing; consider all the case study findings about Mr. Monroe woven throughout this chapter. When answering the following questions, begin drawing conclusions and see how the pieces of assessment must work together to create an environment for personalized, appropriate, and accurate care.

- What are some causes of constipation that would immediately be apparent in this case?
- What health-promotion activities is Mr. Monroe already doing to stay healthy?
- What assessments might the nurse perform in addition to the screening examination?

Key Points

- Adults heal more slowly because of slower growth of new cells.
- Loss of vision can significantly affect daily activities including dressing, grooming, and ambulating safely.
- Allow older adults extra time to answer subjective data questions.
- Special challenges to interviewing older adults include hearing, visual, language, and cognitive impairments.
- Geriatric syndromes include nutritional changes, mobility impairment, falls, polypharmacy, and skin breakdown.
- Common symptoms of older adults include urinary incontinence, sleep problems, pain, cognitive changes, depression, and elder abuse.
- The skin of the older adult has increased wrinkling and is thinner, less elastic, and drier. Pressure ulcers in any of the following areas should be staged and interventions begun immediately: sacral and ischial areas, greater trochanteric area, heels.
- Senile ptosis, dry or red eyes, smaller and slower pupillary responses and difficulty with glare are common ocular findings.
- Loss of hearing is a common finding in the older adult.
- Abnormal findings in the mouth include pallor, malodorous breath, poor dentition, and candida.
- The older adult has a less elastic chest wall, decreased respiratory muscle strength, loss of alveolar recoil, and increased residual volume.
- Arterial walls are less elastic and stiffer, causing increased systolic blood pressure, increased ventricular wall hypertrophy, decreased coronary blood flow, reduced cardiac output, and increased circulating catecholamines.
- Arrythmias, especially atrial fibrillation, are common in older adults but should be considered abnormal.
- Gastrointestinal changes include slowed peristalsis, reduced hepatic flow, and decreased metabolism of drugs on the first pass.
- Common normal neurological findings include decreased upward gaze, slowed coordination, slowed gait, decreased reflexes, decreased strength and impaired sensation.
- The older adult should be assessed for depression, dementia, Parkinson's and signs of cerebrovascular accident.
- Older adults often lose height and lean body mass.
- Large nodules in the distal interphalangeal joints are Heberden nodes and enlargements of the proximal interphalangeal joints are Bouchard nodes, common with arthritis.
- Kidney function decreases with age, causing a decreased glomerular filtration rate, decreased creatinine clearance, and inability to conserve sodium.
- Endocrine changes include decreased growth hormone, decreased adrenal hormones, decreased response of the immune system, and increased glucose intolerance.
- Common nursing diagnoses for older adults include risk for falling, risk for skin breakdown, urinary incontinence, altered sleep pattern, confusion, adult failure to thrive, disturbed sensory perception, and imbalanced nutrition.

Review Questions

1. Which of the following findings are considered a normal change in the skin with aging?
   A. Solar lentigines (liver spots)
   B. Actinic keratoses
   C. Loss of subcutaneous fat
   D. Photoaging

2. Which of the following statements is true with aging?
   A. The lens becomes smaller and less dense.
   B. The tympanic membrane becomes more flexible and retracted.
   C. Changes in the inner ear can interfere with sound discrimination.
   D. Increased pupillary responses lead to difficulty in light accommodation.

3. When working with a frail older adult, the nurse knows that it is best to
   A. fill in silences to avoid discomfort
   B. address all questions to the patient's family
   C. try to gain all information directly from the patient's memory
   D. ask the question in lay terms rather than medical terms

4. The nurse assesses for geriatric syndromes, which are
   A. the interaction of multiple diagnoses that contribute to these problems
   B. the exacerbation of chronic conditions such as CHF or COPD
   C. conditions in which older adults may not mount an immune response
   D. decreases in growth hormones and steroids that reduce functional status

5. The DETERMINE nutritional screening is an abbreviated assessment of risk factors that
   A. indicate that the patient is at high nutritional risk
   B. identify older adults who may require a more comprehensive assessment
   C. calculate BMI and classify patients as obese versus malnourished
   D. describe food frequency and microelements that may be lacking in the diet

6. What is the best question for the nurse to assess medication use in the older adult living in the community?
   A. "What medications are you taking?"
   B. "What is the schedule for your medications?
   C. "Do you understand why you are taking all of your medications?

7. The nurse asks the patient to immediately state three words as part of the mini mental status examination. This is a measure of which of the following?
  A. Orientation
  B. Registration
  C. Recall
  D. Attention

8. Which of the following patients should the nurse see first?
  A. Unilateral changes in vision
  B. Ectropian of the lower lid
  C. Presbyopoia
  D. Senile ptosis

9. The nurse auscultates a loud murmur. The nurse should also assess for which of the following?
  A. Coarse rhonchi and purulent sputum
  B. Irregular heartbeat and pulse deficit
  C. Crackles in the lungs and leg edema
  D. Abdominal distention and liver tenderness

10. The patient has findings of cognitive decline, minimal to no intake of nutrition, neglect of the home environment and finances. The nurse labels this diagnosis as
  A. disturbed sensory perception
  B. impaired individual coping
  C. imbalanced nutrition, less than body requirements
  D. adult failure to thrive

References

Amella, E. J. (2004). Presentation of illness in older adults: If you think you know what you're looking for, think again. *American Journal of Nursing, 104,* 40–52.

Arterburn, D. E., Crane, P. K., & Sullivan, S. D. (2004). The coming epidemic of obesity in elderly Americans. *Journal of the American Geriatrics Society, 52,* 1907–1912.

Bance, M. (2007). Hearing and aging. *Canadian Medical Association Journal, 176*(7), 925–927.

Bergstrom, N., Braden, B. J., Laguzza, A., & Holman, V. (1987). The Braden scale for preventing pressure sore risk. *Nursing Research, 36*(4), 205–210.

Bernhard, D., & Laufer, G. (2008). The aging cardiomyocyte: a mini-review. *Gerontology, 54*(1), 24–31.

Boyce, J. M., & Shone, G. R. (2006). Effects of ageing on smell and taste. *Postgraduate Medicine, 82,* 249–241.

Braden, B. & Bergstrom, M. (1989). Clinical utility of the Braden scale for predicting pressure sore risk. *Advances in Skin and Wound Care, 2*(3), 44–51.

Brodie, S. E. (2003). Aging and disorders of the eye. In R. C. Tallis & H. M. Fillit (Eds.), *Brocklehurst's textbook of geriatric medicine and gerontology* (6th ed., pp. 735–747). London, UK: Churchill Livingstone.

Bulecheck, G. B., Butcher, H. K., & McCloskey Dochterman (2008). *Nursing interventions classification (NIC)* (5th ed.) St Louis, MO: Mosby.

Byrd, L. (2008). Making a stand against malignant melanoma. *Geriatric Nursing, 29*(3), 174.

CDC (Centers for Disease Control and Prevention). (2010). *Basic information bout skin cancer.* Retrieved June 24, 2010, from http://www.cdc.gov/cancer/skin/basic_info/

Centers for Disease Control and Prevention and Merck Foundation. (2007). *The state of aging and health in America.* Whitehouse Station, NJ: The Merck Company Foundation.

Chahal, H. S., & Drake, W. M. (2007). The endocrine system and aging. *Journal of Pathology, 211*(2), 173–180.

Defloor, T. & Grypdonck, M. F. H. (2005). Pressure ulcers: Validation of two risk assessment scales. *Journal of Clinical Nursing, 14*(3), 373–382.

DeoLeo, D., & Spathonis, K. (2003). Suicide and euthanasia in later life. *Aging: Clinical and Experimental Research, 15*(2), 99–110.

Elmadfa, I., & Meyer, A. L. (2008). Body composition, changing physiological functions and nutrient requirements of the elderly. *Annals of Nutrition and Metabolism, 52*(Suppl 1), 2–5.

Felson, D. T. (2004). An update on the pathogenesis and epidemiology of osteoarthritis. *Radiologic Clinics of North America, 42*(1), 1–9.

Fisher, G. J., Kang, S., Varani, J., Bata-Csorgo, Z., Wan, Y., Datta, S., et al. (2002). Mechanisms of photoaging and chronological skin aging. *Archives of Dermatology, 138*(11), 1462–1470.

Folstein, M. F., Folstein, S. E., & McHugh, P. R. (1975). "Mini-mental state" a practical method for grading the cognitive state of patients for the clinician. *Journal of Psychiatric Research, 12,* 189–198.

Foster, T. C. (2006). Biological markers of age-related memory deficits: Treatment of senescent physiology. *CNS Drugs, 20*(2), 153–166.

Guay, D. R., Artz, M. B., Hanlon, J. T., & Schmader, K. (2003). The pharmacology of aging. In R. C. Tallis & H.M. Fillit (Eds.). *Brocklehurst's textbook of geriatric medicine and gerontology* (6th ed.). London: Churchill-Livingston.

Ham, R., Sloane, P., Warshaw, G, Bernard, M. A., & Flaherty, E. (2007). *Primary care geriatrics: A case-based approach* (5th ed.). St Louis, MO: Mosby, Inc.

Hastings, S. N., Whitson, H. E., Jama, L., Purser, J. L., et al. (2009). *57*(10), 1856–1861. Published Online: August 20, 2009.

Healthy people 2010: What are its goals? (n.d.). Retrieved July 7, 2010, from http://www.healthypeople.gov/About/goals.htm

Hemenway, M. (2006). Skin cancer: Skin color doesn't matter. *EastWest Magazine.* Retrieved June 8, 2008, from http://www.eastwestmagazine.com/content/view/39/40.

Hendrich, A. L., et al. (2003). Validation of the Hendrich II Fall Risk Model: A large concurrent case/control study of hospitalized patients. *Applied Nursing Research, 16,* 9–21.

Huffman, G. B. (2002). Evaluating and treating unintentional weight loss in the elderly. *American Family Physician, 65*(4), 551–553.

Hybels, C. F., & Blazer, D. G. (2003). Epidemiology of late life mental disorders. *Clinics in Geriatric Medicine, 19*(4), 663–696.

Jette, A. M. (1987). The functional status index: reliability and validity of a self-report functional disability measure. *Journal of Rheumatology, 15*(suppl):15–21.

Kane, R. L., Ouslander, J. G., & Abrass, I. B. (2004). *Essentials of clinical geriatrics* (5th ed.). New York, NY: McGraw Hill.

Karagiozis, H., Gray, S., Sacco, J., Shapiro, M. & Kawas, C. (1998). The direct assessment of functional abilities (DAFA): A comparison to an indirect measure of instrumental activities of daily living. *Gerontologist, 38*(1), 113–121.

Katz, S., et al. (1963). Studies of illness in the aged: The index of ADL, A standardized measure of biological and psychosocial functioning, *JAMA, 185*, 94–101.

Kresevic, D. M., & Mezey, M. (2003). Assessment of function. In M. Mezey, et al. (Eds.), *Geriatric nursing protocols for best practice* (2nd ed., pp. 31–46). New York, NY: Springer Publishing.

Kung, H., Hoyart, D., Xu, J., & Murphy, S. (2008). Deaths: Final data for 2005. *National Vital Statistics Report, 56*, 10, 1–16.

Lach, H., & Smith, C. (2007). Assessment: Focus on function. In A. Linton & H. Lach, *Matteson & McConnells' gerontological nursing concepts and practice* (3rd ed.). St Louis, MO: Saunders, Elsevier.

Lamb, E. J., O'Riordan, S. E., & Delaney, M. P. (2003). Kidney function in older people: Pathology, assessment, and management. *Clinical Chimica Acta, 334*(1–2), 25–40.

Lawton, M. P., & Brody, E. M. (1969). Assessment of older people: Self-maintaining and instrumental activities of daily living. *Gerontologist, 9*(3), 179–186.

Linton, A., & Lach, H. (2007). *Matteson & McConnells' gerontological nursing concepts and practice* (3rd ed.). St Louis, MO: Saunders, Elsevier.

Mahoney, F. I., & Barthel, D. W. (1965). Functional evaluation: The Barthel index. *Maryland State Medical Journal, 14*, 61–65.

Makrantonaki, E., & Zouboulis, C. C. (2007). Molecular mechanisms of skin aging: State of the art. *Annals of the NY Academy of Sciences, 1119*, 40–50.

Mathias, S., Nayak, U. S., & Isaacs, B. (1986). Balance in elderly patients: The get up and go test. *Archives of Physical Medicine in Rehabilitation, 67*(6), 387–389.

Miller, C. (2008). Communication difficulties in hospitalized older adults with dementia. *American Journal of Nursing*, 108 (3), 58–66.

Miller, J. (2007). Parkinson's disease. In R. Ham, P. Sloane, G. Warshaw, Bernard, M. A., & Flaherty, D. (Eds.), *Primary care geriatrics: A case-based approach* (5th ed.). St Louis, MO: Mosby, Inc.

Moorhead, S., Johnson, M., & Mass, M. (2007). *Nursing Outcomes Classification* (*NOC*) (4th ed.). Philadelphia, PA: Mosby.

Morse, J. M. (2006). The modified Morse Fall Scale. *International Journal of Nursing Practice, 12*(3), 174–175.

Morse, J. M., Tylko, S. J., & Dixon, H. A. (1987). Characteristics of the fall-prone patient. *Gerontologist, 27*(4), 516–522.

National Institute of Deafness and Communication Disorders. (2010). *Quick statistics*. Retrieved June 24, 2010, from http://www.nidcd.nih.gov/health/statistics/quick.htm

North American Nursing Diagnosis Association. (2009). *Nursing diagnoses, 2009–2011 Edition: Definitions and classifications* (*NANDA NURSING DIAGNOSIS*). West Sussex UK: John Wiley & Sons.

Ostechega, Y., Paulose-Ram, R., Dillon, C. F., & Hughes, J. P. (2007). Prevalance of peripheral arterial disease and risk factors in persons aged 60 and older: Data from the National Health and Nutrition Examination survey 1999-2004. *Journal of the American Geriatric Society, 55*(4), 583–589.

Peterson, M. D., Rhea, M. R., Sen, A., & Gordon, P. M. (2010). Resistance exercises for musculoskeletal strength in older adults: A metaanalysis. *Ageing Research Reviews, 9*(3), 226–237.

Porth, C. M. (2007). *Pathophysiology: Altered states of health* (7th ed.). Philadelphia: Lippincott.

Posner, B. M., Jette, A. M., Smith, K.W., & Miller, D. R. (1993). Nutrition and health risks in the elderly: The nutrition screening initiative. *Journal of American Public Health, 83*(7), 927–978.

Schober-Flores, C. (2001). The sun's damaging effects. *Dermatology Nursing, 13*(4), 279–286.

Sharma G., & Goodwin, J. (2006). Effect of aging on respiratory system physiology and immunology. *Clinical Interventions in Aging, 1*(3), 253–260.

Sheikh, J. A., & Yesavage, J. A. (1986). Geriatric Depression Scale (GDS): Recent findings and development of a shorter version. In T. L. Brink (Ed.), *Clinical gerontology: A guide to assessment and intervention* (pp. 165–176). New York, NY: Howarth Press.

Soriano, T. A., DeCherrie, L. V., & Thomas, D. C. (2007). Falls in the community-dwelling older adult: a review for primary-care providers. *Clinical Interventions in Aging, 2*(4), 545–554.

Stevens, J. A. (2006). Fatalities and injuries from falls amoung older adults in the US 1993–2003 and 2001–2005. *Morbidity and Mortality Weekly Report, 55*(45), 1–32.

Stitt, W. Z., & Gilchrest, B. A. (2003). Skin diseases and old age. In R. C. Tallis & H. M. Fillit (Eds), *Brocklehurst's textbook of geriatric medicine and gerontology* (6th ed.). London, UK: Churchill Livingstone.

Stratton, R. J., King, C. L., Stroud. M. A., Jackson, A. A., & Elia, M. (2006). Malnutrition Universal Screening Tool predicts mortality and length of hospital stay in acutely ill elderly. *British Journal of Nutrition, 95*(2), 325–330.

Thomas, J. M., Isenring, E., & Kellett, E. (2007). Nutritional status and length of stay in patients admitted to an Acute Assessment Unit. *Journal of Human Nutrition and Diet, 20*(4), 320–328.

Tobias, J. H., & Sharif, M. (2002). Aging and the musculoskeletal system. In R. C. Tallis & H. M. Fillit (Eds). *Brocklehurst's textbook of geriatric medicine and gerontology* (6th ed.). London, UK: Churchill Livingstone.

U.S. Preventative Services Task Force (USPSTF). (2010). Retrieved March 11, 2010, from http://www.ahrq.gov/clinic/USpstf/uspstopics.htm.

Wright, J. (2000). The FIM™. The Center for Outcome Measurement in Brain Injury. Retrieved July 27, 2008, from http://222.tbims.org/combi/FIM.

Yesavage, J. A., Brink, T. L., & Rose, T. (1982). Development and validation of a geriatric depression screening scale: A preliminary report. *Journal of Psychiatric Research, 17*, 37–49.

The Jensen suite offers these additional resources to enhance learning and facilitate understanding of this chapter:

- thePoint on line resource, http//thepoint.lww.com/Jensen1E
- Student CD-ROM included with the book
- *Laboratory Manual for Nursing Health Assessment: A Best Practice Approach*
- *Pocket Guide for Nursing Health Assessment: A Best Practice Approach*

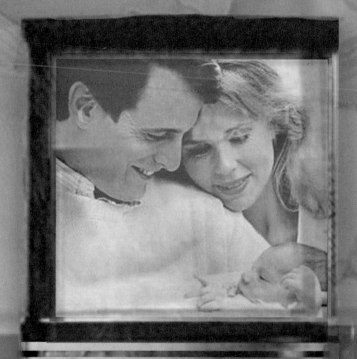

Putting it All Together

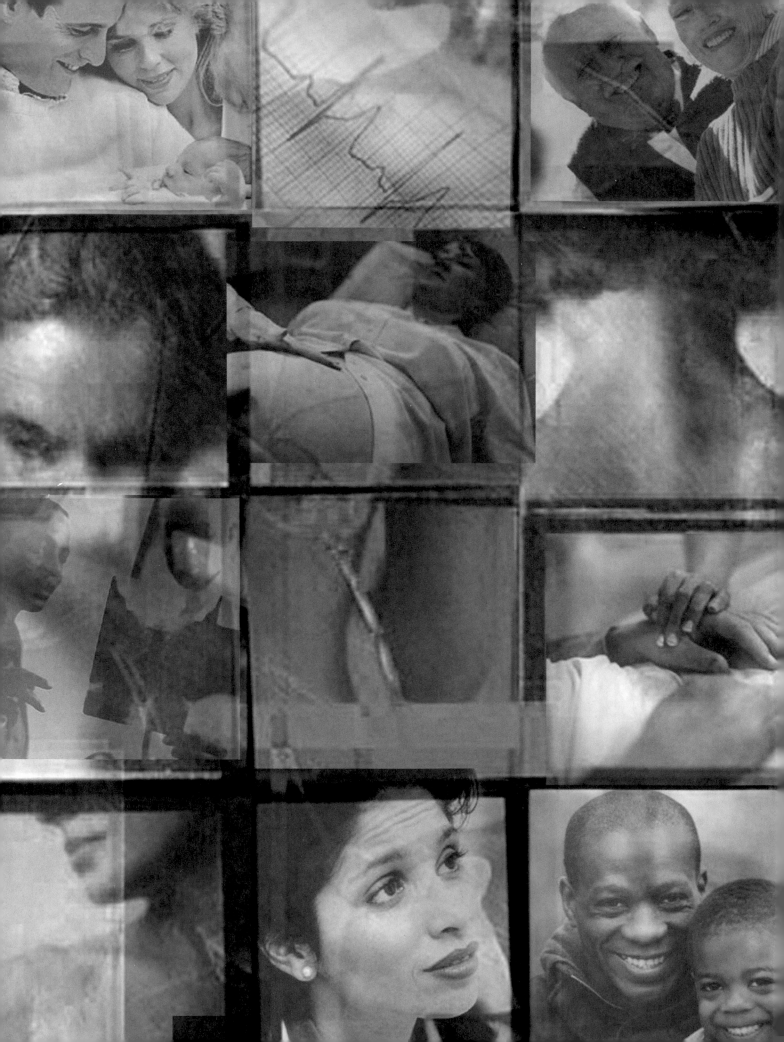

31

Head-to-Toe Assessment of the Adult

Learning Objectives

1 Identify the rationale for a comprehensive, screening, or focused health assessment depending on the patient situation and setting.

2 Collect subjective data, including history and risk assessment.

3 Identify teaching opportunities for health promotion and risk reduction.

4 Collect objective data by completing a head-to-toe physical assessment.

5 Individualize the health assessment, considering the condition, age, gender, and culture of the patient.

6 Identify normal and abnormal findings from inspection, palpation, percussion, and auscultation during the head-to-toe assessment.

7 Document and communicate data using appropriate medical terminology.

8 Use subjective and objective data to analyze findings and plan interventions.

9 Use assessment findings to identify patterns and problems, set outcomes, and initiate a plan of care.

*D*orothy Jane Suleri, 44 years old, is admitted with diarrhea, obesity, ulcerative colitis, abdominal pain, rosacea, fatigue, and anemia. Her current problem is bleeding related to the colitis, for which she uses prescribed medications. She has had three bloody stools today. She is married with two children, 15 and 13 years old.

As you read through the chapter, consider the following questions:

- How will the nurse individualize the admitting history to focus on Mrs. Suleri?
- How will the nurse focus the physical assessments considering Mrs. Suleri's diagnosis?
- How will the nurse use the assessment information to develop a plan of care?

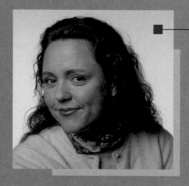

This chapter outlines a comprehensive assessment by a registered nurse. Although the chapter describes some typical assessments, it is important to keep in mind that adaptations are wide ranging, depending on the patient's status, clinical setting, and standards of practice. Beginning nurses learn the range of assessment skills, but the application of how and when to use these skills occurs in the clinical setting. The nurse combines sensitive history taking with accurate and thorough physical assessment techniques by beginning with a firm foundation of evidence and scientific knowledge. With experience and support, patient assessment becomes an art. The most important thing is to develop a consistent, logical technique organized in a way that is comfortable for the nurse and individualized and focused on the patient.

The comprehensive health assessment integrates all body systems; findings help the nurse form an overall impression of the patient and his or her condition. Complete subjective data collection includes data related to the patient's history and risk factors. The nurse typically collects these once and then gathers focused data more frequently. Comprehensive assessment also includes collection of objective and physical assessment data beginning at the head and ending at the toes. This arrangement provides a practical organizational framework, facilitating efficient movement for the nurse and energy conservation for the patient. The nurse usually also collects objective data once and then either collects focused data, or, in the case of an acute or critically ill patient, may repeat the head-to-toe examination. After gathering all data, the nurse then reorganizes it according to body system, problem, or diagnosis. He or she detects patterns and identifies findings in associated systems. The nurse analyzes assessment data by using critical thinking to identify problems and then plan and evaluate care. Therefore, an accurate history (subjective data) and physical assessment (objective data) create an essential foundation for complete and individualized care.

This chapter also covers specific assessments to use for a hospitalized patient: admitting, screening, and focused. In addition, the content also introduces specialized assessment steps completed by the nurse practitioner.

Acute Assessment

The nurse constantly assesses and observes the patient.

⚠ SAFETY ALERT 31.1

If skin color is cyanotic or pale, breathing is difficult, posture is strained, facial expression is anxious, and overall appearance indicates distress, the nurse focuses on the immediate problem. Other cues that indicate an unstable condition in a patient are difficulty managing the airway; high or low respirations, pulse, or blood pressure; acute change in mental status; seizure; new onset of chest pain; or any other concerns by the nurse (Offner, et al., 2007).

In cases like those just described, the nurse gathers pertinent subjective and objective assessment data related to the problem to assist with identifying the cause and intervening promptly. The patient may be treated as more data is collected. It may be necessary to request additional nursing assistance, contact the primary provider, or activate a rapid response. The nurse immediately reports any concerns.

Subjective Data Collection

Subjective data collection involves assessing present problems, taking health history, and evaluating risk factors. The nurse gives the patient time and encouragement to tell his or her story and experience of health or illness. Doing so provides an opportunity for the patient to express concerns; it often forms the foundation for a therapeutic relationship. If the patient is anxious, the nurse acknowledges that it is common for patients to feel uncomfortable at times; the patient is given permission to disclose only information with which he or she is comfortable. Additionally, the nurse informs the patient that the information is confidential except in situations where there is concern about safety or harm.

If the patient is stable, the nurse may perform the history first and then complete the physical examination. Alternatively, the nurse may thread collection of subjective data throughout the physical examination (eg, asking about cough when auscultating the lungs). After reviewing the patient chart, the nurse formulates a list of initial problems or topics to discuss, including health promotion and risk-reduction assessment. The history is usually performed with the patient clothed, because most patients are more comfortable when covered.

Areas for Health Promotion/*Healthy People*

An important purpose of the health history is to gather information to promote health and provide health teaching. Health-promotion activities focus on preventing disease, identifying problems early, and reducing complications of existing or established diagnoses. They also serve to reinforce existing healthy habits and encourage refinements to approaches the patient already is practicing.

Patient education, health promotion, and risk reduction are some of the most important roles in nursing. The nurse weaves relevant topics into conversation during health history collection and follow-up teaching sessions. Nurses promote patient education and healthy behaviors as they apply the nursing process. The topics in Table 31-1 are national goals related to the primary care setting that can guide individual health goals.

Assessment of Risk Factors

Assessment of risk factors involves collecting comprehensive subjective data, including demographic information and other data from the chart, history of present problem, past health history, family history, review of systems, psychosocial history, functional status, ADLs, and growth/development. After collecting and analyzing all these data, the nurse determines potential and actual risk factors for the patient

Table 31.1 Healthy People Goals for Primary Care

Goal	Patient Education Topics
Increase the proportion of persons appropriately counseled about health behaviors.	Review healthy diet, regular exercise, weight reduction, and recommended screenings.
Increase the proportion of persons who have a specific source of ongoing care.	Encourage patient to have regular visits for health promotion and screening.
Increase the proportion of adults with diabetes who have at least an annual foot examination.	Remind patients with diabetes to get foot checks annually.
Increase the proportion of HIV-infected adolescents and adults who receive testing, treatment, and prophylaxis consistent with current Public Health Service treatment guidelines.	Discuss safe-sex practices and encourage patients who are at risk to get testing.
Increase the proportion of adults who are vaccinated annually against influenza and ever vaccinated against pneumococcal disease.	Supply flyers and reminders for patients; supply low-cost vaccine for patients.

Source: *Healthy people 2010: What are its goals?* (n.d.). Retrieved July 7, 2010, from http://www.healthypeople.gov/About/goals.htm

and uses this information to plan specific screening, health promotion, and patient teaching activities.

The U.S. Preventive Services Task Force (USPSTF, 2006) recommends that primary providers discuss priority screening services with patients and offer them (Table 31-2). Screening and resulting teaching (see the section "Demographic Data") are primary prevention services that nurses offer as part of their professional responsibilities. The nurse assesses risk factors according to the individual's risks (eg, injury in a teenager, genetic diseases in a pregnant woman). Cancer screening, dental caries prevention for preschoolers, Rh incompatibility screening for pregnant women, and

behavioral counseling for a healthy diet are included as primary prevention activities. These screenings are essential in maintaining high-level wellness.

Demographic Data

Initially the nurse begins with common chart items, such as demographic information, primary problems, and a medication list, along with allergies. The nurse reviews this chart before meeting the patient to avoid repetitive questions. He or she compares the medication list with home medications stated by the patient. Additionally, the nurse validates the problem list and medications with the patient. If areas are inconsistent or

Table 31-2 Screening and Health Promotion Activities from USPSTF

Recommendation	Adults		Special Populations	
	Men	Women	Pregnant Women	Children
Alcohol misuse screening and behavioral counseling interventions, counseling to prevent tobacco use and tobacco-caused disease	X	X	X	
Screening for asymptomatic bacteriuria, Rh (D) incompatibility screening			X	
Breast cancer, cervical cancer, osteoporosis in postmenopausal women screening		X		
Prevention of dental caries in preschool children, screening for visual impairment in children younger than age 5 years				X
Depression screening, colorectal cancer screening, screening for Type II diabetes mellitus in adults, behavioral counseling in primary care to promote a healthy diet, screening for high blood pressure and lipid disorders, screening for obesity in adults	X	X		
Gonorrhea, hepatitis B virus infection, syphilis infection, chlamydial infection screening; behavioral interventions to promote breastfeeding		X	X	
HIV screening	X	X	X	X

unclear, the nurse obtains additional information, notifies the primary provider, and reconciles the differences.

Figure 31-1 illustrates how the nurse implements this in the clinical setting, using information related to Ms. Suleri as presented in the case study. The assessment is a screening or RN assessment. The following data are obtained from the chart during the preinterview phase.

History of Present Problem

The patient interview begins with a focus on the primary problem. The nurse asks about the reason for the visit and history of the present problem. He or she evaluates the reasons for the visit by asking, "Tell me why you came in today." At this point, the nurse obtains a history of the present illness by assessing pain or discomfort using the following parameters:

- Location: "Where does it hurt?"
- Duration: "When did it start?" How long has it lasted?"
- Intensity: "On a scale of 1 to 10 how do you rate your pain?"
- Quality: "Tell me what it feels like."
- Alleviating/aggravating factors: "What makes it better? Worse?"

- Pain goal: "What level of pain is acceptable to you?"
- Functional goal: "What would you like to be able to do if you were not in pain?

Past Health History

The nurse assesses past health history to provide context for how the current problem might be related. He or she assesses findings considering the information previously reviewed in the chart. For example, the nurse might say, "I'm going to ask you some questions about your health history. I noticed that your chart says that you have an allergy to Zofran. Tell me about that." This is a way of verifying information and obtaining further details. Some examples of categories for the past medical and family history include the following:

- **Assess for allergies.** Include iodine, shellfish, and latex. Also assess the patient's reaction including rash, hives, anaphylaxis, uticaria, pruritis, gastrointestinal (GI) upset, nausea, vomiting, or diarrhea. Validate answers with the information in the chart. Include reaction.
- **Obtain past history of illness.** Include medical, surgical, and obstetric history.

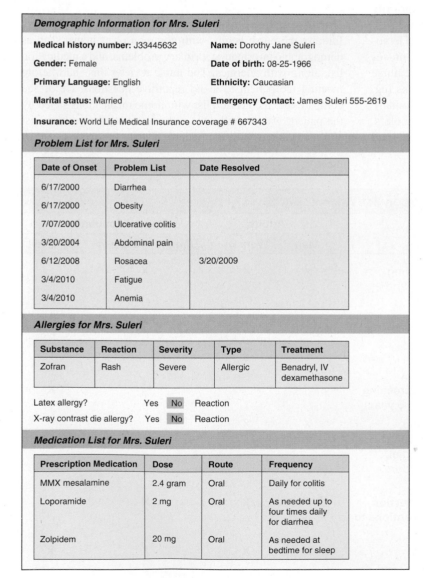

Demographic Information for Mrs. Suleri

Medical history number: J33445632	**Name:** Dorothy Jane Suleri
Gender: Female	**Date of birth:** 08-25-1966
Primary Language: English	**Ethnicity:** Caucasian
Marital status: Married	**Emergency Contact:** James Suleri 555-2619

Insurance: World Life Medical Insurance coverage # 667343

Problem List for Mrs. Suleri

Date of Onset	Problem List	Date Resolved
6/17/2000	Diarrhea	
6/17/2000	Obesity	
7/07/2000	Ulcerative colitis	
3/20/2004	Abdominal pain	
6/12/2008	Rosacea	3/20/2009
3/4/2010	Fatigue	
3/4/2010	Anemia	

Allergies for Mrs. Suleri

Substance	Reaction	Severity	Type	Treatment
Zofran	Rash	Severe	Allergic	Benadryl, IV dexamethasone

Latex allergy?   Yes   No   Reaction
X-ray contrast die allergy?   Yes   No   Reaction

Medication List for Mrs. Suleri

Prescription Medication	Dose	Route	Frequency
MMX mesalamine	2.4 gram	Oral	Daily for colitis
Loporamide	2 mg	Oral	As needed up to four times daily for diarrhea
Zolpidem	20 mg	Oral	As needed at bedtime for sleep

Figure 31.1 Problem list for Mrs. Suleri.

- **Obtain list of medications.** Include over-the-counter drugs, herbals, and supplements (medications listed in the chart and double checked and reconciled with patient).
- **Assess family history.** What was the condition? Who had it?
- **Assess childhood illnesses and immunizations.** Include influenza, pneumococcal, and PPD (TB test).
- **Obtain information on most recent screening assessments.** These include TB, vision or hearing screening, and mammograms.
- **Evaluate mental health and psychiatric history.** Medications may provide clues to mental health issues, such as antidepressants.

Review of Systems

The nurse reviews the body systems using lay language focused on the following common symptoms (or the patient may complete a form; see Chapter 3). The nurse documents findings, however, using medical terminology (Fig. 31-2).

- **General survey:** Fever, chills, weight loss, weight gain, fatigue
- **Nutrition:** Nausea, loss of appetite, vomiting, indigestion, problems swallowing or chewing
- **Skin, hair, and nails:** Rash, itch, lesions, nails, hygiene practices, hair loss
- **Head and neck:** Headaches, dizziness, syncope, seizures, enlarged lymph nodes
- **Eyes:** Glasses, contacts, blurry vision, double vision, loss of vision, swelling, tearing or dry eyes, date of last vision examination
- **Ears:** Hearing loss, pressure, earache
- **Nose, mouth, throat:** Congestion, sore throat, voice change, usual dental care, last dental visit
- **Thorax and lungs:** Shortness of breath, wheezing, cough
- **Heart:** Fast or slow pulse, heart murmur, chest pain, pounding or fluttering in chest, swelling in feet, rings tighter than usual
- **Peripheral vascular:** Cramping, pain, numbness in extremities
- **Breast:** Pain, tenderness, discharge, lump, date of last self breast examination

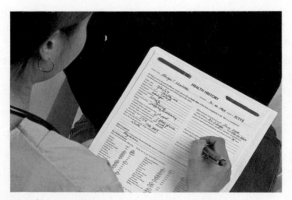

Figure 31.2 The nurse carefully documents findings from the health history in the patient's chart, using medical terminology.

- **Abdominal/gastrointestinal:** Frequency of bowel movements and description, bloody stool, diarrhea, constipation, soiling of clothes, hemorrhoids
- **Abdominal/genitourinary (GU):** Frequency and description of urine, difficulty or burning with urination, blood in urine, urination at night, urgency, increased frequency, wetting of clothes, feeling of incomplete emptying or dribbling
- **Musculoskeletal:** Mobility, pain, stiffness, spasm, tremor, gait, impaired balance, foreign bodies or implants
- **Neurological:** Headache, one-sided weakness, memory loss, confusion
- **Genitalia, female:** Vaginal discharge, pain with menstruation, excessive bleeding with menstruation, last menstrual period (LMP), pain with sexual intercourse
- **Genitalia, male:** Discharge, pain, swelling, lumps, trauma, erectile dysfunction
- **Endocrine:** Excessive thirst, increased urination, hair loss, skin changes, hot flashes
- **Mental health:** Anxiety, depression, abnormal thoughts, difficulty sleeping
- **Summary:** How would you say that your health is in general?

Psychosocial History. The nurse assesses psychosocial, spiritual, and cultural history, language of choice, and need for interpreter. He or she may ask "Do you have any special religious, spiritual, or cultural needs? Would you like an interpreter?" The nurse assesses use of tobacco, alcohol, and recreational drugs by asking directly "Do you use tobacco, alcohol, or other substances?" He or she assesses for safety and domestic violence by asking "Because violence is so common in many people's lives, I ask all patients about it routinely. Are you in a relationship with a person who physically or sexually hurts or threatens you?"

Functional Health Status. As time allows, and as the relationship is established the nurse also can obtain information about the patient's functional health status. For these questions, it is best to prioritize and weave one or two questions into care. See Chapter 3.

Activities of Daily Living. Additionally nurses assess ability to perform self-care activities, or **activities of daily living** (**ADLs**; see Chapter 3). These include behaviors such as eating, dressing, and grooming. Nurses score these items based on whether patients are totally independent, need assistance from a person or device such as a cane, or are dependent on others. See also Chapter 3.

Growth and Development

Assessment of developmental stage occurs over time, as the nurse works with the patient. Some things to consider when working with patients across the lifespan are the psychosocial development described by Erikson (1963). The nurse will also assess developmental milestones or stage of development in children. Refer to Chapter 9 for more information.

Risk Assessment and Health-Related Patient Teaching

Risk assessment and screening help identify a potential problems so that health care providers can give the patient information to influence behavioral choices. Potential or actual problems requiring health teaching are identified. The most important focus areas for health-related patient teaching involve ensuring adequate nutrition, increasing physical activity, maintaining weight, and reducing stress. Avoidance of behaviors that contribute to disease (eg, smoking, overuse of alcohol) is important as well. Another teaching point is childhood immunizations and pneumococcal and influenza vaccines.

Injury prevention involves interventions such as recommending bicycle helmets, avoiding drinking and driving, and using seatbelts. Primary prevention of disease and promotion of health are priorities for increased quality and quantity of life. An additional specialized focus area is promotion of health during pregnancy and breastfeeding. Maintaining health during pregnancy is vital for both mother and fetus. Teaching regarding importance of prenatal appointments and screenings and promotion of breastfeeding are key topics.

Focused Health History Related to Common Symptoms

In addition to the overall review of systems and general health promotion, the nurse focuses questions on concerns specific to the patient. In this way, the patient is viewed as a person with multiple areas affected by the health status. These questions are related to the primary problems and concerns for the patient, included in each system-specific chapter.

Therapeutic Dialogue: Collecting Subjective Data

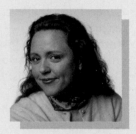

Mrs. Suleri, introduced at the beginning of this chapter, is a 44-year-old mother of two children admitted with bloody diarrhea. The nurse uses professional communication techniques to gather subjective data from her. The following conversations give two examples of interview styles during the middle of the interview used by different nurses. One style is more effective than the other.

Less Effective

Nurse: So I bet that your kids are missing you at home.

Mrs. Suleri: Yeah, I usually drive them to soccer practice and ballet.

Nurse: I have kids. How old are yours?

Mrs. Suleri: They are 13 and 15. Busy ages. They aren't old enough to drive yet but have a lot of activities.

Nurse: Yeah, mine aren't there yet. They are only 5 and 8 years old. What schools did yours go to?

Mrs. Suleri: Heritage Elementary and now they are in Lincoln Middle School. How about yours?

Nurse: Mine are in Washington Elementary. It's a pretty good school.

More Effective

Nurse: How does your family depend upon you for things, and how are they coping with your illness?

Mrs. Suleri: Thanks for asking. Usually I take the kids to soccer practice and ballet. My husband is a backup but he works late so this has been a stress on all of us. I've been so tired lately that I haven't been able to keep up.

Nurse: Do you generally feel rested and ready for activities after sleeping?

Mrs. Suleri: Not really, I'm exhausted (pause) and I barely can make it to work.

Nurse: How is this hospital stay affecting your work?

Mrs. Suleri: I've been missing a lot.

Nurse: Because many people have financial concerns related to their hospital stay, I usually ask about that. Would you like to see a social worker about any financial concerns?

Mrs. Suleri: Actually I would. Talking with someone might put my mind at ease about paying for this.

Critical Thinking Challenge

- How did the professional role of the two nurses differ?
- Why did the more effective nurse gain more information than the less effective?
- How might you ask the question about finances, which can be a sensitive subject?

Objective Data Collection

Pulling together a smooth and organized physical assessment is challenging. It is important to practice and develop a pattern of assessment that eventually becomes automatic to avoid skipping or repeating items. The nurse links together sections of the assessment according to the body part being examined, even if they are related to different body systems. For example, while the patient stands, the nurse assesses sensory and motor neurological function, musculoskeletal range of motion, and peripheral vascular pulses.

Equipment

- Cotton swabs
- Drapes, gown
- Examining gloves
- Nasal speculum
- Ophthalmoscope/otoscope
- Reflex hammer
- Blood-pressure cuff
- Scale with height measure
- Stethoscope
- Thermometer
- Tongue blade
- Watch with second hand
- Optional: Vision charts
- **If specimens are needed:**
  - Vaginal speculum
  - Lubricant
  - Culture media
  - Glass slides
  - KOH
  - Hemoccult testing cards and solution
  - Pap smear spatula

Preparation

Following completion of the health history previously described, the nurse explains the process for the physical examination, from head to toe and including auscultation of heart and lung sounds, auscultation and palpation of the abdomen, and screening for neuromuscular problems. Because some assessments may be uncomfortable (eg, breast, gynecological), the nurse asks the patient for permission to perform them. Additionally, the nurse asks the patient if he or she prefers to have a third person in the room or, if appropriate, a same gender nurse. The nurse explains that the patient will be draped and modesty will be a priority; only the body part being examined will be exposed.

The nurse asks if the patient would like to empty the bladder, because pressure during abdominal palpation may elicit the urge to void. He or she instructs the patient to

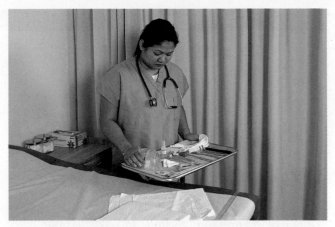

Figure 31.3 The nurse is setting up the examination room for a head-to-toe physical assessment.

change into a gown that ties in back. At this point, the nurse obtains the necessary equipment and leaves the room so that the patient can change (Fig. 31-3). He or she instructs the patient to sit on the examination table after finishing undressing. Upon return, the nurse washes and warms the hands to avoid chilling the patient and asks the patient about comfort level and room temperature. If the patient is cold, an additional blanket may be used. The nurse encourages the patient to ask questions about the assessment techniques and findings.

Patients may be seen because of abnormal findings, so it is important to be honest when there are difficulties, such as, "Your blood pressure is a little high. We can talk more about that after we're finished." Instead of giving false reassurances, the nurse instead provides objective data. Nevertheless, the nurse avoids sharing conclusions before collecting all data, because the initial problem list may change during the interaction. The nurse evaluates the response of the individual and family to actual or potential health problems and also performs assessments related to the direct care role.

Comprehensive Physical Examination

The physical examination begins with height, weight, and vital signs if not previously obtained. Next, is the head-to-toe assessment, with the nurse moving efficiently and reducing the number of movements for the patient. It is important to consider how to remember each of these steps by combining items or developing cues to remember them. As a beginner, a pocket guide might be helpful so that at the end the nurse can review it for any forgotten items. The nurse can review this before leaving the patient's room so it is not necessary to return asking for more information. Reviewing findings with the patient at the end provides closure before leaving.

Technique and Normal Findings	Abnormal Findings
Wash hands or use gel. Wipe stethoscope.	

Vital Signs

Obtain temperature. *35.8°C–37.3°C*	Hypothermia, hyperthermia
Obtain pulse. *60–100 bpm*	Tachycardia, bradycardia, irregular rate. If irregular take apical pulse.
Obtain respirations. *12–20/min*	Bradypnea, tachypnea, hyperventilation, Cheyne-Stokes, apnea.
Obtain blood pressure. *Systolic 100–120/diastolic 60–80 mm Hg.*	Hypertension, hypotension, auscultatory gap. Perform orthostatic BP and P if indicated. BP that stays 120–139/80–89 is considered *prehypertension;* above this level (140/90 mm Hg or higher) is high (hypertension; AHA, 2009).
Obtain oxygen saturation level. *92%–100%*	<92%.

General Survey

Inspect overall skin color. *Pink.*	Pallor, jaundice, flushing, cyanosis (central vs. peripheral), erythema, ruddy, mottled
Evaluate breathing effort. *No dyspnea*	Dyspnea, head of bed elevated, tripod position
Observe appearance. *Appears stated age*	Appears older than stated age
Assess mood. *Patient is calm, pleasant, and cooperative. Appropriate affect.*	Flat or inappropriate affect, depression, elation, euphoria, anxiety, irritable, labile.
Observe nutritional status. *Appears well nourished.*	Appears poorly nourished, overweight, or obese.
Evaluate personal hygiene. *Good personal hygiene.*	Poor personal hygiene
Assess posture. *Posture erect.*	Slouching, bent to one side
Observe for physical deformities. *No obvious physical deformities.*	Obvious physical deformity present
Perform safety check. *Call bell within reach; bedside stand positioned; ID band correct; IVs, medications, tubes, and drains intact.*	Unsafe environment, medications or IVs not verified.

Skin

Inspect skin with each corresponding body area. Inspect color; check for rashes and lesions. *Skin pink, no cyanosis. No telangiectasia, erythema, or papules.*	Changes in skin pigmentation. If there are lesions or rashes, identify configuration. Note any infections (eg, cellulitis). Infestations include scabies, lice, and fleas.
Palpate for moisture, temperature, texture, turgor, and edema. *Skin warm, slightly dry, and intact. Good turgor on upper extremities; no edema, lesions, or tenderness.*	Growths or tumors are abnormal. Describe any wounds or incisions including size, depth, color, exudate, and wound borders.

Head

Evaluate facial structures. *Symmetrical structures without edema, deformities, or lesions. Patent nares.*	Asymmetry, edema, deformities, ptosis, lesions. Absence of "sniff," deviated septum, polyps, drainage.

Technique and Normal Findings (continued)	Abnormal Findings (continued)
Observe facial expression. *Appropriate to situation.*	Anxious, facial grimace; facial droop, asymmetry.
Inspect hair, scalp. *Straight hair with normal distribution. Hair supple and thick. Scalp pink and smooth without pests, flaking, lesions, or tenderness.* Palpate cranium, temporal artery, and temporomandibular joint (TMJ). *Normocephalic, head midline. Temporal artery 2–3+ bilaterally, nontender. TMJ moves freely, without crepitus or tenderness.*	Facial asymmetry may indicate damage to CN VII or a serious condition such as *stroke*. Enlarged bones or tissues are associated with *acromegaly*. A puffy "moon" face is associated with *Cushing's syndrome*. Increased facial hair in females may be a sign of *Cushing's syndrome* or *endocrinopathy*. Periorbital edema is seen with *congestive heart failure* and *hypothyroidism* (*myxedema*).
Assess cranial nerve (CN) V, motor strength and light touch, three facial branches. *Strong contraction of muscles and senses light touch on forehead, cheek, and chin.*	Decreased or dulled sensation, weakness, or asymmetric movements are abnormal findings associated with CN V.
Assess CN V and VII: squeeze eyes shut, wrinkle forehead, clench teeth, smile, puff cheeks. *Facial movements are strong and symmetrical.*	A weak blink from facial weakness may result from paralysis of CN V or VII.
Inspect lids, lashes, and brows. *No ptosis, lid lag, discharge, or crusting. Even lash distribution. Brows with hair loss on outer third.*	Depressed or absent corneal response is common in contact lens wearers.

Mouth and Throat

Inspect mouth with light and tongue blade. Inspect inside lips, buccal mucosa, gums, teeth, hard/soft palates, uvula, tonsils, pharynx, tongue and floor of mouth (APRN may use light from otoscope). *Lips, mucosa, gums, palates are pink and smooth. Floor of mouth intact, moist, smooth. Pharynx pink, intact. Tongue pink and rough. No lesions or tenderness. Teeth white, intact with good occlusion.*	Lesions, sponginess, or edema; bleeding gums; missing or discolored teeth; malocclusion; inflammation or tenderness of ducts.
Grade tonsils. *Tonsils 0–2+. Pink with no discharge or lesions.*	Swollen glands or tonsils (grade 3+ to 4+).
Note mobility of uvula when patient says "ahh." *Uvula midline and rises symmetrically.*	Uvula asymmetrical or enlarged.
Assess CN XII; look for symmetry of tongue when extended. *Tongue at midline and extends symmetrically.*	A tongue that deviates to one side is common with *stroke*.

Eyes

Assess near and distant vision if appropriate. *Reads newsprint accurately. Snellen test 20/20.*	<20/20 corrected. Vision blurred. Note use of glasses, contact lenses, or assistive devices.
Inspect conjunctiva and sclera. *Pink, moist conjunctiva; white sclera.*	Sclera yellow with *jaundice*. Conjunctiva pink with *inflammation*.
Inspect cornea, iris, and anterior chamber. *Cornea and lens are clear.* Assess CNs III, IV, VI and extraocular movements (EOMs). *EOMs intact, no nystagmus.* Assess visual fields, peripheral vision. *Visual fields equal to the examiner's.*	A narrow angle indicates *glaucoma*. Cloudiness of the lens can indicate *cataract*, which is associated with increased age, smoking, alcohol intake, and sunlight exposure. Risk factors for cataracts are primarily environmental.

(text continues on page 930)

Technique and Normal Findings (continued)	Abnormal Findings (continued)
Darken room. Obtain light. Assess CN II. *Pupils equal, round, and reactive to light and accommodation (PERRLA L 6–4, R 6–4).*	Asymmetry, pinpoint, or "blown" pupils; describe measure of pupil and response to light.
Perform ophthalmoscope examination: check red reflex, disc, vessels, and macula. Move to opposite side of patient. *Red reflex symmetric. Discs cream-colored with sharp margins. Retina pink. No hemorrhages or exudates; no arteriolar narrowing. Macula yellow.*	Lack of *red reflex* may need urgent follow up. If a white pupil reflex (leukokoria) is elicited, then an urgent ophthalmologic referral is required. Disease or trauma (eg, *retinoblastoma, hyphema, toxocariasis, retinal detachment*) often causes a white pupil reflex. Blood vessels can be directly observed in the retina. Systemic diseases are often reflected in the blood vessels and can be directly observed in the eye.
Ears	
Turn on lights. Inspect ear alignment. *Ears aligned properly.* Palpate auricle, lobe, and tragus. *Ears are without lesions, crusting, masses, or tenderness.*	Microtia, macrotia, edema, cartilage pseudomonas infection, carcinoma on auricle, cyst, and frost bite are abnormal findings.
Change to otoscope head. Perform otoscope examination of canal and tympanic membrane. Move to opposite side of patient. *Canals with small amount of moist yellow cerumen. Tympanic membranes intact, gray, and translucent; light reflex and body landmarks present.*	Redness, external swelling, and discharge indicate *external otitis.* Obstructed canal can be by either foreign body or cerumen.
Assess CN VIII hearing. *Whispered words heard bilaterally.*	Unable to repeat whispered words.
Obtain tuning fork. Perform Rinne's test (on mastoid) if the patient has hearing loss. *Air conduction > bone conduction.*	Bone conduction longer or the same as air conduction is evidence of *conductive hearing loss.*
Perform Weber's test (at midline of skull) if patient has hearing loss. *No lateralization.*	Unilateral identification of the sound indicates *sensorineural loss* in the ear that the patient did not hear the sound or had reduced perception.
Nose and Sinuses	
Inspect external nose. *Midline, no flaring or crusting.*	Asymmetry, swelling, or bruising may result from trauma or occur with lesions or growths.
Assess nostril patency. *Patent bilaterally.*	Unable to sniff because of *deviated septum* or *obstructed nares.*
Perform otoscopic examination of mucosa, turbinates, and septum. *Nasal mucosa pink, intact; no polyps. No drainage. Turbinates and septum intact and symmetrical.*	Infection, inflammation of nasal mucosa may be present with *viral, bacterial, or allergic rhinitis.*
Palpate frontal and maxillary sinuses. *No frontal or maxillary sinus tenderness.*	Redness and swelling over the sinuses may represent *acute infection, abscess, or mucocele.*
Neck	
Inspect symmetry. *Neck symmetrical, moves freely without crepitus.*	Neck asymmetrical or with crepitus
Test flexion, extension, lateral bending, rotation, range of motion (ROM), and strength. *Full ROM, strength 4–5+ bilaterally.*	Reduced neck ROM is <4+.

Technique and Normal Findings (continued)	Abnormal Findings (continued)
Palpate tracheal position midline. *Trachea at midline.*	Deviated trachea.
Palpate carotid pulse. *Carotid pulse 2–3+ bilaterally.*	Carotid pulses may be reduced from *carotid stenosis.*
Inspect jugular veins. *No jugular venous distention (JVD).*	Jugular veins may be either flat or distended.
Palpate preauricular, postauricular, occipital, and posterior cervical chains. *They are not palpable or tender.*	Lymph nodes are not freely movable or are tender.
Palpate tonsillar, submandibular, submental, and anterior cervical chains. *They are not palpable or tender.*	
Palpate supraclavicular nodes. *They are not palpable or tender.*	

Neurological

Assess mental status and level of consciousness. *Patient is alert. Eyes open spontaneously.*	Agitated, asleep, lethargic, obtunded, restless, stuporous. Use coma scale if reduced (eye opening, verbal, motor). Does not respond to stimuli or pain; decorticate rigidity, decerebrate rigidity, or no response to pain.
Assess orientation. *Oriented × 3.*	Alert and oriented × 2 (person and place). A&O × 1 (person), disoriented × 3. Can also assess orientation to situation (A&O × 4).
Assess ability to follow commands. *Follows directions.*	Unable to follow commands, such as squeeze my hand, or sit up.
Evaluate short- and long-term memory. *Immediate, recent, and distant memory intact.*	Immediate, recent or distant memory impaired; describe specific details.
Assess speech. *Speech clear.*	Speech difficult to understand.
Assess hearing. *Hears voices and responds appropriately.*	Difficulty understanding spoken words. Hard of hearing. Note hearing aids or assistive devices.

Upper Extremities

Evaluate circulation, movement, and sensation (CMS). Assess hands and joints. Evaluate nails on upper extremities. *CMS intact. Nails smooth without clubbing. Joints without swelling or deformity.*	Decreased CMS, including color, temperature; capillary refill >3 seconds, pulses, decreased movement, decreased sensation and paresthesia. Nails are breakable, cracking, inflamed, jagged, bitten, and clubbing.
Perform hand grasp for ROM and muscle strength. *4–5+ muscle strength symmetrical.*	Decreased ROM, swelling, or nodules in joints. Muscle strength asymmetrical or 0–3+
Musculoskeletal and Neurological. Perform finger-to-nose test if indicated. *Smooth and intact.*	*Ataxia* is an unsteady, wavering movement with inability to touch the target. During rapid alternating movements, lack of coordination is *adiadochokinesia.*
Test rapid alternating movements if indicated. *Smooth and intact.*	
Test stereognosis if indicated. *Patient identifies key or other object.*	Inability to identify objects correctly (*astereognosis*) may result from damage to the sensory cortex caused by *stroke.*
Test graphesthesia if indicated. *Patient identifies the number 8 or another number.*	Cortical sensory function may be compromised following a *stroke.*

(text continues on page 932)

Anterior Thorax

Assess breathing effort, rate, rhythm, and pattern; position to breathe. *Breathes easily, with symmetrical expansion and contraction*	Dyspnea, orthopnea, paroxysmal nocturnal dyspnea. Rhythm regular, sitting straight upright or using tripod position to breathe.
Inspect chest shape and skin. *A:P to transverse ratio 1:2 symmetrical. Skin intact.* If patient is on an examination table, move to front of patient. Inspect costovertebral angle, configuration, and pulsations. *No pulsations visible. No dyspnea, retractions, or accessory muscle use.*	Barrel chest, funnel chest, pigeon chest, thoracic kyphoscoliosis.
Auscultate breath sounds. *Bronchovesicular sounds midline, vesicular in lung periphery. Lung sounds clear.*	Diminished or absent breath sounds, bronchial or bronchovesicular sounds in lung periphery. Describe adventitious sounds (crackles, gurgles, wheezes, stridor, pleural rub). Are they inspiratory or expiratory? Do they clear with coughing? Where specifically do you hear them?
Assess for cough, inspect sputum. *No cough or sputum.*	Cough (brassy, harsh, loose, productive) present. Sputum (color, consistency, amount) present.
Inspect precordium. *Point of maximal impulse (PMI) may be visible or absent.*	PMI lateral to midclavicular line (MCL); heaves or thrills.
Assess heart rate, rhythm, murmurs, and extra sounds. *Heart rate and rhythm regular. No gallops, murmurs, or rubs.*	Tachycardia, bradycardia, irregular rhythm, murmurs (systolic vs. diastolic), extra sounds (S3, S4, friction rub).
Auscultate heart with bell at apex and left sternal border with patient lying down. Auscultate heart with diaphragm in aortic, pulmonic, left sternal border, tricuspid, mitral with patient on left side. *Heart rate and rhythm regular; no murmurs, gallops, or rubs.*	If rhythm is irregular, identify if the irregularity has a pattern or is totally irregular. For example, every third beat missed would be a regular irregular rhythm. No detectable pattern is characteristic of *atrial fibrillation*, common in older adults. Murmurs, rubs, or gallops are abnormal in adults.
Palpate chest for fremitus, thrill, heaves, and PMI. *Tactile fremitus symmetrical; no thrill, heave, or lift. Cardiac impulse nonpalpable.*	Asymmetrical fremitus may occur with unilateral disease (eg, lung tumor). Thrills, heaves, and lifts indicate turbulence over a valve and are abnormal.
Percuss anterior chest from apex to base and sides. *Lung fields resonant with dullness over heart area.*	Dull lung percussion indicates increased consolidation as with *pneumonia.*
Auscultate carotid artery. *No bruit.*	Bruits over the carotid indicate *carotid artery stenosis.*

Female Breasts

Inspect the breasts. Have patient raise arms overhead, press hands together, and lean forward. *No retraction or dimpling; symmetrical movement.*	Retraction, dimpling, or discharge may indicate *breast cancer.*
Palpate breasts and nipple for discharge. *No lesions or masses; no discharge. Nontender.*	
Palpate axillary nodes. *Axillary nodes not palpable, nontender.*	Positive nodes may indicate *breast cancer*, especially if immovable or tender.

Abdomen

Inspect abdomen. *Abdomen symmetrical, rounded, or flat. Smooth, intact skin without lesions or rashes. Peristalsis and pulsations evident in thin patients. Flat, round umbilicus.*	Scars, striae, ecchymosis, lesions, prominent dilated veins, rashes, marked pulsation. Red, everted, enlarged, or tender umbilicus.

Technique and Normal Findings (continued)	Abnormal Findings (continued)
Auscultate bowel sounds. *Bowel sounds present all quadrants.*	Hypoactive, hyperactive, or absent bowel sounds.
Auscultate aorta, renal, and femoral arteries with bell. *No bruit.*	Venous hum, friction rub, or bruits are abnormal arterial sounds.
Percuss abdomen in all quadrants and for gastric bubble. *Abdomen tympanic in all quadrants. Gastric bubble percussed 6th left intercostal space (ICS) at MCL.*	Abdomen dull or flat.
Percuss liver margin at right MCL. *Liver border above ribs at right MCL.*	Liver margin below ribs.
Percuss spleen. *Spleen percussed in 10th left ICS posterior to midaxillary line.*	Spleen that deviates downward and medially.
Palpate abdominal tenderness, distention in all quadrants. *Nontender, soft.* Palpate liver, spleen, and kidneys. *Liver lower border less than one finger below costal border at right MCL. Spleen and kidneys nonpalpable.*	Large masses, hard, tenderness with guarding or rigidity, rebound tenderness. Liver palpable more than one finger below costal border at right MCL.
Palpate aorta, femoral pulses, and inguinal lymph nodes or hernias. *Aorta palpable, smooth. Femoral pulses 2–3+. No inguinal nodes or hernias.*	An enlarged aorta (>3 cm) or one with lateral pulsations that are palpable can indicate *abdominal aortic aneurysm.*
Evaluate swallowing, chewing, aspiration risk, special diet. *Eats >75% of meal without difficulty.*	Dysphagia, impaired chewing, impaired swallowing, medically prescribed diet, tube feedings, significant weight gain/loss.
Ask about nausea, vomiting, constipation, diarrhea. *No N/V/D.*	Nausea, vomiting, constipation, or diarrhea. Describe characteristics of emesis (eg, coffee grounds, blood).
Inspect stool; record last bowel movement. Ask about passing flatus. *Last BM within patient's normal, soft and brown. Passing flatus.*	Dark stool may indicate blood in it. If hemorrhoids are present, the stool may be normal but have bright red blood coating it.
Inspect urine color, character, and amount with voiding. *Urine clear, yellow, and >30 ml/ hour.*	Urine dark, bloody, red, with sediment, cloudy, or <30 mL/hr.

Lower Extremities

Inspect skin and nails for symmetry, edema, veins, and lesions. *Toenails white and smooth. Skin intact, slightly pale, and symmetrical, without edema, varicose veins, or lesions.*	Note areas of pressure on heels and if they blanch with pressure. Lesions, ulcers, varicosities, edema. Mottled, ruddy, reddened or flaky skin. Note indurations with infection or inflammation.
Palpate dorsalis pedis pulses bilaterally. Palpate popliteal pulse and posterior tibial pulse. *Pulses 2–3+.*	Diminished or absent pulses. If present, obtain Doppler for assessment. Bounding (4+) pulses are also abnormal.
Assess capillary refill on both feet. *Brisk capillary refill <3 seconds.*	Capillary refill >3 seconds
Inspect and palpate edema on ankle, shin. *No edema.*	1+ barely perceptible (2 mm) 2+ moderate (4 mm) 3+ moderate (6 mm) 4+ severe (>8 mm)

(text continues on page 934)

Technique and Normal Findings (continued)	Abnormal Findings (continued)
Palpate for tenderness and temperature. *Feet warm, no tenderness.*	Tenderness to palpation, feet cool or cold.
Palpate lower extremities and joints from hips to toes. *No tenderness or swelling.*	
Observe ROM of joints. *Full joint ROM.*	Limited or reduced ROM.
Test muscle strength on feet, observe for symmetry. Test muscle strength in hips, knees, and ankles. *Strength 4–5+.*	Strength 0–3+
Test sensation. *Appropriately identifies when touched.*	Loss of sensation
Obtain reflex hammer. Perform deep tendon reflexes— patellar, Achilles, and Babinski. *Patellar, Achilles DTRs 2+; Babinski negative.*	If reflexes are 3–4+ they are brisker than normal. If they are 1+–0 they are diminished or absent. A positive Babinski indicates a poor neurological outcome.

Posterior Thorax

Move behind patient. Palpate thyroid. *Thyroid borders palpable, no enlargement, nodules, or masses noted.*	Thyroid enlargement or masses can be seen more easily when the patient swallows and while illuminating the neck with a tangential light.
Inspect skin, symmetry, configuration, and observe respirations. *Chest symmetrical, oval, without barrel chest. AP: transverse ratio 1:2. Respirations 20 without dyspnea.*	In barrel chest, which can accompany *COPD*, the transverse: AP ratio approximates 1:1, giving the chest a round appearance.
Palpate spine and scapulae. *Spine straight, without scoliosis, kyphosis, or lordosis. Scapulae symmetrical.*	Skeletal scoliosis and kyphosis can limit respiratory excursion. Asymmetry and paradoxical respirations occur in flail chest.
Assess tactile fremitus. *Tactile fremitus symmetrical.*	Increased tactile fremitus over an area indicates increased consolidation.
Percuss posterior chest from apex to base to sides. *Lung fields resonant.*	Dullness occurs with increased consolidation; hyper-resonance occurs with hyper-inflation as in *COPD*.
Test flank tenderness (kidney). *No tenderness to indirect percussion.*	Kidney tenderness is present with *urinary tract infection*.
Auscultate breath sounds. *Breath sounds clear.*	Coarse breath sounds are abnormal. Crackles, gurgles (ronchii), and wheezing are abnormal adventitious sounds.
Inspect lower back, buttocks (redness, symmetry). *No redness, breakdown.*	Any redness, especially over pressure areas, is a concern. Scoliosis, lordosis, and kyphosis are abnormal spine findings.
Inspect spine. *Spine straight, skin intact.*	

Gait and Balance/Fall Risk

Evaluate fall risk: history of falling, secondary diagnosis, ambulatory aid, IV therapy, gait, and mental status. *Scores at low risk on fall scale.*	Gait abnormalities include hesitancy, unsteadiness, staggering, reaching for external support, high stepping, foot scraping, inability to raise the foot completely off the floor, persistent toe or heel walking, excessive pointing of toes inward or outward, asymmetry of step height or length, limping, stooping, wavering, shuffling, waddling, excessive swinging of shoulders or pelvis, and slow or rapid speed.

Musculoskeletal and Neurological

Perform heel-to-shin test for coordination. *Smooth, coordinated movement*. Have patient stand. Note muscle strength and coordination when moving. *Moves easily in the environment*.

The dominant side usually has slightly better coordination. Poor coordination may be from pain, injury, deformity, or *cerebellar disorders*. Coordination is often tested during assessment of the musculoskeletal system, but it is actually an assessment of the neurological system.

Observe spinal alignment, hip level, gluteal and knee folds. *Spine straight, posture erect*. Assess spine flexion, extension, lateral bending, and rotation. *Full ROM in spine*.

Scoliosis or low back pain may cause the patient to lean forward or to the side when standing or sitting.

Ask patient to walk on heels and then toes, and then to stand on one foot and then the other. *Good balance and coordination*.

Skin Breakdown

Evaluate risk for skin breakdown: sensory perception, moisture, activity, mobility, nutrition, friction, and shear. *Scores at low risk for skin breakdown*.

The Braden scale scores patients from 1 to 4 in six subscales: sensory perception, moisture, activity, mobility, nutrition, and friction (Braden & Bergstrom, 1989). High scores place the patient at high risk.

Wounds, Drains, Devices

Assess intravenous, drainage, catheter, suction. *Wound healing, drains intact, catheter draining well, suction on. IV site clean, dry intact without erythema or tenderness*.

Pressure ulcers may be deep tissue, Stage I, Stage II, Stage III, Stage IV, or unstagable (NPUAP, 2007). Stages I and II are partial thickness into the dermis. Stages III and IV are full thickness. Wound drainage is classified as serous (clear), sanguineous (bloody), serosanguineous (mixed), fibrinous (sticky yellow), or purulent (pus). Note any signs or symptoms of infection.

Male Genitalia

Obtain gloves and hemoccult card. *No redness, discharge skin intact*. Palpate the scrotum for tenderness, lumps, and masses. *No tenderness, lumps, or masses*.

Assess for inguinal hernia. *No hernia*.

Abnormal genital hair findings are no hair, patchy growth, or distribution in a female or triangular pattern with base over the pubis. Observe for infestations such as *pediculosis, scabies,* or parasites. Look for inflammation, lesions, or dermatitis. *Candidiasis* infections cause crusty, multiple, red, round erosions and pustules; this infection is associated with immunological deficiencies. *Tinea curis* (commonly referred to as "jock itch") is a fungal infection on the patient's groin and upper thighs. It appears with large red, scaly patches that are extremely itchy. Tinea cruris rarely involves the scrotum.

Female Genitalia

Obtain gloves, speculum, gel, and hemoccult card. Inspect perineal and perianal areas. *No redness or tenderness, skin intact*.

Symptoms of herpes simplex virus 2 include vulvar or vaginal pain, flu-like symptoms (eg, chills, fever), sores on the vulva or genital region, scattered vesicles along the labia, matching vesicles on the labia reflecting "kissing" lesions, surface ulcerations or crusted healing lesions, and inguinal lymphadenopathy.

Insert speculum. Inspect cervix and vaginal walls. *Vaginal walls pink, no lesions. Cervix pink, round, no discharge*. Obtain specimens. Remove speculum. *No infections, Pap test negative*.

(text continues on page 936)

Technique and Normal Findings (continued)	Abnormal Findings (continued)
Perform bimanual examination of cervix, uterus, and adnexa. *No pain when moving the cervix, uterus midline; no enlargement, masses or tenderness. Adnexa and ovaries smooth, no masses or tenderness.*	
Rectum	
Inspect perianal area. *No redness or tenderness; skin intact.* With lubricated finger, palpate rectal wall (and prostate in male). *No hemorrhoids, fissures, lesions, masses, or tenderness. Rectal wall intact. Male: prostate smooth and round.* Obtain stool sample for occult blood. *Stool soft and brown.*	Look for thrombosed hemorrhoids, rectal fissures, or hard stool. Hemorrhoids can be classified as external or internal. Hemorrhoids are usually caused by constant or excessive straining upon defecation.
Closure	
• Summarize findings for patient. "Does this sound accurate?" • Assess room for safety (bedside table, lights, call light, toileting). "Do you have any concerns?" • Assess for questions or further needs. "Is there anything else I can do?" • Wash hands or use hand gel when leaving.	Summarizing findings provides closure and ensures accurate conclusions. Asking an open-ended question allows the patient to add any other information that might have been overlooked. Assessing for safety is of primary importance. Always assess the patient and environment for risks. Follow up on care planning and interventions for the next visit.

 ## Lifespan and Cultural Considerations

The complete RN assessment needs adaptations for the age, gender, and cultural background of the patient. A woman's body changes during pregnancy, and fetal growth needs to be assessed (see Chapter 27). A newborn requires a special assessment to evaluate breathing, circulation, and alertness (see Chapter 28). The child may need to be examined while sitting in a parent's lap. An adolescent will need privacy and a safe place to express concerns (see Chapter 29). The older adult may fatigue easily and need to have the assessment divided over several time periods (see Chapter 30). Some men or women, especially in some cultures, prefer to have a health care provider of the same gender (see Chapter 11). A translator may be used when the patient has limited English. Lifespan and cultural consideration are included when providing individualized and holistic care.

Documenting Abnormal Findings

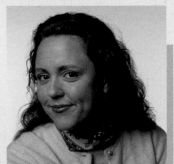

Mrs. Suleri's primary problem is related to the bleeding caused by ulcerative colitis. Other issues that can be clustered and further assessed include diarrhea from ulcerative colitis, pain from cramping, anemia from blood loss, fatigue from anemia, and nutritional status related to obesity and dietary intake. Focusing on these problems, the nurse notes the following findings.

Inspection: Five dark brown liquid stools over 12 hours totaling 500 cm³. Hemoccult positive for blood. Reports abdominal pain primarily in lower quadrants. Rates pain as 5 on a 1–10 scale. Describes it as a cramping, gnawing sensation that comes in waves but never completely goes away, rates it as 2/10 when best. Skin color pale, P 110 beats/min, BP 112/ 80 mm Hg, last hemoglobin 10 g/dL (low) and hematocrit 31% (low). Intake for past 12 hours 800 mL and output 860 mL. Weight 92 kg, down 1.5 kg from yesterday. Abdomen protuberant.

Auscultation: Bowel sounds hyperactive in all four quadrants.

Palpation: Abdomen soft but tender to light palpation. Facial grimace present, guarding abdomen.

Percussion: Abdomen tympanic.

Hospital Assessment

The nurse in the hospital performs a comprehensive assessment of the patient on admission. This assessment is more detailed and complete than screening and focused assessments that evaluate progress toward a goal later in the stay. The comprehensive admitting, screening, and focused assessments are important in establishing and maintaining documentation of current findings.

Comprehensive Admitting Assessment

The nurse performs the initial hospital assessment and documents results in the patient chart. It includes collection of both subjective and objective data. Subjective assessment of risk factors, common symptoms, and health history are the same as previously described; however, the hospital nurse may need to gather history from secondary sources such as the chart or relatives to avoid fatiguing the acutely ill patient. The general survey and vital signs are also the same. Risks for falling and skin breakdown are added because of the hospital environment.

Because acuity of the hospitalized patient is often increased, the nurse prioritizes which data to collect related to the presenting problems and performs a basic screening of other body systems. He or she uses clinical judgment about which items to include and to omit. Techniques are adapted based on the individual patient situation. The admitting assessment is usually documented in a separate area of the patient chart, and may include input from other health care professionals. Refer to Chapter 5 for a common admitting assessment on the hospitalized patient in a systems format.

Initial patient history and head-to-toe physical examination may take 30 or more minutes to complete, but subsequent assessments are shorter because they focus on problem areas rather than the entire body. It is important to make this assessment comfortable and smooth with practice. The assessment is adapted to the patient, in a style that is professional yet personal and individualized. The nurse also allows some time for documentation of findings and analysis of data. In addition to positive findings, it is essential to document absence of findings because, in the legal world, "if it's not documented, it's not done." For example, if the patient develops acute confusion, it is important for the nurse to look back in the chart and see "no confusion" to identify this change in status as significant.

Some time is also needed for patient teaching, validation of problems, mutual goal setting, and discussion of an action plan. This way the nurse knows the patient and his or her concerns well, and agrees on an action plan to establish a trusting and lasting relationship. Creating and maintaining an intimate and professional therapeutic relationship to make a difference in the outcomes is one of the most important and satisfying elements in the process.

Table 31-3	Basic RN Screening Assessment
System	**Normal Findings**
Pain	0 on pain scale
Resp	On room air Breath sounds clear to auscultation Respiration unlabored and symmetrical
CV	Pulse regular No edema VS stable
Neuro	Responds appropriately Speech clear Moves all extremities
GI	Bowel sounds present Tolerates prescribed diet Abdomen soft, nontender, nondistended Passing flatus Last BM _____
GU	Continent Urine output adequate Urine clear yellow
M/S	Moves all extremities without difficulty Activity at expected level
Skin/mucosa	Skin warm, dry and intact Mucous membranes pink and moist Skin color within patient's normal Sacrum and heels skin intact
Safety	Low fall risk, environmental check Double check IVs, tubes, drains
Psych/social	Patient calm and interactive

Screening Hospital Assessment

Because of the complications of immobility and being in a hospital environment, the nurse performs a short screening assessment at the beginning of each shift. He or she does so for all patients. This assessment typically takes 5 to 10 minutes to provide a basis for comparison in the event of a sudden change in condition. This screening enables the nurse to identify patient acuity; need for immediate treatment, teaching, or discharge planning; and care priorities. See Table 31-3 for a typical beginning-of-shift screening assessment for a patient with normal findings. The nurse completes and documents this assessment on an assessment form.

Focused Hospital Assessment

The RN working in a hospital also performs a focused assessment on each patient, which can take anywhere from 1 minute when assessing one or two items, to 10 to 20 minutes for a more complete review of complex problems (Fig. 31-4). Therefore, the nurse must prioritize information. Usually an abnormal finding or diagnosis triggers the need for a more complete and focused assessment. The nurse also uses clinical judgment to determine which data are most important.

Initially the beginning nurse may need to consult with a more experienced nurse, but with experience typical patterns emerge. These assessments are individualized to the specific patients. Trends of improving or declining status are identified, treatment is modified, and other health care providers are consulted for changes in the patient's orders or need for further diagnostic testing. The documenting abnormal findings example above illustrates how the assessment is focused on the individual patient's problems.

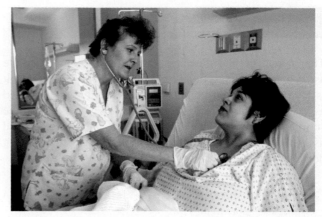

Figure 31.4 Re-assessments in hospital settings focus on key areas for ongoing evaluation. One example would be assessing the lungs in a postpartum woman.

Table 31-4	Common Nursing Diagnoses Applied to Mrs. Suleri		
Diagnosis and Related Factors	**Point of Differentiation**	**Assessment Characteristics**	**Nursing Interventions**
Diarrhea related to inflammatory changes of the bowel	Loose, unformed, and watery stools	Three or more loose liquid stools per day, abdominal cramps, hyperactive bowel sounds, urgency to use toilet	Observe and document stool characteristics. Provide medications as ordered.* Ensure adequate hydration and electrolyte replacements.*
Acute pain related to cramping in ulcerative colitis	Unpleasant sensory and emotional experience arising from actual or potential tissue damage	Increases in vital signs, restlessness, moaning, crying, hypervigilance, irritability, sighing, guarding behavior, positioning, verbal report	Complete pain assessment. Provide medications as ordered,* distraction, relaxation, massage, use of heat or cold pack.
Fatigue related to low hemoglobin and hematocrit and inability to sleep	Overwhelming exhaustion; decreased capacity for physical and mental work	Decreased performance, drowsiness, inability to maintain usual routine or to feel restored and energetic after usual sleep	Monitor labs. Provide periods of rest by clustering care. Gradually increase activity as tolerated. Gather resources for home care and daily activities such as house cleaning.
Ineffective coping related to repeat episodes of diarrhea and financial stressors	Inability to accurately appraise the stressors, inadequate choices of responses, inability to use resources	Inability to meet role expectations, sleep disturbance, fatigue, destructive behavior, verbalization of inability to cope	Accurately assess stressors and effectiveness of coping methods. Identify additional resources available. Allow time for patient to express feelings.

*Collaborative interventions.

Evidence-Based Critical Thinking

Common Laboratory and Diagnostic Testing

Many patients in primary care settings and most hospitalized patients have a standard set of screening tests done to identify common problems. Electrolytes are measured to identify problems with balances.

⚠ *SAFETY ALERT 31.2*

Serum potassium level may affect nerve or heart cell conduction, leading to arrhythmias and potentially cardiac arrest. Potassium must be maintained within normal limits and abnormalities must be corrected promptly.

Serum sodium can be a reflection of sodium intake, but is more likely a reflection of having too much or too little water, therefore diluting or concentrating the sodium. The red blood cells, hemoglobin, and hematocrit reflect the blood's oxygen-carrying capacity. Many patients also receive a chest x-ray that can identify areas of infection, collapse, or fluid. Routine urinalysis may be ordered to identify if there is an infection, blood, or sediment. Additional tests depend on the individual patient's problems. It is important for the nurse to be able to recognize the significance of abnormal test results.

Diagnostic Reasoning

Nursing diagnoses must be individualized to the patient and his or her current conditions. These include both actual diagnoses and those for which the patient is at risk. Table 31-4 provides a comparison of nursing diagnoses, abnormal findings, and interventions for Mrs. Suleri (NANDA-I, 2009).

Analyzing Findings

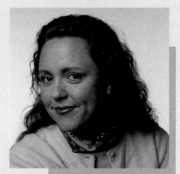

The nurse analyzes findings and synthesizes information to initiate a plan of care. The nursing thinking is shown in progress notes, in this case, using the SOAP format. The subjective and objective data are from the assessment that the nurse has performed. The analysis then leads to a preliminary plan of care.

Subjective: "I've been having about 10 bloody stools a day, and I'm just exhausted. This pain and cramping have just really gotten to me."

Objective: Reports abdominal pain primarily in lower quadrants. Rates pain as 5 on a 1–10 scale. Describes it as a cramping, gnawing sensation that comes in waves but never completely goes away, rates it as 2/10 when best. Soaking in her bathtub and staying quiet seem to alleviate the pain. Stress, coffee, increased activity, and the end of the day make it worse. Hopes to achieve pain of 2/10 at peak and reduction in cramping. Functional goal is to return to normal activities at home, including cooking meals and transporting children, and also return to work. Concerned about financial issues. Facial grimace present, guarding abdomen.

Assessment: Pain related to ulcerative colitis exacerbation as evidenced by pain 5/10, facial grimace and guarding. Risk for ineffective coping because of illness and financial concerns.

Plan: Provide medication for pain as ordered. Teach relaxation techniques as a nonpharmacological pain measure. Limit mobility and provide rest. Allow periods of sleep at night. Assess foods that are preferred. Contact social work to evaluate need for additional resources.

T. Sazi, RN

Critical Thinking Challenge

- What other assessment should be gathered based upon the number of bloody stools?
- Are there other items that the nurse may want to assess based upon the pain level?
- What other body systems might be affected based upon the known assessments?

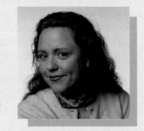

Collaboration with Other Health Care Providers

In many facilities, nurses initiate referrals for based on assessment findings. Social workers help patients to cope with and solve issues related to family and personal problems. Some social workers help clients who face a disability, life-threatening disease, inadequate housing, unemployment, financial concern, or substance abuse. Social workers also assist families with domestic conflicts, such as child or spousal abuse. In the hospital setting they assist with financial issues, patient placement, and funding for placements and resources after discharge.

Mrs. Suleri has been experiencing many of the problems outlined above; therefore, a social work consult is indicated. The following conversation illustrates how the nurse might organize the data and make recommendations about the patient's situation.

Situation: Hello, Margie (the social worker for the unit). I'm taking care of Mrs. Suleri today. Do you know her? (Margie replies no.)

Background: She is a 44-year-old woman who was admitted with bleeding related to her ulcerative colitis. She is married and has two children ages 15 and 13 years old.

Assessment: She is currently employed but has been missing a lot of work because of her colitis. She's worried about caring for her family as she has two young teenagers. She also is worried about her finances and medical bills as her insurance only covers 80% of the hospital bill.

Recommendations: Do you think that you would be able to see her in the next day or so to talk with her about resources?

Critical Thinking Challenge

- What other assessments might the nurse make based upon Mrs. Suleri's role in the family?
- How might her additional stressors be affecting her physiological health?
- What other nursing diagnoses might be considered regarding her psychological health?

Pulling It All Together: Reflection and Critical Thinking

The nurse uses assessment data to formulate a nursing care plan with patient outcomes and interventions for Mrs. Suleri. Outcomes are specific to the patient, realistic to achieve, measurable, and have a time frame for meeting the outcome. The interventions are actions that the nurse performs, based on evidence and practice guidelines. After these interventions are completed, the nurse re-evaluates Mrs. Suleri and documents the findings in the chart to show progress toward the patient outcome. The nurse uses critical thinking and judgment to continue or revise the diagnosis, outcomes, or interventions. This is often in the form of a care plan or case note similar to the one seen below.

Nursing Diagnosis	Patient Outcomes	Nursing Interventions	Rationale	Evaluation
Fatigue related to anemia as evidenced by low hematocrit, hemoglobin, pale, tired	Patient will explain an energy conservation plan to offset effects of fatigue.	Assess severity of fatigue on a 0–10 scale. Evaluate adequacy of nutrition and sleep patterns. Collaborate with provider to treat anemia.	Fatigue is discomfort that can be rated using a numeric scale. A commonly suggested treatment is rest. Fatigue is related to the anemia from bleeding.	Patient stated that she has not been sleeping well because of cramping, pain, and frequent stools at night. Will plan to provide medication for diarrhea and sleeping tonight. Would like to have sign on the door asking to not be woken up. Taking 50% of meals at this time.

Sources: NANDA-I (2009); Bulechek, et al. (2008); Moorhead, et al.(2007).

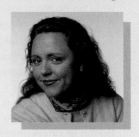

Using the previous steps of diagnostic reasoning, organizing, and prioritizing, consider all the case study findings woven throughout this chapter. When answering the following questions, begin drawing conclusions and see how the pieces of assessment must work together to create an environment for personalized, appropriate, and accurate care.

- How will the nurse individualize the admitting history to focus it on Mrs. Suleri?
- How will the nurse focus the physical assessments considering Mrs. Suleri's diagnosis?
- How will the nurse use the assessment information to develop a plan of care?

Key Points

- Health assessment is individualized considering the condition, age, gender, and culture of the patient.
- Nurses adapt assessments depending on scope of practice, clinical setting, and patient situation.
- Indications of unstable status that necessitate intervention include cyanosis or pallor, dyspnea, strained posture, anxious facial expression, distressed appearance, difficulty managing the airway, extremely high or low pulse or blood pressure, acute change in mental status, or new onset of chest pain.
- Subjective data collection includes health promotion, risk factors, history of present problem, past medical and family history, personal and social history, and assessment of common symptoms.
- Objective data collection is organized by body area, moving from head to toes for efficiency.
- Inspection, palpation, percussion, and auscultation are techniques used during the head-to-toe assessment.
- Nurses document and communicate assessment data using appropriate medical terminology.
- Assessment occurs during all phases of the nursing process.
- An accurate and complete health assessment is the foundation for appropriate holistic and individualized nursing care.

Review Questions

1. The nurse performs the first assessment on the hospitalized patient and documents it in the chart as the
   A. sporadic assessment
   B. functional assessment
   C. focused assessment
   D. admitting assessment

2. A patient is anxious, dyspneic, pale, and using accessory muscles to breathe. Vital signs are T 37°C, P 126 beats/min, R 40 breaths/min, and BP 122/74 mm Hg. The type of assessment that the nurse would perform is
   A. acute assessment
   B. general survey
   C. health history
   D. objective assessment

3. The nurse assesses a patient presenting with nausea, vomiting, and diarrhea. When the focused assessment is performed, the nurse performs the following techniques:
   A. Auscultate lungs, auscultate heart, auscultate abdomen
   B. Evaluate for dehydration, assess skin turgor, auscultate lungs
   C. Auscultate abdomen, palpate abdomen, evaluate for dehydration
   D. Palpate abdomen, percuss abdomen, auscultate heart

4. After being given report and gathering data from the chart, the nurse will assess a group of four patients. Which one will the nurse assess first?
   A. 32-year-old man with an open wound and receiving antibiotics
   B. 66-year-old woman 2 days postoperatively following ankle surgery
   C. 45-year-old man with HIV and *Pneumocystis pneumonia* with dyspnea
   D. 88-year-old woman with confusion and stroke 4 days ago

5. The nurse gathers subjective data related to the history of the present problem. Items that are included are
   A. onset, location, duration, character, aggravating/ associated factors, relieving factors, temporal factors, severity
   B. asymmetry, borders, color, diameter
   C. heart rate, respiratory effort, response, color
   D. eye opening, verbal response, motor response

6. The nurse usually performs a complete physical examination with elements in the following order:
   A. Face, heart, legs, arms
   B. Head, abdomen, lungs, legs
   C. Eyes, heart, abdomen, legs
   D. Ears, back, lungs, arms

7. A patient develops a sudden onset of acute chest pain. In addition to a complete description of the symptoms, what objective assessment is a priority?
   A. Pulse, blood pressure, peripheral pulses
   B. Heart sounds, rate, and rhythm
   C. Circulation, sensation, and movement
   D. Murmurs, rubs, and gallops

8. A 50-year-old patient is seen in the clinic for an annual physical examination and screening. The patient has no known health problems. This type of care is referred to as
   A. primary prevention
   B. promotion prevention
   C. tertiary prevention
   D. healthy prevention

9. The nurse assesses if the patient outcome, "Patient drinks 1 L every shift" has been met. This is called
   A. assessment
   B. planning
   C. implementation
   D. evaluation

10. Auscultation is one of the most important components of which body systems?
    A. Reproductive, neurological, integumentary
    B. Cardiovascular, pulmonary, gastrointestinal
    C. Pulmonary, gastrointestinal, neurological
    D. Gastrointestinal, neurological, reproductive

References

American Heart Association. (2009). *About high blood pressure*. Retrieved March 18, 2009, from http://www.americanheart.org/presenter.jhtml?identifier=468

Braden, B. & Bergstrom, M. (1989). Clinical utility of the Braden scale for predicting pressure sore risk. *Advances in Skin and Wound Care, 2*(3), 44–51.

Bulechek, G. B., Butcher, H. K., & McCloskey Dochterman. (2008). *Nursing Interventions Classification (NIC)* (5th ed.) St. Louis, MO: Mosby.

Erikson, E. H. (1963). *Childhood and society* (2nd ed.). New York: W.W. Norton & Co.

Healthy people 2010: What are its goals? (n.d.). Retrieved January 7, 2007, from http://www.healthypeople.gov/About/goals.htm

Moorhead, S., Johnson, M., & Mass, M. (2007). *Nursing Outcomes Classification (NOC)* (4th ed.). Philadelphia: Mosby.

National Pressure Ulcer Advisory Panel (NPUAP). (2007). *Pressure ulcer stages*. Retrieved June 24, 2010, from http://www.npuap.org/pr2.htm

North American Nursing Diagnosis Association. (2009). *Nursing diagnoses, 2009–2011 Edition: Definitions and classifications (NANDA NURSING DIAGNOSIS)*. West Sussex UK: John Wiley & Sons.

Offner, P. J., Heit, J., & Roberts, R. (2007). Implementation of a rapid response team decreases cardiac arrest outside of the intensive care unit. *Journal of Trauma, 62*(5), 1223–1227; discussion 1227–1228.

USPSTF. (2006). *Guide to clinical preventative services*. Retrieved August 16, 2007, from http://www.ahrq.gov/clinic/pocketgd/gcps1.htm#ref1

The Jensen suite offers these additional resources to enhance learning and facilitate understanding of this chapter:

- thePoint on line resource, http//thepoint.lww.com/Jensen1E
- Student CD-ROM included with the book
- *Laboratory Manual for Nursing Health Assessment: A Best Practice Approach*
- *Pocket Guide for Nursing Health Assessment: A Best Practice Approach*

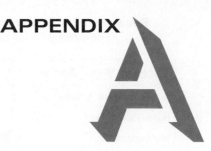

Immunization Reference Charts

Recommended Immunization Schedule for Persons Aged 0 Through 6 Years—United States • 2010
For those who fall behind or start late, see the catch-up schedule

Vaccine ▼ Age ▶	Birth	1 month	2 months	4 months	6 months	12 months	15 months	18 months	19–23 months	2–3 years	4–6 years
Hepatitis B[1]	HepB	HepB			HepB						
Rotavirus[2]			RV	RV	RV[2]						
Diphtheria, Tetanus, Pertussis[3]			DTaP	DTaP	DTaP	*see footnote*[3]	DTaP				DTaP
Haemophilus influenzae type b[4]			Hib	Hib	Hib[4]	Hib					
Pneumococcal[5]			PCV	PCV	PCV	PCV				PPSV	
Inactivated Poliovirus[6]			IPV	IPV		IPV					IPV
Influenza[7]						Influenza (Yearly)					
Measles, Mumps, Rubella[8]						MMR		*see footnote*[8]			MMR
Varicella[9]						Varicella		*see footnote*[9]			Varicella
Hepatitis A[10]						HepA (2 doses)				HepA Series	
Meningococcal[11]										MCV	

Range of recommended ages for all children except certain high-risk groups

Range of recommended ages for certain high-risk groups

This schedule includes recommendations in effect as of December 15, 2009. Any dose not administered at the recommended age should be administered at a subsequent visit, when indicated and feasible. The use of a combination vaccine generally is preferred over separate injections of its equivalent component vaccines. Considerations should include provider assessment, patient preference, and the potential for adverse events. Providers should consult the relevant Advisory Committee on Immunization Practices statement for detailed recommendations: **http://www.cdc.gov/vaccines/pubs/acip-list.htm**. Clinically significant adverse events that follow immunization should be reported to the Vaccine Adverse Event Reporting System (VAERS) at **http://www.vaers.hhs.gov** or by telephone, **800-822-7967**.

1. **Hepatitis B vaccine (HepB).** (Minimum age: birth)
   At birth:
   - Administer monovalent HepB to all newborns before hospital discharge.
   - If mother is hepatitis B surface antigen (HBsAg)-positive, administer HepB and 0.5 mL of hepatitis B immune globulin (HBIG) within 12 hours of birth.
   - If mother's HBsAg status is unknown, administer HepB within 12 hours of birth. Determine mother's HBsAg status as soon as possible and, if HBsAg-positive, administer HBIG (no later than age 1 week).
   After the birth dose:
   - The HepB series should be completed with either monovalent HepB or a combination vaccine containing HepB. The second dose should be administered at age 1 or 2 months. Monovalent HepB vaccine should be used for doses administered before age 6 weeks. The final dose should be administered no earlier than age 24 weeks.
   - Infants born to HBsAg-positive mothers should be tested for HBsAg and antibody to HBsAg 1 to 2 months after completion of at least 3 doses of the HepB series, at age 9 through 18 months (generally at the next well-child visit).
   - Administration of 4 doses of HepB to infants is permissible when a combination vaccine containing HepB is administered after the birth dose. The fourth dose should be administered no earlier than age 24 weeks.
2. **Rotavirus vaccine (RV).** (Minimum age: 6 weeks)
   - Administer the first dose at age 6 through 14 weeks (maximum age: 14 weeks 6 days). Vaccination should not be initiated for infants aged 15 weeks 0 days or older.
   - The maximum age for the final dose in the series is 8 months 0 days.
   - If Rotarix is administered at ages 2 and 4 months, a dose at 6 months is not indicated.
3. **Diphtheria and tetanus toxoids and acellular pertussis vaccine (DTaP).** (Minimum age: 6 weeks)
   - The fourth dose may be administered as early as age 12 months, provided at least 6 months have elapsed since the third dose.
   - Administer the final dose in the series at age 4 through 6 years.
4. ***Haemophilus influenzae* type b conjugate vaccine (Hib).** (Minimum age: 6 weeks)
   - If PRP-OMP (PedvaxHIB or Comvax [HepB-Hib]) is administered at ages 2 and 4 months, a dose at age 6 months is not indicated.
   - TriHiBit (DTaP/Hib) and Hiberix (PRP-T) should not be used for doses at ages 2, 4, or 6 months for the primary series but can be used as the final dose in children aged 12 months through 4 years.
5. **Pneumococcal vaccine.** (Minimum age: 6 weeks for pneumococcal conjugate vaccine [PCV]; 2 years for pneumococcal polysaccharide vaccine [PPSV])
   - PCV is recommended for all children aged younger than 5 years. Administer 1 dose of PCV to all healthy children aged 24 through 59 months who are not completely vaccinated for their age.
   - Administer PPSV 2 or more months after last dose of PCV to children aged 2 years or older with certain underlying medical conditions, including a cochlear implant. See *MMWR* 1997;46(No. RR-8).
6. **Inactivated poliovirus vaccine (IPV)** (Minimum age: 6 weeks)
   - The final dose in the series should be administered on or after the fourth birthday and at least 6 months following the previous dose.
   - If 4 doses are administered prior to age 4 years a fifth dose should be administered at age 4 through 6 years. See *MMWR* 2009;58(30):829–30.
7. **Influenza vaccine (seasonal).** (Minimum age: 6 months for trivalent inactivated influenza vaccine [TIV]; 2 years for live, attenuated influenza vaccine [LAIV])
   - Administer annually to children aged 6 months through 18 years.
   - For healthy children aged 2 through 6 years (i.e., those who do not have underlying medical conditions that predispose them to influenza complications), either LAIV or TIV may be used, except LAIV should not be given to children aged 2 through 4 years who have had wheezing in the past 12 months.
   - Children receiving TIV should receive 0.25 mL if aged 6 through 35 months or 0.5 mL if aged 3 years or older.
   - Administer 2 doses (separated by at least 4 weeks) to children aged younger than 9 years who are receiving influenza vaccine for the first time or who were vaccinated for the first time during the previous influenza season but only received 1 dose.
   - For recommendations for use of influenza A (H1N1) 2009 monovalent vaccine see *MMWR* 2009;58(No. RR-10).
8. **Measles, mumps, and rubella vaccine (MMR).** (Minimum age: 12 months)
   - Administer the second dose routinely at age 4 through 6 years. However, the second dose may be administered before age 4, provided at least 28 days have elapsed since the first dose.
9. **Varicella vaccine.** (Minimum age: 12 months)
   - Administer the second dose routinely at age 4 through 6 years. However, the second dose may be administered before age 4, provided at least 3 months have elapsed since the first dose.
   - For children aged 12 months through 12 years the minimum interval between doses is 3 months. However, if the second dose was administered at least 28 days after the first dose, it can be accepted as valid.
10. **Hepatitis A vaccine (HepA).** (Minimum age: 12 months)
    - Administer to all children aged 1 year (i.e., aged 12 through 23 months). Administer 2 doses at least 6 months apart.
    - Children not fully vaccinated by age 2 years can be vaccinated at subsequent visits
    - HepA also is recommended for older children who live in areas where vaccination programs target older children, who are at increased risk for infection, or for whom immunity against hepatitis A is desired.
11. **Meningococcal vaccine.** (Minimum age: 2 years for meningococcal conjugate vaccine [MCV4] and for meningococcal polysaccharide vaccine [MPSV4])
    - Administer MCV4 to children aged 2 through 10 years with persistent complement component deficiency, anatomic or functional asplenia, and certain other conditions placing them at high risk.
    - Administer MCV4 to children previously vaccinated with MCV4 or MPSV4 after 3 years if first dose administered at age 2 through 6 years. See *MMWR* 2009;58:1042–3.

The Recommended Immunization Schedules for Persons Aged 0 through 18 Years are approved by the Advisory Committee on Immunization Practices (**http://www.cdc.gov/vaccines/recs/acip**), the American Academy of Pediatrics (**http://www.aap.org**), and the American Academy of Family Physicians (**http://www.aafp.org**).

Department of Health and Human Services • Centers for Disease Control and Prevention

CS207330-A

Recommended Immunization Schedule for Persons Aged 7 Through 18 Years—United States • 2010
For those who fall behind or start late, see the schedule below and the catch-up schedule

Vaccine ▼ Age ▶	7–10 years	11–12 years	13–18 years
Tetanus, Diphtheria, Pertussis[1]		Tdap	Tdap
Human Papillomavirus[2]	see footnote 2	HPV (3 doses)	HPV series
Meningococcal[3]	MCV	MCV	MCV
Influenza[4]	Influenza (Yearly)		
Pneumococcal[5]	PPSV		
Hepatitis A[6]	HepA Series		
Hepatitis B[7]	Hep B Series		
Inactivated Poliovirus[8]	IPV Series		
Measles, Mumps, Rubella[9]	MMR Series		
Varicella[10]	Varicella Series		

Range of recommended ages for all children except certain high-risk groups

Range of recommended ages for catch-up immunization

Range of recommended ages for certain high-risk groups

This schedule includes recommendations in effect as of December 15, 2009. Any dose not administered at the recommended age should be administered at a subsequent visit, when indicated and feasible. The use of a combination vaccine generally is preferred over separate injections of its equivalent component vaccines. Considerations should include provider assessment, patient preference, and the potential for adverse events. Providers should consult the relevant Advisory Committee on Immunization Practices statement for detailed recommendations: **http://www.cdc.gov/vaccines/pubs/acip-list.htm**. Clinically significant adverse events that follow immunization should be reported to the Vaccine Adverse Event Reporting System (VAERS) at **http://www.vaers.hhs.gov** or by telephone, **800-822-7967**.

1. **Tetanus and diphtheria toxoids and acellular pertussis vaccine (Tdap).** (Minimum age: 10 years for Boostrix and 11 years for Adacel)
   - Administer at age 11 or 12 years for those who have completed the recommended childhood DTP/DTaP vaccination series and have not received a tetanus and diphtheria toxoid (Td) booster dose.
   - Persons aged 13 through 18 years who have not received Tdap should receive a dose.
   - A 5-year interval from the last Td dose is encouraged when Tdap is used as a booster dose; however, a shorter interval may be used if pertussis immunity is needed.

2. **Human papillomavirus vaccine (HPV).** (Minimum age: 9 years)
   - Two HPV vaccines are licensed: a quadrivalent vaccine (HPV4) for the prevention of cervical, vaginal and vulvar cancers (in females) and genital warts (in females and males), and a bivalent vaccine (HPV2) for the prevention of cervical cancers in females.
   - HPV vaccines are most effective for both males and females when given before exposure to HPV through sexual contact.
   - HPV4 or HPV2 is recommended for the prevention of cervical precancers and cancers in females.
   - HPV4 is recommended for the prevention of cervical, vaginal and vulvar precancers and cancers and genital warts in females.
   - Administer the first dose to females at age 11 or 12 years.
   - Administer the second dose 1 to 2 months after the first dose and the third dose 6 months after the first dose (at least 24 weeks after the first dose).
   - Administer the series to females at age 13 through 18 years if not previously vaccinated.
   - HPV4 may be administered in a 3-dose series to males aged 9 through 18 years to reduce their likelihood of acquiring genital warts.

3. **Meningococcal conjugate vaccine (MCV4).**
   - Administer at age 11 or 12 years, or at age 13 through 18 years if not previously vaccinated.
   - Administer to previously unvaccinated college freshmen living in a dormitory.
   - Administer MCV4 to children aged 2 through 10 years with persistent complement component deficiency, anatomic or functional asplenia, or certain other conditions placing them at high risk.
   - Administer to children previously vaccinated with MCV4 or MPSV4 who remain at increased risk after 3 years (if first dose administered at age 2 through 6 years) or after 5 years (if first dose administered at age 7 years or older). Persons whose only risk factor is living in on-campus housing are not recommended to receive an additional dose. See *MMWR* 2009;58:1042–3.

4. **Influenza vaccine (seasonal).**
   - Administer annually to children aged 6 months through 18 years.
   - For healthy nonpregnant persons aged 7 through 18 years (i.e., those who do not have underlying medical conditions that predispose them to influenza complications), either LAIV or TIV may be used.
   - Administer 2 doses (separated by at least 4 weeks) to children aged younger than 9 years who are receiving influenza vaccine for the first time or who were vaccinated for the first time during the previous influenza season but only received 1 dose.
   - For recommendations for use of influenza A (H1N1) 2009 monovalent vaccine. See *MMWR* 2009;58(No. RR-10).

5. **Pneumococcal polysaccharide vaccine (PPSV).**
   - Administer to children with certain underlying medical conditions, including a cochlear implant. A single revaccination should be administered after 5 years to children with functional or anatomic asplenia or an immunocompromising condition. See *MMWR* 1997;46(No. RR-8).

6. **Hepatitis A vaccine (HepA).**
   - Administer 2 doses at least 6 months apart.
   - HepA is recommended for children aged older than 23 months who live in areas where vaccination programs target older children, who are at increased risk for infection, or for whom immunity against hepatitis A is desired.

7. **Hepatitis B vaccine (HepB).**
   - Administer the 3-dose series to those not previously vaccinated.
   - A 2-dose series (separated by at least 4 months) of adult formulation Recombivax HB is licensed for children aged 11 through 15 years.

8. **Inactivated poliovirus vaccine (IPV).**
   - The final dose in the series should be administered on or after the fourth birthday and at least 6 months following the previous dose.
   - If both OPV and IPV were administered as part of a series, a total of 4 doses should be administered, regardless of the child's current age.

9. **Measles, mumps, and rubella vaccine (MMR).**
   - If not previously vaccinated, administer 2 doses or the second dose for those who have received only 1 dose, with at least 28 days between doses.

10. **Varicella vaccine.**
    - For persons aged 7 through 18 years without evidence of immunity (see *MMWR* 2007;56[No. RR-4]), administer 2 doses if not previously vaccinated or the second dose if only 1 dose has been administered.
    - For persons aged 7 through 12 years, the minimum interval between doses is 3 months. However, if the second dose was administered at least 28 days after the first dose, it can be accepted as valid.
    - For persons aged 13 years and older, the minimum interval between doses is 28 days.

The Recommended Immunization Schedules for Persons Aged 0 through 18 Years are approved by the Advisory Committee on Immunization Practices (**http://www.cdc.gov/vaccines/recs/acip**), the American Academy of Pediatrics (**http://www.aap.org**), and the American Academy of Family Physicians (**http://www.aafp.org**). Department of Health and Human Services • Centers for Disease Control and Prevention

CS207330-A

Recommended Adult Immunization Schedule
UNITED STATES · 2010
Note: These recommendations *must* be read with the footnotes that follow containing number of doses, intervals between doses, and other important information.

Figure 1. Recommended adult immunization schedule, by vaccine and age group

VACCINE ▼ AGE GROUP▶	19–26 years	27–49 years	50–59 years	60–64 years	≥65 years
Tetanus, diphtheria, pertussis (Td/Tdap)[1,*]	Substitute 1-time dose of Tdap for Td booster; then boost with Td every 10 yrs				Td booster every 10 yrs
Human papillomavirus (HPV)[2,*]	3 doses (females)				
Varicella[3,*]	2 doses				
Zoster[4]				1 dose	
Measles, mumps, rubella (MMR)[5,*]	1 or 2 doses		1 dose		
Influenza[6,*]	1 dose annually				
Pneumococcal (polysaccharide)[7,8]	1 or 2 doses				1 dose
Hepatitis A[9,*]	2 doses				
Hepatitis B[10,*]	3 doses				
Meningococcal[11,*]	1 or more doses				

*Covered by the Vaccine Injury Compensation Program.

For all persons in this category who meet the age requirements and who lack evidence of immunity (e.g., lack documentation of vaccination or have no evidence of prior infection)	Recommended if some other risk factor is present (e.g., on the basis of medical, occupational, lifestyle, or other indications)

No recommendation

Report all clinically significant postvaccination reactions to the Vaccine Adverse Event Reporting System (VAERS). Reporting forms and instructions on filing a VAERS report are available at www.vaers.hhs.gov or by telephone, 800-822-7967.

Information on how to file a Vaccine Injury Compensation Program claim is available at www.hrsa.gov/vaccinecompensation or by telephone, 800-338-2382. To file a claim for vaccine injury, contact the U.S. Court of Federal Claims, 717 Madison Place, N.W., Washington, D.C. 20005; telephone, 202-357-6400.

Additional information about the vaccines in this schedule, extent of available data, and contraindications for vaccination is also available at www.cdc.gov/vaccines or from the CDC-INFO Contact Center at 800-CDC-INFO (800-232-4636) in English and Spanish, 24 hours a day, 7 days a week.

Use of trade names and commercial sources is for identification only and does not imply endorsement by the U.S. Department of Health and Human Services.

Figure 2. Vaccines that might be indicated for adults based on medical and other indications

VACCINE ▼ INDICATION ►	Pregnancy	Immuno-compromising conditions (excluding human immunodeficiency virus [HIV])[3-6,13]	HIV infection[3-6,12,13] CD4+ T lympho-cyte count <200 cells/µL	HIV infection ≥200 cells/µL	Diabetes, heart disease, chronic lung disease, chronic alcoholism	Asplenia[12] (including elective splenectomy and persistent complement component deficiencies)	Chronic liver disease	Kidney failure, end-stage renal disease, receipt of hemodialysis	Health-care personnel
Tetanus, diphtheria, pertussis (Td/Tdap)[1,*]	Td	Substitute 1-time dose of Tdap for Td booster; then boost with Td every 10 yrs							
Human papillomavirus (HPV)[2,*]		3 doses for females through age 26 yrs							
Varicella[3,*]	Contraindicated			2 doses					
Zoster[4]	Contraindicated			1 dose					
Measles, mumps, rubella (MMR)[5,*]	Contraindicated			1 or 2 doses					
Influenza[6,*]	1 dose TIV annually								1 dose TIV or LAIV annually
Pneumococcal (polysaccharide)[7,8]	1 or 2 doses								
Hepatitis A[9,*]	2 doses								
Hepatitis B[10,*]	3 doses								
Meningococcal[11,*]	1 or more doses								

*Covered by the Vaccine Injury Compensation Program.

For all persons in this category who meet the age requirements and who lack evidence of immunity (e.g., lack documentation of vaccination or have no evidence of prior infection)

Recommended if some other risk factor is present (e.g., on the basis of medical, occupational, lifestyle, or other indications)

No recommendation

These schedules indicate the recommended age groups and medical indications for which administration of currently licensed vaccines is commonly indicated for adults ages 19 years and older, as of January 1, 2010. Licensed combination vaccines may be used whenever any components of the combination are indicated and when the vaccine's other components are not contraindicated. For detailed recommendations on all vaccines, including those used primarily for travelers or that are issued during the year, consult the manufacturers' package inserts and the complete statements from the Advisory Committee on Immunization Practices (www.cdc.gov/vaccines/pubs/acip-list.htm).

The recommendations in this schedule were approved by the Centers for Disease Control and Prevention's (CDC) Advisory Committee on Immunization Practices (ACIP), the American Academy of Family Physicians (AAFP), the American College of Obstetricians and Gynecologists (ACOG), and the American College of Physicians (ACP).

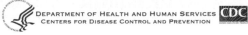

DEPARTMENT OF HEALTH AND HUMAN SERVICES
CENTERS FOR DISEASE CONTROL AND PREVENTION

CDC

Footnotes

Recommended Adult Immunization Schedule—UNITED STATES · 2010

For complete statements by the Advisory Committee on Immunization Practices (ACIP), visit www.cdc.gov/vaccines/pubs/ACIP-list.htm.

1. Tetanus, diphtheria, and acellular pertussis (Td/Tdap) vaccination

Tdap should replace a single dose of Td for adults aged 19 through 64 years who have not received a dose of Tdap previously.

Adults with uncertain or incomplete history of primary vaccination series with tetanus and diphtheria toxoid-containing vaccines should begin or complete a primary vaccination series. A primary series for adults is 3 doses of tetanus and diphtheria toxoid-containing vaccines; administer the first 2 doses at least 4 weeks apart and the third dose 6–12 months after the second; Tdap can substitute for any one of the doses of Td in the 3-dose primary series. The booster dose of tetanus and diphtheria toxoid-containing vaccine should be administered to adults who have completed a primary series and if the last vaccination was received ≥10 years previously. Tdap or Td vaccine may be used, as indicated.

If a woman is pregnant and received the last Td vaccination ≥10 years previously, administer Td during the second or third trimester. If the woman received the last Td vaccination <10 years previously, administer Tdap during the immediate postpartum period. A dose of Tdap is recommended for postpartum women, close contacts of infants aged <12 months, and all health-care personnel with direct patient contact if they have not previously received Tdap. An interval as short as 2 years from the last Td is suggested; shorter intervals can be used. Td may be deferred during pregnancy and Tdap substituted in the immediate postpartum period, or Tdap can be administered instead of Td to a pregnant woman.

Consult the ACIP statement for recommendations for giving Td as prophylaxis in wound management.

2. Human papillomavirus (HPV) vaccination

HPV vaccination is recommended at age 11 or 12 years with catch-up vaccination at ages 13 through 26 years.

Ideally, vaccine should be administered before potential exposure to HPV through sexual activity; however, females who are sexually active should still be vaccinated consistent with age-based recommendations. Sexually active females who have not been infected with any of the four HPV vaccine types (types 6, 11, 16, 18 all of which HPV4 prevents) or any of the two HPV vaccine types (types 16 and 18 both of which HPV2 prevents) receive the full benefit of the vaccination. Vaccination is less beneficial for females who have already been infected with one or more of the HPV vaccine types. HPV4 or HPV2 can be administered to persons with a history of genital warts, abnormal Papanicolaou test, or positive HPV DNA test, because these conditions are not evidence of prior infection with all vaccine HPV types.

HPV4 may be administered to males aged 9 through 26 years to reduce their likelihood of acquiring genital warts. HPV4 would be most effective when administered before exposure to HPV through sexual contact.

A complete series for either HPV4 or HPV2 consists of 3 doses. The second dose should be administered 1–2 months after the first dose; the third dose should be administered 6 months after the first dose.

Although HPV vaccination is not specifically recommended for persons with the medical indications described in Figure 2, "Vaccines that might be indicated for adults based on medical and other indications," it may be administered to these persons because the HPV vaccine is not a live-virus vaccine. However, the immune response and vaccine efficacy might be less for persons with the medical indications described in Figure 2 than in persons who do not have the medical indications described or who are immunocompetent. Health-care personnel are not at increased risk because of occupational exposure, and should be vaccinated consistent with age-based recommendations.

3. Varicella vaccination

All adults without evidence of immunity to varicella should receive 2 doses of single-antigen varicella vaccine if not previously vaccinated or the second dose if they have received only 1 dose, unless they have a medical contraindication. Special consideration should be given to those who 1) have close contact with persons at high risk for severe disease (e.g., health-care personnel and family contacts of persons with immunocompromising conditions) or 2) are at high risk for exposure or transmission (e.g., teachers; child-care employees; residents and staff members of institutional settings, including correctional institutions; college students; military personnel; adolescents and adults living in households with children; nonpregnant women of childbearing age; and international travelers).

Evidence of immunity to varicella in adults includes any of the following: 1) documentation of 2 doses of varicella vaccine at least 4 weeks apart; 2) U.S.-born before 1980 (although for health-care personnel and pregnant women, birth before 1980 should not be considered evidence of immunity); 3) history of varicella based on diagnosis or verification of varicella by a health-care provider (for a patient reporting a history of or presenting with an atypical case, a mild case, or both, health-care providers should seek either an epidemiologic link with a typical varicella case or to a laboratory-confirmed case or evidence of laboratory confirmation, if it was performed at the time of acute disease); 4) history of herpes zoster based on diagnosis or verification of herpes zoster by a health-care provider; or 5) laboratory evidence of immunity or laboratory confirmation of disease.

Pregnant women should be assessed for evidence of varicella immunity. Women who do not have evidence of immunity should receive the first dose of varicella vaccine upon completion or termination of pregnancy and before discharge from the health-care facility. The second dose should be administered 4–8 weeks after the first dose.

4. Herpes zoster vaccination

A single dose of zoster vaccine is recommended for adults aged ≥60 years regardless of whether they report a prior episode of herpes zoster. Persons with chronic medical conditions may be vaccinated unless their condition constitutes a contraindication.

5. Measles, mumps, rubella (MMR) vaccination

Adults born before 1957 generally are considered immune to measles and mumps.

Measles component: Adults born during or after 1957 should receive 1 or more doses of MMR vaccine unless they have 1) a medical contraindication; 2) documentation of vaccination with 1 or more doses of MMR vaccine; 3) laboratory evidence of immunity; or 4) documentation of physician-diagnosed measles.

A second dose of MMR vaccine, administered 4 weeks after the first dose, is recommended for adults who 1) have been recently exposed to measles or are in an outbreak setting; 2) have been vaccinated previously with killed measles vaccine; 3) have been vaccinated with an unknown type of measles vaccine during 1963–1967; 4) are students in postsecondary educational institutions; 5) work in a health-care facility; or 6) plan to travel internationally.

Mumps component: Adults born during or after 1957 should receive 1 dose of MMR vaccine unless they have 1) a medical contraindication; 2) documentation of vaccination with 1 or more doses of MMR vaccine; 3) laboratory evidence of immunity; or 4) documentation of physician-diagnosed mumps.

A second dose of MMR vaccine, administered 4 weeks after the first dose, is recommended for adults who 1) live in a community experiencing a mumps outbreak and are in an affected age group; 2) are students in postsecondary educational institutions; 3) work in a health-care facility; or 4) plan to travel internationally.

Rubella component: 1 dose of MMR vaccine is recommended for women who do not have documentation of rubella vaccination, or who lack laboratory evidence of immunity. For women of childbearing age, regardless of birth year, rubella immunity should be determined and women should be counseled regarding congenital rubella syndrome. Women who do not have evidence of immunity should receive MMR vaccine upon completion or termination of pregnancy and before discharge from the health-care facility.

Health-care personnel born before 1957: For unvaccinated health-care personnel born before 1957 who lack laboratory evidence of measles, mumps, and/or rubella immunity or laboratory confirmation of disease, health-care facilities should consider vaccinating personnel with 2 doses of MMR vaccine at the appropriate interval (for measles and mumps) and 1 dose of MMR vaccine (for rubella), respectively.

During outbreaks, health-care facilities should recommend that unvaccinated health-care personnel born before 1957, who lack laboratory evidence of measles, mumps, and/or rubella immunity or laboratory confirmation of disease, receive 2 doses of MMR vaccine during an outbreak of measles or mumps, and 1 dose during an outbreak of rubella.

Complete information about evidence of immunity is available at www.cdc.gov/vaccines/recs/provisional/default.htm.

6. Seasonal Influenza vaccination

Vaccinate all persons aged ≥50 years and any younger persons who would like to decrease their risk of getting influenza. Vaccinate persons aged 19 through 49 years with any of the following indications.

Medical: Chronic disorders of the cardiovascular or pulmonary systems, including asthma; chronic metabolic diseases, including diabetes mellitus; renal or hepatic dysfunction, hemoglobinopathies, or immunocompromising conditions (including immunocompromising conditions caused by medications or HIV); cognitive, neurologic or neuromuscular disorders; and pregnancy during the influenza season. No data exist on the risk for severe or complicated influenza disease among persons with asplenia; however, influenza is a risk factor for secondary bacterial infections that can cause severe disease among persons with asplenia.

Occupational: All health-care personnel, including those employed by long-term care and assisted-living facilities, and caregivers of children aged <5 years.

Other: Residents of nursing homes and other long-term care and assisted-living facilities; persons likely to transmit influenza to persons at high risk (e.g., in-home household contacts and caregivers of children aged <5 years, persons aged ≥50 years, and persons of all ages with high-risk conditions).

Healthy, nonpregnant adults aged <50 years without high-risk medical conditions who are not contacts of severely immunocompromised persons in special-care units may receive either intranasally administered live, attenuated influenza vaccine (FluMist) or inactivated vaccine. Other persons should receive the inactivated vaccine.

7. Pneumococcal polysaccharide (PPSV) vaccination

Vaccinate all persons with the following indications.

Medical: Chronic lung disease (including asthma); chronic cardiovascular diseases; diabetes mellitus; chronic liver diseases, cirrhosis; chronic alcoholism; functional or anatomic asplenia (e.g., sickle cell disease or splenectomy [if elective splenectomy is planned, vaccinate at least 2 weeks before surgery]); immunocompromising conditions including chronic renal failure or nephrotic syndrome; and cochlear implants and cerebrospinal fluid leaks. Vaccinate as close to HIV diagnosis as possible.

Other: Residents of nursing homes or long-term care facilities and persons who smoke cigarettes. Routine use of PPSV is not recommended for American Indians/Alaska Natives or persons aged <65 years unless they have underlying medical conditions that are PPSV indications. However, public health authorities may consider recommending PPSV for American Indians/Alaska Natives and persons aged 50 through 64 years who are living in areas where the risk for invasive pneumococcal disease is increased.

8. Revaccination with PPSV

One-time revaccination after 5 years is recommended for persons with chronic renal failure or nephrotic syndrome; functional or anatomic asplenia (e.g., sickle cell disease or splenectomy); and for persons with immunocompromising conditions. For persons aged ≥65 years, one-time revaccination is recommended if they were vaccinated ≥5 years previously and were younger than aged <65 years at the time of primary vaccination.

9. Hepatitis A vaccination

Vaccinate persons with any of the following indications and any person seeking protection from hepatitis A virus (HAV) infection.

Behavioral: Men who have sex with men and persons who use injection drugs.

Occupational: Persons working with HAV-infected primates or with HAV in a research laboratory setting.

Medical: Persons with chronic liver disease and persons who receive clotting factor concentrates.

Other: Persons traveling to or working in countries that have high or intermediate endemicity of hepatitis A (a list of countries is available at wwwn.cdc.gov/travel/contentdiseases.aspx).

Unvaccinated persons who anticipate close personal contact (e.g., household contact or regular babysitting) with an international adoptee from a country of high or intermediate endemicity during the first 60 days after arrival of the adoptee in the United States should consider vaccination. The first dose of the 2-dose hepatitis A vaccine series should be administered as soon as adoption is planned, ideally ≥2 weeks before the arrival of the adoptee.

Single-antigen vaccine formulations should be administered in a 2-dose schedule at either 0 and 6–12 months (Havrix), or 0 and 6–18 months (Vaqta). If the combined hepatitis A and hepatitis B vaccine (Twinrix) is used, administer 3 doses at 0, 1, and 6 months; alternatively, a 4-dose schedule, administered on days 0, 7, and 21–30 followed by a booster dose at month 12 may be used.

10. Hepatitis B vaccination

Vaccinate persons with any of the following indications and any person seeking protection from hepatitis B virus (HBV) infection.

Behavioral: Sexually active persons who are not in a long-term, mutually monogamous relationship (e.g., persons with more than one sex partner during the previous 6 months); persons seeking evaluation or treatment for a sexually transmitted disease (STD); current or recent injection-drug users; and men who have sex with men.

Occupational: Health-care personnel and public-safety workers who are exposed to blood or other potentially infectious body fluids.

Medical: Persons with end-stage renal disease, including patients receiving hemodialysis; persons with HIV infection; and persons with chronic liver disease.

Other: Household contacts and sex partners of persons with chronic HBV infection; clients and staff members of institutions for persons with developmental disabilities; and international travelers to countries with high or intermediate prevalence of chronic HBV infection (a list of countries is available at wwwn.cdc.gov/travel/contentdiseases.aspx).

Hepatitis B vaccination is recommended for all adults in the following settings: STD treatment facilities; HIV testing and treatment facilities; facilities providing drug-abuse treatment and prevention services; health-care settings targeting services to injection-drug users or men who have sex with men; correctional facilities; end-stage renal disease programs and facilities for chronic hemodialysis patients; and institutions and nonresidential daycare facilities for persons with developmental disabilities.

Administer or complete a 3-dose series of HepB to those persons not previously vaccinated. The second dose should be administered 1 month after the first dose; the third dose should be administered at least 2 months after the second dose (and at least 4 months after the first dose). If the combined hepatitis A and hepatitis B vaccine (Twinrix) is used, administer 3 doses at 0, 1, and 6 months; alternatively, a 4-dose schedule, administered on days 0, 7, and 21–30 followed by a booster dose at month 12 may be used.

Adult patients receiving hemodialysis or with other immunocompromising conditions should receive 1 dose of 40 μg/mL (Recombivax HB) administered on a 3-dose schedule or 2 doses of 20 μg/mL (Engerix-B) administered simultaneously on a 4-dose schedule at 0, 1, 2 and 6 months.

11. Meningococcal vaccination

Meningococcal vaccine should be administered to persons with the following indications.

Medical: Adults with anatomic or functional asplenia, or persistent complement component deficiencies.

Other: First-year college students living in dormitories; microbiologists routinely exposed to isolates of *Neisseria meningitidis*; military recruits; and persons who travel to or live in countries in which meningococcal disease is hyperendemic or epidemic (e.g., the "meningitis belt" of sub-Saharan Africa during the dry season [December through June]), particularly if their contact with local populations will be prolonged. Vaccination is required by the government of Saudi Arabia for all travelers to Mecca during the annual Hajj.

Meningococcal conjugate vaccine (MCV4) is preferred for adults with any of the preceding indications who are aged ≤55 years; meningococcal polysaccharide vaccine (MPSV4) is preferred for adults aged ≥56 years. Revaccination with MCV4 after 5 years is recommended for adults previously vaccinated with MCV4 or MPSV4 who remain at increased risk for infection (e.g., adults with anatomic or functional asplenia). Persons whose only risk factor is living in on-campus housing are not recommended to receive an additional dose.

12. Selected conditions for which *Haemophilus influenzae* type b (Hib) vaccine may be used

Hib vaccine generally is not recommended for persons aged ≥5 years. No efficacy data are available on which to base a recommendation concerning use of Hib vaccine for older children and adults. However, studies suggest good immunogenicity in patients who have sickle cell disease, leukemia, or HIV infection or who have had a splenectomy. Administering 1 dose of Hib vaccine to these high-risk persons who have not previously received Hib vaccine is not contraindicated.

13. Immunocompromising conditions

Inactivated vaccines generally are acceptable (e.g., pneumococcal, meningococcal, influenza [inactivated influenza vaccine]) and live vaccines generally are avoided in persons with immune deficiencies or immunocompromising conditions. Information on specific conditions is available at www.cdc.gov/vaccines/pubs/acip-list.htm.

Answers to Review Questions

For full rationales for each question, visit http://thepoint.lww.com/Jensen1e. At the same site, you can also find recommended guidance for responding to the book's case studies as well.

Chapter 1: The Nurse's Role in Health Assessment
1. B. 2. C. 3. A. 4. A. 5. D. 6. A. 7. D. 8. C. 9. D. 10. A.

Chapter 2: The Interview and Therapeutic Dialogue
1. A. 2. C. 3. D. 4. C. 5. A. 6. C. 7. D. 8. C. 9. C. 10. D.

Chapter 3: The Health History
1. A. 2. A. 3. C. 4. C. 5. A. 6. D. 7. A. 8. C. 9. B. 10. A.

Chapter 4: Techniques of Physical Examination and Equipment
1. B. 2. A. 3. D. 4. C. 5. D. 6. B. 7. C. 8. A. 9. C. 10. A.

Chapter 5: Documentation and Interdisciplinary Communication
1. A. 2. A, B, C, D. 3. C. 4. A and B. 5. D. 6. A. 7. C. 8. B. 9. D. 10. D.

Chapter 6: General Survey and Vital Signs Assessment
1. The apical pulse is close to the left nipple. 2. Rate, rhythm, force (amplitude), and elasticity. 3. C. 4. C. 5. B. 6. D. 7. A. 8. C. 9. B. 10. A, B, and C.

Chapter 7: Pain Assessment
1. A. 2. C. 3. D. 4. B. 5. A. 6. B. 7. B. 8. A. 9. C. 10. D.

Chapter 8: Nutrition Assessment
1. D. 2. A. 3. D. 4. C. 5. D. 6. A. 7. B. 8. C. 9. D. 10. C.

Chapter 9: Assessment of Developmental Stages
1. C. 2. A. 3. B. 4. D. 5. C. 6. D. 7. C. 8. B. 9. A. 10. A.

Chapter 10: Mental Health Assessment
1. A. 2. D. 3. B. 4. D. 5. C. 6. C. 7. D. 8. A. 9. C. 10. D.

Chapter 11: Assessment of Social, Cultural, and Spiritual Health
1. D. 2. A. 3. B. 4. C. 5. B. 6. C. 7. A. 8. D. 9. C. 10. D.

Chapter 12: Assessment of Human Violence
1. D. 2. A. 3. B. 4. C. 5. D. 6. B. 7. A. 8. A. 9. D. 10. A.

Chapter 13: Skin, Hair, and Nails Assessment
1. C. 2. D. 3. B. 4. A. 5. B. 6. D. 7. A. 8. A. 9. C. 10. A. 11. B.

Chapter 14: Head and Neck with Lymphatics Assessment
1. A. 2. B. 3. B. 4. C. 5. D. 6. C. 7. D. 8. B. 9. B. 10. C.

Chapter 15: Eyes Assessment
1. B. 2. A. 3. D. 4. C. 5. B. 6. D. 7. A. 8. C. 9. B. 10. B.

Chapter 16: Ears Assessment
1. A. 2. D. 3. A, B, C, and D. 4. A and C. 5. C. 6. A. 7. D. 8. B. 9. D. 10. A, B, and C.

Chapter 17: Nose, Sinuses, Mouth, and Throat Assessment
1. C. 2. C. 3. A. 4. D. 5. A. 6. B. 7. D. 8. B. 9. C. 10. A.

Chapter 18: Thorax and Lungs Assessment
1. B. 2. A. 3. A. 4. D. 5. D. 6. C. 7. B. 8. A, B, C, and D. 9. B. 10. B.

Chapter 19: Heart and Neck Vessels Assessment
1. A. 2. C. 3. A. 4. D. 5. D. 6. C. 7. D. 8. A. 9. A. 10. D.

Chapter 20: Peripheral Vascular and Lymphatic Assessment
1. C. 2. B. 3. B. 4. C. 5. C. 6. B. 7. A. 8. D. 9. A. 10. B.

Chapter 21: Breasts and Axillae Assessment
1. B, C. 2. D. 3. A. 4. C. 5. B. 6. C. 7. D. 8. A. 9. A. 10. C.

Chapter 22: Abdominal Assessment
1. C. 2. B. 3. B. 4. D. 5. C. 6. C. 7. B. 8. A. 9. D. 10. A.

Chapter 23: Musculoskeletal Assessment
1. B. 2. D. 3. A. 4. C. 5. A. 6. B. 7. C. 8. B. 9. D. 10. A. 11. C.

Chapter 24: Neurological Assessment
1. B. 2. A. 3. D. 4. B. 5. D. 6. A. 7. B. 8. B. 9. A. 10. B.

Chapter 25: Male Genitalia and Rectal Assessment
1. B. 2. D. 3. B. 4. C. 5. B. 6. A. 7. B. 8. A. 9. D. 10. D.

Chapter 26: Female Genitalia and Rectal Assessment
1. B. 2. D. 3. A. 4. D. 5. C. 6. B. 7. D. 8. A. 9. B. 10. D.

Chapter 27: Pregnant Women
1. C. 2. C. 3. D. 4. C. 5. C. 6. A. 7. B. 8. B. 9. D. 10. C.

Chapter 28: Newborns and Infants
1. B. 2. C. 3. A. 4. B. 5. B. 6. D. 7. C. 8. D. 9. D. 10. C.

Chapter 29: Children and Adolescents
1. D. 2. B. 3. A. 4. C. 5. B. 6. B. 7. D. 8. C. 9. D. 10. A.

Chapter 30: Older Adults
1. C. 2. C. 3. D. 4. A. 5. B. 6. C. 7. B. 8. A. 9. C. 10. D.

Chapter 31: Head-to-Toe Assessment of the Adult
1. D. 2. A. 3. C. 4. C. 5. A. 6. C. 7. A. 8. A. 9. D. 10. B.

ILLUSTRATION CREDIT LIST

CHAPTER 1

Figure 1.2A & B, 1.7: Photo by B. Proud.

Figure 1.3: Travis, J. W., & Ryan, R. S. (2004). *The wellness workbook* (3rd ed.). New York, NY: Celestial Arts.

Figure 1.4: Pender, N. J., Murdaugh, C. L., Parsons, M. A. (2006). *Health promotion in nursing practice* (5th ed. ©, p. 50). Reprinted by permission of Pearson Education, Inc., Upper Saddle River, NJ.

CHAPTER 2

Case Figure: Photo by A. Powdrill, Getty Images®.

Figures 2.2A and 2.4: Photo by B. Proud.

CHAPTER 4

Figures 4.1, 4.2, 4.4, 4.5, and 4.12: Photo by B. Proud.

CHAPTER 5

Figures 5.3, 5.5, and 5.7: Photo by B. Proud.

Figure 5.6: Courtesy of Nazareth Hospital, Philadelphia, PA.

CHAPTER 6

Figures 6.2, 6.4, 6.5, 6.6, and 6.7: Photo by B. Proud.

Table 6.7: *Cardiac Output, Viscocity, Elasticity of Vessel Walls:* Asset provided by Anatomical Chart Co.; *Circulating Blood Volume:* Fleisher, G. R., Ludwig, S., & Baskin, M. N. (2004). *Atlas of pediatric emergency medicine.* Philadelphia, PA: Lippincott Williams & Wilkins.

Table 6.11: *Achondroplastic Dwarfism:* Sadler, T. (2003). *Langman's medical embryology* (9th ed. Image Bank). Baltimore: Lippincott Williams & Wilkins; *Acromegaly:* McConnell, T.H. (2007). *The nature of disease pathology for the health professions.* Philadelphia, PA: Lippincott Williams & Wilkins; *Gigantism:* Gagel R. F., & McCutcheon, I. E. (1999). Images in Clinical Medicine. *New England Journal of Medicine, 340,* 524. Copyright © 2003. Massachusetts Medical Society; *Obesity, Anorexia Nervosa:* Biophoto Associates/Photo Researchers, Inc.

CHAPTER 7

Figure 7.6: Adapted from McCaffery, M., & Pasero, C. (1999). *Pain: Clinical manual* (2nd ed., p. 37). St. Louis, MO: C. V. Mosby.

Figure 7.7: Copyright © 1991, Charles S. Cleeland, PhD.

Figure 7.8: Hockenberry, M. J., & Wilson, D. (2009). *Wong's essentials of pediatric nursing* (8th ed.). St. Louis, MO: C. V. Mosby. Used with permission. Copyright Mosby.

CHAPTER 8

Figure 8.1: U.S. Department of Health.

Figure 8.2: Used with permission from Hark, L. & Darwin, D. Jr. (1999). Taking a nutrition history: A practical approach for family physicians. *The American Family Physician, 59*(6), 1521–1523.

Figure 8-4: From Baer, H. J., Blum, R. E., Helaine R. H., et al. (2005). Use of a food frequency questionnaire in American Indian and Caucasian pregnant women: A validation study. *BMC Public Health, 5,* 135. Retrieved from http://www.biomedcentral.com/content/pdf/1471-2458-5-135.pdf on May 12, 2009.

Table 8-8: *Alopecia, Bitot's Spots, Magenta Tongue:* Ostler, H. B., Maibach, H. I., Hoke, A. W., & Schwab, I. R. (2004). *Diseases of the eye and skin: A color atlas.* Philadelphia, PA: Lippincott Williams & Wilkins; *Follicular Keratosis:* Tasman, W., & Jaeger, E. (2001). *The Wills eye hospital atlas of clinical ophthalmology* (2nd ed.). Lippincott Williams & Wilkins; *Genu Varum:* Courtesy of Shriners Hospitals for Children, Houston, TX.

CHAPTER 9

Figure 9.4: Jeffrey Greenberg/Photo Researchers, Inc.

Figure 9.5A: Bill Aron/Photo Researchers, Inc.

Figure 9.5B: Lawrence Migdale/Photo Researchers, Inc.

CHAPTER 11

Figure 11.1: Adapted from Andrews, M. M. & Boyle, J. S. (2008). *Transcultural concepts in nursing care* (5th ed.). Philadelphia: Lippincott Williams & Wilkins.

Figure 11.2: Anderson, E. T., & McFarlane, J. (2011). *Community as partner: Theory and practice in nursing* (6th ed.). Philadelphia, PA: Wolters Kluwer Health/Lippincott Williams & Wilkins.

CHAPTER 13

Figures 13.5A, B, 13.8, 13.13A, B, C: Goodheart, H. P. (2008). *Goodheart's photoguide of common skin disorders* (3rd ed.). Philadelphia, PA: Lippincott Williams & Wilkins.

Fig. 13.6: Photo by B. Proud.

Fig 13.10: Courtesy of Philip Siu, MD.

Fig 13.14: From O'Doherty, N. (1979). *Atlas of the newborn.* Philadelphia, PA: JB Lippincott.

Table 13.2: *A, C, D, E:* Goodheart, H. P. (2008). *Goodheart's photoguide of common skin disorders* (3rd ed.). Philadelphia, PA: Lippincott Williams & Wilkins; *B:* Courtesy of Art Huntley, M.D., University of California at Davis.

Table 13.9: *Pallor, Café-au-lait Macules:* Fleisher, G. R., Ludwig, W., & Baskin, M. N. (2004). *Atlas of pediatric emergency medicine.* Philadelphia, PA: Lippincott Williams & Wilkins; *Pigmented Macules:* Robinson, H. B. G., & Miller A. S. (1990). *Colby, Kerr, and Robinson's color atlas of oral pathology.* Philadelphia, PA: JB Lippincott; *Hirsutism:* (2008). *Goodheart's photoguide of common skin disorders* (3rd ed.). Philadelphia, PA: Lippincott Williams & Wilkins; *Malar Rash:* McConnell, T. H. (2007). *The nature of disease pathology for the health professions.* Philadelphia, PA: Lippincott Williams & Wilkins; *Pallor of Fingers:* Effeney, D. J. & Stoney, R. J. (1993). *Wylie's atlas of vascular surgery: Disorders of the extremities.* Philadelphia, PA: Lippincott Williams & Wilkins.

Table 13.10: *Macule, Patch, Papule, Plaque, Wheal, Lipoma, Vesicle, Bulla, Pustule, Cyst:* (2008). *Goodheart's photoguide of common skin disorders* (3rd ed.). Philadelphia, PA: Lippincott Williams & Wilkins.

Table 13.11: *Atrophy, Keloid, Scale, Lichenification, Excoriation, Erosion, Fissure, Ulcer:* (2008). *Goodheart's Photoguide of Common Skin Disorders* (3rd ed.). Philadelphia, PA: Lippincott Williams & Wilkins; *Scar:* Weber, J. & Kelley, J. (2003). *Health assessment in nursing* (2nd ed.). Philadelphia, PA: Lippincott Williams & Wilkins; *Crust:* McConnell T. H. (2007). *The nature of disease pathology for the health professions.* Philadelphia, PA: Lippincott Williams & Wilkins.

Table 13.12: *Annular, Iris, Linear, Polymorphous, Serpiginous, Nummular, Umbilicated, Verrucaform:* (2008). *Goodheart's photoguide of common skin disorders* (3rd ed.). Philadelphia, PA: Lippincott Williams & Wilkins; *Filiform:* Ostler, H. B., Maibach, H. I., Hoke, A. W., & Schwab, I. R. (2004). *Diseases of the eye and skin: a color atlas.* Philadelphia, PA: Lippincott Williams & Wilkins.

Table 13.13: *Asymmetric, Diffuse, Discrete, Generalized, Grouped, Localized, Satellite, Symmetric, Zosteriform:* (2008). *Goodheart's photoguide of common skin disorders* (3rd ed.). Philadelphia, PA: Lippincott Williams & Wilkins; *Confluent:* Bickley, L. S. (2009). *Bates' guide to physical examination and history taking* (10th ed.). Philadelphia, PA: Lippincott Williams & Wilkins.

Table 13.14: *Pustular Acne, Cystic Acne, Warts, Cellulitis, Impetigo, Herpes Simplex (Cold Sores), Measles (Rubeola), Pityriasis Rosea, Roseola, Candida, Tinea Corporis, Tinea Versicolor:* (2008). *Goodheart's photoguide of common skin disorders* (3rd ed.). Philadelphia, PA: Lippincott Williams & Wilkins.

Table 13.15: *Psoriasis, Eczema, Contact Dermatitis, Urticaria, Allegic Drug Reaction, Insect Bites, Seborrhea:* (2008). *Goodheart's photoguide of common skin disorders* (3rd ed.). Philadelphia, PA: Lippincott Williams & Wilkins.

Table 13.16: *Lice (Pediculosis) A & B, Scabies, Ticks:* (2008). *Goodheart's Photoguide of Common Skin Disorders* (3rd ed.). Philadelphia, PA: Lippincott Williams & Wilkins.

Table 13.17: *Moles or Nevi, Skin Tags, Lentigo, Actinic Keratosis, Basal Cell Carcinoma, Squamous Cell Carcinoma, Malignant Melanoma, Kaposi's Sarcoma:* (2008). *Goodheart's Photoguide of Common Skin Disorders* (3rd ed.). Philadelphia, PA: Lippincott Williams & Wilkins; *Lipoma:* Image provided by Steadman's.

Table 13.18: *Hemangioma:* O'Doherty, N. (1979). *Atlas of the newborn.* Philadelphia, PA: JB Lippincott; *Nevus Flammeus:* From Sauer G. C., & Hall J. C. (1996). *Manual of skin diseases* (7th ed.). Philadelphia, PA: Lippincott-Raven; *Venous Lake:* (2008). *Goodheart's Photoguide of Common Skin Disorders* (3rd ed.). Philadelphia, PA: Lippincott Williams & Wilkins, 2008.

Table 13.19: *Petechiae:* McConnell, T. H. (2007). *The nature of disease pathology for the health professions.* Philadelphia, PA: Lippincott Williams & Wilkins; *Purpura, Ecchymosis:* (2008). *Goodheart's Photoguide of Common Skin Disorders* (3rd ed.). Philadelphia, PA: Lippincott Williams & Wilkins; *Hematoma, Laceration, Puncture Wound:* From Fleisher, G.

R., Ludwig, S., Baskin, M. N. (2004). *Atlas of pediatric emergency medicine*. Philadelphia, PA: Lippincott Williams & Wilkins; *Avulsion:* Dr. P. Marazzi/Photo Researchers, Inc.

Table 13.20: *Stage I, Stage II, Stage III, Stage IV:* Nettina, S. M. (2001). *The Lippincott manual of nursing practice* (7th ed.). Philadelphia, PA: Lippincott Williams & Wilkins.

Table 13.21: *Venous Ulcer (Vascular), Arterial Ulcer (Vascular):* Nettina, S. M. (2001). *The Lippincott manual of nursing practice* (7th ed.). Philadelphia, PA: Lippincott Williams & Wilkins, 2001.

Table 13.24: *Longitudinal Ridging, Onycholysis, Pitted Nails, Yellow Nails, Half-and-half Nails, Dark Longitudinal Streaks:* (2008). *Goodheart's Photoguide of Common Skin Disorders* (3rd ed.). Philadelphia, PA: Lippincott Williams & Wilkins; *Koilonychia, Clubbing, Splinter Hemorrhages:* Image provided by Steadman's; *Beau's Lines:* Bickley, L. S. (2009). *Bates' guide to physical examination and history taking* (10th ed.). Philadelphia, PA: Lippincott Williams & Wilkins.

Table 13.25: *Alopecia Areata, Traction Alopecia, Trichotillomania:* (2008). *Goodheart's photoguide of common skin disorders* (3rd ed.). Philadelphia, PA: Lippincott Williams & Wilkins; *Hirsutism:* Image provided by Steadman's.

CHAPTER 14

Table 14.5: *Hydrocephalus, Fetal Alcohol Syndrome:* Gold, D. H., Weingeist, T. A. (2001). *Color atlas of the eye in systemic disease*. Baltimore, MD: Lippincott Williams & Wilkins; *Cretinism (Congenital Hypothyroidism):* Centers for Disease Control and Prevention Public Health Image Library.

Table 14.6: *Acromegaly:* Willis, M. C. (2002). *Medical terminology: A programmed learning approach to the language of health care*. Baltimore, MD: Lippincott Williams & Wilkins; *Bell's Palsy, Cerebral Vascular Accident (Stroke), Myxedema:* Dr. P. Marazzi/Photo Researchers, Inc.; *Cushing's Syndrome:* Ostler, H. B., Maibach, H. I., Hoke, A. W., & Schwab, I. R. (2004). *Diseases of the eye and skin: A color atlas*. Philadelphia, PA: Lippincott Williams & Wilkins; *Scleroderma:* Gold, D. H., & Weingeist, T. A. (2001). *Color atlas of the eye in systemic disease*. Baltimore, MD: Lippincott Williams & Wilkins; *Goiter:* Scott Camazine/Photo Researchers, Inc.

CHAPTER 15

Figures 15.15, 15.27, 15.28, and 15.29: Tasman, W., & Jaeger, E. (2001). *The Wills eye hospital atlas of clinical ophthalmology* (2nd ed.). Philadelphia, PA: Lippincott Williams & Wilkins.

Figures 15.17, 15.32: Gold, D. H., & Weingeist, T. A. (2001). *Color atlas of the eye in systemic disease*. Baltimore, MD: Lippincott Williams & Wilkins.

Figure 15.19: Fleisher, G. R., Ludwig, S., & Baskin, M. N. (2004). *Atlas of pediatric emergency medicine*. Philadelphia, PA: Lippincott Williams & Wilkins.

Figure 15.20: Courtesy of Terri Young, MD.

Figures 15.22, 15.23, 15.24: Bickley, L. S. (2009). *Bates' guide to physical examination and history taking* (10th ed.). Philadelphia, PA: Lippincott Williams & Wilkins.

Table 15.7: *Nystagmus:* Bickley, L. S. (2009). *Bates' guide to physical examination and history taking* (10th ed.). Philadelphia, PA: Lippincott Williams & Wilkins; *Esotropia:* Courtesy of

Dean John Bonsall, MD, FACS; *Exotropia, Vertical Deviation:* Tasman, W., & Jaeger, E. (2001). *The Wills eye hospital atlas of clinical ophthalmology* (2nd ed.). Philadelphia, PA: Lippincott Williams & Wilkins.

Table 15.8: *Jaundice, Cataract:* Rubin, E., & Farber, J. L. (1999). *Pathology* (3rd ed.). Philadelphia, PA: Lippincott Williams & Wilkins; *Iris Nevus, Blepharitis, Bacterial Conjunctivitis, Glaucoma, Amblyopia, Hordeolum (Stye):* Tasman, W., & Jaeger, E. (2001). *The Wills eye hospital atlas of clinical ophthalmology* (2nd ed.). Philadelphioa, PA: Lippincott Williams & Wilkins; *Hyphema, Allergic Conjunctivitis:* Fleisher, G. R., Ludwig, S., & Baskin, M. N.. *Atlas of pediatric emergency medicine*. Philadelphia, PA: Lippincott Williams & Wilkins; *Chalazion:* Bickley, L. S. (2009). *Bates' guide to physical examination and history taking* (10th ed.). Philadelphia, PA: Lippincott Williams & Wilkins; *Exophthalmos:* Goodheart, H. P. (2008). *Photoguide of common skin disorders* (3rd ed.). Philadelphia, PA: Lippincott Williams & Wilkins; *Osteogenesis Imperfecta:* Ostler, H. B., Maibach, H. I., Hoke, A. W., & Schwab, I. R. (2004). *Diseases of the eye and skin: A color atlas*.

Table 15.9: *Horner's Syndrome, Adie's Pupil, Mydriasis (Dilated Fixed Pupil), Oculomotor (CN III) Nerve Damage:* Tasman, W., & Jaeger, E. (2001). *The Wills eye hospital atlas of clinical ophthalmology*. (2nd ed.). Philadelphia, PA: Lippincott Williams & Wilkins; *Key Hole Pupil (Coloboma):* Courtesy of Brian Forbes, MD; *Miosis (Small Fixed Pupil):* Gold, D. H., & Weingeist, T. A. (2001). *Color atlas of the eye in systemic disease*. Baltimore, MD: Lippincott Williams & Wilkins.

Table 15.10: *AMD, Retinopathy, Retinitis Pigmentosa:* Tasman, W., & Jaeger, E. (2001). *The Wills eye hospital atlas of clinical ophthalmology* (2nd ed.). Philadelphia, PA: Lippincott Williams & Wilkins; *Copper Wiring:* McConnell, T.H. (2007). *The nature of disease pathology for the health professions*. Philadelphia, PA: Lippincott Williams & Wilkins.

CHAPTER 16

Figure 16.16: Moore, K. L., & Dalley, A. F. (1999). *Clinically oriented anatomy* (4th ed.). Baltimore, MD: Lippincott Williams & Wilkins.

Figure 16.17: Mills S. E. (2007). *Histology for pathologists* (3rd ed.). Philadelphia, PA: Lippincott Williams & Wilkins.

Figure 16.20: Bickley, L. S. (2009). *Bates' guide to physical examination and history taking* (10th ed.). Philadelphia, PA: Lippincott Williams & Wilkins.

Table 16.4: *Microtia:* Biophoto Associates/Photo Researchers, Inc.; *Macrotia:* Saturn Stills/Photo Researchers, Inc.; *Edematous Ears, Cartilage Staphyloccous or Pseudomonas Infection:* Ostler, H. B., Maibach, H. I., Hoke, A. W., & Schwab, I. R. (2004). *Diseases of the eye and skin: a color atlas; Carcinoma on Auricle:* (2008). *Goodheart's photoguide of common skin disorders* (3rd ed.). Philadelphia, PA: Lippincott Williams & Wilkins, 2008; *Cyst:* Young, E. M. Jr., Newcomer, V. D., & Kligman, A. M. (1993). *Geriatric dermatology: color atlas and practitioner's guide*. Philadelphia, PA: Lea & Febiger; *Tophi:* Weber, J. & Kelley, J. (2003). *Health assessment in nursing* (2nd ed.). Philadelphia, PA: Lippincott Williams & Wilkins.

Table 16.5: *TM Rupture:* Courtesy of Michael Hawke, MD, Toronto, Canada; *Acute Otitis*

Media: Moore, K. L., & Dalley, A. F. II. (1999). *Clinically oriented anatomy* (4th ed.). Baltimore, MD: Lippincott Williams & Wilkins; *Scarred TM:* Weber, J., & Kelley, J. (2003). *Health assessment in nursing* (2nd ed.). Philadelphia, PA: Lippincott Williams & Wilkins; *Foreign Body:* Dr P. Marazzi / Photo Researchers, Inc.

CHAPTER 17

Figure 17.1: Moore, K. L., & Dalley, A. F. II. (2008). *Clinically oriented anatomy* (6th ed.). Baltimore, MD: Lippincott Williams & Wilkins.

Figures 17.6, 17.15: Bickley, L. S. (2009). *Bates' guide to physical examination and history taking* (10th ed.) Philadelphia, PA: Lippincott Williams & Wilkins.

Figures 17.16, 17.20, 17.28: (2008). *Goodheart's photoguide of common skin disorders* (3rd ed.). Philadelphia, PA: Lippincott Williams & Wilkins.

Figure 17.21: Fleisher, G. R., Ludwig, W., & Baskin, M. N. (2004). *Atlas of pediatric emergency medicine*. Philadelphia, PA: Lippincott Williams & Wilkins.

Figure 17.23: Courtesy of Seth Zwillenberg.

Figure 17.24: Langlais, R. P., & Miller, C. S. (1992). *Color atlas of common oral diseases*. Philadelphia, PA: Lea & Febiger. Used with permission.

Figure 17.30: Robinson, H. B. G., & Miller, A. S. (1990). *Colby, Kerr, and Robinson's color atlas of oral pathology*. Philadelphia, PA: JB Lippincott.

Table 17.7: *Epistaxis (Nosebleed):* Ian Boddy/Photo Researchers, Inc.; *Nasal Polyps:* Handler, S. D., & Myer, C. M. (1998). *Atlas of ear, nose and throat disorders in children* (p 59). Ontario, Canada: BC Decker; *Deviated Septum:* Moore, K. L., & Dalley, A. F. II. (2008). *Clinically oriented anatomy* (6th ed.). Baltimore, MD: Lippincott Williams & Wilkins; *Perforated Septum, Foreign Body:* Dr P. Marazzi/Photo Researchers, Inc.

Table 17.8: *Cleft Lip/Palate:* Rubin, E., & Farber, J. L. (1999). *Pathology* (3rd ed.). Philadelphia, PA: Lippincott Williams & Wilkins; *Bifid Uvula:* Courtesy of Paul S. Matz, MD; *Acute Tonsillitis or Pharyngitis:* BSIP/Photo Researchers, Inc.; *Strep Throat:* Centers for Disease Control and Prevention Public Health Image Library.

Table 17.9: *Herpes Simplex Virus, Candidasis, Leukoplakia, Black Hairy Tongue, Carcinoma:* (2008). *Goodheart's photoguide of common skin disorders* (3rd ed.). Philadelphia, PA: Lippincott Williams & Wilkins.

Table 17.10: *Baby Bottle Tooth Decay:* Fleisher, G. R., Ludwig, S., & Baskin, M. N. (2004). *Atlas of pediatric emergency medicine*. Philadelphia, PA: Lippincott Williams & Wilkins; *Dental Caries:* Langlais, R. P., & Miller, C. S. (1992). *Color atlas of common oral diseases*. Philadelphia, PA: Lea & Febiger. Used with permission; *Gingival Hyperplasia:* Courtesy of Dr. James Cottone; *Ankyloglossia (Tongue Tie):* Courtesy of Paul S. Matz, MD.

CHAPTER 18

Figure 18.1: Moore, K. L., & Dalley, A. F. II. (2008). *Clinically oriented anatomy* (6th ed.). Baltimore, MD: Lippincott Williams & Wilkins.

Figures 18.4, 18.5, 18.6, 18.7, 18.8: Bickley, L. S. (2009). *Bates' guide to physical examination and history taking* (10th ed.). Philadelphia, PA: Lippincott Williams & Wilkins.

Figures 18.11, 18.12, 18.13, 18.14, 18.15: Photos by B. Proud.

CHAPTER 19

Figures 19.4, 19.17: Photo by B. Proud.

Figure 19.15: Bickley, L. S. (2009). *Bates' guide to physical examination and history taking* (10th ed.). Philadelphia, PA: Lippincott Williams & Wilkins.

CHAPTER 20

Table 20.4: *Acute Arterial Occlusion:* Nettina, S. M. (2001). *The Lippincott manual of nursing practice* (7th ed.). Philadelphia, PA: Lippincott Williams & Wilkins; ***Abdominal Aortic Aneurysm:*** Moore, K. L., & Dalley, A. F. II. (2008). *Clinically oriented anatomy* (6th ed.). Baltimore, MD: Lippincott Williams & Wilkins; ***Raynaud's Phenomenon and Raynaud's Disease:*** Marks, R. (1987). *Skin disease in old age.* Philadelphia, PA: JB Lippincott.

Table 20.5: *Chronic Venous Insufficiency, Neuropathy:* Marks, R. (1987). *Skin disease in old age.* Philadelphia, PA: JB Lippincott; ***Deep Vein Thrombosis:*** Dr. P. Marazzi/Photo Researchers, Inc.; ***Thrombophlebitis:*** Biophoto Associates/ Photo Researchers, Inc.; ***Lymphedema:*** Rubin, E., & Farber, J. L. (1999). *Pathology* (3rd ed.). Philadelphia, PA: Lippincott Williams & Wilkins.

CHAPTER 21

Figures 21.2A, 21.3: Moore, K. L., & Dalley, A. F. II. (2008). *Clinically oriented anatomy* (6th ed.). Baltimore, MD: Lippincott Williams & Wilkins.

Figure 21.4: Courtesy of Esther K. Chung, MD.

Figures 21.6, 21.9A–D, 21.11, 21.12A-C, 21.13: Photo by B. Proud.

Figures 21.10, 21.14: Mulholland, M. W., & Maier, R. V. (2006). *Greenfield's surgery scientific principles and practice* (4th ed.). Philadelphia, PA: Lippincott Williams & Wilkins.

Table 21.6: *Carcinoma 1, Carcinoma 2:* Mulholland, M. W., & Maier, R. V. (2006). *Greenfield's surgery scientific principles and practice* (4th ed.). Philadelphia, PA: Lippincott Williams & Wilkins; ***Paget Disease, Mastitis:*** (2005). *Atlas of infectious diseases of the female genital tract.* Philadelphia, PA: Lippincott Williams & Wilkins; ***Mastectomy:*** Steve Percival/Photo Researchers, Inc.; ***Gynecomastia:*** Courtesy of Christine Finck, MD.

CHAPTER 22

Figures 22.7, 22.8, 22.9, 22.13, 22.14: Photo by B. Proud.

Table 22.7: *Acute Abdomen 1, Acute Abdomen 2, Abdominal Aortic Aneurysm:* Photo by B. Proud; ***Appendicitis (Rovsing's Sign), Acute Cholecystitis:*** Berg, D. & Worzala, K. (2006). *Atlas of adult physical diagnosis.* Philadelphia, PA: Lippincott Williams & Wilkins; ***Obturator Sign:*** Bickley, L. S. (2009). *Bates' guide to physical examination and history taking* (10th ed.). Philadelphia, PA: Lippincott Williams & Wilkins.

CHAPTER 23

Case Figure: Joe Sohm/Photo Researchers, Inc.

Goniometer: Oatis, C. A. (2004). *Kinesiology - The mechanics and pathomechanics of human movement.* Baltimore, MD: Lippincott Williams & Wilkins.

Figures 23.13, 23.25: Bickley, L. S. (2009). *Bates' guide to physical examination and history taking* (10th ed.). Philadelphia, PA: Lippincott Williams & Wilkins.

Figures 23.24, 23.26A-C: Photo by B. Proud.

Figures 23.27A, B, 23.28 A, B, and 23.31: Moore, K. L., & Dalley, A. F. II. (2008). *Clinically*

oriented anatomy (6th ed.). Baltimore, MD: Lippincott Williams & Wilkins.

Table 23.10: *Bulge Test:* Bickley, L. S. (2009). *Bates' guide to physical examination and history taking* (10th ed.). Philadelphia, PA: Lippincott Williams & Wilkins; ***McMurray's Test, Thomas Test, LeSegue's Test, Drawer Sign, Trendelenburg Test:*** Berg, D. & Worzala, K. (2006). *Atlas of adult physical diagnosis.* Philadelphia, PA: Lippincott Williams & Wilkins.

Table 23.15: *Atrophy, Joint Effusions, Epicondylitis:* Bickley, L. S. (2009). *Bates' guide to physical examination and history taking* (10th ed.). Philadelphia, PA: Lippincott Williams & Wilkins; ***Joint Dislocation, Polydactyly, Swan Neck and Boutonniere Deformity, Syndactyly, Ulnar Deviation:*** Strickland, J. W., & Graham, T. J. (2005). *Master techniques in orthopedic surgery: The hand* (2nd ed.). Philadelphia, PA: Lippincott Williams & Wilkins; ***Rheumatoid Arthritis:*** Gold, D. H., & Weingeist, T. A. (2001). *Color atlas of the eye in systemic disease.* Baltimore, MD: Lippincott Williams & Wilkins; ***Rotator Cuff Tear, Bursitis, Ganglion Cyst, Dupuytren's Contracture, Heberden's and Bouchard's Nodes, Carpal Tunnel Syndrome:*** Berg, D. & Worzala, K. (2006). *Atlas of adult physical diagnosis.* Philadelphia, PA: Lippincott Williams & Wilkins; ***Genu Valgum:*** Courtesy of Bettina Gyr, MD; ***Congenital Hip Dislocation:*** Bucholz, R. W., & Heckman, J. D. (2001). *Rockwood and Green's fractures in adults* (5th ed.). Philadelphia, PA: Lippincott Williams & Wilkins; ***Herniated Nucleus Pulposus:*** Daffner R. H. (2007). *Clinical radiology the essentials* (3rd ed.). Philadelphia, PA: Lippincott Williams & Wilkins; ***Talipes Equinovarus:*** Courtesy of J Adams; ***Acute Rheumatoid Arthritis:*** Image provided by Stedman's; ***Ankylosing Spondylitis:*** McConnell, T. H. (2007). *The nature of disease pathology for the health professions.* Philadelphia, PA: Lippincott Williams & Wilkins.

CHAPTER 24

Figures 24.12, 24.18, 24.21, 24.23A–C: Bickley, L. S. *Bates' guide to physical examination and history taking* (10th ed.). Philadelphia, PA: Lippincott Williams & Wilkins.

Figure 24.17: Photo by B. Proud.

Table 24.11: *Paralysis:* Centers for Disease Control and Prevention Public Image Library; ***Dystonia:*** Fleisher, G. R., Ludwig, W., Baskin, M. N. (2004). *Atlas of pediatric emergency medicine.* Philadelphia, PA: Lippincott Williams & Wilkins.

CHAPTER 25

Figure 25.2: Moore, K. L., & Dalley, A. F. II. (2008). *Clinically oriented anatomy* (6th ed.). Baltimore, MD: Lippincott Williams & Wilkins.

Figures 25.8, 25.9, 25.10, 25.11, Box 25.3: Photos by B. Proud.

Table 25.6: *Phimosis, Paraphimosis, Hypospadias:* Courtesy of T. Ernesto Figueroa; ***Balanitis:*** Fleisher, G. R., Ludwig, S., & Baskin, M. N. (2004). *Atlas of pediatric emergency medicine.* Philadelphia, PA: Lippincott Williams & Wilkins; ***Epispadias:*** MacDonald, M. G., Seshia M. M. K., et al. (2005). *Avery's neonatology pathophysiology & management of the newborn* (6th ed.). Philadelphia, PA: Lippincott Williams & Wilkins.

Table 25.7: *Scabies Infection, Syphilis:* Goodheart, H. P. (2008). *Goodheart's photoguide of common skin disorders* (3rd ed.). Philadelphia, PA: Lippincott Williams & Wilkins; ***Chlamydia:***

Image from Rubin, E. & Farber, J. L. (1999). *Pathology* (3rd ed.). Philadelphia, PA: Lippincott Williams & Wilkins; ***Gonorrhea:*** Sanders, C. V. & Nesbitt, L. T. (1995). *The skin and infection.* Baltimore, MD: Williams & Wilkins.

Table 25.8: *Testicular Torsion, Varicocele:* Courtesy of T. Ernesto Figueroa, MD.

Table 25.9: *Rectal Polyp, Carcinoma of the Rectum and Anus:* Mulholland, M. W., Maier, R. V., et al. (2006). *Greenfield's surgery scientific principles and practice* (4th ed.). Philadelphia, PA: Lippincott Williams & Wilkins; ***Rectal Prolapse:*** Courtesy of Mary L. Brandt, MD; ***Prostatitis:*** Image from Rubin, E. & Farber, J. L. (1999). *Pathology* (3rd ed.). Philadelphia, PA: Lippincott Williams & Wilkins.

CHAPTER 26

Equipment Box, Figures 26.5B, 26.6, 26.9, 26.12, 26.16, 26.18A, 26.19A: Photo by B. Proud.

Figures 26.7, 26.14, 26.15: Berg, D. & Worzala, K. (2006). *Atlas of adult physical diagnosis.* Philadelphia, PA: Lippincott Williams & Wilkins.

Table 26.5: *Candidiasis:* Goodheart, H. P. (2008). *Goodheart's photoguide of common skin disorders* (3rd ed.). Philadelphia, PA: Lippincott Williams & Wilkins; ***Bacterial Vaginosis, Chlamydia, Gonorrhea, Trichomoniasis, Condylomata Acuminatum:*** Sweet, R. L., Gibbs, R. S. (2005). *Atlas of infectious diseases of the female genital tract.* Philadelphia, PA: Lippincott Williams & Wilkins.

Table 26.6: *Pediculosis, Chancre, Abscess of the Bartholin's Gland:* Sweet, R. L., Gibbs, R. S. (2005). *Atlas of infectious diseases of the female genital tract.* Philadelphia, PA: Lippincott Williams & Wilkins; ***Urethral Caruncle:*** Courtesy of Allan R. De Jong, MD; ***Contact Dermatitis:*** Courtesy of George A. Datto, III, MD.

CHAPTER 27

Case Figure: Lawrence Migdale/Photo Researchers, Inc.

Figure 27.7A: Goodheart, H. P. (2008). *Goodheart's photoguide of common skin disorders* (3rd ed.). Philadelphia, PA: Lippincott Williams & Wilkins.

CHAPTER 28

Figure 28.3: Ballard, J. L., Khoury, J. C., Wedig, K., et al. (1991). New Ballard score, expanded to include extremely premature infants. *J Pediatr, 119,* 417–423.

Figure 28.11: MacDonald, M. G., Seshia, M. M. K., et al. (2005). *Avery's neonatology pathophysiology & management of the newborn* (6th ed.). Philadelphia, PA: Lippincott Williams & Wilkins.

Table 28.7: *Pediculosis Capitis:* Courtesy of Hans B. Kersten, MD; ***Tinea Corporis,**** **Scabies, Café-au-Lait Spots:*** Fleisher, G. R., Ludwig, S., Baskin, M. N. (2004). *Atlas of pediatric emergency medicine.* Philadelphia, PA: Lippincott Williams & Wilkins; ***Staphylococcal Scalded Skin Syndrome:*** Courtesy of Gary Marshall, MD; ***Molluscum Contagiosum, Bullous Impetigo, Allergic Contact Diaper Dermatitis, Eczema:*** Goodheart, H. P. (2008). *Goodheart's photoguide of common skin disorders* (3rd ed.). Philadelphia, PA: Lippincott Williams & Wilkins; ***Intertrigo, Lichen Simplex Chronicus:*** Sauer G. C., & Hall J. C. (1996). *Manual of skin diseases* (7th ed.). Philadelphia, PA: Lippincott-Raven; ***Irritant Diaper Dermatitis, Candidal Diaper Dermatitis:*** Courtesy of Jan E. Drutz, MD.

INDEX

Page numbers followed by b indicate boxes; those followed by f indicate figures; those followed by t indicate tables.